D0741964

ESSENTIALS OF SKELETAL RADIOLOGY

Volume One

Second Edition

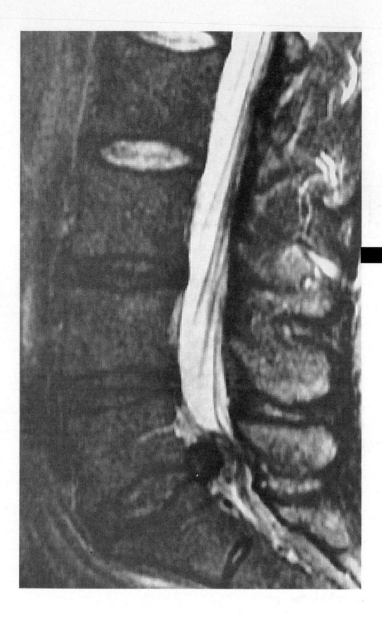

Volume One

ESSENTIALS OF SKELETAL RADIOLOGY

Second Edition

Terry R. Yochum

B.S., D.C., D.A.C.B.R., F.C.C.R. (C), F.I.C.C.

Director
Rocky Mountain Chiropractic Radiological Center
Denver, Colorado

Adjunct Professor of Radiology
Los Angeles College of Chiropractic

Instructor
Skeletal Radiology
Department of Radiology
University of Colorado School of Medicine
Denver, Colorado

Formerly:
Senior Lecturer
Department of Diagnostic Sciences
Division Head
Department of Radiology
Phillip Institute of Technology—School of Chiropractic
Melbourne, Australia

Professor and Chairman
Department of Radiology
Logan College of Chiropractic
St. Louis, Missouri

Assistant Professor of Radiology
National College of Chiropractic
Lombard, Illinois

Lindsay J. Rowe

M. App. Sc. (Chiropractic), M.D., D.A.C.B.R., F.C.C.R. (C), F.A.C.C.R. (AUS), F.I.C.C.

Department of Medical Imaging
John Hunter Hospital
Newcastle, Australia

Senior Lecturer
Centre for Chiropractic
Macquarie University
Sydney, Australia

Adjunct Faculty
School of Chiropractic
Royal Melbourne Institute of Technology University
Melbourne, Australia

Post Graduate Faculty
Northwestern Chiropractic College
Minneapolis, Minnesota
Canadian Memorial Chiropractic College
Toronto, Canada

Formerly:
Associate Professor and Chairman
Department of Radiology
Northwestern Chiropractic College
Minneapolis, Minnesota

Associate Professor and Chairman
Department of Radiology
Canadian Memorial Chiropractic College
Toronto, Canada

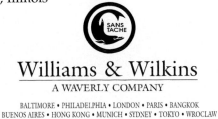

Williams & Wilkins

A WAVERLY COMPANY

BALTIMORE • PHILADELPHIA • LONDON • PARIS • BANGKOK
BUENOS AIRES • HONG KONG • MUNICH • SYDNEY • TOKYO • WROCLAW

Editor: John P. Butler
Managing Editor: Karen K. Gulliver
Production Coordinator: Barbara J. Felton
Copy Editing and Production: University Graphics Production Services
Designer: Wilma E. Rosenberger
Illustration Planner: Wayne Hubbel/Joanne Och
Cover Designer: Wilma E. Rosenberger
Typesetter: University Graphics, Inc.
Printer: Cadmus Journal Services
Binder: Maple Press

Copyright © 1996 Williams & Wilkins

351 West Camden Street
Baltimore, Maryland 21201-2436 USA

Rose Tree Corporate Center
1400 North Providence Road
Building II, Suite 5025
Media, Pennsylvania 19063-2043 USA

All rights reserved. This book is protected by copyright. No part of this book may be reproduced in any form or by any means, including photocopying, or utilized by any information storage and retrieval system without written permission from the copyright owner.
First Edition 1987

Printed in the United States of America

Library of Congress Cataloging-in-Publication Data

Yochum, Terry R.
Essentials of skeletal radiology / Terry R. Yochum, Lindsay J.
    Rowe. — 2nd ed.
        p.   cm.
    Includes bibliographical references and index.
    ISBN 0-683-09330-4
    1.   Human skeleton—Radiography.   I.   Rowe, Lindsay J.   II.   Title.
      [DNLM: 1.   Bone and Bones—Radiography.   WE 225 Y54e 1996]
    RC930.5.E85   1996
    616.71'07572—dc20
    DNLM/DLC
    for Library of Congress   95-33501
                                                                              CIP

The Publishers have made every effort to trace the copyright holders for borrowed material. If they have inadvertently overlooked any, they will be pleased to make the necessary arrangements at the first opportunity.

98 99
3 4 5 6 7 8 9 10

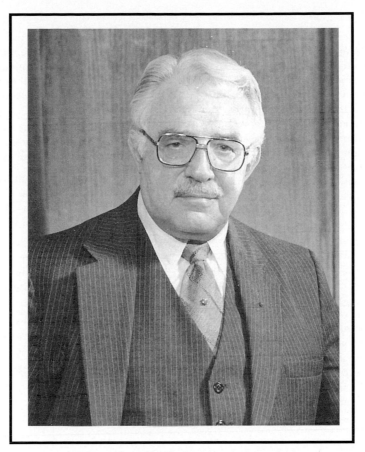

Joseph (Jozias) Janse, D.C.
(1909–1985)

In a profession now 100 years old, a few giants rise above the crowd. While each giant stands with unique distinction, a common underlying principle unites them. Longfellow captured the essence:

> The heights of great men reached and kept
> Were not attained by sudden flight,
> But they, while their companions slept,
> Were toiling upward through the night.
> Henry Wadsworth Longfellow
> "The Ladder of St. Augustine"

Through the hectic hallowed halls of college, first as a student, then resident, and finally as a faculty member, Dr. Joseph Janse was before us as the example of dedication and commitment to a cause. He was more than a college president (National College of Chiropractic 1945–1983). He was more than a person of international renown in politics, education, research and chiropractic. Foremost, he was a teacher! Always concerned, "Did you get that?" he would ask, arms raised, elbows bent and a stiffened right forefinger pointing toward heaven. You would think he was asking a higher power if they understood what he was explaining until he brought his eyes back to focus on his students. He studied their faces waiting for the lights to go on inside. The English language never received such an exercise as when he spoke. Uncommon words pierced reality and definitions always followed with clear examples that even his grandchildren could understand. An artisan of the highest order, no one could experience his tutelage without being edified while being educated.

From his humble beginnings in Holland, Joe Janse experienced poverty and hard times. Supported by the toils of a dedicated father and mother, two older sisters, one of whom hired out at an early age, and an older brother hampered with a severe kyphoscoliosis of the spine, "Jozias" never complained because they were no worse off than anyone else. The family migrated to Utah after converting to Mormonism in Holland. Father Pieter left in advance of the family by nearly a year to work and earn their passage to the New World. Their new-found religion instilled lasting values of self-worth, compassion without prejudice and added an eternal perspective to life. Coupled with forced frugality associated with near frontier farm life, hard work, and a keen desire for excellence, Joe excelled in school. He returned to Europe for three years as a self-supported missionary for the Mormon church. Upon his return he sought direction for his secular life.

Janse's mother had experienced severe migraine headaches and relief came only from the hands of a chiropractor. Intrigued, young Joe investigated. Soon convinced that chiropractic had a place, he enrolled at the National School of Chiropractic (Chicago). The Utah town folk, including prominent church leaders whom he respected, discouraged the decision. Undaunted, J.J. (as so many affectionately called him) excelled as a student and was invited to join the faculty after his graduation and marriage in 1938. For the next seven years he would excite and guide his students in the field of chiropractic. He served as Dean of Students and stories abound regarding his willingness to help individuals with their studies, their dissections, and their manipulative techniques.

By 1945, the business manager of the school (the president had passed away) asked Janse to assume the role of president and was charged to lead the college out of proprietorship into a non-profit status, a bold move at the time. In the 1950's Dr. Janse was brought up short by a talented lawyer challenging the validity of chiropractic education because of the absence of an educational standard developed and maintained by a nationally recognized accrediting body. As a result, Janse pioneered the creation of the Council on Chiropractic Education (CCE) and led the charge to gain accreditation from the North Central Accrediting Association in 1974. He also pioneered, with his close friend Dr. Fred W. Ilii, the early research on the movement of the sacroiliac joints. This work served as a foundation for additional study to document true movement of these joints and describe their relationship to gait and posture. He generated the motivation for the development of specialty councils and specialty certification boards on a national level and was one of the first three board certified chiropractic radiologists. He placed the school in deep debt to finance a new campus in Lombard, Illinois, in the 1960's and then proceeded to become the most prolific fund-raiser in the history of the National College to meet the financial challenge. A beautiful campus, debt free, now stands as a monument to his dedicated stewardship, leadership and untiring efforts.

Some memorable quotes come to mind when we, as two of his many students, think back to the times of his motivational lectures on life's principles and chiropractic philosophy. When asked, "What is it that you do?", Janse would respond, "I am a chiropractor, nothing more, but incidentally, my friend, nothing less." Perhaps his most memorable quote came from Rudyard Kipling which speaks of the great spirit of understanding and fellowship that Joseph Janse held for his chiropractic colleagues:

> Here's to the men and women of my own breed,
> Good or bitter bad, as though they may be,
> At least they hear the things I hear,
> And see the things I see.

The accolades could continue, but the legacy is clear. His inspiring example allowed no room for mediocrity or compromise. His commitment to excellence remains unparalleled. How well he is represented by one of his favorite poems:

> Oh for the silent doer of the deed,
> One who is happy with the deed's own reward,
> One who in people's plight of night
> Has solitary certitude of that which is right.

Similarly, the creators of this book and its revisions have been driven to bring to pass a text worthy of his emulation. We dedicate the product of our labors to the life of Dr. Joseph Janse in the hope that its readers may come to understand the value of "toiling upward through the night."

Terry R. Yochum
Lindsay J. Rowe

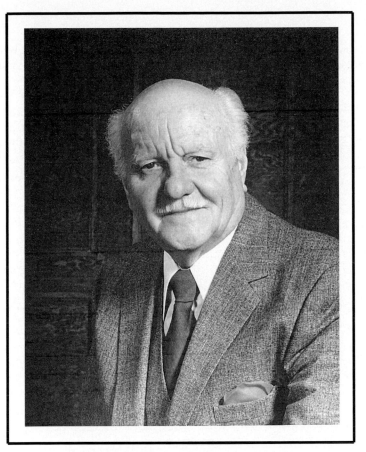

Kenneth E. Yochum, D.C.
(1914–1989)

Few children have the privilege of entering the same profession as their father. I consider it a real honor to be a second generation chiropractor following in my father's footsteps. Kenneth Emil Yochum, D.C., my father and best friend, provided the impetus to enter this great profession of chiropractic.

Kenneth E. Yochum was a resident of South St. Louis, Missouri. He graduated from Cleveland High School in 1933 and the Missouri Chiropractic College in 1939. He practiced in South St. Louis at the Wilmington Chiropractic Clinic for 45 years. Dr. Yochum presented many lectures at the National College of Chiropractic and Logan College of Chiropractic in the area of clinical practice, nutrition, and the Nimmo technique. He had a keen interest in orthopedics and nutrition, with a special love for radiology. In 1980, Dr. Yochum was honored to be invited to present a lecture for the International College of Chiropractic in Melbourne and Sydney, Australia. He was one of the first five certified instructors in the receptor tonus (RT) technique (Nimmo technique), a topic which he frequently lectured on.

Dr. Yochum's untimely death in 1989 deprived his family of his love and guidance, and many students of his great clinical expertise. Kenneth E. Yochum was a man of great character and integrity who always put the best interest of his patients before any personal need or gain. What a privilege it was to have been raised in a chiropractic family with such a great role model as a father and leader in the chiropractic profession. He lived his life by a number of spirited commitments. I can remember him saying many times, "Son, right is right and wrong is nobody." He spent his life attempting to always do the right thing for his patients and family. A leader in his community in every way, he stood as the pillar of his practice and family. So many times he told me that "chiropractic was worth making a difference for—extend yourself to make it better." His most memorable quotation involves living one's life as a reflective leader. He said that I, as his son, should "make dust—not eat dust." How thankful I am to have had a father who cared so much about the chiropractic profession and his family to have extended himself so sincerely, seemingly at every turn within his personal life.

A motivated student of radiology and an excellent radiographic technician, he produced radiographs of the finest quality in his clinical practice in St. Louis. In fact, his name follows many films in both the first and second editions of this book, cases which came directly from his practice.

Kenneth E. Yochum was a very proud man and this was reflected in all aspects of his professional and personal life. His commitment to excellence was untiring and that driving spirit was given to me by this great man. His influence upon my life still continues. He is greatly missed by the entire Yochum family and it is befitting that the second edition of the Yochum and Rowe textbook be dedicated to his memory.

Terry R. Yochum

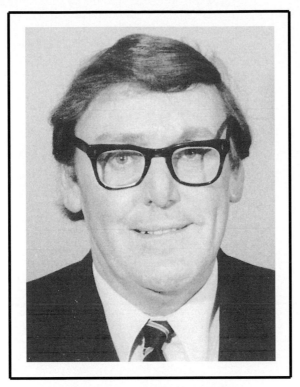

Bryan Hartley, M.D.
(1926–1984)

Within a lifetime, a few select individuals will significantly affect the life of another. For both of us, Bryan Hartley, M.D., was one of those individuals. He was a person who seemed to achieve whatever he wanted in life: an extraordinary professional career, diversified personal interests, and close ties with family and friends. Bryan was born at Aldershot, England, in 1926 and studied medicine at Guy's Hospital Medical School in London. He was appointed house surgeon at the Royal Infirmary, Edinburgh, in 1950, following which he emigrated to Australia. He became a flight lieutenant in the R.A.A.F. medical branch and was a Fulbright traveling scholar. He was appointed medical officer in the Northern Territory Medical Services and continued his medical training at the Royal Perth Hospital in Western Australia and was a resident medical officer at General Hospital in Tasmania.

Bryan Hartley's early postgraduate training appointments alternated between the fields of surgery and radiology. He held appointments in surgery at the Union Memorial Hospital in Baltimore, Maryland; Launceston General Hospital in Tasmania; the Royal Children's Hospital in Melbourne, Victoria; and as Surgeon Superintendent at the Lyell District Hospital, Tasmania. His appointments in radiology were at the Launceston General Hospital, St. Vincent's Hospital, Melbourne, and the Royal Hobart Hospital in Tasmania. After a short appointment in Rome as a radiologist for the Department of Immigration, Bryan returned to Melbourne to become the director of the Department of Radiology at the Repatriation General Hospital and held this position until 1981. At that time, he accepted a position as staff radiologist in the Department of Radiology at the Austin Hospital also in Melbourne, the post he occupied until his death.

In his chosen career of medicine, Bryan Hartley excelled in both surgery and radiology, holding specialist qualifications in both fields. This interest in surgery was of considerable advantage to him in radiology, as it enabled him to see a diagnostic problem in its proper clinical perspective. A unique combination of clinical understanding, experience, and aptitude for clear expression made Bryan an outstanding teacher for his many students, residents, and colleagues. His boundless enthusiasm and wry humor provided for stimulating and informative discussions on almost any topic. His opinions were highly valued, particularly in patient evaluation and treatment.

For both of us, it was Bryan who, by example, provided the stimulus for developing our knowledge and abilities and advancing the standards of our profession. His influence on our careers is reflected not only in the use of his personal case material in this text, but more importantly in the knowledge, expertise, and teaching methods he so freely shared with us. His untimely death in 1984 now deprives us and others of the opportunity of sharing his special gifts. He is survived by his wife, Beverley, and their children, Lynne and John.

In gratitude we have dedicated the first edition of this book to Bryan Hartley, M.D.

Terry R. Yochum
Lindsay J. Rowe

Foreword to the Second Edition

I have known the two authors of this text for many years and, as stated in their Preface, although they currently are separated physically by thousands of miles, they both remain extremely focused and dedicated to the specialty of musculoskeletal imaging and to teaching what they know to others. Through clear and concise writing, an organized and logical approach, and the use of selected high quality images, their passion for this subspecialty and their abilities as teachers are readily apparent. Simply, they love what they do and it shows. As an author myself, I recognize the energy and commitment that are required in the preparation of a book of this size. The task mandates that they do little else during a period of months and, even, years and that they sacrifice family responsibilities and recreational time to read and organize available literature and sort through innumerable radiographic examples to choose the ones whose message is most vivid. The only reward is the satisfaction derived from a job well done and from the belief that others will profit from their efforts.

Terry and Lindsay, from different countries and now from different scientific specialties, have, through their extraordinary effort, expressed their knowledge and beliefs in the form of words, phrases, sentences, and paragraphs, coupled with high quality images, which when read and viewed will lead you through the intricacies of musculoskeletal imaging and will provide the insight necessary for appropriate treatment of your patients. Their text is comprehensive, covers technical aspects, and provides a summary of various categories of disease that affect the musculoskeletal tissues. Spend the time necessary to master the principles outlined in this text and you will be a better health provider for your efforts.

I congratulate Terry and Lindsay for their considerable effort.

Donald Resnick, M.D.
Professor of Radiology
University of California, San Diego
Chief of Osteoradiology Section
Veterans Affairs Medical Center
San Diego, California

Foreword to the Second Edition

Diagnostic imaging has a prominent role in the care of patients with musculoskeletal complaints. While x-rays retain considerable importance in the diagnosis of fractures, arthritis, dysplasias, and other conditions characterized by gross changes in bone morphology, radiography continues to give way to advanced computer-assisted imaging technologies. These newer technologies reveal bony and soft tissue anatomy in great detail, and some techniques can show abnormalities of physiology and metabolism. Computed tomography and magnetic resonance imaging have broad applicability and may be combined with more invasive procedures such as arthrography and percutaneous needle biopsy. To utilize properly the tools of diagnostic imaging, a high level of sophistication is required. High costs and concern about litigation have added to the complexity of the decision-making process.

The first edition of Yochum and Rowe's *Essentials of Skeletal Radiology* addressed the need for current knowledge about diagnostic imaging. In the new edition, the authors have expanded and updated their work, retaining their no-nonsense writing style and their sharp eye for illustration. Of particular interest is the completely rewritten chapter on diagnostic imaging of the musculoskeletal system. Sections devoted to each imaging technology include the historical background, a glossary of specialized terminology (helpful when consulting with the radiologist), a concise explanation of underlying physical principles, diagrams of equipment, and descriptions of medicolegal implications. The discussions of indications and contraindications for particular examinations are pragmatic and useful, and go beyond rote lists and simplistic algorithms. Frequently asked questions are explicitly raised and answered, and extensive case illustrations drive the points home. The non-radiologist practitioner must understand how radiological images are generated and interpreted in order to make an informed choice among the many options. Like the first edition, this book will become virtually indispensable for many practitioners.

Felix S. Chew, M.D.
Department of Radiology
Massachusetts General Hospital
Harvard Medical School
Boston, Massachusetts

Foreword to the Second Edition

Success is not searching for you. You must do the seeking.
Destiny is not a matter of choice; it is not a thing to be waited for,
it is a thing to be achieved!

William Jennings Bryan

As a mountaineer scrambles up the final ascent of a high peak, exhilarating breaths of anticipation come with labored intensity. Muscles persist in aching and cramping. Headache throbs signal severe oxygen depletion as icy winds blow at a sunburned, chapped face. What, you say? ". . . the pain and suffering is worth the view!" If that be the case, why is the summit experience often limited to just enough time for a few quick pictures, a light snack, some liquid, and back down you go? Nay my friend, there is more to it than just the view.

The reward for supreme sacrifice and effort is both tangible and intangible. The tangible—recognition, praise, money, and prestige—are easily dismissed as the sole motivation for total commitment. It is the intangible, the unmeasurable, that spins the inner turbines and generates the necessary energy required to scale the peak. A sense of fulfillment, a feeling of self-worth knowing that one is able to excel beyond the limits of one's self, a supreme achievement—is the secret victory.

Once the peak is conquered, why do it again? How can it be as challenging or rewarding the second time around? Why a second edition of *Essentials of Skeletal Radiology,* one of the most widely published texts in the 100-year history of radiology and **the** mostly widely used radiology text in the 100-year history of chiropractic? How can one improve on a classic?

Multiple ascents of the same peak are rendered challenging by scaling new and more difficult routes, climbing under different and less optimal conditions, climbing with new partners, testing new equipment, and recognizing that the passage of time brings new knowledge. In the ever-changing world of diagnostic imaging, new and improved technology carries our vision beyond what our imaginations saw when the first edition was produced. With the power of this new vision, many new concepts need to be teased out and organized while old patterns of thought must be re-evaluated and validated. In this text, the new application of advanced imaging for early detection of bone injury is but one example of how Terry and Lindsay have placed this edition on the cutting edge of knowledge.

Contributions from new, invited authors have added a bright dimension to this edition. When scaling a wall, a team of climbers must know and trust every movement of the persons to whom they are tied. An improper anchoring, a slip, or a fall, could spell disaster for everyone. Yet with a master climber as anchor person on the team, even if partners slip, the team is held secure. Rest assured, dear reader, the quality of this text would never be compromised to allow for mediocrity. The Yochum mark of perfection is found on every page and we reap the benefit of the polishing teamwork of Terry and Lindsay and their co-participants. This level of quality is not bought with honoraria and royalties, but with blood, sweat, and tears. Perhaps such a colorful mixture has contributed to the bright hues found throughout the text.

Finally, the descent can be as treacherous as the ascent. Fatigue, boredom, mineral depletion, and lack of focus open opportunities for mistakes through carelessness. When the text is written and put to page proofs, even with the sophisticated technology of today, errors creep in. Thus, every word and every picture must be examined and re-read on every page to assure, "All is well!" The novice would say, "Tis the easier portion. The work has been done." Try it! Scrupulous hours of final proofing with a keen-focus on the work at hand is as challenging as the creative work at the beginning of the project. No one person can do it all alone. But the tenacity of Dr. Yochum for perfection in production assures that this second edition is as close to flawless as humanly possible. He would be the first to acknowledge all those who came to his assistance, and rightfully so. But without his forceful encouragement, the level of quality would not be as it is. As his daddy, Dr. Ken Yochum used to always say, "Son, right's right and wrong's nobody!"

Finally, we must consider the hero who never makes it to the mountain summit; sees only pictures of the view, hears the climber's complaints, endures sleepless nights, but still has energy to calm and encourage when needed and to retreat when prudent. Without the loving support of a wife like Inge, there never would have been a second edition, or a first edition. Or even a Dr. Yochum as we know him today, to be shared with the chiropractic profession, the radiology profession, the baseball profession, and the swing dance profession. To them both I host these words as a momento to their achievements:

> The heights of great men reached and kept,
> Were not attained by sudden flight,
> But, they, while their companions slept,
> Were toiling upward through the night.
> Henry Wadsworth Longfellow, ''The Ladder of St. Augustine''

Reed B. Phillips, DC, DACBR, PhD
President
Los Angeles College of Chiropractic
Whittier, California

Foreword to the Second Edition

I was quite delighted to have the opportunity to review Drs. Yochum and Rowe's first publication of *Essentials of Skeletal Radiology*. Today, I am even happier to recommend this new edition to those who are interested in and fascinated with skeletal imaging.

Terry and Lindsay are wonderful teachers, and this second edition displays their characteristic way of presenting difficult material in a simplified form that promotes not only understanding, but also retention.

Their transmitted knowledge of MRI contained in chapter 6, Diagnostic Imaging of the Musculoskeletal System, is especially enjoyable and the reader is capable of rapid digestion of the material. They have distilled a complex array of information not only on how MRI works (as good a job as I've ever seen) but also shows superb images that display this pathology succinctly and explain how, and when or when not to obtain them.

The chapters follow a solid, logical progression that first-time readers will appreciate. For our newer colleagues in radiology, the chapters on Principles of Radiologic Interpretation and Report Writing in Skeletal Radiology will be especially helpful.

If anyone is interested in mnemonics for skeletal radiology this book is a goldmine for providing the tools necessary in learning how to quickly recall a lot of material. Terry and Lindsay really piqued my interest here, and I'm sure the reader will enjoy the lessons.

This revision represents a tremendous amount of work. The quality is evident in the writing as well as the case selections. Anyone interested in skeletal radiology will truly enjoy this book because the authors grasp the complexities of the subject and are able to stress what really is important. This book represents the state of the art in skeletal radiology.

M. Bruce Farkas, D.O., J.D.
Professor of Radiology (Retired)
Chicago College of Osteopathic Medicine
Chief, Radiology Military Entrance and Processing Station
Chicago, Illinois

Foreword to the First Edition

Although there are a number of excellent books dealing with skeletal radiology, the addition of these volumes to the literature is more than welcome. The unique format and the approach taken by Drs. Yochum and Rowe should make this book particularly valuable as a reference source. Happily, the material is also very readable and should serve as an excellent textbook. As an educator I am especially pleased to have the chapter dealing with *principles of radiological interpretation* included since this material in detail is not found elsewhere.

The compilation of this material indeed represents a monumental effort. Contributions of case material from doctors of various disciplines worldwide not only augments the extensive material Drs. Yochum and Rowe and the other authors have compiled but also speaks to the esteem in which the authors are held and the increasing cooperation among the several healing arts.

The ultimate reward for a teacher is to see his students excell. As Dr. Yochum's chief I take pride in his accomplishments and those of Dr. Rowe, his former student. The results of their efforts in compiling this work will stand as a tribute to unceasing dedication and excellence in their chosen field. I deem it a privilege to be a contributor to this work. I expect that *Essentials of Skeletal Radiology* will be the benchmark for publications by doctors of chiropractic and will find a place among the standard works in skeletal radiology.

Joseph W. Howe, D.C., D.A.C.B.R., F.I.C.C., Fellow, A.C.C.R.
Professor and Chairman
Radiology Department
Los Angeles College of Chiropractic
Whittier, California

Foreword to the First Edition

I have known Drs. Yochum and Rowe for many years. When they visited Dr. William E. Litterer in Elizabeth, New Jersey, it was not uncommon for us to spend many hours in front of the view boxes viewing and sharing interesting cases, many of which now appear in this text.

Both authors possess a unique quality that I refer to as a passion for knowledge. It is because of this thirst for knowledge and a willingness to share information that this book has become a reality.

Essentials of Skeletal Radiology is an excellent book that can serve as both a core textbook and a reference text. Although originally written for the chiropractic profession, I would recommend this book to anyone interested in skeletal radiology.

I congratulate Drs. Yochum and Rowe for a job well done.

Steven P. Brownstein, M.D.
Chief of Computed Tomography Section
East Orange Veterans Administration Hospital
East Orange, New Jersey

Associate Attending Professor of Radiology
University Hospital
Newark, New Jersey

Clinical Assistant Professor of Radiology
New Jersey University Medical and Dental School
Newark, New Jersey

Foreword to the First Edition

Radiology is such a dynamic medical specialty. We students of the field have amassed a wealth of information since the first x-rays were taken in the nineteenth century. Those of us who have been around radiology for more than a few years have seen tremendous improvements in our imaging departments. We have not only many ways to produce an image but also many ways to capture and view the image we want. And we can do it with less radiation to the patient or no radiation at all. This delightful growth in radiology parallels the careers of the two accomplished doctors who are the authors of this fine text. I have had the privilege of watching these two charming and interesting fellows as their careers began to bloom and focus on radiology. They possess an insatiable thirst for radiology and a special propensity for skeletal radiology. They have studied and traveled around the globe not only to improve their knowledge, but also to share their expertise with fellow students and radiologists.

This book represents a tremendous compilation of material. Terry and Lindsay say it all in a rare flow of concise reading, fine charts, and excellent radiographs. This is a gem, a quality jewel of a book that we all will enjoy using and telling friends, students, practitioners and fellow radiologists, ''Pick up Yochum and Rowe's *Essentials of Skeletal Radiology*.''

M. Bruce Farkas, D.O.
Professor of Radiology
Chicago College of Osteopathic Medicine
Chicago, Illinois

Preface to the Second Edition

Essentials of Skeletal Radiology is now into its second decade with the release of this second edition. It is an honor to have the release of this revised edition coincide with the centenary of Roentgen's revolutionary discovery. Although we live in different countries, share common distractions and duties with professional activities, family and the events of life, the rekindling of this team's chemistry has rapidly brought the second edition to its full fruition.

The acceptance and success of the first edition has been overwhelming and unexpected. We believed in our work and were aware of its merits. What we did not fully perceive was the magnitude of the need for this text. Throughout the world we have been startled at the impact of this publication. So many books lay tattered and torn as testimony to its use. Copies have been stolen for destinations unknown and even illegal counterfeit copies have surfaced. The number of citations of the book in many subsequent publications has been extremely encouraging.

Criticisms have been few, but have always been interpreted by us as constructive. The good reviews, encouraging comments from colleagues, and acceptance into the teaching curricula of many institutions, including chiropractic and medical schools, reflect a groundswell of fulfilling a real need in the clinical community in the United States and internationally. This is the impetus for this subsequent edition.

A second edition is like original art being retouched. Though there is always the risk of spoiling it, the challenge of constructing a revision that is better than the first provided the inspiration for this second edition. Incorporating the technological explosion of the imaging revolution (which the first edition has lived through) into this next generation of pages has provided a unique dilemma. Our efforts have been directed at containing the size of this text to maintain its usefulness in the classroom, while attempting to provide a comprehensive review that incorporates these recent imaging advances. In some chapters this required complete re-writing in order to reflect these quantum changes.

A number of changes have been made in this second edition, though the basic fabric of the book remains essentially the same. Structurally, color has been added to enhance readability and accentuate important points. Most of the diagrams have been highlighted to emphasize the key radiologic features. Headings and figure captions similarly have been selectively colored. The method of presentation under progressive headings of *general considerations, clinical features, pathologic features, radiologic features* and *treatment and prognosis* has been maintained. The *capsule summary* remains an integral component. A key addition has been the *medicolegal implications* section that follows many of the conditions discussed. This was designed to assist in important therapeutic and management decisions and reflects the increasing emphasis that diagnostic imaging has assumed in clinical practice. The use of *algorithms* in Chapter 5 will significantly impact the treatment of many patients. Additionally, a special section on *mnemonics* appears as an Appendix at the end of each volume as a unique learning aid for all students of radiology.

Many favorable comments have been relayed to us regarding how the references in the first edition have been used as the basis for various research and other scientific articles and case reports. For this second edition the vast amount of relevant literature was systematically reviewed with only those of significant merit being used. All owners of this second edition, whether student, teacher, researcher or practitioner, should find these additions of significant assistance with their endeavors.

The photographic reproductions and diagrams have always been listed as one of the most attractive characteristics of the book. New diagrams have been added and improvements on existing ones have been made, such as the well-known regional distribution body skeleton which has incorporated new localizing symbols to identify most common and less common sites for involvement. Radiographs are difficult to read, even when viewing high quality originals with subtle features often converting into highly significant clinical ramifications. We have selectively removed some images from the first edition and replaced them with new ones. We have also continued with the teaching principle of placing arrows on images to correlate with the descriptive caption to direct all readers to important facets of the case. In general, the case material has been augmented with bone scans, CT, and MR imaging to reflect the technological revolution in musculoskeletal diagnosis. A quick glance at Chapter 6 demonstrates these efforts.

The most common question asked of any author in a second edition is, "Are there any differences from the first edition?" This text has undergone significant structural and content changes. Each chapter has been revised, some more extensively than others. Despite this, there has been a vigilant effort to maintain the hallmark features and core material of the first edition so familiarity in this second edition will be evident. As we outlined in the preface of the first edition, the emphasis has been placed on constructing a clear and concise presentation. As with the first edition, this text is meant to be used for at least three purposes: as a *teaching text* aimed at all those who seek knowledge and expertise in musculoskeletal disorders; as a *reference text* when information is sought; and, as a *clinical aid* to assist you with those patients who seek your care. In this regard, we encourage you to read this text carefully and use it for its intended purposes.

The eye does not see what the brain does not know.

Terry R. Yochum
Lindsay J. Rowe

Preface to the First Edition

The conception of this textbook, *Essentials of Skeletal Radiology*, began in 1980 in Melbourne, Australia. A set of unique circumstances brought an American radiology professor (TRY) and an Australian radiology resident (LJR) together. Both felt the frustration of utilizing multiple texts from which to teach and to learn about disorders that afflict the human skeleton. A tentative table of contents and a sample chapter were submitted to Williams & Wilkins for review. In 1982, at the November Radiological Society of North America (RSNA) meeting in Chicago, a formal contract to create this textbook was agreed upon. We ventured into this project essentially not knowing how much time and effort would actually be required. We began with enthusiasm and optimism in different countries, Dr. Yochum in Australia and Dr. Rowe in Canada, and later joined forces in the United States.

The initial tasks were to catalogue the photographed case material we already had and to seek out from diverse sources that which we did not have but felt should be included in a comprehensive text. The magnitude of this aspect alone is represented by the final selection of some 2500 illustrative cases from a collective pool of more than 7000. All of this without a single word yet written!

After the accumulation of the resource material, the creation of the text, beginning in January 1984, was another journey into the unknown. Every word was initially **handwritten,** amassing some 10,000 pages of raw manuscript. At completion we filled 30 computer discs and gained a unique appreciation for the amazing properties of word processing. We sympathize with authors who have compiled even larger and more complex texts in years past without such technology available to them. Thorough review of the copy edited manuscript was followed by proofreading the voluminous galleys and page proofs and compiling the comprehensive index.

An explanation of the title, *Essentials of Skeletal Radiology*, may help to clarify the book's purpose and scope. The word "essentials" was selected as the fundamental guiding concept throughout the compilation of this work. From the vast and overwhelming body of knowledge of skeletal disorders we have extracted the core facts and brought them together into a single unique source. It is the desire and intent of the authors that through this endeavor the process of learning and understanding the radiology of skeletal disorders will become somewhat easier for all, from the student of radiology to the experienced clinician. We have combined these "essentials" with our own personal observations sometimes interpreted as experience. Our intent for this work is that it perform as a textbook. A textbook, as defined by Webster, is "a book containing the principles of a subject, used as a basis for instruction." Practically interpreted, a textbook serves as a foundation and provides the framework upon which one should add his or her own "experience."

To serve this purpose the book has been carefully constructed around a clear and concise mode of presentation. The subject of each chapter was thoughtfully selected and placed in a logical sequence, beginning with the technology of producing diagnostic skeletal radiographs and interpreting the depicted normal radiographic anatomy. Following this, the many diverse congenital anomalies and normal skeletal variants are presented both in text and pictorial atlas format. Then follow the radiographic measurements and the biomechanically related disorders of the musculoskeletal system: scoliosis, spondylolisthesis and spinal stenosis. These precede an introductory chapter into the principles of radiographic interpretation of the more complex pathological entities. This chapter is a keystone to comprehending the basic principles of radiographic diagnosis of the skeleton. The chapters that follow deal with the seven categories of bone disease: skeletal dysplasias, trauma, arthritic disorders, tumor and tumor-like processes, infection, vascular and hematologic disorders, and nutritional, metabolic and endocrine disorders. This forms the nucleus of the pathologic aspect of this text. The last three chapters cover often-neglected aspects of skeletal radiology: report writing, radiographic artifacts, and a pictorial atlas of vertebral names.

The methodology of presentation we have chosen is to break down the subject material into logical headings. Initially a discussion of *general* and occasionally *historical considerations* of each disorder is given. Under the next heading of *clinical features* we have accurately outlined the physical and laboratory abnormalities demonstrated with each condition. Specific details have been included that relate to clinical presentation, incidence, age, sex, location, and any distinctive physical characteristics. The *pathologic features* offer a fundamental presentation covering etiology, pathogenesis, and histopathologic abnormalities basic to the radiographic signs. The *radiologic features* have formed the major emphasis of discussion for each disorder, and the essential roentgenographic signs are stressed. The understanding of these signs is augmented by photographic reproductions of many actual radiographs, as well as illustrative line drawings. Wherever possible, *treatment* and *prognosis* have been discussed. A highlight of the text is an outline of the core material of the chapter in a concise *capsule summary*. The summaries are distinguished by a different typeface and by their placement within shaded blocks. Their purpose is to provide a quick and easy reference source.

A comprehensive bibliography from many health disciplines has been integrated within the text to substantiate the facts presented and to provide resources to stimulate further investigation.

The large number of case studies and illustrations reflects our desire to depict visually the essential roentgenographic signs of even the most complex skeletal disorders. The captions describe details to be noted in the illustrations. Aspects of particular importance are indicated by arrows on the figures. Additionally, important facts are reinforced with a *comment* section at the conclusion of the caption.

The comprehensive index was compiled with considerable thought and effort. The page numbers of the primary discussion of the selected disorder are printed in bold type to facilitate the reader's search.

In conclusion, this text is meant to be read from cover to cover and also to be used as a reference source. Use this book as it is intended—to help you master the knowledge and perfect the skill of interpreting skeletal radiographs so that you might better evaluate, understand and treat your patients.

Terry R. Yochum
Lindsay J. Rowe

Acknowledgments

The release of *Essentials of Skeletal Radiology* in 1987 was a dream fulfilled for both of us. We had hardly blinked an eye and the publishers were requesting us to consider a second edition, a monumental task that took approximately two and one-half years in production and publication once we actually began the process. A task of this magnitude is never accomplished without significant support from numerous people assisting in many different ways.

Our contributing authors have provided a distinct and unique contribution to this second edition and we wish to recognize their efforts:

Michael S. Barry, D.C., D.A.C.B.R.
Gary M. Guebert, D.C., D.A.C.B.R.
Bryan Hartley, M.D.
Norman W. Kettner, D.C., D.A.C.B.R.
Claude Pierre-Jerome, M.D.
Margaret A. Seron, D.C., D.A.B.C.O., D.A.C.B.R.
David P. Thomas, M.D.

Their assistance in four chapters of this edition is greatly appreciated.

We would also like to thank Leon L. Wiltse, M.D., Long Beach Memorial Hospital, Long Beach, California, and Lyle J. Micheli, M.D., Children's Hospital, Harvard Medical School, Department of Orthopedics, Boston, Massachusetts, for their expert review and editing of Chapter 5, "The Natural History of Spondylolysis and Spondylolisthesis."

Chapter 6 entitled "Diagnostic Imaging of the Musculoskeletal System" represents a new addition to the second edition of this textbook. We wish to acknowledge and offer special thanks to Felix S. Chew, M.D., Assistant Professor of Radiology, Massachusetts General Hospital, Harvard Medical School, Boston, Massachusetts, for his editorial expertise and review of Chapter 6. In order to publish a chapter on special imaging covering the musculoskeletal system, unique and interesting case material was necessary. We wish to thank Steven P. Brownstein, M.D., James L. Qualle, M.D., Kenneth B. Reynard, M.D., and Frank E. Seidelmann, D.O., for their very timely assistance in filling our "wish list" for the necessary material to promptly complete this unique new chapter.

A special thank you to those physicians who have graciously provided the forewords for the second edition:

Felix S. Chew, M.D.
M. Bruce Farkas, D.O., J.D.
Reed B. Phillips, D.C., D.A.C.B.R., PhD.
Donald Resnick, M.D.

Several people were involved at varying levels in the editorial process of the production of the second edition of this textbook. Special thanks is offered to Drs. Todd A. Ryan and John L. Golden, radiology residents from Logan College of Chiropractic, who worked diligently to help finalize Chapter 6. Our sincere gratitude extends to a longtime friend, Dr. Gary M. Guebert, for his excellent work on Chapter 3 and his assistance in finalizing Chapter 6. Thanks also to the graduating class of August 1996 at Logan College of Chiropractic who provided Dr. Guebert with reference assistance in the finalization of Chapter 3.

The seemingly constant proofreading process appears as a never-ending exercise in the production of a manuscript this size. Unique support in this area came from talented friends and colleagues like Craig Lincoln, D.C., John K. Hyland, D.C., D.A.C.B.R., D.A.B.C.O., and Jeffrey R. Thompson, D.C., D.A.C.B.R., Jolie Haug, D.C., a unique and dedicated chiropractor, proofread and provided editorial assistance to us for the entire first edition and then, shortly after her return from China, once again blessed us with additional editorial assistance in the finalization of Chapter 6. Special thanks to all for their distinctive and creative talents.

Simple phone calls to our good friends, John A.M. Taylor, D.C., D.A.C.B.R., and Beverly L. Harger, D.C., D.A.C.B.R., while we were looking for unique technical artifacts for Chapter 16 proved fruitful. At a moment's notice they provided the case material necessary to fill the gaps in this technical arena. Thanks so much for your support and case material.

Special thanks to Michael L. Manco-Johnson, M.D., F.A.C.R., Professor of Radiology and Medicine, Chairman of the Department of Radiology, University of Colorado Health Science Center, Denver, Colorado, and Ray F. Kilcoyne, M.D., Professor of Radiology, Vice-Chairman of the Department of Radiology, University of Colorado Health Science Center, Denver, Colorado, for allowing the case material that has circulated through the various departments at the University to be photographed and utilized in this second edition. Thanks also to the many radiology residents who have secured unique skeletal radiology cases for our teaching file and, in particular, this second edition. Many of those residents' names appear scattered throughout various chapters following their case material.

Chapter 8 ("Skeletal Dysplasias") of this book provided a particular challenge in upgrading the case material. Children's Hospital, Department of Radiology, Denver, Colorado, was most cooperative in allowing us to photograph their skeletal teaching file. These cases are dispersed throughout the textbook, particularly in the area of dysplasias. Thanks specifically to John D. Strain, M.D., Chairman of the Department of Radiology, Children's Hospital, Denver, Colorado for assisting us in obtaining this case material.

There are some line drawing illustrations that have been repeated from Chapter 6 in the first edition which were admirably produced by Marshall N. Deltoff, D.C., D.A.C.B.R. We have repeated these line drawings in Chapter 6 and appreciate the opportunity to do so. Many of the new line drawings in this text have been executed by Mr. Frank Pryor, Pryority Graphics, Lakewood, Colorado. These new line drawings are scattered throughout the various chapters, with the majority being found in Chapter 6. Thanks for a job well done on these medical illustrations.

The majority of the new photographs for this second edition were skillfully processed and perfected by The Pro Lab, Inc., Denver, Colorado. Special thank you to William E. Inman, Diane Belfour, Susan Hill, Mark A. Eirhart, Don Markham, Michael T. Lung, Kimberly Berger, Roy Nieto, and Sharon Sternberg. All of these wonderful people helped in moving the negatives, along with black and white prints, back and forth from the laboratory and my office under very difficult time constraints. The quality of their work is exemplified by the end product, specifically the many new photographic additions, particularly the complete revision and all new photographs in Chapter 6.

Thanks also to the medical illustrations department of Washington University, St. Louis, Missouri, and Yuji Oishi, M.D., Denver, Colorado, for providing some of the photographic reproductions in Chapters 3 and 6.

To the staff of Williams & Wilkins, and to our Editor, John Butler, we are most thankful for their support in bringing this manuscript to final publication. Special thanks to George Stamathis, President, Barbara Felton, Production Coordinator, and, to Wayne Hubbel, Illustration Planner, for his outstanding work on perfecting the illustrations in this second edition. Also, thank you to Wilma Rosenberger, Designer, and Karen Gulliver, Managing Editor, for her excellent review of the manuscript.

Finally, our gratitude is expressed to Joseph Janse, D.C., and Kenneth E. Yochum, D.C., in our dual dedications.

Terry R. Yochum
Lindsay J. Rowe

With a deep sense of gratitude, I wish to thank my devoted companion, Inge. This tremendous woman also happens to be my wife. Her understanding, support, and unconditional love fashioned the vehicle that carried me as I traveled the road of this second edition. Special thanks and love to my children, Kimberley Ann, Philip Andrew, and Alicia Marie. They are the three little joys of my life who readily forgave all of their father's frequent absences during the project. Special thanks to my most devoted follower, Cecelia Yochum, my mother who gave me life and continues to nurture and encourage.

To my professional acquaintances who have inspired and influenced me throughout my career, I wish to acknowledge:

- Dr. M. Bruce Farkas, who helped me greatly in the beginning of my career.
- Dr. Joseph W. Howe, after whom a progeny of radiology diplomates emerged.
- Dr. Joseph Janse, a name which is practically an eponym for modern chiropractic.
- Dr. William E. Litterer, who spares no detail and forgets no face.
- Dr. Reed B. Phillips, a critical thinker, man of integrity and my very best friend.
- Dr. Donald B. Tomkins, who is remembered for knowledge tempered by wisdom.
- Dr. James F. Winterstein, who inspires his colleagues with creative impulse.

For the development and production of this book I express sincere gratitude to:

- my associate, Michael Sean Barry, D.C., D.A.C.B.R., who, at great personal sacrifice, has coauthored three chapters in this edition. His physical and intellectual support were exceptional and continued through finalization of all chapters. Our friendship has been strengthened as a result of his Herculean effort.
- Leah Barry, for releasing her husband Michael to devote many hours beyond the call of duty, especially in the final four months of the project.
- one of my most outstanding residents, devoted friends, and colleague, Gary M. Guebert, D.C., D.A.C.B.R. Special thanks for his outstanding work on the revision of Chapter 3, "Congenital Anomalies and Normal Skeletal Variants." His additional assistance in helping finalize Chapter 6 was an exemplary effort and greatly appreciated.
- Connie Jones, R.T.(R), my close friend, employee of thirteen years, medical radiographer, and hard-working compatriot. She has never missed a day's work and has supported me through both editions of this textbook!
- Kim Kochevar, for her efforts in holding things together in our busy radiology practice while I diverted my attention to the text's revision.
- Debbie Schlosser, for the time she freely gave when her energy was needed to type and repeatedly edit the manuscript. Her efforts to bring it to perfection were unparalleled.

I express particular thanks to three very distinguished individuals:

- Mr. Kent S. Greenawalt, President of Foot Levelers, Inc., Roanoke, Virginia.
- Mr. Calvin Kleinman, President of Bennett X-ray, Corp., Copiague, New York.
- Dr. Reed B. Phillips, President, Los Angeles College of Chiropractic, Whittier, California.

These dear friends were never too busy to receive a late night phone call or to be a sounding board for my concerns and woes. They carried me over hard, rocky places as I proceeded down a road not well traveled.

The inspiration to upgrade the second edition of this text came from the many doctors who have attended my lectures from coast to coast, and I wish to thank them for providing me this motivation.

And finally, to my coauthor, friend, and colleague, Dr. Lindsay J. Rowe. His succinct, instructive writing is an expression of his advanced talents as a great academic and clinical radiologist. It is a privilege to share and coauthor this book with him.

Terry R. Yochum

Arising from the entanglements in the development of this second edition comes the support and encouragement from many without whom such a work does not happen. One feeds on their energy and kind words usually without realization until there is time to reflect.

In the mirror I see my good friend and colleague James R. Brandt, DC, MSc, FACO, whose clock in life never stops and who winds mine whenever it runs out. From afar his insightful judgements, clarity of thought, and enthusiasm generated inertia to see the project through to completion. His eloquent and timely notes have colored my life and served as impromptu smiling devices in times of need.

To Michael Buna, BSc, DC, support is a small word that embodies his constant inquiring mind and yearning to see this next edition become a tangible reality. For Kevin Schwager, BAppSc (Chiro), who took the time to check on my progress at any hour of any day I am grateful for his backing, reminders and distractions. In my friend Lise Janelle, DC, her zest for life and commitment to the enhancement of the lives of others I found inspiration to contribute to yet another project that potentially could amplify the health for all that seek our care.

Thanks to Wayne Minter, BEcon, BAppSc (Chiro), for those words of wisdom and devices of life for survival over the past years and ensuring that the future included this next edition. From Shane Carter, BAppSc (Chiro), came those convenient notes and words of encouragement echoed from afar that fortuitously arrived uncannily when they were most needed. To Roy Logan, DC, having entrusted to me some of his wisdom and whose parting words to me in this life were to finish this work I can truly say, "yes I have." More recently my reacquaintance with Brian Nook, DC, CCSP, and Timothy Mick, DC, DACBR, gave me new meaning to what is true friendship and spurred my efforts onward. My close friends Pat and John Zapitello have motivated me by their understanding and kind thoughts. To the students I have taught past, present, and future I am indebted to you for providing the groundwork in developing and molding this work.

Over the years since the first edition was released my travels have taken me to many places where so many friends, colleagues, and students have encouraged me to see a second edition through. Support from those patients who have either written, telephoned, or spoken to me personally I thank you for your kind words and inspiration to help others. I hope you all smile when you read these simple words. Even if your names do not appear in print your faces will always remain indelibly imprinted into my own occipital cortex.

For the photographs generated here in Australia Pat Leyland and Bruce Turnbull of the Medical Communications Unit, University of Newcastle, have been committed to technical excellence and fostering friendship along the way. The computer wizardry of Michael Murray has only been exceeded by his friendship, which I am glad to enjoy.

From my interactions with the team at Williams & Wilkins I have witnessed them being expedient and enthusiastic in their individual tasks. They have perpetuated the ethic from the first edition for excellence in technical quality, attention to detail and encouragement performed in the spirit of friendly goodwill. Through the difficulties encountered they have remained firmly committed to these ideals for which I acknowledge John Butler, Barbara Felton, Karen Gulliver, Wayne Hubbel, Linda Napora, Jonathan Pine, Tim Satterfield, and George Stamathis.

In my family giants walk this earth in soft ways, not disturbing those they meet but enhancing life for all that they touch. My work belongs to them. To my sister, Robyn Cunningham, the strength of my admiration for her open heart and listening ear is only clouded by my inability to express it. To Robert, my dad, and Dorothy, my mum, my emotional dictionary lies open as they quietly bring balance and a sense of meaning to my life. I record my debt to my spotted friends, Oscar and Jezebel, who smile on command, have kept my feet warm, and remain acutely aware of where the clock hands were as I toiled the time away. Thanks to Moet for looking through the window and keeping an eye on me while I worked.

For my coauthor Terry R. Yochum, BS, DC, DACBR, it has as always been a stimulating and rewarding experience to rekindle the chemistry, share the turmoil of the mixture, and be part of the genesis of something new and innovative. To live and breathe the same energy, enthusiasm, and dedication for the enhancement of our fellow human beings in this project has been a privilege and an honor.

Lindsay J. Rowe

Contributing Authors

Norman W. Kettner, D.C., D.A.C.B.R., F.I.C.C.

Chairman, Department of Radiology
Logan College of Chiropractic
Chesterfield, Missouri

Professor, Clinical Science Division
Logan College of Chiropractic
Chesterfield, Missouri

Margaret A. Seron, D.C., D.A.B.C.O., D.A.C.B.R.

Private Radiology Practice
Denver, Colorado

Postgraduate Faculty Member
Los Angeles College of Chiropractic
Whittier, California

formerly:
Assistant Professor of Radiology
Los Angeles College of Chiropractic
Whittier, California

David P. Thomas, M.D.

formerly:
Head, Department of Radiology
Austin Hospital
Melbourne, Australia

Contents

VOLUME ONE

VOLUME TWO

Abbreviations of Attained Degrees

B. App. Sc. (Chiro)
Bachelor of Applied Science (Chiropractic)
This is the chiropractic qualification issued by the Royal Melbourne Institute of Technology—
School of Chiropractic, Melbourne, Australia

B.S.
Bachelor of Science

C.C.S.P.
Certified Chiropractic Sports Physician

D.C.
Doctor of Chiropractic

D.A.B.C.O.
Diplomate of the American Board of Chiropractic Orthopedists

D.A.C.B.N.
Diplomate of the American Chiropractic Board of Nutrition

*D.A.C.B.R.
Diplomate of the American Chiropractic Board of Radiology

D.A.C.B.R. (Hon.)
Honorary Diplomate of the American Chiropractic Board of Radiology

D.A.C.B.S.P.
Diplomate of the American Chiropractic Board of Sports Physicians

D.O.
Doctor of Osteopathy

D.P.M.
Doctor of Podiatric Medicine

Ed.D.
Doctor of Education

F.A.C.C.R. (Aus)
Fellow of the Australian Chiropractic College of Radiology (Australia)

F.A.C.O.
Fellow of the Academy of Chiropractic Orthopedists

*F.C.C.R.(C)
Fellow Chiropractic College of Radiologists (Canada)

*Fellow, A.C.C.R.
Fellow American Chiropractic College of Radiology

F.I.C.C.
Fellow of the International College of Chiropractors

J.D.
Juris Doctor

*M.D.
Doctor of Medicine

M.I.R.
Member of the Institute of Radiography

M.Sc. or M.S.
Master of Science

Ph.D.
Doctor of Philosophy

R.T. (R.)
Radiological Technologist (Radiology)

*Physicians referred to in this text holding these degrees are radiologists.

Skeletal Radiology:
A Historical Perspective

Lindsay J. Rowe and Terry R. Yochum

All disciplines within the health sciences have undergone radical changes as new technologies have evolved, and radiology is no exception. In the 100 years since the discovery of x-rays in 1895, the first crude pieces of equipment and vague shadows have been replaced by sophisticated machines that produce exquisitely detailed images. So explosive have the technological gains been that radiology is no longer limited to utilizing x-rays for the diagnosis of disease. Advancements in technology have expanded the scope of diagnostic radiology to include the imaging capabilities of ultrasonic waves, radioisotopes, computers, and magnetic fields.

The history of the development of radiology is long and intricate. As with so many other significant advancements in science, x-rays were discovered accidentally. In 1895, Wilhelm Conrad Roentgen, a professor at the University of Würzburg in Germany, was working on experiments in his laboratory. (Fig. A) He was investigating the properties of an early cathode ray tube, called a Crookes' tube, which accelerated electrons in a manner similar to today's x-ray apparatus. While conducting a stream of electrons from the cathode through the evacuated tube, he noticed that a plate covered with barium platinocyanide located at some

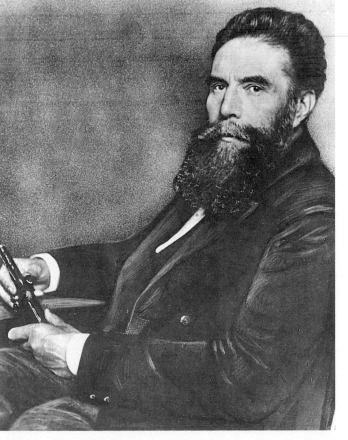

Figure A. WILHELM CONRAD ROENTGEN. Professor at the University of Würzburg in Germany, winner of the first Nobel Prize for Physics in 1901 for his discovery of the x-ray.

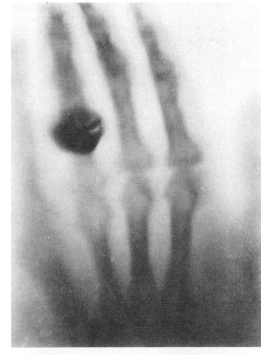

Figure B. ROENTGEN'S FIRST RADIOGRAPH. Professor Roentgen's historic first radiograph of his wife's hand taken November 8, 1895, in Würzburg, Germany. (Courtesy of Deutsches Rontgen-Museum, Remscheid-Lennep, West Germany)

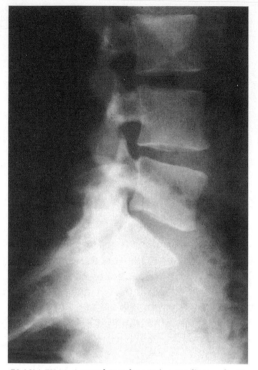

Figure C.   PLAIN FILM. Lateral Lumbar Spine Radiograph. Bony detail is well demonstrated. The space for the intervertebral discs can be appreciated though no details of disc integrity, internal structure or adjacent neural relations can be determined.

distance away began to fluoresce. Not knowing what to call these invisible rays from the Crookes' tube that induced fluorescence he named them "x-rays," "X" standing for the unknown quantity. Roentgen then feverishly began experimenting and defining their characteristics, and in little more than a month he had described all the major properties of the x-ray as they are recognized today. Professor Roentgen produced the first clinical radiograph, an image of his wife's hand, on November 8, 1895, (Fig. B) and first reported his findings on December 8, 1895, to the Würzburg Physico-Medical Society. In recognition of his discovery he received the first Nobel Prize for Physics in 1901. Others soon recognized the potential role of the x-ray in industry and the health care professions. Examples of the earliest diagnostic x-rays are those made in 1896 by Pupin of a hand imbedded with multiple shotgun pellets, those made by Frost of a fractured wrist, and a case of osteosarcoma imaged by Manell.

Thereafter, a global technological revolution began. Pupin developed the first intensifying screen, and Edison, the first fluoroscope, to mention only two developments. In 1921, Potter and Bucky introduced a moving grid mechanism. Sausser, a chiropractor, in 1934, was the first to produce a single exposure, anteroposterior full spine radiograph. The cumulative result of all of these refinements was the production of diagnostic images of improved quality, which depicted abnormalities directing more effective treatment. (Figs. C–E)

These early advancements were tempered with the recognition of the harmful nature of radiation. Many severe and often fatal injuries occurred to those who pioneered the research in

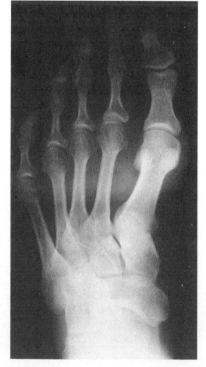

Figure D.   PLAIN FILM. Dorsiplantar View of the Foot. Observe the filtration of the forefoot and toes used to obtain a uniform exposure.

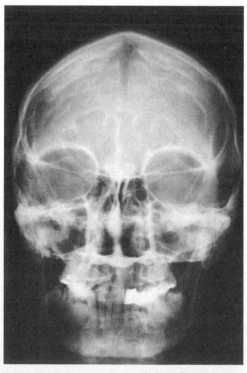

Figure E.   PLAIN FILM. Posteroanterior Skull Radiograph. The complexity of the anatomy requires careful attention to detail and anatomic landmarks. Supplemental imaging such as CT or MRI clarifies not only these structures but also provides depiction of clinically important intracranial structures.

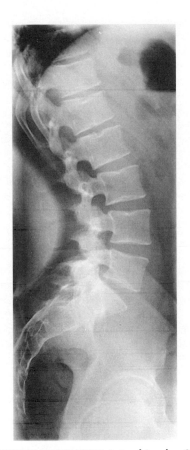

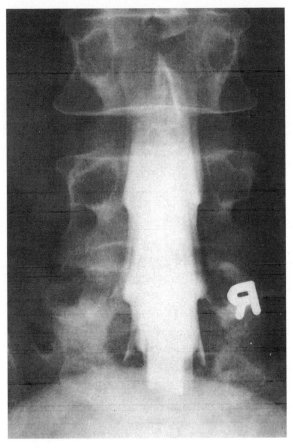

Figure F.   BALANCING FILTRATION. Lateral Lumbar Spine Radiograph. A single exposure standing lateral radiograph from the lower sacrum to the T11 level has been achieved by the placement of a number of aluminum filters in the primary beam at the collimator. These include 2 mm to the level of the iliac crest, a curved tapered filter into the lumbar lordosis to enhance detail of the spinous processes and neural arch, and a curved filter conforming to the diaphragmatic contour to eliminate overexposure of the lower thoracic segments. (Courtesy of Lloyd Wingate, DC, Dapto, Australia)

Figure G.   METRIZAMIDE LUMBAR MYELOGRAM. Placement of water soluble contrast media into the subarachnoid space allows demonstration of the normal cauda equina, dural sleeves, and caudal sac.

radiology. As a result, the use of the x-ray came under close bureaucratic scrutiny and control. Despite these complications and in the face of increasingly poor publicity, the usefulness of this new diagnostic tool could not be ignored, and innovations in imaging technology continued aimed at dose reduction, personnel and patient protection and improved image quality. In more recent times the use of rare earth screens, balancing filtration, and high frequency generators have been among the significant advancements. (Fig. F)

The dynamics of joint motion have been extensively investigated with various imaging methods. Spinal mechanics have been depicted with single views performed at the extremes of motion (dynamic or stress radiography) and with compression-distraction forces. Obtaining simultaneous views at 90° to each other (biplanar radiography) has been employed for complex computer analysis of motion patterns. Continuous spinal and peripheral joint motion can be observed with fluoroscopy and videotaped for retrospective analysis (videofluoroscopy).

The use of radiopaque contrast media within hollow organs and body spaces improved the accuracy of diagnostic evaluation. Introduction of radiopaque substances into the subarachnoid

space of the spine (myelography) provided information not previously available, especially in regard to intraspinal and intervertebral disc lesions. (Figs. G and H) Injection of the nucleus pulposus of the intervertebral disc which can be performed in conjunction with CT (discography, CT discography) provides a morphological evaluation of disc integrity, and a clinical provocational tool for isolating a discogenic cause of spinal pain syndromes. In the skeletal system, an opaque medium placed into the joint space of a peripheral or spinal facet articulation (arthrography) allows demonstration of cartilage, synovium, and ligamentous structures. (Fig. I) Introduction of contrast into a peripheral lymphatic vessel will opacify both lymphatic channels and lymph nodes (lymphangiogram). Contrast can also be injected into sinus infection or pilonidal tracts to trace their course (sinugram). (Fig. J) In some bone lesions, such as simple bone cysts, details of their internal structure can be identified.

The inherent lack of sensitivity of conventional radiography was countered by the administration of selective radioisotopes (nuclear medicine) that seek out specific tissues and areas of cellular activity. In skeletal disorders the administration of isotopes such as technetium-99m and gallium provides information on bone activity (bone scan) not recognizable with conventional procedures. These are usually performed as a triphasic study consisting of an initial "flow" study, a "blood pool," and a "delayed"

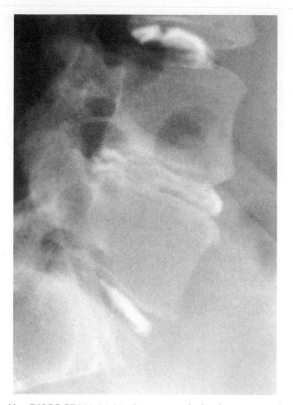

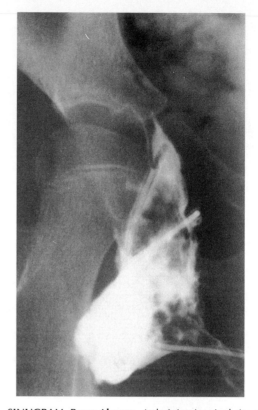

Figure H.   DISCOGRAM. L3-L5. Contrast media has been injected into the nucleus pulposus at three levels. Only the L3 disc is normal in morphology, with both L4 and L5 demonstrating migration of contrast posteriorly and anteriorly through discal tears. (Courtesy of Inger F. Villadsen, DC, Newcastle, Australia)

Figure J.   SINUGRAM. Psoas Abscess. A draining inguinal sinus was cannulated and opaque contrast media was introduced. Observe the tracking of the contrast cephalad outlining the course of the sinus which proved later to be continuous with a tuberculous infective focus in the spine at the L2-L3 level.

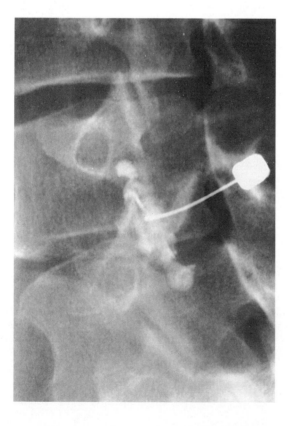

Figure I.   FACET ARTHROGRAM. L4-L5. Under fluoroscopic guidance a needle has been placed into the facet joint space which has been injected with a contrast agent. This reveals the integrity of the joint capsule and identifies correct needle placement prior to injection of a local anesthetic, irritant or anti-inflammatory agent for diagnostic or therapeutic purposes.

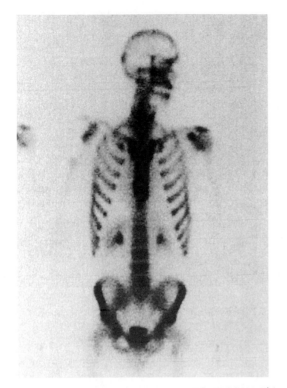

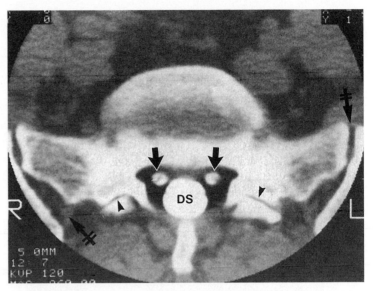

Figure M.   CONTRAST ENHANCED (MYELOGRAM) COMPUTED TO-MOGRAM OF THE S1 LEVEL. The dural sac (*DS*) and the S1 spinal nerve roots (arrows) are accurately depicted. Additionally the lumbosacral (arrowheads) and sacroiliac (crossed arrows) articulations are demonstrated.

Figure K.   FULL BODY DELAYED NUCLEAR BONE SCAN. This study is designated as "delayed" since the image is obtained some hours later following intravenous injection of the isotope. This is usually preceded by an immediate post-injection study and within minutes another set of images obtained to evaluate capillary "pooling." The delayed study demonstrates the normal uptake of radioactive isotope in metabolically active areas of the skeleton shown as dark regions ("hot spots"), requiring only a 3–5% change in activity to be detectable. (Courtesy of Nuclear Medicine Department, M.D. Anderson Hospital, Houston, Texas)

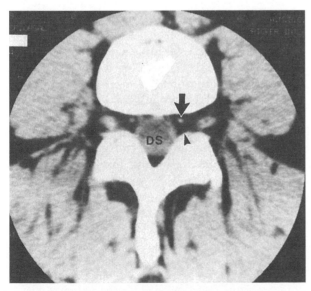

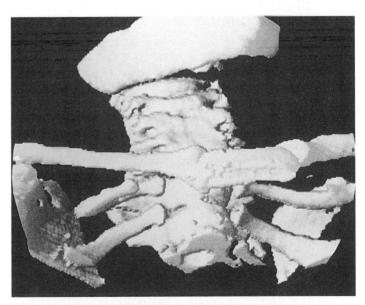

Figure N.   THREE DIMENSIONAL COMPUTED TOMOGRAPHY. Thoracic Outlet. The image has been reconstructed from thin axial images and then tilted to allow visualization of the relations of the bony thorax. Soft tissues could similarly be detected by selecting a different "window" setting. (Courtesy of Kenneth B. Heithoff, MD, Minneapolis, Minnesota)

Figure L.   COMPUTED TOMOGRAM OF THE L4 LEVEL. Observe the exquisite details of the dural sac (*DS*), nerve roots (arrow), perineural fat (arrowhead), paravertebral musculature and bony confines.

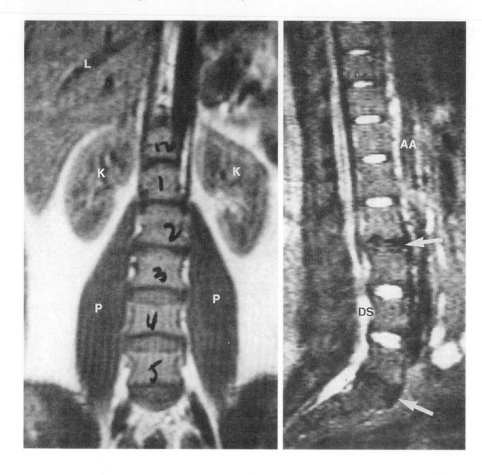

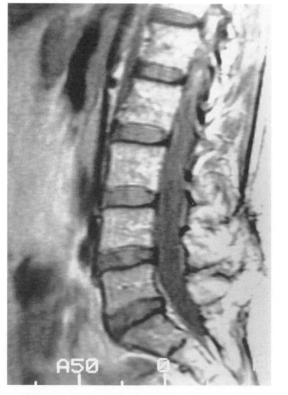

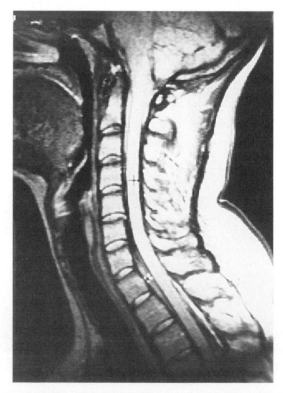

Figure O.   CORONAL AND SAGITTAL MAGNETIC RESONANCE IMAGE (MRI) OF THE ABDOMEN AND SPINE. Details of the posterior abdomen can be defined including the liver (*L*), kidneys (*K*), and psoas muscles (*P*). The dural sac (*DS*) and the abdominal aorta (*AA*) are also visible. Note the low signal intensity of the discs at L2 and L5 (arrows) representing degenerative dehydration; and the Schmorl's node affecting the inferior endplate of the L2 vertebral body.

Figure P.   SAGITTAL MAGNETIC RESONANCE IMAGE OF THE LUMBAR SPINE. Exquisite anatomic detail is depicted including the cauda equina, vertebral bodies, and intervertebral discs. (Courtesy of Kenneth B. Heithoff, MD, Minneapolis, Minnesota)

Figure Q.   SAGITTAL MAGNETIC RESONANCE IMAGE (MRI) OF THE CERVICAL SPINE. A normal study.

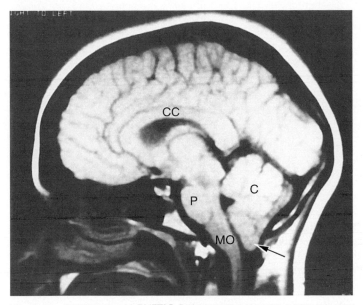

Figure R. SAGITTAL MAGNETIC RESONANCE IMAGE (MRI) OF THE BRAIN. This view clearly shows the normal pons (*P*), medulla oblongata (*MO*), cerebellum (*C*), and corpus callosum (*CC*). Observe the cerebellar tonsils below the foramen magnum (arrow)—Arnold-Chiari malformation type II.

study. (Fig. K) This has been particularly important in the early detection of many skeletal disorders. The combination of computed tomograms with nuclear medicine has added a third dimension to musculoskeletal imaging (Single Photon Emission Computed Tomography, SPECT).

In the early 1970's, computed tomograms (CT scans, CAT scans) were first produced combining the technology of the computer with the advances in x-ray technology. With refinements in machine and computer technology, exquisite sectional images are now produced in almost every anatomic plane. Computed tomograms have had a particular impact on the evaluation of spinal and neurological diseases (Figs. L and M) Three dimensional images depict anatomy and abnormalities in exquisite detail. (Fig. N) More recently the use of strong magnetic fields (Magnetic Resonance Imaging, MRI) has revolutionized body imaging capabilities and the identification of abnormalities previously unrecognizable. (Figs. O–S) The use of gadolinium enhanced MRI delivers information on vascularity and the inflammatory nature of a lesion. Ultrasound has had some limited applications in musculoskeletal disorders, providing some limited information that can assist in management of soft tissue lesions. Ultrasound screening for pediatric hip dysplasia has been a particularly notable contribution to early identification of a common problem that has considerable delayed morbidity if undetected.

In spite of all these technological advances, many fundamental principles of imaging remain unchanged. The plain film radiograph still forms the foundation for a large portion of the diagnostic investigations in clinical practice, especially in the evaluation of skeletal disorders. This is demonstrated with an example

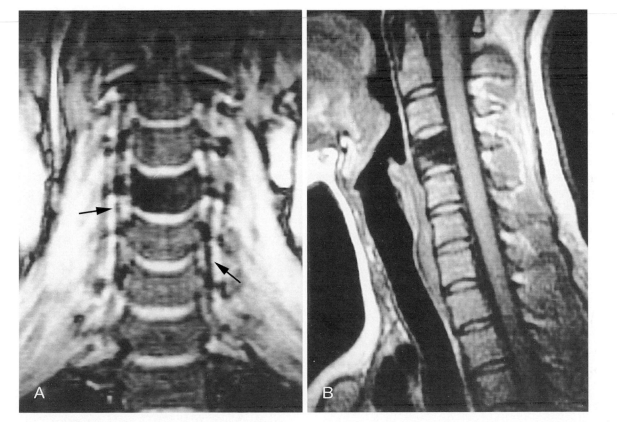

Figure S. A. CORONAL PROJECTION MAGNETIC RESONANCE IMAGE OF THE CERVICAL SPINE. B. SAGITTAL MAGNETIC RESONANCE IMAGE OF THE CERVICAL SPINE. Observe the low signal intensity of the C4 vertebral body on this T2-weighted MRI scan. This has occurred as a result of significant marrow replacement, etiology unknown (vertebral artery (VA)—(arrows). (Courtesy of Todd M. Aordkian, DC, Astoria, New York)

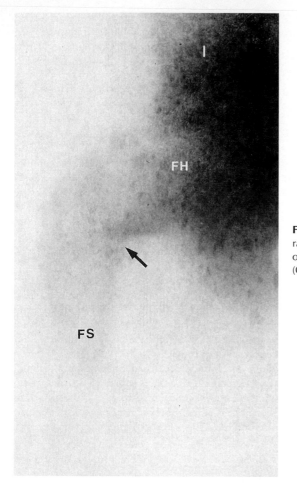

Figure T.   RADIOGRAPHIC ANTIQUE: FRACTURED FEMUR FROM 1897. Despite the crude radiographic image observe the ilium (*I*), femoral head (*FH*), and femoral shaft (FS). Careful observation reveals an acute angular deformity of the femoral neck due to a fracture (arrow). (Courtesy of Michael L. Davis, DC, Conroe, Texas)

from the past. (Fig. T) The depicted radiograph was taken in 1897 at the John Sealy Hospital in Galveston, Texas, just 2 years after Roentgen's discovery of x-rays. In 1976 the patient, Mrs. Minne Powell Bowers, consulted a chiropractor in Conroe, Texas, for evaluation of a low back complaint. When questioned about prior x-rays, she stated that she had fallen at the age of 14 and her father, a medical doctor, had decided to transport her from Willis, Texas, to Galveston in a horse drawn wagon to have her hip pain evaluated with this new "x-ray" procedure. Mrs. Bowers brought on her next visit to the chiropractor the radiograph pictured in

Figure T. Although the radiograph has aged and lacks technical clarity, careful observation of the image reveals an acute angular deformity of the femoral neck due to a displaced fracture. Even today, some 100 years later, the initial diagnostic examination of choice for a similar case is still the same: *the plain film radiograph.*

For examinations of the skeleton, there is no modality to match the time and cost-effectiveness of the plain film radiograph. It is from this "plain film" perspective that *Essentials of Skeletal Radiology* has been written and integrated with examples of more complex sophisticated imaging technologies.

ESSENTIALS OF SKELETAL RADIOLOGY

Volume Two

Second Edition

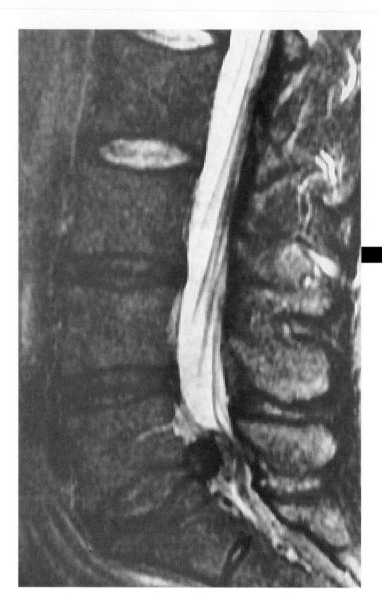

Volume Two

ESSENTIALS OF SKELETAL RADIOLOGY

Second Edition

Terry R. Yochum

B.S., D.C., D.A.C.B.R., F.C.C.R. (C), F.I.C.C.

Director
Rocky Mountain Chiropractic Radiological Center
Denver, Colorado

Adjunct Professor of Radiology
Los Angeles College of Chiropractic

Instructor
Skeletal Radiology
Department of Radiology
University of Colorado School of Medicine
Denver, Colorado

Formerly:
Senior Lecturer
Department of Diagnostic Sciences
Division Head
Department of Radiology
Phillip Institute of Technology—School of Chiropractic
Melbourne, Australia

Professor and Chairman
Department of Radiology
Logan College of Chiropractic
St. Louis, Missouri

Assistant Professor of Radiology
National College of Chiropractic
Lombard, Illinois

Lindsay J. Rowe

M. App. Sc. (Chiropractic), M.D., D.A.C.B.R., F.C.C.R. (C), F.A.C.C.R. (AUS), F.I.C.C.

Department of Medical Imaging
John Hunter Hospital
Newcastle, Australia

Senior Lecturer
Centre for Chiropractic
Macquarie University
Sydney, Australia

Adjunct Faculty
School of Chiropractic
Royal Melbourne Institute of Technology University
Melbourne, Australia

Post Graduate Faculty
Northwestern Chiropractic College
Minneapolis, Minnesota
Canadian Memorial Chiropractic College
Toronto, Canada

Formerly:
Associate Professor and Chairman
Department of Radiology
Northwestern Chiropractic College
Minneapolis, Minnesota

Associate Professor and Chairman
Department of Radiology
Canadian Memorial Chiropractic College
Toronto, Canada

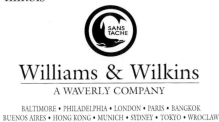

Williams & Wilkins
A WAVERLY COMPANY

BALTIMORE • PHILADELPHIA • LONDON • PARIS • BANGKOK
BUENOS AIRES • HONG KONG • MUNICH • SYDNEY • TOKYO • WROCLAW

1

Radiographic Positioning and Normal Anatomy

Lindsay J. Rowe and Terry R. Yochum

INTRODUCTION

In the 100 years since the discovery of the "X" ray by Wilhelm Conrad Roentgen in 1895 attempts to accurately depict the skeleton have undergone little change. (1) What was true in 1895 in terms of positioning and anatomy remains true today, with only the technical aspects undergoing significant modification. (2,3)

The purpose of this first chapter is to provide a foundation for the chapters that follow. It is composed of two parts—radiographic positioning and normal anatomy. These are synthesized to allow the reader to be able to perform the examination and comprehend the normal anatomy demonstrated on the obtained radiograph. For each projection a concise description of the positioning parameters is given, supplemented with photographs demonstrating the actual position. In addition, the resulting radiograph is shown and labeled, along with relevant anatomic and radiographic specimens, to augment understanding.

More detailed and specialized texts should be consulted for views not included in this chapter. (4–7)

In radiology, as in other clinical disciplines, to understand and recognize the abnormal a thorough knowledge and familiarity with the normal is mandatory. Of equal importance is the technologic process involved in producing the radiograph, since it is the quality of the image on which the accuracy of the interpretation is largely based. (8) To produce radiographs of inadequate technical quality is to handicap the interpretation, which ultimately compromises patient care. It is for these reasons that the student of radiology and the health care practitioner who utilizes skeletal radiographic procedures must master these two aspects of the discipline.

RADIOGRAPHIC POSITIONING

Format of Presentation

Each projection to follow is described in a standard format for simplicity and easy reference. The various parameters for each projection are concisely provided under various headings.

Basic Projections. List of routine views.

Optional Projections. List of nonroutine views.

Demonstrates. The structures shown on the projection are listed.

Measure. The anatomy that is measured for calculating the exposure factors. This is usually the area through which the central ray will pass.

kVp. The optimum kVp and range is stated for the body part being examined. (Table 1.1) kVp values are recommended throughout this chapter for the purpose of creating a diagnostic radiograph of adequate contrast and should be applicable to most current film-screen combinations. Those readers utilizing detail (extremity) rare earth screens may experience underexposed radiographs if values less than 55 kVp are routinely used, because of the diminished light output of the crystals at this relatively low energy level. For these practitioners a kVp value of 55 or greater should be used for the production of those radiographs.

Film Size. As a guide, the film size is given; however, clinical discretion should be applied according to the size of the body part under examination.

Grid. Extremities measuring under 10 cm; lateral, flexion/extension, and oblique cervicals; and chest films may all be done without a grid. All other projections should use a grid. A minimum grid ratio of 10:1 is recommended, while a 12:1 ratio is considered optimal.

Tube-Film Distance (TFD). This is often referred to as the focal-film distance (FFD) and is the distance between the tube and

1

Table 1.1 Optimum Kilovolts Peak (kVp)*	
Region	kVp
Skull	85
Sinuses	85
Cervical spine	80
Thoracic spine	90
Lumbar spine	
Anteroposterior	85
Lateral	90
Pelvis	80
Sacrum	80
Coccyx	80
Full Spine	90
Hip	80
Knee	60
Ankle	55
Foot	55
Toes	55
Shoulder	75
Clavicle	70
Acromioclavicular	70
Elbow	55
Wrist	55
Hand	55
Fingers	55
Thumb	55
Ribs	80
Chest	110
Abdomen	
Soft tissue	100
Calcific densities	70

*These kVp ranges can be lowered by 10 with 100 kHz high frequency.

film. While a 40-inch TFD is traditionally offered, faster film/screen combinations make it practical to use 60 to 80 inches for some exposures.

Tube Tilt. The angulation of the tube in relation to the head (cephalad) and feet (caudad).

Patient Position. The postural attitude of the patient when the radiograph is obtained (e.g., upright, recumbent, seated).

Part Position. The position of the body part that is being radiographed (flexion, extension, supination, etc.).

Central Ray (CR). The theoretical center of the radiographic beam as defined by the position of the light localizer cross-markings from the collimator.

Collimation. Limiting the irradiated film size is a practical decision based on the patient and film size. However, the smallest size compatible with the body component should be obtained and collimation never should exceed the film size. Collimation is instrumental in reducing radiation dose to the patient and improving imaging quality.

Side Marker. Appropriate side markers should be placed, preferably in the corner of the radiographic field, so as not to obstruct any anatomic details.

Breathing Instructions. The patient is told either to stop breathing (arrested respiration), take a deep breath in and hold it (suspended deep inspiration), or let the breath out and hold it (suspended expiration). These respirations may be partial or complete. Occasionally, a breathing technique is utilized to intentionally blur obscuring overlying anatomy.

Clinicoradiologic Correlations. Key clinically important radiologic features are highlighted. This typically follows the "ABCs" format—**A**lignment, **B**one, **C**artilage (joints), and **S**oft tissue.

Positioning Terminology

Equipment-Related Factors. The equipment described in this chapter will only be dealt with briefly.

Radiographic Series. In any body location a minimum of two views perpendicular to each other must be performed on initial evaluation. A series is the set of radiographs obtained on a particular body area. A "scout" radiograph is a single view taken for the sole purpose of obtaining a general, nonspecific overview of the body part, which is later followed by more specific projections.

Spot Projections. These are isolated, closely collimated views of a particular region, to more closely evaluate an area that is not well seen on routine views or that may be abnormal.

Film Identification. Each film must be identified with the patient's name, date of exposure, and clinic where taken.

Bucky. The bucky is the mechanism for housing and moving the grid. Generally, the surface the patient contacts during the exposure is often referred to as the "bucky". Motion induced by the bucky on the grid eliminates the appearance of grid lines on the film. An exposure time of less than 0.2 seconds may "freeze" the grid and create grid lines. The bucky is used on thicker body parts to improve image quality. For examinations of the chest and thinner body parts less than 10 cm a grid need not be used, since the scatter radiation generated is relatively small. Lateral cervical spine views taken at 200 cm (72 inches) also can be performed nongrid since the air-gap between the neck and film allows for scattered rays to not reach the film. Nonbucky techniques significantly reduce the radiation exposure required to produce a diagnostic image.

Grid. When x-rays penetrate and enter the body, they interact with atoms by ejecting orbital electrons, displacing orbital electrons to another shell, or altering the electrical charge of the atomic nucleus. The net result is an alteration of the electrical charge of the atom (*ionizing radiation*). Following any of these interactions, x-rays of lower energy are produced that have an altered path (*scattered radiation*). These create an overall decrease in image quality by graying the densities (fog). (9)

A grid functions to eliminate this scattered radiation and prevent its reaching the film. The structure of a grid consists of lead strips separated by a radiolucent material. The scattered x-rays tend to be multidirectional and do not easily pass between the lead strips as do the primary (undiverted) rays. The end result is that there is an overall decrease in film fog, which increases film contrast and image quality. (8,9)

Use of a grid necessarily increases the patient dose and is therefore not necessary for body parts less than 10 cm in thickness and for air-gap techniques such as lateral cervical views.

Tube. This is the apparatus where the x-rays are produced and emitted toward the patient.

Tube Tilt. The angle of the beam is occasionally altered to better depict certain anatomic details. A general rule with tube tilt is for every 5° of angulation the tube should be moved 1 inch closer to the patient; otherwise, the film may be underexposed.

Tube-Film Distance (TFD). This is the measured distance between the tube and film.

Collimator. This is a cube-shaped structure on the outside of the x-ray tube that can be manipulated to reduce the field size of the emitted radiation. Placed inside the collimator is a light source that produces a light beam that accurately simulates the exiting radiation. On this light beam intersecting lines that represent the center of the emission can be easily identified.

kVp (Kilovolts Peak).   This is the potential difference created between the cathode (filament) and anode during the exposure. It is responsible for the speed that electrons will have when they interact at the anode. This determines the "strength" of the emitted x-rays, which translates into the ability to pass through the body (penetration). Therefore, kVp is the main determinant of beam quality and alters the film's scale of contrast (gray scale). (9,10) As body thickness increases, generally, so does the kVp. In this chapter optimum kVps are given for each body region.

mAs (Milliampere Seconds).   This is the number of electrons generated per second and determines the density (film blackness) of the image. A linear relationship exists between film density and mAs that allows simpler computation when presented with performing a retake of an over- or underexposed radiograph. (9,10)

Lead Blockers.   These are usually used to block part of a cassette during an exposure to protect that portion of film from scatter radiation so that it can be used for multiple projections on the same film. This is commonly used in examinations of the extremities on the same piece of film.

Markers (Fig. 1.1).   For oblique and lateral views the general rule is to identify the side closest to the film, placing the marker so that it does not obstruct important anatomy. Many types of markers are available. At a minimum, on anteroposterior views the right or left side should be identified, and on laterals and obliques the side closest to the film is marked. Specialized projections such as stress studies of the spine can be identified with the addition of an arrow to show the direction of patient motion.

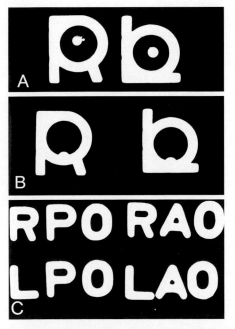

Figure 1.1.   EXAMPLES OF RADIOGRAPHIC MARKERS. A. Mitchell Markers. Note the central position of the mercury ball, indicating the horizontal position of the cassette. **B. Upright Markers.** The mercury ball has now gravitated inferiorly, indicating the vertical position of the cassette. **C. Oblique Markers. RPO:** Right posterior oblique; **LPO:** Left posterior oblique; **RAO:** Right anterior oblique; **LAO:** Left anterior oblique.

Upright and recumbent studies can be identified by the appropriate word, arrow, or a mercury ball inside the marker.

Filtration (Fig. 1.2).   The placement of aluminum and/or aluminum-copper filters (added filtration) at the collimator considerably reduces the amount of low-energy x-rays reaching the patient. In addition to reducing patient radiation dose, filters (sectional filtration) can be used to compensate for varying body thicknesses. This is especially the case in the thoracic and lumbar spine. The effect is to eliminate overexposure of thinner body parts, creating a more homogeneous density radiograph. (9,11)

Relative Exposure.   Radiographs are assessed according to film density (film blackness). Assuming an optimal kVp, an overexposed film will appear exceedingly dark because of too much mAs, while an underexposed film will be too light because of too little mAs.

Object Density.   If an area on a radiograph appears black, it is termed radiolucent; if it appears to be whiter, then it is called radiopaque.

Patient-Related Factors

Patient Position (Fig. 1.3).   Various terms are commonly used to describe the patient's body position in relation to the x-ray beam.

1. Posteroanterior (PA). The x-ray beam enters the posterior surface and exits the anterior surface.
2. Anteroposterior (AP). The x-ray beam enters the anterior surface and exits the posterior surface.
3. Lateral (L). Right lateral (RL) indicates that the right side of the patient is in contact with the film. Left lateral (LL) indicates the left side of the patient is in contact with the film.
4. Right anterior oblique (RAO). The right anterolateral surface of the body is closest to the film.
5. Left anterior oblique (LAO). The left anterolateral surface of the body is closest to the film.
6. Right posterior oblique (RPO). The right posterolateral surface of the body is closest to the film.
7. Left posterior oblique (LPO). The left posterolateral surface of the body is closest to the film.
8. Upright (erect). The patient stands for the film.
9. Recumbent. The patient lies down for the film.
10. Lateral decubitus. The patient lies on one side, with the beam passing through horizontally.
11. Seated. Sitting on a chair, with the unaffected body parts placed outside the path of the x-ray beam.

Patient Variability.   Various differences in body type, position, and bone density alter certain aspects of the technology involved in producing optimum radiographs.

1. Obese patients. Although the overall dimensions of the body part may be increased, fat is of relatively low radiodensity and may cause inadvertent overexposure. For this reason, recumbent projections will compress the body tissues and provide a better radiographic exposure. A reduction in kVp will help to improve film contrast.
2. Muscular patients. As muscle mass increases, this can be compensated for by an increase in kVp of approximately 10 from the original optimum kVp settings.
3. Pediatric patients. To ensure a proper exposure, younger patients must be appropriately immobilized. In the extremities routine bilateral views for comparison are discouraged. They should only be performed when specifically indicated.

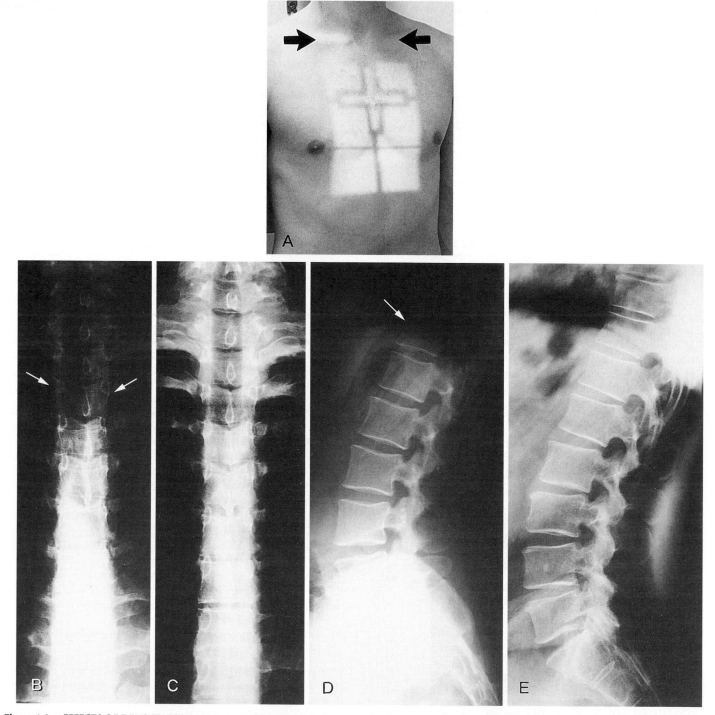

Figure 1.2.   EFFECTS OF DENSITY EQUALIZING FILTRATION. A. Anteroposterior Thoracic Spine: Filtration. Observe the filtered region (arrows). The filter is placed on the collimator. **B. Anteroposterior Thoracic Spine: Without Filtration.** Note the overexposed upper thoracic spine (arrows) and the underexposed lower thoracic spine. **C. Anteroposterior Thoracic Spine: With Filtration.** The entire thoracic spine is of a uniform density. **D. Lateral Lumbar Spine: Without Filtration.** The lumbosacral junction is underexposed, the thoracolumbar region is overexposed (arrow). **E. Lateral Lumbar Spine: With Filtration.** Observe that the density from the upper sacrum through to the lower thoracic vertebrae are uniformly exposed. Numerous filters have been utilized; lower lung fields, iliac crests, and for the spinous processes. (Courtesy of Felix G. Bauer, DC, DACBR(Hon), Sydney, Australia)

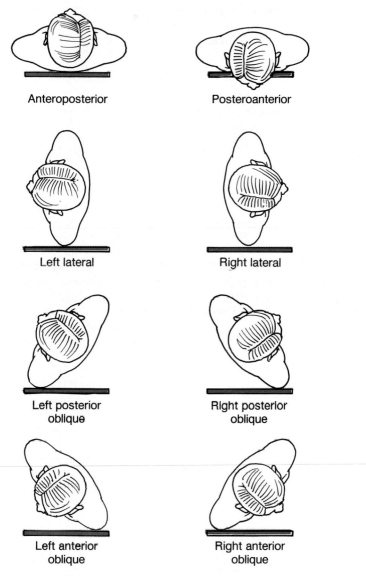

Anteroposterior

Posteroanterior

Left lateral

Right lateral

Left posterior oblique

Right posterior oblique

Left anterior oblique

Right anterior oblique

Figure 1.3.   RADIOGRAPHIC POSITIONS.

4. Upright and recumbent projections. The body thickness alters with changes in postural position. A measurement obtained in the upright position will not be accurate for determining exposure factors in the recumbent position because of tissue compression.
5. Bone density changes. Decreased bone density (osteopenia) is frequently associated with various disorders. Under these conditions, and with increasing age (senile osteoporosis), a reduction in the mAs of approximately 25% may avoid overexposure. Conversely, in disorders of increased bone density the mAs should be increased by approximately 25%.
6. Traumatized patient. Under no circumstances should optimal patient positioning take priority over patient safety. Attempts to position the truly injured patient may exacerbate the injury, with potentially catastrophic results in some instances.

Motion.   Causes of motion include inadequate stabilization of the respective body part, misinstruction of the patient, long exposure time, and patient discomfort. All such factors should be controlled as much as possible.

Patient Protection.   In general, only the area of interest should be in the x-ray beam. All other body parts should be positioned outside the primary beam or be protected. To reduce patient exposure to primary radiation, collimation to film size (or smaller) must be performed. A pregnant woman should not be irradiated unless the clinical circumstances are life threatening. The risk of irradiating an early stage developing fetus can be reduced by appropriate patient questioning and application of the 10-day rule. (12)

Gonadal Shielding.   In general, every attempt to reduce gonadal radiation must be made. Various methods for gonadal shielding have been devised, which require accurate placement. In examinations of the hips or pelvis, especially in females, shields should not be used if the suspected pathology would be obscured. Female patients following complete hysterectomy or who are postmenopausal do not require gonadal shielding.

The Bureau of Radiological Health recommends that gonadal shielding be used in three particular instances: (a) when gonads lie within the primary x-ray field or within close proximity (about 5 cm); (b) if the clinical objective of the examination will not be compromised; and (c) if the patient has a reasonable reproductive potential. (13)

Measurement. Measuring calipers are used to determine the thickness of the body part traversed by the central ray. On the basis of this measurement, the exposure may then be calculated.

Relationship Terms

Cephalad. Toward the head.
Caudad. Toward the feet.
Proximal. Toward the center of the body.
Distal. Toward the periphery of the body.
Lateral. Toward the right or left side of the body.
Medial. Toward the middle of the body.
Flexion. The angle between body parts is decreased.
Extension. The angle between body parts is increased.
Adduction. Movement of the body part toward the midline.
Eversion. Outward movement of the foot or ankle. Plantar surface faces medially.
Inversion. Inward movement of the foot or ankle. Plantar surface moved laterally.
Supination. Palm up.
Pronation. Palm down.

Patient Preparation. Before examination of a particular body part, various steps should be performed.

1. Removal of all clothing and putting on a gown, if necessary.
2. Removal of all metallic objects or dental appliances within the radiographic field. (Table 1.2)
3. Evacuation of the bowel or bladder, if the abdomen, sacrum, or coccyx is being examined.

Breathing Instructions. In most projections respiration is transiently halted to prevent motion of the body part (arrested respiration). On occasion breathing may assist in blurring out overlying structures such as the ribs on a lateral thoracic spine study. Suspended deep inspiration is used for chest and thoracic exposures to depress the diaphragm, while suspended expiration is used in abdominal films to elevate the diaphragm.

Table 1.2 Common Artifacts of Various Body Regions

SKULL	Hairpins, wigs, false teeth, eyeglasses, necklaces, earrings, bizarre hair styles.
CERVICAL SPINE	Hairpins, wigs, false teeth, eyeglasses, necklaces, earrings, bizarre hair styles, clothing.
THORACIC SPINE	Necklaces, brassieres, clothing.
LUMBAR SPINE	Orthopedic supports, brassieres, underwear, pants with objects in the pockets.
PELVIS, HIPS, AND SHOULDERS	Orthopedic supports, brassieres, underwear, pants with objects in the pockets.
WRIST AND HAND	Watches, rings, bracelets, orthopedic supports.
ANKLE AND FOOT	Shoes, socks, orthopedic supports.

RADIOGRAPHIC ANATOMY

In radiographic evaluations of the skeleton, the major structures demonstrated are the bones, joints, and surrounding soft tissues (muscle, viscera, skin). A more in-depth discussion of these features is to be found in Chapter 7. The basic background details related to this chapter will be presented.

Skeletal Anatomy

Osteology. Osteology is the study of bones. (6,7,14) There are a total of 206 separate bones, divided into the axial and appendicular skeleton. (Table 1.3) The axial skeleton consists of 80 bones, which include the skull, vertebral column, ribs, and sternum. The appendicular skeleton consists of 126 bones, which include the upper and lower extremities, as well as the shoulder and pelvic girdles.

These bones are frequently referred to according to their shape—long, short, flat, or irregular.

Long Bones. These bones are located in the appendicular skeleton. Typical examples include the femur, tibia, humerus, and radius.

Each long bone can be divided into six components—the epiphysis, physis, metaphysis, diaphysis, apophysis, and periosteum.

1. Epiphysis. This is the expanded end of a long bone, which is covered by articular cartilage and contains articular cortex and underlying supporting bone. Its prime function is related to supporting joint movement.
2. Physis (growth plate). In growing immature bones, this region is cartilaginous and is responsible for enchondral bone growth. Radiographically, the physis will appear as a radiolucent band at the base of the epiphysis.
3. Metaphysis. The expanded area beneath the growth plate that tapers into the normal caliber of the shaft is called the me-

Table 1.3. Total Number of Bones by Region

Axial Skeleton		Appendicular Skeleton	
SKULL		SHOULDER GIRDLES	
Cranium	8	Clavicle	2
Facial bones	14	Scapula	2
HYOID	1	UPPER EXTREMITIES	
AUDITORY OSSICLES	6	Humerus	2
VERTEBRAL COLUMN		Ulna	2
Cervical	7	Radius	2
Thoracic	12	Carpals	16
Lumbar	5	Metacarpals	10
Sacrum	1	Phalanges	28
Coccyx	1	PELVIC GIRDLE	
THORAX		Innominate	2
Sternum	1	LOWER EXTREMITIES	
Ribs	24	Femur	2
Total	80	Tibia	2
		Fibula	2
		Patella	2
		Tarsals	14
		Metatarsals	10
		Phalanges	28
		Total	126

taphysis. It is the greatest metabolic region of bone and is responsible for forming the long bone shape during growth.

4. Diaphysis (shaft). This is the narrowest and longest portion of the bone. Its main function is mechanical support and housing for the bone marrow.

5. Apophysis (e.g., greater tuberosity, lesser trochanter). An apophysis is a bony site for attachment of ligaments or tendons and is usually seen as a protuberance beyond the bone contour.

6. Periosteum. This is a soft tissue envelope around and attached to the entire circumference of the bone. Notably, it is not located within the joint. Its function is to maintain the caliber of the bone by appositional bone growth. Radiographically, the periosteum is not visible unless it is mechanically elevated or chemically irritated, which will result in external periosteal new bone formation.

In addition to these divisions, the structure of a long bone comprises two distinct components—compact bone and cancellous bone. Compact bone is recognized on the radiograph as a thick, white outer bone shell, which is called the cortex. The cortex has two divisions—an outer cortex and the inner cortex, often referred to as the endosteum. Notably, cortical thickness is greatest in the middle portion of the bone and gradually tapers toward the end of the bone. At the metaphysis the cortex is sharply attenuated from a thick band to a thin line. Internal to the cortex lies the medullary cavity, which is traversed by thin trabeculae (cancellous or spongy bone).

Short Bones. These are small, cube-shaped bones (e.g., the wrist and ankle).

Flat Bones. These are rich in marrow and are characterized by their broad surfaces. The cortical thickness is relatively large and the medullary space is interposed. In the skull the cortices are called tables and the medullary space the diploe.

Irregular Bones. Bones that do not conform to any particular shape are massed together in this category. These include bones of the cranial base and the vertebrae. Vertebral segments have a number of named components that are readily identifiable by imaging via plain films, computed tomograms (CT), and magnetic resonance images (MRI).

1. Vertebral body (centrum). The shape, size, and configuration of the vertebral body differs in various regions of the spine. It is composed of an outer cortical shell and houses trabeculae, which resist the biomechanical stresses of weight bearing and movement. The presence of blood and marrow elements encased within a tight bony shell and trabecular network is an effective component for a vertebral body under load.

2. Vertebral endplates. The upper and lower surfaces are relatively linear and are designated the superior and inferior endplates, respectively. They are comprised of cortical bone and are perforated with numerous tiny vascular holes. On the discal surface is supported a thin layer of hyaline cartilage. The interface of the intervertebral disc and cartilage-bony endplate is often referred to as the *discovertebral junction.*

3. Pedicle. Two pedicles arise at each segment from either the posterior or posterolateral surface of the vertebral body. All pedicles arise from the upper half of each vertebral body and contribute to the bony confines of the intervertebral foramen. These structures are extremely strong and readily identified on radiographs and are sometimes referred to as the "eyes" of the vertebral segment.

4. Articular process. On each vertebra there are four articular processes—two inferior (IAP) and two superior (SAP). In the cervical spine they are fused into a single bony block referred to as the *articular pillar.* On the posterior edge of the lumbar SAP a small bump is referred to as the mammillary process. Secondary ossification centers are located on the tips of each articular process.

The distal surfaces of the articular processes are smooth zones called *facets,* which are the site for coverage by articular cartilage. An opposing SAP and IAP form the *facet joint.* Joints formed in this manner have been subject to widespread variation in nomenclature, including posterior joints, facet joints, apophyseal joints, zygapophyseal, or just the "Z" joints. The anatomically correct term is the *zygapophyseal joint.*

5. Pars interarticularis. Anatomically this exists as part of the lamina near its point of attachment to the pedicle. As the term suggests it is the part lying between the superior and inferior articular processes. It runs obliquely upward from the lateral laminar margin to its medial border. Externally there are no markers for its accurate identification and therefore it is more of an abstract zone than a true landmark.

6. Transverse process (TVP). Projecting from the junction of the lamina and pedicle is this distinctive tapered bony bar of variable length. At its distal end is a small secondary growth center that, especially at L1, is prone to nonunion. The L3 vertebra usually exhibits the longest transverse process of all lumbar segments.

7. Lamina. Paired flat sheets of bone project from the pedicles obliquely to fuse in the midline, thereby demarcating the posterior margin or "roof" of the spinal canal. The union with the spinous process in the midline completes the formation of the neural arch into a ringlike structure. This spinolaminar junction is visible radiographically and is an extremely useful anatomic landmark.

8. Spinous process (SP). From the junction of the two opposing lamina the central blade of the spinous process begins (spinolaminar junction). SPs are directed slightly caudad and at their tips are teardrop in shape in the thoracic and lumbar spines. Cervical spinous processes are characteristically bifid.

Arthrology. Arthrology is the study of joints (articulations). (6,7,14) Articulations can be categorized by two classifications—joint motion or articular histology.

Joint Motion. Three types are recognized—synarthroses, amphiarthroses, and diarthroses.

1. Synarthroses. Fixed, immobile joints. Examples include the skull sutures and growth plates.

2. Amphiarthroses. Slightly movable joints. Examples include intervertebral discs and symphysis pubis.

3. Diarthroses. Freely movable joints. Examples include the hips and shoulder joints.

Articular Histology. This classification emphasizes the tissue type found in the joint space and is especially useful in understanding joint disease. Three histologic types of joints are identified—fibrous, cartilaginous, and synovial. Essentially, these are equivalent to the joint motion classification, with fibrous tissue being present in synarthroses, cartilage within amphiarthroses, and synovial tissue within diarthroses.

Radiologic Features.   A joint is readily identified by a smooth, regular, lucent articular space and opposing parallel bony surfaces. For a joint to be adequately demonstrated, the x-ray beam must pass through the same plane as the joint surfaces.

HIGH-FREQUENCY TECHNOLOGY: REGULATORY CHANGES AND THE FUTURE

As society evolves toward a managed health care environment, all health care providers and patients will undergo adaptation as the changing tide of reform ebbs and flows. Stricter regulations and guidelines are imminent as policies, practices, personnel, and equipment come under increasing scrutiny. Radiologic procedures receive considerable attention in this movement because of their contribution to health expenditures and potential public health hazards.

In the United States in 1991 the New York State Department of Health (NYSDOH) adopted the Radiation Safety–Quality Assurance Program, which placed surprisingly stringent performance requirements on the medical and chiropractic professions. (15) NYSDOH stipulated immediate and mandatory compliance with the program's guidelines, which contained two major objectives—to reduce radiation exposure and to optimize diagnostic image quality. (16) The New York model has in many ways set a precedent that other states have adopted with more sure to follow. It is most likely that internationally similar guidelines will be established.

Implementation of such a program is clearly demonstrated by the adoption by the United States Federal Government in 1992 of the Mammographic Quality Standards Act (MQSA), which took effect in October 1994. (17) This Act seeks to establish the authority for the regulation of mammography and radiologic equipment. All personnel, facilities, and equipment must be certified by an independent accreditation board established by federal authorities. Numerous states have instigated monitoring and enforce maximum dose levels for specified anatomic views. (18) A specific restriction in the act is the prohibited use of single-phase radiographic systems. The mandated standard for mammographic use is high-frequency, low-dose equipment.

While both the NYSDOH Program and MQSA are primarily directed at the medical profession, these regulations foreshadow changes anticipated in chiropractic and other health professions across the United States and potentially internationally. Single-phase equipment has been until recent times the traditional diagnostic apparatus in use, but is now considered inefficient, delivering unacceptably high radiation doses. Over 95% of medical imaging is performed with either high-frequency or three-phase equipment. (19) Health care providers utilizing single-phase equipment must be aware of the legislative acts already in place and the future trends in control of radiographic equipment, which will virtually ensure that high-frequency or three-phase machinery will be the only type to use. Three-phase equipment tends to be expensive because of high installation costs with a specific, incoming power line being required.

Single-phase radiographic equipment utilizes only the peak of the single, incoming power wave to generate diagnostic x-rays. Longer exposure times are required to produce enough x-rays to form the final diagnostic image. In addition, a greater proportion of lower energy x-rays are produced that are absorbed by the patient and that do not contribute significantly to the final image. High-frequency equipment uses the principle of overlapping incoming power waves to place their peaks close to each other to minimize the fluctuations in energy from wave to wave ("ripple"). The results are significantly reduced times for exposure and diminished radiation doses. As an example, an AP lumbar projection with high-frequency technology can result in almost a 50% reduction in mAs when compared with single-phase equipment. (8) Unlike three-phase equipment, no expensive special installation costs are required for high-frequency equipment.

The measure of high-frequency generators is the *kilohertz* (kHz). The actual frequency begins at 39 kHz, with the *gold standard* considered to be 100 kHz. (20) At this frequency ripple is small, producing an efficient, largely homogeneous x-ray beam. The major benefits are short exposure times, accurate timing of exposures, and reduced patient dose.

When equipment is being purchased, careful attention should be given to the kilohertz range to ensure that it lies in the range of 39 to 100 kHz. In general, the higher the kilohertz rating, the greater the benefits. As high-frequency technology displaces outdated, single-phase equipment, more remanufactured units will become available in the marketplace. Purchasing new or remanufactured secondhand, single-phase equipment is to be discouraged because of the impending legislative changes and high-radiation doses as outlined previously.

MEDICOLEGAL IMPLICATIONS
Radiographic Technology

- A rationale for obtaining the study should be established. (21–23) Obtaining radiographs should not be a "screening" procedure without the clinical expectation for finding an abnormality that will significantly alter patient management. Obtaining a radiographic history of previous studies performed and their location may assist in deciding what and whether to x-ray.

- Adequate views must be obtained. A minimum of frontal (AP, PA) and lateral projections of the region is required. (24)

- Supplemental views such as oblique and spot views should be obtained when clinically indicated or when abnormal findings are found on an initial study. (24)

- Reexamination by x-ray must be substantiated by clear criteria. Practitioners run the same risks for taking too many films, taking not enough films, taking them too often, or not taking them often enough. Other than scoliosis, there are few postural alterations that indicate a need to repeat a radiographic examination to evaluate therapeutic progress. Indicators for reexamination include an intervening complication (neoplasia, trauma, fever, rigors, weight loss, drug or alcohol use, surgery), appearance of abnormal clinical examination findings, failure to respond to therapy within 4 to 6 weeks, and an unexplained deterioration in the condition.

- Contraindications to a particular study should be identified. Examples include pregnancy with lumbar-pelvic studies; and odontoid abnormalities, vertigo, or vertebrobasilar ischemia with cervical flexion-extension studies.

- Patient preparation should be rigorously conducted. (21) This includes removal of potential artifacts such as metallic objects (clasps, necklaces, earrings, etc.) and practicing of the procedures to assist compliance and reduce motion artifacts.

- Optimum image quality is paramount. Films must exhibit collimation and must be properly exposed, free of artifacts, processed accurately, and properly identified. (25) This is one of the most common sources for antagonistic medicolegal action. (26) Measurement of the patient and accurate calculation of exposure factors are crucial to diminishing retakes. (21)

- Adequate demonstration of desired anatomy is vitally important. Poor positioning fails to demonstrate structures accurately and hinders the diagnostic process. Inclusion of the clinically important area on the radiograph should be made.

- Gonadal shielding should be used whenever possible, unless it obscures a pelvic structure that is deemed clinically important such as the sacroiliac joint. Females in menopause or who have undergone a hysterectomy do not require gonadal shielding. (12) In males gonadal shielding has few contraindications.

- A log book should be kept documenting the date of the study, views performed, measurement of the patient, TFD, kVp, mAs, and screen type with a space for comments to be made on image quality.

- The facility, the equipment, and the operator should be appropriately licensed and certified. All equipment should be functional and present no hazard to the safety of the operator or the patient. Equipment should be modern and preferably state-of-the-art such as high-frequency generators and rare earth screens. (27)

**SKULL
Lateral Projection**

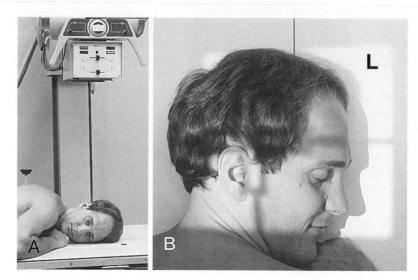

Figure 1.4.   LATERAL SKULL. A. Patient Position. B. Collimation and Central Ray.

Demonstrates: Lateral cranial structures closest to the bucky (temporal, parietal), sella turcica, sphenoid sinus, occipitocervical junction, and calvarium. (1–4)

Measure: At the central ray.

kVp: 85 (80 to 90).

Film Size: 10 × 12 inches (24 × 30 cm).

Grid: Yes.

TFD: 40 inches (102 cm).

Tube Tilt: None.

Patient Position: Semiprone.

Part Position: Head is in true lateral position against the bucky. The infraorbital meatal line is parallel with the long edge of the cassette, and the interpupillary line is perpendicular.

CR: Passes 3/4 inch superior and 3/4 inch anterior to the external auditory meatus.

Collimation: To the patient's skull size.

Side Marker: Side closest to the film placed in a corner.

Breathing Instructions: Suspended expiration.

Clinicoradiologic Correlations: Both right and left laterals should be performed routinely. (4)

1. *Alignment:* A well-positioned lateral should show superimposition of the mandibular rami, orbital roofs, and sella turcica. The tip of the dens should lie not more than 8 mm above the plane from the hard palate to the occipital convexity (McGregor's line). (See Chapter 2)
2. *Bone:* The vascular markings off the middle meningeal artery should not be confused with a fracture line. (4) The sclerotic density of the skull base may mimic bone pathology.
3. *Cartilage:* The atlantodental interspace should be inspected.
4. *Soft tissue:* The palate and retropharyngeal tissues should be perused for evidence of swelling or abnormal density.

Normal Anatomy (Figure 1.4C)

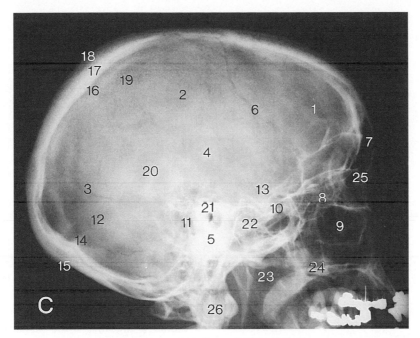

Figure 1.4.   C. Radiograph, Lateral Skull.

1. Frontal bone.
2. Parietal bone.
3. Occipital bone.
4. Squamous portion, temporal bone.
5. Petrous portion, temporal bone.
6. Middle meningeal artery.
7. Frontal sinus.
8. Ethmoid sinus.
9. Maxillary sinus.
10. Sphenoid sinus.
11. Mastoid air cells.
12. Transverse venous sinus.
13. Sella turcica.

14. Internal occipital protuberance (IOP).
15. External occipital protuberance (EOP).
16. Inner table.
17. Diploe.
18. Outer table.
19. Parietal star (diploic venous confluence).
20. Pinna of the ear.
21. Internal auditory meatus.
22. Temporomandibular joint.
23. Nasopharynx.
24. Hard palate.
25. Orbit.
26. Odontoid process.

BASIC
*Lateral (right and left)
Posteroanterior Caldwell
Anteroposterior Towne's

SKULL
Lateral Projection

OPTIONAL
Vertex

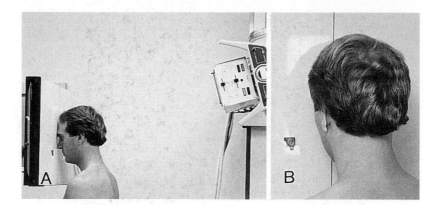

Figure 1.5. PA CALDWELL, SKULL. A. Patient Position. B. Collimation and Central Ray.

Demonstrates: Frontal bone, frontal sinus, ethmoid sinus, orbits, sphenoid wings, petrous ridges, and internal auditory canals. (1–4)

Measure: Through the central ray.

kVp: 85 (80 to 90).

Film Size: 10 × 12 inches (24 × 30 cm).

Grid: Yes.

TFD: 40 inches (102 cm) (must correct for tube tilt).

Tube Tilt: 15° caudad.

Patient Position: Prone or upright.

Part Position: Frontal bone in contact with the bucky. Remove all lateral head tilt and rotation. The orbitomeatal line should be perpendicular to the cassette.

CR: Exits through the nasion.

Collimation: To skull size.

Side Marker: In open space away from the cranium.

Breathing Instructions: Suspended expiration.

Clinicoradiologic Correlations:

1. *Alignment:* The nasal septum and calcified pineal gland should be midline. If the pineal is displaced, this may indicate an intracranial mass.
2. *Bone:* Done upright, this is a useful projection in the evaluation of sinus disease. Orbital detail is superior in this projection in comparison with the straight posteroanterior view without tube tilt.
3. *Cartilage:* No joints are clearly depicted.
4. *Soft tissue:* Aeration of the sinuses, the thickness of the mucosal lining, and evidence of air-fluid levels should be noted.

BASIC
Lateral (right and left)
*Posteroanterior
Caldwell
Anteroposterior Towne's

SKULL
Posteroanterior Caldwell Projection

OPTIONAL
Vertex

Normal Anatomy (Figure 1.5C)

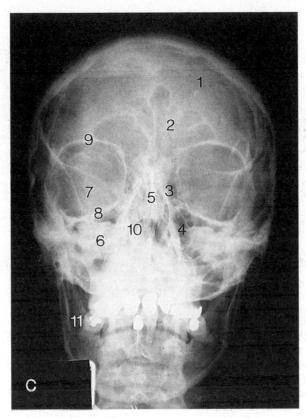

Figure 1.5.   C. Radiograph, PA Skull (Caldwell).

BASIC
Lateral (right and left)
*Posteroanterior
Caldwell
Anteroposterior Towne's

SKULL
Posteroanterior Caldwell Projection

OPTIONAL
Vertex

1. Frontal bone.
2. Frontal sinus.
3. Ethmoid sinus.
4. Maxillary sinus.
5. Nasal septum.
6. Petrous ridge.

7. Greater wing of sphenoid.
8. Infraorbital rim.
9. Supraorbital rim.
10. Nasal turbinates.
11. Mandible.

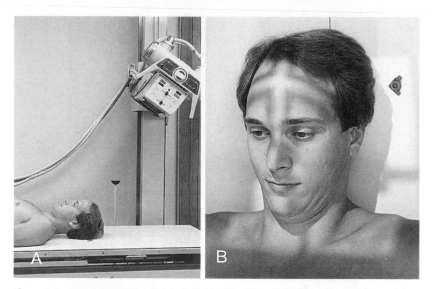

Figure 1.6. AP TOWNE'S, SKULL. A. Patient Position. B. Collimation and Central Ray.

Demonstrates: Occipital bone, petrous pyramids, posterior foramen magnum, dorsum sellae, posterior clinoids, zygomatic arches, and mandibular condyle. (1–4)
Measure: Through the central ray.
kVp: 85 (80 to 90).
Film Size: 10 × 12 inches (24 × 30 cm).
Grid: Yes.
TFD: 40 inches (102 cm) (must correct for tube tilt).
Tube Tilt: 35° caudad.
Patient Position: Supine or upright.
Part Position: Centered, with removal of lateral head tilt and rotation. Infraorbital meatal line is perpendicular to the cassette.
CR: Passes through the midline at the external auditory meatus.

Collimation: To skull size.
Side Marker: In open space at film corner.
Breathing Instructions: Suspended expiration.
Clinicoradiologic Correlations:

1. *Alignment:* The dorsum sellae and posterior clinoid processes should project into the anterior portions of the foramen magnum.
2. *Bone:* The occipital bone is best demonstrated as are the petrous ridges, auditory meati, zygoma, and mandibular condyle.
3. *Cartilage:* The temporomandibular joint is poorly demonstrated.
4. *Soft tissue:* The pineal gland should lie in the midline.

SKULL
Anteroposterior Towne's Projection

Normal Anatomy (Figure 1.6C)

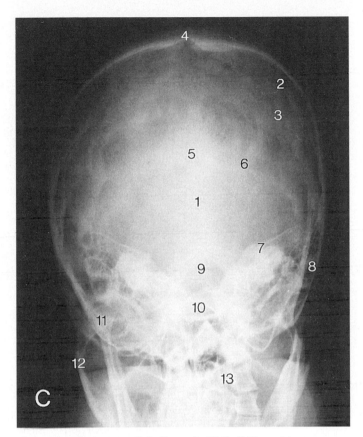

Figure 1.6.   C, Radiograph, AP Skull (Towne's).

1. Occipital bone.
2. Parietal bone.
3. Lambdoidal suture.
4. Sagittal suture.
5. Internal occipital protuberance.
6. Transverse venous sinus.
7. Petrous pyramids.

8. Mastoid air cells.
9. Foramen magnum.
10. Dorsum sellae.
11. Mandibular condyle.
12. Zygomatic arch.
13. Cervical pillar.

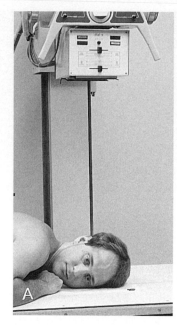

Figure 1.7. LATERAL PARANASAL SINUSES. A. Patient Position.

BASIC
*Lateral
Waters

PARANASAL SINUSES
Lateral Sinus and Facial Bones Projection

OPTIONAL
Submentovertical

Demonstrates: Maxilla, hard palate, maxillary sinus, ethmoid sinus, sphenoid sinus, frontal sinus, and orbits. (1–4)

Measure: Between left and right lateral canthus.

kVp: 85 (80 to 90).

Film Size: 8 × 10 inches (18 × 24 cm).

Grid: Yes.

TFD: 40 inches (102 cm).

Tube Tilt: None.

Patient Position: Semiprone or upright, with head turned to lateral position.

Part Position: Head is turned to a true lateral position. The midsagittal plane is parallel to the cassette, and the interpupillary line is perpendicular.

CR: At the lateral canthus of the eye.

Collimation: To the film.

Side Marker: Side closest to the film, near a corner.

Breathing Instructions: Suspended expiration.

Clinicoradiologic Correlations: Upright films are preferred to demonstrate fluid levels within the sinuses.

1. *Alignment:* The palate should lie parallel to the film.
2. *Bone:* Details of the maxillary, frontal, ethmoid, and sphenoid sinuses are well shown.
3. *Cartilage:* The temporomandibular joint is occasionally demonstrated.
4. *Soft tissue:* Air-fluid levels are indicators of sinus disease, which may be fluid, pus, or blood.

Normal Anatomy (Figure 1.7B)

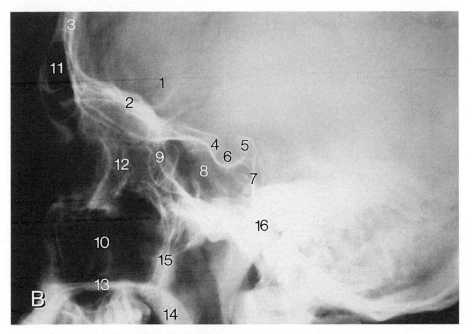

Figure 1.7.   B. Radiograph, Lateral Paranasal Sinuses.

1. Vascular impression of middle meningeal artery.
2. Orbital plate, frontal bone.
3. Frontal bone.
4. Tuberculum sellae and anterior clinoids.
5. Posterior clinoids.
6. Sella turcica.
7. Clivus (dorsum sellae).
8. Sphenoid sinus.

9. Ethmoid sinus.
10. Maxillary sinus.
11. Frontal sinus.
12. Frontal process, zygoma.
13. Hard palate.
14. Soft palate.
15. Posterior wall, maxillary sinus.
16. Petrous portion, temporal bone.

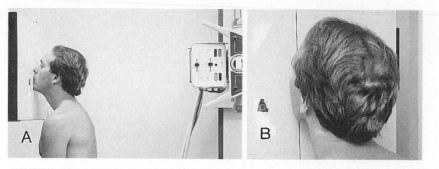

Figure 1.8. WATER'S PROJECTION, PARANASAL SINUSES. A. Patient Position. B. Collimation and Central Ray.

Demonstrates: Maxillary sinuses, ethmoid sinuses, frontal sinuses, orbits, and zygomatic arches. (1–4)

Measure: Through the central ray.

kVp: 85 (80 to 90).

Film Size: 8 × 10 inches (18 × 24 cm).

Grid: Yes.

TFD: 40 inches (102 cm).

Tube Tilt: None.

Patient Position: Prone or upright (posteroanterior).

Part Position: Midline, with no lateral head tilt or rotation. The head is extended such that the canthomeatal line is elevated 37° relative to the central ray.

CR: Should exit just below the nares.

Collimation: To film size.

Side Marker: In open space.

Breathing Instructions: Suspended expiration.

Clinicoradiologic Correlations: Can be done with the mouth open, to visualize the sphenoid sinus, or closed. Upright positioning is preferred to demonstrate fluid levels within the sinuses.

1. *Alignment:* The nasal septum should lie in the midline.
2. *Bone:* The bony outlines of the orbits and maxillary sinuses are well shown.
3. *Cartilage:* The temporomandibular joint can be identified.
4. *Soft tissue:* Air-fluid levels within the maxillary sinus may be fluid, pus, or blood. This is a decisive view in orbital trauma to detect "blowout" fractures.

BASIC
Lateral
Waters

PARANASAL SINUSES
Water's Projection

OPTIONAL
Submentovertical

Normal Anatomy (Figure 1.8C)

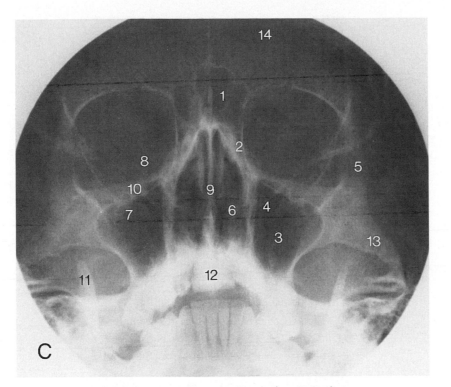

Figure 1.8.   C. Radiograph, Water's Sinus Projection.

1. Frontal sinus.
2. Ethmoid sinus.
3. Maxillary sinus (antrum).
4. Supraorbital fissure.
5. Frontal process, zygoma.
6. Inferior turbinate.
7. Greater wing of sphenoid.
8. Lesser wing of sphenoid.
9. Nasal septum,
10. Infraorbital foramen.
11. Coronoid process, mandible.
12. Top incisors.
13. Zygomatic arch.
14. Frontal bone.

BASIC
Lateral
*Waters

PARANASAL SINUSES
Water's Projection

OPTIONAL
Submentovertical

CERVICAL SPINE

Anteroposterior Lower Cervical Spine Projection

BASIC
*AP Lower cervical
AP open mouth
Lateral
Obliques*

OPTIONAL
*Flexion
Extension
Pillar
Moving jaw*

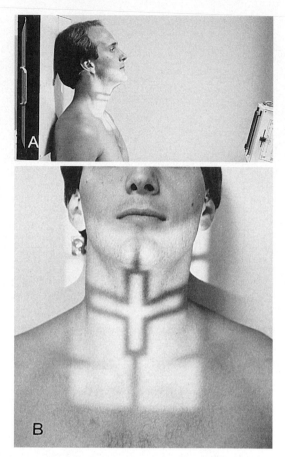

Figure 1.9. ANTEROPOSTERIOR LOWER CERVICAL SPINE. A. Patient Position. B. Collimation and Central Ray.

Demonstrates: Lower five cervical vertebrae (especially vertebral bodies, von Luschka joints, and spinous processes), the upper two or three thoracic vertebrae and ribs, medial border of the clavicles, lung apices, trachea, and neck muscles. (1–4)

Measure: At C4 level (apex of thyroid cartilage).

kVp: 80 (75 to 85).

Film Size: 8 × 10 inches (18 × 24 cm), or 10 × 12 inches (24 × 30 cm).

Grid: Yes.

TFD: 40 inches (102 cm) (must correct for tube tilt).

Tube Tilt: 15° cephalad, dependent on lordosis.

Patient Position: Upright or supine. Necklaces should be removed.

Part Position: Center cervical spine to the midline of the bucky. Extend head so that a line from the lower edge of the chin to the base of the occiput is perpendicular to the film.

CR: Thyroid cartilage (C4).

Collimation: To film size, with an 8-inch wide collimation used so that the lung apices are included. Include the lower margin of the mandible.

Side Marker: Indicate left or right lateral to the midportion of the neck.

Breathing Instructions: Suspended expiration.

Clinicoradiologic Correlations: If the cervical lordosis is reduced, the cephalad tube angulation should also be decreased to allow the rays to pass through the intervertebral disc spaces. It may be helpful to expose and develop the lateral radiograph first, to better approximate the angle of the lower disc spaces.

1. *Alignment:* Note the alignment of the spinous processes; a sharp intersegmental discrepancy (widened interspinous space, rotation) may indicate facet dislocation. (5)
2. *Bone:* All structures should be identified; spinouses, laminae, pedicles, transverse processes, articular pillars, vertebral body and uncinate process. Identify T1 by the transverse processes being oriented cephalad. Trace the upper ribs and clavicles.
3. *Cartilage:* Recognize each intervertebral disc space and uncovertebral joint. The facet joints can be recognized as lying at the apex of the convexity of the undulating contour of the articular pillars. Note the costal joints.
4. *Soft tissue:* The trachea should be midline and uniform in caliber except for the laryngeal constriction (vocal cords). The lung apices should be equally aerated.

Normal Anatomy (Figure 1.9C–E)

BASIC
*AP Lower cervical
AP open mouth
Lateral
Obliques

CERVICAL SPINE

Anteroposterior Lower Cervical Spine Projection

OPTIONAL
Flexion
Extension
Pillar
Moving jaw

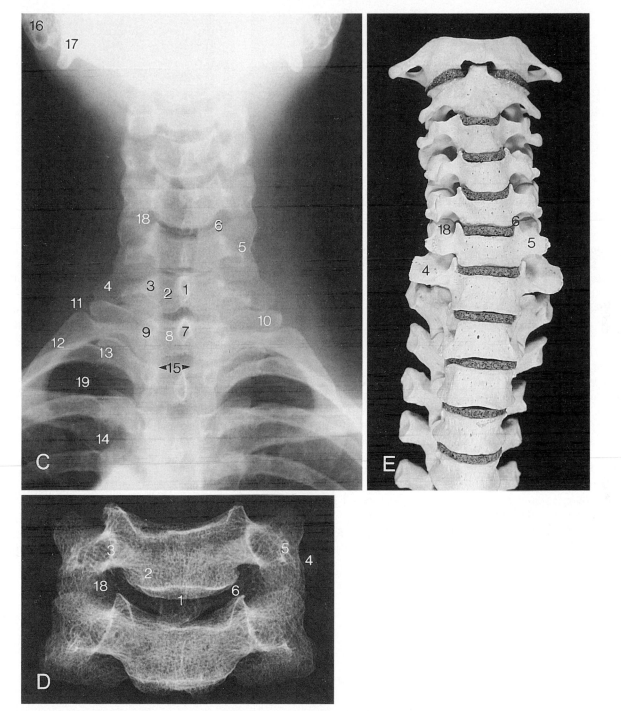

Figure 1.9.   C. Radiograph, Anteroposterior Lower Cervical. D. Specimen Radiograph (C7-T1). E. Anatomic Specimen Cervical Spine.

1. C7 spinous process.
2. C7 lamina.
3. C7 pedicle.
4. C7 transverse process.
5. C6 articular pillar.
6. C5-C6 von Luschka joint (uncinate process and fossa).
7. T1 spinous process.
8. T1 lamina.
9. T1 pedicle.
10. T1 transverse process.

11. First costotransverse joint.
12. First rib.
13. Second costotransverse joint.
14. Medial clavicle.
15. Trachea.
16. Mastoid process.
17. Angle of mandible.
18. C5 intervertebral foramen.
19. Lung apex.

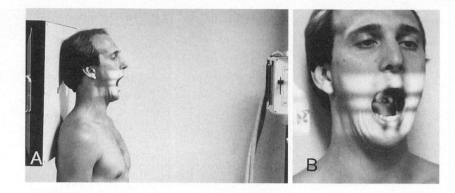

Figure 1.10.   ANTEROPOSTERIOR OPEN MOUTH, CERVICAL SPINE. A. Patient Position. B. Collimation and Central Ray.

Demonstrates: Upper two cervical vertebrae and occipital condyles. (6,7)

Measure: At C4 level.

kVp: 80 (75 to 85).

Film Size: 8 × 10 inches (18 × 24 cm).

Grid: Yes.

TFD: 40 inches (102 cm).

Tube Tilt: None.

Patient Position: Upright or supine. Dentures if worn should be removed.

Part Position: Center cervical spine to the midline of the bucky. The head is positioned so that the lower border of the upper incisors and the tips of the mastoid processes are in the same plane perpendicular to the film. The patient's mouth is opened as wide as possible.

CR: Directed to the midpoint of the open mouth, through the uvula.

Collimation: Below patient's eyes, include mastoid processes laterally and exclude the symphysis menti.

Side Marker: Place appropriate marker inferior to mastoid process at film edge.

Breathing Instructions: Suspended expiration.

Clinicoradiologic Correlations: Due to close collimation, it is suggested that the mAs be increased by at least 50%, and occasionally, a doubling of the mAs may be necessary to ensure adequate exposure. Dental appliances should be removed for this projection. A combination open mouth and lower cervical projection can be obtained with an extended exposure time, while moving the jaw and providing appropriate head stabilization (Ottenello's projection). (8,9) If the head is extended the occiput overlies the atlantoaxial joint; if the head is flexed the incisors cover the joint.

1. *Alignment:* The atlas lateral mass should not overlap the lateral margin of the axis. The lateral atlantodental interspaces should be equidistant. The dens should not be tilted more than 5° otherwise a fracture may be present. (10)
2. *Bone:* All bony landmarks must be identified; atlas (lateral mass, anterior and posterior arch, transverse foramen and transverse process), mastoid process, and the axis (odontoid process, pedicle, lamina, spinous process, transverse foramen and process).
3. *Cartilage:* Two joint complexes can be delineated; atlanto-occipital and atlantoaxial joints.
4. *Soft tissue:* The tongue is frequently visible overlying the axis.

BASIC
AP *lower cervical*
*AP *open mouth*
Lateral
Obliques

CERVICAL SPINE
Anteroposterior Open Mouth Projection

OPTIONAL
Flexion
Extension
Pillar
Moving jaw

Normal Anatomy (Figure 1.10C and D)

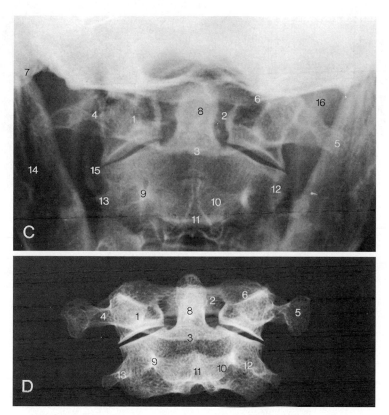

BASIC
AP lower cervical
*AP open mouth
Lateral
Obliques

CERVICAL SPINE
Anteroposterior Open Mouth Projection

OPTIONAL
Flexion
Extension
Pillar
Moving jaw

Figure 1.10.   C. Cervical Radiograph, Anteroposterior Open Mouth. D. Specimen Radiograph (C1-C2).

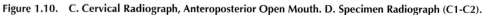

1. Atlas lateral mass.
2. Atlas anterior arch.
3. Atlas posterior arch.
4. Atlas transverse foramen.
5. Atlas transverse process.
6. Atlanto-occipital joint.
7. Mastoid process.
8. Odontoid process.

9. Axis pedicle.
10. Axis lamina.
11. Axis spinous process.
12. Axis transverse foramen.
13. Axis transverse process.
14. Mandible.
15. Tongue.
16. Styloid process.

BASIC
AP lower cervical
AP open mouth
*Lateral
Obliques

CERVICAL SPINE
Neutral Lateral Projection

OPTIONAL
Flexion
Extension

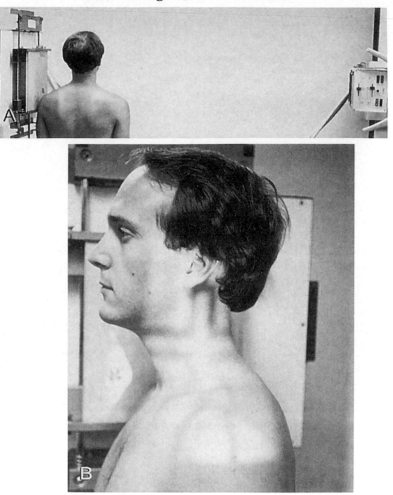

Figure 1.11.   NEUTRAL LATERAL CERVICAL SPINE. A. Patient Position. B. Collimation and Central Ray.

Demonstrates: Cervical spine, soft tissues of the neck, and the base of the skull. (1–4,11,12)
Measure: At C6 level (base of neck).
kVp: 80 (75 to 85).
Film Size: 8 × 10 inches (18 × 24 cm), or 10 × 12 inches (24 × 30 cm).
Grid: No. Use vertical cassette holder.
TFD: 72 inches (183 cm).
Tube Tilt: None.
Patient Position: Upright lateral, either standing or sitting. Place the convex side of a scoliosis next to the film. Earrings and necklaces removed.
Part Position: Shoulder in contact with cassette holder. Head and neck in true lateral position. Relax and drop shoulders as much as possible (patient may hold weights).
CR: C4. Center film to CR.
Collimation: Superior to inferior collimation to the top of the ear and tip of the shoulder.
Side Marker: Side closest to the bucky is marked, just below the mandible.
Breathing Instructions: Suspended full expiration.
Clinicoradiologic Correlations: All seven vertebrae must be visible. If the C7 vertebra is not visualized this can be overcome by; (a) increasing the exposure and doing a spot projection, (b) having the patient hold weights during the ex-

posure, or (c) performing a "swimmer's" lateral of the cervicothoracic junction. Occasionally, computed tomography may be the only means of demonstrating the C7 vertebra.

1. *Alignment:* Four visual lines of alignment should be checked; the anterior and posterior vertebral bodies, spinolaminar lines and tips of the spinous processes. Measure the atlantodental interspace (ADI) at less than 3 mm in adults and less than 5 mm in children.
2. *Bone:* All bony landmarks should be ascertained; atlas (posterior tubercle and arch, anterior arch and tubercle, lateral masses), axis (dens, axis body, lamina, spinous), and C3-C7 levels (body, articular pillar and facet, lamina, transverse process, spinous process, spinolaminar junction).
3. *Cartilage:* The intervertebral discs, facets, and atlantodental joints should be identified and assessed for joint space and smooth articular contours.
4. *Soft tissue:* The prevertebral spaces should be measured and smooth anterior borders (retropharyngeal interspace at C2; <7 mm, retrotracheal interspace at C6; <22 mm). The calcified thyroid cartilage can be identified. The air spaces of the nasopharynx, pharynx, and trachea are usually identifiable.

Normal Anatomy (Figure 1.11C–E)

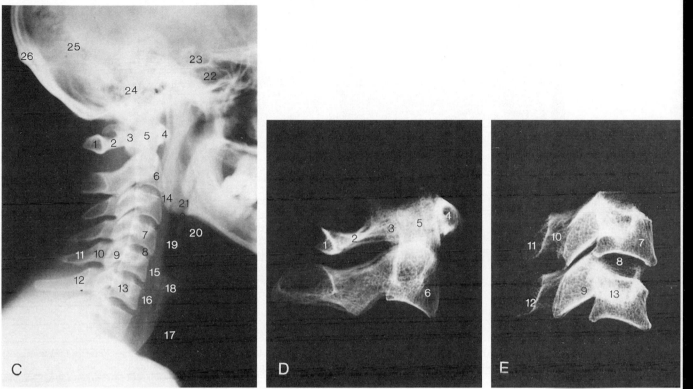

Figure 1.11. C. Radiograph, Neutral Lateral Cervical. D. Specimen Radiograph, Atlantoaxial Segments. E. Specimen Radiograph, Lower Cervical Segment (C4-C5).

1. Atlas posterior tubercle.
2. Atlas posterior arch.
3. Atlas lateral masses.
4. Atlas anterior arch.
5. Odontoid process.
6. Axis body.
7. C4 body.
8. C4 intervertebral disc.
9. C5 articular pillar and facet.
10. C5 lamina.
11. C5 spinous process.
12. C5 spinolaminar junction.
13. C5 transverse process.

14. Retropharyngeal interspace (RPI).
15. Retrolaryngeal interspace (RLI).
16. Retrotracheal interspace (RTI).
17. Trachea.
18. Thyroid cartilage and larynx.
19. Pharynx.
20. Hyoid bone.
21. Angle of mandible.
22. Sphenoid sinus.
23. Sella turcica.
24. Mastoid air cells.
25. Lambdoidal suture.
26. External occipital protuberance (EOP).

BASIC
AP lower cervical
AP open mouth
*Lateral
Obliques

CERVICAL SPINE
Neutral Lateral Projection

OPTIONAL
Flexion
Extension

BASIC
AP lower cervical
AP open mouth
Lateral
*Obliques

CERVICAL SPINE
Oblique Projection

OPTIONAL
Flexion
Extension
Pillars
Moving jaw

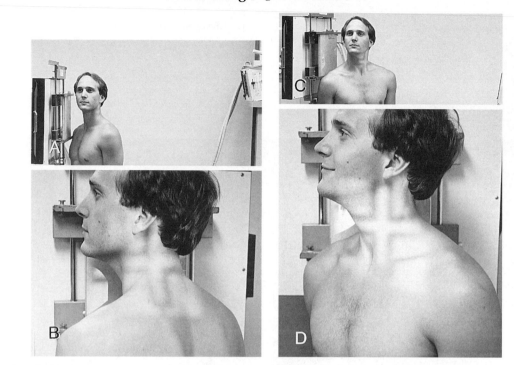

Figure 1.12. OBLIQUES, CERVICAL SPINE. A. Patient Position, Anterior Obliques. B. Collimation and Central Ray, Anterior Obliques. C. Patient Position, Posterior Obliques. D. Collimation and Central Ray, Posterior Obliques.

Demonstrates: Intervertebral foramina, von Luschka joints, apophyseal joints, and pedicles. (1–4,13,14)
Measure: At C6 level (base of neck).
kVp: 80 (75 to 85).
Film Size: 8 × 10 inches (18 × 24 cm).
Grid: No. Use nonbucky cassette holder.
TFD: 72 inches (183 cm) (must correct for tube tilt).
Tube Tilt: 15°: (a) Anterior obliques—caudad. (b) Posterior obliques—cephalad.
Patient Position: Upright or recumbent.
Part Position: (a) *Anterior obliques*: Facing the bucky, the body is rotated 45° away. The head is then rotated to be parallel with the plane of the bucky, and the chin is jutted out slightly. (Fig. 1.12A and B) (b) *Posterior obliques*: Facing the tube, the body is rotated 45° away. The head is then rotated to be parallel with the plane of the bucky, and the chin is jutted out slightly. (Fig. 1.12C and D)
CR: C4 level.
Collimation: Top and bottom of the film, with tight lateral collimation.
Side Marker: Under the mandible on posterior obliques; behind spine on anterior obliques when using right or left markers. RPO and LPO or RAO and LAO markers can be placed anywhere outside of the field of interest.
Breathing Instructions: Suspended full expiration.

Clinicoradiologic Correlations: In circumstances where these films cannot be performed at 72 inches, they can be done at 60 inches with the bucky, which does compromise detail and increase patient dose. Posterior obliques demonstrate the contralateral foramina (e.g., RPO—left foramina), while anterior obliques demonstrate the ipsilateral structures (e.g., RAO—right foramina. With posterior obliques rotating the patient to 55° may enhance depiction of the lower cervical segments. (15)

1. *Alignment:* The laminae in profile should be vertically aligned. The alignment of the opposing facet surfaces should be parallel.
2. *Bone:* This is a key demonstration of cervical pedicles since on AP and lateral views they are obscured.
3. *Cartilage:* Facet and uncovertebral joints should be assessed with smooth contours. The disc space is not usually well determined.
4. *Soft tissue:* The key structures are the intervertebral foramina, which are round-oval in configuration and have smooth contours. Their borders should be traced (pedicle, facet joints, vertebral body, and uncovertebral joints). Degenerative spurs may narrow the foramen from the facet or uncovertebral joints, while a neurofibroma may expand the foramen.

Normal Anatomy (Figure 1.12E)

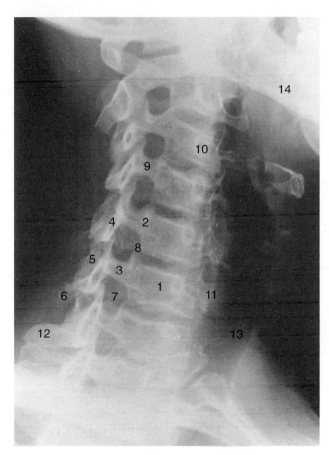

1. C6 vertebral body.
2. C5 transverse process.
3. C6 pedicle.
4. C5 lamina.
5. C6 articular pillar.
6. C6 spinous process.
7. C6-C7 intervertebral foramen.
8. C5-C6 von Luschka joint.
9. C4 pedicle.
10. C3 pedicle.
11. C6 transverse process.
12. First rib.
13. Trachea.
14. Mandible.

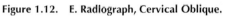

Figure 1.12. E. Radiograph, Cervical Oblique.

BASIC
AP lower cervical
AP open mouth
Lateral
*Obliques

CERVICAL SPINE
Oblique Projection

OPTIONAL
Flexion
Extension
Pillars
Moving Jaw

BASIC
AP lower cervical
AP open mouth
Lateral
Obliques

CERVICAL SPINE
Flexion/Extension Projection

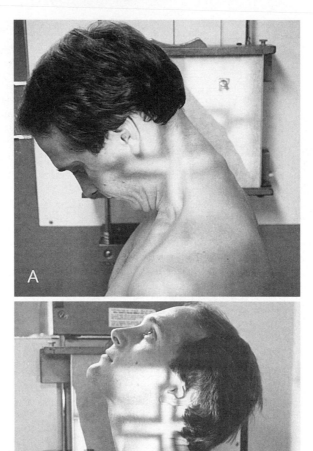

Figure 1.13. FLEXION-EXTENSION CERVICAL SPINE. A. Patient Position, Collimation and Central Ray, Flexion. B. Patient Position, Collimation and Central Ray, Extension.

Demonstrates: As per neutral lateral, but additionally evaluates patterns of intersegmental motion and ligamentous instability.

Measure: At the C4 level.

kVp: 80 (75 to 85).

Film Size: 8 × 10 inches (18 × 24 cm), 10 × 12 inches (24 × 30 cm).

Grid: No. Use nonbucky cassette holder.

TFD: 72 inches (183 cm).

Tube Tilt: None.

Patient Position: True lateral position aligned to the bucky midline.

Part Position: (a) *Flexion*: Tuck chin, then flex the head forward as far as possible; (b) *Extension*: Elevate the chin, then extend the head backward as far as possible.

CR: At the C4 level.

Collimation: To the film size.

Side Marker: Mark side closest to the film, below the chin in extension and behind the head in flexion.

Breathing Instructions: Suspended expiration.

Clinicoradiologic Correlations: Contraindications to these studies include vertebrobasilar ischemia, postural vertigo, fracture-dislocations, odontoid lesions, or significant neurologic deficits. The neutral lateral projection should be evaluated and the patient carefully examined before these exposures are taken. (16,17) Special attention to eliminating patient motion is necessary, since the patient is placed in a stressed position. Flexion/extension films are often used in cases of trauma and, may be part of a seven-view examination (AP open mouth, AP lower cervical, neutral lateral, right and left obliques, and flexion/extension views), called a *Davis series.* (18)

1. *Alignment:* Four visual lines of alignment should be checked; the anterior and posterior vertebral bodies, spinolaminar lines, and tips of the spinous processes. Measure the atlantodental interspace (ADI) at less than 3 mm in adults and less than 5 mm in children.

Normal Anatomy (Figure 1.13C and D)

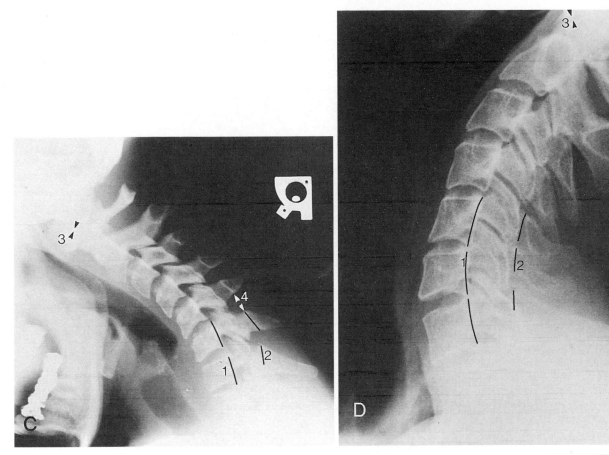

Figure 1.13.   C. Radiograph, Flexion Cervical. D. Radiograph, Extension Cervical.

Review the structures seen in the neutral lateral position.

Alignment and Motion Patterns:

1. Posterior vertebral bodies
(George's line).
2. Spinolaminar junction lines
(posterior cervical line—PCL).
3. Atlantodental interspace (ADI).
4. Interspinous spaces.

BASIC
AP lower cervical
AP open mouth
Lateral
Obliques

CERVICAL SPINE
Flexion/Extension Projection

BASIC
AP lower cervical
AP open mouth
Lateral
Obliques

CERVICAL SPINE
Articular Pillars Projection

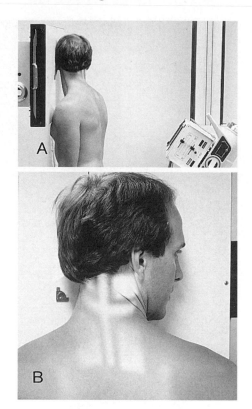

Figure 1.14.   POSTEROANTERIOR ARTICULAR PILLARS, CERVICAL SPINE. A. Patient Position. B. Collimation and Central Ray.

Demonstrates: Articular processes and apophyseal joints. Both sides must be done for comparison. (1–4,19,20)
Measure: At C4 level.
kVp: 80 (75 to 85).
Film Size: 8 × 10 inches (18 × 24 cm).
Grid: Yes.
TFD: 40 inches (102 cm) (must correct for tube tilt).
Tube Tilt: 35° cephalad.
Patient Position: PA.
Part Position: Rotate head 45 to 50° away from side of interest.
CR: Direct the CR through the C5 vertebra. CR enters neck at superior margin of thyroid cartilage and 1 inch lateral to midline on the side of interest. Center film to CR.
Collimation: Top and bottom of film, side 4 inches wide.

Side Marker: Place appropriate marker, marking side opposite head rotation.
Breathing Instructions: Suspended expiration.
Clinicoradiologic Correlations: This view can be taken anteroposterior, with caudad tube tilt.

1. *Alignment:* The facet joints alignment can be judged by the congruity of the joint surfaces and their alignment at the lateral margins.
2. *Bone:* The shape and height of each pillar can be assessed. Fractures of the articular pillars are frequently only observed on these special pillar projections. (17)
3. *Cartilage:* Integrity of the facet joints can be evaluated by noting the joint cavity and the smooth articular surfaces.
4. CT is the best means to image a pillar fracture.

BASIC
AP lower cervical
AP open mouth
Lateral
Obliques

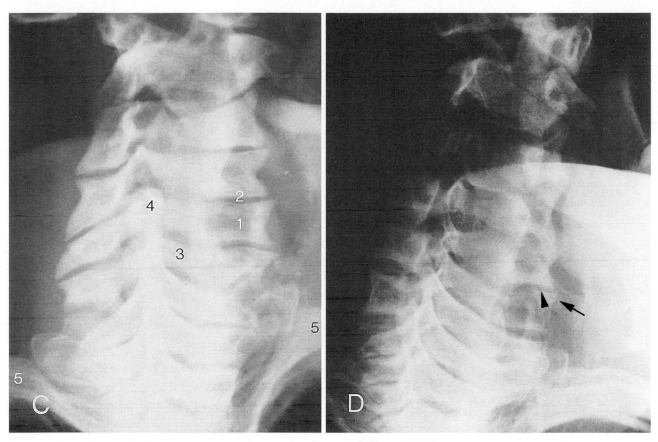

Figure 1.14.   C. Cervical Radiograph, Posteroanterior Articular Pillars. D. Fractured C7 Pillar. The pillar view shows offset laterally (arrow) and at the articular surface of the superior articular facet (arrowhead). No fracture was evident on any other views, highlighting the value of this special pillar projection. (Courtesy of Thomas M. Goodrich, DC, DACBR, Indianapolis, Indiana)

1. C5 articular pillar.
2. C4-C5 apophyseal joint.
3. C6 lamina.

4. C5 spinous process.
5. First rib.

THORACIC SPINE
Anteroposterior Projection

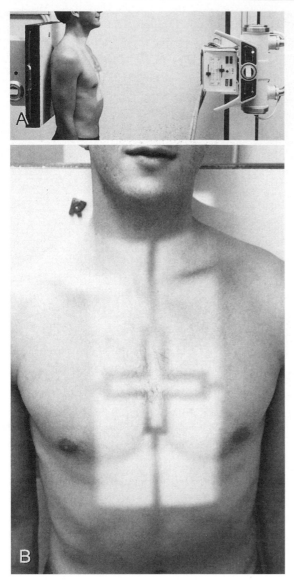

Figure 1.15. ANTEROPOSTERIOR THORACIC SPINE. A. Patient Position. B. Collimation and Central Ray.

Demonstrates: Thoracic spine, posterior rib heads, lung fields, and mediastinum. (1–3)

Measure: At T6 level.

kVp: 80 (75 to 85).

Film Size: 7 × 17 inches (18 × 43 cm), or 14 × 17 inches (35 × 43 cm) if significant scoliosis is present.

Grid: Yes.

TFD: 40 inches (102 cm).

Tube Tilt: None.

Patient Position: Upright or supine with hips and knees flexed.

Part Position: Align midsagittal plane of the body to the central ray, with no rotation.

CR: Place the top of the cassette 2 inches above the C7 spinous process. Center CR to film (CR will enter approximately 3 inches inferior to sternal angle).

Collimation: 7 × 17 inches (18 × 43 cm) film—collimate to film size. 14 × 17 inches (35 × 43 cm) film—collimate to area of interest.

Side Marker: Place appropriate marker in one of the top corners, preferably above the level of the clavicles.

Breathing Instructions: Suspended inspiration to depress the diaphragm.

Clinicoradiologic Correlations: A compensating filter should be used, if available, from the midthoracic to upper thoracic spine.

1. *Alignment:* Scoliosis is common in the thoracic spine and should be identified (cause-congenital, idiopathic, etc.) and accurately described (e.g., side of convexity, end and apex vertebrae, rotational component).
2. *Bone:* Each vertebra should have its individual components identified; transverse processes, pedicles, spinous process, inferior and superior endplates, and intervertebral disc space. The ribs, sternum, and medial clavicles can be delineated. The T1 transverse processes are oriented cephalad.
3. *Cartilage:* The intervertebral, costotransverse, and costovertebral joints should be identified.
4. *Soft tissue:* The key landmarks are the paraspinal lines. These occur bilaterally from approximately T8 to the diaphragm and represent the pleural interface between the lung and paraspinal soft tissues. (4)

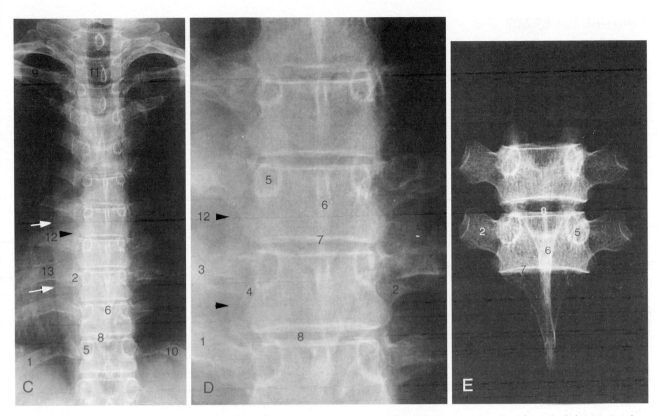

Figure 1.15.   C. Radiograph, Anteroposterior Thoracic Spine. D. Spot Radiograph, Anteroposterior Thoracic Spine. E. Specimen Radiograph, Thoracic Segments.

1. Rib.
2. Transverse process.
3. Costotransverse joint.
4. Costovertebral joint.
5. Pedicle.
6. Spinous process.
7. Inferior endplate.

8. Intervertebral disc space.
9. Clavicle.
10. Diaphragm.
11. Trachea.
12. Paraspinal line (arrowheads).
13. Aorta (arrows).

BASIC
*AP
Lateral

THORACIC SPINE
Anteroposterior Projection

OPTIONAL
Swimmer's lateral
Obliques

THORACIC SPINE
Lateral Projection

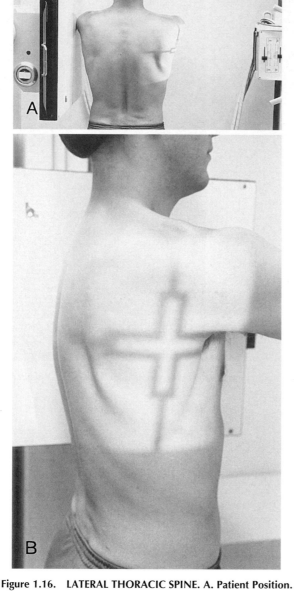

Figure 1.16. LATERAL THORACIC SPINE. A. Patient Position. B. Collimation and Central Ray.

Demonstrates: Thoracic spine, ribs, lung fields, and heart. (1,2,5)

Measure: At T6 level, under the axilla adjacent to the scapula.

kVp: 90 (85 to 95).

Film Size: 7 × 17 inches (18 × 43 cm), or 14 × 17 inches (35 × 43 cm) if kyphosis is increased.

Grid: Yes.

TFD: 40 inches (102 cm).

Tube Tilt: None.

Patient Position: Lateral recumbent or upright lateral.

Part Position: Align mid axillary plane to central ray.

CR: Place the top of the cassette 2 inches above the C7 spinous process. Center CR to film (CR will enter approximately 3 inches inferior to sternal angle).

Collimation: 7 × 17 inches (18 × 43 cm) film—collimate to film size. 14 × 17 inches (35 × 43 cm) film—collimate to area of interest.

Side Marker: Place appropriate marker in film corner behind spine.

Breathing Instructions: Suspended inspiration to depress diaphragm.

Clinicoradiologic Correlations: The overlying rib structures can be obliterated from the film by allowing shallow respiration during an extended exposure time (approximately 1 second). Care must be taken to reduce motion of the spinal column by allowing only shallow, quiet respiration and careful patient instruction. A compensating filter should be used from the mid to lower thoracic spine.

1. *Alignment:* The thoracic kyphosis is assessed as to degree and pattern of curvature. The posterior bodies should be aligned.
2. *Bone:* All components of each vertebra should be identified: vertebral body, endplates, pedicle, intervertebral foramen, and apophyseal joint. Rib elements can also be determined. Note that the axillary border of the scapula is superimposed over the upper thoracic vertebral bodies.
3. *Cartilage:* Each intervertebral disc gradually diminishes in height from caudad (T12) to cephalad (T1). Apophyseal joints can usually be identified in the lower thoracic spine.
4. *Soft tissue:* The diaphragm is readily discerned as an arc of soft tissue density curving anteriorly. Typically the right hemidiaphragm is higher than the left. The posterior margin of the heart is formed by the left ventricle and left atrium. Linear branching opacities of the pulmonary vasculature emanate from the hilar region of the lung.

Normal Anatomy (Figure 1.16C–E)

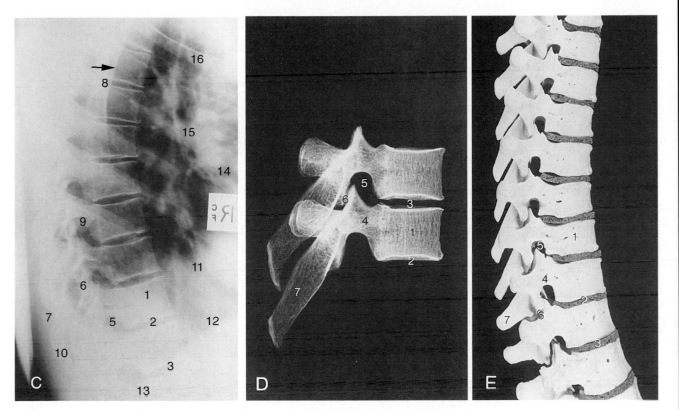

Figure 1.16. C. Radiograph, Lateral Thoracic Spine. D. Specimen Radiograph, Thoracic Segments. E. Anatomic Specimen, Thoracic Spine.

1. Vertebral body.
2. Endplate. (arrowhead)
3. Intervertebral disc.
4. Pedicle.
5. Intervertebral foramen.
6. Apophyseal joint.
7. Spinous process.
8. Axillary margin, scapula (arrow).
9. Rib head.
10. Posterior rib.
11. Lateral rib.
12. Diaphragm.
13. Posterior costophrenic sulcus.
14. Heart.
15. Lung hilus.
16. Trachea.

THORACIC SPINE
Lateral Cervicothoracic Junction (Swimmer's Projection)

BASIC
AP
Lateral

OPTIONAL
*Swimmer's lateral
Obliques*

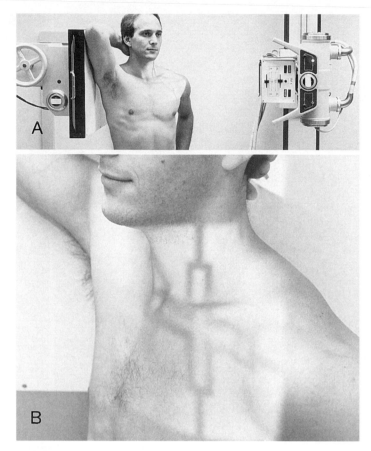

Figure 1.17. LATERAL CERVICOTHORACIC JUNCTION. A. Patient Position. B. Collimation and Central Ray.

Demonstrates: Lower cervical and upper thoracic vertebrae, especially the vertebral bodies and intervertebral discs. (6,7)

Measure: As for lateral thoracic, at the T6 level, under the axilla adjacent to the scapula.

kVp: 90 (85 to 95).

Film Size: 10 × 12 inches (24 × 30 cm).

Grid: Yes.

TFD: 40 inches (102 cm).

Tube Tilt: None.

Patient Position: Upright or recumbent lateral position. Rotate the posterior body 10 to 20° toward the bucky. The arm closest to the bucky is flexed, with the hand placed on the top or behind the head. The arm closest to the tube is extended, with the hand placed over the hip.

CR: Passes just anterior to the tube-side shoulder through the sternal notch.

Collimation: To film size.

Side Marker: In top corner of film, posterior to the cervical spinous processes.

Breathing Instructions: Suspended expiration to accentuate shoulder depression.

Clinicoradiologic Correlations: The *swimmer's* lateral is useful following cervicothoracic trauma and in broad-shouldered individuals. (7) A caudal angulation of 5° may assist in separating the overlying shoulders. Care must be taken in cases of trauma since positioning for this view may accentuate any intersegmental instability at the cervicothoracic junction. (8)

1. *Alignment:* Alignment of the posterior vertebral bodies must be evaluated.
2. *Bone:* Meticulous scrutiny of the lower cervical and upper thoracic vertebrae is required to find evidence of fracture, especially compression fractures of the vertebral bodies and fractures of the spinous processes.
3. *Cartilage:* Check the alignment of the facet joints and note any evidence for dislocation.
4. *Soft tissue:* The retrotracheal space should be measured for any evidence of soft tissue swelling with the space normally less than 22 mm.

Normal Anatomy (Figure 1.17C)

BASIC
AP
Lateral

THORACIC SPINE
Lateral Cervicothoracic Junction (Swimmer's Projection)

OPTIONAL
*Swimmer's lateral
Obliques

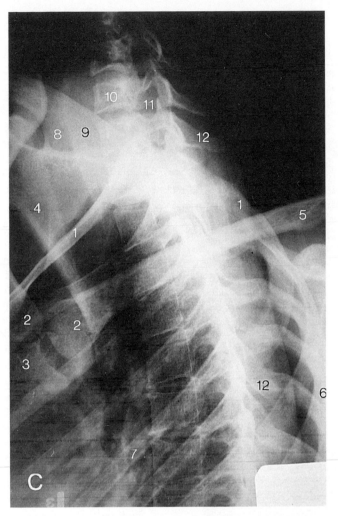

Figure 1.17.   C. Lateral Cervicothoracic Radiograph, "Swimmer's" Projection.

1. First rib.
2. Medial clavicle.
3. Manubrium.
4. Scapula.
5. Distal clavicle.
6. Posterior ribs.

7. Lateral ribs.
8. Trachea.
9. Retrotracheal space.
10. C6 vertebral body.
11. C6 intervertebral foramen.
12. Spinous process (C7, T5).

BASIC
*AP
Lateral
Obliques
AP spot

LUMBAR SPINE
Anteroposterior Lumbopelvic Projection

OPTIONAL
Lateral lumbosacral spot
Flexion
Extension
Lateral bending

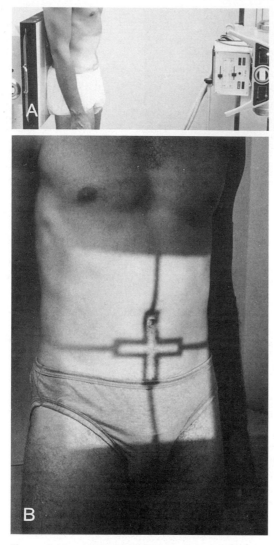

**Figure 1.18. ANTEROPOSTERIOR LUMBOPELVIC.
A. Patient Position. B. Collimation and Central Ray.**

Demonstrates: Lumbar vertebrae, pelvis, hips, proximal femora, and soft tissues of the abdomen. (1–4)

Measure: At L4-L5 level.

kVp: 85 (80 to 90).

Film Size: 14 × 17 inches (35 × 43 cm).

Grid: Yes.

TFD: 40 inches (102 cm).

Tube Tilt: None.

Patient Position: Upright or supine.

CR: 1 1/2 inches below the iliac crest level. Center film to CR.

Collimation: 14 × 17-inch field.

Side Marker: Place appropriate side marker at one of the upper film corners.

Breathing Instructions: Suspended expiration.

Clinicoradiologic Correlations: For the AP lumbosacral view without the full pelvis, use 14 × 17 inch (35 × 43 cm) or 7 × 17 inch (18 × 43 cm) film, collimated laterally to include sacroiliac joints, with the CR at the level of the iliac crests. In obese patients a supine view is preferred to compress the abdomen and reduce the time of exposure. Use gonad shielding when appropriate. Posteroanterior (PA) views can be used to take advantage of the diverging beam passing directly through the vertebral endplates although pathological details of the pelvis will be compromised. (5)

1. *Alignment:* Note the presence of any scoliosis and any pelvic obliquity. If the pelvis is included, use lines (Shenton's, iliofemoral, Skinner's, Klein's) and angles (acetabular, femoral) to determine normality.
2. *Bone:* All vertebral components should be located, including the neural arch (spinous process, lamina, pedicle, articular processes, transverse processes, pars interarticularis) and vertebral bodies (endplates, centrum). The sacrum, ilium, and lower ribs should also be observed.
3. *Cartilage:* The intervertebral disc spaces, facet joints, sacroiliac, pubic, and hip joints should be assessed for joint-space thickness and integrity of the articular surfaces.
4. *Soft tissue:* The psoas shadow is readily seen as a pyramid-shaped soft tissue density originating at T12-L1 and diverging laterally into the pelvis. Less than 40% of normal patients will exhibit clear definition of both psoas shadows; the left psoas is twice as commonly seen as the right. (6) In scoliosis less than 30% will have a psoas visible (being most common on the convex side and rare on the concave side). (6)

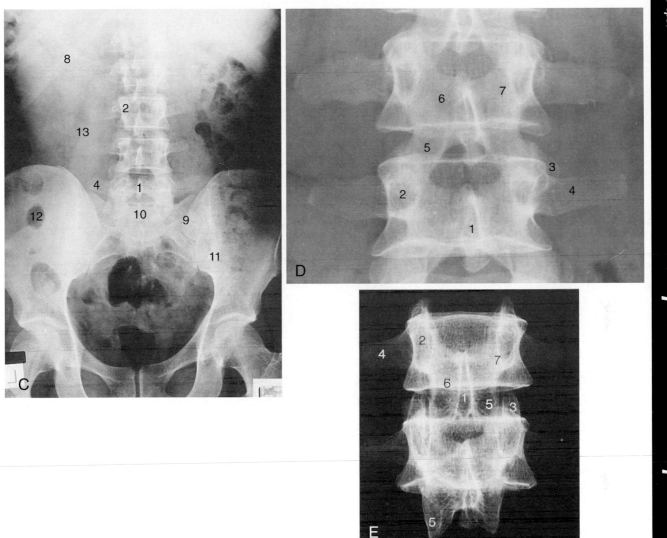

Figure 1.18. C. Radiograph, Anteroposterior Lumbopelvic. D. Spot Radiograph, Anteroposterior Lumbar Spine. E. Specimen Radiograph, Lumbar Segments.

1. Spinous process.
2. Pedicle.
3. Superior articular process.
4. Transverse process.
5. Inferior articular process.
6. Lamina.
7. Pars interarticularis (isthmus).

8. Twelfth rib.
9. Sacral ala.
10. First sacral tubercle.
11. Sacroiliac joint.
12. Descending colon.
13. Psoas muscle.

BASIC
*AP
Lateral
Obliques
AP spot

LUMBAR SPINE
Anteroposterior Lumbopelvic Projection

OPTIONAL
Lateral lumbosacral spot
Flexion
Extension
Lateral bending

LUMBAR SPINE
Lateral Lumbosacral Projection

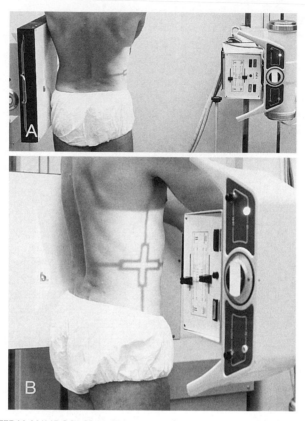

Figure 1.19.   LATERAL LUMBOSACRAL SPINE. A. Patient Position. B. Collimation and Central Ray.

Demonstrates: Lumbar vertebrae, sacrum, coccyx, and soft tissues of the pelvis, abdomen, and lower chest. (1,2,7,8)
Measure: Males—1 inch below the iliac crests. Females—1 inch below the iliac crests and 1 inch above the iliac crests, then average the two.
kVp: 90 (85 to 95).
Film Size: 7 × 17 inches (18 × 43 cm), or 14 × 17 inches (35 × 43 cm) if lordosis is increased, or with obese patients.
Grid: Yes.
TFD: 40 inches (102 cm).
Tube Tilt: None.
Patient Position: Upright lateral or lateral recumbent.
CR: 1 inch above the iliac crest level, with the vertical central ray passing halfway between the ASIS and PSIS. Center film to CR.
Collimation: Top and bottom of film, side collimation to accommodate the lordosis.
Side Marker: Place appropriate marker in a film corner or within the lordosis away from the spine.
Breathing Instructions: Suspended expiration, to elevate the diaphragm to visualize the lower thoracic spine.
Clinicoradiologic Correlations: In patients with a large discrepancy between the measurements above and below the

iliac crests, a compensating filter should be used. Use gonad shielding when appropriate. If scoliosis is present, the convexity should be directed toward the bucky.

1. *Alignment:* Observe the lordosis, sacral base angle, intervertebral disc angles, and gravity weight bearing lines. Each posterior vertebral body margin (posterior body line) should be in alignment.
2. *Bone:* Each vertebral segment should have its components identified; vertebral body, endplates, neural arch (pedicles, articular processes, spinous process, pars interarticularis), and intervertebral foramen. Observe the landmarks of the sacrum, including the sacral base and promontory.
3. *Cartilage:* The facet joints and intervertebral discs are well seen at all levels.
4. *Soft tissue:* The hemidiaphragms curve anteriorly over the thoracolumbar junction. Colonic gas and in erect postures the air fluid level in the fundus of the stomach (magenblasse) are often visible. Calcified aortic atherosclerotic plaques are commonly observed anterior to the L3 and L4 vertebral body margins.

Normal Anatomy (Figure 1.19C and D)

BASIC
Anteroposterior
*Lateral
Obliques
Anteroposterior spot

LUMBAR SPINE
Lateral Lumbosacral Projection

OPTIONAL
Lateral lumbosacral spot
Flexion
Extension
Lateral bending

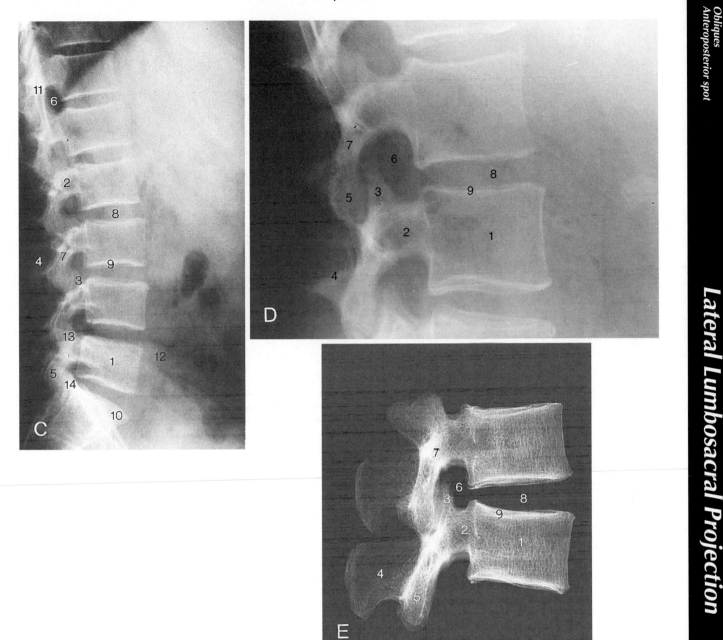

Figure 1.19. C. Radiograph, Lateral Lumbosacral Spine. D. Spot Radiograph, Lateral Lumbar Spine. E. Specimen Radiograph, Lumbar Segments.

1. Vertebral body.
2. Pedicle.
3. Superior articular process.
4. Spinous process.
5. Inferior articular process.
6. Intervertebral foramen (IVF).
7. Pars interarticularis (isthmus).
8. Intervertebral disc.
9. Vertebral endplate.
10. Sacral promontory.
11. Twelfth rib.
12. Iliac crest.
13. Apophyseal (facet) joint.
14. Superior articulating processes, sacrum.

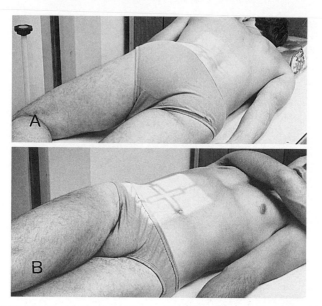

Figure 1.20. OBLIQUES, LUMBAR SPINE. A. Patient Position, Collimation and Central Ray, Anterior Oblique. B. Patient Position, Collimation and Central Ray, Posterior Oblique.

LUMBAR SPINE
Oblique Projection

Demonstrates: The *scotty dog*—transverse process, pedicle, articulating processes, facet joints, pars interarticularis, and laminae. Also provides an additional view of the vertebral body and abdominal soft tissues. (1,2,9,10)

Measure: At the central ray at L3.

kVp: 80 (75 to 85).

Film Size: 10 × 12 inches (24 × 30 cm).

Grid: Yes.

TFD: 40 inches (102 cm).

Tube Tilt: None.

Patient Position: Upright or recumbent.

Part Position: (a) *Anterior oblique*: Semiprone, with the body rotated 45°. On the side elevated, flex the knee and elbow to support the position. Align the spine to the central ray. (Fig. 1.20A) (b) *Posterior oblique*: Semisupine, with the body rotated 45°. Arm along table lays at patient's side. The elevated arm crosses the body to grasp the edge of the table. (Fig. 1.20B)

CR: (a) *Anterior oblique*: 1 inch lateral to L3 spinous process. (b) *Posterior oblique*: 1 inch above the iliac crest and 2 inches medial to the ASIS.

Collimation: Top to bottom, to film size, and 8 inches from side to side.

Side Marker: For anterior obliques, place marker behind the spine; for posterior obliques, place the side marker in front of the spine.

Breathing Instructions: Suspended expiration.

Clinicoradiologic Correlations: Anterior obliques show greater structural detail because the lumbar lordosis compliments the diverging x-ray beam. Both right and left obliques must be routinely taken.

1. *Alignment:* The facet joints from L1-L5 form virtually a straight line. The joint surfaces of each facet should be parallel to each other and aligned at their edges (Hadley's "S" curve).
2. *Bone:* The pars interarticularis is clearly seen and should be inspected for a defect ("collar" sign) or a healed defect. (11) The remainder of the *scotty dog* at each level should be identified—especially the pedicle, which is a favored site for bone malignancy.
3. *Cartilage:* The key structure to analyze is the facet joints for arthritis (loss of joint space), anomalies and dislocations. (12)

OPTIONAL
Lateral
Lumbosacral spot
Flexion
Extension
Lateral bending

Normal Anatomy (Figure 1.20C and D)

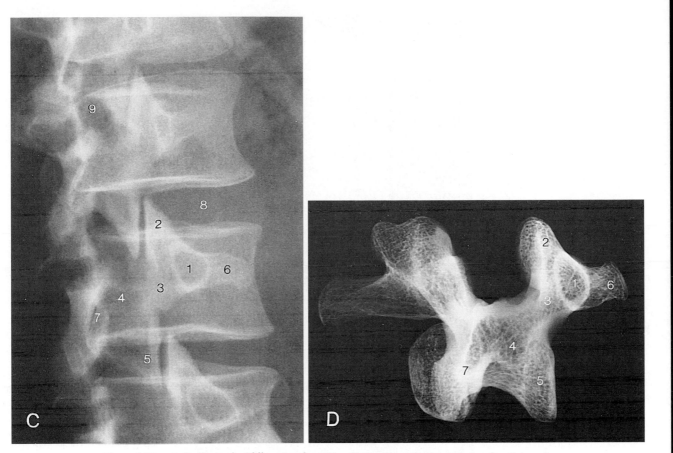

Figure 1.20.   C. Radiograph, Oblique Lumbar Spine. E. Specimen Radiograph, Lumbar Segment.

1. Pedicle.
2. Superior articular process.
3. Pars interarticularis (isthmus).
4. Lamina.
5. Inferior articular process.

6. Transverse process.
7. Spinous process.
8. Intervertebral disc.
9. Interlaminar space.

OPTIONAL
Lateral
Lumbosacral spot
Flexion
Extension
Lateral bending

BASIC
Anteroposterior
Lateral
Obliques
*Anteroposterior spot

LUMBAR SPINE
Anteroposterior Lumbosacral Spot Projection

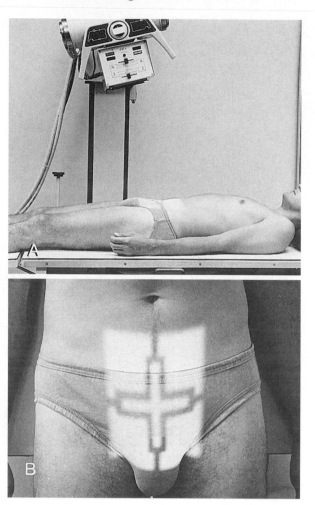

Figure 1.21. **ANTEROPOSTERIOR LUMBOSACRAL SPOT. A. Patient Position. B. Collimation and Central Ray.**

Demonstrates: L5 vertebra and disc, upper sacrum, and sacroiliac joints. (1,2,13–15)

Measure: Through the central ray.

kVp: 85 (80 to 90).

Film Size: 8 × 10 inches (18 × 24 cm) anteroposterior, or 10 × 12 inches (24 × 30 cm) posteroanterior.

Grid: Yes.

TFD: 40 inches (102 cm) (must correct for tube tilt).

Tube Tilt: 20° cephalad or to coincide with the plane of the sacral base.

Patient Position: Upright or supine.

Part Position: Supine or erect. Center lumbosacral spine to midline of film.

CR: Enter midline at the level of the inferior aspect of the ASIS (halfway between the umbilicus and the pubic articulation). Center film to CR.

Collimation: To film size.

Side Marker: Place appropriate marker in the corner of the film.

Breathing Instructions: Suspended expiration.

Clinicoradiologic Correlations: For a posteroanterior lumbosacral spot projection done upright or prone, the tube is tilted caudad (20°), with the CR passing through the L5 spinous process. Often referred to as the *tilt-up* view.

1. *Alignment:* The relationship of L5 to the sacral base can be assessed.
2. *Bone:* The sacrum is well demonstrated on this view. The three key landmarks are the sacral pedicles, sacral body endplates, and cortical margins of each sacral foramen (*arcuate* or *foraminal* lines). (16) Frequently lumbosacral transitional segments, defects in the L5 pars interarticularis, and abnormalities of the pedicle or facet are shown on this view. (11,17)
3. *Cartilage:* This is the optimum view for sacroiliac evaluation, since oblique views seldom demonstrate these joints clearly. (17–21) Note in the lower two thirds synovial portion of the joint the uniform joint cavity and smooth articular cortex. Details of the L5-S1 disc and facet joints can be distinguished.

OPTIONAL
Lateral
Lumbosacral spot
Flexion
Extension
Lateral bending

Normal Anatomy (Figure 1.21C)

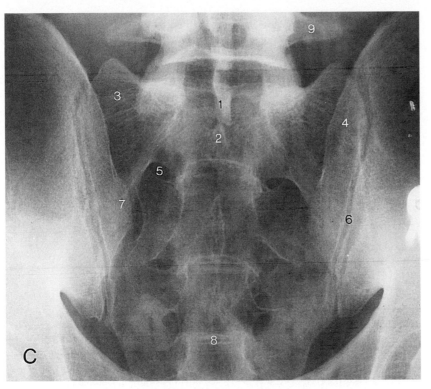

Figure 1.21. C. Radiograph, Anteroposterior Lumbosacral Spot.

1. Spinous process of L5.
2. First sacral tubercle.
3. Sacral ala.
4. Medial posterior ilium.
5. First sacral foramina.

6. Sacroiliac joint.
7. Posterior superior iliac spine (PSIS).
8. Sacral endplate.
9. Transverse process of L5.

OPTIONAL
Lateral
Lumbosacral spot
Flexion
Extension
Lateral bending

LUMBAR SPINE
Lateral Lumbosacral Spot Projection

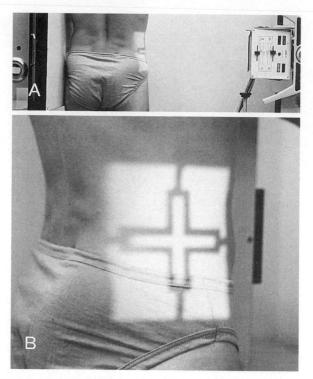

Figure 1.22.   LATERAL LUMBOSACRAL SPOT. A. Patient Position. B. Collimation and Central Ray.

Demonstrates: L5 vertebra and disc, upper sacrum, and adjacent soft tissues. (1,2,22)
Measure: 1 inch below the iliac crests.
kVp: 90 (85 to 95).
Film Size: 8 × 10 inches (18 × 24 cm).
Grid: Yes.
TFD: 40 inches (102 cm).
Tube Tilt: None.
Patient Position: Upright lateral or lateral recumbent.

Part Position: True lateral position, with CR entering midway between ASIS and PSIS.
CR: 1 inch below the iliac crest level. Center film to CR.
Collimation: 8 × 10 inches (24 × 30 cm).
Side Marker: Place appropriate side marker in film corner.
Breathing Instructions: Suspended expiration.
Clinicoradiologic Correlations: This is a supplemental view obtained when the lumbosacral joint is underexposed on the routine lateral lumbar film. (23,24)

OPTIONAL
*Lateral
Lumbosacral spot
Flexion
Extension
Lateral bending

Normal Anatomy (Figure 1.22C)

BASIC
Anteroposterior
Lateral
Obliques
Anteroposterior spot

LUMBAR SPINE
Lateral Lumbosacral Spot Projection

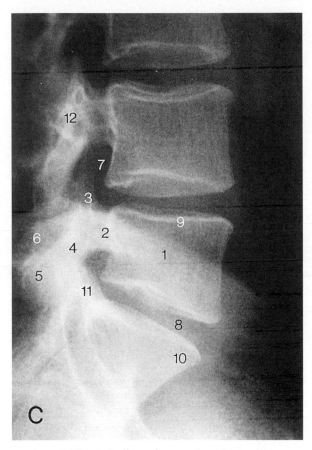

Figure 1.22. C. Radiograph, Lateral Lumbosacral Spot.

1. Body.
2. Pedicle.
3. Superior articular process.
4. Pars interarticularis (isthmus)
5. Inferior articular process.
6. Lamina.

7. Intervertebral foramina.
8. Intervertebral disc.
9. Vertebral endplate.
10. Sacral promontory.
11. Superior articular process of the sacrum.
12. Transverse process.

OPTIONAL
*Lateral
Lumbosacral spot
Flexion
Extension
Lateral bending

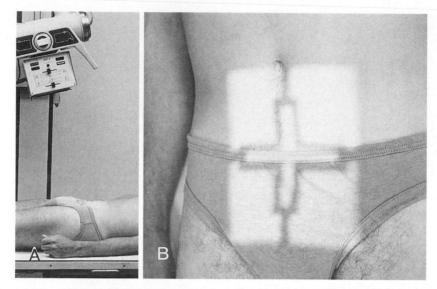

Figure 1.23. ANTEROPOSTERIOR SACRUM. A. Patient Position. B. Collimation and Central Ray.

Demonstrates: Sacrum, sacroiliac joints, coccyx, and lumbosacral joint. (1–5)

Measure: At CR.

kVp: 80 (75 to 85).

Film Size: 10 × 12 inches (24 × 30 cm).

Grid: Yes.

TFD: 40 inches (102 cm) (must correct for tube tilt).

Tube Tilt: 15° cephalad. Tilt will depend on sacral position. Ultimately, the central ray should be perpendicular to the body of the sacrum.

Patient Position: Supine or upright.

Part Position: Patient is centered to the midline.

CR: Midway between the pubic symphysis and the umbilicus. Center film to central ray.

Collimation: 10 × 12 inch field.

Side Marker: Place appropriate marker.

Breathing Instructions: Suspended expiration.

Clinicoradiologic Correlations: A preceding enema and voiding of the bladder should be performed to reduce the confusing overlying densities of gas, feces, and urine. (4)

1. *Alignment:* The relationship of L5 to the sacral base can be assessed.
2. *Bone:* The sacrum is well demonstrated on this view. The three key landmarks are the sacral pedicles, sacral body endplates, and cortical margins of each sacral foramen (*arcuate* or *foraminal* lines). (5,6) Frequently lumbosacral transitional segments, defects in the L5 pars interarticularis, and abnormalities of the pedicle or facet are shown on this view. (6,7)
3. *Cartilage:* This is the optimum view for sacroiliac evaluation, since oblique views seldom demonstrate these joints clearly. (7,8) Note in the lower two thirds synovial portion of the joint the uniform joint cavity and smooth articular cortex. Details of the L5-S1 disc and facet joint can be distinguished.

Normal Anatomy (Figure 1.23C and D)

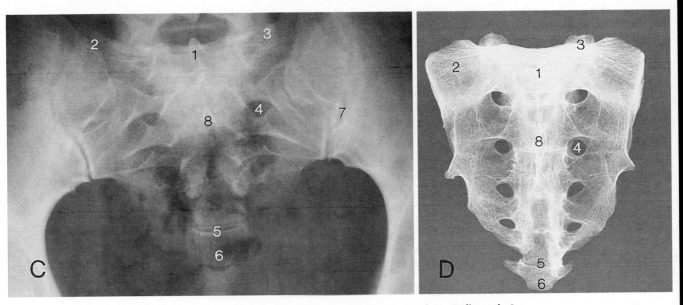

Figure 1.23. C. Radiograph, Anteroposterior Sacrum. D. Specimen Radiograph, Sacrum.

1. First sacral tubercle.
2. Sacral ala.
3. Superior articular process of the sacrum.
4. Second sacral foramen.

5. Sacral/coccygeal junction.
6. Coccyx.
7. Sacroiliac joint.
8. Third sacral tubercle.

Positioning (Figure 1.24A and B)

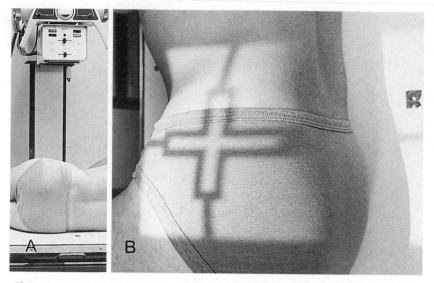

Figure 1.24.   LATERAL SACRUM. A. Patient Position. B. Collimation and Central Ray.

Demonstrates: Sacrum, lumbosacral joint, and coccyx. (1–4)

Measure: At CR.

kVp: 80 (75 to 85).

Film Size: 10 × 12 inches (24 × 30 cm).

Grid: Yes.

TFD: 40 inches (102 cm).

Tube Tilt: None.

Patient Position: Lateral recumbent or upright.

Part Position: Place patient in the lateral position, with the hips and knees flexed for support, if recumbent. Center the sacrum over the midline of the table.

CR: At the ASIS level, 2 inches anterior to the posterior sacral surface. Center the film to central ray.

Collimation: 10 × 12 inch field.

Side Marker: Place appropriate marker in film corner.

Breathing Instructions: Suspended expiration.

Clinicoradiologic Correlations: The complex anatomy of the sacrum makes structural identification difficult in this projection. Careful attention to systematic evaluation will assist in determining these structures.

1. *Alignment:* Note the position of the coccyx in relation to the sacrum, which is subject to wide variation and does not correlate with coccygodynia. (9,10) Similarly, note the sacral base angle.
2. *Bone:* Identify the sacral base, promontory, crest and canal. Follow the continuous scalloped contour of the anterior and posterior surfaces. Note the relative lucency of each sacral body from the superimposed foramina.
3. *Cartilage:* Check the lumbosacral disc, rudimentary sacral discs and the sacrococcygeal joint.
4. *Soft tissue:* The soft tissue area between the sacrum and rectum (presacral space) should be measured normally at less than 2 cm. A space greater than 2 cm is a sign of rectal or sacral disease associated with a soft tissue mass (tumor, infection, etc.).

Normal Anatomy (Figure 1.24C and D)

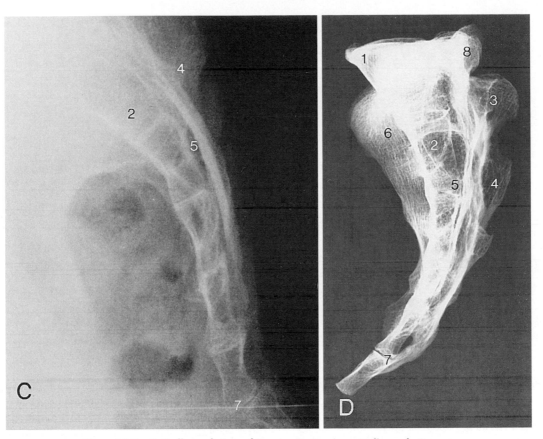

Figure 1.24.   C. Radiograph, Lateral Sacrum. D. Specimen Radiograph, Sacrum.

1. Sacral promontory.
2. Second sacral segment.
3. First sacral tubercle.
4. Sacral crest.

5. Sacral canal.
6. Auricular surface.
7. Sacrococcygeal joint.
8. Superior articular process, sacrum.

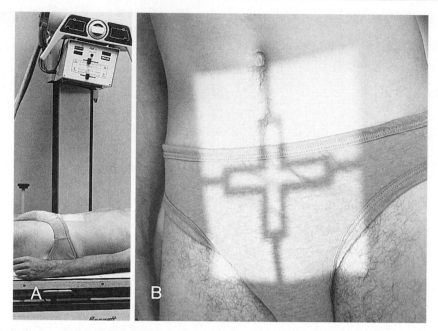

Figure 1.25. ANTEROPOSTERIOR COCCYX. A. Patient Position. B. Collimation and Central Ray.

Demonstrates: Coccyx and lower sacrum. (1–3)
Measure: At the CR.
kVp: 80 (75 to 85).
Film Size: 8 × 10 inches (18 × 24 cm).
Grid: Yes.
TFD: 40 inches (102 cm) (must correct for tube tilt).
Tube Tilt: 10° caudad. Tilt will depend on coccygeal position. Ultimately, the central ray should be perpendicular to the ventral surface of the coccyx.
Patient Position: Supine or upright.
Part Position: Centered to the bucky.
CR: Enters at a point 2 1/2 inches above the symphysis pubis. Center film to central ray.
Collimation: 5 × 5 inch field.
Side Marker: Place appropriate marker.
Breathing Instructions: Suspended expiration.

Clinicoradiologic Correlations: Patient preparation such as voiding of the bladder and an enema to remove overlying, confusing gas and fecal shadows should be performed. It may be helpful to expose and develop the lateral radiograph first, to most accurately determine the necessary tube tilt for the AP spot projection.

1. *Alignment:* There is wide variation in alignment of the coccyx either at the sacrococcygeal joint or between coccygeal segments. (4,5)
2. *Bone:* Evaluate the lower sacrum by tracing its lateral margins, sacral body endplates and foraminal lines. Identify the sacral hiatus and cornu of the first coccygeal segment.
3. *Cartilage:* The sacrococcygeal and intercoccygeal joints can be seen.

Normal Anatomy (Figure 1.25C and D)

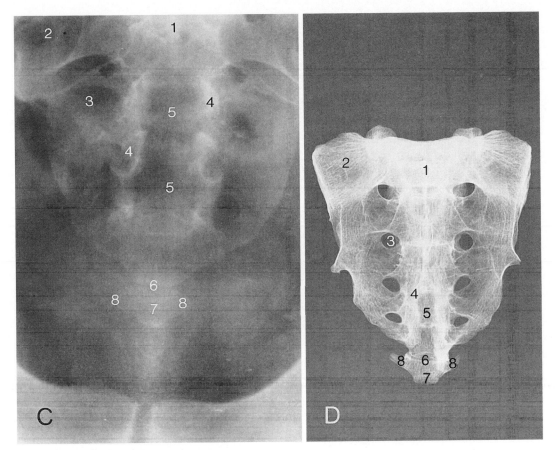

Figure 1.25. C. Radiograph, Anteroposterior Coccyx. D. Specimen Radiograph, Sacrum and Coccyx.

1. First sacral tubercle.
2. Sacral ala.
3. Second sacral foramen.
4. Sacral pedicle.

5. Sacral hiatus.
6. Sacrococcygeal junction.
7. Coccyx.
8. Cornu of the coccyx.

Positioning (Figure 1.26A and B)

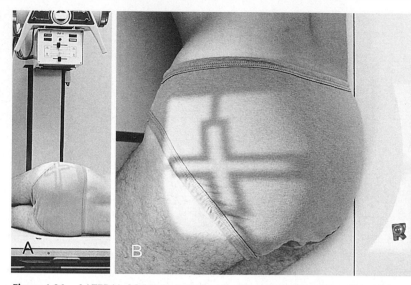

Figure 1.26.   LATERAL COCCYX. A. Patient Position. B. Collimation and Central Ray.

COCCYX
Lateral Projection

Demonstrates: Coccyx and lower sacrum. (1–3)
Measure: At the CR.
kVp: 80 (75 to 85).
Film Size: 8 × 10 inches (18 × 24 cm).
Grid: Yes.
TFD: 40 inches (102 cm).
Tube Tilt: None.
Patient Position: Lateral recumbent or upright lateral.
Part Position: Lateral position, with the coccyx centered over the midline of the bucky.
CR: Directed through the sacrococcygeal junction, 2 inches anterior to the posterior body surface. Center film to central ray.
Collimation: 8 × 8 inch field.

Side Marker: Place appropriate marker.
Breathing Instructions: Suspended expiration.
Clinicoradiologic Correlations: Mobility of the coccyx can be demonstrated by seated and recumbent studies, which can on occasions be linked with coccygodynia. (5)

1. *Alignment:* Note the position of the coccyx in relation to the sacrum, which is subject to wide variation and does not correlate with coccygodynia or posttraumatic subluxation. (4,5)
2. *Bone:* The number of coccygeal segments varies considerably.
3. *Cartilage:* The sacrococcygeal joint is identified as the first separated level of the lower sacrum.

Normal Anatomy (Figure 1.26C and D)

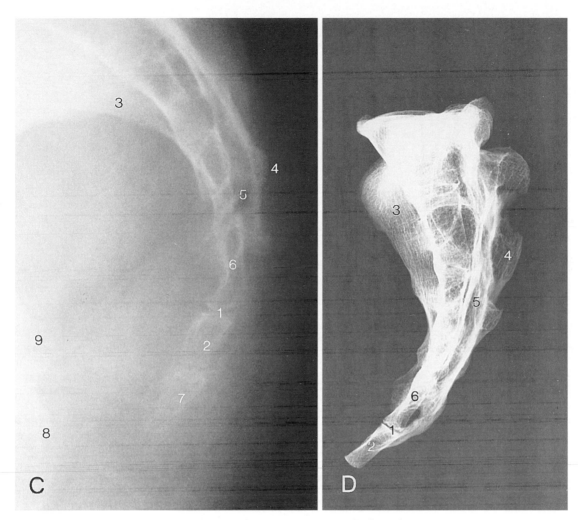

Figure 1.26. C. Radiograph, Lateral Coccyx. D. Specimen Radiograph, Sacrum and Coccyx.

1. Sacrococcygeal joint.
2. First coccygeal segment.
3. Auricular surface.
4. Sacral crest.
5. Sacral canal.

6. Fifth sacral segment.
7. Distal coccygeal segment.
8. Ischial tuberosity.
9. Ischial spine.

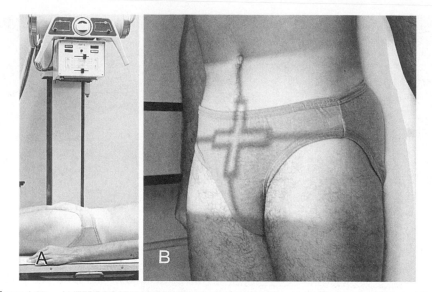

Figure 1.27. ANTEROPOSTERIOR PELVIS. A. Patient Position. B. Collimation and Central Ray.

PELVIS
Anteroposterior Projection

Demonstrates: Both innominates, sacrum, and coccyx, as well as the proximal femora. (1–5)

Measure: At the CR.

kVp: 80 (75 to 85).

Film Size: 14 × 17 inches (35 × 43 cm) crosswise.

Grid: Yes.

TFD: 40 inches (102 cm).

Tube Tilt: None.

Patient Position: Supine or upright.

Part Position: Center the midsagittal plane of the body to the midline. Internally rotate the feet about 15° (heels apart and big toes together), and use sandbags to stabilize.

CR: Midway between the symphysis pubis and iliac crest. Center film to central ray.

Collimation: 14 × 17 inches.

Side Marker: Place appropriate marker at film corner.

Breathing Instructions: Suspended expiration.

Clinicoradiologic Correlations: If the feet are not internally rotated, the femoral necks will appear foreshortened, and their anatomic details and relationships will be obscured. (6)

1. *Alignment:* Trace the cortex of the pelvic inlet from left to right, noting any disruptions at the sacroiliac, acetabular, and pubic regions. Follow the inferior margin of the superior pubic ramus and note the smooth continuity with the medial femoral neck (Shenton's line). Note the smooth contour from the lateral ilium across the acetabulum onto the lateral femoral neck (iliofemoral line). These visual guidelines should be compared bilaterally for symmetry.

2. *Bone:* Identify all structures systematically, including the ilium, pubis, ischium, proximal femur, sacrum, and lumbosacral spine.

3. *Cartilage:* All joints (sacroiliac, symphysis pubis, hip, lumbosacral) are inspected for alignment, joint space, and articular contours.

4. *Soft tissue:* Identify the bladder outline and at its lateral margins the fat line of the obturator internus muscle. Note the gas within the colon identified by haustrations.

Normal Anatomy (Figure 1.27C)

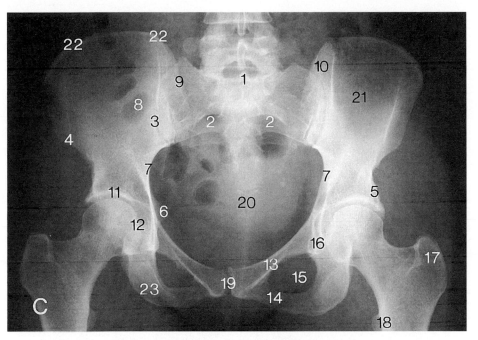

Figure 1.27.   C. Radiograph, Anteroposterior Pelvis.

1. First sacral tubercle.
2. Anterior sacral foramina.
3. Sacroiliac Joint.
4. Anterior superior iliac spine (ASIS).
5. Anterior inferior iliac spine (AIIS).
6. Ischial spine.
7. Pelvic brim.
8. Gas in the colon overlying the iliac fossa.
9. Sacral ala.
10. Posterior surface of the ilium.
11. Acetabular rim.
12. Fovea capitus centralis of the femoral head.
13. Superior pubic ramus.
14. Inferior pubic ramus.
15. Obturator foramen.
16. Inferior edge of the acetabular fossa (Kohler's teardrop).
17. Greater trochanter of the femur.
18. Lesser trochanter of the femur.
19. Pubic symphysis.
20. First coccygeal segment.
21. Iliac fossa.
22. Iliac crest.
23. Ischial tuberosity.

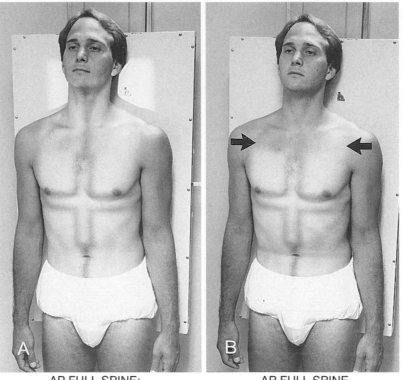

AP FULL SPINE:
WITHOUT FILTRATION

AP FULL SPINE
WITH FILTRATION

Figure 1.28.   ANTEROPOSTERIOR FULL SPINE. A. Patient Position, Collimation and Central Ray without Compensating Filtration.
B. Patient Position, Collimation and Central Ray with Compensating Filtration.

Demonstrates: Pelvis and lumbar, thoracic, and cervical spine. (1–4)

Measure: Anteroposterior at the lumbosacral joint.

kVp: 90 (85 to 95).

Film Size: 14 × 36 inches (14 × 91 cm).

Grid: Yes.

TFD: 84 inches (200 cm) optimum; no less than 72 inches (183 cm).

Tube Tilt: None.

Patient Position: Upright.

Part Position: Spine centered to bucky. Film placed 1 inch below inferior gluteal fold.

CR: To the film.

Collimation: To exclude the eyes and include the ischial tuberosities. Laterally to the ASIS bilaterally.

Side Marker: Appropriate marker adjacent to and above the shoulder.

Breathing Instructions: Suspended expiration.

Clinicoradiologic Correlations: Unless strict technical parameters are adhered to (high frequency generators, patient selection, immobilization, high grid ratio, tight collimation, filtration, rare earth screens, etc.) single- exposure, full-spine radiography should be avoided. (5) (Fig. 1.28C and D) The large area of exposure requires all structures included on the film to be adequately interpreted, including soft tissues.

Patients with anteroposterior measurements greater than 28 cm should not have a single, anteroposterior, full-spine projection. (Fig. 1.28B) Use gonad shielding when appropriate. A compensating filter such as the Baulin system should be used to prevent overexposure to the upper third of the film. (5–10) Lateral, full-spine radiographs have significantly reduced film quality and can only be used for postural analysis, not for pathologic evaluation. (11) Wherever possible sectional studies are preferred to single, full-spine lateral exposures.

1. *Alignment:* Observe for pelvic unleveling, scoliosis, intersegmental rotation, lateral wedging, or listhesis.
2. *Bone:* All skeletal structures must be evaluated, including each vertebral segment, pelvis, ribs, and shoulder girdles.
3. *Cartilage:* All joints (sacroiliac, pubic, discs, facets, costal, etc.) need to be studied carefully, despite their less than adequate demonstration.
4. *Soft tissue:* Many paraspinal structures are included and need to be carefully assessed: abdomen—psoas, kidney, liver, spleen, gas shadows, etc; chest—paraspinal lines, lung fields, heart, great vessels, etc.; and neck—trachea, vasculature, and muscles.

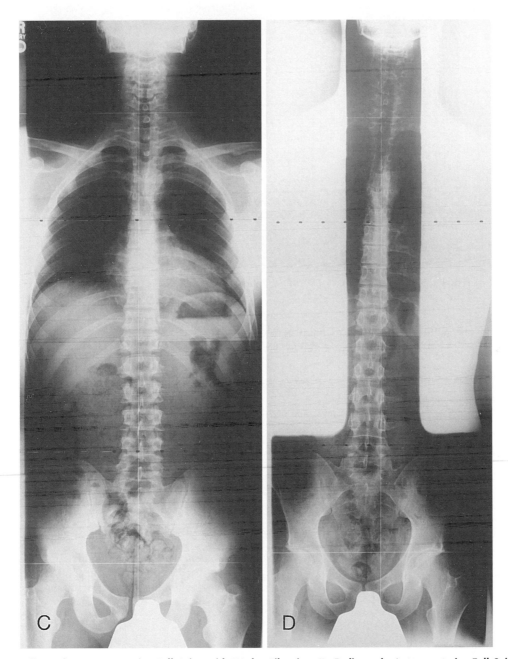

Figure 1.28. C. Radiograph, Anteroposterior Full Spine with Wedge Filtration. D. Radiograph, Anteroposterior Full Spine with Wedge Filtration and "T" Collimation. COMMENT: Both **C** and **D** were male patients with an A-P measurement of 24 cm. Technical parameters were 76 kVp, 50 mAs using a 1200-speed system (Kodak Lanex Fast Screens, T-Mat H Film) 72-inch FFD and utilizing a Bennett 100-kilohertz high frequency generator x-ray machine. (Courtesy of Todd A. Ryan, M.Ed., DC, Logan College of Chiropractic, Chesterfield, Missouri)

Positioning (Figure 1.29A and B)

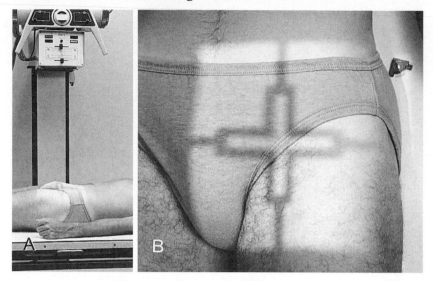

Figure 1.29.   ANTEROPOSTERIOR HIP. A. Patient Position. B. Collimation and Central Ray.

Demonstrates: Acetabulum, adjacent pelvis, joint space, femoral head, neck, trochanters, and proximal diaphysis. (1–5)

Measure: At the CR.

kVp: 80 (75 to 85).

Film Size: 10 × 12 inches (24 × 30 cm).

Grid: Yes.

TFD: 40 inches (102 cm).

Tube Tilt: None.

Patient Position: Supine or upright.

Part Position: The leg is internally rotated 15°. (4) The femoral neck is centered to the midline.

CR: Make an imaginary line between the ASIS and symphysis pubis, and locate its midpoint. From the midpoint, move away from the umbilicus 2 inches to locate the center point.

Collimation: 10 × 12 inch field.

Side Marker: Place appropriate marker in film corner.

Breathing Instructions: Suspended expiration.

Clinicoradiologic Correlations: In bilateral hip studies a crosswise film of suitable size can be used and positioned appropriately. Generally, for children under 12 years of age both hips are done for comparison. If the feet are not internally rotated, the femoral necks will appear foreshortened, and their anatomic details and relationships will be obscured. (5) Use gonadal shielding when appropriate.

1. *Alignment:* Apply the lines and measurements of the hip (Shenton's line, iliofemoral line, femoral angle, Skinner's line, Klein's line, etc.; see Chapter 2).
2. *Bone:* Identify all structures systematically, including the ilium, pubis, ischium, and proximal femur.
3. *Cartilage:* At the hip note the joint space (superior-4 mm, axial-4 mm, and medial-8 mm) and smooth articular contours. Do not mistake the fovea capitus for a bone lesion.
4. *Soft tissue:* Identify the bladder outline and at its lateral margins the fat line of the obturator internus muscle. Note the fat lines of the gluteus medius and psoas.

Normal Anatomy (Figure 1.29C and D)

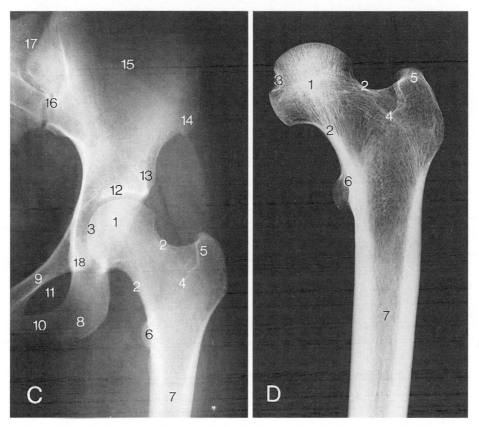

Figure 1.29. C. Radiograph, Anteroposterior Hip. D. Specimen Radiograph, Proximal Femur.

1. Femoral head.
2. Femoral neck.
3. Fovea capitus centralis of the femoral head.
4. Intertrochanteric crest.
5. Greater trochanter.
6. Lesser trochanter.
7. Shaft of the femur.
8. Ischial tuberosity.
9. Superior pubic ramus.

10. Inferior pubic ramus.
11. Obturator foramen.
12. Acetabular rim.
13. Anterior inferior iliac spine (AIIS).
14. Anterior superior iliac spine (ASIS).
15. Iliac fossa.
16. Sacroiliac joint.
17. Sacral ala.
18. Inferior acetabular fossa (Kohler's teardrop).

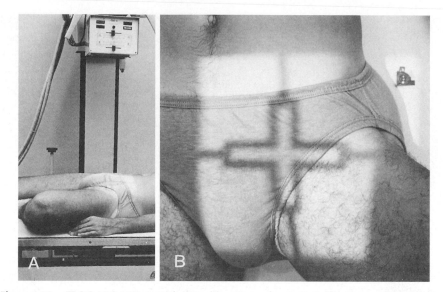

Figure 1.30. FROG-LEG HIP. A. Patient Position (Recumbent). B. Collimation and Central Ray.

Demonstrates: Acetabulum, adjacent pelvis, joint space, femoral head, neck, trochanters, and proximal diaphysis. (1–3,5,6)

Measure: At the CR.

kVp: 80 (75 to 85).

Film Size: 10 × 12 inches (24 × 30 cm).

Grid: Yes.

TFD: 40 inches (102 cm).

Tube Tilt: None.

Patient Position: Supine or upright.

Part Position: The femoral neck is centered to the midline of the table. The hip and knee are flexed until the foot reaches the level of the opposite knee. The flexed lower extremity is then abducted as far as possible.

CR: Make an imaginary line between the ASIS and symphysis pubis, and locate its midpoint. From this midpoint, move away from the umbilicus 2 inches to locate the center point.

Collimation: 10 × 12 inch field.

Side Marker: Place appropriate marker in film corner.

Breathing Instructions: Suspended expiration.

Clinicoradiologic Correlations: A bilateral frog-leg view can be obtained with the cassette placed crosswise. Generally, for children under 12 years of age both hips are taken for comparison. Use gonadal shielding when appropriate. This view is vital for proper diagnosis of many hip conditions, especially fracture, slipped epiphysis, and Perthe's disease.

A modification of the supine technique may enable a satisfactory radiograph obtained in the upright position (*Appa's view*). (Fig. 1.30C and D) The patient grasps a stabilizing object and places the hip into a flexed, abducted, and externally rotated position. The CR is directed to 2 inches below the midinguinal point.

1. *Alignment:* Use Shenton's and Klein's line in this position.
2. *Bone:* Structures of the acetabulum and proximal femur are depicted in a different plane.
3. *Cartilage:* The hip joint space is well depicted.
4. *Soft tissue:* The tissues of the buttock and hip are shown in profile.

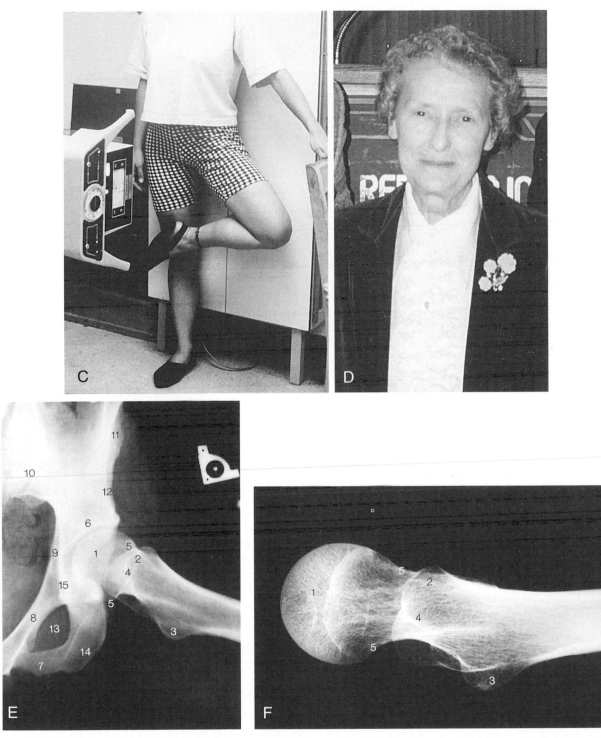

Figure 1.30.   C. Frog-Leg Patient Positioning (Erect, "Appa's View"). D. Appa L. Anderson DC, DACBR (With such a first name, "Ap-Pa" it's clear she was destined to become a radiologist.) E. Radiograph, Frog-Leg Hip. F. Specimen Radiograph, Proximal Femur.

1.   Femoral head.
2.   Greater trochanter.
3.   Lesser trochanter.
4.   Intertrochanteric line.
5.   Femoral neck.
6.   Acetabular rim.
7.   Inferior pubic ramus.
8.   Superior pubic ramus.

9.   Pelvic rim.
10.   Sacroiliac joint.
11.   Anterior superior iliac spine (ASIS).
12.   Anterior inferior iliac spine (AIIS).
13.   Obturator foramen.
14.   Ischial tuberosity.
15.   Inferior acetabular fossa (Kohler's teardrop).

KNEE
Anteroposterior Projection

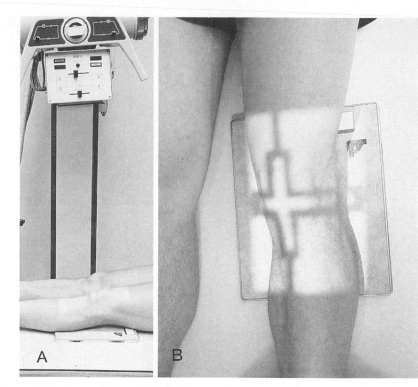

Figure 1.31.   ANTEROPOSTERIOR KNEE. A. Patient Position. B. Collimation and Central Ray.

Demonstrates: Distal femur, proximal tibia and fibula, femorotibial joint space, and patella. (1–3)

Measure: At the CR.

kVp: 60 (55 to 65).

Film Size: 8 × 10 inches (18 × 24 cm).

Grid: Yes, if the knee measures more than 10 cm; below 10 cm, a nongrid technique is used.

TFD: 40 inches (102 cm) (must correct for tube tilt).

Tube Tilt: 5° cephalad (central ray coincident with tibial surface).

Patient Position: Supine or upright.

Part Position: Internally rotate the leg slightly so that the knee is in a true anteroposterior position. Sandbag the ankle and foot.

CR: 1 cm inferior to the apex of the patella. Center film to CR.

Collimation: Collimate to area of radiographic interest.

Side Marker: Place appropriate marker at film corner.

Clinicoradiologic Correlations: This view can also be performed upright, which frequently identifies joint space nar-

rowing and/or instability when non-weight-bearing views appear normal. (4,5) Performed upright, posteroanterior with 10° of caudal tube tilt and the knees flexed to 45° may show these changes even more dramatically. (6)

1. *Alignment:* The lateral femorotibial components should be vertically aligned.
2. *Bone:* All components of the distal femur (femoral shaft, medial and lateral epicondyles, medial and lateral condyles, intercondylar notch, adductor tubercle), proximal tibia (intercondylar eminences, medial and lateral condyles), fibula (head and neck of the fibula, styloid process), and patella (superior and inferior poles) need to be located.
3. *Cartilage:* Medial and lateral femorotibial joint compartments should be equal in width with smooth articular contours.

Normal Anatomy (Figure 1.31C and D)

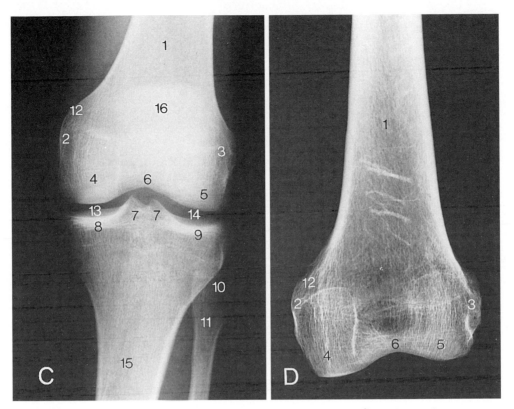

Figure 1.31. C. Radiograph, Anteroposterior Knee. D. Specimen Radiograph, Distal Femur.

1. Femoral shaft.
2. Medial epicondyle.
3. Lateral epicondyle.
4. Medial condyle.
5. Lateral condyle.
6. Intercondylar notch.
7. Intercondylar eminences (tibial spines).
8. Medial condyle of the tibia.
9. Lateral condyle of the tibia.
10. Head of the fibula.
11. Neck of the fibula.
12. Adductor tubercle.
13. Medial joint space.
14. Lateral joint space.
15. Tibial shaft.
16. Patella.

BASIC
*Anteroposterior
Lateral
Intercondylar
Tangential

KNEE
Anteroposterior Projection

OPTIONAL
Obliques

KNEE
Lateral Projection

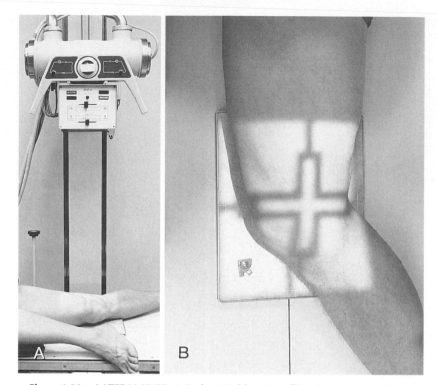

Figure 1.32.   LATERAL KNEE. A. Patient Position. B. Collimation and Central Ray.

Demonstrates: Distal femur, proximal tibia and fibula, patella, and patellofemoral and tibiofemoral joint spaces. (1–3,7,8)

Measure: At the CR.

kVp: 60 (55 to 65).

Film Size: 8 × 10 inches (18 × 24 cm).

Grid: Yes. Can be done nonbucky if part measures less than 10 cm.

TFD: 40 inches (102 cm).

Tube Tilt: Optional. 5° cephalad may be used to superimpose the inferior aspects of the medial and lateral femoral condyles.

Patient Position: Lateral recumbent.

Part Position: Place the patient on the table with the side of the leg being examined down. Flex the lower leg about 45° to traction the patella in place. Cross the opposite leg over the leg being examined and support, if necessary, to prevent pelvic rotation. Center the long axis of the femur to the midline of the film. Only when the posterior surface of the buttocks is perpendicular to the film will a true lateral view of the distal femur be assured.

CR: Enters 1 cm distal to the medial epicondyle. Center the film to central ray.

Collimation: By film size.

Side Marker: Place appropriate marker in film corner.

Clinicoradiologic Correlations: A cross table lateral with the knee fully extended may demonstrate fat/fluid levels (lipohemarthrosis) as evidence of an often unrecognized intraarticular fracture.

1. *Alignment:* The position of the patella is assessed.
2. *Bone:* All components of the distal femur (femoral shaft, medial and lateral condyles, intercondylar notch), proximal tibia (intercondylar eminences, medial and lateral condyles), fibula (head and neck), and patella (superior and inferior poles) need to be located.
3. *Cartilage:* Evaluate the patellofemoral, femorotibial, and tibiofibular joints for joint space and smooth articular cavities.
4. *Soft tissue:* Identify the infrapatellar (Hoffa's fat-pad) and suprapatellar fat-pads. Note the density and outline of the popliteal fossa and the location of the fabella.

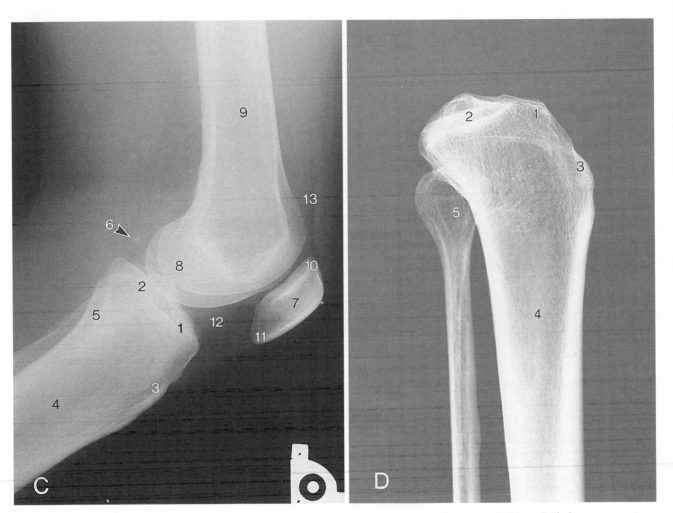

Figure 1.32.   C. Radiograph, Anteroposterior Knee. D. Specimen Radiograph, Proximal Tibia and Fibula.

1. Anterior intercondylar area.
2. Posterior intercondylar area.
3. Tibial tuberosity.
4. Tibial shaft.
5. Head of fibula.
6. Fabella (sesamoid bone in the head of the lateral gastrocnemius tendon).
7. Patella.
8. Condyles (medial and lateral).
9. Femoral shaft.
10. Superior pole, patella.
11. Inferior pole, patella.
12. Infrapatellar fat (Hoffa's fat-pad).
13. Suprapatellar fat.

BASIC
Anteroposterior
*Lateral
Intercondylar
Tangential

KNEE
Lateral Projection

OPTIONAL
Obliques

BASIC
Anteroposterior
Lateral
*Intercondylar
Tangential

KNEE

Intercondylar (Tunnel) Projection

OPTIONAL
Oblique

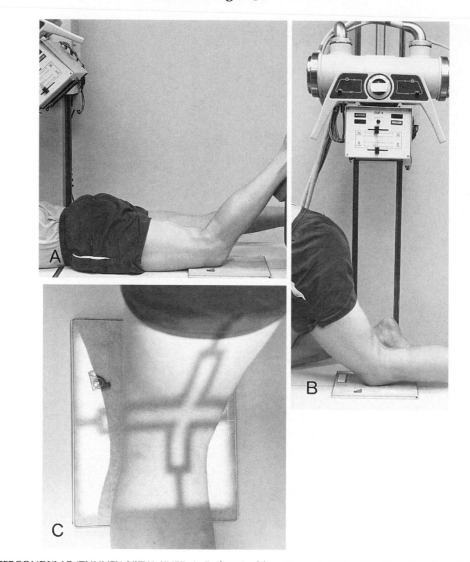

Figure 1.33. INTERCONDYLAR (TUNNEL) VIEW, KNEE. A. Patient Position, Prone. B. Patient Position, Kneeling. C. Collimation and Central Ray, Kneeling.

Demonstrates: Intercondyloid fossa, distal femur, proximal tibia, tibial eminences, proximal fibula, and joint space. (1–3,9,10)

Measure: At the CR.

kVp: 60 (55 to 65).

Film Size: 8 × 10 inches (18 × 24 cm).

Grid: Yes. Can be done nonbucky if the knee measures less than 10 cm.

TFD: 40 inches (102 cm) (must correct for tube tilt).

Tube Tilt: 45° caudal angulation with the prone position.

Patient Position: Prone or kneeling.

Part Position: (a) *Prone:* The patient is prone on the table. The knee is flexed approximately 45°, with the lower leg and ankle supported. (Fig. 1.33A) (b) *Kneeling:* The patient is on the table in the kneeling position. The patient then leans forward so that the shaft of the femur will form a 25° angle with the central ray. (Fig. 1.33B) The unaffected knee is brought forward so that the majority of the weight of the torso is on this knee. It can also be taken while the patient is sitting with the knee flexed. (11)

CR: (a) *Prone:* The central ray is angled 25° caudad and enters the knee joint at the popliteal depression. Center film to the central ray. (b) *Kneeling:* No tube tilt is used, and the central ray passes through the knee joint. Center film to the central ray.

Collimation: Collimate closely.

Side Marker: Place appropriate marker in film corner.

Clinicoradiologic Correlations: This view depicts the intercondylar notch, which is a common site for intraarticular loose bodies to hide.

Normal Anatomy (Figure 1.33D and E)

BASIC
Anteroposterior
Lateral
*Intercondylar
Tangential

KNEE
Intercondylar (Tunnel) Projection

OPTIONAL
Oblique

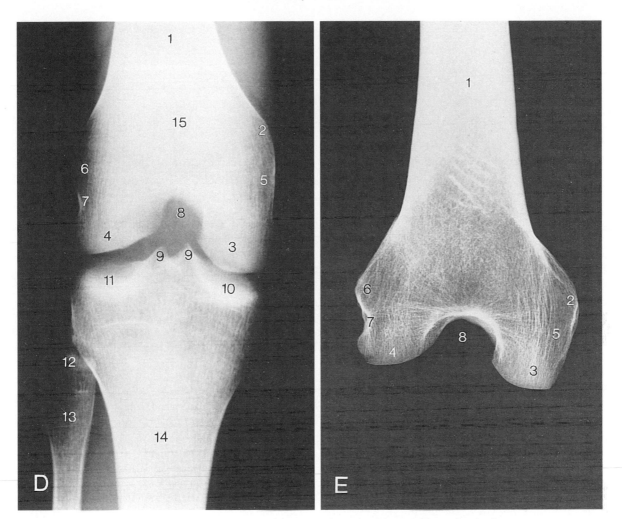

Figure 1.33. D. Radiograph, Intercondylar Projection. E. Specimen Radiograph, Distal Femur.

1. Femoral shaft.
2. Adductor tubercle.
3. Medial condyle.
4. Lateral condyle.
5. Medial epicondyle.
6. Lateral epicondyle.
7. Popliteal groove.
8. Intercondylar notch.
9. Intercondylar eminences (tibial spines).
10. Medial condyle, tibia.
11. Lateral condyle, tibia.
12. Styloid process, fibula.
13. Neck of fibula.
14. Tibial shaft.
15. Patella.

KNEE
Tangential (Skyline, Sunrise) Projection

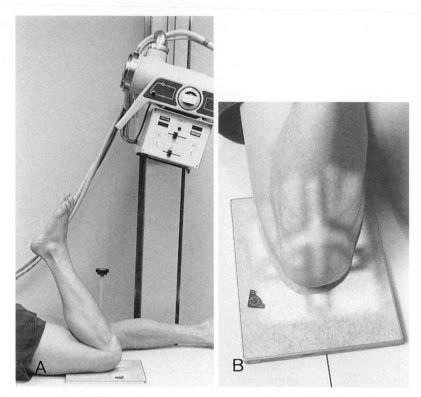

Figure 1.34.   TANGENTIAL VIEW, KNEE. A. Patient Position. B. Collimation and Central Ray.

Demonstrates: Patella and patellofemoral joint space. (1–3,12–15)

Measure: At the CR.

kVp: 60 (55 to 65).

Film Size: 8 × 10 inches (18 × 24 cm).

Grid: Yes. May be done non grid if part measures less than 10 cm.

TFD: 40 inches (102 cm) (must correct for tube tilt).

Tube Tilt: 10° cephalad.

Patient Position: Prone.

Part Position: The knee is fully flexed. If the patient is unable to fully flex the knee, angle the central ray cephalad so that a 45° angle exists between the lower leg and the central ray.

CR: Set the central ray between the patella and the femoral condyles. Center film to central ray.

Collimation: 4 × 4 inch field.

Side Marker: Place appropriate marker in film corner.

Clinicoradiologic Correlations: This is particularly useful in the assessment of the patella position, patellofemoral joint, the retropatellar surface, and the femoral groove. (6)

1. *Alignment:* The apex of the patellar articular surface lies directly above the deepest part of the femoral groove.
2. *Bone:* Details of the patella (medial and lateral facets, apex) and articular surface of the femur can be determined. The superior surface of the patella is often irregular and perforated by numerous vascular grooves.
3. *Cartilage:* Note the depth of the joint space; the ratio of the joint space at the patellar apex to the lateral depth is usually 1 or less.

Normal Anatomy (Figure 1.34C and D)

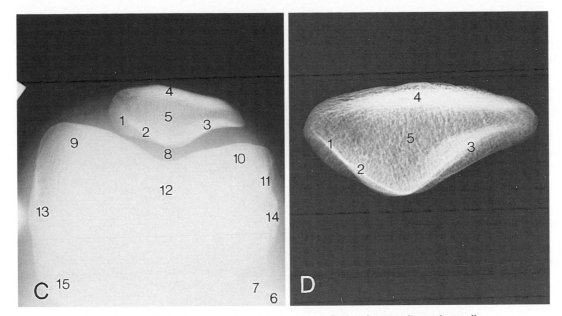

Figure 1.34.   C. Radiograph, Tangential View, Knee. D. Specimen Radiograph, Patella.

1. Odd facet of the patella.
2. Medial facet of the patella.
3. Lateral facet of the patella.
4. External cortical surface of the patella.
5. Patella.
6. Head of the fibula.
7. Tibiofibular articulation.
8. Patellofemoral articulation.

9. Medial condyle.
10. Lateral condyle.
11. Popliteal groove.
12. Intercondylar notch. (femoral groove)
13. Medial epicondyle.
14. Lateral epicondyle.
15. Adductor tubercle.

BASIC
Anteroposterior
Lateral
Intercondylar
*Tangential

KNEE
Tangential (Skyline, Sunrise) Projection

OPTIONAL
Oblique

BASIC
*Anteroposterior
Medial oblique
Lateral

ANKLE
Anteroposterior Projection

OPTIONAL
Stress studies

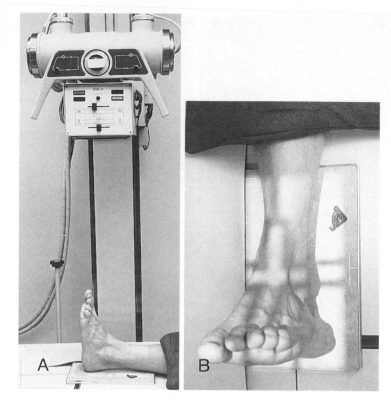

Figure 1.35. ANTEROPOSTERIOR ANKLE. A. Patient Position. B. Collimation and Central Ray.

Demonstrates: Distal tibia and fibula, talus, and ankle joint. (1–3)

Measure: Anteroposterior at the ankle mortise.

kVp: 55 (50 to 60).

Film Size: 10 × 12 inches (24 × 30 cm). Divide in half; the other half is for the medial oblique.

Grid: No.

TFD: 40 inches (102 cm).

Tube Tilt: None.

Patient Position: Supine.

Part Position: The ankle is slightly dorsiflexed so that the plantar surface of the foot is perpendicular to the film. Internally rotate the lower leg so that a line through the malleoli is parallel with the film surface.

CR: Center halfway between the medial and lateral malleolus.

Collimation: Collimate to a 6 × 10 inch field.

Side Marker: Place appropriate marker in film corner.

Clinicoradiologic Correlations: If the foot is not dorsiflexed, the tibiotalar joint space will not be clearly visualized (3); however, in subtle fractures of the talar dome plantar flexion will often demonstrate the fracture site. (4)

1. *Alignment:* The opposing articular surfaces of the tibia (plafond) and talar dome should be parallel but may diverge up to 6°. (5)
2. *Bone:* Landmarks of the distal tibia (plafond, medial and posterior malleolus), fibula, and talar dome should be identified.
3. *Cartilage:* Examine for congruence of the entire joint space from medial to lateral.
4. *Soft tissue:* Note the close proximity of the overlying skin line to the underlying malleoli.

BASIC
*Anteroposterior
Medial oblique
Lateral

ANKLE
Anteroposterior Projection

OPTIONAL
Stress Studies

Normal Anatomy (Figure 1.35C and D)

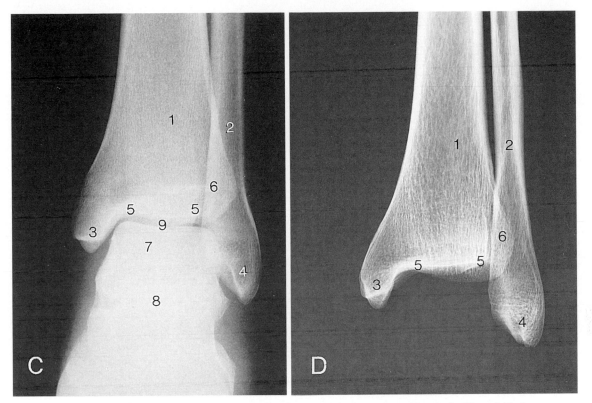

Figure 1.35. C. Radiograph, Anteroposterior Ankle. D. Specimen Radiograph, Distal Tibia and Fibula.

1. Tibla.
2. Fibula.
3. Medial malleolus, tibia.
4. Lateral malleolus, fibula.
5. Plafond of the tibia.

6. Lateral surface of the tibia.
7. Dome of the talus.
8. Neck of the talus.
9. Posterior malleolus.

BASIC
Anteroposterior
*Medial oblique
Lateral

ANKLE
Medial Oblique Projection

OPTIONAL
Stress views

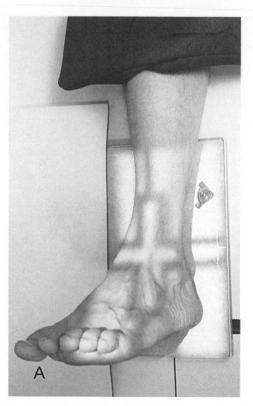

Figure 1.36.   MEDIAL OBLIQUE ANKLE. A. Patient Position, Collimation and Central Ray.

Demonstrates: Distal tibia and fibula, talus, and ankle joint. (1–3,6)

Measure: Anteroposterior at the ankle mortise.

kVp: 55 (50 to 60).

Film Size: 1/2 of a 10 × 12 inches (24 × 30 cm). Divide in half; the other half is used for the anteroposterior projection.

Grid: No.

TFD: 40 inches (102 cm).

Tube Tilt: None.

Patient Position: Supine.

Part Position: The ankle is slightly dorsiflexed so that the plantar surface of the foot is perpendicular to the film. The lower leg is then internally rotated so that the intermalleolar line forms an angle of 35 to 45° with the film.

CR: Center halfway between the medial and lateral malleolus. Center film to central ray.

Collimation: Collimate to a 6 × 10 inch field.

Side Marker: Place appropriate marker in film corner.

Clinicoradiologic Correlations: This is an important view in the assessment of the posttraumatic ankle for detecting subtle fractures of the distal fibula, posterior tibia, talar dome, and base of the fifth metatarsal.

1. *Alignment:* The opposing articular surfaces of the tibia and talar dome should be parallel, but may diverge up to 6°. (5)
2. *Bone:* Landmarks of the distal tibia (plafond, medial and posterior malleolus), fibula, and talar dome should be identified.
3. *Cartilage:* Examine for congruence of the entire joint space from medial to lateral.
4. *Soft tissue:* Note the close proximity of the overlying skin line to the underlying malleoli.

Normal Anatomy (Figure 1.36B)

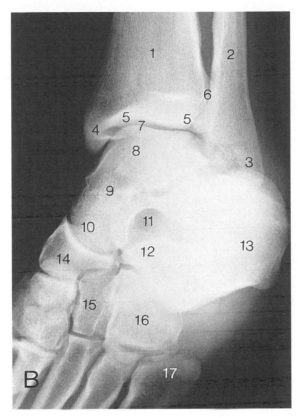

Figure 1.36.   B. Radiograph, Medlal Oblique Ankle.

1. Tibia.
2. Fibula.
3. Lateral malleolus, fibula.
4. Medial malleolus, tibia.
5. Plafond of the tibia.
6. Lateral surface of the tibia.
7. Posterior malleolus.
8. Body of the talus.
9. Neck of the talus.
10. Head of the talus.
11. Sinus tarsi (sulcus calcanei).
12. Anterior tubercle, calcaneus.
13. Calcaneus.
14. Navicular.
15. Lateral cuneiform.
16. Cuboid.
17. Fifth metatarsal base.

BASIC
Anteroposterior
*Medial oblique
Lateral

ANKLE
Medial Oblique Projection

OPTIONAL
Stress views

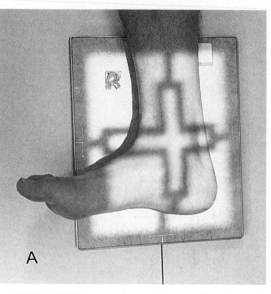

Figure 1.37. LATERAL ANKLE. A. Patient Position, Collimation and Central Ray.

ANKLE
Lateral Projection

Demonstrates: Distal tibia and fibula, ankle joint talus, and calcaneus. (1–3,7,8)
Measure: Transversely through the malleoli.
kVp: 55 (50 to 60).
Film Size: 8 × 10 inches (18 × 24 cm).
Grid: No.
TFD: 40 inches (102 cm).
Tube Tilt: None.
Patient Position: Lateral recumbent.
Part Position: The lateral surface of the ankle is in contact with the film, with the foot slightly dorsiflexed. Cross the opposite leg over the leg being examined, and support the opposite knee to avoid rotation of the ankle.
CR: Directed to the medial malleolus. Center film to the central ray.
Collimation: 8 × 10 inch field.

Side Marker: Place appropriate marker in film corner.
Clinicoradiologic Correlations: The posterior tibial lip is a frequent site of fracture and can be best demonstrated in an off-lateral projection, with slight external rotation of the foot. (8)

1. *Alignment:* Note the position of the tibia on the talus.
2. *Bone:* Trace the outlines of individual bones noting their individual named parts.
3. *Cartilage:* Isolate the tibiotalar, talocalcaneal, and talonavicular joints.
4. *Soft tissue:* Posterior to the tibia there is a triangular radiolucent region of the pre-Achilles fat-pad. At the talotibial anterior joint margin a small fat-pad can occasionally be located. Note the thickness of the skin overlying the calcaneus posteriorly and on the plantar surface.

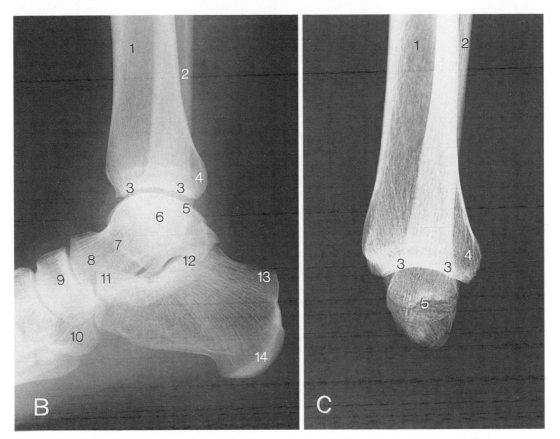

Figure 1.37.   B. Radiograph, Lateral Ankle. C. Specimen Radiograph, Distal Tibia and Fibula.

1. Tibia.
2. Fibula.
3. Plafond of the tibia.
4. Posterior malleolus, tibia.
5. Lateral malleolus, fibula.
6. Talar dome.
7. Neck of talus.
8. Head of talus.
9. Navicular.
10. Cuboid.
11. Anterior tubercle, calcaneus.
12. Middle tubercle, calcaneus.
13. Posterior tubercle, calcaneus.
14. Posterior surface, calcaneus.

BASIC
Anteroposterior
Medial oblique
*Lateral

ANKLE
Lateral Projection

OPTIONAL
Stress views

BASIC
*Dorsiplantar
Medial oblique
Lateral

FOOT
Dorsiplantar Projection

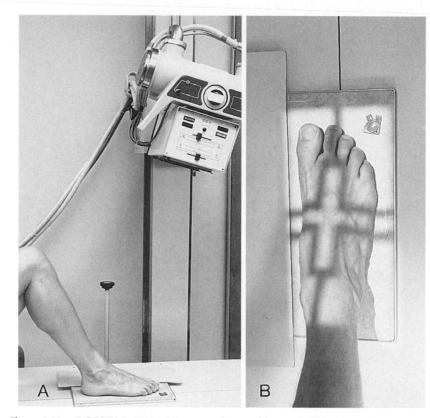

Figure 1.38.   DORSIPLANTAR FOOT. A. Patient Position. B. Collimation and Central Ray.

Demonstrates: Phalanges, metatarsals, cuneiforms, cuboid, and navicular. (1–5)

Measure: Through the tarsometatarsal junction at the base of the third metatarsal.

kVp: 55 (50 to 60).

Film Size: 10 × 12 inches (24 × 30 cm). Divide in half lengthwise.

Grid: No.

TFD: 40 inches (102 cm) (must correct for tube tilt).

Tube Tilt: 10° cephalad.

Patient Position: Supine, with knee flexed, or standing.

Part Position: The knee is flexed so that the plantar surface of the foot is resting on the film.

CR: Centered to base of third metatarsal. Center film to the central ray.

Collimation: 5 × 12 inch exposure field.

Side Marker: Place appropriate marker in corner of film.

Clinicoradiologic Correlations: A compensating filter can be used to prevent overexposure of the metatarsal heads and toes, filtering from the midshaft of the metatarsals dis-

tally. Tube tilt improves visualization of the intertarsal and tarsometatarsal articulations. Weight-bearing views of the foot may have some biomechanical value.

1. *Alignment:* A number of relationships can be assessed: (a) Hallux abductus angle—the angle between the shafts of the first metatarsal and proximal phalanx (0 to 15°). (b) Intermetatarsal angle—angle between the first and second metatarsal shafts (14°). (c) Metatarsal angle—tangential lines drawn along the articular surfaces of the first to second and fifth to second metatarsal heads (140°). (6)
2. *Bone:* All bones displayed should be identified. Note that there are only two phalanges at the first ray, which also has two sesamoid bones on the plantar surface of the first metatarsal head.
3. *Cartilage:* Identify all joints and note the width of the joint cavity and the smooth articular surfaces. The articulations of the cuneiforms and cuboid are often not well seen on this view.

Normal Anatomy (Figure 1.38C and D)

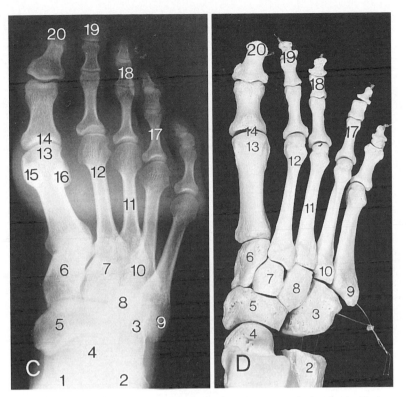

Figure 1.38.   C. Radiograph, Dorsiplantar Foot. D. Anatomic Specimen, Foot.

BASIC
*Dorsiplantar
Medial oblique
Lateral

FOOT
Dorsiplantar Projection

1.   Medial malleolus, tibia.
2.   Calcaneus.
3.   Cuboid.
4.   Head of talus.
5.   Navicular.
6.   First cuneiform (medial).
7.   Second cuneiform (intermediate).
8.   Third cuneiform (lateral).
9.   Base of fifth metatarsal (styloid process).
10.   Base of fourth metatarsal.

11.   Shaft of third metatarsal.
12.   Neck of second metatarsal.
13.   Head of first metatarsal.
14.   First metatarsal phalangeal articulation.
15.   Medial sesamoid in tendon of flexor hallucis brevis.
16.   Lateral sesamoid in tendon of flexor hallucis brevis.
17.   Proximal phalanx of the fourth toe.
18.   Middle phalanx of the third toe.
19.   Distal phalanx of the second toe.
20.   Distal ungual tuft of the first toe.

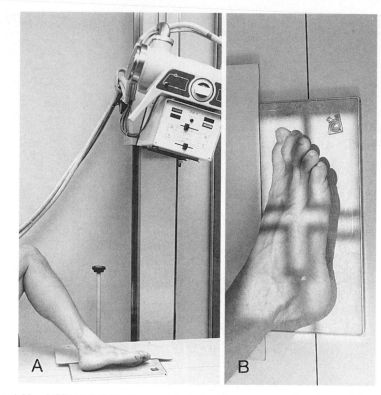

Figure 1.39. MEDIAL OBLIQUE FOOT. A. Patient Position. B. Collimation and Central Ray.

BASIC
Dorsiplantar
*Medial oblique
Lateral

FOOT
Medial Oblique Projection

Demonstrates: Phalanges, metatarsals, cuboid, third cuneiform, navicular, and distal calcaneus. (1–7)
Measure: Tarsometatarsal junction at the base of the third metatarsal.
kVp: 55 (50 to 60).
Film Size: 10 × 12 inches (24 × 30 cm). Divide in half lengthwise.
Grid: No.
TFD: 40 inches (102 cm).
Tube Tilt: 10° cephalad.
Patient Position: Supine, with knee flexed, or standing.
Part Position: Begin with the knee flexed so that the foot rests flat on the film. The leg is rotated medially so that the plantar surface of the foot forms an angle of approximately 35° with the plane of the film, the fifth digit being elevated from the film surface.
CR: Center to the base of the third metatarsal. Center film to the central ray.
Collimation: 5 × 12 inch field size.
Side Marker: Place appropriate marker in film corner.
Clinicoradiologic Correlations: This view adds to the dorsiplantar view specifically in rotating the metatarsals to show a different surface and separates out the intertarsal joints.

Normal Anatomy (Figure 1.39C and D)

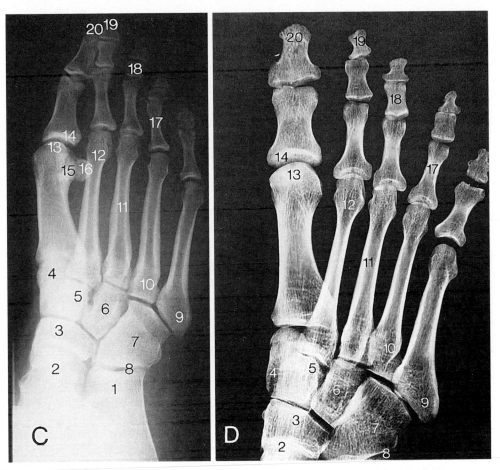

Figure 1.39. C. Radiograph, Medial Oblique Foot. D. Anatomic Specimen, Foot.

1. Calcaneus.
2. Head of talus.
3. Navicular.
4. First cuneiform (medial).
5. Second cuneiform (intermediate).
6. Third cuneiform (lateral).
7. Cuboid.
8. Calcaneocuboid joint.
9. Base of fifth metatarsal (styloid process).
10. Base of fourth metatarsal.
11. Shaft of third metatarsal.
12. Neck of second metatarsal.
13. Head of first metatarsal.
14. First metatarsal phalangeal articulation.
15. Bipartite medial sesamoid in tendon of flexor hallucis brevis.
16. Lateral sesamoid in tendon of flexor hallucis brevis.
17. Proximal phalanx of the fourth toe.
18. Middle phalanx of the third toe.
19. Distal phalanx of the second toe.
20. Distal ungual tuft of the first toe.

BASIC
Dorsiplantar
Medial Oblique
Lateral

FOOT
Medial Oblique Projection

Positioning (Figure 1.40A and B)

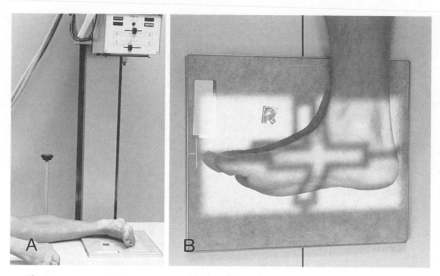

Figure 1.40. LATERAL FOOT. A. Patient Position. B. Collimation and Central Ray.

Demonstrates: Distal tibia and fibula, tarsals, ankle joint, metatarsals, and phalanges. (1–5)

Measure: Navicular to fifth metatarsal.

kVp: 55 (50 to 60).

Film Size: 8 × 10 inches (18 × 24 cm), or 10 × 12 inches (24 × 30 cm) for large feet.

Grid: No.

TFD: 40 inches (102 cm).

Tube Tilt: None.

Patient Position: Lateral recumbent or standing.

Part Position: Cross the unaffected leg over and forward for patient stability. The affected foot is placed in true lateral projection, with the fifth metatarsal in contact with the film. The plantar surface should be perpendicular to the film.

CR: At the navicular.

Collimation: To the film.

Side Marker: Place appropriate marker in film corner.

Clinicoradiologic Correlations: Weight-bearing views of the feet may have some biomechanical value for assessing the longitudinal arch.

1. *Alignment:* Angles can be assessed (calcaneus; Boehler's). (5)
2. *Bone:* The calcaneus, cuboid, and fifth metatarsal are clearly shown in profile.
3. *Cartilage:* Many joint details are obscured in this view. Trace each individual bone and identify its articulations.
4. *Soft tissue:* The pre-Achilles fat- and heel-pads can be identified.

Normal Anatomy (Figure 1.40C)

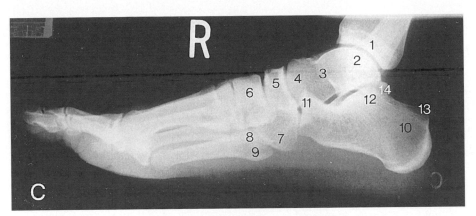

Figure 1.40.   C. Radiograph, Lateral Foot.

1. Tibia.
2. Dome of talus.
3. Neck of talus.
4. Head of talus.
5. Navicular.
6. Cuneiforms (superimposed on each other).
7. Cuboid.
8. Base of fifth metatarsal.
9. Styloid process, fifth metatarsal.
10. Calcaneus.
11. Anterior tubercle, calcaneus.
12. Middle tubercle, calcaneus.
13. Posterior tubercle, calcaneus.
14. Os trigonum.

BASIC
Dorsiplantar
Medial oblique
Lateral

FOOT
Lateral Projection

BASIC
*Dorsiplantar
Oblique

TOES
Dorsiplantar Projection

OPTIONAL
Axial (sesamoids)

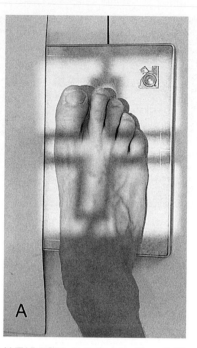

Figure 1.41.   DORSIPLANTAR TOES. A. Patient Position, Collimation and Central Ray.

Demonstrates: Phalanges, distal metatarsals, and interphalangeal and metatarsophalangeal joints. (1–4)

Measure: At the proximal interphalangeal joints. For the great toe, at the interphalangeal joint.

kVp: 55 (50 to 60).

Film Size: 8 × 10 inches (18 × 24 cm) divided into halves; the other half is used for the oblique.

Grid: No.

TFD: 40 inches (102 cm).

Tube Tilt: None.

Patient Position: Supine or sitting on the table top.

Part Position: The knee is flexed so the foot is placed flat on the film.

CR: At the proximal interphalangeal joint.

Collimation: If a general evaluation of the toes is required, all of the toes should be exposed. If a specific toe is being evaluated, then appropriate collimation should be performed.

Side Marker: Appropriate marker in film corner.

Clinicoradiologic Correlations: These structures are best evaluated on a separate film from the foot to ensure improved exposure and detail. If a selected toe is involved, it should be radiographed in sequential "around the clock" views (AP, PA, oblique, and lateral).

1. *Alignment:* Note any deviation of the digits (flexion, axial). A common variant is fusion of the fifth distal interphalangeal joint.
2. *Bone:* Each phalanx is examined noting their diaphyseal constriction, expanded articular ends and ungual tuft.
3. *Cartilage:* Because of flexion of the digits all phalangeal joints may not be observed. Note how the metatarsophalangeal joints have relatively wide joint spaces.
4. *Soft tissue:* Carefully follow the skin outlines of each digit.

Normal Anatomy (Figure 1.41B and C)

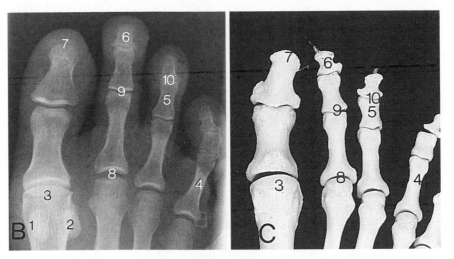

Figure 1.41.   B. Radiograph, Dorsiplantar Toes. C. Anatomic Specimen, Toes.

1. Medial sesamoid bone in tendon of flexor hallucis brevis.
2. Lateral sesamoid bone in tendon of flexor hallucis brevis.
3. First metatarsal head.
4. Proximal phalanx, fourth toe.
5. Middle phalanx, third toe.

6. Distal phalanx, second toe.
7. Distal ungual tuft, first toe.
8. Metatarsal phalangeal joint, second toe.
9. Interphalangeal joint.
10. Distal interphalangeal joint, third toe.

BASIC
*Dorsiplantar
Oblique

TOES
Dorsiplantar Projection

OPTIONAL
Axial (sesamoids)

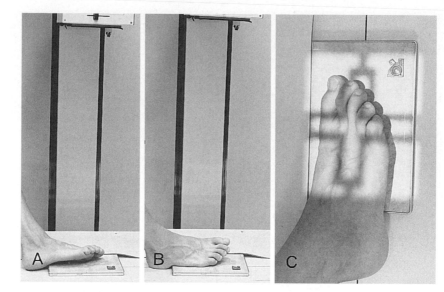

Figure 1.42.   OBLIQUE TOES. A. Patient Position, Toes 1-3. B. Patient Position, Toes 4 and 5. C. Collimation and Central Ray.

TOES
Oblique Projection

Demonstrates: Phalanges, distal metatarsals, and interphalangeal and metatarsophalangeal joints. (1–4)

Measure: At interphalangeal joints.

kVp: 55 (50 to 60).

Film Size: 8 × 10 inches (18 × 24 cm) divided into halves; the other half is used for the dorsiplantar view.

Grid: No.

TFD: 40 inches (102 cm).

Tube Tilt: None.

Patient Position: Supine or sitting on the tabletop.

Part Position: The knee is flexed so the foot is placed flat on the film. (a) *Toes 1, 2, and 3.* Elevate the fifth metatarsal region so the foot forms a 45° angle with the film. (Fig. 1.42A) (b) *Toes 4 and 5.* Elevate the great toe region so the foot forms a 45° angle with the film. (Fig. 1.42B)

CR: At the proximal interphalangeal joint.

Collimation: If a general evaluation of the toes is required, all of the toes should be exposed. If a specific toe is being evaluated, then appropriate collimation should be performed.

Side Marker: Appropriate marker in film corner.

Clinicoradiologic Correlations: These structures are best evaluated on a separate film from the foot to ensure improved exposure and detail. If a selected toe is involved, it should be radiographed in sequential "around the clock" views (AP, PA, oblique, and lateral).

1. *Alignment:* Note any deviation of the digits (flexion, axial). A common variant is fusion of the fifth distal interphalangeal joint.
2. *Bone:* Each phalanx is examined noting their diaphyseal constriction, expanded articular ends and ungual tuft. The hallux sesamoids are often seen in profile though are best shown on an axial projection. (4)
3. *Cartilage:* Because of flexion of the digits all phalangeal joints may not be observed. Note how the metatarsophalangeal joints have relatively wide joint spaces.
4. *Soft tissue:* Carefully follow the skin outlines of each digit.

Normal Anatomy (Figure 1.42D and E)

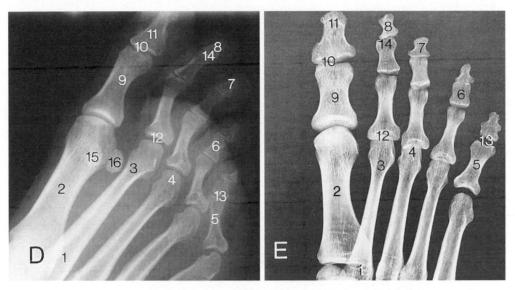

Figure 1.42.   D. Radiograph, Oblique Toes. E. Specimen Radiograph, Toes.

1. Base of second metatarsal.
2. Shaft of first metatarsal.
3. Neck of second metatarsal.
4. Head of third metatarsal.
5. Proximal phalanx, fifth toe.
6. Middle phalanx, fourth toe.
7. Distal phalanx, third toe.
8. Distal tuft (ungual), second toe.
9. Proximal phalanx, first toe.
10. Interphalangeal joint, first toe.
11. Distal phalanx, first toe.
12. Metatarsal phalangeal articulation, second toe.
13. Proximal interphalangeal joint, fifth toe.
14. Distal interphalangeal joint, second toe.
15. Medial sesamoid bone in the tendon of flexor hallucis brevis.
16. Lateral sesamoid bone in the tendon of flexor hallucis brevis.

BASIC
Dorsiplantar
*Oblique

TOES
Oblique Projection

OPTIONAL
Axial (sesamoids)

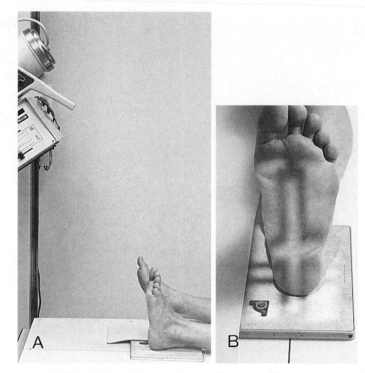

Figure 1.43.   AXIAL CALCANEUS. A. Patient Position. B. Collimation and Central Ray.

Demonstrates: Calcaneus. (1,2)
Measure: Through the central ray.
kVp: 55 (50 to 60).
Film Size: 8 × 10 inches (18 × 24 cm) divided into halves; the other half is used for the lateral projection.
Grid: No.
TFD: 40 inches (102 cm) (must correct for tube tilt).
Tube Tilt: 35 to 40° cephalad.
Patient Position: Supine, with legs extended.
Part Position: Foot is dorsiflexed such that the plantar surface is perpendicular to the film.

CR: 2 inches up from the back of the heel.
Collimation: To the size of the calcaneus (approximately 5 × 5 inches).
Side Marker: Appropriate side marker in film corner.
Clinicoradiologic Correlations: A looped strap can be placed around the ball of the foot and grasped by the patient, to maintain dorsiflexion of the foot. Specific views of the calcaneus are required for proper evaluation. The axial view depicts the body and its posterior aspect.

Normal Anatomy (Figure 1.43C and D)

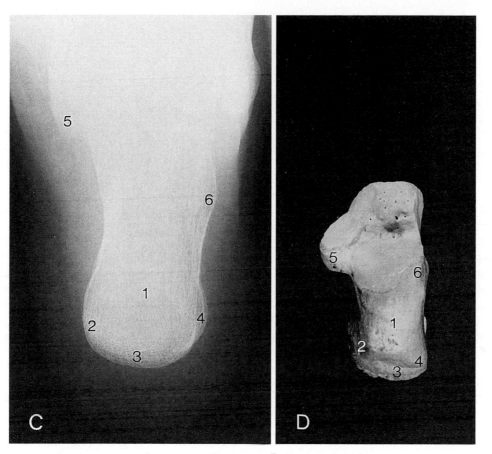

Figure 1.43.   C. Radiograph, Axial Calcaneus. D. Anatomic Specimen, Calcaneus.

1. Calcaneus.
2. Medial process, calcaneus.
3. Tuberosity, calcaneus.

4. Lateral process, calcaneus.
5. Sustentaculum tali, calcaneus.
6. Trochlear process, calcaneus.

Positioning (Figure 1.44A)

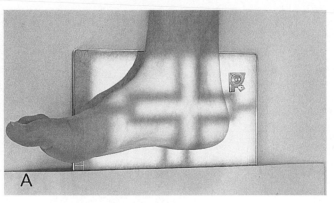

Figure 1.44.   LATERAL CALCANEUS. A. Patient Position, Collimation and Central Ray.

Demonstrates: Calcaneus, talus, subtalar joints, and Achilles tendon. (1,2)
Measure: At the CR.
kVp: 55 (50 to 60).
Film Size: 8 × 10 inches (18 × 24 cm) divided into halves; the other half is used for the axial projection.
Grid: No.
TFD: 40 inches (102 cm).
Tube Tilt: None.
Patient Position: Lateral recumbent.
Part Position: The unaffected leg is crossed over and anterior for patient stability. The lateral side of the foot contacts the film, with the plantar surface perpendicular to the film.
CR: Midcalcaneus (1 1/2 inches up from the plantar surface of the heel and 2 inches from the posterior surface of the heel).

Collimation: To the calcaneus size (5 × 5 inches).
Side Marker: Appropriate side marker in film corner.
Clinicoradiologic Correlations: The calcaneus and its articulations in this projection are seen optimally.

1. *Alignment:* Boehler's angle should be carefully measured.
2. *Bone:* All bones and their components should be identified.
3. *Cartilage:* The tibiotalar, talocalcaneal (subtalar), talonavicular, and calcaneocuboid joints should be isolated, their joint spaces defined, and their smooth surfaces noted. The subtalar joint is usually partially obscured in its midportion.
4. *Soft tissue:* The pre-Achilles fat- and heel-pads can be identified.

Normal Anatomy (Figure 1.44B and C)

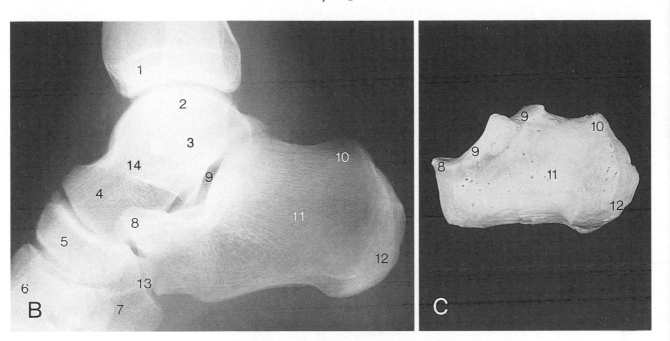

Figure 1.44.   B. Radiograph, Lateral Calcaneus. C. Anatomic Specimen, Calcaneus.

1. Tibia.
2. Dome of the talus.
3. Body of the talus.
4. Head of the talus.
5. Navicular.
6. Cuneiforms (superimposed on each other).
7. Cuboid.

8. Anterior tuberosity of the calcaneus.
9. Subtalar joint.
10. Posterior tuberosity of the calcaneus.
11. Calcaneus.
12. Posterior surface of the calcaneus.
13. Calcaneocuboid Joint.
14. Neck of the talus.

BASIC
*Internal rotation
External rotation
Abduction (baby arm)

SHOULDER
Anteroposterior Internal Rotation Projection

OPTIONAL
Transaxial

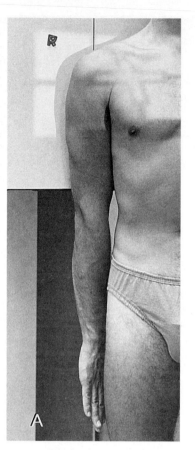

Figure 1.45. ANTEROPOSTERIOR INTERNAL ROTATION, SHOULDER. A. Patient Position, Collimation and Central Ray.

Demonstrates: Proximal humerus, scapula, clavicle, rib cage, and lung. (1–6)
Measure: Between the coracoid process and scapula.
kVp: 75 (70 to 80).
Film Size: 10 × 12 inches (24 × 30 cm) vertical.
Grid: Yes.
TFD: 40 inches (102 cm).
Tube Tilt: None.
Patient Position: Upright or supine.
Part Position: The patient is rotated to be at 30° to the bucky. The coracoid is centered to the bucky and the arm internally rotated until the elbow epicondyles are perpendicular to the film.
CR: Through the coracoid process.
Collimation: To film size.
Side Marker: Appropriate marker placed at film corner above humeral head.
Breathing Instructions: Suspended expiration.
Clinicoradiologic Correlations: If the trunk is not rotated, a clear view of the glenohumeral joint will not be obtained.

A comfortable positioning alternative for the patient with an acute shoulder is to allow 90° of elbow flexion, then rest the forearm against the abdomen.

1. *Alignment:* Check that there is a smooth transition from the medial humerus across the glenoid fossa to the axillary border of the scapula. Also note the alignment across the acromioclavicular joint and the acromiohumeral distance.
2. *Bone:* Specifically outline the greater and lesser tuberosities.
3. *Cartilage:* The joint space of the glenohumeral articulation may not be clearly seen, but the anterior cavity can usually be discerned. Note the acromioclavicular joint for the depth of the space and the usually smooth articular margins.
4. *Soft tissue:* Carefully look around the greater tuberosity for evidence of abnormal soft tissue calcification. Screen the lung fields for any abnormal mass.

Normal Anatomy (Figure 1.45B and C)

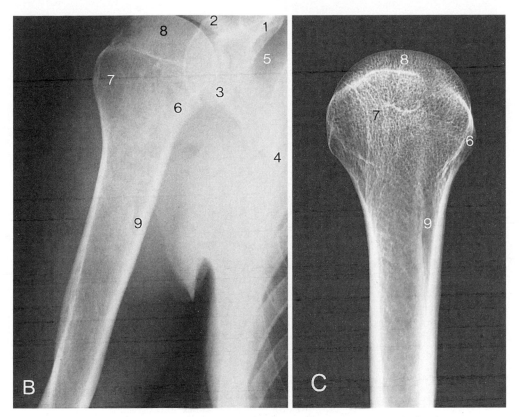

Figure 1.45. B. Shoulder Radiograph, Anteroposterior Internal Rotation. C. Anatomic Specimen, Humerus.

1. Coracoid process, scapula.
2. Acromion, scapula.
3. Glenoid fossa.
4. Axillary border, scapula.
5. Subscapular fossa.

6. Lesser tuberosity, humerus.
7. Greater tuberosity, humerus.
8. Humeral head.
9. Pectoralis groove.

BASIC
*Internal rotation
External rotation
Abduction (baby arm)

SHOULDER
Anteroposterior Internal Rotation Projection

OPTIONAL
Transaxial

BASIC
Internal rotation
External rotation
Abduction

SHOULDER
Anteroposterior External Rotation Projection

OPTIONAL
Transaxial

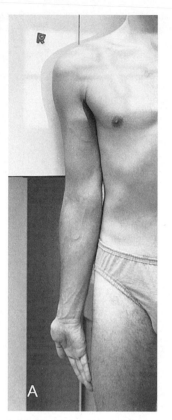

Figure 1.46.   ANTEROPOSTERIOR EXTERNAL ROTATION, SHOULDER. A. Patient Position, Collimation and Central Ray.

Demonstrates: Proximal humerus (especially the greater tuberosity), scapula, clavicle, rib cage, and lung. (1–6)
Measure: Between the coracoid process and scapula.
kVp: 75 (70 to 80).
Film size: 10 × 12 (24 × 30 cm) vertical.
Grid: Yes.
TFD: 40 inches (102 cm).
Tube Tilt: None.
Patient Position: Upright or supine.
Part Position: The patient is rotated to be at 30° to the bucky. The coracoid is centered to the bucky and the arm externally rotated until the elbow epicondyles are parallel to the film.
CR: To the coracoid process.
Collimation: To film size.
Side Marker: Appropriate marker placed at film corner above humeral head.
Breathing Instructions: Suspended expiration.
Clinicoradiologic Correlations: This is an especially useful view to demonstrate calcific tendinitis and fractures of the greater tuberosity. (7) Greater external rotation may be assured by allowing 90° of elbow flexion, with the patient maximally externally rotating the forearm.

1. *Alignment:* Check that there is a smooth transition from the medial humerus across the glenoid fossa to the axillary border of the scapula. Also note the alignment across the acromioclavicular joint and the acromiohumeral distance. Elevation of the humerus within the glenoid is a sign of rotator cuff tendon tear.
2. *Bone:* Specifically outline the greater tuberosity, which is shown in profile.
3. *Cartilage:* The joint space of the glenohumeral articulation may not be clearly seen, but the anterior cavity can usually be discerned. Note the acromioclavicular joint for the depth of the space and the usually smooth articular margins.
4. *Soft tissue:* Carefully look around the greater tuberosity for evidence of abnormal soft tissue calcification. Screen the lung fields for any abnormal mass. (Fig. 1.46C)

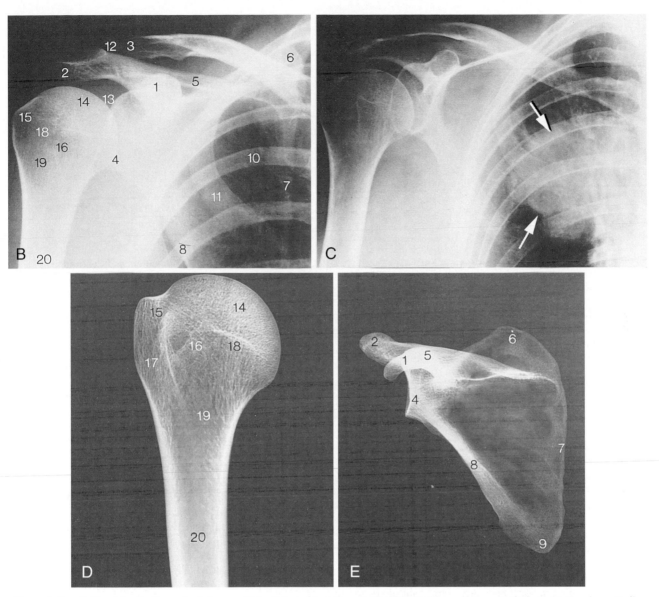

Figure 1.46.   B. Shoulder Radiograph, Anteroposterior External Rotation. C. Shoulder Radiograph, Lung Pathology. D. Specimen Radiograph Humerus. E. Specimen Radiograph Scapula. COMMENT: This case demonstrates why at least in one view of the shoulder the lung field should be included and screened for a mass (arrows). (Courtesy of Robert L. Wohlert, DC, Iowa Falls, Iowa)

1. Coracoid process, scapula.
2. Acromion, scapula.
3. Distal clavicle.
4. Glenoid fossa.
5. Spine of scapula.
6. Superior angle, scapula.
7. Vertebral border, scapula.
8. Axillary border, scapula.
9. Inferior angle, scapula.
10. Posterior rib.
11. Anterior rib.
12. Acromioclavicular joint.
13. Glenohumeral articulation.
14. Humeral head.
15. Greater tuberosity, humerus.
16. Lesser tuberosity, humerus.
17. Intertubercular groove, humerus.
18. Anatomical neck, humerus.
19. Surgical neck, humerus.
20. Shaft of the humerus.

BASIC
Internal rotation
*External rotation
Abduction

SHOULDER
Anteroposterior External Rotation Projection

OPTIONAL
Transaxial

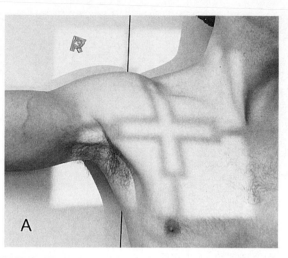

Figure 1.47. ANTEROPOSTERIOR ABDUCTION VIEW, SHOULDER. A. Patient Position, Collimation, and Central Ray.

Demonstrates: Proximal humerus, scapula (especially the coracoid and acromion), acromioclavicular joint, upper rib cage, clavicle, and lung apex. (1–5)

Measure: Between Coracoid process + scapula.

kVp: 75 (70 to 80).

Film size: 10 × 12 inches (24 × 30 cm) horizontal.

Grid: Yes.

TFD: 40 inches (102 cm).

Tube Tilt: None.

Patient Position: Upright or spine.

Part Position: The patient's back is flat to the bucky. The arm is abducted to 90°, the elbow flexed to 90°, the palm of the hand faces the x-ray tube.

CR: At the midclavicular line at the level of the coracoid process.

Collimation: To film size.

Side Marker: Appropriate side marker at film corner above humerus.

Breathing Instructions: Suspended expiration.

Clinicoradiologic Correlations: An attempt should be made to include the upper thorax to the spine. Attention should be directed to the lung apex to rule out pulmonary pathology and to the C7 vertebra to rule out a cervical rib on the resulting radiograph.

1. *Alignment:* Check that there is a smooth transition from the medial humerus across the glenoid fossa to the axillary border of the scapula. Also note the alignment across the acromioclavicular joint and the acromiohumeral distance. Elevation of the humerus within the glenoid is a sign of rotator cuff tendon tear, which is accentuated in this view greater than any other projection. (8)

2. *Bone:* Specifically outline the greater tuberosity, which is shown in profile.

3. *Cartilage:* The joint space of the glenohumeral articulation may not be clearly seen, but the anterior cavity can usually be discerned. Note the acromioclavicular joint for the depth of the space and the usually smooth articular margins.

4. *Soft tissue:* Carefully look around the greater tuberosity for evidence of abnormal soft tissue calcification. Screen the lung fields for any abnormal mass. (Fig. 1.46C)

BASIC
Internal rotation
External rotation
Abduction (baby arm)

SHOULDER
Abduction (Baby Arm) Projection

OPTIONAL
Transaxial

Normal Anatomy (Figure 1.47B)

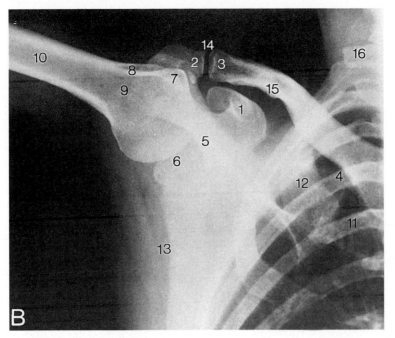

Figure 1.47.   B. Radiograph, Abduction View, ("Baby Arm") Shoulder.

1. Coracoid process, scapula.
2. Acromion, scapula.
3. Distal clavicle.
4. Superior angle, scapula.
5. Spine of scapula.
6. Glenoid fossa.
7. Greater and lesser tuberosities superimposed.
8. Intertubercular groove, humerus.

9. Surgical neck, humerus.
10. Shaft, humerus.
11. Posterior rib.
12. Anterior rib.
13. Axillary border, scapula.
14. Acromioclavicular joint.
15. Conoid tubercle, clavicle.
16. Transverse process, T1.

BASIC
Internal rotation
External rotation
*Abduction (baby arm)

SHOULDER
Abduction (Baby Arm) Projection

OPTIONAL
Transaxial

BASIC
Anteroposterior
(cephalad angulation)
Posteroanterior
(caudad angulation)

CLAVICLE
Posteroanterior Projection

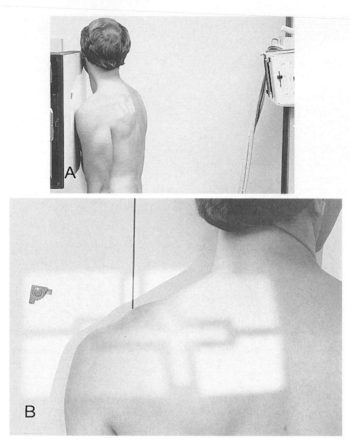

Figure 1.48.   POSTEROANTERIOR VIEW, CLAVICLE. A. Patient Position. B. Collimation and Central Ray.

Demonstrates: Clavicle, upper ribs, scapula, and lung. (1–3)

Measure: At coracoid process.

kVp: 70 (65 to 75).

Film Size: 10 × 12 inches (24 × 30 cm).

Grid: Yes.

TFD: 40 inches (102 cm) (must correct for tube tilt).

Tube Tilt: (a) *Posteroanterior:* 10° caudad. (b) *Anteroposterior:* 10° cephalad.

Patient Position: Upright.

Part Position: (a) *Posteroanterior:* Facing the bucky, with no body rotation, but the head is turned away from the side being evaluated. Midpoint of the clavicle is centered to the midline of the bucky. (b) *Anteroposterior:* Facing the tube, with no body rotation. Midpoint of the clavicle is centered to the midline of the bucky.

CR: (a) *Posteroanterior:* Through the midclavicle and 1 inch above the level of the clavicle at the patient's back. (b) *Anteroposterior:* Through the midclavicle.

Collimation: Top to bottom, 8 inches; side to side, 12 inches.

Side Marker: Appropriate marker above the humeral head.

Breathing Instructions: Suspended expiration.

Clinicoradiologic Correlations: The posteroanterior projection is preferred for anatomic detail and in kyphotic patients.

1. *Alignment:* Observe the position of the clavicle with the acromion and sternum, as well as the acromiohumeral and coracoclavicular spaces.
2. *Bone:* Trace and identify all bony components depicted.
3. *Cartilage:* The sternoclavicular, acromioclavicular, glenohumeral, and costal joints can all be identified.
4. *Soft tissue:* Note the skin line of the trapezius muscle. A thin, soft tissue line following the superior surface of the clavicle is usually visible ("companion shadow").

Normal Anatomy (Figure 1.48C and D)

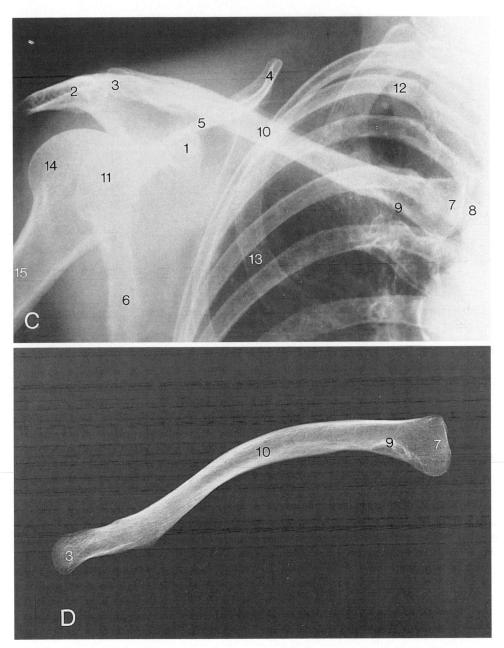

BASIC
Anteroposterior
(cephalad angulation)
*Posteroanterior
(caudad angulation)

CLAVICLE
Posteroanterior Projection

Figure 1.48.   C. Radiograph, Posteroanterior Clavicle. D. Specimen Radiograph, Clavicle.

1. Coracoid process, scapula.
2. Acromion, scapula.
3. Distal clavicle.
4. Superior angle, scapula.
5. Superior border, scapula.
6. Axillary border, scapula.
7. Medial clavicle.
8. Sternoclavicular joint.

9. Rhomboid fossa.
10. Midportion, clavicle.
11. Glenoid fossa.
12. Posterior rib.
13. Anterior rib.
14. Humeral head.
15. Shaft of the humerus.

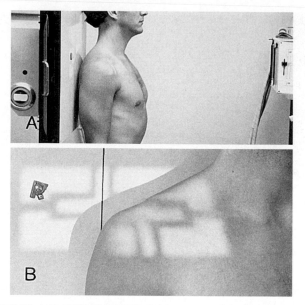

Figure 1.49. ANTEROPOSTERIOR, ACROMIOCLAVICULAR JOINT. A. Patient Position. B. Collimation and Central Ray.

Demonstrates: Distal clavicle and acromioclavicular joint. (1–3)

Measure: At the coracoid process; use half the mAs as calculated from the shoulder exposure factors.

kVp: 70 (65 to 75).

Film Size: 8 × 10 inches (18 × 24 cm) horizontal.

Grid: Yes.

TFD: 40 inches (102 cm) (must correct for tube tilt).

Tube Tilt: 5° cephalad.

Patient Position: Upright.

Part Position: Anteroposterior position, with no body rotation and the acromioclavicular joint centered to the bucky. The same position is done with and without the patient holding 10 to 15-pound weights. (4)

CR: Through the acromioclavicular joint.

Collimation: To the film.

Side Marker: Appropriate marker placed in upper film corner above the humeral head.

Breathing Instructions: Suspended expiration.

Clinicoradiologic Correlations: The purpose of comparing non-weight-bearing and weight-bearing views is to attempt to assess the integrity of the acromioclavicular and costoclavicular ligaments. (5–6) Bilateral anteroposterior comparison in a single exposure is discouraged, unless appropriate shielding of the thyroid is utilized.

1. *Alignment:* There should be a smooth transition across the acromioclavicular joint with the distal clavicle aligned with the acromion.
2. *Bone:* Carefully scrutinize the length of the clavicle noting the normal curved contour of the bone and the fluctuations in cortical thickness and bone density distally.
3. *Cartilage:* The acromioclavicular joint space is variable in depth, sometimes being capacious in young patients. The distal clavicular surface is often noticeably concave. (5)
4. *Soft tissue:* The lung apex should be checked bilaterally for aeration and symmetry.

Normal Anatomy (Figure 1.49C)

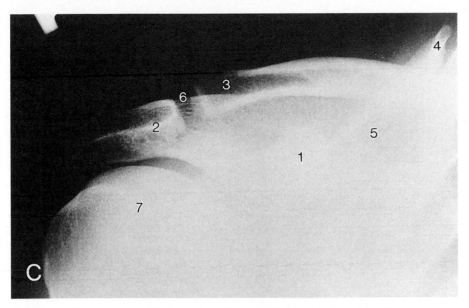

Figure 1.49.   C. Radiograph, Anteroposterior Acromioclavicular Joint.

1. Coracoid process, scapula.
2. Acromion, scapula.
3. Distal clavicle.
4. Superior angle, scapula.

5. Superior border, scapula.
6. Acromioclavicular joint.
7. Humeral head.

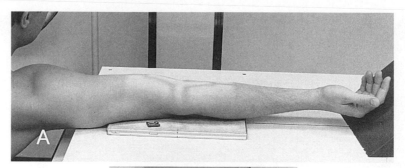

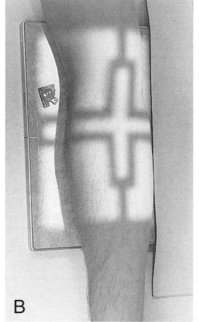

Figure 1.50.   ANTEROPOSTERIOR, ELBOW. A. Patient Position. B. Collimation and Central Ray.

Demonstrates: Distal humerus, proximal ulna, proximal radius, and elbow joint. (1–3)

Measure: Anteroposterior through the elbow at the epicondyles.

kVp: 55 (50 to 60).

Film Size: 10 × 12 inches (24 × 30 cm) divided in half; the other half used for the medial oblique projection.

Grid: No.

TFD: 40 inches (102 cm).

Tube Tilt: None.

Patient Position: Seated, with body rotated away from the table.

Part Position: Arm fully extended, and the hand supinated. If the elbow cannot be extended, two APs are done, one with the forearm on the film and the second with the humerus on the film.

CR: To the elbow, between and 1 inch below the level of the epicondyles.

Collimation: To the arm.

Side Marker: Appropriate marker adjacent to the humerus at the film edge.

Clinicoradiologic Correlations: All three bones of the elbow are clearly visible. Because of the complexity of the joint, multiple views should be obtained. Lead vinyl must be placed beneath the cassette to reduce primary and secondary radiation to the patient.

1. *Alignment:* The axial relationships should be assessed. (See Chapter 2) Note that the radial head is aligned with the capitellum and that the olecranon lies within the olecranon fossa of the humerus.
2. *Bone:* Structural details and landmarks of all three bones need to be identified.
3. *Cartilage:* Note uniform joint space and the undulating surface contour of the joint containing the convex surface of the capitellum and more angular configuration of the trochlea.

BASIC
*Anteroposterior
Medial oblique
Lateral
Tangential

ELBOW
Anteroposterior Projection

OPTIONAL
Radial head

BASIC
*Anteroposterior
Medial oblique
Lateral
Tangential

ELBOW
Anteroposterior Projection

OPTIONAL
Radial head

Normal Anatomy (Figure 1.50C and D)

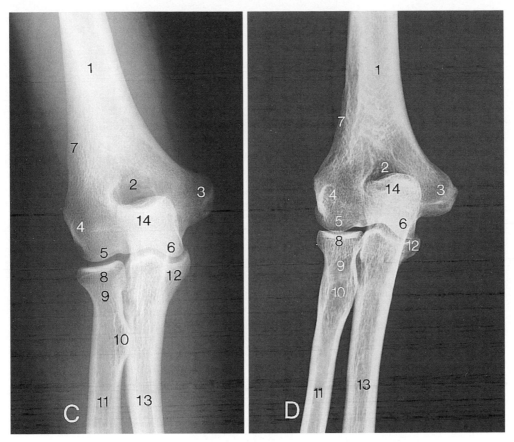

Figure 1.50.   C. Radiograph, Anteroposterior Elbow. D. Specimen Radiograph, Elbow.

1. Shaft of the humerus.
2. Olecranon fossa, ulna.
3. Medial epicondyle, humerus.
4. Lateral epicondyle, humerus.
5. Capitellum, humerus.
6. Trochlea, humerus.
7. Supracondylar ridge, humerus.
8. Radial head.
9. Neck of the radius.
10. Radial tuberosity.
11. Shaft of the radius.
12. Coronoid process, ulna.
13. Ulna.
14. Olecranon process, ulna.

ELBOW
Medial Oblique Projection

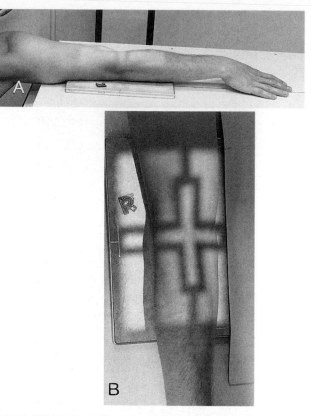

Figure 1.51. MEDIAL OBLIQUE, ELBOW. A. Patient Position. B. Collimation and Central Ray.

Demonstrates: Distal humerus, proximal ulna, proximal radius, and elbow joint. (1–3)

Measure: At the CR.

kVp: 55 (50 to 60).

Film Size: 10 × 12 inches (24 × 30 cm) divided in half; the other half is used for the anteroposterior projection.

Grid: No.

TFD: 40 inches (102 cm).

Tube Tilt: None.

Patient Position: Seated, with body rotated away from the table.

Part Position: Arm fully extended, and the forearm pronated.

CR: 1 inch below the epicondyles.

Collimation: To the arm.

Side Marker: Appropriate marker adjacent to the humerus at the film edge.

Clinicoradiologic Correlations: The elbow is projected in a different plane, which is especially useful for depicting the radial head, coronoid process of the ulna, and medial epicondyle. Lead vinyl must be placed beneath the cassette to reduce primary and secondary radiation to the patient.

1. *Alignment:* Note that the radial head is aligned with the capitellum and that the olecranon lies within the olecranon fossa of the humerus.
2. *Bone:* Structural details and landmarks of all three bones need to be identified.
3. *Cartilage:* The trochlea component of the joint is slightly better seen.

Normal Anatomy (Figure 1.51C)

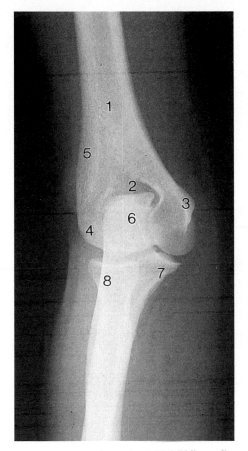

Figure 1.51. C. Radiograph, Medial Oblique Elbow.

1. Shaft of the humerus.
2. Olecranon fossa, humerus.
3. Medial epicondyle, humerus.
4. Lateral epicondyle, humerus.

5. Supracondylar ridge.
6. Olecranon process, ulna.
7. Coronoid process, ulna.
8. Radial head.

ELBOW
Lateral Projection

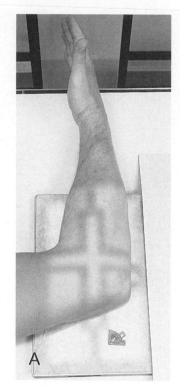

Figure 1.52.   LATERAL VIEW, ELBOW. A. Patient Position, Collimation and Central Ray.

Demonstrates: Distal humerus, proximal ulna, proximal radius, and elbow joint. (1–3)

Measure: At the CR.

kVp: 55 (50 to 60).

Film Size: 10 × 12 inches (24 × 30 cm) divided in half; the other half is used for the tangential projection.

Grid: No.

TFD: 40 inches (102 cm).

Tube Tilt: None.

Patient Position: Seated, with the body rotated away from the table.

Part Position: Elbow flexed to 90°, with the ulnar surface of the forearm flat on the film. The hand is in the true lateral position. The humerus must also be parallel to the film plane.

CR: Mid elbow joint, just anterior to the lateral epicondyle.

Collimation: To the arm, 10 inches along the forearm axis and 6 inches top to bottom.

Side Marker: Appropriate marker placed in the corner of the film adjacent to the olecranon.

Clinicoradiologic Correlations: This is a useful view in the evaluation of the posttraumatic elbow for fracture. A modified lateral view (radial head-capitellum view) with the tube angled 45° toward the radial head better depicts the radial head, capitellum and coronoid process. (4) Lead vinyl must be placed beneath the cassette to reduce primary and secondary radiation to the patient.

1. *Alignment:* The plane of the radius passes through the middle of the capitellum (radiocapitellar line). Note that the humeral condyles are slightly angled forward in relation to the plane of the humeral shaft.
2. *Bone:* Structural details and landmarks of all three bones need to be identified.
3. *Cartilage:* Identify the radiohumeral and humeroulnar articulations.
4. *Soft tissue:* Anterior and posterior to the distal humeral surfaces are pericapsular fat-pads which are normally imperceptible, though the anterior fat-pad can occasionally be just visible. If displaced away from the humerus because of hemarthrosis (positive fat-pad sign), then in up to 90% of cases an intraarticular fracture will be present, most commonly of the radial head. The supinator fat line can normally be identified close and parallel to the radius.

Normal Anatomy (Figure 1.52B and C)

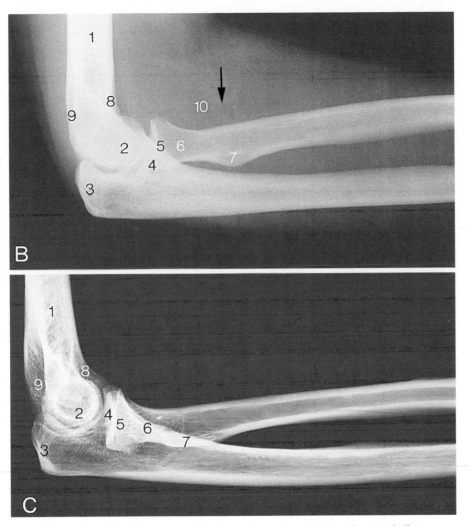

Figure 1.52.   B. Radiograph, Lateral Elbow. C. Specimen Radiograph, Lateral Elbow.

1.   Shaft of the humerus.
2.   Capitellum and trochlea superimposed.
3.   Olecranon process, ulna.
4.   Coronoid process, ulna.
5.   Radial head.

6.   Neck of the radius.
7.   Radial tuberosity.
8.   Coronoid fossa, humerus.
9.   Olecranon fossa, humerus.
10.   Supinator fat line (arrow).

ELBOW
Tangential (Jones) Projection

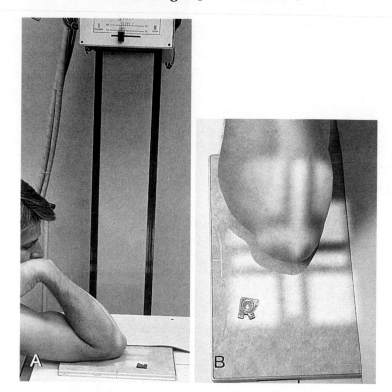

Figure 1.53.   TANGENTIAL, ELBOW. A. Patient Position. B. Collimation and Central Ray.

Demonstrates: Olecranon, ulnar groove, trochlea, and radial head. (1–3,5)

Measure: 2 inches above the olecranon tip.

kVp: 55 (50 to 60).

Film Size: 10 × 12 inches (24 × 30 cm) divided in half; the other half is used for the lateral projection.

Grid: No.

TFD: 40 inches (102 cm).

Tube Tilt: None.

Patient Position: Elbow is fully flexed and the humerus is placed parallel to the film.

CR: 2 inches above the olecranon tip.

Collimation: 6 × 6 inches.

Side Marker: Appropriate marker in film corner adjacent to the olecranon.

Clinicoradiologic Correlations: The selective visualization of the olecranon/trochlear joint compartment is useful in the detection of intraarticular loose bodies and degenerative osteophytes. The ulnar groove in which lies the ulnar nerve is also well seen. Lead vinyl must be placed beneath the cassette to reduce primary and secondary radiation to the patient.

1. *Alignment:* Assess the relationship of the olecranon with the humerus.
2. *Bone:* The articular surface of the humerus and olecranon process are best seen.
3. *Cartilage:* The olecranon-trochlea joint is demonstrated.

Normal Anatomy (Figure 1.53C)

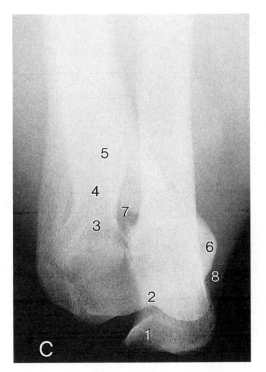

Figure 1.53. C. Radiograph, Tangential Elbow.

1. Olecranon process.
2. Trochlea.
3. Head of the radius.
4. Neck of the radius.
5. Tuberosity, radius.
6. Medial epicondyle, humerus.
7. Olecranon fossa.
8. Ulnar groove.

BASIC
Anteroposterior
Medial oblique
Lateral
*Tangential

ELBOW
Tangential (Jones) Projection

OPTIONAL
Radial head

WRIST
Posteroanterior Projection

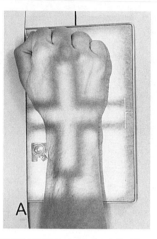

Figure 1.54. POSTEROANTERIOR WRIST. A. Patient Position, Collimation and Central Ray.

Demonstrates: Carpal bones and joints, distal radius, and ulna. (1–4)

Measure: Posteroanterior at the level of the wrist.

kVp: 55 (50 to 60).

Film Size: 10 × 12 inches (24 × 30 cm) divided into quarters; the other quarters are used for the other basic projections.

Grid: No.

Tube Tilt: None.

Patient Position: Seated.

Part Position: Forearm pronated, with a loosely closed fist and the wrist flat on the film.

CR: To the midcarpal region.

Collimation: To the wrist (approximately 6 inches).

Side Marker: Appropriate marker at film corner.

Clinicoradiologic Correlations: The closed fist allows closer wrist/film contact and may accentuate any ligamentous disruption within the carpus, especially the scapholunate space. The scapholunate space is best depicted with 10° of tube tilt from the ulna toward the radius. (5) Lead vinyl should be placed beneath the cassette to reduce primary and secondary radiation to the patient.

1. *Alignment:* Three arcs can be followed within the carpus: (a) proximal surface, scaphoid-lunate-triquetrum; (b) distal surface, scaphoid-lunate-triquetrum; (c) proximal surface, capitate-hamate. (6)
2. *Bone:* All carpal bones, proximal metacarpals, and distal radius and ulna should be identified. The ulna is 1 to 2 mm shorter than the radius. The hook of the hamate is a distinctive landmark.
3. *Cartilage:* The joint spaces between the carpal bones is 1 to 2 mm. (6) The distal radioulnar joint is visible with a joint space also of 1 to 2 mm.
4. *Soft tissue:* A fat line (navicular fat stripe) can be seen running parallel to the scaphoid in over 90% of wrist radiographs. (7) If absent or displaced, there usually is an associated fracture of the scaphoid.

Normal Anatomy (Figure 1.54B and C)

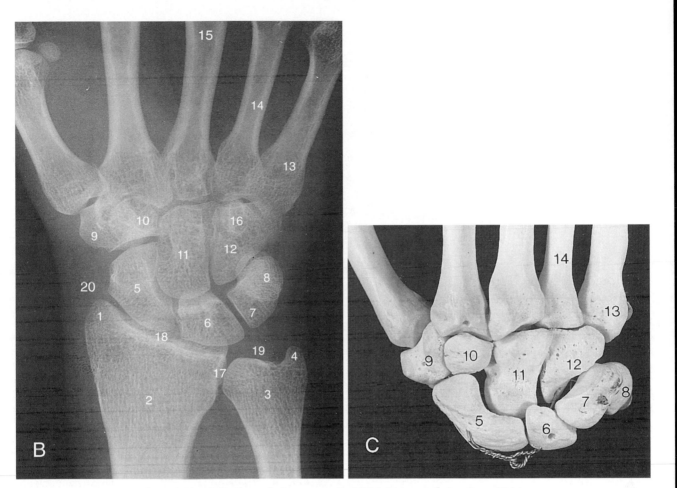

Figure 1.54. B. Radiograph, Posteroanterior Wrist. C. Anatomic Specimen, Wrist.

1. Styloid process, radius.
2. Metaphysis, distal radius.
3. Metaphysis, distal ulna.
4. Styloid process, ulna.
5. Scaphoid.
6. Lunate.
7. Triquetrum.
8. Pisiform.
9. Trapezium.
10. Trapezoid.
11. Capitate.
12. Hamate.
13. Base, fifth metacarpal.
14. Shaft, fourth metacarpal.
15. Neck, third metacarpal.
16. Hook of the hamate.
17. Radioulnar joint.
18. Radiocarpal joint.
19. Ulnocarpal joint.
20. Navicular fat stripe.

BASIC
*Posteroanterior
Posteroanterior ulnar flexion
Medial oblique
Lateral

WRIST
Posteroanterior Projection

OPTIONAL
Carpal tunnel
Scaphoid
Lateral oblique (pisiform)

WRIST

Posteroanterior Ulnar Flexion Projection

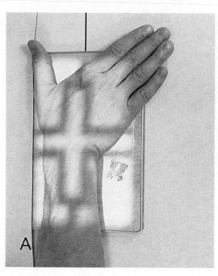

Figure 1.55.   POSTEROANTERIOR ULNAR FLEXION, WRIST. A. Patient Position, Collimation and Central Ray.

Demonstrates: Carpal bones and joints, distal radius, and ulna. (1–4) The view is especially good for assessing the scaphoid. (8,9)

Measure: Posteroanterior at the level of the wrist.

kVp: 55 (50 to 60).

Film Size: 10 × 12 inches (24 × 30 cm) divided into quarters; the other quarters are used for the other basic projections.

Grid: No.

TFD: 40 inches (102 cm).

Tube Tilt: None.

Patient Position: Seated.

Part Position: Forearm pronated, the wrist moved into ulnar deviation and placed flat on the film.

CR: To the midcarpal region.

Collimation: To the wrist (approximately 6 × 5 inches).

Side Marker: Appropriate marker at film corner.

Clinicoradiologic Correlations: This view enhances visualization of scaphoid fractures by distracting the fracture line. Lead vinyl must be placed beneath the cassette to reduce primary and secondary radiation to the patient.

1. *Alignment:* Three arcs can be followed within the carpus: (a) proximal surface, scaphoid-lunate-triquetrum; (b) distal surface, scaphoid-lunate-triquetrum; (c) proximal surface, capitate-hamate (6). There is radial rotation of the proximal carpal row.

2. *Bone:* All carpal bones, proximal metacarpals, and distal radius and ulna should be identified. The ulna is 1 to 2 mm shorter than the radius. The hook of the hamate is a distinctive landmark. Careful scrutiny of the radial surface of the scaphoid for fracture should be done.

3. *Cartilage:* The joint spaces between the carpal bones is 1 to 2 mm. (6) The distal radioulnar joint is visible with a joint space also of 1 to 2 mm. Within the ulnar compartment lies the triangular cartilage.

4. *Soft tissue:* A fat line (navicular fat stripe) can be seen running parallel to the scaphoid in over 90% of wrist radiographs. (7) If absent or displaced, there usually is an associated fracture of the scaphoid.

Normal Anatomy (Figure 1.55B)

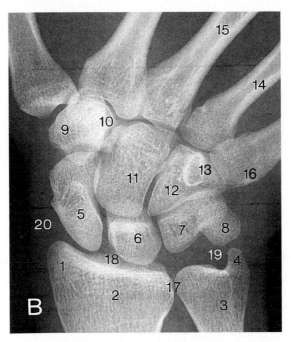

Figure 1.55.   B. Radiograph, Posteroanterior Ulnar Flexion, Wrist.

1. Styloid process, radius.
2. Metaphysis, distal radius.
3. Metaphysis, distal ulna.
4. Styloid process, ulna.
5. Scaphoid.
6. Lunate.
7. Triquetrum.
8. Pisiform.
9. Trapezium.
10. Trapezoid.

11. Capitate.
12. Hamate.
13. Hook of the hamate.
14. Shaft, fourth metacarpal.
15. Shaft, third metacarpal.
16. Base, fifth metacarpal.
17. Radioulnar joint.
18. Radiocarpal joint.
19. Ulnocarpal joint.
20. Navicular fat stripe.

BASIC
Posteroanterior
**Posteroanterior ulnar flexion*
Medial oblique
Lateral

WRIST
Posteroanterior Ulnar Flexion Projection

OPTIONAL
Carpal tunnel
Scaphoid
Lateral oblique (pisiform)

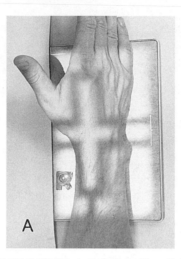

Figure 1.56.   MEDIAL OBLIQUE WRIST. A. Patient Position, Collimation and Central Ray.

BASIC
Posteroanterior
Posteroanterior ulnar flexion
*Medial oblique
Lateral

WRIST
Medial Oblique Projection

OPTIONAL
Carpal tunnel
Scaphoid
Lateral oblique (pisiform)

Demonstrates: Carpal bones and joints, distal radius, and ulna. (1–4,10)

Measure: Laterally, between radial and ulnar styloid processes.

kVp: 55 (50 to 60).

Film Size: 10 × 12 inches (24 × 30 cm) divided into quarters; the other quarters are used for the other basic projections.

Grid: No.

TFD: 40 inches (102 cm).

Tube Tilt: None.

Patient Position: Seated.

Part Position: Forearm semipronated so the dorsum of the wrist is 45° to the film (see oblique hand).

CR: To the midcarpal area.

Collimation: To the wrist (approximately 6 × 5 inches).

Side Marker: Appropriate marker at film corner.

Clinicoradiologic Correlations: This view is an integral component of wrist evaluation. Lead vinyl must be placed beneath the cassette to reduce primary and secondary radiation to the patient.

1. *Alignment:* The first metacarpal-trapezium alignment is shown, as well as within the carpus.
2. *Bone:* The dorsal surfaces of the triquetrum and hamate are seen. The distal pole and waist of scaphoid, distal radius, and metacarpal bases are well depicted.
3. *Cartilage:* A number of joints are shown clearly; the distal radioulnar articulation, trapezium, trapezoid, scaphoid, capitate, and lunate.

Normal Anatomy (Figure 1.56B and C)

BASIC
Posteroanterior
Posteroanterior ulnar flexion
*Medial oblique
Lateral

WRIST
Medial Oblique Projection

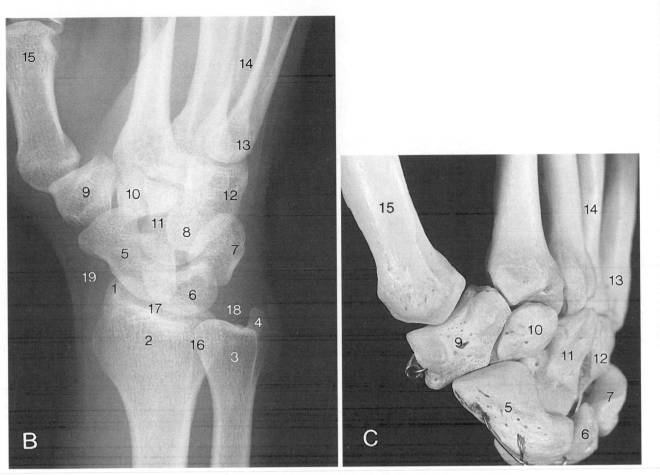

Figure 1.56.   B. Radiograph, Medial Oblique Wrist. C. Anatomical Specimen, Wrist.

1. Styloid process, radius.
2. Metaphysis, distal radius.
3. Metaphysis, distal ulna.
4. Styloid process, ulna.
5. Scaphoid.
6. Lunate.
7. Triquetrum.
8. Pisiform.
9. Trapezium.
10. Trapezoid.

11. Capitate.
12. Hamate.
13. Base, fifth metacarpal.
14. Shaft, fourth metacarpal.
15. Shaft, first metacarpal.
16. Radioulnar joint.
17. Radiocarpal joint.
18. Ulnocarpal joint.
19. Navicular fat stripe.

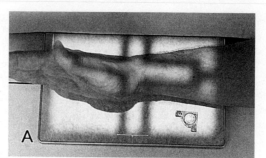

Figure 1.57.   LATERAL WRIST. A. Patient Position, Collimation and Central Ray.

BASIC
Posteroanterior
Posteroanterior ulnar flexion
Medial oblique
*Lateral

WRIST
Lateral Projection

OPTIONAL
Carpal tunnel
Scaphoid
Lateral oblique (pisiform)

Demonstrates: Carpal bones, distal radius, and ulna. (1–4)

Measure: Laterally, between the radial and ulnar styloids.

kVp: 55 (50 to 60).

Film Size: 10 × 12 inches (24 × 30 cm) divided into quarters; the other quarters are used for the other basic projections.

Grid: No.

TFD: 40 inches (102 cm).

Tube Tilt: None.

Patient Position: Seated.

Part Position: Forearm is in true lateral position.

CR: To the midcarpal area.

Collimation: To the wrist (approximately 6 × 5 inches).

Side Marker: Appropriate marker at film corner.

Clinicoradiologic Correlations: This view is especially useful in determining the relationships of the carpal bones (especially the lunate) and distal radius following trauma. Lead vinyl should be placed beneath the cassette to reduce primary and secondary radiation to the patient.

1. *Alignment:* The plane through the long axes of the radius, lunate, capitate, and third metacarpal usually does not deviate more than 10°. The articular surface of the distal radius is tilted ventrally 10 to 15°. The distal radius projects 1 to 3 mm beyond the ulna.
2. *Bone:* The lunate, distal radius, and ulna are well depicted. The dorsal surface of the triquetrum can also be identified.
3. *Cartilage:* The radiolunate and capitate-lunate joints are readily identified.
4. *Soft tissue:* The fat line of the pronator quadratus is usually seen lying close to and parallel to the distal radius. Practically all fractures of the distal radius result in displacement or obliteration of the pronator quadratus fat line. (11)

Normal Anatomy (Figure 1.57B)

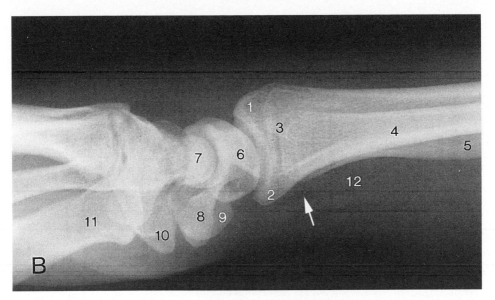

Figure 1.57. B. Radiograph, Lateral Wrist.

1. Posterior lip, radius.
2. Anterior lip, radius.
3. Styloid process, ulna.
4. Shaft of the radius.
5. Shaft of the ulna.
6. Lunate.

7. Capitate.
8. Scaphoid.
9. Pisiform.
10. Trapezium.
11. Base, first metacarpal.
12. Fat line, pronator quadratus (arrow).

BASIC
Posteroanterior
Posteroanterior ulnar flexion
Medial oblique
Lateral

WRIST
Lateral Projection

OPTIONAL
Carpal tunnel
Scaphoid
Lateral oblique (pisiform)

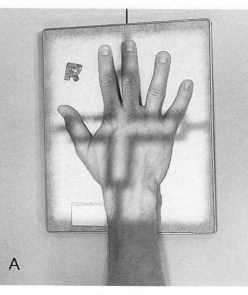

Figure 1.58.   POSTEROANTERIOR, HAND. A. Patient Position, Collimation and Central Ray.

HAND
Posteroanterior Projection

BASIC
*Posteroanterior
Oblique*

OPTIONAL
Norgaard's (Ball catcher's)

Demonstrates: Carpals, metacarpals, phalanges, and joints. (1–3)
Measure: Posteroanterior through metacarpals.
kVp: 55 (50 to 60).
Film Size: 8 × 10 inches (18 × 24 cm).
Grid: No.
TFD: 40 inches (102 cm).
Tube Tilt: None.
Patient Position: Seated.
Part Position: Hand is placed palm down on the film.
CR: Third metacarpal head.
Collimation: To hand size.
Side Marker: Appropriate marker at film corner.
Clinicoradiologic Correlations: Examination of the hand should consist of a minimum of three views—PA, PA oblique, and lateral. Lead vinyl must be placed beneath the cassette to reduce primary and secondary radiation to the patient.

1. *Alignment:* Each phalanx and metacarpal for a single digit is called a *ray* in which all components should be aligned. The long axes of each individual ray should diverge uniformly from the adjacent ray(s). Note the gradual shortening of each metacarpal so that the third to fifth heads are aligned tangentially.
2. *Bone:* Each metacarpal exhibits a base, shaft, and head. At the head small grooves occur laterally referred to as *valleculae.* Identify each phalanx noting the same components. Note the thumb has only two phalanges and sesamoid bones at the metacarpophalangeal joint. Small vascular channels are frequently seen at the distal aspect of the phalanges as thin, oblique, radiolucent lines.
3. *Cartilage:* Multiple joints are visible and each needs to be evaluated for joint space and articular cortex.
4. *Soft tissue:* The skin line over each digit should be followed observing any deviation, especially near a joint as evidence of swelling. Note the contour of the distal finger tip, and in good quality films identify the nail.

Normal Anatomy (Figure 1.58B and C)

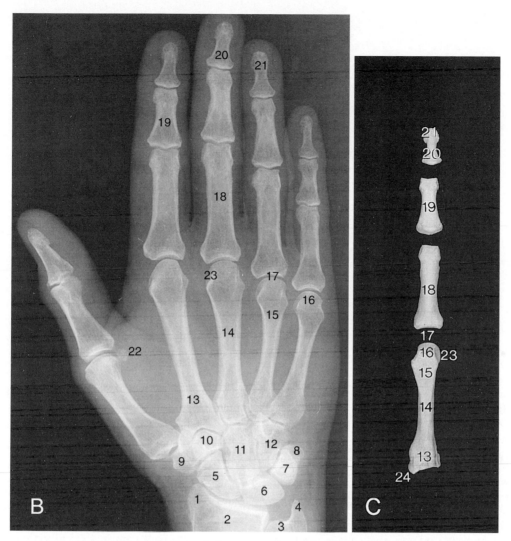

Figure 1.58.   B. Radiograph, Posteroanterior Hand. C. Anatomic Specimen.

1. Styloid process, radius.
2. Metaphysis, radius.
3. Metaphysis, ulna.
4. Styloid process, ulna.
5. Scaphoid.
6. Lunate.
7. Triquetrum.
8. Pisiform.
9. Trapezium.
10. Trapezoid.
11. Capitate.
12. Hamate.

13. Metacarpal base.
14. Metacarpal shaft.
15. Metacarpal neck.
16. Metacarpal head.
17. Metacarpophalangeal joint.
18. Proximal phalanx.
19. Middle phalanx.
20. Distal phalanx.
21. Distal (ungual) tuft.
22. Sesamoid bone (flex. pollicus brevis, adductor pollicus).
23. Vallecula, metacarpal head.
24. Metacarpal styloid process.

BASIC
*Posteroanterior
Oblique

HAND
Posteroanterior Projection

OPTIONAL
Norgaard's (Ball catcher's)

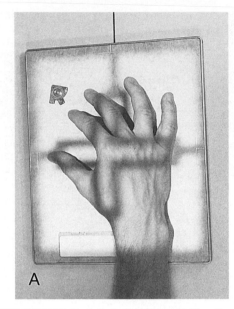

Figure 1.59.   OBLIQUE HAND. A. Patient Position, Collimation and Central Ray.

Demonstrates: Carpals, metacarpals, phalanges, and joints. (1–4)

Measure: Through the CR.

kVp: 55 (50 to 60).

Film Size: 8 × 10 inches (18 × 24 cm).

Grid: No.

TFD: 40 inches (102 cm).

Tube Tilt: None.

Patient Position: Seated.

Part Position: Hand is semipronated to be 45° to the film. For stability, the fingers are flexed to touch the film and to be projected free from each other (see oblique wrist), or they may be placed on a foam-rubber positioning aid.

CR: Between the second and third metacarpal heads.

Collimation: To hand size.

Side Marker: Appropriate marker at film corner.

Clinicoradiological Correlations: The oblique film is especially useful in depicting fractures of the metacarpals. Lead vinyl must be placed beneath the cassette to reduce primary and secondary radiation to the patient.

1. *Alignment:* Trace each metacarpal noting the curved inferior surface and slight ventral tilt of the head.
2. *Bone:* Each metacarpal exhibits a base, shaft and head. At the head small grooves occur laterally and are referred to as *valleculae*. Identify each phalanx noting the same components. Note the thumb has only two phalanges, and sesamoid bones at the metacarpophalangeal joint are often very well seen in this projection. Small vascular channels are frequently seen at the distal aspect of the phalanges as thin oblique radiolucent lines.
3. *Cartilage:* Multiple joints are visible, and each needs to be evaluated for joint space and articular cortex.

BASIC
Posteroanterior
*Oblique

HAND
Oblique Projection

OPTIONAL
Norgaard's (Ball catcher's)

Normal Anatomy (Figure 1.59B)

BASIC
Posteroanterior
*Oblique

HAND
Oblique Projection

OPTIONAL
Norgaard's (Ball catcher's)

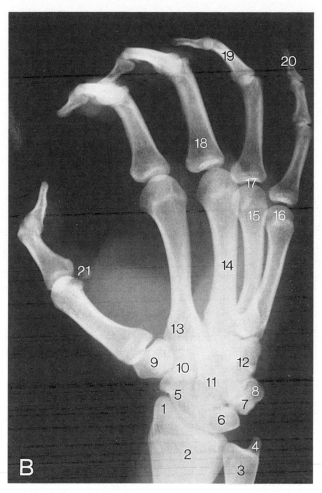

Figure 1.59.   B. Radiograph, Oblique Hand.

1. Styloid process, radius.
2. Metaphysis, radius.
3. Metaphysis, ulna.
4. Styloid process, ulna.
5. Scaphoid.
6. Lunate.
7. Triquetrum.
8. Pisiform.
9. Trapezium.
10. Trapezoid.
11. Capitate.
12. Hamate.
13. Base, second metacarpal.
14. Shaft, third metacarpal.
15. Neck, fourth metacarpal.
16. Head, fifth metacarpal.
17. Metacarpophalangeal joint.
18. Proximal phalanx.
19. Middle phalanx.
20. Distal phalanx.
21. Sesamoid bones (flex. pollicus brevis, add. pollicus). (arrow)

BASIC
*Posteroanterior
*Oblique
*Lateral

FINGERS
Posteroanterior, Oblique, and Lateral Projections

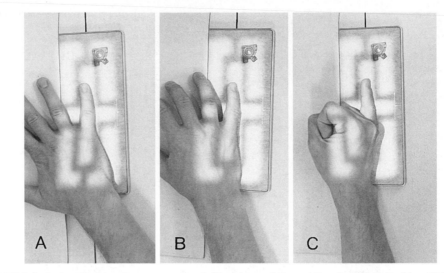

Figure 1.60.   FINGERS. A. Patient Position Posteroanterior, Collimation and Central Ray. B. Patient Position Oblique, Collimation and Central Ray. C. Patient Position Lateral, Collimation and Central Ray.

Demonstrates: Phalanges, metacarpal heads, and interphalangeal joints. (1–4)

Measure: At metacarpal head.

kVp: 55 (50 to 60).

Film Size: 8 × 10 inches (18 × 24 cm) divided into thirds; the other divisions are used for the other basic views.

Grid: No.

TFD: 40 inches (102 cm).

Tube Tilt: None.

Patient Position: Seated.

Part Position: (a) *Posteroanterior*: Hand prone, with affected finger centered. (Fig. 1.60A) (b) *Oblique*: Hand semiprone to 45° with the film, fingers slightly flexed and spread apart. (Fig. 1.60B) (c) *Lateral*: Hand in true lateral position, affected finger extended and the remaining fingers flexed. (Fig. 1.60C)

CR: At the proximal interphalangeal joint.

Collimation: To include only the affected digit.

Side Marker: Appropriate marker in film corner adjacent to fingertip.

Clinicoradiologic Correlations: In lateral projection the finger should be parallel to the film to adequately show the interphalangeal joints and small chip fractures. Lead vinyl must be placed beneath the cassette to reduce primary and secondary radiation to the patient.

1. *Alignment:* The plane through the long axes of each phalanx and metacarpal usually does not deviate more than 10° in the extended position.
2. *Bone:* If the fingers were flexed individually, the phalanges are well seen. In the lateral position superimposition of the metacarpals largely obscures them, though 10° of pronation will show the second and third metacarpals, while 10° of supination shows the fourth and fifth metacarpals.
3. *Cartilage:* The interphalangeal and metacarpophalangeal joints are visible.
4. *Soft tissue:* The skin line over each digit should be followed observing any deviation, especially near a joint as evidence of swelling. Note the contour of the distal finger tip, and in good quality films identify the nail.

Normal Anatomy (Figure 1.60D–G)

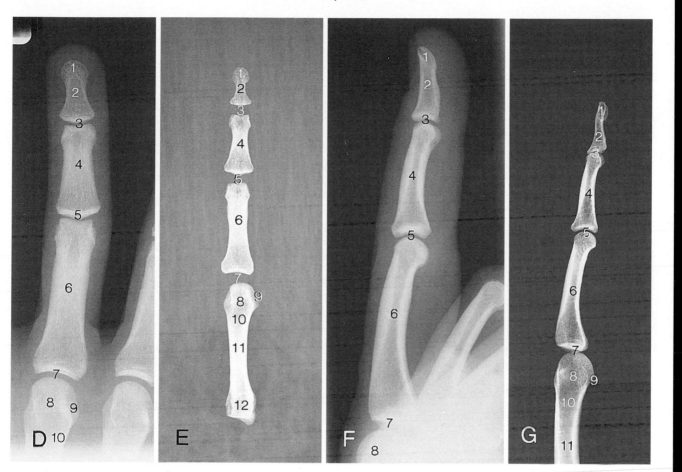

BASIC
*Posteroanterior
*Oblique
*Lateral

FINGERS

Posteroanterior, Oblique, and Lateral Projections

Figure 1.60. **D. Radiograph, Posteroanterior Finger. E. Specimen Radiograph, Posteroanterior. F. Radiograph, Lateral Finger. G. Specimen Radiograph, Lateral Finger.**

1. Distal (ungual) tuft.
2. Distal phalanx.
3. Distal interphalangeal joint.
4. Middle phalanx.
5. Proximal interphalangeal joint.
6. Proximal phalanx.

7. Metacarpophalangeal joint.
8. Head, metacarpal.
9. Vallecula.
10. Neck, metacarpal.
11. Shaft, metacarpal.
12. Base, metacarpal.

Positioning (Figure 1.61A and B)

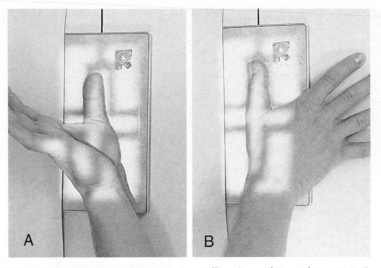

Figure 1.61. THUMB. A. Patient Position Anteroposterior, Collimation and Central Ray. B. Patient Position Lateral.

THUMB

Anteroposterior and Lateral Projections

Demonstrates: Phalanges, first metacarpal, trapezium, scaphoid, and intervening joints. (1–4)

Measure: At the metacarpophalangeal joint.

kVp: 55 (50 to 60).

Film Size: 8 × 10 inches (18 × 24 cm) divided into halves.

Grid: No.

TFD: 40 inches (102 cm).

Tube Tilt: None.

Patient Position: Seated.

Part Position: (a) *Anteroposterior*: The hand is rotated internally until the posterior surface of the thumb contacts the film. (Fig 1.61A) (b) *Lateral*: The hand is placed prone and the thumb brought to a lateral position. This is assisted by slightly flexing of the metacarpophalangeal joints. (Fig 1.61B)

CR: Through the first metacarpophalangeal joint.

Collimation: To thumb size.

Side Marker: Appropriate marker at film corner adjacent to thumb tip.

Clinicoradiologic Correlations: Depiction of the thumb on routine hand views is inadequate, particularly for the base of the first metacarpal and its joint.

1. *Alignment:* Considerable mobility exists at the first metacarpotrapezium joint, which should not be mistaken as subluxation.
2. *Bone:* Identify all bony components of the thumb.
3. *Cartilage:* The interphalangeal and first metacarpotrapezium joints are evaluated for joint space and articular contours.
4. *Soft tissue:* The apparent increased soft tissue density of the thenar pad should not be confused with soft tissue swelling.

Normal Anatomy (Figure 1.61C–E)

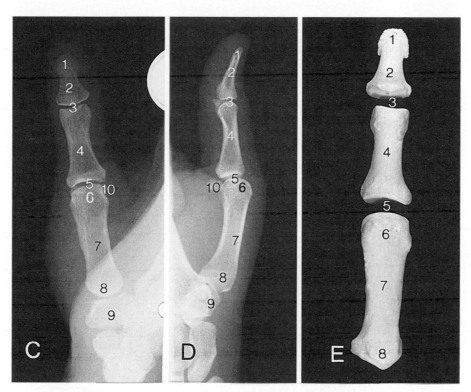

Figure 1.61. C. Radiograph, Anteroposterior Thumb. D. Radiograph, Lateral Thumb. E. Anatomic Specimen.

1. Distal (ungual) tuft.
2. Distal phalanx.
3. Distal interphalangeal joint.
4. Proximal phalanx.
5. Metacarpophalangeal joint.

6. Metacarpal head.
7. Metacarpal shaft.
8. Metacarpal base.
9. Trapezium.
10. Sesamoid bones (flexor pollicus brevis, adductor pollicus).

BASIC
*Anteroposterior
*Lateral

THUMB
Anteroposterior and Lateral Projections

OPTIONAL
Oblique

BASIC
*Anteroposterior or
Posteroanterior (above or
below diaphragm)
*Anterior oblique (45°)
*Posterior oblique (45°)

RIBS
Anteroposterior and Posteroanterior Projections

OPTIONAL
Tangential

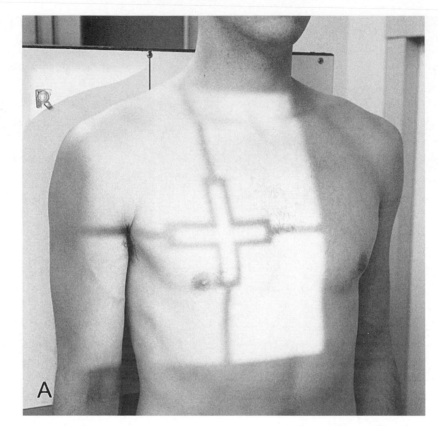

Figure 1.62. ANTEROPOSTERIOR AND POSTEROANTERIOR RIBS. A. Patient Position, Collimation and Central Ray.

Demonstrates: Ribs, anterior and posterior. (1–5)
Measure: Anteroposterior chest at CR.
kVp: 80 (75 to 85) (low for ribs above diaphragm: high for ribs below diaphragm).
Film Size: 14 × 17 inches (35 × 43 cm).
Grid: Yes.
TFD: 40 inches (102 cm).
Tube Tilt: None.
Patient Position: Upright or recumbent.
Part Position: (1) *Anteroposterior*: If rib lesion is posterior, centered to the bucky. (2) *Posteroanterior*: If rib lesion is anterior, centered to the bucky.
CR: To the area of complaint.
Collimation: To the film.
Side Marker: Appropriate marker at film corner.
Breathing Instructions: Above diaphragm rib projection, suspended full inspiration. Below diaphragm rib projection, suspended full expiration.
Clinicoradiologic Correlations: Multiple oblique views at varying angles may be necessary to demonstrate rib frac-

tures. If the suspected lesion is located anteriorly, the obliques are taken PA; if posterior, they are taken anteroposterior. Because of normal overlying anatomy the positioning, exposure, and interpretation of rib radiographs is extremely difficult.

1. *Alignment:* Compare the intercostal spaces for symmetry, tracing them from posterior to anterior.
2. *Bone:* Posteriorly the rib is narrowed, gradually widening and becoming thinner anteriorly. Note the inferior margins, especially at the seventh to twelfth ribs, is often irregular and may even appear absent.
3. *Cartilage:* Identify the costotransverse and costovertebral joints. Note the gradual transition of the anterior ribs into the costal cartilages, which are frequently calcified.
4. *Soft tissue:* Look systematically at the lung fields; aeration, vascularity, cardiovascular silhouette, diaphragms, costophrenic-angles and observe for any masses.

Normal Anatomy (Figure 1.62B–E)

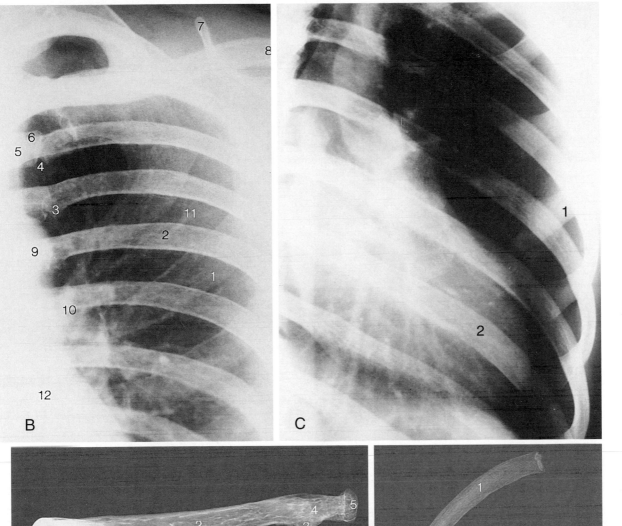

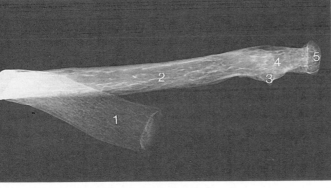

Figure 1.62. B. Radiograph, Anteroposterior Ribs. C. Radiograph, Oblique Ribs. D and E. Specimen Radiographs.

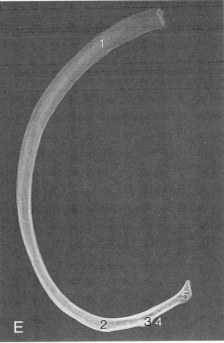

1. Anterior rib.
2. Posterior rib.
3. Rib tubercle.
4. Costotransverse joint.
5. Rib head.
6. Transverse process.
7. Superior angle, scapula.
8. Distal clavicle.
9. Transverse aorta.
10. Pulmonary artery.
11. Peripheral pulmonary vessel.
12. Heart.

BASIC
*Anteroposterior or
Posteroanterior (above or
below diaphragm)
Anterior oblique (45°)
Posterior oblique (45°)

RIBS
Anteroposterior and Posteroanterior Projections

OPTIONAL
Tangential

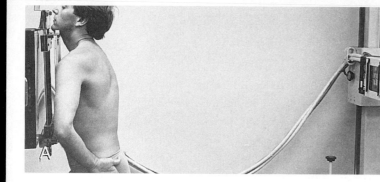

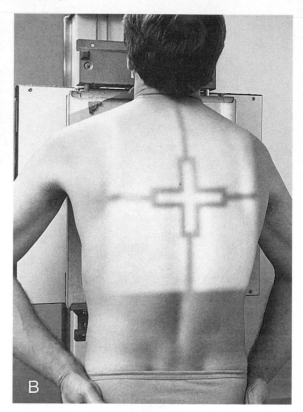

Figure 1.63. POSTEROANTERIOR CHEST. A. Patient Position. B. Collimation and Central Ray.

Demonstrates: Lung fields, heart, great vessels, ribs, shoulder girdles, thoracic spine, and upper abdomen. (1–4)

Measure: Anteroposterior at greatest diameter in full, deep inspiration.

kVp: 110 (100 to 120).

Film Size: 14 × 17 inches (35 × 43 cm).

Grid: No.

TFD: 72 inches (183 cm).

Tube Tilt: None.

Patient Position: Upright.

Part Position: Posteroanterior, chin elevated, hands placed over buttocks, and shoulders rolled forward. Thoracic spine centered to the midline of the bucky. Cassette positioned so that its superior border is 2 inches above the shoulders.

CR: To the film.

Collimation: To the film.

Side Marker: Appropriate marker in film corner above shoulder.

Breathing Instructions: Suspended deep inspiration.

Clinicoradiologic Correlations: To evaluate if a full inspiratory breath has been achieved, seven anterior ribs or ten posterior ribs should be visible above the diaphragm. Expiration chest radiography is a useful supplemental view when evaluating for pneumothorax.

1. *Alignment:* Rotational malposition is assessed by the relative positions of the medial clavicles to the thoracic spine. Observe for scoliosis, elevated shoulder, diaphragm, and mediastinal-cardiovascular silhouette positions.

2. *Bone:* Evaluate the bony thorax; shoulder girdles, spine, and ribs.

3. *Cartilage:* The joints of the shoulder girdles (glenohumeral, acromioclavicular, sternoclavicular), spine (discs) and ribs (costotransverse, costovertebral) can also be identified.

4. *Soft tissue:* Look systematically at the lung fields; aeration, vascularity, minor fissure, trachea and bronchi, cardiovascular silhouette, diaphragms, costophrenic angles and observe for any masses. Outline visible structures of the upper abdomen (liver, colonic gas, stomach air bubble).

BASIC
*Posteroanterior
Lateral

CHEST
Posteroanterior Projection

OPTIONAL
Lordotic
Oblique

Normal Anatomy (Figure 1.63C)

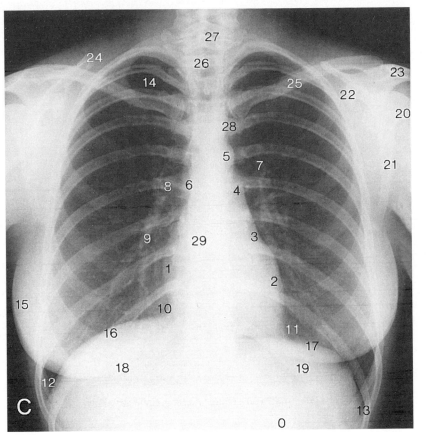

Figure 1.63. **C. Radiograph, Posteroanterior Chest.**

BASIC
*Posteroanterior
Lateral

CHEST
Posteroanterior Projection

OPTIONAL
Lordotic
Oblique

1. Right atrial border.
2. Left ventricular border.
3. Left atrial border.
4. Pulmonary trunk.
5. Transverse aorta (aortic knob).
6. Ascending aorta.
7. Left pulmonary hilus.
8. Right pulmonary hilus.
9. Right pulmonary vessel.
10. Right cardiophrenic angle.
11. Left cardiophrenic angle.
12. Right costophrenic angle.
13. Left costophrenic angle.
14. Right apex.
15. Breast.
16. Right hemidiaphragm.
17. Left hemidiaphragm.
18. Liver.
19. Gastric air bubble (magenblasse).
20. Humeral head.
21. Axillary border, scapula.
22. Coracoid process, scapula.
23. Acromion, scapula.
24. Superior angle, scapula.
25. Clavicle.
26. Spinous process, T2.
27. Tracheal air shadow.
28. Manubrium.
29. Thoracic spine.

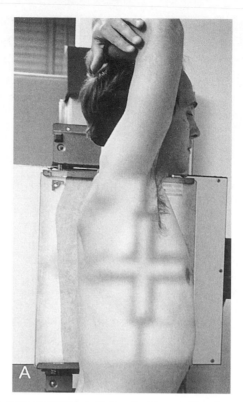

Figure 1.64.   LATERAL CHEST. A. Patient Position, Collimation and Central Ray.

Demonstrates: Lung fields, heart, great vessels, ribs, sternum, and thoracic spine. (5–7)
Measure: Transversely, under the axilla, at the T6 level.
kVp: 110 (100 to 120).
Film Size: 14 × 17 inches (35 × 43 cm).
Grid: No.
TFD: 72 inches (183 cm).
Tube Tilt: None.
Patient Position: Upright.
Part Position: Left lateral position, with no rotation. Both arms elevated and crossed on top of the head. Cassette position is 2 inches above the shoulders.
CR: To the film.
Collimation: To patient size.
Side Marker: Left marker placed anterior to the sternum or behind the upper thoracic spine.
Breathing Instructions: Suspended deep inspiration.

Clinicoradiologic Correlations: Left laterals are routinely performed to reduce cardiac magnification.

1. *Alignment:* Measure the degree of kyphosis present. Observe the contour of the sternum.
2. *Bone:* Evaluate the bony thorax; shoulder girdles, spine, and ribs.
3. *Cartilage:* The joints of the shoulder girdles (glenohumeral), spine (discs, facets), and ribs (costotransverse, costovertebral) can also be identified.
4. *Soft tissue:* Look systematically at the lung fields; aeration, vascularity, fissures (major, minor), trachea and bronchi, cardiovascular silhouette, diaphragms, costophrenic angles and observe for any masses. Outline visible structures of the upper abdomen (liver, colonic gas, stomach air bubble).

Normal Anatomy (Figure 1.64B)

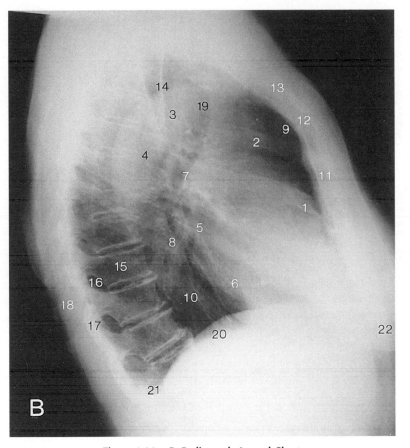

Figure 1.64.   B. Radiograph, Lateral Chest.

1.   Right ventricular border.
2.   Ascending aorta.
3.   Aortic arch.
4.   Descending aorta.
5.   Left atrial border.
6.   Left ventricular border.
7.   Hilus.
8.   Pulmonary vessels.
9.   Retrosternal space.
10. Retrocardiac space.
11. Body of sternum.

12. Manubriosternal joint.
13. Manubrium.
14. Axillary borders, scapulae.
15. Vertebral body.
16. Intervertebral foramen.
17. Posterior rib.
18. Spinous process.
19. Trachea.
20. Diaphragm.
21. Posterior costophrenic sulcus.
22. Breast shadow.

CHEST
Lordotic Projection

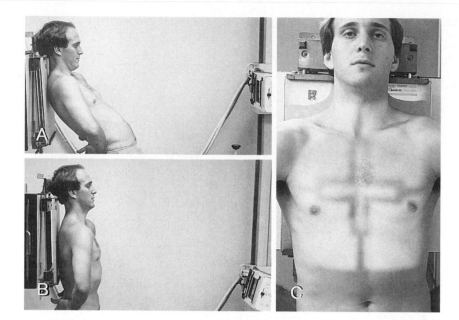

Figure 1.65. LORDOTIC, CHEST. A. Patient Position, Anteroposterior Patient Tilt. B. Patient Position, Anteroposterior Tube Tilt. C. Collimation and Central Ray.

Demonstrates: Lung apices, right middle lobe, and lingula segments. (8–11)

Measure: Through the CR.

kVp: 110 (100 to 120).

Film Size: 14 × 17 inches (35 × 43 cm).

Grid: No.

TFD: (a) 72 inches (183 cm); no tilt; (b) 72 inches (must correct for tube tilt; 66 inches).

Tube Tilt: (a) No tilt. (b) 30° cephalad.

Patient Position: Upright.

Part Position: (a) *Anteroposterior Patient Tilt*: Patient stands one foot from the bucky and leans back, with shoulders, neck, and back of the head against bucky. (Fig.1.65A) (b) *Anteroposterior Tube Tilt*: Alternatively, the patient stands straight upright and tube is angled cephalad 30°. The film is placed 2 inches above the shoulders. (Fig. 1.65B and C)

CR: To the film.

Collimation: To the film.

Side Marker: Appropriate marker at film corner above the shoulder.

Breathing Instructions: Suspended full inspiration.

Clinicoradiologic Correlations: This is an optional view utilized in the evaluation of lung disease involving the apices, middle lobe, and lingula. (12,13)

1. *Alignment:* Note if the trachea is displaced and the symmetry of clavicular orientation.
2. *Bone:* The bones of the shoulder girdle (humerus, clavicle, scapula) and cervicothoracic spines can be identified.
3. *Cartilage:* The joints of the upper ribs and shoulder girdle can be seen.
4. *Soft tissue:* The lung fields are assessed for symmetry of aeration or masses, vascularity, fissure, and trachea position, especially of the upper and middle lobes, as well as the lingula.

Normal Anatomy (Figure 1.65D)

BASIC
Posteroanterior
Lateral

CHEST
Lordotic Projection

OPTIONAL
*Lordotic
Oblique

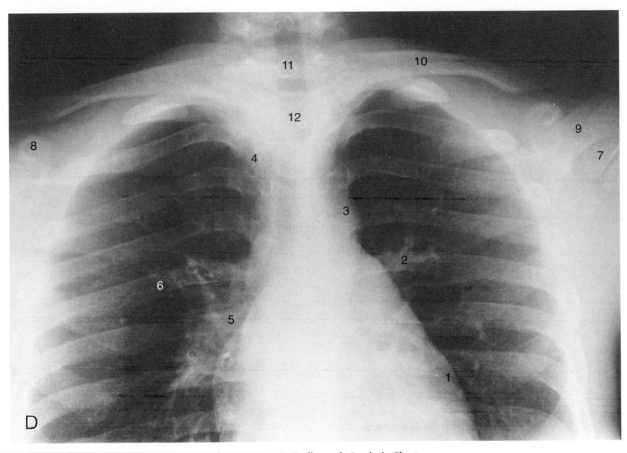

Figure 1.65.   D. Radiograph, Lordotic Chest.

1. Left ventricular border.
2. Left pulmonary vessels.
3. Aortic arch (aortic knob).
4. Superior vena cava.
5. Right pulmonary vessels.
6. Posterior rib.

7. Humeral head.
8. Coracoid process.
9. Acromion process.
10. Clavicle.
11. T1 vertebra.
12. Trachea.

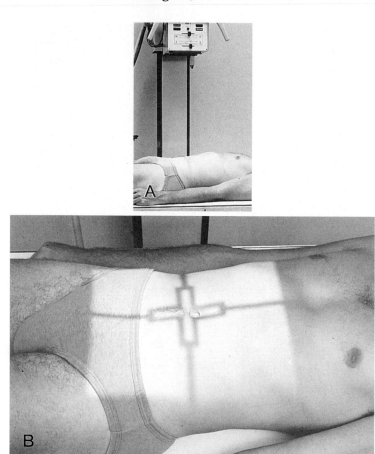

Figure 1.66.   ANTEROPOSTERIOR ABDOMEN. A. Patient Position. B. Collimation and Central Ray.

Demonstrates: Kidneys, urinary bladder, liver, spleen, large bowel, psoas shadow, pelvis, lumbar spine, and lower ribs. (1–4)

Measure: At the iliac crest.

kVp: (a) 70 (65 to 75) for calcific densities; (b) 100 (95 to 105) for soft tissue detail.

Film Size: 14 × 17 inches (35 × 43 cm).

Grid: Yes.

TFD: 40 inches (102 cm).

Tube Tilt: None.

Patient Position: Supine.

Part Position: Spine positioned to the midline.

CR: At the top of the iliac crests.

Collimation: To film size.

Side Marker: Appropriate marker in top corner of film.

Breathing Instructions: Suspended expiration.

Clinicoradiologic Correlations: Obese patients should be examined posteroanterior to compress the body tissues and decrease the time of exposure. Exceptionally tall patients may be exposed during a deep inspiration to ensure the abdominal contents from diaphragm to pubic symphysis are included on the radiograph.

1. *Alignment:* Note for scoliosis, the position of the liver, the lower level of the right kidney, the gastric air bubble, and the distribution of bowel gas.
2. *Bone:* The spine, pelvis, sacrum, and lower ribs can all be identified.
3. *Cartilage:* Joints, including the disc spaces, sacroiliac, pubic, hips, and lower costals, can all be seen.
4. *Soft tissue:* Many soft tissue outlines can be determined; kidneys, urinary bladder, liver, spleen, large bowel, stomach, and psoas shadow.

Normal Anatomy (Figure 1.66C)

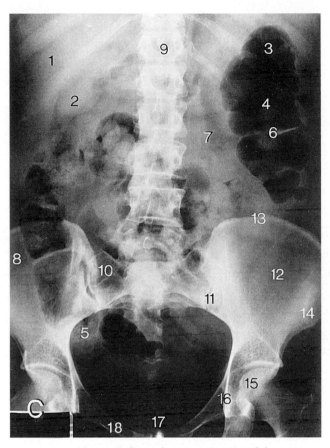

Figure 1.66.   C. Radiograph, Anteroposterior Abdomen.

1. Liver.
2. Right kidney.
3. Gas in splenic flexure.
4. Solid feces in colon.
5. Semifluid feces in colon.
6. Haustra, descending colon.
7. Psoas margin.
8. Flank stripe.
9. T12 vertebral body.

10. Sacral ala.
11. Sacroiliac joint.
12. Iliac fossa.
13. Iliac crest.
14. Anterior superior iliac spine (ASIS).
15. Femoral head.
16. Kohler's teardrop.
17. Symphysis pubis.
18. Superior pubic ramus.

REFERENCES

INTRODUCTION

1. **Roentgen WC:** *Ueber eine neue Art von Strahlen.* I, Sitzungsber, Phys-med. Gesellsch, Wuzburg, 1985. English translation in *Science,* February, 1896.
2. **Grigg ERN:** *The Trail of the Invisible Light,* Springfield, IL, Charles C Thomas, 1965.
3. **Eastman TR:** *History of radiographic technique.* Appl Radiol 7:97, 1978.
4. **Clark KC:** *Positioning in Radiography,* ed 9. Vols 1 and 2, London, Ilford Limited, William Heinemann Medical Books, 1974.
5. **Merrill V:** *Atlas of Roentgenographic Positions and Standard Radiologic Procedures.* ed 4. Vols 1, 2 and 3. St. Louis: CV Mosby, 1975.
6. **Meschan I:** *An Atlas of Anatomy Basic to Radiology.* Philadelphia, Lea & Febiger, 1975.
7. **Meschan I:** *Radiographic Positioning and Related Anatomy,* ed 2. Philadelphia, WB Saunders, 1978.
8. **Guebert GM, Pirtle OL, Yochum TR:** *Essentials of Diagnostic Imaging.* St. Louis, Mosby-Year Book , 1995.
9. **Christensen E, Curry T, Dowdy J:** *An Introduction to the Physics of Diagnostic Radiology,* ed 3. Philadelphia, Lea & Febiger, 1984.
10. **Eastman TR:** *Technique charts: The key to radiographic quality.* Radiol Technol 46:365, 1975.
11. **Sherman R, Bauer F:** *X-ray X-pertise-from A-X.* Ft. Worth, TX, Parker Chiropractic Research Foundation, 1982.
12. **Howe JW, Yochum TR:** *X-ray, pregnancy, and therapeutic abortion: A current perspective.* ACA J Chiro April 1985.
13. *Gonad shielding in diagnostic radiology.* Bureau of Radiological Health, Rockville, MD, Pub No. (FDA)75-8024, 1975.
14. **Warwick R, Williams PL:** *Gray's Anatomy,* ed 35. (British). Philadelphia, WB Saunders, 1973.
15. *New York State Department of Health.* March 15, 1992 (letter).
16. *New York State Department of Health.* A guide for radiation safety-quality assurance program, 1992.
17. US Federal Government. Mammography Quality Standards Act. *HR6182:1,* 1992.
18. *Conference of Radiation Control Program Directors. Survey.* 1992.
19. *Medical Imaging.* April 57, 1994 (editorial).
20. **Curry TS, Dowdey JE, Murray RC:** *Christensen's Introduction to the Physics of Diagnostic Radiology,* ed 5. Philadelphia: Lea and Febiger, 1990.
21. **Mootz RD, Meeker RD:** *Minimizing radiation exposure to patients in chiropractic practice.* ACA J Chiro April 65, 1989.
22. **Phillips RB:** *Plain film radiology in chiropractic.* J Manipulative Physiol Ther 15(1):47, 1992.
23. **Modic MT, Herzog RJ:** *Spinal imaging modalities. What's available and who should order them?* Spine 19(15):1764, 1994.
24. **Schultz G, Phillips RB, Cooley J, et al:** *Diagnostic imaging of the spine in chiropractic practice: Recommendations for utilization.* Chiro J Austr 22(4):141, 1992.
25. **Rueter FG, Conway BJ, McCrohan JL, et al:** *Radiography of the lumbosacral spine: Characteristics of examinations performed in hospitals and other facilities.* Radiology 185:43, 1992.
26. **Guebert GM, Kettner NW, Yochum TR:** *Limiting professional liability: Improving x-ray quality.* Appl Diagn Imag 1(2):9, 1989.
27. **Guebert GM, Kettner NW, Yochum TR:** *The chiropractor's guide to radiographic technology.* Appl Diagn Imag 1(4):29, 1989.

SKULL

1. **Taveras J, Wood E:** *Diagnostic Neuroradiology,* ed 2, Vol 1. Baltimore, Williams & Wilkins, 1976.
2. **Weathers RM, Lee A:** *Radiologic examination of the skull.* Radiol Clin North Am 12:215, 1974.
3. **Potts DG:** *A system of skull radiography.* Radiology 94:25, 1970.
4. **Masters SJ:** *Evaluation of head trauma: Efficacy of skull films.* AJR 135:539, 1980.

PARANASAL SINUSES

1. **Macmillan AS Jr:** *Techniques in paranasal sinus radiography.* Semin Roentgenol 3:115, 1968.
2. **Yanagisawa E, Smith HW:** *Normal radiographic anatomy of the paranasal sinuses.* Otolaryngol Clin North Am 6:429, 1973.
3. **Waters CA:** *A modification of the occipitofrontal position in roentgen examination of the accessory nasal sinuses.* Arch Radiol Ther 20:15,1915.
4. **Spillman R:** *Early history of roentgenology of the sinuses.* AJR 54:643,1945.

CERVICAL SPINE

1. **Christenson PC:** *The radiologic study of the normal spine. Cervical, thoracic, lumbar, and sacral.* Radiol Clin North Am 15:133, 1977.
2. **Bumstead HD:** *Routine examination of the cervical spine.* Xray Techn 27:247, 1955.
3. **Hadley LA:** *Roentgenographic studies of the cervical spine.* AJR 52:173, 1944.
4. **DeLuca SA, Rhea JA:** *Radiographic anatomy of the cervical vertebrae.* Med Radiogr Photogr 56:18, 1980.

5. **Scher AT:** *The value of the anteroposterior radiograph in "hidden" fractures and dislocations of the lower cervical spine.* S Afr Med J 55:221, 1979.
6. **Apuzzo ML, Weiss MH, Heiden JS:** *Transoral exposure of the atlantoaxial region.* Neurosurg 3:201, 1978.
7. **George AW:** *Method for more accurate study of injuries to the atlas and axis.* Boston Med Surg J 181:395, 1919.
8. **Ottonello P:** *New method for roentgenography of the entire cervical spine in ventrodorsal projection.* Rev Radiol Fis Med 2:291, 1930.
9. **Jacobs LG:** *Roentgenography of the second cervical vertebra by Ottonello's method.* Radiology 31:412, 1938.
10. **Thomeir WC, Brown DC, Mirvis SE:** *The laterally tilted dens: A sign of subtle odontoid fracture on plain film radiography.* AJNR 11:605, 1990.
11. **Hinck VC, Hopkins CE:** *Measurement of the atlanto-dental interval in the adult.* AJR 84:945, 1960.
12. **Penning L:** *Prevertebral hematoma in cervical spine injury. Incidence and etiologic significance.* AJR 136:553, 1981.
13. **Marks JL, Parks SL:** *A simplified position for demonstrating the cervical intervertebral foramina.* AJR 63:575, 1950.
14. **Boylston BF:** *Oblique roentgenographic views of the cervical spine in flexion and extension: An aid in the diagnosis of cervical subluxations and obscure dislocations.* J Bone Joint Surg (Am) 39:1302, 1957.
15. **Marcelis S, Seragini FC, Taylor JAM, et al:** *Cervical spine: comparison of 45° and 55° anteroposterior oblique radiographic projections.* Radiology 188:253, 1993.
16. **Weir DC:** *Roentgenographic signs of cervical injury.* Clin Orthop 109:9, 1975.
17. **Miller MD, Gehweiler JA, Martinex S, et al:** *Significant new observations on cervical spine trauma.* AJR 130:659, 1978.
18. **Davis AG:** *Injuries of the cervical spine.* JAMA 127 (3):149, 1945.
19. **Hagen DE:** *Introduction to the pillar projection of the cervical spine.* Radiol Technol 35:239, 1964.
20. **Smith GR, Abel MS:** *Visualization of the posterolateral elements of the upper cervical vertebrae in the anteroposterior projection.* Radiology 115:219, 1975.

THORACIC SPINE

1. **Christenson PC:** *The radiologic study of the normal spine. Cervical, thoracic, lumbar, and sacral.* Radiol Clin North Am 15:133, 1977.
2. **Fuchs AW:** *Thoracic vertebrae.* Radiogr Clin Photogr 17:2, 1941.
3. **Scher AT:** *The diagnostic value of the anteroposterior radiograph for thoracolumbar injuries.* S Afr Med J 58:415, 1980.
4. **Dalton CJ, Schwartz SS:** *Evaluation of the paraspinal line in roentgen examination of the thorax.* Radiology 66:195, 1954.
5. **Guerreiro G:** *Lateral roentgenographic examination of the thoracic spine.* J Bone Joint Surg (Am) 32:192, 1950.
6. **Clarke EK:** *Visualization of the first and second dorsal and the fifth lumbar vertebrae in lateral or slightly semilateral positions.* X ray Techn 12:5, 1940.
7. **Scher A, Vambeck V:** *An approach to the radiological examination of the cervicodorsal junction following injury.* Clin Radiol 28:243, 1977.
8. **Davis JW:** *Cervical injuries-perils of the swimmer's view: Case report.* J Trauma 29:891, 1989.

LUMBAR SPINE

1. **Lumbar vertebrae.** Radiogr Clin Photgr 18:2, 1942.
2. **Cornwell WS:** *Some aspects of radiography of the lumbar vertebrae.* X ray Techn 14:77, 1942.
3. **Scavone JG, Latchaw RF, Weidner WA:** *Anteroposterior and lateral radiographs: an adequate lumbar spine examination.* AJR 136:715, 1981.
4. **Abel MS, Smith GR:** *Visualization of the posterolateral elements of the lumbar vertebrae in the anteroposterior projection.* Radiology 122:824, 1977.
5. **Tsuno MM, Shu GJ:** *Posteroanterior versus anteroposterior lumbar spine radiology.* J Manipulative Physiol Ther 13(3):144, 1990.
6. **Bloom RA, Gheorghiu D, Verstandig A et al:** *The psoas sign in normal subjects without bowel preparation: the influence of scoliosis on visualization.* Clin Radiol 41:204, 1990.
7. **Hickey PM:** *Lateral roentgenology of the spine.* AJR 4:101, 1917.
8. **Boyland KG:** *True lateral positioning of the lumbar spine and pelvis.* Radiography 13:44, 1947.
9. **Etter L, Carabello NC:** *Roentgen anatomy of oblique views of the lumbar spine.* AJR 61:699, 1949.
10. **Brown RC, Evans ET:** *What causes the "eye of the scotty dog" in the oblique projection of the lumbar spine?* AJR 118:435, 1972.
11. **Libson E, Bloom RA:** *Anteroposterior angulated view.* Radiology 149:315, 1983.
12. **Pathria M, Sartoris DJ, Resnick D:** *Osteoarthritis of the facet joints: accuracy of oblique radiographic assessment.* Radiology 164:227, 1987.
13. **Ferguson AB:** *The clinical and roentgenographic interpretation of lumbosacral anomalies.* Radiology 22:548, 1934.
14. **Horowitz T, Smith MR:** *An anatomical, pathological, and roentgenological study of the intervertebral joints of the lumbar spine and of the sacroiliac joints.* AJR 43:173, 1940.
15. **Logroscino D:** *Das huftgelenk und das sakroiliakalgelenk in gunstiger rontgenographischer projektion.* Rontgenpraxis 8:433, 1936.
16. **Jackson H, Burke JT:** *The sacral foramina.* Skeletal Radiol 11:282, 1984.
17. **Yochum TR, Guebert GM, Kettner NW:** *The tilt-up view: A closer look at the lumbosacral junction.* Appl Diagn Imag 1(6):49, 1989.

18. **Darling BC:** *The sacroiliac joint: its diagnosis as determined by x-ray.* Radiology 3:486, 1924.
19. **Kamieth H:** *What do spot films of the sacroiliac joint accomplish? Pathology of the sacroiliac joint.* Radiol Clin 26:139, 1957.
20. **Johannsen A, Jepsen OL, Winge J:** *Radiological and scintigraphical examination of the sacroiliac joints in the diagnosis of sacroiliitis.* Dan Med Bull 21:246, 1974.
21. **Resnick D, Niwayama G, Goergen T:** *Comparison of abnormalities of the sacroiliac joint in degenerative disease and ankylosing spondylitis.* AJR 128:189, 1977.
22. **William PC, Wigby PE:** *Technique for the roentgen examination of the lumbosacral articulation.* AJR 33:511, 1935.
23. **Curran JT:** *New approach to positioning for lumbosacral junction in lateral projection.* Radiol Technol 46:294, 1975.
24. **Eisenberg RL, Akin JR, Hedgcock MW:** *Single, well-centered lateral view of lumbosacral spine: Is a coned view necessary?* AJR 133:711, 1979.

SACRUM

1. **Christenson PC:** *The radiologic study of the normal spine. Cervical, thoracic, lumbar, and sacral.* Radiol Clin North Am 15:133, 1977.
2. **Hoing M:** *A new technic of coccyxography.* Xray Techn 7:68, 1935.
3. **Zochert RW:** *The sacrum and coccyx: Location and technic for radiography.* Xray Techn 4:118, 1933.
4. **Turner ML, Mulhern CB, Dalinka MK:** *Lesions of the sacrum: Differential diagnosis and radiological evaluation.* JAMA 245:275, 1981.
5. **Amorosa JK, Wintraub S, Amorosa LF, et al:** *Sacral destruction: Foraminal lines revisited.* AJR 145:773, 1985.
6. **Jackson H, Burke JT:** *The sacral foramina.* Skeletal Radiol 11:282, 1984.
7. **Yochum TR, Guebert GM, Kettner NW:** *The tilt-up view: A closer look at the lumbosacral junction.* Appl Diagn Imag 1(6):49, 1989.
8. **Resnick D, Niwayama G, Goergen T:** *Comparison of abnormalities of the sacroiliac joint in degenerative disease and ankylosing spondylitis.* AJR 128:189, 1977.
9. **Postacchini F, Massobrio M:** *Idiopathic coccygodynia. Analysis of fifty one operative cases and a radiographic study of the normal coccyx.* J Bone Joint Surg (Am) 65:1116, 1983.
10. **Maigne JY, Guedj S, Straus C:** *Idiopathic coccygodynia.* Spine 19:930, 1994.

COCCYX

1. **Christenson PC:** *The radiologic study of the normal spine. Cervical, thoracic, lumbar, and sacral.* Radiol Clin North Am 15:133, 1977.
2. **Hoing M:** *A new technic of coccyxography.* Xray Techn 7:68, 1935.
3. **Zochert RW:** *The sacrum and coccyx: Location and technic for radiography.* Xray Techn 4:118, 1933.
4. **Postacchini F, Massobrio M:** *Idiopathic coccygodynia. Analysis of fifty one operative cases and a radiographic study of the normal coccyx.* J Bone Joint Surg (Am) 65:1116, 1983.
5. **Maigne JY, Guedj S, Straus C:** *Idiopathic coccygodynia.* Spine 19:930, 1994.

PELVIS

1. **Bridgman CF:** *Radiography of the hip bone.* Med Radiogr Photogr 28:38, 1952.
2. **Liliequist B:** *Roentgenologic examination of the acetabular part of the os coxae.* Acta Radiol Diagn 4:289, 1966.
3. **Armbuster TG, et al:** *The adult hip: An anatomic study. Part I: The bony landmarks.* Radiology 128:1, 1978.
4. **Katz JF:** *Precise identification of radiographic acetabular landmarks.* Clin Orthop 141:166, 1979.
5. **Bowerman JW, Sena JM, Chang R:** *The teardrop shadow of the pelvis: Anatomy and clinical significance.* Radiology 143:659, 1982.
6. **Mitton KL, Auringer EM:** *Roentgenological study of the femoral neck.* AJR 66:639, 1951.

FULL SPINE

1. **Farren J:** *Routine radiographic assessment of the scoliotic spine.* Radiography 47(556):92, 1981.
2. **Davies WG:** *Radiography in the treatment of scoliosis and in leg lengthening. II. Radiography in scoliosis.* Radiography 26(311):349, 1960.
3. **Sausser WS:** *Achievement—Entire body x-ray technic perfected.* ACA J Chiro 4(2):17, 1935.
4. **Young LW, Oestreich AE, Goldstein LA:** *Roentgenology in scoliosis: Contribution to evaluation and management.* AJR 108:778, 1970.
5. **Taylor JAM:** *Full-spine radiography: A review.* J Manipulative Physiol Ther 16:460, 1993.
6. **Field TJ, Buehler MT:** *Improvements in chiropractic full spine radiography.* J Manipulative Physiol Ther 4:21, 1981.
7. **Cartwright PH:** *The Baulin filtration system: Its effectiveness in patient dose control in chiropractic radiography.* Christchurch, NZ: National Radiation Laboratory, Report NZL 1980/12, 1982.
8. **Merkin JJ, Sportelli L:** *The effects of two new compensating filters on patient exposure in chiropractic full spine radiography.* J Manipulative Physiol Ther 5:25, 1982.
9. **Gray JE, Hoffman AD, Peterson NA:** *Reduction of radiation exposure during radiography for scoliosis.* J Bone Joint Surg (Am) 65:5, 1983.
10. **Bhatnagar JP:** *X-ray doses to patients undergoing full-spine radiographic examination.* Radiology 138:231, 1981.
11. **Greko PJ:** *Evaluation of quality of lateral full spine radiographs: A statistical study.* J Manipulative Physiol Ther 15:217, 1992.

HIP

1. **Bridgman CF:** *Radiography of the hip joint.* Med Radiogr Photogr 26:2, 1950.
2. **Bridgman CF:** *Radiography of the hip joint.* Med Radiogr Photogr 27:2, 1951.
3. **Bridgman CF:** *Radiography of the hip joint.* Med Radiogr Photogr 28:38, 1952.
4. **Hooper AC, Ormond DJ:** *A radiographic study of hip rotation.* Ir J Med Sci 144:25, 1975.
5. **Armbuster TG, et al:** *The adult hip: An anatomic study. Part I: The bony landmarks.* Radiology 128:1, 1978.
6. **Mitton KL, Auringer EM:** *Roentgenological study of the femoral neck.* AJR 66:639, 1951.

KNEE

1. **Larsen RM:** *Radiography of extremities.* Xray Techn 12:215, 1941.
2. **Harris J:** *Radiography of the lower limb.* Radiography 31:235, 1965.
3. **Funke T:** *Radiography of the knee joint.* Med Radiogr Photogr 36:1, 1960.
4. **Leach RE, Gregg T, Ferris JS:** *Weight-bearing radiography in osteoarthritis of the knee.* Radiology 97:265, 1970.
5. **Thomas R, Resnick D, Alazraki N, et al:** *Compartmental evaluation of osteoarthritis of the knee: A comparative study of available diagnostic modalities.* Radiology 116:585, 1975.
6. **Rosenburg TD, Paulos LE, Parker RD, et al:** *The forty-five degree posteroanterior flexion weight-bearing radiograph of the knee.* J Bone Joint Surg (Am) 70:1479, 1988.
7. **Vaughan FMA:** *Lateral knees.* Radiography 16:75, 1950.
8. **Alexander OM:** *Routine lateral radiography of the knee and ankle joints.* Radiography 17:10, 1951.
9. **Camp JD, Coventry MB:** *Use of special views in roentgenography of the knee joint.* US Naval Med Bull 42:56, 1944.
10. **Holmblad EC:** *Postero-anterior x-ray view of the knee in flexion.* JAMA 109:1196, 1937.
11. **Turner GW, Burns CB, Previtte RG:** *Erect positions for "tunnel" views of the knee.* Radiol Technol 55:640, 1983.
12. **Settegast:** *Typische roentgenbilder von normalen menschen.* Lahmanns Med Atlanten 5:211, 1921.
13. **Hughston JC:** *Subluxation of the patella.* J Bone Joint Surg (Am) 50:1003, 1968.
14. **Laurin CA, Dussault R, Levesque HP:** *The tangential x-ray investigation of the patello-femoral joint: X-ray technique, diagnostic criteria, and their interpretation.* Clin Orthop 144:16, 1979.
15. **Wiberg G:** *Roentgenographic and anatomic studies on the femoropatellar joint.* Acta Orthop Scan 12:319, 1941.
16. **Rowe LJ:** *Imaging of the Knee.* In: A.L. Logan ed.: *The Knee. Clinical Applications.* Aspen Publishers, Gaithersburg, 1994.

ANKLE

1. **Larsen RM:** *Radiography of extremities.* X-ray Technol 12:215, 1941.
2. **Harris J:** *Radiography of the lower limb.* Radiography 31:235, 1965.
3. **Goergen TG, Danzig LA, Resnick D, et al:** *Roentgenographic evaluation of the tibiotalar joint.* J Bone Joint Surg (Am) 59:874, 1977.
4. **Thompson JP, Loomer RL:** *Osteochondral lesions of the talus in a sports medicine clinic. A new radiographic technique and surgical approach.* Am J Sports Med 12(6):460, 1984.
5. **Rowe LJ:** *Imaging of the Ankle.* In: A.L. Logan, ed.: *The Foot and Ankle. Clinical Applications,* Aspen Publishers, Gaithersburg, 1995.
6. **Hutter CG Jr, Scott W:** *Tibial torsion.* J Bone Joint Surg (Am) 31:511, 1949.
7. **Alexander OM:** *Routine lateral radiography of the knee and ankle joints.* Radiography 17:10, 1951.
8. **Mandell J:** *Isolated fracture of the posterior tibial lip at the ankle as demonstrated by an additional projections, the "poor" lateral view.* Radiology 101:319, 1971.

FOOT

1. **Larsen RM:** *Radiography of extremities.* Xray Techn 12:215, 1941.
2. **Harris J:** *Radiography of the lower limb.* Radiography 31:235, 1965.
3. **Meschan I:** *Radiology of the normal foot.* Semin Roentgenol 15:327, 1970.
4. **Graham D, Rorrison J:** *Radiography of the tarsal bones.* Radiography 28:156, 1962.
5. **Santora PJ:** *Anteroposterior view of the ankle joint and foot.* AJR 45:127, 1941.
6. **Rowe LJ:** *Imaging of the Ankle.* In: A.L. Logan, ed.: *The Foot and Ankle. Clinical Applications,* Aspen Publishers, Gaithersburg, 1995.
7. **Piotrowski Brother D:** *Oblique view of the ankle joint and foot.* AJR 45:127, 1938.

TOES

1. **Larsen RM:** *Radiography of extremities.* Xray Techn 12:215, 1941.
2. **Harris J:** *Radiography of the lower limb.* Radiography 31:235, 1965.
3. **Meschan I:** *Radiology of the normal foot.* Semin Roentgenol 5:327, 1970.
4. **Rowe LJ:** *Imaging of the Ankle.* In: A.L. Logan, ed.: *The Foot and Ankle. Clinical Applications,* Aspen Publishers, Gaithersburg, 1995.

CALCANEUS

1. **Burdick AV:** *Calcaneus.* Xray Techn 23:276, 1952.
2. **Harris RI, Beath T:** *Etiology of peroneal spastic flat foot.* J Bone Joint Surg (Br) 30:624, 1948.

SHOULDER

1. **Lawrence WS:** *New position in radiographing the shoulder joint.* AJR 2:728, 1915.
2. **Freedman E:** *Radiography of the shoulder.* Radiogr Clin Photogr 10:8, 1934.
3. **Jones ML:** *Radiographic examination of the shoulder.* Xray Techn 7:104, 1936.
4. **Blackett CW, Healy TR:** *Roentgen studies of the shoulder.* AJR 37:760, 1937.

5. **Knutsson F:** *An axial projection of the shoulder joint.* Acta Radiol 30:214, 1948.
6. **Stripp WJ:** *Radiographs of the scapulothoracic region.* Xray Focus 4:8, 1963.
7. **ViGario GD, Keats TE:** *Localization of calcific deposits in the shoulder.* AJR 108:806, 1970.
8. **Bloom RA:** *The active abduction view: A new manoeuvre in the diagnosis of rotator cuff tears.* Skeletal Radiol 20:255, 1991.

CLAVICLE

1. **Quesada F:** *Technique for the roentgen diagnosis of fractures of the clavicle.* Surg Gynecol Obstet 42:424, 1926.
2. **Stripp WJ:** *The clavicle and the acromioclavicular joint.* Xray Focus 4:21, 1963.
3. **Zanca P:** *Shoulder pain: Involvement of the acromioclavicular joint. Analysis of 1000 cases.* AJR 112:493, 1971.

ACROMIOCLAVICULAR JOINTS

1. **Alexander OM:** *Radiography of the acromioclavicular joint.* Radiography 54:139, 1948.
2. **Alexander OM:** *Radiography of the acromioclavicular articulation.* Med Radiogr Photogr 30:34, 1954.
3. **Zanca P:** *Shoulder pain: Involvement of the acromioclavicular joint. Analysis of 1000 cases.* AJR 112:493, 1971.
4. **Rockwood CA, Green DP:** *Fractures,* vol I, Philadelphia, JB Lippincott, 1975.
5. **Bossart PJ:** *Lack of efficacy of "weighted" radiographs in diagnosing acute acromioclavicular separation.* Ann Emerg Med 17:20, 1988.
6. **Keats TE, Pope TL Jr:** *The acromioclavicular joint: normal variation and the diagnosis of dislocation.* Skeletal Radiol 17:159, 1988.

ELBOW

1. **Buxton D:** *A radiographic survey of normal joints: The elbow joint.* Br J Radiol 29:395, 1924.
2. **Rogers LF:** *Fractures and dislocations of the elbow.* Semin Roentgenol 13:97, 1978.
3. **Holly EW:** *Radiography of the radial head.* Med Radiogr Photogr 32:13, 1956.
4. **Greenspan A, Norman A:** *Radial head-capitellum view: An expanded imaging approach to elbow injury.* Radiology 164:272, 1987.
5. **Jones R:** *A note on the treatment of injuries about the elbow.* Prov Med J 14:28, 1895.

WRIST

1. **Buxton D:** *A radiographic survey of normal joints: The wrist joint and hand.* Br J Radiol 32:199, 1927.
2. **Roderick JF:** *The roentgenographic examination of the carpus.* Xray Techn 18:8, 1946.
3. **Alexander OM:** *Radiography of the wrist.* Radiology 4:181, 1938.
4. **DeSmet AA, Martin NL, Fritz SL, et al:** *Radiographic projections for the diagnosis of arthritides of the hands and wrists.* Radiology 139:577, 1981.
5. **Kindynis P, Resnick D, Kang HS, et al:** *Demonstration of the scapholunate space with radiography.* Radiology 175:278, 1990.
6. **Gilula LA:** *Carpal injuries: Analytic approach and case exercises.* AJR 133:503, 1979.
7. **Terry DW Jr, Ramin JE:** *The navicular fat stripe. A useful roentgen feature for evaluating wrist trauma.* AJR 124:25, 1975.
8. **Bridgman CF:** *Radiography of the carpal navicular bone.* Med Radiogr Photogr 25:104, 1949.
9. **Fodor J, Malott JC:** *Radiography of the carpal navicular.* Radiol Technol 52:175, 1980.
10. **Lewis RW:** *Oblique views in roentgenography of the wrist.* AJR 50:119, 1943.
11. **MacEwan DW:** *Changes due to trauma in the fat plane of the pronator quadratus muscle: A radiologic sign.* Radiology 82:879, 1964.

HAND

1. **Buxton D:** *A radiographic survey of normal joints: The wrist joint and hand.* Br J Radiol 32:199, 1927.
2. **DeSmet AA, Martin NL, Fritz SL, et al:** *Radiographic projections for the diagnosis of arthritides of the hands and wrist.* Radiology 139:577, 1981.
3. **Yeh HC, Wolf BS:** *Radiographic anatomical landmarks of the metacarpophalangeal joints.* Radiology 122:353, 1977.
4. **Gramiak R:** *Oblique radiography of the hands.* Med Radiogr Photogr 42:28, 1966.

FINGERS

1. **Buxton D:** *A radiographic survey of normal joints. The wrist joint and hand.* Br J Radiol 32:199, 1927.
2. **DeSmet AA, Martin NL, Fritz SL, et al:** *Radiographic projections for the diagnosis of arthritides of the hands and wrists.* Radiology 139:577, 1981.
3. **Yeh HC, Wolf BS:** *Radiographic anatomical landmarks of the metacarpophalangeal joints.* Radiology 122:353, 1977.
4. **Reichmann S, Deichgraber E, Strid KG, et al:** *Soft-tissue radiography of finger joints.* Acta Radiol 15:439, 1974.

THUMB

1. **Buxton D:** *Radiographic survey of normal joints: The wrist joint and hand.* Br J Radiol 32:199, 1927.
2. **DeSmet AA, Martin NL, Fritz SL, et al:** *Radiographic projection for the diagnosis of arthritides of the hands and wrists.* Radiology 139:577, 1981.
3. **Kaye JJ:** *Fractures and dislocations of the hand and wrist.* Semin Roentgenol 13:109, 1978.
4. **Jones RP, Leach RE:** *Fracture of the ulnar sesamoid bones of the thumb.* Am J Sports Med 8:446, 1980.

RIBS

1. **Bartsch GW:** *Radiographic examination of the ribs.* Xray Techn 14:18, 1942.
2. **Rogers NJS:** *A technique of x-ray examination of the ribs.* Radiography 9:7, 1943.
3. **Bridgeman CF, Holly EW, Zariquiey MO:** *Radiography of the ribs and costovertebral joints.* Med Radiogr Photogr 32:38, 1956.
4. **Hohmann D, Gasteiger W:** *Roentgen diagnosis of the costovertebral joints.* Fortschr Roentgenstr 112:783, 1970.
5. **Morris L, Bailey J:** *A simple method to demonstrate the ribs and sternum.* Clin Radiol 21:320, 1970.

CHEST

1. **Pesauera GS:** *The evolution of chest roentgenographic technique.* AJR 40:405, 1938.
2. **Kattan KR, Wiot JF:** *How was this roentgenogram taken, AP or PA,* AJR 117:843, 1973.
3. **Bauer RG:** *High kilovoltage chest radiography with an air gap.* Radiol Technol 42:10, 1970.
4. **Kattan K:** *High kilovoltage oblique roentgenography of the chest; its advantage in differential diagnosis of the lung and pleura.* Dis Chest 50:605, 1966.
5. **Proto AV, Speckman JM:** *The left lateral radiograph of the chest.* Med Radiogr Photogr 55:30, 1979.
6. **Riggs W Jr, Parvey L:** *Differences between right and left lateral chest radiographs.* AJR 127:997, 1976.
7. **Bachman DM, Ellis K, Austin JH:** *The effects of minor degrees of obliquity on the lateral chest radiograph.* Radiol Clin N Am 16:465, 1978.
8. **Bray HA:** *A suggestion for improving the visibility of the apical field on the chest radiogram.* AJR 8:602, 1921.
9. **Lavner G, Copelman B:** *The anteroposterior lordotic projection in the roentgenographic examination of the lungs.* Radiology 43:135, 1944.
10. **Zinn B, Monroe J:** *The lordotic position in fluoroscopy and roentgenography of the chest.* AJR 75:682, 1956.
11. **Jacobson G, Sargent EN:** *Apical roentgenographic views of the chest.* AJR 104:822, 1968.
12. **Baum F, Black LT:** *The importance of the apical roentgenogram in pulmonary tuberculosis.* Am Rev Tuber 12:228, 1925.
13. **Flaxman AJ:** *Apical tuberculosis with roentgen technique.* Am Rev Tuber 54:1, 1946.

ABDOMEN

1. **Williams FH:** *X-ray examination of the abdomen.* Boston Med Surg J 23, 1900.
2. **Kelly JF, Dowell DH:** *The value of the preliminary film without opaque media in the diagnosis of abdominal conditions.* Radiology 29:104, 1937.
3. **Miller RE:** *The technical approach to the acute abdomen.* Semin Roentgenol 8:267, 1973.

2

Measurements in Skeletal Radiology

Lindsay J. Rowe and Terry R. Yochum

INTRODUCTION

Since the time of the first roentgen image, measurements have been used to evaluate normal and abnormal skeletal relationships. Many measurements have been determined through astute observation and appropriate statistical evaluation.

In all analytical assessments of skeletal spatial relationships, the outcome is dependent on the quality of the radiographic data collected and on its correct interpretation. Any attempt to measure and quantify the human frame has inherent, uncontrolled error. The major errors arising in the mensuration process include (a) image unsharpness, (b) projectional geometric distortion, (c) inconsistency in patient positioning, (d) individual anatomic vari-

ation, (e) imprecision in locating standard reference points, and (f) observer error. (1–4)

Additional confusion exists around the issues of clinical interpretation of measurements and their application to treatment protocols. This is highlighted in the spine and pelvis, where small measurements derived from various systems of analysis have often exerted a strong influence on treatment regimes. Among the various systems of analysis, there appears to be little correlation in the results obtained. (1,5–7) Many measurements have been used to evaluate spinal segmental motion abnormalities from static radiographs, which inadequately reflect motion biomechanics.

In general, any measurement is meaningless unless it is performed accurately and correlated clinically. (8,9) Too often it is the x-ray that is treated, not the patient. To rely on a radiographic measurement as the sole criterion for a particular treatment method is a frail approach to patient care.

In this chapter each measurement is described according to *synonyms, optimum projections, normal values, special considerations,* and *significance.* Whenever numerical data are given, they have been rounded for simplicity. Unless otherwise stated, the measurements are film image sizes and are not corrected for true anatomic dimensions. References to the literature are included so the reader may seek further information.

MEDICOLEGAL IMPLICATIONS
Radiographic Measurements

- The application of standard lines and measurements to radiographs often allows the detection of subtle abnormalities and assists in avoiding misdiagnosis.

- Comparison of studies is facilitated. This may allow regression or progression of the disorder to be recognized and the response to therapy quantified.

- Inherent errors in skeletal measurements are well recognized and must be minimized. The major errors arising in the mensuration process include (a) image unsharpness (image quality), (b) projectional geometric distortion, (c) inconsistency in patient positioning, (d) individual anatomic variation, (e) imprecision in locating standard reference points, and (f) observer error. (1–4)

- Knowledge of the normal range within a population for age and sex must be known as well as the significance of an abnormal measurement.

- Applying a measurement or line analysis system does not replace a pathologic evaluation of radiographs. Measurements and lines should only be applied after the film has been pathologically evaluated. No films should be obtained purely for a line or angular analysis.

- Accurate measurements cannot be made on poor quality or poorly positioned radiographs.

- Drawing on radiographs should be only done with a medium that can be readily removed without defacing the image if the need arises. Lines and angles should be marked on radiographs as sparingly as is clinically practicable.

- Any measurement made should not be the sole criterion for a diagnosis or for establishing a treatment regime. All measurements must be correlated clinically.

CORRECTION OF GEOMETRIC DISTORTION

Numerous methods can be used to determine the anatomic dimensions demonstrated on a given radiograph. These include nomograms and algebraic formulations. (1,2) The roentgen image is always larger than the true anatomic size because of the effect of diverging rays on a structure not in close contact with the film.

To algebraically arrive at the correct object size (*O*), three values must be known: (Fig. 2.1)

1. Film image dimension (cm) (*I*)
2. Target film distance (cm) (*D*)
3. Object film distance (cm) (*d*)

Initially, a correction factor (*CF*) is calculated:

$$CF = \frac{D - d}{D}$$

The film image dimension (*I*) is then multiplied by this correction factor:

$$O = I \times CF$$

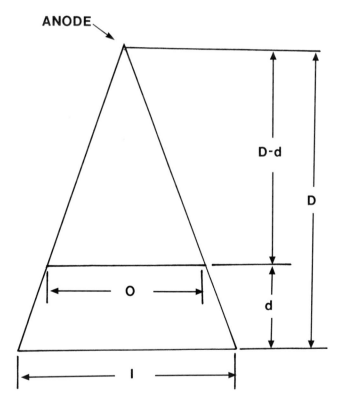

Figure 2.1.   GEOMETRIC DISTORTION IN IMAGE PRODUCTION.

SKULL

VASTINE-KINNEY METHOD OF PINEAL GLAND LOCALIZATION

Synonyms.   None.
Technique
Projection. Lateral skull.
Landmarks. The pineal gland must be visible as a result of calcium deposition before four measurements are made: (1) (Fig. 2.2)

A. The greatest distance from the pineal gland to the inner table of the frontal bone
B. The greatest distance from the pineal gland to the inner aspect of the occipital bone
C. The greatest distance from the pineal gland to the inner table of the skull vertex
D. The greatest distance from the pineal gland to the posterior margin of the foramen magnum

Normal Measurements. Measurements A and B are used to assess anterior or posterior pineal displacement, while measurements C and D are used to assess superior or inferior displacement.

1. *Anteroposterior position.* Measurement A is plotted against the sum of A and B and should fall within the specified range.
2. *Superoinferior position.* Measurement C is plotted against the sum of C and D and also should fall within a specified range. (2)

Special Considerations. An alternative and more accurate method for pineal gland localization is the Pawl-Walter method. (3)

Significance.   A pineal shift may be due to a space-occupying mass, such as a tumor, hemorrhage, or localized atrophic cerebral disease.

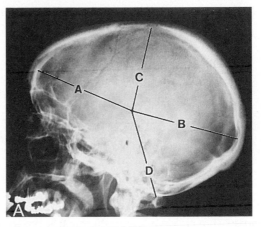

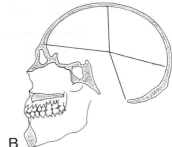

Figure 2.2.   VASTINE-KINNEY METHOD OF PINEAL LOCALIZATION (see text).

SELLA TURCICA SIZE

Synonyms.   Pituitary fossa size.
Technique
Projection. Lateral skull.
Landmarks. Two measurements are made—the greatest antero-posterior diameter and the greatest vertical diameter. The antero-posterior value is the widest distance between the anterior and posterior surfaces of the pituitary fossa. The vertical dimension is between the fossa floor and the plane between the opposing surfaces of the anterior and posterior clinoid processes. (4,5) (Fig. 2.3)

Normal Measurements. The anteroposterior dimension averages about 11 mm with a normal range of 5 to 16 mm. The vertical measurement averages about 8 mm with a normal range of 4 to 12 mm. (4–6) (Table 2.1) In children these values will be progressively smaller with decreasing chronologic age.

Table 2.1. Normal Values of Sella Turcica Size			
	Average (mm)	Minimum (mm)	Maximum (mm)
Anteroposterior	11	5	16
Vertical	8	4	12

Special Considerations. All lateral flexion and rotation of the skull should be eliminated in order for these measurements to be accurate.

Significance.   The finding of a small sella is of debatable significance. (7) However, an enlarged sella may be associated with a pituitary neoplasm, empty sella syndrome, extrapituitary mass (neoplasm, aneurysm), or may even be a normal variant.

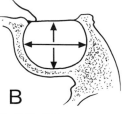

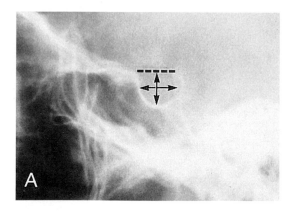

Figure 2.3. LATERAL MEASUREMENTS OF THE SELLA TURCICA (see text).

BASILAR ANGLE

Synonyms.   Welcker's basilar angle, Martin's basilar angle, sphenobasilar angle.
Technique
Projection. Lateral skull.
Landmarks. Three points are located, joined together by two lines, and the subsequent angle is measured. The three points are the nasion (frontal-nasal junction), the center of the sella turcica (midpoint between the clinoid processes), and the basion (anterior margin of the foramen magnum). (Fig. 2.4)

Normal Measurements. The average normal angle subtended by these two lines is 137° with a normal variation of 123 to 152°. (8) (Table 2.2)

Table 2.2. Normal Values of the Basilar Angle		
Average (°)	Minimum (°)	Maximum (°)
137	123	152

Significance.   The measurement is an index of the relationship between the anterior skull and its base. The angle will increase beyond 152° in platybasia, where the base is elevated in relation to the rest of the skull. This may or may not be associated with basilar impression. The deformity may be congenital (isolated impression, occipitalization) or acquired (Paget's disease, rheumatoid arthritis, fibrous dysplasia).

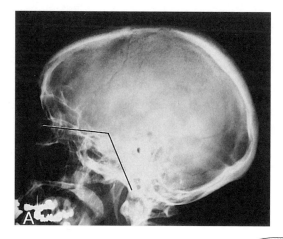

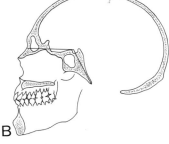

Figure 2.4.   BASILAR ANGLE (see text).

MCGREGOR'S LINE

Synonyms.   Basal line.

Technique

Projection. Lateral skull, lateral cervical.

Landmarks. A line is drawn from the posterosuperior margin of the hard palate to the most inferior surface of the occipital bone. (9) The relationship of the odontoid apex to this line is then examined. (Fig. 2.5)

Normal Measurements. In 90% of individuals the odontoid apex should not lie above this line more than 8 mm in males and 10 mm in females. (9) In children under the age of 18 years, these maximum values diminish with decreasing chronologic age.

Special Considerations. Of all methods used to evaluate for basilar impression on the lateral projection, McGregor's line appears to be the most accurate and reproducible. (10)

Significance.   An abnormal superior position of the odontoid is indicative of basilar impression. Common precipitating causes include platybasia, atlas occipitalization, and bone-softening diseases of the skull base, such as Paget's disease, osteomalacia, and fibrous dysplasia. Occasionally, rheumatoid arthritis may also precipitate this deformity.

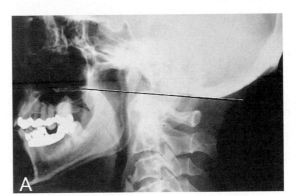

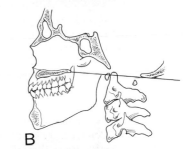

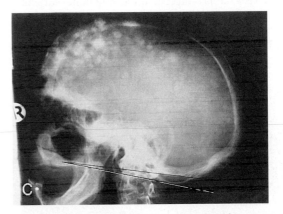

Figure 2.5.   McGREGOR'S LINE. A and B. Normal McGregor's Line (see text). **C. Abnormal McGregor's Line. (m)** Note the tip of the odontoid (retouched) is well above the line due to basilar invagination from Paget's disease.

CHAMBERLAIN'S LINE

Synonyms. Palato-occipital line.

Technique

Projection. Lateral skull, lateral cervical.

Landmarks. A line is constructed from the posterior margin of the hard palate to the posterior aspect of the foramen magnum. The relationship of this line to the tip of the odontoid process is then assessed. (11) (Fig. 2.6)

Normal Measurements. In the majority of patients the tip of the odontoid process should not project above this line; however, a normal variation of 3 mm above this line may occur. (8) A measurement of 7 mm or more is definitely abnormal.

Special Considerations. This relationship can also be evaluated on lateral cervical views but is best done on lateral skull films, preferably with tomography. To locate the posterior aspect of the foramen magnum, identify the inner table of the occipital bone and follow it anteriorly and observe for an oblique cortical white line crossing the diploe to merge with the outer table. This should be found slightly posterior to the plane of the atlas spinolaminar junction.

Significance. An abnormal superior position of the odontoid is indicative of basilar impression. Common precipitating causes include platybasia, atlas occipitalization, and bone- softening diseases of the skull base, such as Paget's disease, osteomalacia, and fibrous dysplasia. Occasionally, rheumatoid arthritis may also precipitate this deformity.

MACRAE'S LINE

Synonyms. Foramen magnum line.

Technique

Projection. Lateral skull.

Landmarks. A line is drawn between the anterior (basion) and posterior (opisthion) margins of the foramen magnum. Two assessments are then made in relation to this line: (1) the occipital bone, and (2) the odontoid process. (Fig. 2.7)

Normal Measurements. The inferior margin of the occipital bone should lie at or below this line. Additionally, a perpendicular line drawn through the odontoid apex should intersect this line in its anterior quarter. (10,12)

Special Considerations. A true lateral view with no lateral flexion distortion should be obtained in order for this positional line to be applied.

Significance. If the inferior margin of the occipital bone is convex in a superior direction and/or lies above this line, then basilar impression is present. Predisposing causes include platybasia, occipitalization, rheumatoid arthritis, and such bone-softening diseases as Paget's disease, osteomalacia, and fibrous dysplasia. If the odontoid apex does not lie in the ventral quarter of this line, a dislocation of the atlanto-occipital joint or a fracture or dysplasia of the dens may be present.

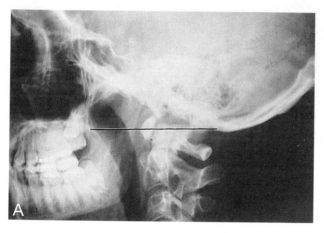

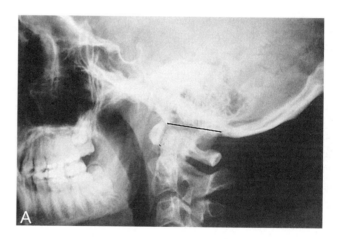

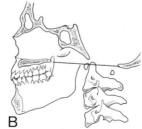

Figure 2.6. CHAMBERLAIN'S LINE (see text).

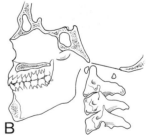

Figure 2.7. MACRAE'S LINE (see text).

DIGASTRIC LINE

Synonyms.   Biventor line.
Technique
Projection. Anteroposterior open mouth.
Landmarks. The digastric groove medial to the base of the mastoid process is located on each side, and a line is drawn between them. The vertical distance to the odontoid apex and atlanto-occipital joints is then measured. (Fig. 2.8)

Normal Measurements. The digastric line-odontoid apex average measurement is 11 mm but may range between 1 mm and 21 mm. The odontoid should not project above this line. The digastric line–atlanto-occipital joint average measurement is 12 mm with a normal range between 4 mm and 20 mm. (10,13) (Table 2.3)

Table 2.3. Normal Digastric Line Values			
	Average (mm)	Minimum (mm)	Maximum (mm)
Digastric-Odontoid	11	1	21
Digastric-CI-OCC Joint	12	4	20

Special Considerations. Tomographic evaluation is the most accurate method to use to obtain clear visualization of the necessary anatomic landmarks.

Significance.   Both measurements will decrease in basilar impression due to platybasia, occipitalization, and bone-softening diseases like Paget's disease, osteomalacia, and fibrous dysplasia.

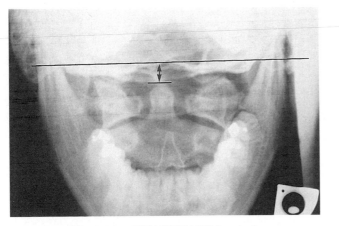

Figure 2.8.   DIGASTRIC LINE (see text).

HEIGHT INDEX OF KLAUS

Synonyms.   None.
Technique
Projection. Lateral skull, lateral cervical spine.
Landmarks. A line is drawn from the tuberculum sellae to the internal occipital protuberance. The vertical distance between this line and the apex of the odontoid is measured. (14) (Fig. 2.9)

Normal Measurements. (Refer to Table 2.4)

Table 2.4. Normal Values for the Height Index of Klaus	
Average (mm)	Minimum (mm)
40–41	30

Significance.   A measurement less than 30 mm indicates basilar impression. Values between 30 and 36 mm reflect a tendency toward basilar impression. (10,14) The wide range of normal variation casts doubt upon the usefulness of this measurement. (12)

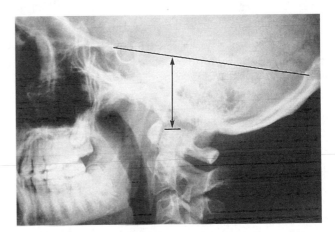

Figure 2.9.   HEIGHT INDEX OF KLAUS (see text).

BOOGARD'S LINE AND ANGLE

Synonyms. None.
Technique
Projection. Lateral skull, lateral cervical spine.
Landmarks.

Boogard's line: A line is drawn connecting the nasion to the opisthion. (15) (Fig. 2.10A)

Boogard's angle: A line is drawn between the basion and opisthion (MacRae's line). A second line is drawn from the dorsum sellae to the basion along the plane of the clivus. The angle between these two lines is measured. (15) (Fig. 2.10B)

Normal Measurements.

Boogard's line: The basion should lie below this line.
Boogard's angle: (Refer to Table 2.5)

Table 2.5. Normal Values for Boogard's Angle		
Average (°)	Minimum (°)	Maximum (°)
122	119	135

Significance. Both measurements will be altered in basilar impression—the basion will be above Boogard's line, and the angle will be greater than 135°.

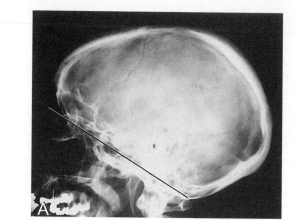

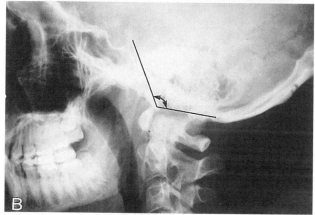

Figure 2.10.   A. BOOGARD'S LINE. B. BOOGARD'S ANGLE (see text).

ANTERIOR ATLANTO-OCCIPITAL DISLOCATION MEASUREMENT

Synonyms.   Power's index.
Technique
Projection. Lateral cervical spine, lateral skull.
Landmarks. Four osseous landmarks are located—the basion, opisthion, and the anterior and posterior arches of the atlas. Two measurements are then made:

1. The distance between the basion and the posterior arch at the spinolaminar junction (B–P).

2. The distance between the opisthion and the posterior margin of the anterior arch (O–A).

The ratio of these two measurements (B–P:O–A) is then calculated. (16) (Fig. 2.11)

Normal Measurements. In the normal individual the ratio is always less than one.

Special Considerations. This relationship can only be assessed when there are no associated fractures or dislocations of the atlas and odontoid process.

Significance.   When the ratio is equal to or greater than one, then an anterior atlanto-occipital dislocation probably exists.

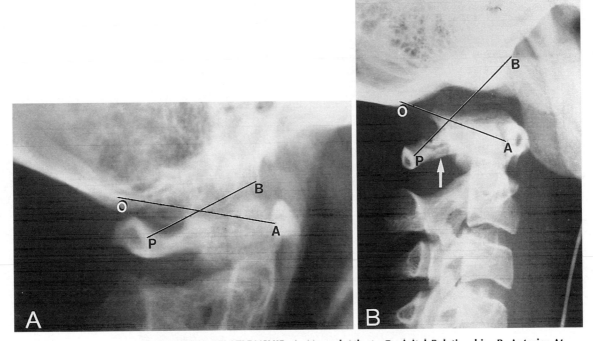

Figure 2.11.   ATLANTO-OCCIPITAL RELATIONSHIP. A. Normal Atlanto-Occipital Relationship. B. Anterior Atlanto-Occipital Dislocation (see text). Observe the posterior arch fracture of C1 (arrow). (Courtesy of Steven B. Wasserman, DC, Long Beach, California)

CERVICAL SPINE

ATLANTODENTAL INTERSPACE

Synonyms. Atlas-odontoid space, predental interspace, atlas-dens interval.

Technique

Projection. Lateral neutral, flexion-extension cervical spine.

Landmarks. The distance measured is between the posterior margin of the anterior tubercle and the anterior surface of the odontoid. (Fig. 2.12)

Normal Measurements. A small, insignificant difference exists between males and females. The measurement is slightly increased in normal children. (1,2) (Table 2.6) The shape of the interspace will alter in flexion to be a "V" configuration, while in extension an inverted "V" pattern will be visible. (3,4)

Special Considerations. Flexion is the optimum view to assess the interspace, since in this position the most stress is placed on the transverse ligament of the atlas.

Significance. There are numerous disorders that may alter the interspace. A decreased space is to be expected with advancing age because of degenerative joint disease of the atlantodental joint. A more significant change is an abnormally widened space with reduction in the neural canal size. (5) The most frequent causes include trauma, occipitalization, Down's syndrome, pharyngeal infections (Grisel's disease), and inflammatory arthropathies, such as ankylosing spondylitis, rheumatoid arthritis, psoriatic arthritis, and Reiter's syndrome. (5,6)

Table 2.6.	Normal Values of the Atlantodental Interspace	
	Minimum (mm)	Maximum (mm)
Adults	1	3
Children	1	5

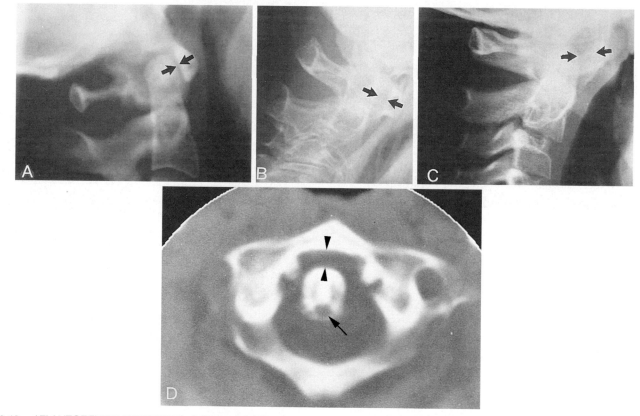

Figure 2.12.   ATLANTODENTAL INTERSPACE. A. Normal Adult Atlantodental Interspace. The interspace measures less than 3 mm (arrows). **B. Abnormal Atlantodental Interspace.** On flexion, a patient with rheumatoid arthritis exhibits anterior translation of the atlas by 5 mm (arrows). **C. Normal Childhood Atlantodental Interspace.** The interspace measures less than 5 mm (arrows). **D. CT Scan, Abnormal Atlantodental Interspace.** In this patient with rheumatoid arthritis, the atlantodental interspace is increased (arrowheads). Note the erosion at the posterior surface of the odontoid at the site of synovial tissue beneath the transverse ligament (arrow).

METHOD OF BULL

Synonyms.   None.

Technique

Projection. Lateral skull, lateral cervical.

Landmarks. Two lines are drawn and the resultant angle measured. The first line is drawn from the posterior aspect of the hard palate to the posterior margin of the foramen magnum (Chamberlain's line). The second line is drawn through the midpoints of the anterior and posterior tubercles of the atlas (atlas plane line). The angle formed posteriorly is then measured. (7) (Fig. 2.13)

Normal Measurements. The posterior angle formed by these two lines should be 13°. If this angle is greater than 13°, it is abnormal. (2)

Special Considerations. The accuracy of this measurement is affected in individuals with acute neck pain due to muscular spasm.

Significance.   The angle will increase if the odontoid is tilted posteriorly because of congenital malformation or fracture displacement. In some individuals the atlas may be altered in position, which changes this angle even in the absence of odontoid abnormality.

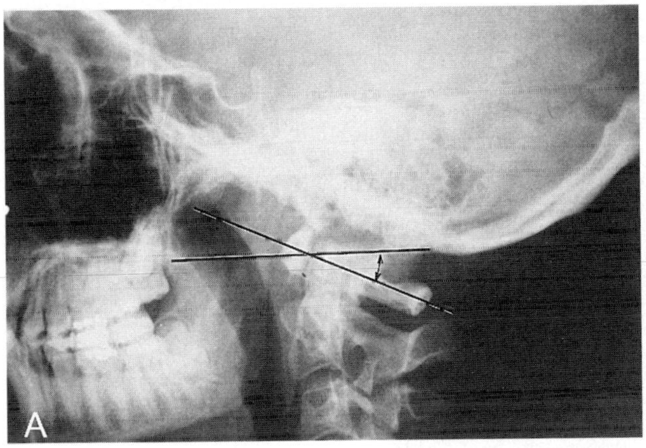

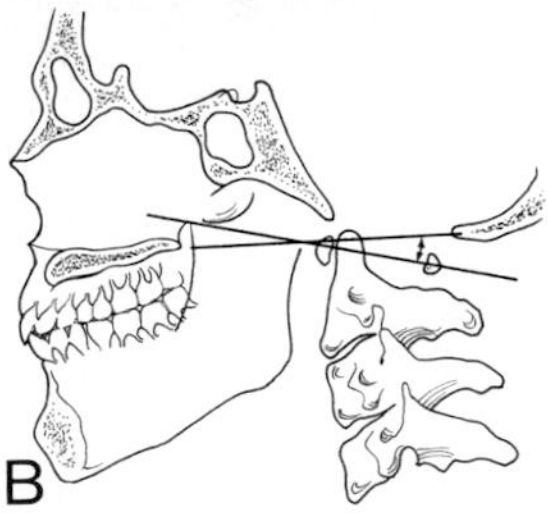

GEORGE'S LINE

Synonyms.   Posterior vertebral alignment line, posterior body line.

Technique

Projection. Lateral cervical.

Landmarks. The posterior vertebral body surfaces are connected with a continuous line that traverses the intervertebral disc. A straight line cannot be drawn because of the normal concavity of the posterior surface. The key landmarks are the alignment of the superior and inferior posterior body corners. (Fig. 2.14)

Normal Measurements. Normally, there is a smooth vertical alignment of each posterior body corner.

Special Considerations. Flexion and extension films are especially useful in determining disruptions in George's line. (8,9) The posterior body line can be incorporated with other complex measuring systems to assess stability. (10,11) Care should be taken to eliminate positional rotation, since this will create a projectional disruption of the line at consecutive levels ("stair stepping"). This line can be applied throughout the entire spine.

Significance.   In 1919 George called attention to the relevance of ascertaining alignment in order to detect posttraumatic cervical injuries. (12,13) Proper alignment of the posterior vertebral bodies signified no fracture, dislocation, or ligamentous laxity. In burst fractures of the vertebral body a posteriorly displaced fragment of bone will lie behind the line. (14,15) If an anterolisthesis or retrolisthesis is present, then this may be a radiologic sign of instability due to fracture, dislocation, ligamentous laxity, or degenerative joint disease.

Figure 2.13.   METHOD OF BULL (see text).

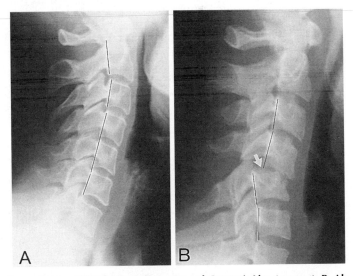

Figure 2.14.   GEORGE'S LINE. A. Normal George's Line (see text). **B. Abnormal George's Line.** Due to traumatic bilateral facet dislocation (arrow).

POSTERIOR CERVICAL LINE

Synonyms.   Spinolaminar junction line, arch-body line.
Technique
Projection. Lateral cervical (neutral, flexion, extension).
Landmarks. The cortical white line of the spinolaminar junction is first identified at each level C1 to C7. Each spinolaminar junction will be curved anteriorly slightly from superior to inferior. For consistency, the most anterior part of the convexity will be compared between levels. (Fig. 2.15)

Normal Measurements. When each spinolaminar junction point is joined, a smooth arclike curve results. At the C2 level, the spinolaminar junction line in children should not be more than 2 mm anterior to this line.

Significance.   If the drawn curve is discontinuous at any level, then an anterior or posterior displacement may be present. This line is especially useful in the detection of subtle odontoid fractures and atlantoaxial subluxation (anterior), which otherwise may be easily overlooked. (16) A disruption in the middle to lower cervical spine may also be a sign of anterolisthesis, retrolisthesis, or frank dislocation.

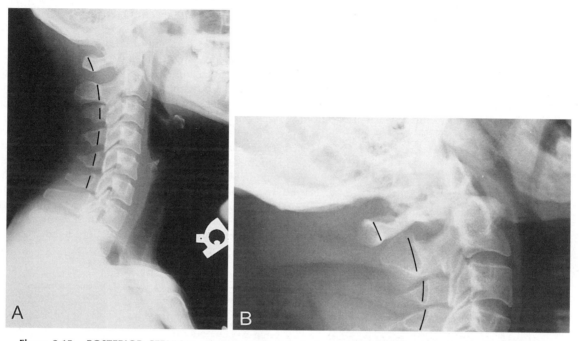

Figure 2.15.   POSTERIOR CERVICAL LINE. A. Normal Posterior Cervical Line (see text). **B. Abnormal Posterior Cervical Line.** Due to posterior displacement of the atlas secondary to os odontoideum.

SAGITTAL DIMENSION OF THE CERVICAL SPINAL CANAL

Synonyms. None.

Technique

Projection. Lateral cervical (neutral, flexion, extension).

Landmarks. The sagittal diameter is measured from the posterior surface of the midvertebral body to the nearest surface of the same segmental spinolaminar junction line. (17) (Fig. 2.16)

Normal Measurements. These will vary according to the cervical level. (18) (Table 2.7) Values will alter in children. (17,19)

Table 2.7.   Normal Sagittal Diameter of the Cervical Spinal Canal

Level	Average (mm)	Minimum (mm)	Maximum (mm)
C1	22	16	31
C2	20	14	27
C3	18	13	23
C4	17	12	22
C5	17	12	22
C6	17	12	22
C7	17	12	22

Significance. Narrowing of the canal (stenosis) may be present when the measurement is less than 12 mm, which can be assessed on plain film and on computed tomography (CT) and magnetic resonance imaging (MRI). (20) If degenerative posterior osteophytes are present, the measurement can be made from their tip to examine the magnitude of the stenotic effect. The degree of stenosis from these spurs is best measured on extension films. (18) An abnormally widened canal may be associated with a spinal cord neoplasm or syringomyelia.

The most accurate measurement is by the ratio of the sagittal dimension of the canal and vertebral body (canal–body ratio, Pavlov's ratio). (21,22) A ratio of less than 0.82 is significant for spinal stenosis. (21) The benefit of this method is that it removes the effects of radiographic magnification.

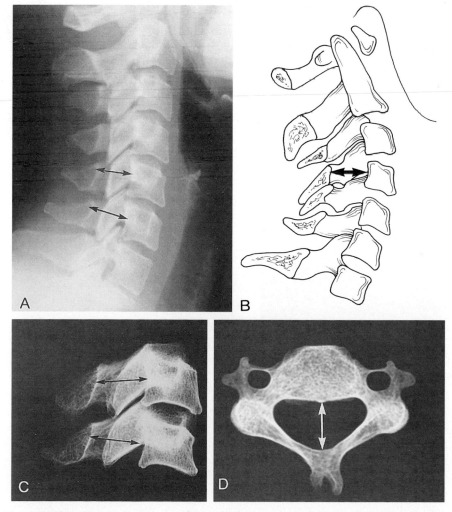

Figure 2.16.   CERVICAL SPINAL CANAL. A and B. Sagittal Dimensions of the Cervical Spinal Canal (arrows) (see text). **C and D.** Dry specimen correlation demonstrating the distance being evaluated (arrows).

ATLANTOAXIAL ALIGNMENT

Synonyms. Spread of the atlas.
Technique
Projection. Anteroposterior open mouth, cervical spine.
Landmarks. The lateral margins of the atlas lateral masses are compared to the opposing lateral corner of the axis articular surface. (Fig. 2.17)
Normal Measurements. These two landmarks should be in vertical alignment.
Significance. If the lateral margin of the atlas lateral mass lies lateral to the lateral axis margin, this may be a radiologic sign of Jefferson's fracture, odontoid fracture, alar ligament instability, or rotatory atlantoaxial subluxation. (23,24) If there is overhang of the lateral mass in combination with a laterally tilted dens of more than 5°, there is at least a 70% probability a fracture of the odontoid is present. (25) In children up to 4 years of age, overhang of the atlas may be a normal variant resulting from accelerated growth of the atlas ("pseudospread"). (24,26)

CERVICAL GRAVITY LINE

Synonyms. None.
Technique
Projection. Lateral cervical spine (neutral).
Landmarks. A vertical line is drawn through the apex of the odontoid process. (27) (Fig. 2.18)
Normal Measurements. This line should pass through the seventh cervical body.
Significance. The line allows a gross assessment of where the gravitational stresses are acting at the cervicothoracic junction.

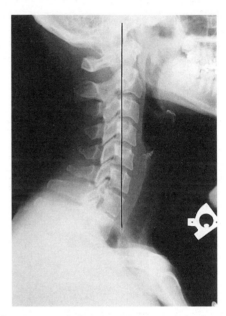

Figure 2.18. CERVICAL GRAVITY LINE (see text).

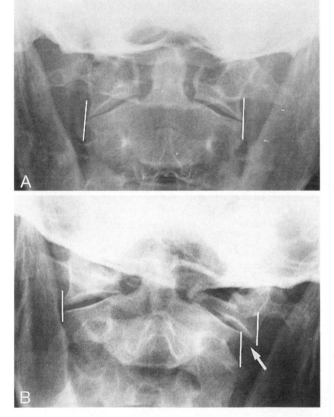

Figure 2.17. ATLANTOAXIAL ALIGNMENT. A Normal Atlantoaxial Alignment. B. Abnormal Atlantoaxial Alignment. (arrow) Due to Jefferson's fracture of the atlas.

CERVICAL LORDOSIS

Synonyms.   Angle of the cervical curve, cervical (lordotic) angle.

Technique
Projection. Cervical spine, neutral.
Landmarks. Numerous methods have been devised. (28-35) Some are described here.

Depth of cervical curve. (32) A line is drawn from the superior posterior aspect of the odontoid to the posterior inferior corner of the seventh cervical vertebra. The greatest transverse distance between this line and the posterior vertebral bodies is measured. (Fig. 2.19A)

Method of Jochumsen. (33) A line is drawn from the anterior border of the atlas anterior tubercle to the anterosuperior corner of the seventh cervical body. The distance from this line to the anterior border of the fifth cervical body is then measured. (Fig. 2.19B)

Angle of cervical curve. (34) Two lines are drawn, one through and parallel to the inferior endplate of the seventh cervical body, the other through the midpoints of the anterior and posterior tubercles of the atlas (atlas plane line). Perpendiculars are then constructed to the point of intersection, and the resultant angle is measured. (Fig. 2.19C)

Method of Gore. (28) A line is drawn through the posterior surface of the C2 body and another through the posterior surface of the C7 vertebral body. The angle formed by these two lines is measured.

Method of Drexler. (35) This is a laborious but accurate method. Each individual segment is assessed by drawing lines along the body endplates and measuring the resultant angle. The lordosis value is the cumulative total of each intersegmental measurement.

Normal Measurements. (Table 2.8)
Special Considerations. The position of the head is a critical factor in determining the lordosis. If the chin is lowered, tucked downward, or retracted 1 inch, the effect is to straighten the lordosis. (36-38)

Table 2.8. Normal Values of Cervical Lordosis

Method	Average	Minimum	Maximum
Depth (mm)	12	7	17
Jochumsen (mm)	3–8	1	9
Angle (°)	40	35	45
Drexler (°)	40	16	60

Significance.   Many authors have stressed the lack of correlation between altered cervical curvature and clinical symptomatology and its limitations as a prognostic indicator. (31,39) However, a reduced or reversed curve may be observed following trauma, muscle spasm, and degenerative spondylosis. (31,32,36,37,40) In patients with myelopathy due to degenerative stenosis, response to laminectomy is diminished when the lordosis is reversed or straightened. (41)

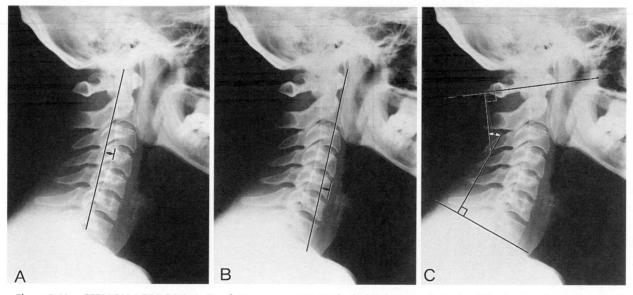

Figure 2.19.   CERVICAL LORDOSIS. A. Depth Measurement. B. Method of Jochumsen. C. Angle of the Cervical Curve (see text).

STRESS LINES OF THE CERVICAL SPINE

Synonyms.   Ruth Jackson's lines.
Technique
Projection. Lateral cervical spine (flexion, extension).
Landmarks. On each film two lines are constructed. The first line is drawn along the posterior surface of the axis. The second line is drawn along the posterior surface of the seventh cervical body until it intersects the axis line. (40) (Fig. 2.20)

Normal Measurements.

1. *Flexion.* These lines normally should intersect at the level of the C5-C6 disc or facet joints.
2. *Extension.* These lines normally should intersect at the level of the C4-C5 disc or facet joints.

Significance.   The value of these lines has not been established. The intersection point represents the focus of stress when the cervical spine is placed in the respective positions. (40) Their point of intersection does not appear to correlate with the level of degenerative disc disease. (42) Muscle spasm, joint fixation, and disc degeneration may alter the stress point.

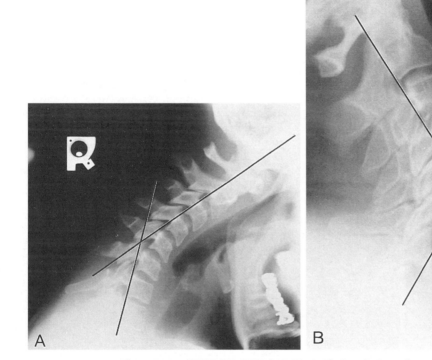

Figure 2.20.   CERVICAL STRESS LINES. A. Flexion. B. Extension (see text).

PREVERTEBRAL SOFT TISSUES

Synonyms.   Retropharyngeal interspace (RPI), retrolaryngeal interspace (RLI), retrotracheal interspace space (RTI).

Technique

Projection. Lateral cervical (neutral, flexion, extension).

Landmarks. The soft tissue in front of the vertebral bodies and behind the air shadow of the pharynx, larynx, and trachea is measured. The bony landmarks are the anterior arch of the atlas, the inferior corners of the axis and C3, the superior corner of C4, and the inferior corners of C5, C6, and C7. (43,44) At C2-C3 this is called the retropharyngeal interspace; behind the larynx, the retrolaryngeal interspace (C4-C5); and behind the trachea (C5-C7), the retrotracheal interspace. (Fig. 2.21)

Normal Measurements. These will vary according to the level being measured and the position of the patient at the time of the exposure. (43,44) (Table 2.9)

Special Considerations. The values at the C4 and C5 levels may alter depending on the position of the larynx, which may change with swallowing, screaming, axial rotation, and lateral flexion. (44) There is no difference between sexes, and the values are not altered significantly by radiographic magnification. (44) Patients larger than 180 lb (82 kg) may have a space 1 mm more than the normal range, while patients over 70 years of age have spaces of 1 mm less than normal. (44) No more than 1 mm change occurs in the measurement between flexion and neutral. (43) Anterior degenerative osteophytes may cause deflection of the pharyngeal contour.

Significance.   Any soft tissue mass may increase these measurements. These include posttraumatic hematoma, retropharyngeal abscess, or neoplasm from the adjacent bone and soft tissue structures.

Table 2.9.	Normal Cervical Prevertebral Soft Tissue Values		
Level	Flexion (mm)	Neutral (mm)	Extension (mm)
C1	11	10	8
C2	6	5	6
C3	7	7	6
C4	7	7	8
C5	22	20	20
C6	20	20	19
C7	20	20	21

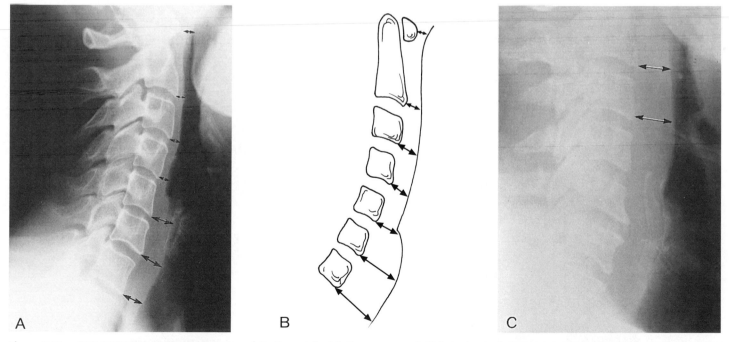

Figure 2.21.   PREVERTEBRAL SOFT TISSUE. A and B. Prevertebral Soft Tissues (arrows) (see text). **C. Abnormal Retropharyngeal Soft Tissue Measurement.** This is due to hematoma formation following cervical trauma (arrows). (Courtesy of Norman W. Kettner, DC, DACBR, St. Louis, Missouri)

THORACIC SPINE

COBB METHOD OF SCOLIOSIS EVALUATION

Synonyms.   Cobb-Lippman method.
Technique
Projection. Anteroposterior spine.
Landmarks.

End vertebrae. There are two, one each located at the superior and inferior extremes of the scoliosis. They are defined as the last segment that contributes to the spinal curvature. They appear as the last segment at the extreme ends of the scoliosis, where the endplates tilt to the side of the curvature concavity.

Endplate lines. On the superior end vertebra, a line is drawn through and parallel to the superior endplate. On the inferior end vertebra, a line is constructed in a similar manner through and parallel to the inferior endplate.

Perpendicular lines. At right angles to both endplate lines, lines are drawn to intersect, and their resultant angle is measured. (Fig. 2.22)

Special Considerations. This is the preferred method in scoliosis assessment. In those with double scoliotic curves each component should be measured. Care should be taken to ensure that common landmarks are utilized in progressive evaluations. Interobserver errors in measurement range up to 10°, which is a problem, since progression of a scoliosis of 5° between two successive radiographs is considered significant when deciding on therapeutic options. (1–3)

Significance.   This procedure was introduced by Lippman in 1935 and popularized later by Cobb. (4) Essentially, curvatures less than 20° require no bracing or surgical intervention; however, if curvatures less than 20° are present in a patient between 10 and 15 years of age, careful monitoring should be implemented to assess for progression of 5° or more in any 3-month period. (1,5) Curves between 20 and 40° should be braced to prevent progression in the growth period. Surgical intervention may be contemplated for cosmetic reasons, underlying anomaly, curvature progression in an immature spine, or curvature in excess of 40°. (See Chapter 4)

RISSER-FERGUSON METHOD OF SCOLIOSIS EVALUATION

Synonyms.   None.
Technique
Projection. Anteroposterior spine.
Landmarks.

1. *End vertebrae.* Same as described under the Cobb method.
2. *Apical vertebra.* This vertebral segment is the most laterally placed in the curve and usually is the most rotated.
3. *Vertebral body center.* For each end vertebra and apical segment, diagonals are drawn from opposing corners of the body to locate the body center.
4. *Connecting line.* Two lines are constructed connecting the body centers of the apical segment with each end vertebra, and the resultant angle is measured. (Fig. 2.23)

Special Considerations. This method gives values approximately 25% below those of the Cobb method (10°), and some investigators have advocated its use in larger curves, but this practice is to be discouraged. (6) (See Chapter 4)

Significance.   Ferguson first introduced this methodology in the early 1920s and later published his findings in the 1930s and 1940s. (7,8) Like the Cobb method, this assesses the degree of scoliosis and provides data used in the therapeutic decision process.

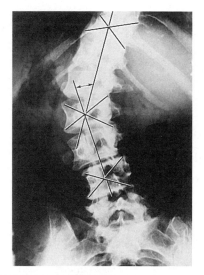

Figure 2.23.   RISSER-FERGUSON METHOD OF SCOLIOSIS EVALUATION (see text).

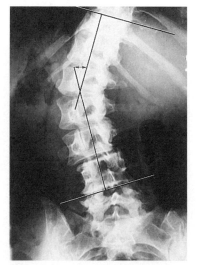

Figure 2.22.   COBB METHOD OF SCOLIOSIS EVALUATION (see text).

THORACIC KYPHOSIS

Synonyms.   None.
Technique
Projection. Lateral thoracic spine.
Landmarks. A line is drawn parallel to and through the superior endplate of the first thoracic vertebral body. A similar line is drawn through the inferior endplate of the twelfth thoracic vertebral body. Perpendicular lines to these endplate lines are then constructed, and the resultant angle is measured at the intersection of the lines. (Fig. 2.24)

Normal Measurements. These will vary according to age and sex. (9) (Tables 2.10, 2.11)

Table 2.10.   Degree of Normal Kyphosis in Females by Age

| Age | Kyphosis (°) | | | |
	Mean	SD	Minimum	Maximum
2–9	24	7	8	36
10–19	26	7	11	41
20–29	27	8	7	40
30–39	28	9	10	42
40–49	33	7	21	50
50–59	41	10	22	53
60–69	45	8	34	54
70–79	42	9	30	56

Table 2.11.   Degree of Normal Kyphosis in Males by Age

| Age (yr) | Kyphosis (°) | | | |
	Mean	SD	Minimum	Maximum
2–9	21	8	5	40
10–19	25	8	8	39
20–29	26	8	13	48
30–39	29	8	13	49
40–49	30	7	17	44
50–59	33	6	25	45
60–69	35	5	25	62
70–79	41	8	32	66

Special Considerations. Frequently, the vertebral bodies at the ends of the thoracic spine will not be clearly visible. In these circumstances the first visible segment will suffice but may alter the angular value. Interobserver errors in measurement up to 11° are common. (2) Physiologic anterior vertebral body wedging accounts for the natural kyphotic curvature of the thoracic spine. (10,11) This normal anterior wedging for each vertebral body is approximately 4 to 5° or 2 to 3 mm. (11–14) The wedging increases by almost 1 mm for each successive level, with approximately 45° of thoracic kyphosis accounted for by this wedging. (11)

Significance.   The kyphosis may be altered in many disorders. An increased kyphosis may be seen in old age, osteoporosis, Scheuermann's disease, congenital anomalies, muscular paralysis, and even cystic fibrosis. (9,15) The degree of kyphosis increases with age, and the rate of increase is greater in females than in males. (16)

A reduction in the kyphosis (straight back syndrome) may alter the dynamics of intracardiac blood flow and manifest as an apparent cardiac murmur. (17,18)

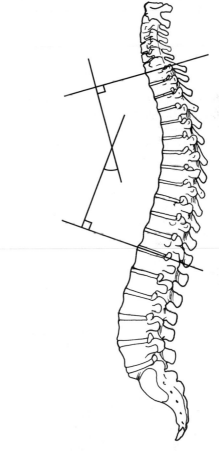

Figure 2.24.   THORACIC KYPHOSIS MEASUREMENT (see text).

THORACIC CAGE DIMENSION

Synonyms.   Straight back syndrome evaluation.
Technique
Projection. Lateral chest.
Landmarks. The distance between the posterior sternum and anterior surface of the eighth thoracic vertebral body is measured. (Fig. 2.25)
Normal Measurements. The sagittal dimension will normally vary slightly. (18) (Table 2.12)

Table 2.12.	Normal Sagittal Dimensions of the Thoracic Cage		
	Average (cm)	Minimum (cm)	Maximum (cm)
Male	14	11	18
Female	12	9	15

Significance.   A measured sagittal dimension below 13 cm in males and below 11 cm in females may indicate the presence of the straight back syndrome. (Table 2.13) If an abnormal measurement is found, the chest should be auscultated for a cardiac murmur. If detected, an organic cause should be searched for, although one may not be found. The decreased anteroposterior diameter may create such a murmur by creating cardiac compression and altered intracardiac hemodynamics. (17,18)

Table 2.13.	Sagittal Dimensions in the Straight Back Syndrome		
	Average (cm)	Minimum (cm)	Maximum (cm)
Male	11	9	13
Female	10	8	11

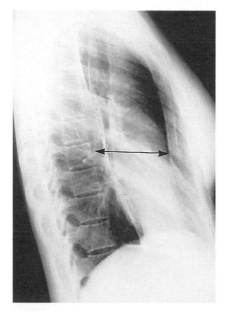

Figure 2.25.   SAGITTAL THORACIC CAGE DIMENSION IN STRAIGHT BACK SYNDROME (arrows) (see text).

LUMBAR SPINE

INTERVERTEBRAL DISC HEIGHT

Synonyms.   None.
Technique
Projection. Lateral, lumbar spine.
Landmarks. A number of methodologies have been described, but only two are presented. (1,2)

Hurxthal method. (3) The distance between the opposing endplates at the midpoint between the anterior and posterior vertebral body margins is measured. (Fig. 2.26A)
Farfan's method. (4) The anterior and posterior disc heights are measured and expressed as a ratio to disc diameter. These two ratios are then reduced to a ratio of each other. (Fig. 2.26B)

$$\text{Anterior Height Ratio (AHR)} = \frac{\text{Anterior Height (A)}}{\text{Diameter (D)}}$$

$$\text{Posterior Height Ratio (PHR)} = \frac{\text{Posterior Height (P)}}{\text{Diameter (D)}}$$

$$\text{Disc Height (DH)} = \frac{\text{AHR}}{\text{PHR}}.$$

Normal Measurements. Considerable variation exists in disc height, according to the lumbar interspace being assessed.
Special Considerations. Where segmental rotation exceeds 40° or lateral flexion is greater than 20°, these methods become unreliable.
Significance.   Disc spaces can be altered in many conditions. The most common causes for a decreased disc height include disc degeneration, postsurgery, postchemonucleolysis, infection, and congenital hypoplasia. There is poor correlation between loss of disc height and the focus for low back pain. (2,5)

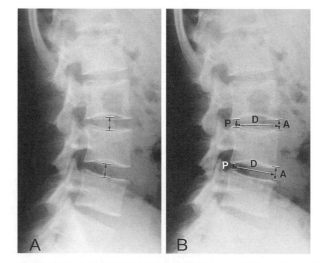

Figure 2.26.   INTERVERTEBRAL DISC HEIGHT MEASUREMENT. A. Hurxthal Method (arrows) (see text). **B. Farfan Method** (arrows) (see text).

LUMBAR INTERVERTEBRAL DISC ANGLES

Synonyms. None.
Technique
Projection. Lateral lumbar spine.
Landmarks. Lines are drawn through and parallel to each lumbar body endplate, the lines being extended posteriorly until they intersect. The angles formed at each interspace are then measured. (Fig. 2.27)
Normal Measurements. These vary according to the lumbar level. (6) (Table 2.14)

Table 2.14. Normal Lumbar Intervertebral Disc Angles	
Disc Level	**Average Angle (°)**
L1	8
L2	10
L3	12
L4	14
L5	14

Special Considerations. An alternative method of measurement includes the vertebral bodies in the calculation. (7)

Significance. The mean angular values will be altered in conditions of antalgia, muscular imbalance, and improper posture. These measurements may be of assistance in distinguishing the origins of low back pain. In facet syndrome the angles may be increased, while in acute discal injuries a reduction in the angle may be seen. (7)

LUMBAR LORDOSIS

Synonyms.   Lumbar curve, lumbar spinal angle, lumbar angle.
Technique
Projection. Lateral lumbar spine.
Landmarks. A line is drawn through and parallel to the superior endplate of the first lumbar segment. A second line is drawn through the superior endplate of the first sacral segment. Perpendiculars are then erected, and the angle at their intersection measured. (Fig. 2.28)
Normal Measurements. A wide variation exists within normal individuals. However, an average appears to be approximately 50 to 60°. (6,7)
Special Considerations. Some investigators prefer to use the inferior endplate of the fifth lumbar body in order to eliminate the effects of an altered sacral position. (8)
Significance.   The significance of an altered lumbar curve has not been delineated. A wide spectrum of opinions have been expressed, from it being of no importance (9) to it being a prime consideration as it relates to low back pain. (7,10–13) An increase in lordosis tends to move the nucleus pulposus anteriorly; the significance of this finding is unclear. (14) There is no difference in lordosis between whites and blacks. (15)

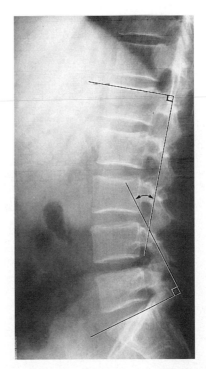

Figure 2.28.   LUMBAR LORDOSIS MEASUREMENT (see text).

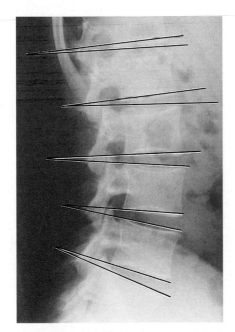

Figure 2.27.   LUMBAR INTERVERTEBRAL DISC ANGLES (see text).

LUMBOSACRAL LORDOSIS ANGLE

Synonyms.   None.
Technique
Projection. Lateral lumbar spine.
Landmarks. Two lines are drawn, and the angle formed is measured.

1. The centers of the third and fifth lumbar bodies are located by intersecting diagonal lines from opposing corners for each of the two vertebra. A line is then constructed joining the midpoints of these two bodies.
2. The midpoint of the first sacral segment is located in a similar manner, and a second line is then drawn between the fifth lumbar and first sacral midpoints.
3. The angle formed posteriorly is measured. (Fig. 2.29)

Normal Measurements. A wide variation in this angle exists. (16) (Table 2.15)

Table 2.15. Normal Values of the Lumbosacral Lordosis		
Average (°)	Minimum (°)	Maximum (°)
146	124	162

Special Considerations. There appear to be small changes in this angle between the recumbent and upright positions.
Significance.   The role of an excessive or diminished lumbosacral lordosis angle has not been adequately assessed; however, this is a measurement that can be applied when the upper lumbar segments are not included in the field of study.

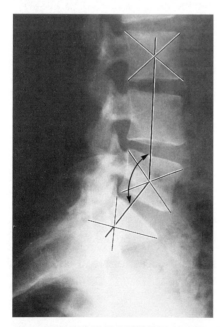

Figure 2.29.   LUMBOSACRAL LORDOSIS ANGLE (see text).

SACRAL INCLINATION

Synonyms.   Sacral tilt angle.
Technique
Projection. Lateral sacrum, lumbar spine.
Landmarks. Two lines are drawn:

1. A tangential line parallel to and through the posterior margin of the first sacral segment and
2. A vertical line intersecting the tangential sacral line. The angle formed is then measured. (Fig. 2.30)

Normal Measurements. A wide variation occurs. (16) (Table 2.16)

Table 2.16. Normal Sacral Inclination		
Average (°)	Minimum (°)	Maximum (°)
46	30	72

Significance.   This measurement can be used in the assessment of sacral position and provides additional data on the static mechanics of the low lumbar spine.

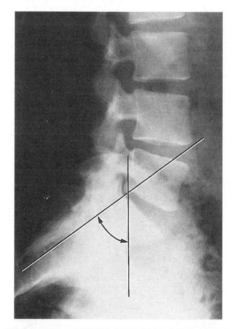

Figure 2.30.   SACRAL INCLINATION (see text).

LUMBOSACRAL ANGLE

Synonyms.   Sacral base angle, Ferguson's angle.
Technique
Projection. Lateral lumbar, lumbosacral.
Landmarks. Two lines are drawn and the resultant angle measured.

1. A horizontal line is made parallel to the bottom edge of the film.
2. An oblique line is drawn through and parallel to the sacral base. (17–19) (Fig. 2.31)

Normal Measurements. A wide normal variation is encountered. (20) (Table 2.17) The value will also increase from the recumbent to upright positions by 8 to 12°.

Table 2.17.	Normal Lumbosacral Angle Values			
	Average (°)	One SD	Minimum (°)	Maximum (°)
Upright	41	±7	26	57

Significance.   There is no consensus of opinion on the exact role and significance of either a decreased or increased lumbosacral angle. (13,21-23) An increased angle has been implicated as a mechanical factor in producing low back pain by increasing shearing and compressive forces on the lumbosacral posterior joints. (17,24,25) An increased sacral base angle does not appear to be associated with an increased incidence of spondylolisthesis. (26)

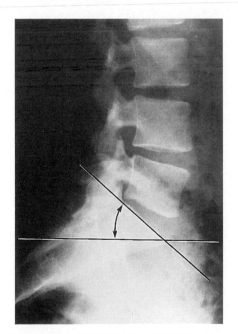

Figure 2.31.   LUMBOSACRAL ANGLE (see text).

LUMBOSACRAL DISC ANGLE

Synonyms.   Sacrovertebral disc angle.
Technique
Projection. Lateral lumbar, lumbosacral spine.
Landmarks. A line is drawn parallel and through the inferior endplate of the fifth lumbar and superior endplate of the first sacral segment. The angle formed by these lines is then measured. (17) (Fig. 2.32)

Normal Measurements. The normal range appears to be between 10 and 15°. (7,27)

Significance.   An increase in the lumbosacral disc angle more than 15° has been linked to the presence of low back pain due to facet impaction. (27) Also there may be a decrease in the value in the presence of acute disc herniation at the fifth lumbar disc. (7) An increased lumbosacral disc angle does not appear to be associated with an increased incidence of spondylolisthesis. (26)

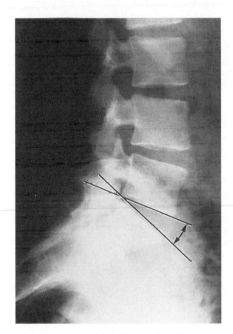

Figure 2.32.   LUMBOSACRAL DISC ANGLE (see text).

STATIC VERTEBRAL MALPOSITIONS

Synonyms.   Static intersegmental subluxations.
Technique
Projection. Anteroposterior and lateral spine.
Landmarks. Numerous terms are applied to describe static vertebral malpositions: (28) (Fig. 2.33)

1. *Flexion.* The endplates of the opposed segments diverge posteriorly in the lateral view.
2. *Extension* (Fig. 2.33A). The endplates of the opposed segments converge more than normal posteriorly in the lateral view.
3. *Lateral flexion* (Fig. 2.33B). The endplates of the opposed segments diverge laterally on one side and converge on the other side in the anteroposterior view.
4. *Rotation* (Fig. 2.33C). The pedicles will be asymmetrical in shape, and the spinous may be deviated in the anteroposterior view.
5. *Anterolisthesis* (Fig. 2.33D). An anterior displacement of one vertebral body in relation to the vertebra below.
6. *Retrolisthesis* (Fig. 2.33D). A posterior displacement of one vertebral body in relation to the vertebra below.
7. *Laterolisthesis* (Fig. 2.33C). A sideways displacement of one vertebral body in relation to the vertebra below.

Special Considerations. This classification system and terminology can be used for the entire vertebral column. The position of the superior vertebra is always described relative to the subadjacent vertebra; i.e., there is a retrolisthesis of C4 upon C5.

Significance.   These various interbody disrelationships may be related to degenerative processes, antalgia, or abnormal mechanics; however, the recognition of these displacements does not necessarily confirm a clinically significant finding.

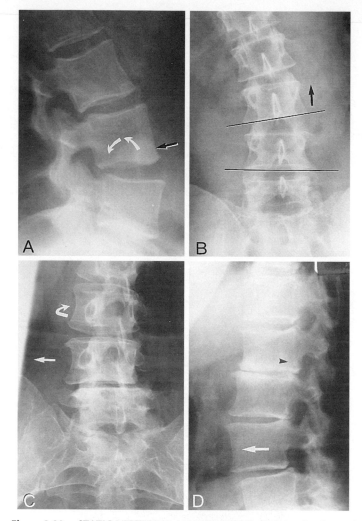

Figure 2.33.   STATIC VERTEBRAL MALPOSITIONS. A. Extension (curved arrows). Of incidental notation, observe the domed sclerosis at the antero-inferior aspect of the L3 vertebral body (arrow). This has been called hemispherical spondylosclerosis. **B. Lateral Flexion** (arrow). **C. Laterolisthesis** (arrow), **Rotation** (curved arrow). **D. Anterolisthesis** (arrow), **Retrolisthesis** (arrowhead).

LUMBAR GRAVITY LINE

Synonyms. Ferguson's weight-bearing line, Ferguson's gravitational line.

Technique

Projection. Lateral lumbar.

Landmarks. The center of the third lumbar body is located by intersecting diagonals from opposing body corners. A vertical line is then constructed through this point, and the relationship to the upper sacrum is assessed. (17,18,29) (Fig. 2.34)

Normal Measurements. According to Ferguson the center of gravity of the trunk passes through the center of the third lumbar body and continues vertically to intersect the sacral base. (17,18)

Special Considerations. This original description was performed on recumbent lateral lumbar projections; however, some studies suggest that the patient position, whether upright or recumbent, is irrelevant. (7) Some investigators use the intersection point through the L5 vertebra as the reference point. (30)

Significance. If this line passes anterior to the sacrum by more than 10 mm (½ in) an increase in shearing stresses in an anterior direction between the lumbosacral apophyseal joints may be occurring. (17) Conversely, it has been suggested that a posterior shift in this gravity line may be an indicator of increased weight-bearing forces on these same lumbosacral joints which may also be active in the production of low back pain. (10,11,24) Increased stress on the pars interarticularis may also be incurred from this posterior shift in weight bearing, although a direct relationship to the formation of spondylolysis has not been demonstrated, only inferred. (25)

MACNAB'S LINE

Synonyms. None.

Technique

Projection. Lateral lumbar.

Landmarks. A line is drawn through and parallel to the inferior endplate at the level to be evaluated. The relationship of the adjacent tip of the superior articular process of the vertebra below is then assessed. (Fig. 2.35)

Normal Measurements. The line should lie above the tip of the adjacent superior articular process. (31)

Significance. If the line intersects the superior articulating process, facet imbrication (subluxation) may be present. The effect of these facets overriding each other is to mechanically infringe on the size of the intervertebral foramen and lateral recess. The reliability of this line, however, has not been documented. (7) It should be noted that the original description of this line was with respect to recumbent radiographs, and its application to weight-bearing films is uncertain. The relevance of this line is doubtful given the high incidence in asymptomatic individuals. (29,32)

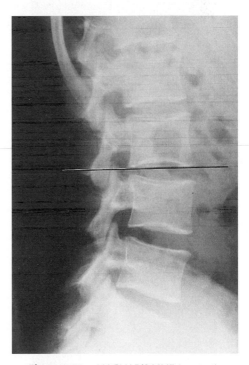

Figure 2.35.   MACNAB'S LINE (see text).

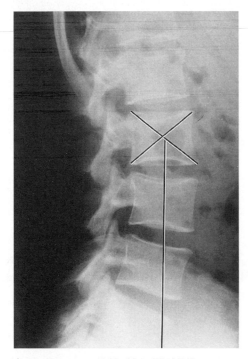

Figure 2.34.   LUMBAR GRAVITY LINE (see text).

HADLEY'S "S" CURVE

Synonyms. None.

Technique

Projection. Oblique, anteroposterior lumbar spine.

Landmarks. A curvilinear line is constructed along the inferior margin of the transverse process and down along the inferior articular process to the apophyseal joint space. The line is then continued across the articulation to connect with the outer edge of the opposing superior articular process. (33,34) (Fig. 2.36)

Normal Measurements. The resultant configuration of this line will look like the letter "S." The key region of the "S" is the normally smooth transition across the joint space.

Significance. An abrupt interruption in the smooth contour of this line may indicate facet imbrication (subluxation), though displacements as great as 3 mm may not be visible on plain film examination. (35,36) A localized, wide facet joint has been linked with disc derangement. (37)

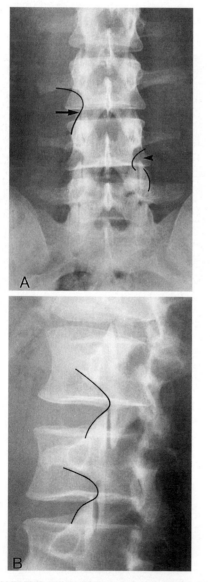

VAN AKKERVEEKEN'S MEASUREMENT OF LUMBAR INSTABILITY

Synonyms. None.

Technique

Projection. Lateral lumbar spine (neutral, flexion, extension).

Landmarks. Two lines are drawn through and parallel to opposing segmental endplates until they intersect posteriorly. The distance from the posterior body margins to the point of intersection is then measured. Alternatively, the displacement can be assessed by measuring the offset in the opposing body corners. (Fig. 2.37)

Normal Measurements. There should be less than 1.5 mm displacement, as determined by either measurement method. (38)

Special Considerations. This evaluation is best performed on the extension film, when the most stress is applied to the lower lumbar discs.

Significance. If there is greater than 1.5 mm difference in measurement, then it is likely that nuclear, annular, and posterior ligament damage at the displaced segment is present. Other investigators have cited 3 mm displacement to be of clinical significance. (39)

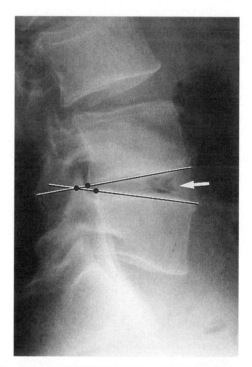

Figure 2.37.   VAN AKKERVEEKEN'S MEASUREMENT DEMONSTRATING INTERSEGMENTAL INSTABILITY (see text). Observe the vacuum phenomenon within the L4 disc (arrow).

Figure 2.36.   HADLEY'S "S" CURVE. A. Anteroposterior Normal (arrow), **Anteroposterior Abnormal** (arrowhead). **B. Oblique Normal** (see text).

DEGENERATIVE LUMBAR SPINAL INSTABILITY—FLEXION/EXTENSION

Synonyms. Horizontal displacement measurement.
Technique
Projection. Lateral lumbar, with flexion and extension.
Landmarks. The landmarks apply on both flexion and extension. Two methods of assessment can be made—gross and accurate mensuration. (40)

1. *Gross assessment.* The alignment of the posterior lumbar bodies is examined by visually observing the relationship of the opposing posterior body corners (George's line).
2. *Accurate measurement—horizontal displacement.* The posterior body corners of each body are located. At each segment the superior corners are joined by a line. At the segment that is normal, a line is drawn parallel to the posterior corner line through the posterior corner of the displaced segment above. The interspace between these two lines is then measured, which represents the displaced distance (DD). To remove the effects of radiographic magnification, measure the width of the unstable vertebral body (W) and express the horizontal disrelationship measurement as a percentage (HD%).

$$HD\% = \frac{DD}{W} \times 100$$

3. *Accurate measurement—angular displacement.* A line is drawn perpendicular to the posterior corner line at opposing body surfaces, and the subtended angle measured.

Normal Measurements. During flexion and extension, there should be no detectable anterior or posterior translation of the vertebral bodies in relation to each other. This is assessed by noting the alignment of the posterior body corners in both flexion and extension. (Fig. 2.38) Additionally, only one posterior corner of each vertebra should be seen.

Significance. If anterior or posterior displacement is seen on flexion or extension, it indicates degenerative or traumatically induced instability. A similar phenomenon has been demonstrated on traction-compression radiography. (41) (See Chapter 5)

More specifically, if anterior displacement is seen during flexion, this denotes laxity of the posterior ligamentous complex (interspinous, supraspinous, capsular, flaval ligaments, and annular disc fibers). Conversely, a posterior displacement during extension implies an anterior ligamentous complex failure (anterior longitudinal ligament and annular disc fibers). These may frequently occur together as a manifestation of total segmental ligamentous failure.

There has been poor correlation between abnormal findings and clinical symptoms. (42) The combination of sagittal translation and increased posterior opening can be associated with debilitating symptoms. (43) In spondylolisthesis greater than 12°, dynamic angulation or 8% translation on flexion-extension is considered evidence of instability. (44)

Another sign of instability during flexion/extension is the recognition of intersegmental rotation. This can be identified by the observation of two posterior body corners at one segment and implies posterior joint ligamentous instability.

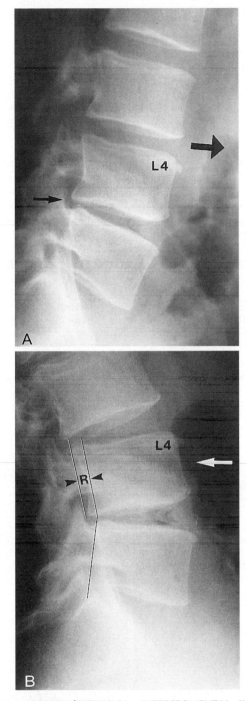

Figure 2.38.   FLEXION/EXTENSION INTERSEGMENTAL INSTABILITY EVALUATION. A. Flexion. Note the alignment at the fourth lumbar level (arrow). **B. Extension.** Note the degree of retrolisthesis (*R*) indicative of extension instability (arrow).

DEGENERATIVE LUMBAR INSTABILITY—LATERAL BENDING

Synonyms. None.

Technique

Projection. Lateral bending, lumbar spine.

Landmarks. Three structures are evaluated—the vertebral body margins, pedicles, and spinous process. (40) (Fig. 2.39)

Normal Measurements. On normal lateral bending, the following should be noted:

1. *Vertebral body alignment.* No lateral segmental displacement (shear) should be seen, and the disc space should be less on the concave side.
2. *Pedicle position.* Each segment should show progressive rotation as evidenced by the altered shape of the pedicle contour along the concave side of the induced curve.
3. *Spinous position.* Similarly, the normal rotational segmental coupling will be shown by gradual spinous deviation of each successive segment into the concavity of the curve.

Significance. If there is lateral segmental displacement (shear), it usually indicates laxity of the discal ligaments and is a sign of degenerative lumbar instability.

Abnormalities in normal posterior joint coupling movements, where there is a lack of or even complete reversal of rotatory motion (paradoxical motion), indicate ligamentous laxity of the posterior joints or altered joint mechanics. There has been poor correlation between abnormal findings and clinical symptoms. (42)

LATERAL-BENDING SIGN

Synonyms. None.

Technique

Projection. Right and left lateral bending, lumbar spine.

Landmarks. Transverse lines are drawn on each segment through either of two locations: (a) the tips of the superior articulating process or (b) the superior border of the pedicles. (Fig. 2.40)

Normal Measurements. On each lateral-bending study the constructed lines will converge toward the bending side in a gradually increasing manner from the lumbosacral junction up. (40)

Significance. In the presence of appropriate clinical symptoms, a localized segmental failure to laterally flex may indicate the presence of a posterolateral (axillary) disc herniation. (45) However, altered biomechanical function of the posterior joints may produce an identical radiographic appearance. (40)

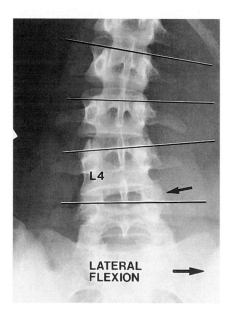

Figure 2.40.   LATERAL-BENDING SIGN. Observe the failure of intersegmental lateral flexion at the fourth lumbar segment (arrow) due to a posterolateral disc herniation.

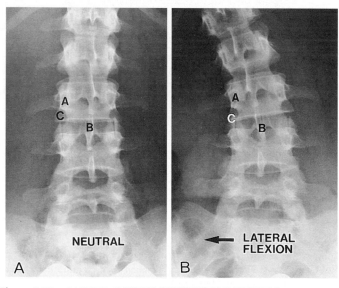

Figure 2.39.   LATERAL FLEXION INSTABILITY EVALUATION. A. Neutral Position. Three structures are observed: (*A*) pedicle position and configuration; (*B*) spinous position; and (*C*) adjacent vertebral margin alignment. **B. Lateral Flexion.** The changes in these structures from the neutral to lateral flexion position are assessed.

MEYERDING'S GRADING METHOD IN SPONDYLOLISTHESIS

Synonyms. None.
Technique
Projection. Lateral lumbar, lumbosacral.
Landmarks. The superior surface of the first sacral segment is divided into four equal divisions. The relative position of the posterior-inferior corner of the fifth lumbar body to these segments is then made. (46) (Fig. 2.41)

Normal Measurements. The posterior-inferior corner of the fifth lumbar body should be aligned with the posterior-superior corner of the first sacral segment.

Special Considerations. The same assessment can be applied to other spinal levels by dividing the superior endplate of the segment below the spondylolisthesis into four. In spondylolisthesis, greater than 12° dynamic angulation or 8% translation on flexion-extension views is considered evidence of instability. (44)

Significance. The degree of anterolisthesis of the affected vertebral body can be categorized according to the division in which the posterior-inferior corner of the body lies. These are designated into "grades":

Grade 1. The posterior-inferior corner is aligned within the first division.
Grade 2. The posterior-inferior corner is aligned within the second division.
Grade 3. The posterior-inferior corner is aligned within the third division.
Grade 4. The posterior-inferior corner is aligned within the fourth division. If the vertebral body has completely slipped beyond the sacral promontory, then this is called "spondyloptosis."

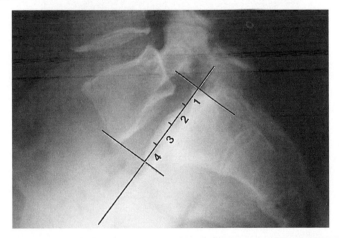

Figure 2.41. MEYERDING'S CLASSIFICATION OF SPONDYLOLIS-THESIS.

ULLMANN'S LINE

Synonyms. Garland-Thomas line, right-angle test line.
Technique
Projection. Lateral lumbar, lumbosacral.
Landmarks. Two lines are drawn: (1) parallel to and through the sacral base and (2) perpendicular to the first line at the anterior margin of the sacral base. The relationship of the fifth lumbar body to this perpendicular line is then assessed. (46–48) (Fig. 2.42)

Normal Measurements. The fifth lumbar body should lie posterior to or just contact this perpendicular line.

Significance. If the anterior margin of the fifth lumbar body crosses the perpendicular line, then anterolisthesis may be present. This is a useful line in detecting the presence of spondylolisthesis when there is poor visualization of the pars region. Application of this line must be interpreted in light of lumbar biomechanics; e.g., if there is a significant loss of the lumbar lordosis, a false positive finding may be present.

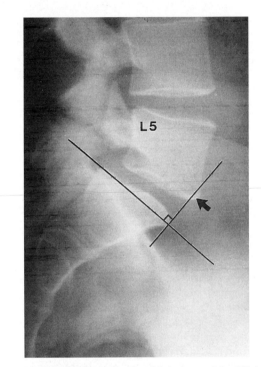

Figure 2.42. ULLMANN'S LINE. Spondylolisthesis of the fifth lumbar segment demonstrated by the intersection of the line with the fifth lumbar body (arrow).

INTERPEDICULATE DISTANCE

Synonyms.   Coronal dimension of the spinal canal.

Technique

Projection. Anteroposterior cervical, thoracic, and lumbar spines.

Landmarks. The shortest distance between the inner convex cortical surfaces of the opposing segmental pedicles is measured. (Fig. 2.43)

Normal Measurements. These vary according to each spinal level and the patient's age. (49) (Table 2.18)

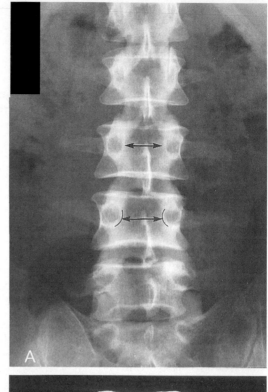

Table 2.18.	Normal Adult Interpediculate Distances		
Spinal Level	Average (mm)	Minimum (mm)	Maximum (mm)
C3	28	25	31
C4	29	26	32
C5	29	26	33
C6	29	26	33
C7	28	24	32
T1	24	20	28
T2	20	17	24
T3	19	16	22
T4	18	15	21
T5	17	14	21
T6	17	14	20
T7	17	14	20
T8	18	15	21
T9	18	15	21
T10	19	15	22
T11	20	18	24
T12	23	19	27
L1	25	21	29
L2	26	21	30
L3	26	21	31
L4	27	21	33
L5	30	23	36

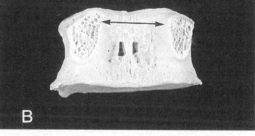

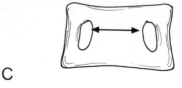

Significance.   This is a useful measurement applied in the evaluation of spinal stenosis, congenital malformation, and intraspinal neoplasms. In stenosis the minimum measurement is exceeded, but for accurate delineation it is best used in combination with other measurements, such as the sagittal canal dimension (Eisenstein) and size of the vertebral body (canal/body ratio). The maximum interpediculate distance may be increased due to pedicular erosion from an expanding spinal cord tumor (Elseberg-Dyke sign). (50)

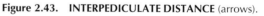

Figure 2.43.   INTERPEDICULATE DISTANCE (arrows).

EISENSTEIN'S METHOD FOR SAGITTAL CANAL MEASUREMENT

Synonyms.   None.
Technique
Projection. Lateral lumbar spine.
Landmarks. For each lumbar level, except the fifth, the sagittal canal diameter can be determined by measuring between two points.

1. *Articular process line.* A line is drawn to connect the tips of the superior and inferior articular processes at each level.
2. *Posterior body margin.* The measurement point is on the posterior body margin at the midpoint between the superior and inferior endplate. (Fig. 2.44)
3. *Sagittal canal measurement.* This is obtained by determining the distance between the posterior body and articular process line.

For determining the sagittal canal dimension of the fifth lumbar segment, measurement is made between the spinolaminar junction line and posterior body. (51)

Normal Measurements. No single measurement should be less than 15 mm, (51) though some have suggested 14 mm to be minimum value. (52)

Special Considerations. The actual lowest anatomic measurement found on cadaver specimens has been 12 mm. (51)

Significance.   A measurement below 15 mm may indicate the presence of spinal stenosis. This appears to be the single most reliable measurement on plain radiographs in the assessment of spinal stenosis. (51) However, before definitive diagnosis is made, appropriate clinical studies and CT must be performed. (52)

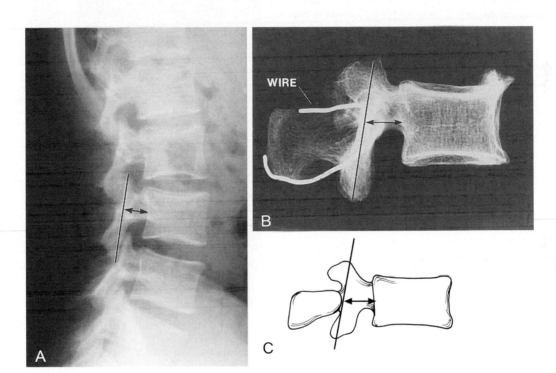

Figure 2.44.   EISENSTEIN'S METHOD FOR SAGITTAL CANAL MEASUREMENT. A (see text). **B and C.** Note that the line will closely approximate the posterior limits of the canal (metal wire).

CANAL/BODY RATIO

Synonyms.   Spinal index.

Technique

Projection. Anteroposterior and lateral lumbar spine.

Landmarks. Four measurements are made, two per film, for each spinal segment. (53,54) (Fig. 2.45)

1. *Interpediculate distance* (A). This is the smallest distance between each pedicle.
2. *Sagittal canal dimension* (B). The method of Eisenstein is applied. A line is drawn from the tips of the superior and inferior articular processes, and adjacent to the midpoint on the posterior body margin the sagittal distance is measured.
3. *Transverse body dimension* (C). The width of the vertebral body on the anteroposterior film is measured at the midpoint between the endplates.
4. *Sagittal body dimension* (D). The length of the vertebral body on the lateral film is measured at the midpoint between the endplates.

Normal Measurements. These four measurements are combined to provide an index of the canal size in relation to vertebral body size. This is derived by:

$$\frac{\text{Interpediculate Dimension} \times \text{Sagittal Canal Dimension}}{\text{Transverse Body Dimension} \times \text{Sagittal Body Dimension}}$$

that is,

$$\text{Canal/Body Ratio} = \frac{A \times B}{C \times D}$$

The normal range will vary according to the lumbar level. (53) (Table 2.19)

Table 2.19. Normal Lumbar Canal-Body Ratios		
	Minimum	Maximum
L3	1:3.0	1:6.0
L4	1:3.0	1:6.0
L5	1:3.2	1:6.5

Significance.   The higher the ratio, the smaller the spinal canal, which is an indicator of possible spinal stenosis; however, this method of spinal canal assessment has been shown to be unreliable. (51)

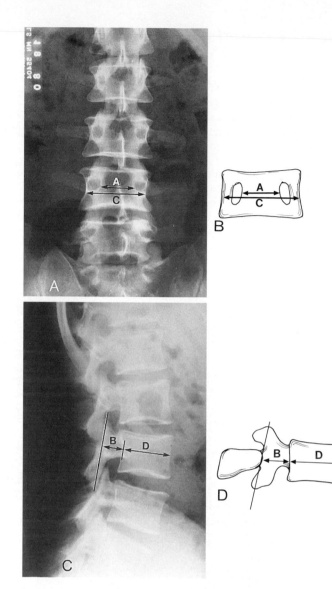

Figure 2.45.   CANAL/BODY RATIO. A. Anteroposterior Measurements. Interpediculate distance (*A*) and transverse body dimension (*C*). **B. Lateral Measurements.** Sagittal canal dimension (*B*) and sagittal body dimension (*D*).

INTERCRESTAL LINE

Synonyms. None.
Technique
Projection. Anteroposterior lumbar spine.
Landmarks. A transverse line is drawn connecting the iliac crests. The relationship of the bodies and discs of the fifth and fourth lumbar segments to this line is then made. (55) (Fig. 2.46)

Normal Measurements. The relative position of these two segments within the pelvis is variable; however, the most stable position appears to be where the line intersects through the bottom half of the fourth lumbar body or disc. It is usually lower in females. (56)

Significance. This line, along with other skeletal parameters, may be a useful indicator in predicting the level where the most biomechanical stress is occurring in the lumbar spine and the level at which degenerative changes are most likely to occur. (55) It is not, however, a reliable predictor for predisposing to back pain. (5,56) The criteria for probable L4-L5 degeneration are:

1. A high intercrestal line passing through the upper half of L4
2. Long transverse processes on L5
3. Rudimentary rib
4. Transitional vertebra

The criteria for predicting probable L5-S1 degeneration are:

1. An intercrestal line passing through the body of L5
2. Short transverse processes on L5
3. No rudimentary rib
4. No transitional vertebra

LENGTH OF LUMBAR TRANSVERSE PROCESSES

Synonyms. None.
Technique
Projection. Anteroposterior lumbar spine.
Landmarks. A vertical line is drawn through the tip of the third lumbar transverse process. This is done bilaterally. The relationship of the fifth lumbar transverse process to this line is then assessed. (55) (Fig. 2.47)

Normal Measurements. Considerable variation in the length of the fifth lumbar transverse occurs.

Significance. If the fifth lumbar transverse process is short, then this may be an inherent structural instability factor at the lumbosacral junction. Conversely, a long transverse process can be seen as a stabilizing factor at this level. The length of this transverse process can be used in combination with other parameters to predict segmental instability (see intercrestal line).

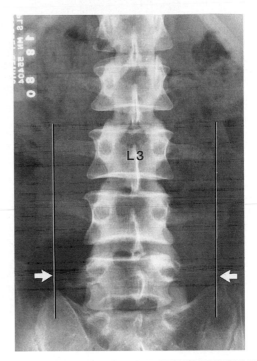

Figure 2.47. LENGTH OF THE LUMBAR TRANSVERSE PROCESSES (see text).

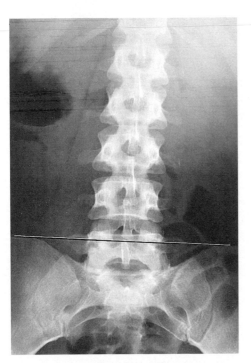

Figure 2.46.   INTERCRESTAL LINE (see text).

LOWER EXTREMITY

TEARDROP DISTANCE

Synonyms.   Medial joint space of the hip.
Technique
Projection. Anteroposterior pelvis, hip.
Landmarks. The distance between the most medial margin of the femoral head and outer cortex of the pelvic teardrop is measured. (1–3) (Fig. 2.48)

Table 2.20. Normal Teardrop Distances		
Average (mm)	Minimum (mm)	Maximum (mm)
9	6	11

Normal Measurements. (Refer to Table 2.20)

Significance.   If the teardrop distance exceeds 11 mm or if there is more than a 2-mm discrepancy from right to left (Waldenstrom's sign), then hip disease is most likely present. Left to right discrepancies of >1 mm will be present in 90% of hip joint effusions. (2) This is an especially sensitive sign in early Legg-Calvé-Perthes disease and may also be seen in septic arthritis or other inflammatory diseases. (1,2)

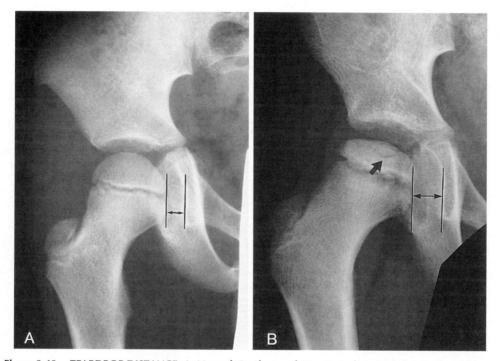

Figure 2.48.   TEARDROP DISTANCE. A. Normal. B. Abnormal, Due to Early Legg-Calvé-Perthes Disease. Observe the "crescent" sign in the femoral capital epiphysis (arrow).

HIP JOINT SPACE WIDTH

Synonyms. None.
Technique
Projection. Anteroposterior, hip.
Landmarks. Three measurements are made of the joint cavity. (2) (Fig. 2.49)

1. *Superior joint space.* This is the space between the most superior point on the convex articular surface of the femur and adjacent acetabular cortex.
2. *Axial joint space.* This is the space between the femoral head and acetabulum immediately lateral to the acetabular notch.
3. *Medial joint space (teardrop distance).* This is the space between the most medial surface of the femoral head and opposing acetabular surface.

Normal Measurements. Notably, the superior and axial compartments are approximately equal (4 mm), while the medial space is twice as great (8 mm). (4) (Table 2.21)

Table 2.21.	Normal Hip Joint Space Width		
	Average (mm)	Minimum (mm)	Maximum (mm)
Superior space	4	3	6
Axial space	4	3	7
Medial space	8	4	13

Significance. Various disorders may alter normal values; however, changes within the various compartments may be found in specific entities.

Superior Joint Space. The most common cause for a diminished joint space in this compartment is degenerative joint disease.

Axial Joint Space. Degenerative arthritis and especially inflammatory arthritis, such as rheumatoid arthritis, will diminish this compartment, often with associated loss of joint space in the other compartments.

Medial Joint Space. Narrowing is usually due to degenerative or inflammatory arthritis; however, widening of the compartment is a frequent indicator of hip joint effusion or lateral shift of the femur (Waldenstrom's sign).

ACETABULAR DEPTH

Synonyms. None.
Technique
Projection. Anteroposterior pelvis.
Landmarks. A line is drawn from the superior margin of the pubis at the symphysis joint to the upper outer acetabular margin. The greatest distance from this line to the acetabular floor is measured. (5) (Fig. 2.50)
Normal Measurements. There will be slight variations between males and females. (5) (Table 2.22)

Table 2.22.	Normal Acetabular Depth		
	Average (mm)	Minimum (mm)	Maximum (mm)
Male	13	7	18
Female	12	9	18

Significance. An acetabular depth less than 9 mm in females and 7 mm in males is considered to be shallow and dysplastic, which may be a factor in precipitating degenerative joint disease of the hip.

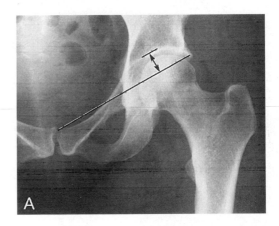
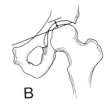

Figure 2.50. DEPTH OF THE ACETABULUM (see text).

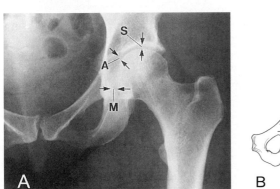
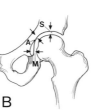

Figure 2.49. WIDTH OF HIP JOINT SPACE: SUPERIOR (*S*), AXIAL (*A*), MEDIAL (*M*). Observe the medial joint space (*M*) is normally twice the width of the other two compartments (see text).

CENTER-EDGE ANGLE

Synonyms.   CE angle, CE angle of Wiberg.
Technique
Projection. Anteroposterior pelvis, hip.
Landmarks. A vertical line is drawn through the center point of the femoral head. Another line is constructed through the femoral head center to the outer upper acetabular margin. The angle formed is then measured. (6) (Fig. 2.51) It can also be measured on CT. (7)
Normal Measurements. (4,6) (Refer to Table 2.23)

Table 2.23.	Normal Center-Edge Angles	
Average (°)	Minimum (°)	Maximum (°)
36	20	40

Significance.   A shallow angle may be related to underlying acetabular dysplasia, which has been linked to the onset of degenerative joint disease. It provides a measure of "coverage" of the femoral head, which means the amount of the acetabulum primarily concerned with weight bearing. (7)

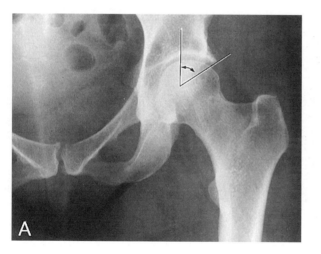

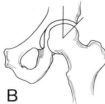

Figure 2.51.   CENTER-EDGE ANGLE (CE ANGLE OF WIBERG) (see text).

SYMPHYSIS PUBIS WIDTH

Synonyms.   None.
Technique
Projection. Anteroposterior pelvis.
Landmarks. The measured distance is between the opposing articular surfaces, halfway between the superior and inferior margins of the joint. (Fig. 2.52)
Normal Measurements. A slight variation exists between males and females. (8) (Table 2.24)

Table 2.24.	Normal Symphysis Pubis Width		
	Average (mm)	Minimum (mm)	Maximum (mm)
Male	6	4.8	7.2
Female	5	3.8	6

Special Considerations. If alignment is being assessed, using the inferior margin appears to be most reliable.
Significance.   Widening of the symphysis may be due to cleidocranial dysplasia, bladder exostrophy, hyperparathyroidism, posttraumatic diastasis, and inflammatory resorption, such as in ankylosing spondylitis, osteitis pubis, and gout.

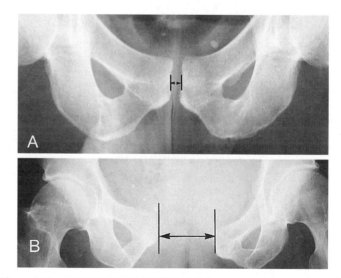

Figure 2.52.   WIDTH OF SYMPHYSIS PUBIS (see text). **A. Normal. B. Abnormal.** Due to traumatic diastasis.

PRESACRAL SPACE

Synonyms. Retrorectal space.
Technique
Projection. Lateral sacrum.
Landmarks. The gray soft tissue density located between the anterior surface of the sacrum and the posterior wall of the rectum is assessed. (Fig. 2.53)
Normal Measurements. There is variation between children and adults. (9,10) (Table 2.25)

Table 2.25.   Normal Presacral Space Measurement

	Average (mm)	Minimum (mm)	Maximum (mm)
Children (1–15 years)	3	1	5
Adults	7	2	20

Significance. An increase in this measurement signifies the presence of an abnormal soft tissue mass. This may be due to sacral destruction (tumor, infection), sacral fracture and associated hematoma, or inflammatory bowel disease, where there is thickening of the intestinal wall.

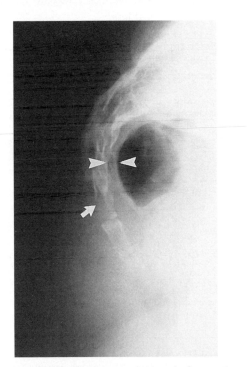

Figure 2.53.   PRESACRAL SPACE (see text). Note the fracture (arrow), which has slightly widened the presacral space (arrowheads).

ACETABULAR ANGLE

Synonyms.   None.
Technique
Projection. Anteroposterior pelvis.
Landmarks. A transverse line is drawn through the right and left triradiate cartilages at the pelvic rim (Y-Y line). A second oblique line connecting the lateral and medial acetabular surfaces is then constructed. The angle of intersection is measured. (11) (Fig. 2.54)
Normal Measurements. Slight variation occurs at different ages, between males and females, as well as between blacks and whites. The presented values are for infants. (11) (Table 2.26)

Table 2.26.   Normal Acetabular Angles in Infants (1 yr)

Average (°)	Minimum (°)	Maximum (°)
20	12	29

Significance. An increased acetabular angle is frequently associated with acetabular dysplasia and congenital hip dislocation. A decreased acetabular angle is seen in Down's syndrome.

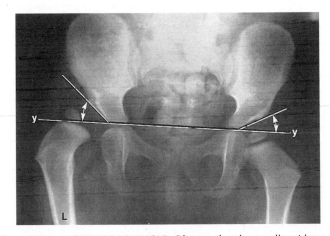

Figure 2.54.   ACETABULAR ANGLE. Observe the abnormally wide angle on the left in association with congenital hip dislocation (see text).

ILIAC ANGLE AND INDEX

Synonyms.   None.
Technique
Projection. Anteroposterior pelvis.
Landmarks. A line is drawn through the triradiate cartilage at the pelvic rim (Y-Y line). A second line is constructed tangential to the most lateral margin of the iliac wing and iliac body. (12) (Fig. 2.55)
Normal Measurements.

1. *Iliac angle.* (Refer to Table 2.27)
2. *Iliac index.* This is the sum of both iliac angles and acetabular angles, divided by 2. (Table 2.28)

Table 2.27.	Normal Iliac Angles		
	Average (°)	Minimum (°)	Maximum (°)
0–3 mo	44	35	58
3–12 mo	55	43	67

Table 2.28.	Normal Iliac Indices		
	Average	Minimum	Maximum
0–3 mo	60	48	87
3–12 mo	81	68	97

Significance.   The iliac index is most useful in the determination of Down's syndrome. When the index is less than 60, Down's syndrome is probable; between 60 and 68, possible; beyond 68, Down's syndrome is unlikely. (13)

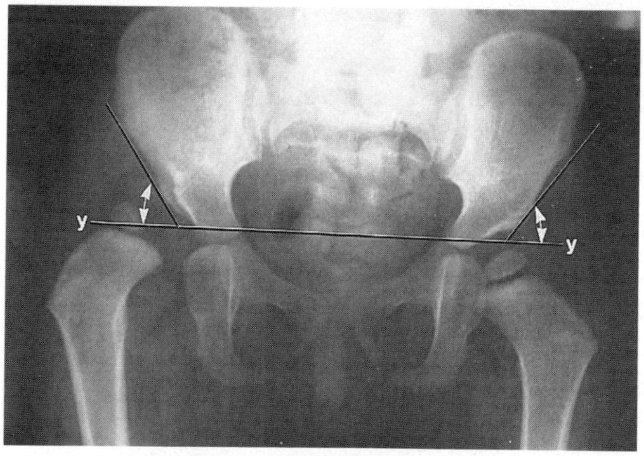

Figure 2.55.   ILIAC ANGLE (see text).

MISCELLANEOUS MEASUREMENTS OF THE GROWING HIP

Synonyms.   None.
Technique
Projection. Anteroposterior pelvis.
Landmarks and Normal Measurements. Numerous lines and angles aid in the assessment of growing hip abnormalities. (14) (Fig. 2.56)

1. *Y-Y line.* A horizontal line is drawn through the triradiate cartilage at its junction with the pelvic rim (cotyloid notch.) This is a base line by which many other angles and lines are derived.
   (a) *Epiphyseal relationship.* The apex of each femoral epiphysis should be equally above the Y-Y line.
   (b) *Diaphyseal interval.* The distance between the top of the diaphysis and the Y-Y line should be bilaterally equal and not less than 6 cm.
   (c) *Pivot point interval.* The distance between the apex of the epiphysis and inner acetabular margin of the ilium should not exceed 16 mm.
   (d) *Vertical line of Ombredanne.* A vertical line to the Y-Y line is constructed through the outer upper acetabular margin. The epiphyseal center should lie below the Y-Y line and medial to this vertical line.
2. *Parallelogram of Kopitz.* A rectangle is constructed by drawing lines between four points—the outer and inner iliac acetabular margins and the corners of the opposing femoral diaphysis. Normally, the angles will be approximately 90° at each corner.

Significance.   The most common cause for alerting the clinician to these relationships is congenital hip dislocation.

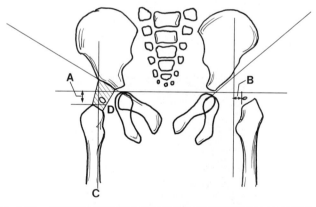

Figure 2.56.   MISCELLANEOUS MEASUREMENTS IN THE ASSESSMENT OF THE GROWING HIP (see text). Diaphyseal interval (*A*), epiphyseal position (*B*), vertical line of Ombredanne (*C*), and the parallelogram of Kopitz (*D*).

MEASUREMENTS OF PROTRUSIO ACETABULI

Synonyms. Kohler's Line.
Technique
Projection. Anteroposterior pelvis, hip.
Landmarks. A line is constructed tangentially to the cortical margin of the pelvic inlet and outer border of the obturator foramen. The relationship of the acetabular floor to this line is assessed. (15,16) (Fig. 2.57)
Normal Measurements. The acetabular floor should not cross this line and usually lies laterally to it.
Significance. If the acetabular floor crosses the line, then protrusio acetabuli is present. The most common causes include an idiopathic form, rheumatoid arthritis, and Paget's disease.

SHENTON'S LINE

Synonyms. Makka's line, Menard's line.
Technique
Projection. Anteroposterior hip, pelvis.
Landmarks. A curvilinear line is constructed along the under-surface of the femoral neck and is continued across the joint to the inferior margin of the superior pubic ramus. (14) (Fig. 2.58)
Normal Measurements. The constructed line should be smooth, especially in the transition zone between the femoral neck and superior pubic ramus. Occasionally, a small portion of the inferior femoral head may just cross the line.
Significance. An interrupted, discontinuous line is useful in the detection of hip dislocation, femoral neck fracture, and slipped femoral capital epiphysis.

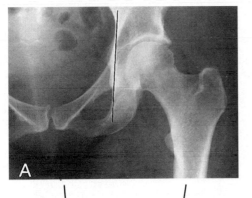
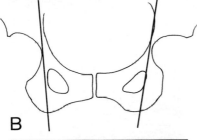
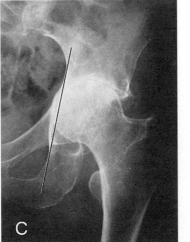

Figure 2.57. KOHLER'S LINE. A and B. Normal Kohler's Line (see text). **C. Protrusio Acetabuli.** Observe the medial displacement of the acetabulum and femoral head in relation to the line as a result of rheumatoid arthritis.

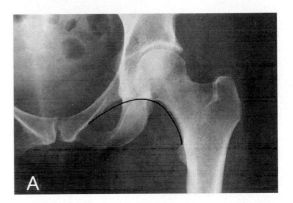
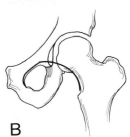
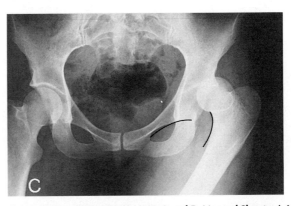

Figure 2.58. SHENTON'S LINE. A and B. Normal Shenton's Line (see text). **C. Hip Dislocation.** Note the interruption in the smooth arc of Shenton's line.

ILIOFEMORAL LINE

Synonyms.   None.
Technique
Projection. Anteroposterior pelvis, hip.
Landmarks. A curvilinear line is constructed along the outer surface of the ilium, across the joint, and onto the femoral neck. (17) (Fig. 2.59)

Normal Measurements. A small portion of the superior femoral head may cause a slight convexity in the line. The most important normal feature is that the line will be bilaterally symmetrical.

Significance.   A discrepancy in symmetry may be due to congenital dysplasia, slipped femoral capital epiphysis, dislocation, and fracture.

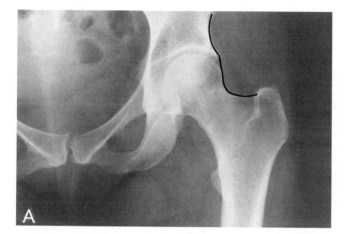

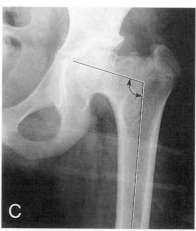

Figure 2.59.   ILIOFEMORAL LINE (see text).

FEMORAL ANGLE

Synonyms.   Femoral angle of incidence, femoral neck angle, Mikulicz's angle.
Technique
Projection. Anteroposterior hip, pelvis.
Landmarks. Two lines are drawn through and parallel to the midaxis of the femoral shaft and femoral neck. The angle subtended is then measured. (18) (Fig. 2.60)

Normal Measurements. Slight variation occurs between males and females. (14) (Table 2.29)

Table 2.29. Normal Femoral Angle	
Minimum (°)	Maximum (°)
120	130

Special Considerations. For accurate depiction of the femoral shaft-neck angle, the foot should be medially rotated 15° at the time of radiographic exposure.

Significance.   A value less than 120° is designated as coxa vara and above 130° as coxa valga.

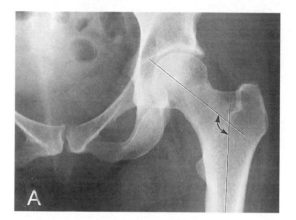

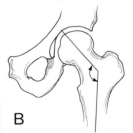

Figure 2.60.   FEMORAL ANGLE. A and B. Normal Femoral Angle (see text). **C. Decreased Femoral Angle (Coxa Vara).**

SKINNER'S LINE

Synonyms. None.
Technique
Projection. Anteroposterior pelvis, hip.

Landmarks. A line is drawn through and parallel to the axis of the femoral shaft. A second line at right angles to the shaft line is constructed tangential to the tip of the greater trochanter. The relationship of the fovea capitus to this trochanteric line is assessed. (19) (Fig. 2.61)

Normal Measurements. The fovea capitus should lie above or at the level of the trochanteric line.

Significance.   If the fovea lies below this line, then this is due to a superior displacement of the femur relative to the femoral head. The most common causes are fracture and those conditions leading to coxa vara.

KLEIN'S LINE

Synonyms.   None.
Technique
Projection. Anteroposterior and frog-leg, hip, or pelvis.

Landmarks. A line is constructed tangential to the outer margin of the femoral neck. The degree of overlap of the femoral head will be apparent. (20) (Fig. 2.62)

Normal Measurements. Comparison should be made with the opposite side, and normally, there will be the same degree of overlap of the femoral head. In most normal hips the outer margin of the femoral head will be lateral to the line.

Special Considerations. This line can be drawn on both the anteroposterior and frog-leg projections.

Significance.   If there is a failure of the femoral head overlap in relation to the line or if there is asymmetry from side to side, then slippage of the femoral capital epiphysis should be suspected. (20)

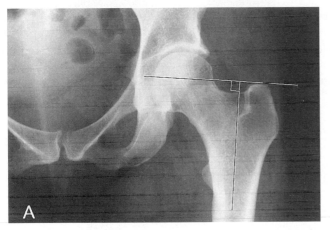

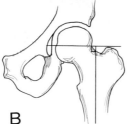

Figure 2.61. SKINNER'S LINE (see text).

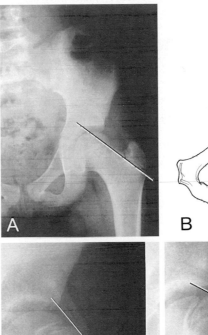

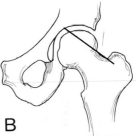

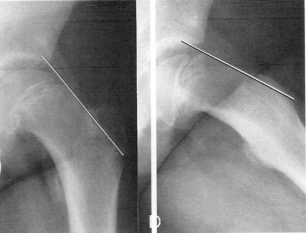

Figure 2.62.   KLEIN'S LINE (see text). **A and B. Normal Adolescent Hip. C and D. Slipped Femoral Capital Epiphysis.** Anteroposterior and frog-leg projection of the hip in slipped femoral capital epiphysis. Note the lack of overlap across the line by the femoral head.

AXIAL RELATIONSHIPS OF THE KNEE

Synonyms. None.
Technique
Projection. Anteroposterior knee.
Landmarks. Four lines and two angles are drawn. (18) (Fig. 2.63)

1. *Femoral shaft line* (A). A line is drawn through and parallel to the midaxis of the femoral shaft.
2. *Tibial shaft line* (B). A line is drawn through and parallel to the midaxis of the tibial shaft.
3. *Femoral condyle line* (C). A line is drawn through and tangential to the articular surfaces of the condyles.
4. *Tibial plateau line* (D). A line is drawn through the medial and lateral tibial plateau margins.
5. *Femoral angle* (FA). This is the angle formed between the femoral shaft and femoral condyle lines.
6. *Tibial angle* (TA). This is the angle formed between the tibial shaft and tibial plateau lines.

Normal Measurements. Slight variation exists between males and females. (Table 2.30)

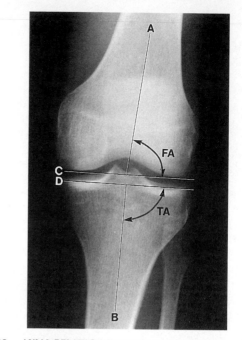

Figure 2.63. AXIAL RELATIONSHIPS OF THE KNEE. Femoral Angle (FA), Tibial Angle (TA) (see text).

Table 2.30. Normal Axial Relationships of the Knee

	Average (°)	Minimum (°)	Maximum (°)
Femoral angle	81	75	85
Tibial angle	93	85	100

Significance. These angles will be altered in fractures and other deformities about the knee.

PATELLAR POSITION

Synonyms. Patella alta evaluation.
Technique
Projection. Lateral knee (semiflexed). (Fig. 2.64A)
Landmarks.

1. *Patellar length* (PL). This is the greatest diagonal dimension between the superior and inferior poles.
2. *Patellar tendon length* (PT). The distance measured is between the insertion points of the posterior tendon surface at the inferior patellar pole and notch at the tibial tubercle. (Fig. 2.64A)

Normal Measurements. Patellar length and patellar tendon length are usually equal to each other. A normal variation up to 20%, however, is considered insignificant. (21)

Significance. When the patellar tendon length is more than 20% greater than the patellar length, *patella alta* is present. (22) This may be found in association with chondromalacia patellae. A low-riding patella (*patella baja*) may be seen in polio, achondroplasia, juvenile rheumatoid arthritis and tibial tubercle transposition.

PATELLAR MALALIGNMENT

Synonyms. Patellar tracking, patellar subluxation, patellofemoral joint incongruence.
Technique
Projection. Tangential knee ("skyline"). (Fig. 2.64B and C)
Landmarks.

1. *Patella apex.* The patella is centered when its apex is directly above the deepest section of the intercondylar sulcus. (23) (Fig. 2.64B)
2. *Sulcus angle.* By drawing lines from the highest points on the medial and lateral condyles to the lowest point of the intercondylar sulcus, an angle is formed. (Fig. 2.64B) Normally, this should be 138 ± 6°. (23,24) Greater measurements (shallow intercondylar groove) predispose to subluxation and dislocation.
3. *Lateral patellofemoral joint index.* The narrowest medial joint space measurement is divided by the narrowest lateral joint space measurement. (Fig. 2.64B) This index is normally less than or equal to 1.0. A value of greater than 1.0 is noted in patients with chondromalacia patellae. (23–27)
4. *Lateral patellofemoral angle.* A line tangential to the femoral condyles is intersected by a line joining the limits of the lateral facet. (23–27) (Fig. 2.64C) The angle is normally open. In patellar subluxation these lines are parallel or open medially.
5. *Lateral patellar displacement.* A line is drawn tangential to the medial and lateral condylar surfaces. A perpendicular line at the medial edge of the femoral condyle normally lies 1 mm or less medial to the patella. (27) (Fig. 2.64C)

Significance. The combined use of these measurements may reveal contributing causes to patellofemoral joint pain syndromes and instability. (22,23)

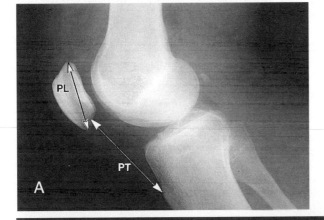

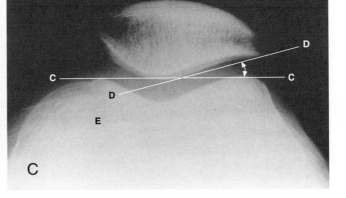

Figure 2.64. PATELLAR RELATIONSHIPS. A. Patellar Position, Lateral Projection. B and C. Tangential Relationships. Patella apex *(C)*, sulcus angle *(A-A:B-B)*, lateral patellofemoral joint index *(C,D)*, lateral patellofemoral angle *(C-C:D-D)*, lateral patellar displacement *(E)*.

AXIAL RELATIONSHIPS OF THE ANKLE

Synonyms.   None.
Technique
Projection. Anteroposterior ankle.
Landmarks. Four lines and two angles are constructed. (18) (Fig. 2.65)

1. *Tibial shaft line* (A). A line is drawn through and parallel to the tibial shaft.
2. *Medial malleolus line* (B). A line is drawn tangential to the articular surface of the medial malleolus.
3. *Lateral malleolus line* (C). A line is drawn tangential to the articular surface of the lateral malleolus.
4. *Talus line* (D). A line is drawn tangential to the articular surface of the talar dome.
5. *Tibial angle* (I). The angle is formed medially between the medial malleolus line and talus line.
6. *Fibular angle* (II). The angle is formed laterally between the lateral malleolus line and talus line.

Normal Measurements. Slight variation occurs between males and females. (18) (Table 2.31)

Table 2.31. Normal Axial Relationships of the Ankle			
	Average (°)	Minimum (°)	Maximum (°)
Tibial angle (I)	53	45	65
Fibular angle (II)	52	43	63

Significance.   These angles will be altered in fractures of the malleoli, ankle mortise instability, and tibiotalar slant deformities. The *tibiotalar joint space* is measured at the lateral and medial joint margins. This should be done on varus-valgus stress studies, on which there should not be more than 3 mm difference between the normal and injured sides. (28) *Talar tilt* is assessed by drawing a line tangential to the talar dome and another line along the adjacent tibial surface. In the neutral position, an angle greater than 6° indicates significant ligamentous injury. On valgus-varus stress views, the normal range is 5 to 23°. More than a 10° difference between right and left also indicates significant ligamentous damage. (29,30) An anterior drawer of 4 mm is indicative also of instability. (31)

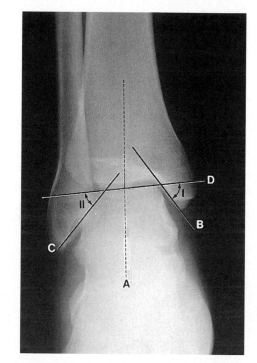

Figure 2.65.   AXIAL RELATIONSHIPS OF THE ANKLE (see text).

HEEL PAD MEASUREMENT

Synonyms. None.

Technique

Projection. Lateral foot, lateral calcaneus (nonweight bearing).

Landmarks. The shortest distance between the plantar surface of the calcaneus and external skin contour is measured. (32) (Fig. 2.66)

Normal Measurements. Variation between sexes does occur. (33) (Table 2.32)

Table 2.32.	Normal Heel Pad Measurement	
	Average (mm)	Maximum (mm)
Male	19	25
Female	19	23

Special Considerations. Blacks may have a slightly larger heel pad distance. (34)

Significance. Increased skin thickness, especially of the heel pad, is a frequent accompanying feature of acromegaly. *Achilles tendon thickness* can be assessed on a lateral view at 1 to 2 cm above the calcaneus and is normally 4 to 8 mm in dimension. (35) Edema from inflammatory arthritis can thicken the ligament.

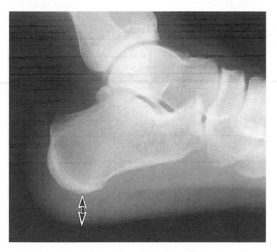

Figure 2.66. HEEL PAD MEASUREMENT (see text).

BOEHLER'S ANGLE

Synonyms. Axial relationships of the calcaneus, tuber angle.

Technique

Projection. Lateral foot, lateral calcaneus.

Landmarks. The three highest points on the superior surface of the calcaneus are connected with two tangential lines. The angle formed posteriorly is then assessed. (Fig. 2.67)

Normal Measurements. The angle formed posteriorly averages between 30 and 35° in most normal subjects but may range between 28 and 40°. Any angle less than 28° is abnormal. (36)

Significance. The most common cause for an angle less than 28° is a fracture with displacement through the calcaneus. Dysplastic development of the calcaneus may also disturb the angle.

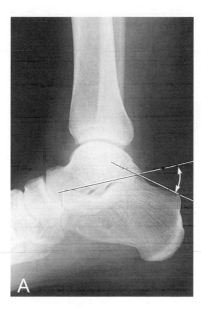

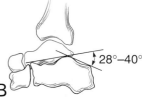

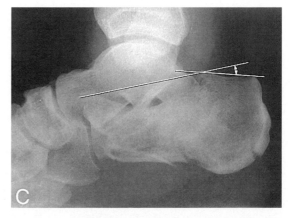

Figure 2.67. BOEHLER'S ANGLE. A and B. Normal Angle. C. Calcaneal Fracture. Observe the decrease in Boehler's angle.

Upper Extremity
AXIAL RELATIONSHIPS OF THE SHOULDER

Synonyms.   Humeral axial angle.
Technique
Projection. Anteroposterior shoulder with external rotation.
Landmarks. (Refer to Fig. 2.68)

1. *Humeral shaft line* (A). A line is drawn through and parallel to the humeral shaft.
2. *Humeral head line* (B). From the apex of the greater tuberosity a line is drawn toward the medial humeral surface at the point where the diaphyseal cortex changes from a band to a line.
3. *Humeral angle* (HA). This is the inferior angle between the humeral shaft and head lines.

Normal Measurements. The average humeral angles are 60° for males and 62° for females. (1)

Significance.   This relationship may be altered following a fracture, especially in the surgical neck.

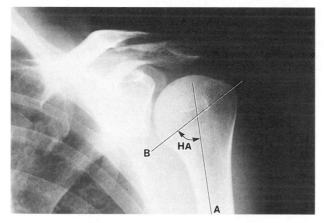

Figure 2.68.   AXIAL RELATIONSHIPS OF THE SHOULDER (see text).

GLENOHUMERAL JOINT SPACE

Synonyms.   None.
Technique
Projection. Anteroposterior shoulder with external rotation.
Landmarks. The measurements are made at the superior, middle, and inferior aspects of the joint. These are combined and averaged. Each distance is ascertained between the opposing articular surfaces. (Fig. 2.69)

Normal Measurements. The average joint space is between 4 and 5 mm. (2)

Significance.   The joint space may be diminished in degenerative arthritis, calcium pyrophosphate dihydrate (CPPD) crystal disease, and posttraumatic arthritis. A widened space is a frequently associated finding of acromegaly and posterior humeral dislocation. (3)

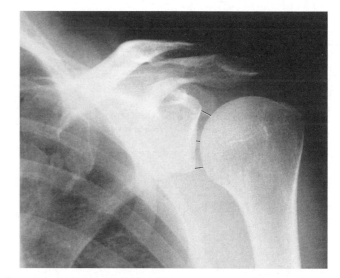

Figure 2.69.   GLENOHUMERAL JOINT SPACE (see text).

ACROMIOHUMERAL JOINT SPACE

Synonyms. None.
Technique
Projection. Anteroposterior shoulder.
Landmarks. The distance between the inferior surface of the acromion and the articular cortex of the humeral head is measured. (Fig. 2.70)
Normal Measurements. (4) (Refer to Table 2.33)

Table 2.33. Normal Acromiohumeral Distance

Average (mm)	Minimum (mm)	Maximum (mm)
9	7	11

Significance. A measurement less than 7 mm is indicative of a rotator cuff tear or degenerative tendinitis due to the unopposed action of the deltoid, (4) allowing superior subluxation of the humerus. A measurement greater than 11 mm may indicate posttraumatic subluxation, dislocation, joint effusion, stroke, or brachial plexus lesions ("drooping shoulder"). (5)

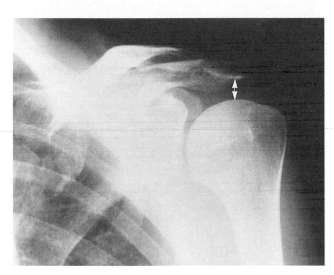

Figure 2.70. ACROMIOHUMERAL SPACE (see text).

ACROMIOCLAVICULAR JOINT SPACE

Synonyms. None.
Technique
Projection. Anteroposterior or posteroanterior shoulder.
Landmarks. The joint space is measured at the superior (S) and inferior (I) borders, and the two values are averaged. (Fig. 2.71)
Normal Measurements. The average joint space is 3 mm, with variation between males and females. There should be no more than 2 to 3 mm difference between the right and left joint spaces. (Table 2.34)

Table 2.34. Normal Acromioclavicular Joint Space

	Average (mm)	Minimum (mm)	Maximum (mm)
Male	3.3	2.5	4.1
Female	2.9	2.1	3.7

Significance. A decreased joint space is seen in degenerative joint disease. An increased joint space may be due to traumatic separation or resorption due to osteolysis in association with hyperparathyroidism or rheumatoid arthritis following trauma.

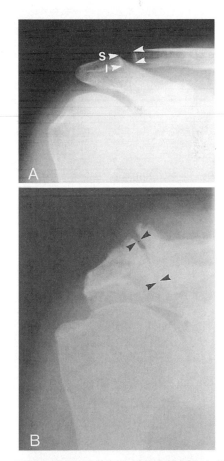

Figure 2.71. ACROMIOCLAVICULAR JOINT SPACE. A. Normal. B. Abnormal. The measurement is abnormally decreased due to degenerative joint disease (arrowheads).

AXIAL RELATIONSHIPS OF THE ELBOW

Synonyms.   None.
Technique
Projection. Anteroposterior elbow.
Landmarks. Three lines and three angles are evaluated. (1) (Fig. 2.72)

1. *Humeral shaft line* (A). A line is drawn through and parallel to the humeral shaft.
2. *Ulnar shaft line* (B). A line is drawn through and parallel to the ulnar shaft.
3. *Humeral articular line* (C). A transverse line is drawn tangentially through the most distal surfaces of the trochlea and capitellum.
4. *Carrying angle* (CA). The angle is formed between the humeral and ulnar shaft lines.
5. *Humeral angle* (HA). The angle is formed between the humeral shaft and articular lines.
6. *Ulnar angle* (UA). The angle is formed between ulnar shaft line and humeral articular line.

Normal Measurements. Slight variations occur between males and females. (Table 2.35)

Table 2.35. Axial Relationships of the Elbow			
	Average (°)	Minimum (°)	Maximum (°)
Carrying angle	169	154	178
Humeral angle	85	72	95
Ulnar angle	84	72	99

Special Considerations. The elbow must be fully extended with no rotation at the humerus.
Significance.   These angles may be altered from fractures or other deformities at the elbow.

RADIOCAPITELLAR LINE

Synonyms.   None.
Technique
Projection. Lateral elbow.
Landmarks. A line is drawn through the center of and parallel to the long axis of the radius and is extended through the elbow joint. (Fig. 2.73)
Normal Measurements. This line should pass through the center of the capitellum in all stages of flexion of the elbow. (6)
Significance.   This assists in determining the presence of radial head subluxation (pulled elbow) or dislocation.

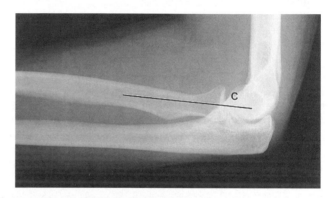

Figure 2.73.   RADIOCAPITELLAR LINE. The radial shaft line passes through the center of the capitellum (*C*) (see text).

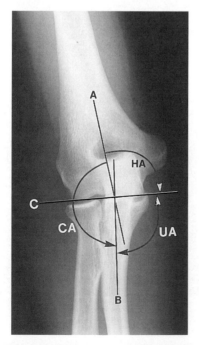

Figure 2.72.   AXIAL RELATIONSHIPS OF THE ELBOW. Carrying angle (*CA*), humeral angle (*HA*), ulnar angle (*UA*) (see text).

AXIAL RELATIONSHIPS OF THE WRIST

Synonyms.   None.
Technique
Projection. Posteroanterior and lateral wrist.

Landmarks of Posteroanterior Relationships. (Fig. 2.74A)

1. *Radioulnar articular line* (A). A tangential line is drawn from the tip of the radial styloid to the base of the ulnar styloid.
2. *Radial shaft line* (B). A line is drawn through and parallel to the shaft of the radius.
3. *Radioulnar angle* (I). The ulnar side angle between the two lines is measured.

Landmarks of Lateral Relationships. (Fig. 2.74B)

1. *Radius articular line* (A). A line is drawn across the most distal points on the articular surface of the radius.
2. *Radial shaft line* (B). A line is drawn through and parallel to the shaft of the radius.
3. *Radius angle* (II). The palmar angle is measured between these two lines.

Normal Measurements. (1) (Refer to Table 2.36)

Table 2.36.   Normal Axial Angles at the Wrist

	Average (°)	Minimum (°)	Maximum (°)
PA radioulnar angle	83	72	95
Lateral radius angle	86	79	94

Significance.   These lines and constructed angles aid in the assessment of radioulnar deformities, especially those due to displaced fractures.

METACARPAL SIGN

Synonyms.   None.
Technique
Projection. Posterior anterior hand.
Landmarks. A line is drawn tangentially through the articular cortex of the fourth and fifth metacarpal heads. (Fig. 2.75)
Normal Measurement. The line should pass distal to or just touch the third metacarpal head. (7)
Significance.   If the line passes through the third metacarpal head this is a frequent sign of gonadal dysgenesis (Turner's syndrome). A fracture deformity may also produce a positive sign.

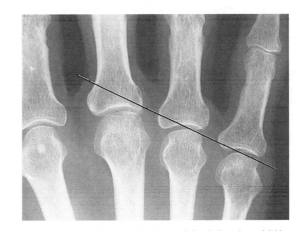

Figure 2.75.   METACARPAL SIGN. Normal third, fourth and fifth metacarpal relationships (see text).

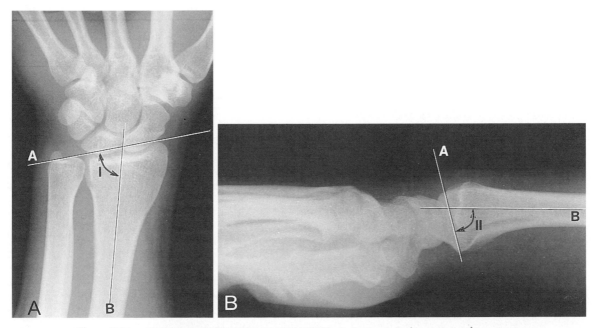

Figure 2.74.   AXIAL RELATIONSHIPS OF THE WRIST. A. Posteroanterior. B. Lateral (see text).

Table 2.37. Lines and Angles of the Skull

Name	Figure Number	Landmarks	Normal Measurements			Significance
			Average	Minimum	Maximum	
Vastine-Kinney	2.2	Pineal gland to inner skull margins: frontal, occipital, vault, and foramen magnum.	Consult standard tables			Intracranial mass or localized atrophy when pineal displaced.
Sella Turcica Size	2.3	Horizontal: Widest diameter. Vertical: Fossa floor—clinoids.	11 mm 8 mm	5 mm 4 mm	16 mm 12 mm	Pituitary and extrapituitary masses enlarge the fossa.
Basilar Angle	2.4	Nasion—center sella turcica. Basion—center sella turcica.	137°	123°	152°	Basilar impression and platybasia widen the angle (>152°).
McGregor's Line	2.5	Hard palate—occiput. Note relative odontoid apex.	Below line		Males: 8 mm Females: 10 mm	Basilar impression when odontoid more than maximum distance above.
Chamberlain's Line	2.6	Hard palate—opisthion.	Below line to 3 mm above		7 mm	Basilar impression when odontoid more than maximum distance above.
MacRae's Line	2.7	Basion—opisthion.	Occipital bone at or below line			Basilar impression when occipital bone above the line.
Digastric Line	2.8	Right and left digastric grooves: (a) Line—odontoid distance. (b) Line—C1/OCC joint distance.	11 mm	1 mm (Odontoid not above the line)	21 mm	Basilar impression when odontoid is above the line.
Height Index of Klaus	2.9	Tuberculum sellae—IOP. Odontoid to line distance.	40–41 mm	30 mm	None	Basilar impression if less than 30 mm.
Boogard's Line	2.10A	Nasion—opisthion.			Basion below line	Basilar impression if basion above the line.
Boogard's Angle	2.10B	Dorsum sella—basion. Basion—opisthion. Angle between lines.	122°	119°	135°	Basilar impression if angle greater than 135°.
Anterior Atlanto-occipital dislocation	2.11	Basion—C1 posterior arch. Opisthion—C1 anterior arch. Ratio of these distances.	Ratio less than one			Atlanto-occipital dislocation where the ratio equal to or greater than one.

Table 2.38. Lines and Angles of the Cervical Spine

Name	Figure Number	Landmarks	Normal Measurements			Significance
			Average	Minimum	Maximum	
Atlantodental interspace (ADI)	2.12	C1 anterior tubercle—odontoid.	(a) Adult (b) Child	1 mm 1 mm	3 mm 5 mm	Transverse ligament rupture or instability. Trauma, Down's, and inflammatory arthritis may increase the measurement.
Method of Bull	2.13	Hard palate—opisthion. C1 anterior arch—C1 posterior arch. Posterior angle measured.			13°	Odontoid malposition if greater than 13°.
George's Line	2.14	Alignment of posterior body margins.	Aligned			A to P vertebral malpositions when line not smooth.
Posterior Cervical Line	2.15	Spinolaminar junction lines.	Aligned			A to P vertebral malpositions when line is not smooth, especially at C1 and C2.
Sagittal Canal Dimension	2.16	Posterior body—spinolaminar junction.	See Table 2.7	12 mm		Spinal stenosis when less than 12 mm. Intraspinal tumor when enlarged.
Atlantoaxial Alignment	2.17	C1 lateral mass—C2 articular pillar margin alignment.	Aligned			Jefferson's or odontoid fractures or alar ligament instability when margins overlap.
Gravity Line	2.18	Vertical line from odontoid apex.	Passes through C7 body			AP displacement is a gross indicator of gravitational stress at the cervicothoracic junction.
Lordosis						
(a) Depth	2.19A	Odontoid apex—post-C7 body. Greatest distance to line.	12 mm	7 mm	17 mm	Role unclear. Decreased following trauma, muscle spasm, spondylosis, and patient tucking the chin at time of exposure.
(b) Jochumsen	2.19B	C1 anterior tubercle—anterior C7 body. Distance to anterior C5 body	3–8 mm	1 mm	9 mm	
(c) Angle	2.19C	Atlas plane line and C7 endplates, then intersecting perpendiculars.	40°	35°	45°	
(d) Drexler		Cumulative total of individual disc angles.	40°	16°	60°	
Stress Lines	2.20	C2 and C7 posterior bodies, and note location of intersection.				Stress point during these movements often altered by muscle spasm, fixation, and spondylosis.
		(a) Flexion	C5–C6 joint			
		(b) Extension	C4–C5 joint			
Prevertebral Soft Tissues	2.21	Anterior bodies—posterior air shadow margins.	See Table 2.9			Soft tissue masses (tumor, infection, hematoma) increase the measurements.
		(a) Retropharyngeal (RPI) (C2–C3–C4)		7 mm		
		(b) Retrolaryngeal (RLI) (C4–C5)		7–20 mm		
		(c) Retrotracheal (RTI) (C5–C7)		20 mm		

Table 2.39. Lines and Angles of the Thoracic Spine

Name	Figure Number	Landmarks	Normal Measurements			Significance
			Average	Minimum	Maximum	
Method of Cobb	2.22	End vertebral endplate lines then intersecting perpendiculars and the angle measured.				Scoliosis evaluation.
Risser-Ferguson	2.23	Centers of end and apical segments joined and the angle measured.				Scoliosis evaluation.
Thoracic Kyphosis	2.24	T1 superior endplate—T12 inferior endplate, then intersecting perpendiculars and the angle measured.	See Tables 2.10, 2.11			Kyphosis evaluation (Scheuermann's, fractures, etc.).
Thoracic Cage Dimension	2.25	Posterior sternum—anterior T8 body.	Male: 14 cm Female: 12 cm	11 cm 9 cm	18 cm 15 cm	Straight back syndrome when the distance is less than 13 cm in males and 11 cm in females.

Table 2.40.   Lines and Angles of the Lumbar Spine

Name	Figure Number	Landmarks	Normal Measurements Average	Minimum	Maximum	Significance
Intervertebral Disc Height						
(a) Hurxthal method	2.26A	Endplate: Endplate distance.	Variable			Decreased disc height (degeneration, surgery, infection).
(b) Farfan method	2.26B	Anterior height divided by disc diameter, posterior height divided by disc diameter, then as ratio to each other.	Variable			Decreased disc height (degeneration, surgery, by disc diameter, then infection).
Intervertebral Disc Angles	2.27	At each disc endplate lines are drawn and the angles are measured.	See Table 2.14			Altered in various mechanical pathologies.
Lordosis	2.28	L1 endplate—S1 endplate; perpendiculars and angle formed.	50–60°			Altered in various mechanical pathologies.
Lumbosacral Lordosis	2.29	Centers of L3, L5, and S1 bodies found and joined, angle measured.	146°	124°	162°	Altered in various mechanical pathologies.
Sacral Inclination	2.30	Posterior surface of S1 to vertical line angle.	46°	30°	72°	Altered in various mechanical pathologies.
Lumbosacral Angle	2.31	Endplate of S1 to horizontal line angle.	41°	26°	57°	Altered in various mechanical pathologies.
Lumbosacral Disc Angle	2.32	Angle between opposing endplates of L5 and S1.	—	10°	15°	Altered in various mechanical pathologies.
Gravity Line (Lumbar)	2.34	A perpendicular line is drawn from the center point of the L3 body.	Intersects sacral base			Altered in various mechanical pathologies.
Macnab's Line	2.35	A line along the inferior endplate.	Should be above superior articular process			Extension malposition, normal variant.
Hadley's "S" Curve	2.36	A line along the inferior surface of the TVP, AP and across the joint.	Smooth across joint			Facet subluxation.
Van Akkerveeken's Measurement	2.37	Endplate lines at opposing segments. Measure from the posterior body to point of intersection.	Equal measurements		1.5 mm difference	Nuclear, annular and posterior ligament damage if more than 1.5 mm difference.
Flexion/Extension	2.38	Amount of displacement on flexion/extension (see text).				Flexion instability: ligamentous failure. Extension instability: Anterior ligamentous failure. Rotation instability: Posterior joint ligamentous failure.
Lateral Bending Instability	2.39	Body alignment.	Aligned			Disc ligament failure if displaced.
		Pedicle position.	Smooth, progressive alteration			Posterior joint ligament laxity.
		Spinous position.	Toward concavity			Posterior joint ligament laxity.
	2.40	Intersegmental wedging.	Gradually increase away from the sacrum			Disc herniation at level failing to laterally flex (lateral bending sign).
Meyerding's Grading	2.41	Sacral base divided into quarters. Relative position of the posterior body of L5 is made.	—			Grading severity of spondylolisthesis.
Ullmann's Line	2.42	Endplate line through S1, perpendicular from sacral promontory.	L5 behind the line			Detection of subtle spondylolisthesis when L5 body crosses perpendicular line.
Interpediculate Distance	2.43	Shortest distance between inner surfaces of opposing pedicles.	See Table 2.18			Widened in intraspinal tumors, Narrowed in spinal stenosis.

Table 2.40.   Lines and Angles of the Lumbar Spine—*Continued*

Name	Figure Number	Landmarks	Normal Measurements			Significance
			Average	Minimum	Maximum	
Eisenstein's Method	2.44	Tips of superior and inferior articular processes joined. Distance between posterior midbody and this line (except at L5).	Variable	15 mm		Spinal stenosis suspected when less than 15 mm.
Canal/Body Ratio	2.45	Canal size (AP, lateral) divided by body size.				
		(a) L3 and L4		1:3.0	1:6.0	>1:6.0 denotes a small canal.
		(b) L5		1:3.2	1:6.5	>1:6.5 denotes a small canal.
Intercrestal Line	2.46	Iliac crests joined. Relative position of L4 and L5 bodies and discs.				May predict level of most stress and subsequent degeneration.
Transverse Process	2.47	Vertical line through L3 TVP. TIP. L5 TVP length assessed relative to this line.				May predict level of most stress and subsequent degeneration.

Table 2.41.   Lines and Angles of the Lower Extremities

Name	Figure Number	Landmarks	Normal Measurements			Significance
			Average	Minimum	Maximum	
Teardrop Distance	2.48	Femoral head—teardrop distance.	9 mm	6 mm	11 mm	Early Perthes or other inflammatory joint disease may widen the space more than 11 mm or create a 2 mm difference from the normal side.
Hip Joint Space Width	2.49	Femoral head—acetabulum distance.				Various joint diseases decrease these distances:
		(a) Superior	4 mm	3 mm	6 mm	Degenerative joint disease.
		(b) Axial	4 mm	3 mm	7 mm	Rheumatoid arthritis.
		(c) Medial	8 mm	4 mm	13 mm	Degenerative and rheumatoid arthritis.
Acetabular Depth	2.50	Superior pubis—outer acetabulum. The distance from the line to the furthest surface is measured.	Male: 13 mm Female: 12 mm	7 mm 9 mm	18 mm 18 mm	A shallow acetabulum exists when the measurement is less than 9 mm in females and 7 mm in males.
Center-Edge Angle	2.51	From the center of the femoral head, vertically, and acetabular edge, lines are drawn. The angle between is measured.	36°	20°	40°	A shallow acetabulum may precipitate degenerative joint disease.
Symphysis Pubis	2.52	The distance between opposing articular surfaces, halfway between the superior and inferior margins.	Male: 6 mm Female: 5 mm	4.8 mm 3.8 mm	7.2 mm 6.0 mm	Diastasis and inflammatory joint disease may widen the joint.
Presacral Space	2.53	Soft tissue density between the rectum and anterior sacral surface.	Child: 3 mm Adult: 7 mm	1 mm 2 mm	5 mm 20 mm	Soft tissue mass (tumor, infection, hematoma), if exceeds maximum distance.
Acetabular Angle	2.54	Y-Y line drawn. Second line from medial to lateral acetabular surfaces. Angle measured.	20°	12°	29°	Congenital hip dislocation widens the angle. Down's syndrome decreases the angle.
Iliac Angle	2.55	Y-Y line drawn. Second line along lateral iliac wing and iliac body.				Combined with acetabular angles to derive iliac index.
Iliac Index		Sum of right and left iliac and acetabular angles, divided by 2.	68°	Below 68°		Down's syndrome possible between 60–80°, and probable below 60°.
Protrusio Acetabuli	2.57	Pelvic inlet—outer obturator. Acetabulum should be lateral to the line.				Protrusio acetabuli (Paget's disease, etc.) when acetabulum is medial to the line.
Shenton's Line	2.58	Smooth curvilinear line along medial femoral neck and superior obturator border.				Femur dislocation or fracture if line is interrupted.
Iliofemoral Line	2.59	Smooth curvilinear line along ilium and onto femoral neck. Should be bilaterally symmetrical.				Asymmetry may denote hip joint abnormality.
Femoral Angle	2.60	Lines through the axis of the femoral shaft and neck.		120°	130°	Coxa vara: Less than 120°. Coxa valga: Greater than 130°.
Skinner's Line	2.61	Femoral shaft line. Perpendicular second line tangential to the tip of the greater trochanter.	Passes through or below fovea capitus			Hip joint abnormality (fracture, varus, etc.) if the line passes above the fovea capitus.
Klein's Line	2.62	Tangential line to outer femoral neck. Head just overlaps laterally.				Slipped epiphysis suspected head does not intersect line.
Axial Relationships of the Knee	2.63	(See text) (a) Femoral angle (b) Tibial angle	81° 93°	75° 85°	85° 100°	Deformities (traumatic, congenital, arthritic) at the knee will alter these angles.

Table 2.41.   Lines and Angles of the Lower Extremities—*Continued*

Name	Figure Number	Landmarks	Average	Minimum	Maximum	Significance
Patellar Malalignment						
Patella Alta	2.64A	Patella length (PL)—patella tendon (PT) ratio.	1:1 (+20%)			Chondromalacia patellae factor if the ratio is exceeded more than 20%.
Patella Apex	2.64B	Apex-intercondylar sulcus	Aligned			Patella subluxation.
Sulcus Angle	2.64B	Surfaces of medial and lateral condyles	138°	132°	144°	Shallow angle (> 144° predisposes to lateral subluxation.
Patellofemoral joint index	2.64B	Medial and lateral joint spaces	1.0			Ratio > 1 in chondromalacia patellae.
Lateral Patellofemoral angle	2.64C	Tangential lines through the femoral condyles and lateral facet of patella	Open angle			If lines parallel or open medially suggests patellar malalignment.
Lateral Patellar Displacement	2.64C	Perpendicular line tangential to the lateral edge of the medial femoral condyle	Tangential to medial edge of patella			Patellar malalignment.
Axial Relationships of the Ankle	2.65	(See text)				
		(a) Tibial angle	53°	45°	65°	
		(b) Fibular angle	52°	43°	63°	
Heel Pad	2.66	Shortest distance between the calcaneus and plantar skin surface.	Male: 19 mm Female: 19 mm		25 mm 23 mm	Acromegaly produces skin overgrowth exceeding the maximum measurement.
Boehler's Angle	2.67	Three superior points joined on the calcaneus. Posterior angle is measured.	30–35°	28°	40°	Calcaneal fractures may reduce the angle to less than 28°.

Table 2.42.   Lines and Angles of the Upper Extremities

Name	Figure Number	Landmarks	Average	Minimum	Maximum	Significance
Axial Relationships of the Shoulder	2.68	Humeral shaft—humeral head angle.	60–62°			Humeral deformities (fractures, congenital, etc.) will alter these values.
Glenohumeral Joint	2.69	Average humeral head—glenoid distance (superior, middle, inferior).	4–5 mm			Degenerative and crystal arthritis diminish the space. Posterior dislocation may widen it.
Acromiohumeral Joint Space	2.70	Acromion—humeral head.	9 mm	7 mm	11 mm	Rotator cuff tear decreases distance. Subluxation and dislocation increases distance.
Acromioclavicular Joint Space	2.71	Average acromion—clavicular distance (superior, inferior).	Male: 3.3 mm Female: 2.9 mm	2.5 mm 2.1	4.1 mm 3.7 mm	Degenerative arthritis decreases distance. Separation and resorption widens distance.
Axial Relationships of the Elbow	2.72	(See text)				
		(a) Carrying angle	169°	154°	178°	Elbow deformities (fractures, congenital, etc.) will alter these values.
		(b) Humeral angle	85°	72°	95°	
		(c) Ulnar angle	84°	72°	99°	
Radiocapitellar Line	2.73	Radius axis line through the elbow joint.	Passes through capitellar center			Radius subluxation/dislocation if line misses the capitellar center.
Axial Relationships of the Wrist	2.74	(See text)				
		(a) PA view: Radioulnar angle	83°	72°	95°	Wrist deformities (traumatic, congenital, etc.) will alter these values.
		(b) Lateral view: Radius angle	86°	79°	94°	
Metacarpal Sign	2.75	Tangential line through the fourth and fifth metacarpal heads. Third head should be proximal to this line.				Turner's syndrome, postfracture deformity.

REFERENCES

INTRODUCTION

1. **Owens EF:** *Line drawing analyses of static cervical x ray used in chiropractic.* J Manipulative Physiol Ther 15(7):442, 1992.
2. **Febbo TA, Morrison R, Valente R:** *Asymmetry of the occipitalcondyles: A computer-assisted analysis.* J Manipulative Physiol Ther 15(9):565, 1992.
3. **Morrissy RT, Goldsmith GS, Hall EC, et al:** *Measurement of the Cobb angle on radiographs of patients who have scoliosis.* J Bone Joint Surg (Am) 72:319, 1990.
4. **Carman DL, Browne RH, Birch JG:** *Measurement of scoliosis and kyphosis radiographs.* J Bone Joint Surg (Am) 72:328, 1990.
5. **Phillips RB:** *An evaluation of the graphic analysis of the pelvis on the AP full spine radiograph.* ACA J Chiro 9(Suppl): 139, December, 1975.
6. **Howe JW:** *Some considerations in spinal x-ray interpretations.* J Clin Chiro Archives 1:75, 1971.
7. **Howe JW:** *Facts and fallacies, myths and misconceptions in spinography.* J Clin Chiro Archives 2:34, 1972.
8. **Coste J, Paolaggi JB, Spira A:** *Reliability of interpretation of plain lumbar spine radiographs in benign, mechanical low-back pain.* Spine 16(4):426, 1991.
9. **Frymoyer JW, Phillips RB, Newberg AH, et al:** *A comparative analysis of the interpretations of lumbar spinal radiographs by chiropractors and medical doctors.* Spine 11(10):1020, 1986.

GEOMETRIC DISTORTION

1. **Ball RP, Golden R:** *Roentgenographic obstetrical pelvicephalometry in erect posture.* AJR 49:731, 1943.
2. **Brown GH:** *Automatic compensation in roentgenographic pelvicephalometry.* AJR 78:1063, 1957.

SKULL

1. **Vastine JH, Kinney KK:** *The pineal shadow as an aid in the localization of brain tumors.* AJR 17:320, 1927.
2. **Dyke CG:** *Indirect signs of brain tumor as noted in routine roentgen examinations. Displacement of the pineal shadow.* AJR 23:598, 1930.
3. **Pawl RP, Walter AK:** *Localization of the calcified pineal body on lateral roentgenograms.* AJR 105:287, 1969.
4. **Camp JD:** *The normal and pathologic anatomy of the sella turcica as revealed at necropsy.* Radiology 1:65, 1923.
5. **Silverman FN:** *Roentgen standards for size of the pituitary fossa from infancy through adolescence.* AJR 78:451, 1957.
6. **DiChiro G, Nelsen KB:** *The volume of the sella turcica.* AJR 87:989, 1962.
7. **Fisher RL, DiChiro G:** *The small sella turcica.* AJR 91:996, 1964.
8. **Poppel MH, Jacobson HG, Duff BK, et al:** *Basilar impression and platybasia in Paget's disease.* Radiology 61:639, 1953.
9. **McGregor M:** *The significance of certain measurements of the skull in the diagnosis of basilar impression.* Br J Radiol 21:171, 1948.
10. **Hinck VC, Hopkins CE, Savara BS:** *Diagnostic criteria of basilar impression.* Radiology 76:572, 1961.
11. **Chamberlain WE:** *Basilar impression (platybasia). A bizarre developmental anomaly of the occipital bone and upper cervical spine, with striking and misleading neurologic manifestations.* Yale J Biol Med 11:487, 1939.
12. **Macrae DL, Barnum AS:** *Occipitalization of the atlas.* AJR 70:23, 1953.
13. **Fischgold H, Metzger J:** *Etude radio-tomographique de l'impression basilaire.* Rev Rhum 19:261, 1952.
14. **Klaus E:** *Rontgendiagnostik der platybasie und basilaren impression. Weitere erfahrungen mit einer neuen untersuchungsmethode.* Fortschr Geb Roentgen 86:460, 1957.
15. **von Torklus D, Gehle W:** *The Upper Cervical Spine,* London, Butterworths, 1972.
16. **Powers B, Miller MD, Kramer RS, et al:** *Traumatic anterior atlanto-occipital dislocation.* Neurosurg 4(1):12, 1979.

CERVICAL SPINE

1. **Hinck VC, Hopkins CE:** *Measurement of the atlanto-dental interval in the adult.* AJR 84:945, 1960.
2. **Locke GR, Gardner JI, Van Epps EF:** *Atlas-dens interval (ADI) in children. A survey based on 200 normal cervical spines.* AJR 97:135, 1966.
3. **Monu J, Bohrer SP, Howard G:** *Some upper cervical norms.* Spine 12:515, 1987.
4. **Bohrer SP, Klein A, Martin W III:** *"V" shaped predens space.* Skeletal Radiol 14:111, 1985.
5. **White KS, Ball WS, Prenger EC, et al:** *Evaluation of the craniocervical junction in Down syndrome: Correlation of measurements obtained with radiography and MR imaging.* Radiology 186:377, 1993.
6. **Yochum TR, Rowe LJ:** *Arthritides of the Upper Cervical Complex.* In: Iczak R, Aspects of Manipulative Therapy, ed 2. New York, Churchill Livingstone, 1985.
7. **Bull JW, Nixon WLB, Pratt RTC:** *The radiological criteria and familial occurrence of primary basilar impression.* Brain 78:229, 1955.
8. **White AA, Southwick WO, Panjabi MM:** *Clinical instability in the lower cervical spine: A review of past and current concepts.* Spine 1:15, 1976.
9. **Wood J, Wagner NO:** *A review of methods for radiographic analysis of cervical sagittal motion.* Chiro Techn 4(3):83, 1992.
10. **Knight RQ:** *Complementary angles. A simplification of sagittal plane rotational assessment in cervical instability.* Spine 18(6):755, 1993.
11. **Henderson DJ, Dorman TM:** *Functional roentgenometric evaluation of the cervical spine in the sagittal plane.* J Manipulative Physiol Ther 8(4):219, 1985.

12. **George AW:** *A method for more accurate study of injuries to the atlas and axis.* Boston Med Surg J 181:13, 1919.
13. **Litterer WE:** *A history of George's line.* ACA J Chiro 39: December, 1983.
14. **Daffner RH, Deeb ZL, Rothfus WE:** *The posterior vertebral body line: Importance in the detection of burst fractures.* AJR 148:93, 1987.
15. **Daffner RH, Deeb ZL, Goldberg AL, et al:** *The radiologic assessment of post traumatic vertebral stability.* Skeletal Radiol 19:103, 1990.
16. **Swischuk LE:** *Anterior displacement of C2 in children: Physiologic or pathologic.* Radiology 122:759, 1977.
17. **Hinck VC, Hopkins CE, Savara BS:** *Sagittal diameter of the cervical spinal canal in children.* Radiology 79:97, 1962.
18. **Wolf BS, Khilnani M, Malis L:** *The sagittal diameter of the bony canal and its significance in cervical spondylosis.* J Mount Sinai Hosp NY 23:283, 1956.
19. **Yousefzadeh DK, El-Khoury GY, Smith WL:** *Normal sagittal diameter and variation in the pediatric cervical spine.* Radiology 144:319, 1982.
20. **Alker G:** *Neuroradiology of cervical spondylotic myelopathy.* Spine 13:850, 1988.
21. **Pavlov H, Torg JS, Robie B, et al:** *Cervical spinal stenosis: Determination with vertebral body ratio method.* Radiology 164:771, 1987.
22. **Torg JS:** *Cervical spine stenosis with cord neuropraxia and transient quadriplegia.* Current Opinions Orthop 5(11):97, 1994.
23. **Shapiro R, Youngberg AS, Rothman SLG:** *The differential diagnosis of traumatic lesions of the occipito-atlanto-axial segment.* Radiol Clin North Am 11(3):505, 1973.
24. **Rowe LJ:** *A clinico-radiologic correlation in cervical trauma-Jefferson's fracture.* J Aust Chiro Assoc 19(5):5, 1989.
25. **Thomeier WC, Brown DC, Mirvis SE:** *The laterally tilted dens: A sign of subtle odontoid fracture on plain film radiography.* AJNR 11:605, 1990.
26. **Suss RA, Zimmerman RD, Leeds NE:** *Pseudospread of the atlas: False sign of Jefferson fracture in young children.* AJR 140:1079, 1983.
27. **Fox MG, Young OG:** *Placement of the gravital line in antero-posterior standing posture.* Research Quart 25:277, 1954.
28. **Gore DR, Sepic SB, Gardner GM:** *Roentgenographic findings of the cervical spine in asymptomatic people.* Spine 11:521, 1986.
29. **Hellsing E, Geigo T, McWilliam J, et al:** *Cervical and lumbar lordosis and thoracic kyphosis in 8-, 11-, and 15-year-old children.* Eur J Orthop 9:129, 1987.
30. **Leach RA:** *An evaluation of the effect of chiropractic manipulative therapy on hypolordosis of the cervical spine.* J Manipulative Physiol Ther 6:17, 1983.
31. **Gay RE:** *The curve of the cervical spine: Variations and significance.* J Manipulative Physiol Ther 16(9): 591, 1993.
32. **Borden AGB, Rechtman AM, Gershon-Cohen J:** *The normal cervical lordosis.* Radiology 74:806, 1960.
33. **Jochumsen OH:** *The curve of the cervical spine.* ACA J Chiro S49: August, 1970.
34. **Jochumsen OH:** *Diagnostics.* J Clin Chiro 2 (4):88, 1969.
35. **Drexler L:** *Rontgenanatomische Untersuchringen uber Form and Krumming der Halswirbelsaule in den Verscchiedenen Lebensaltern,* Stuttgart, Hippokrates, 1962.
36. **Juhl JH, Miller SM, Roberts GW:** *Roentgenographic variations in the normal cervical spine.* Radiology 78:591, 1962.
37. **Fineman S, Borrelli FJ, Rubinstein BM, et al:** *The cervical spine: Transformation of the normal lordotic pattern into a linear pattern in the neutral posture. A roentgenographic depiction.* J Bone Joint Surg (Am) 45:1179, 1963.
38. **Weir DC:** *Roentgenographic signs of cervical injury.* Clin Orthop 109:9, 1975.
39. **Pederson PL:** *A prospective pilot study of the shape of cervical hypolordosis.* J Manipulative Physiol Ther 16(9):591, 1993.
40. **Jackson R:** *The Cervical Syndrome,* ed 4. Springfield, Charles C Thomas, 1977.
41. **Batzdorf U, Batzdorf A:** *Analysis of cervical spine curvature in patients with cervical spondylosis.* Neurosurgery 22:827, 1988.
42. **Bolton PS, Ware AE:** *Degenerative joint disease in the cervical spine of chiropractic patients.* J Aust Chiro Assoc 18:51, 1988.
43. **Penning L:** *Prevertebral hematoma in cervical spine injury: Incidence and etiologic significance.* AJR 136:553, 1981.
44. **Sistrom CL, Southall EP, Peddada SD, et al:** *Factors affecting the thickness of the cervical prevertebral soft tissues.* Skeletal Radiol 22:167, 1993.

THORACIC SPINE

1. **Morrissy RT, Goldsmith GS, Hall EC, et al:** *Measurement of the Cobb angle on radiographs of patients who have scoliosis.* J Bone Joint Surg (Am) 72:319, 1990.
2. **Carman DL, Browne RH, Birch JG:** *Measurement of scoliosis and kyphosis radiographs.* J Bone Joint Surg (Am) 72:328, 1990.
3. **Oda M, Rauh S, Gregory PB, et al:** *The significance of roentgenographic measurement in scoliosis.* J Pediatr Orthop 2:378, 1982.
4. **Cobb JR:** *Outline for the study of scoliosis.* Am Acad Orthop Surg 5:261, 1948.
5. **Keim HA:** *The Adolescent Spine,* New York, Grune & Stratton, 1976.
6. **George K, Rippstein J:** *A comparative study of the two popular methods of measuring scoliotic deformity.* J Bone Joint Surg (Am) 43(6):809, 1961.
7. **Risser JC, Ferguson AB:** *Scoliosis: Its prognosis.* J Bone Joint Surg (Am) 18:667, 1936.
8. **Ferguson AB:** *Roentgen Diagnosis of Extremities and Spine,* New York, Paul B. Hoeber, 1949.
9. **Fon GT, Pitt MJ, Thies AC:** *Thoracic kyphosis. Range in normal subjects.* AJR 134:979, 1980.
10. **Maiman DJ, Pintar FA:** *Anatomy and clinical biomechanics of the thoracic spine.* Clin Neurosurg 38:296, 1992.
11. **Panjabi MM, Takata K, Goel V, et al:** *Thoracic human vertebrae. Quantitative three dimensional anatomy.* Spine 16:888, 1991.
12. **El-Khoury G, Whitten CG:** *Trauma to the upper thoracic spine: Anatomy, biomechanics, and unique imaging features.* AJR 160:95, 1993.

13. Fletcher GH: *Anterior vertebral wedging: Frequency and significance.* AJR 57:232, 1947.
14. Lauridsen KN, De Carvalho A, Andersen AH: *Degree of vertebral body wedging of the dorsolumbar spine.* Acta Radiol 25:29, 1984.
15. Itoi E: *Roentgenographic analysis of posture in spinal osteoporotics.* Spine 16(7):750, 1991.
16. Hellsing E, Gelgo T, McWilliam J, et al: *Cervical and lumbar lordosis and thoracic kyphosis in 8-, 11-, and 15-year-old children.* Eur J Orthop 9:129, 1987.
17. Twigg HL, deLeon AC, Perloff JK, et al: *The straight back syndrome. Radiographic manifestations.* Radiology 88:274, 1967.
18. Yochum TR, Albers VL: *The "straight-back" syndrome.* ACA J Chiro, Radiology Corner, September 1982.

LUMBAR SPINE

1. Pope MH, Hanley EN, Malteri RE, et al: *Measurement of the intervertebral joint space.* Spine 2(4):282, 1977.
2. Dabbs VM, Dabbs LG: *Correlation between disc height narrowing and low-back pain.* Spine 15(12):1366, 1990.
3. Hurxthal LM: *Measurement of anterior vertebral compressions and biconcave vertebrae.* AJR 103:635, 1968.
4. Farfan HF: *Mechanical Disorders of the Low Back,* Philadelphia, Lea & Febiger, 1973.
5. Frymoyer JW, Newberg A, Pope MH, et al: *Spine radiographs in patients with low back pain.* J Bone Joint Surg (Am) 66:1048, 1984.
6. Busche-McGregor M, Naimen J, Grice AS: *Analysis of the lumbar lordosis in an asymptomatic population of young adults.* J Can Chiro Assoc 25:58, 1981.
7. Banks SD: *The use of spinographic parameters in the differential diagnosis of lumbar facet and disc syndromes.* J Manipulative Physiol Ther 6(3):113, 1983.
8. Hildebrandt RW: *Chiropractic Spinography. A Manual of Technology and Interpretation,* ed 2. Baltimore, Williams & Wilkins, 1985.
9. Hansson T, Bigos S, Beecher P, et al: *The lumbar lordosis in acute and chronic low back pain.* Spine 10(2):154, 1985.
10. Adams MA, Hutton WC: *Mechanical factors in the etiology of low back pain.* Orthopedics 5(11):1461, 1982.
11. Drum D: *The posterior gravity line syndrome, recurrent low back pain of postural origin.* J Can Chiro Assoc 12:5, 1968.
12. Kraus H: *The effects of lordosis on the stress in the lumbar spine.* Clin Orthop 117:56, 1976.
13. Bryner P, El Moussali M: *Lumbar spine lordosis in low-back pain: An analysis of radiographs.* Chiro J Aust 22(2):42, 1992.
14. Beattie PF, Brooks WM, Rothstein JM, et al: *Effect of lordosis on the position of the nucleus pulposus in supine subjects. A study using magnetic resonance imaging.* Spine 19(18):2096, 1994.
15. Mosner EA, Bryan JM, Stull MA, et al: *A comparison of actual and apparent lumbar lordosis in black and white adult females.* Spine 14(3):310, 1989.
16. Saraste H, Brostrom LA, Aparisi T, et al: *Radiographic measurement of the lumbar spine.* Spine 10(3):236, 1985.
17. Ferguson AB: *Roentgen Diagnosis of Extremities and Spine,* New York, Paul B. Hoeber, 1949.
18. Ferguson AB: *The clinical and roentgenographic interpretation of lumbosacral anomalies.* Radiology 22:548, 1934.
19. Meschan I, Farrer-Meschan RMF: *Important aspects in the roentgen study of the normal lumbosacral spine.* Radiology 70:637, 1958.
20. Hellems HK, Keats TE: *Measurement of the normal lumbosacral angle.* AJR 113:642, 1971.
21. Jessen AR: *An in depth study of the lumbosacral angle.* ACA J Chiro 65: September, 1971.
22. Splittoff CA: *Lumbosacral junction. Roentgenographic comparisons of patients with and without backaches.* JAMA 152(17):1610, 1953.
23. von Lackum HL: *The lumbosacral region. An anatomical study and some clinical observations.* JAMA 82(14):1109, 1924.
24. Adams MA, Hutton WC: *The effect of posture on the role of the joints in resisting intervertebral compressive force.* J Bone Joint Surg (Br) 62:358, 1980.
25. Jayson MIV: *Compression stresses in the posterior elements and pathologic consequences.* Spine 8(3):338, 1983.
26. Peterson CK, Haas M, Harger BL: *A radiographic study of sacral base, sacrovertebral, and lumbosacral disc angles in persons with and without defects in the pars interarticularis.* J Manipulative Physiol Ther 13(9):491, 1990.
27. Cox JM: *Low Back Pain. Mechanism, Diagnosis, and Treatment,* ed 5. Baltimore, Williams & Wilkins, 1990.
28. *Basic Chiropractic Procedural Manual,* Des Moines, American Chiropractic Association, 1973.
29. Janelle L, Larsen E, Gaillardetz C, et al: *A statistical analysis of preemployment lumbar spine radiographs for structural and postural abnormalities.* Canadian Memorial Chiropractic College, Thesis, 1983.
30. Klaussen K, Rasmussen B: *On the location of the line of gravity in relation to L5 in standing.* Acta Physiol Scand 72:45, 1968.
31. Macnab I: *Backache,* Baltimore, Williams & Wilkins, 1977.
32. Kelly K: *Validity of Macnab's line.* Canadian Memorial Chiropractic College, Thesis, 1985.
33. Hadley LA: *Intervertebral joint subluxation, bony impingement, and foraminal encroachment, with nerve root changes.* AJR 65:377, 1951.
34. Hadley LA: *Anatomico-Roentgenographic Studies of the Spine,* ed 5. Springfield, Charles C Thomas, 1981.

35. Peters RE: *The facet syndrome.* J Austr Chiro Assoc 13(3):15, 1983.
36. Swezey RL, Silverman TR: *Radiographic demonstration of induced vertebral facet displacements.* Arch Phys Med Rehab 52:244, 1971.
37. Abel M: *The unstable apophyseal joint: An early sign of lumbar disc disease.* Skeletal Radiol 2:31, 1977.
38. van Akkerveeken PF, Obrien JP, Park WM: *Experimentally induced hypermobility in the lumbar spine.* Spine 4:236, 1979.
39. Morgan FP, King T: *Primary instability of lumbar vertebrae as a common cause of low back pain.* J Bone Joint Surg (Br) 39:6, 1957.
40. Dupuis PR, Yong-Hing K, Cassidy JD, et al: *Radiologic diagnosis of degenerative lumbar spinal instability.* Spine 10(3):262, 1985.
41. Friberg O: *Lumbar instability: A dynamic approach by traction-compression radiography.* Spine 12(2):119, 1987.
42. Phillips RB, Howe JW, Bustin G, et al: *Stress x-rays and the low back pain patient.* J Manipulative Physiol Ther 13(3):127, 1990.
43. Sato H, Kikuchi S: *The natural history of radiographic instability of the lumbar spine.* Spine 18(14):2075, 1993.
44. Wood KB, Popp CA, Transfeldt EE, et al: *Radiographic evaluation of instability in spondylolisthesis.* Spine 19(15):1697, 1994.
45. Weitz EM: *The lateral bending sign.* Spine 6(4):388, 1981.
46. Meyerding HW: *Spondylolisthesis.* Surg Gynecol Obstet 54:371, 1932.
47. Capener N: *Spondylolisthesis.* Br J Surg 19:374, 1932.
48. Garland LH, Thomas SF: *Spondylolisthesis. Criteria for more accurate diagnosis of true anterior slip of the involved vertebral segment.* AJR 55:275, 1946.
49. Hinck VC, Clark WM Jr, Hopkins CE: *Normal interpediculate distances (minimum and maximum).* AJR 97:141, 1966.
50. Elseberg CA, Dyke CG: *Diagnosis and localization of tumors of spinal cord by means of measurements made on x-ray films of vertebrae, and correlation of clinical and x-ray findings.* Bull Neurol Inst NY 3:359, 1934.
51. Eisenstein S: *Measurements in the lumbar spinal canal in two racial groups.* Clin Orthop Rel Res 115:42, 1976.
52. Weisz GM, Lee P: *Spinal canal stenosis. Concept of spinal reserve capacity: Radiologic measurements and clinical applications.* Clin Orthop Rel Res 179:134, 1983.
53. Jones RAC, Thompson JLG: *The narrow lumbar canal.* J Bone Joint Surg (Br) 50:595, 1968.
54. Williams RM: *The narrow lumbar spinal canal.* Australas Radiol 19:356, 1975.
55. MacGibbon B, Farfan H: *A radiologic survey of various configurations of the lumbar spine.* Spine 4(3):258, 1979.
56. Leboeuf C, Kimber D, White K: *Prevalence of spondylolisthesis, transitional anomalies and low intercrestal line in a chiropractic population.* J Manipulative Physiol Ther 12(3):200, 1989.

LOWER EXTREMITY

1. Eyring EJ, Bjornson DR, Peterson CA: *Early diagnostic and prognostic signs in Legg-Calvé-Perthes disease.* AJR 93:382, 1965.
2. Sweeney JP, Helms CA, Minagi H, et al: *The widened teardrop distance: A plain film indicator of hip joint effusion in adults.* AJR 149:117, 1987.
3. Bowerman JW, Sena JM, Chang R: *The teardrop shadow of the pelvis: Anatomy and clinical significance.* Radiology 143:659, 1982.
4. Armbruster JG, Guerra J, Resnick D, et al: *The adult hip. An anatomic study.* Radiology 128:1, 1978.
5. Murray RO: *The aetiology of primary osteoarthritis of the hip.* Br J Radiol 38:810, 1965.
6. Wiberg G: *Studies on dysplastic acetabula and congenital subluxation of the hip joint—with special reference to the complication of osteoarthritis.* Acta Chir Scand (Suppl 58):1, 1939.
7. Anda S, Terjesen T, Kvistad KA: *Computed tomography measurements of the acetabulum in adult dysplastic hips: Which level is appropriate?* Skeletal Radiol 20:267, 1991.
8. Vix VA, Ryu CY: *The adult symphysis pubis: Normal and abnormal.* AJR 112:517, 1971.
9. Chrispin AR, Fry IK: *The presacral space shown by barium enema.* Br J Radiol 36:319, 1963.
10. Eklöf O, Gierup J: *The retrorectal soft tissue space in children: Normal variations and appearances in granulomatous colitis.* AJR 108:624, 1970.
11. Caffey J: *Contradiction of congenital dysplasia—Predislocation hypothesis of congenital dislocation of hip through study of normal variation in acetabular angles at successive periods in infancy.* Pediatrics (7):632, 1956.
12. Caffey J, Ross S: *Pelvic bones in infantile mongoloidism: Roentgenographic features.* AJR 80:458, 1958.
13. Astley R: *Chromosomal abnormalities in childhood, with particular reference to Turner's syndrome and mongolism.* Br J Radiol 36:2, 1963.
14. Kohler A, Zimmer EA: *Borderlands of the Normal and Early Pathologic in Skeletal Roentgenology,* ed 3. New York, translated by SP Wilk, Grune & Stratton, 1968.
15. Kohler A: *Roentgenology. The Borderlands of the Normal and Early Pathological in the Skiagram,* ed 2. edited by A Turnbull, London, Balliere, Tindall & Cox, 1935.
16. Hubbard MJS: *The measurement of progression in protrusio acetabuli.* AJR 106:506, 1969.
17. Martin HE: *Geometrical-anatomical factors and their significance in the early x-ray diagnosis of hip joint disease in children.* Radiology 56:842, 1951.
18. Keats TE, Teeslink R, Diamond AE, et al: *Normal axial relationships of the major joints.* Radiology 87:904, 1966.
19. Sante LR: *Principles of Roentgenological Interpretation,* ed 8. Ann Arbor, Edwards Bros, 1949.

20. **Klein A, Joplin RJ, Reidy JA, et al:** *Roentgenographic features of slipped capital femoral epiphysis.* AJR 66:361, 1951.
21. **Insall J, Salvati E:** *Patella position in the normal knee joint.* Radiology 101:101, 1971.
22. **Kannus PA:** *Long patella tendon: Radiographic sign of patellofemoral pain syndrome. A prospective study.* Radiology 185:859, 1992.
23. **Rowe LJ:** Imaging of the Knee. In *The Knee. Clinical Applications.* Edited by A.L. Logan. Aspen Publishers, Gaithersburg, 1995.
24. **Merchant AC, Mercer RL, Jacobsen RH, et al.:** *Roentgenologic analysis of patellofemoral joint congruence.* J Bone Joint Surg (Am) 56:1391, 1974.
25. **Hughston JC:** *Subluxation of the patella.* J Bone Joint Surg (Am) 50:1003, 1968.
26. **Wiberg G:** *Roentgenographic and anatomic studies on the femoropatellar joint.* Acta Orthop Scan 12:319, 1941.
27. **Laurin CA, Dussault R, Levesque HP:** *The tangential x-ray investigation of the patello-femoral joint: X-ray technique, diagnostic criteria, and their interpretation.* Clin Orthop 144:16, 1979.
28. **Berquist TH:** *Radiology of the Foot and Ankle.* Raven Press, New York, 1989.
29. **Rubin G, Witten M:** *The talar tilt angle and the fibular collateral ligaments: A method for the determination of talar tilt.* J Bone Joint Surg (Am) 42A:311, 1960.
30. **Christman OD, Snook CA:** *A reconstruction of lateral ligament tears of the ankle: An experimental study and clinical evaluation of seven patients treated by a new modification of the Elmslie procedure.* J Bone Joint Surg (Am) 51:904, 1969.
31. **Gould N, Seligson D, Glassman J:** *Early and late repair of lateral ligaments of the ankle.* Foot Ankle 1:84, 1980.
32. **Steinbach HL, Russell W:** *Measurement of the heel pad as an aid to diagnosis of acromegaly.* Radiology 82:418, 1964.
33. **Kho KM, Wright AD, Doyle FH:** *Heel pad thickness in acromegaly.* Br J Radiol 43:119, 1970.
34. **Puckette SE, Seymour EQ:** *Fallibility of the heel pad thickness in the diagnosis of acromegaly.* Radiology 88:982, 1967.
35. **Resnick DL, Feingold ML, Curd J, et al:** *Calcaneal abnormalities in articular disorders. Rheumatoid arthritis, ankylosing spondylitis, psoriatic arthritis and Reiter's syndrome.* Radiology 125:355, 1977.
36. **Boehler L:** *Diagnosis, pathology, and treatment of fractures of os calcis.* J Bone Joint Surg (Am) 13:75, 1931.

UPPER EXTREMITY

1. **Keats TE, Teeslink R, Diamond AE, et al:** *Normal axial relationship of the major joints.* Radiology 87:904, 1966.
2. **Petersson CJ, Redlund-Johnell I:** *Joint space in normal glenohumeral radiographs.* Acta Orthop Scand 54:274, 1983.
3. **Arndt JH, Sears AD:** *Posterior dislocation of the shoulder.* AJR 94:639, 1965.
4. **Alexander C:** *The acromio-humeral distance in health and disease.* Proc Coll Radiol Aust 3:102, 1959.
5. **Lev-Toaff AS, Karasick D, Rao VM:** *Drooping shoulder—nontraumatic causes of glenohumeral subluxation.* Skeletal Radiol 12:34, 1984.
6. **Storen G:** *Traumatic dislocation of the radial head as an isolated lesion in children. Report of one case with special regard to roentgen diagnosis.* Acta Chir Scand 116:144, 1959.
7. **Archibald RM, Finby N, de Vitto F:** *Endocrine significance of short metacarpals.* J Clin Endocrinol 19:1312, 1959.

3

Congenital Anomalies and Normal Skeletal Variants

Gary M. Guebert, Terry R. Yochum, and Lindsay J. Rowe

INTRODUCTION

Congenital anomalies and normal skeletal variants are a common occurrence in clinical practice. In this chapter a large number of skeletal anomalies of the spine and pelvis are reviewed. Some of the more common skeletal anomalies of the extremities are also presented. Pertinent comments relating to the clinical significance of various anomalies are included.

The second section of this chapter deals with normal skeletal variants. Some of these variants may simulate certain disease processes. In some instances there are no clear-cut distinctions between skeletal variants and anomalies; therefore there may be some overlap of material. The congenital anomalies are presented initially with accompanying text, photos, and references, beginning with the skull and proceeding caudally through the spine to then include the pelvis and extremities. The normal skeletal variants section is presented in an anatomic atlas format without text or references. A full and thorough understanding of these congenital anomalies and skeletal variants will assist the reader in being better prepared to approach the pathologic interpretation of skeletal radiographs.

ANOMALIES OF THE CRANIOVERTEBRAL REGION

OCCIPITALIZATION OF THE ATLAS

Description. Also known as assimilation of C1, Macalister long ago described fusion of the atlas to the base of the occiput. (1) This maldevelopment of the craniovertebral junction repre-

sents the most cephalic "blocked vertebra" encountered in the spine. Embryologically, there is a lack of segmentation and separation of the most caudal occipital sclerotome during the first few weeks of fetal life that results in this deformity of the atlanto-occipital junction.

Generally, young patients will be asymptomatic, and the condition is of radiographic interest only. Symptoms may be caused by compression of the medulla oblongata and proximal spinal cord as the odontoid process protrudes through the foramen magnum. These symptoms include headache, diminished range of motion, visual and auditory abnormalities, neural manifestations in the upper extremities. Older children or young adults may develop degenerative joint changes at the subadjacent, freely articulated segments or possible laxity of the transverse ligament with attendant cord compression. (2)

Occipitalization of C1 may occur as an isolated anomaly, but has been seen in association with platybasia, basilar impression, Arnold-Chiari malformation (type I), atlantoaxial dislocation or instability, Sturge-Weber syndrome, and Klippel-Feil syndrome. (3) When occipitalization occurs in association with basilar impression, symptoms of nuchal pain and vertigo have been reported. (4)

Radiologic Features. The lateral film demonstrates a decreased or nonexistent space between the posterior arch of C1 and the base of the occiput. (Fig. 3.1A–C) On the frontal view, even with the head in optimal position, visualization of the atlanto-occipital joints usually is not possible because of the relative basilar impression that is present, so that the teeth of the maxilla overlie the atlas and axis. Flexion and extension views will demonstrate an absence of motion between the posterior arch of C1 and the lower margin of the occiput. Tomograms in the frontal

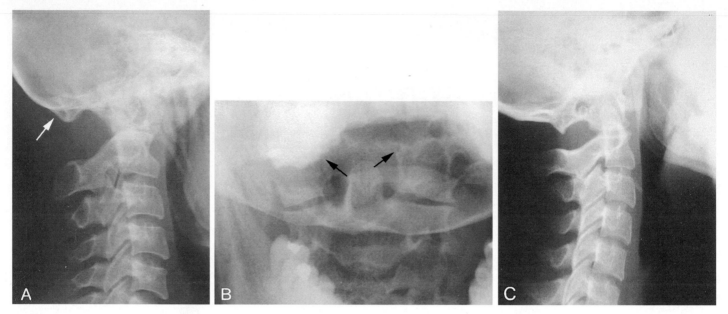

Figure 3.1.   OCCIPITALIZATION OF THE ATLAS. A. Coned Lateral Cervical. Observe the fusion of the posterior arch of C1 to the base of the occiput (arrow). Note the large gap superior to the spinous process of C2. **B. Coned AP Open Mouth**. The fusion of the atlanto-occipital joint can be seen (ar-row). **C. Coned Lateral Cervical**. COMMENT: These patients should have flexion/extension studies performed because of the increased stress placed on adjacent, freely articulated joints. (**A** and **B** Courtesy of Kip LaShoto, DC, Waltham, Massachusetts)

plane demonstrate fusion of one or both atlanto-occipital joints. Computed tomography of the craniovertebral region will optimally demonstrate the osseous abnormalites. MRI is valuable to visualize any neural anomalies that may coexist.

MEDICOLEGAL IMPLICATIONS
Occipitalization of the Atlas

- Occipitalization with basilar invagination may result in catastrophic spinal cord injury with forced cervical extension. (5)
- The vertebral artery may run in the spinal canal below the level of C1 causing lateral C1-C2 punctures to carry more risk. (6)
- Sudden hearing loss has been found with increased incidence in patients with occipitalization. (7)

OCCIPITAL VERTEBRAE

Developmental anomalies of the spine occur with the greatest frequency at transitional areas such as the atlanto-occipital junction or lumbosacral junction. They may occur as isolated defects or in association with other spinal or soft tissue malformations. Development of the occiput begins when the first four somites of the embryo unite to form the basiocciput. The caudal aspect of the fourth somite then fuses with the cranial half of the C1 somite. The disc anlage at this level becomes the apical and alar ligaments.

Failure of normal fusion of the terminal segments of the basiocciput may result in what are called *occipital vertebrae*. If the defective fusion is anterior, the result is called a *third condyle*. Laterally placed anomalies are termed *paracondyloid, paramastoid,* or *epitransverse* processes, depending on their exact anatomic re-

lationships relative to the occiput and atlas. Manifestations of occipital vertebrae also include various other accessory ossicles around the foramen magnum.

THIRD CONDYLE

Description.   The first mention of a third condyle in the radiologic literature is by Hadley in 1948. (1) It results from a failure of fusion of the most caudal occipitoblast, near the midline, resulting in a small bony ossicle near the anteroinferior margin of the foramen magnum. It is also known as *condylus tertius*. Lombardi considers the third condyle to be the most frequent manifestation of occipital vertebrae (2). Generally, this accessory bone is of no clinical significance; however, if large enough, it may restrict head movement.

Radiologic Features.   Small third condyles may be impossible to visualize on lateral plain film radiographs because of the superimposed mastoid processes and the petrous portion of the temporal bone. Larger third condyles may be seen on true lateral radiographs of the upper cervical spine as oval or round bone densities equal in size or smaller than the anterior arch of the atlas. Some are sufficiently large and caudally placed, forming an articulation with the superior aspect of the anterior arch of C1. (Fig. 3.2) A third condyle will not be evident on open mouth radiographs, but conventional tomography or CT evaluation is ideally suited for imaging this anomaly.

EPITRANSVERSE AND PARACONDYLAR PROCESSES

Description.   An epitransverse process may be unilateral or bilateral. It may originate from the transverse process of atlas and will either articulate with the skull near the jugular process or form a solid bony union with the skull base. If, however, the bony process begins at the jugular process of the occiput and projects toward the transverse process of C1, the appropriate name would

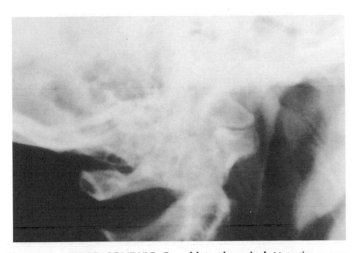

Figure 3.2.   THIRD CONDYLE. Coned lateral cervical. Note the anomalous bone that descends from the skull base to "articulate" with the superior margin of the C1 anterior arch. The presence of the third condyle has deformed the C1 anterior arch. (Courtesy of Gary M. Guebert, DC, DACBR, St. Louis, Missouri)

be a paracondylar process or paramastoid process. (3) The significance of this finding is that a decreased range of motion, particularly lateral flexion, may be perceived at the atlanto-occipital junction. Manipulation of the occiput-C1 articulation would be impossible as the occiput and atlas are effectively fused and move as a unit. Symptoms associated with a paracondylar process include cervical contracture and pain. (4)

Radiologic Features.   The diagnosis of this anomaly may require the use of sophisticated tomography, as the teeth of the maxilla often obstruct the view of this area on well-positioned open-mouth radiographs. (Fig. 3.3A and B) A slightly rotated open-mouth view will shift the molars on the side opposite the direction of head rotation away from the area of interest so that the bony connection between the occiput and the transverse process may be clearly seen. An accessory joint may be present between the anomalous process and the superior aspect of the C1 transverse process, or a solid bony union may be present. (Fig. 3.4A–C) Occasionally, this process will act like a shim and cause a lateral tilt of the head. CT and MRI are excellent for clarifying the exact location and extent of the anomalous process and ruling out neoplasm or other causes for this appearance. (Fig. 3.5A and B)

MEDICOLEGAL IMPLICATIONS
Epitransverse/Paramastoid Process

- Patients with an epitransverse process may be at risk for posttraumatic basal subarachnoid hemorrhage. (5)

ACCESSORY OSSICLES

Description.   A variety of small bone fragments may develop in the ligaments around the foramen magnum. The embryologic evolution of these pieces of bone have been theorized to be expressions of occipital vertebrae, (6) while others consider them to

be examples of secondary ossification within the ligaments around the foramen magnum. (7)

Radiologic Features.   These accessory bones are usually seen above the anterior arch of the atlas as small, round or oval sesamoid-like bones.

PLATYBASIA / BASILAR IMPRESSION

Description.   Platybasia literally means broad base and is the result of congenital maldevelopment of the sphenoid and/or occipital bones. This flattening of the skull base is determined from mensuration performed on lateral skull radiographs. The method of measuring the skull base angle (Martin's basilar angle) has been described in Chapter 2. If this angle is greater than 152°, platybasia exists. Platybasia alone may be clinically insignificant, but it is often found in association with occipitalization of C1 and Klippel-Feil syndrome.

Platybasia should be differentiated from basilar impression, although Chamberlain incorrectly used the terms interchangeably. (1) The term "basilar impression" or "basilar invagination" may be used synonymously. There are two types of basilar impression—primary and secondary.

Primary Basilar Impression.   Primary basilar impression is congenital in origin and is often associated with a variety of vertebral defects such as occipitalization of the atlas, spina bifida occulta of the atlas, odontoid anomalies, agenesis or hypoplasia of the atlas, Klippel-Feil syndrome, and Arnold-Chiari malformation. (2)

Secondary Basilar Impression.   Secondary basilar impression is

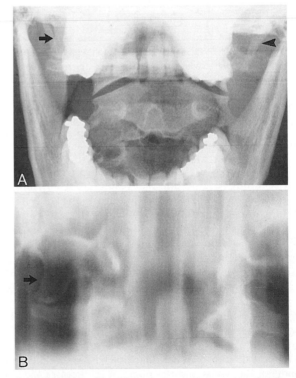

Figure 3.3.   PARACONDYLAR PROCESS. A. AP Open Mouth. Observe the bony protuberance projecting from the paracondylar area directed toward the transverse process of the atlas (arrow). This should not be confused with the slender styloid process of the temporal bone (arrowhead). **B. AP Tomogram.** Tomography clearly shows the paracondylar process (arrow), forming an accessory articulation with the transverse process of C1.

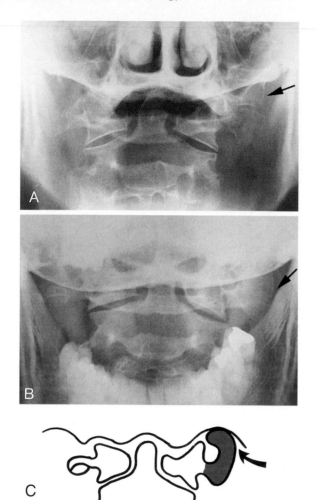

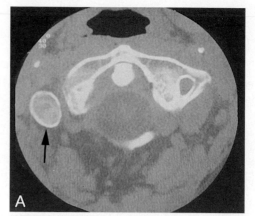

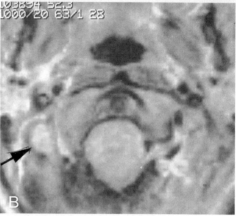

Figure 3.4. EPITRANSVERSE AND PARACONDYLAR PROCESS. A. AP Open Mouth. An epitransverse process (arrow), along with an accessory articulation, is present at the atlas. The clarity of the open-mouth radiograph is the result of two factors: the patient is edentulous, and the patient's jaw was moving intentionally during the exposure. **B. AP Open Mouth.** An osseous bar is noted between the paracondylar area and the transverse process of the atlas, to which it is fully fused (arrow). **C. Schematic Diagram: Epitransverse Process.**

Figure 3.5. EPITRANSVERSE PROCESS. A. The CT bone window demonstrates the osseous bar (arrow) that unites the C1 right transverse process with the occiput. **B.** The axial MRI scan shows a normal marrow signal from within the epitransverse process (arrow). (Courtesy of G. Matt Howard III, DC, Muncie, Indiana)

usually an acquired condition that results from softening of the occipital bone. The weight of the skull causes the occiput to settle around the upper cervical spine so that the distance between the occiput and atlas is reduced, the odontoid process encroaches on the foramen magnum, and there is elevation in the floor of the posterior fossa.

Three bone-softening disorders that are commonly associated with secondary basilar impression are Paget's disease, osteomalacia, and fibrous dysplasia. (2)

Classic symptoms of basilar impression include headache and nystagmus.

Radiologic Features. On a lateral x-ray of the skull, platybasia may be diagnosed when Martin's basilar angle, formed by the plane of the clivus and the plane of the floor of the anterior fossa, is unusually flat (i.e., greater than 152°). (3) There is no evidence of a bone-softening pathology.

Basilar impression will show evidence of elevation of the floor of the posterior fossa and upward convexity of the posterior aspect of the foramen magnum. The apex of the odontoid process may extend above the plane of the foramen magnum, giving a positive finding to Chamberlain's or McGregor's lines. (See Chapter 2.) (Fig. 3.6A and B) Additional signs of the associated bone-softening pathology (e.g., Paget's disease, osteomalacia, fibrous dysplasia) will also be observed. (See Chapters 11 and 14.)

MEDICOLEGAL IMPLICATIONS
Platybasia/Basilar Impression

- Patients with basilar impression often develop pyramidal tract signs, posterior column signs, wasting of the upper limbs, and abnormalities in somatosensory evoked potentials and abnormal brainstem auditory evoked potentials. (4)
- Sudden hearing loss has been found with increased incidence in patients with basilar impression. (3)
- Platybasia has been associated with syringomyelia. The syrinx regressed after odontoid resection. (5)
- Lethal spinal cord injury following hyperextension of the cervical spine has been reported in a patient with basilar impression and occipitalization of C1. (6)

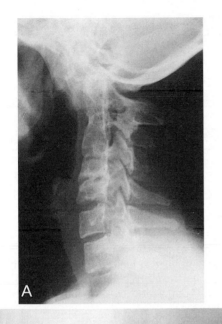

Figure 3.6. BASILAR IMPRESSION. A. Lateral Cervical. The important plain film finding is the lack of interosseous spacing between the occiput and the posterior arch of the atlas. Note, additionally, the congenital malformations affecting the C2-C5 vertebral bodies and neural arches. **B. Lateral Tomogram: Upper Cervical.** The odontoid process (*O*) has projected well above McGregor's line (*M*), proving basilar impression. Patients with this degree of basilar impression often exhibit profound neurologic symptoms.

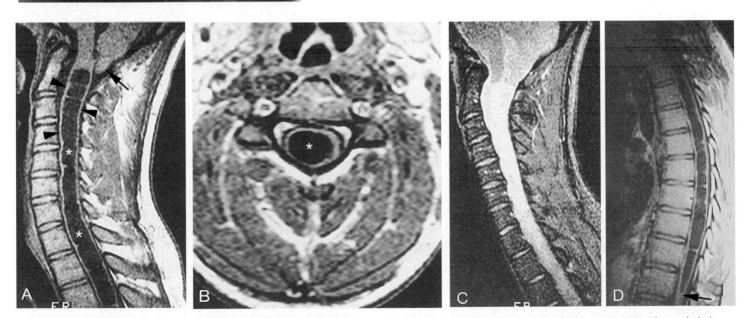

Figure 3.7. ARNOLD-CHIARI TYPE I MALFORMATION WITH HOLO-CORD SYRINX. This 25-year-old male patient presented with cervical spine pain in extension. A thorough neurologic examination revealed a unilateral decreased pinwheel sensation on the right in a shawl-like distribution. **A. MRI, T1-Weighted Sagittal Cervical. B. MRI, T1-Weighted Axial Cervical.** There is caudal displacement of the cerebellar tonsils several millimeters below the foramen magnum (arrow). Observe the large size of the spinal cord (arrowheads) secondary to the huge central canal (*). Note the low signal intensity of the central canal, which contains CSF. The cephalad portion of the syrinx extends to the C1-2 level. **C. MRI, Gradient-Echo Sagittal Cervical.** The low signal intensity CSF becomes hyperintense on this pulse sequence. The thin margins of the spinal cord are obscured by the large amount of CSF within the syrinx. **D. MRI, T1-Weighted Sagittal Thoracic.** The caudal extent of the syrinx terminates in the conus medullaris (arrow). (Courtesy of Mark L. Taylor, DC, Las Vegas, Nevada)

ARNOLD-CHIARI MALFORMATION

Description. In 1891 Chiari (1) and later Arnold (1894) described the morphologic changes of the hindbrain that now bear their names, Arnold-Chiari malformation. The brain changes are characterized by downward displacement or elongation of the brainstem and cerebellar tonsils through the foramen magnum. Hydrocephalus is variably present and mild.

There are two main presentations. Type I Arnold-Chiari malformation patients usually present in adulthood with mild brain changes, mild hydrocephalus, and variable syringomyelia (30 to 56%). Females are predominantly affected 3:2. (2) The presenting symptoms in type I patients are sometimes vague or bizarre and may initially suggest a psychiatric disorder. (3) Common complaints include headache and cervical pain. Type I is also known as tonsilar herniation or tonsilar ectopia.

Type II symptoms are more severe and present in infancy or childhood. Stridor, apnea, and feeding problems may be seen early. Older children may demonstrate nystagmus and cranial nerve palsies. (3) The hydrocephalus is severe. Dorsal kinking of the medulla at the cervicomedullary junction is commonly present, and there is upward displacement of the upper cervical nerves. Spina bifida and meningomyelocele are also associated with type II Arnold-Chiari malformation.

Type III Arnold-Chiari malformation is rare and will not be discussed here.

Associated skeletal abnormalities include occipitalization of the first cervical vertebra, platybasia and basilar impression, cervical block vertebrae, cervical ribs and fused thoracic ribs, and syringomyelia. (2)

Treatment for type I disease is usually posterior fossa and upper cervical decompression (suboccipital craniectomy and cervical laminectomy). If a syrinx is also present, a shunt may be placed within the cavity (spinal myelotomy) to effect spinal cord decompression.

Radiologic Features. Plain radiographs are typically not helpful in making this diagnosis but are capable of showing the associated skeletal malformations. Myelography and CT myelography were used prior to the advent of MRI to make the diagnosis of Arnold-Chiari malformation. MRI currently is the key to making a definitive diagnosis. Low-lying, triangular-shaped cerebellar tonsils and elongation or kinking of the fourth ventricle with a sharp clivoaxial angle are classic findings. Syringomyelia is easily demonstrated by MRI as a spinal cord cavitation. This cavity may be focal, usually cervical or cervicodorsal, or holocord. (Fig. 3.7A and B)

MEDICOLEGAL IMPLICATIONS
Arnold-Chiari Malformation

- Autonomic disturbances such as sexual disorders (reduced potency or impotency), dyspnea, anhidrosis, hyperhidrosis, and constipation have been reported. (4)

- An association between perinatal accidents and syringomyelia has been reported. (5)

- Patients who have decompressive surgery for Arnold-Chiari II malformation may be at risk for postsurgical cervical spine instability. (6)

- An association of progressive scoliosis and syrinx with Arnold-Chiari malformation has been reported. (7)

ANOMALIES OF THE CERVICAL SPINE

ANOMALIES OF THE ATLAS
AGENESIS OF THE C1 POSTERIOR ARCH

Embryology. Ossification of the first cervical vertebra begins about the seventh fetal week at the lateral masses and proceeds perichondrally in a dorsal direction, creating the posterior arch of the atlas. In the second year of life a secondary growth center for the posterior tubercle develops between these neural arches. Complete fusion of the posterior arch should be noted between the third and fifth years. (1)

Description. The basic defect in agenesis of the posterior arch of the atlas is the lack of a cartilage template on which the ossification process builds. Complete or partial agenesis of the posterior arch is rare, and posterior arch defects, by themselves, should not be the cause of neurologic or biomechanical findings unless found in association with other anomalies such as Klippel-Feil syndrome.

Radiologic Features. An absent posterior arch can be easily visualized on standard lateral cervical radiographs by the lack of a bony posterior neural arch. (Fig. 3.8A–C) A commonly associated finding is enlargement of the superior aspect of the second cervical spinous process, which has been referred to as a *megaspinous process*, representing fusion of a rudimentary posterior arch and posterior tubercle of the atlas. (2) (Fig. 3.9A and B) One may also observe increased size of the anterior arch of C1, which is thought to be *stress* related. This is a helpful radiographic sign and suggests a long-standing and probable congenital origin to the defect.

MEDICOLEGAL IMPLICATIONS
Agenesis of the C1 Posterior Arch

- The integrity of the transverse ligament may also be compromised in the maldevelopment process; therefore a cervical flexion radiograph should be performed to evaluate the atlantodental interspace.

SPINA BIFIDA OCCULTA

See discussion under "Anomalies of the Thoracic and Lumbar Spine." (Figs. 3.10 A and B, 3.11, 3.12)

POSTERIOR PONTICLE

Description. A posterior ponticle of the atlas is present when there is a calcification or ossification of the oblique portion of the

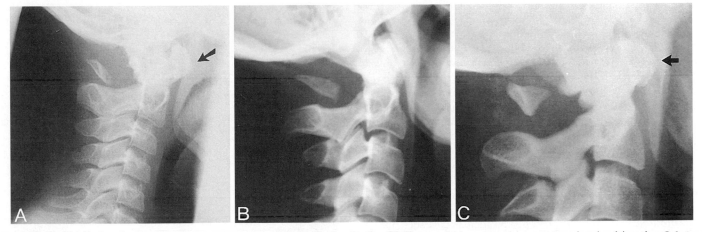

Figure 3.8.   PARTIAL AGENESIS OF THE POSTERIOR ARCH OF THE AT-LAS. A. Lateral Cervical. Observe the agenesis of the posterior arch of the atlas, with the posterior tubercle being present. Stress hypertrophy of the anterior tubercle of the atlas is present (arrow). **B. Lateral Cervical.** Failure of development of the mid portion of the posterior arch of the atlas is noted along with stress enlargement of the anterior tubercle of the atlas. **C. Lateral Cervical.** A focal agenesis of the mid portion of the posterior arch of the atlas is noted. Observe the stress hypertrophy of the anterior tubercle of the atlas (arrow).

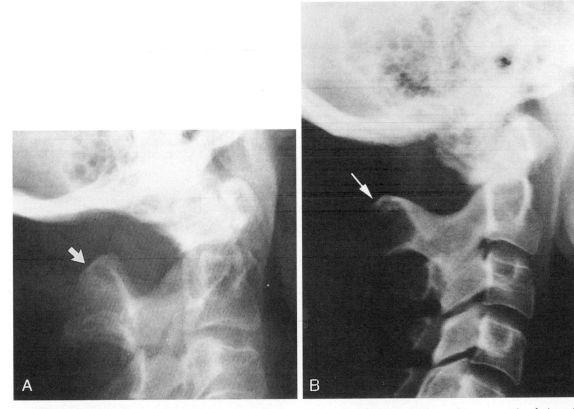

Figure 3.9.   COMPLETE AGENESIS OF THE POSTERIOR ARCH OF THE ATLAS: MEGASPINOUS PROCESS OF C2. A and B. Coned Lateral Cervicals. There is complete agenesis of the posterior arch of the atlas. Observe the "megaspinous" process at C2, representing fusion of the rudimentary posterior arch and posterior tubercle of the atlas (arrow). **(B** Courtesy of John C. Slizeski, DC, Denver, Colorado)

atlanto-occipital ligament that bridges the posterior aspect of the lateral mass and the posterior arch. An arcuate foramen is then formed that transmits the vertebral artery and the first cervical nerve as they pass superior to the posterior arch of C1. It has been given the eponyms "Kimmerly anomaly" (1), "foramen arcuale," "pons posticus," or "posticus ponticus."

This finding is more commonly unilateral and found in approximately 14% of anatomic specimens. It is also suggested to be a vestigial structure in humans, but is commonly found in other primates, particularly cats. (2)

The presence of a posterior ponticle restricts the free movement of the vertebral artery during cervical flexion and extension and causes traction and compression of the artery. The smaller the caliber of the foramen, the greater the restriction of vessel movement. (3)

Radiologic Features. A posterior ponticle is best seen on the lateral x-ray of the cervical spine, forming a partial or complete foramen at the ventral and superior aspect of the vertebral arch. (Fig. 3.13A–D) This calcification may be unilateral or bilateral and is found in approximately 15% of white patients. (1) (Fig. 3.14A

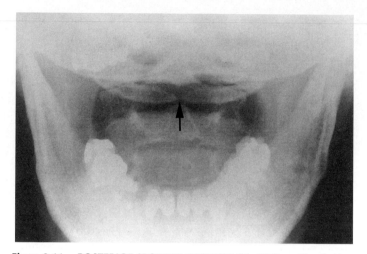

Figure 3.11. POSTERIOR SPONDYLOSCHISIS: C1. AP Open Mouth. Note the variance in this posterior cleft from Figure 3.10 (arrow). (Courtesy of Paul Van Wyk, DC, Denver, Colorado)

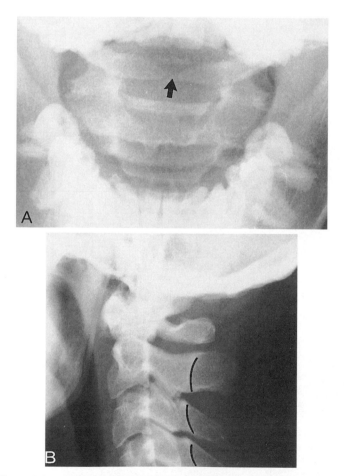

Figure 3.10. POSTERIOR SPONDYLOSCHISIS: C1. A. AP Open Mouth. Observe the radiolucent cleft in the posterior arch of the atlas (arrow) due to failure of fusion of its lateral ossification centers. **B. Coned Lateral Cervical.** Note the artist enhanced lines at C2, C3, and C4, representing the posterior cervical line and the lack of this line at the atlas. Lack of the spinolaminar junction line (posterior cervical line) will probably be the only radiographic sign of posterior spondyloschisis of the atlas on the lateral projection. This defect is also known as posterior rachischisis.

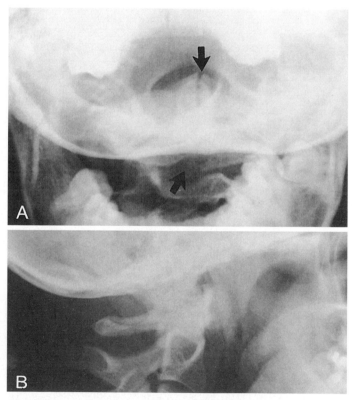

Figure 3.12. ANTERIOR AND POSTERIOR SPONDYLOSCHISIS: C1. A. AP Open Mouth. See the cleft in the anterior arch of C1 (superior arrow), also known as anterior rachischisis, and the obliquely oriented cleft in the posterior arch (inferior arrow). **B. Coned Lateral Cervical.** See how the cleft anterior arch appears enlarged and dysplastic on the lateral view. Also, note the lack of the spinolaminar junction line (posterior cervical line) at C1. (Courtesy of Harry R. Shepard, DC, Marion, Indiana) COMMENT: When anterior and posterior clefts are present the term "split atlas" may be used. (From Lipson SJ, Mazur J: *Anteroposterior spondyloschisis of the atlas revealed by computerized tomography scanning.* J Bone Joint Surg (Am) 60:1104, 1978)

and B) It must be differentiated from an overlying pneumatized mastoid air cell.

MEDICOLEGAL IMPLICATIONS
Posterior Ponticle

- The clinical significance to practitioners of spinal manipulative therapy relates to possible vertebrobasilar insufficiency during rotary manipulations of the cervical spine. (4,5) It would appear that the ponticle may compress or restrict the vertebral artery, which may temporarily diminish blood flow to the base of the brain. This does not occur in the majority of patients with a posterior ponticle. However, proper testing for vertibrobasilar insufficiency must be performed prior to forceful manipulations of the cervical spine when a posterior ponticle is found on x-ray to avoid the potentially catastrophic effects of vertibrobasilar insuf-

ficiency caused by post-manipulative vasospasm or vertebral artery dissection.

- Patients with a posterior ponticle may be at risk for posttraumatic basal subarachnoid hemorrhage. (6)
- The finding of a posterior ponticle has been found in patients with vertebrobasilar insufficiency, Barre-Lieou syndrome (headache, retro-orbital pain, vasomotor disturbance of the face, and recurrent disturbances of vision, swallowing, and phonation caused by alteration of the blood flow in the vertebral arteries and an associated disturbance of the periarterial nerve plexus), and chronic upper cervical syndrome. (2,3)

AGENESIS OF THE ANTERIOR ARCH

Description. Isolated congenital absence of the anterior arch of the atlas is a rare condition. The initial literature account of this condition was in 1886 (1), but further reports are scarce, except for one case in 1972 (2) and two patients in 1986. (3) A case

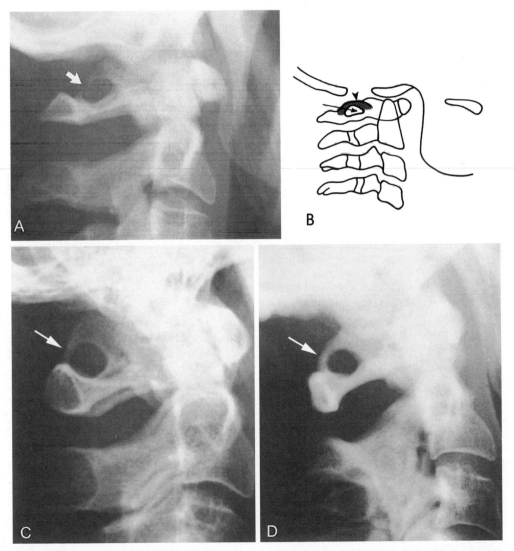

Figure 3.13. POSTERIOR PONTICLE. A. Coned Lateral Cervical. A posterior ponticle of the atlas is noted (arrow). This is an ossification of the atlantooccipital ligament that creates an opening called the arcuate foramen. Its clinical significance is related to vertebrobasilar insufficiency during rotary manipulations. **B. Schematic Diagram**. An arcuate foramen (arrow) is created by a posterior ponticle of the atlas (arrowhead). **C and D.** Note the different patterns of calcification of the posterior ponticle. (**D** Courtesy of Eugene A. Ver Meer, DC, Denver, Colorado)

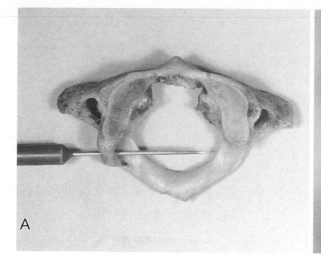

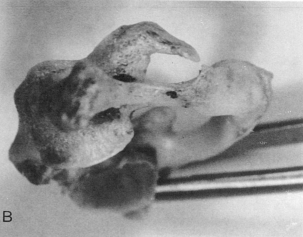

Figure 3.14. POSTERIOR PONTICLE PATHOLOGIC SPECIMEN. A. Superior View. The pointer has been positioned through this unilateral ponticle. **B. Lateral View.** This perspective demonstrates that this ponticle is incomplete and does not fuse to the C1 posterior arch. (Courtesy of Professor J.P. Ellis, St. Louis, Missouri and Marc S. Gottlieb, DC, Raleigh, North Carolina)

of an absence of the anterior arch of C1 and the odontoid process was published, but the patient had extensive rheumatoid arthritis and it is unclear if the missing bones were congenitally absent or were destroyed by the rheumatoid pannus formation. (4) This anomaly has been reported in association with median cleft face syndrome and Pierre-Robin syndrome. (5,6)

Radiologic Features.   Lateral radiographs demonstrate absence of the "D" shaped, corticated anterior arch of the first cervical vertebra. Tomograms or computed tomography (CT) better defines the extent of osseous agenesis. Flexion and extension views may be necessary to determine if hypermobility exists between C1 and C2. Apparently, retrosubluxation of C1 on C2 may be possible.

DOWN'S SYNDROME (MONGOLISM)

Description.   Down's syndrome is the most common autosomal syndrome, occurring once with every 600 births. (1) It is the result of trisomy of the 21st chromosome. Patients affected with Down's syndrome are recognizable at birth, with a decreased anteroposterior diameter of the skull, a small nose with a flat bridge, slanting eyes (epicanthal folds), simian creases, and a protruding tongue. Mental retardation is a constant feature. Various lax ligaments such as spontaneous hip and patellar dislocation have been reported. (2) Leukemia is significantly more common in patients with Down's syndrome than in otherwise normal individuals.

Radiologic Features.   The most clinically significant radiographic finding concerns the integrity of the transverse ligament of the atlas. Up to 20% of these patients are born without a transverse ligament; (3,4) therefore, before cervical spinal manipulative therapy is undertaken, a flexion radiograph must be seen to ensure the stability of the atlantoaxial motion segment. (5) (See Chapter 2.) (Fig. 3.15)

In one report approximately 25% of 38 children with Down's syndrome demonstrated a significantly reduced anteroposterior diameter of the C1 bony ring. This anomaly compounds the problem of atlantoaxial subluxation as the spinal cord would become compressed more quickly. (6)

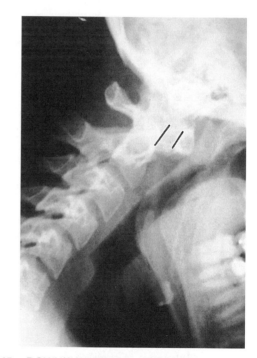

Figure 3.15.   DOWN'S SYNDROME: UPPER CERVICAL INVOLVEMENT. Coned Lateral Cervical. There is a significant increase in the atlantodental interspace (ADI represented by distance between artist enhanced lines) as a result of agenesis of the transverse ligament of the atlas. COMMENT: Up to 20% of patients with Down's syndrome are born without a transverse ligament of the atlas. Upper cervical spinal manipulative therapy is contraindicated until a flexion radiograph of the upper cervical spine has been performed and the atlantodental interspace is proven normal.

Other radiographic findings include a decreased iliac index (see Chapter 2); hypoplasia of the middle phalanx of the fifth finger with clinodactyly; multiple ossification centers for the manubrium; underpneumatization of the paranasal sinuses; decreased anteroposterior diameter of the lumbar vertebral bodies, and either 11 or 13 pairs of ribs. (7) A prominent conoid process of both clavicles may be found. (8)

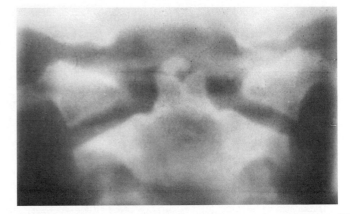

Figure 3.16. OSSICULUM TERMINALE PERSISTENS OF BERGMAN. AP tomogram C1-C2. Observe the failure of union of the cephalic ossification center for the odontoid process tip. A symmetrical "V" shaped lucent cleft helps differentiate this finding from fracture.

MEDICOLEGAL IMPLICATIONS
Down's Syndrome

- In light of the frequency of atlantoaxial subluxation the National Special Olympics Committee has a policy that all participants with Down's syndrome be screened for atlantoaxial instability. (9)

- If the atlantodental interspace measures greater than 4.5 mm, there is sufficient reason to restrict the sporting activities of patients who may incur head or neck trauma. (10)

- Posterior subluxation of the occiput on C1 has been reported to be a common problem in patients with Down's syndrome. (11,12)

- Nonoperative management of Down's syndrome patients with asymptomatic atlantoaxial instability has been recommended because of the high rate of postsurgical complications. (13)

- Adult patients with Down's syndrome are prone to develop cervical myelopathy secondary to cervical spondylosis. (14)

SPINA BIFIDA OCCULTA

See discussion under "Anomalies of the Thoracic and Lumbar Spine."

ANOMALIES OF THE AXIS
OSSICULUM TERMINALE PERSISTENS OF BERGMAN

Description. The cephalic portion of the odontoid process develops a secondary growth center from the first occipital sclerotome that appears about the second year and usually unites at 10 to 12 years of age. (1) Occasionally, this secondary growth center does not unite with the subadjacent odontoid process and remains as a separate ossicle.

Radiologic Features. The x-ray finding of a discrete, round, oval, or diamond-shaped piece of bone at the most cephalic portion of the dens in a patient over the age of 12 years is considered an ossiculum terminale and is a normal variant of development that is of no clinical significance. (Fig. 3.16) It must be differentiated from other anomalies of development of the odontoid process such as an os odontoideum and fracture.

ODONTOID ANOMALIES

Differentiation of the odontoid anomalies (os odontoideum, hypoplasia of the odontoid, or agenesis of the odontoid) is possible by x-ray examination. Most patients with these conditions proceed to develop atlantoaxial instability.

OS ODONTOIDEUM

Description. Anomalies of the odontoid process are considered uncommon (1) and are usually discovered by the principle of "traumatic determinism." This means that the underlying condition predated the injury and is not caused by this current trauma. These anomalies may be associated with Down's syndrome, Klippel-Feil syndrome, Morquio's syndrome, and spondyloepiphyseal dysplasia.

An understanding of the developmental anatomy is necessary because of the potential for significant neurologic damage (e.g., paralysis or death) that may result from a trivial trauma or even spinal manipulative therapy. In os odontoideum the cephalic portion of the odontoid process develops normally from its two lateral ossification centers, but remains ununited with the body of the second cervical vertebra, above the level of the neurocentral synchondrosis. (2) Since the osseous defect is not found at the site of the growth plate (neurocentral synchondrosis), it has been hypothesized that os odontoideum is actually a long-standing and unrecognized fracture nonunion of the base of the odontoid process. (3) Several cases of traumatic atlantoaxial dislocation resulting in os odontoideum have been reported. (4,5) It must be noted that some still consider this entity to constitute an event of congenital nonunion. (6) One report states that the odontoid process forms normally but does not unite to the C2 body because of abnormal motion. (7) The odontoid should fuse to the C2 body by the age 5–7. (7–9) Other articles demonstrate familial os odontoideum and in identical twins. (8,9) The transverse ligament is usually intact, and occasionally in association with this fact the posterior arch of the atlas may be hypoplastic or absent.

Any symptoms the patient may manifest are usually the result of atlantoaxial instability with resultant cord compression (Fig. 3.17A–C); however, if there is compression of the vertebral artery resulting from stretching of the artery during C1 subluxation on C2, then the symptoms may be considerably greater. (10) Increased deep-tendon reflexes, proprioceptive loss, or sphincter incompetence may be encountered. Additionally, compression of the vertebral arteries may result in local thrombosis and vascular occlusion. The thrombus may also serve as a source for emboli to the brain.

Clearly, the combination of os odontoideum with high-velocity injury can produce central cord syndrome or even fatal injury. (11,12)

Radiologic Features. The x-ray diagnosis of os odontoideum in a child below the age of 5 years can be made if there is demonstration of hypermobility of the odontoid process on the body of C2 during flexion and/or extension. In the adult an x-ray diagnosis is certain if a smooth, wide, lucent defect is seen to sep-

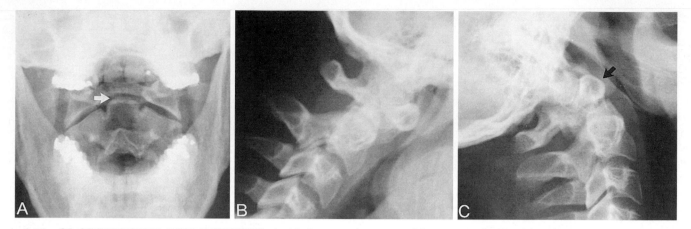

Figure 3.17. OS ODONTOIDEUM WITH INSTABILITY. A. AP Open Mouth. Note the incomplete odontoid process with a wide radiolucent defect (arrow) just above its base. **B. Flexion, Lateral Cervical. C. Extension, Lateral Cervical.** Note the forward excursion of the atlas in flexion and the posterior movement in extension, signifying instability. There is a stress enlargement of the anterior tubercle of the atlas (arrow) as a result of this underlying instability. COMMENT: The presence of a horizontal radiolucent band at the base of the odontoid process may represent Mach lines, an odontoid fracture, or the cleft of an os odontoideum and must always be differentiated.

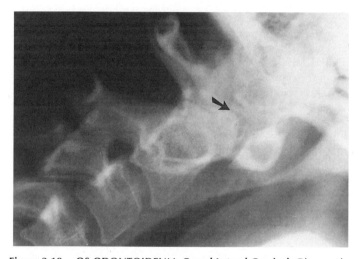

Figure 3.18. OS ODONTOIDEUM. Coned Lateral Cervical. Observe the failure of union of the odontoid process to the base of the body of the axis, as demonstrated by a radiolucent band (arrow). Cortical thickening of the anterior tubercle of the atlas, as well as an angular deformity of the posterior surface of the anterior tubercle, suggests a congenital etiology. (Courtesy of Robert J. Longenecker, DC, DACBR, Irving, Texas)

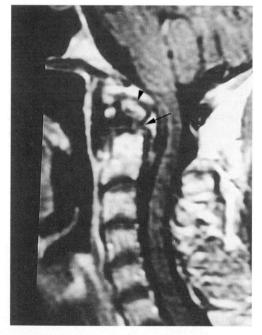

arate the odontoid process from the C2 body at the level of the superior articular processes and there is an associated stress hypertrophy of the anterior tubercle of the atlas. (13,14) (Fig. 3.18) This finding will not be present in the child, as the biomechanical stresses on the anterior arch of the atlas will not have been present for a long enough period to allow the hypertrophy to develop. Os odontoideum must be differentiated from an acute fracture of the odontoid process. (See Chapter 9.) A helpful radiographic sign that may be present and that confirms a developmental defect of the odontoid process is a "molding" of the anterior arch of C1 into the ventral aspect of the odontoid process.

Magnetic resonance imaging is useful in evaluating the spinal cord for angulation, compression, and intramedullary injury (contusion). (15) (Fig. 3.19)

Figure 3.19. OS ODONTOIDEUM: SAGITTAL T1-WEIGHTED MRI. Observe the abrupt change in signal intensity where the failure of fusion occurred causing an os odontoideum (arrow). The secondary ossification center (tip of the dens) can be seen as a brighter signal intensity superior to the stump of the dens (arrowhead). This has permitted posterior subluxation of C1 on C2 and a posterior deformity of the upper cervical spinal cord. Other high-signal structures in the C1-C2 complex include fat posterior to the ossification center. COMMENT: The normal odontoid process also displays a decrease in signal intensity as we move cephalad reflecting the decrease in marrow in its tip. (Courtesy of Steven R. Nokes, MD, Baptist MRI, Little Rock, Arkansas)

MEDICOLEGAL IMPLICATIONS
Os Odontoideum

- Instability of C1 on C2 secondary to os odontoideum carries the risk of damage to the spinal cord or vertebral arteries caused by severe injury. (10)

- A case of a 6-year-old girl with os odontoideum and stroke affecting the posterior circulation of the brain has been reported. (16)

- A pedIatric patient with os odontoideum and atlantoaxial instability and had multiple areas of cerebellar and occipital parietal lobe infarcts has been reported. Surgical stabilization and fusion resulted in normal neurologic function. (17)

- High-velocity, spinal, manipulative techniques are contraindicated in patients with these conditions. Surgical consultation must be considered for patients with progressive instability or neurologic symptoms.

Hypoplastic and Agenetic Odontoid Process

Radiologic Features.   Complete agenesis of the odontoid process, also known as odontoid aplasia, appears to be extremely rare, although its true incidence is unknown. (1) On an open-mouth radiograph, a hypoplastic odontoid process is seen as an abbreviated stump of bone projecting slightly above the C1-C2 articulations. (Fig. 3.20) This anomaly can be diagnosed at birth, on radiographs through the open mouth, as the ossification center for the odontoid process should be present at that time. Flexion and extension radiographs must be performed to rule out instability between C1 and C2. (Fig. 3.21A–C) If instability is demonstrated, high-velocity spinal manipulation is contraindicated, and referral for a surgical opinion concerning arthrodesis is indicated. (Fig. 3.22)

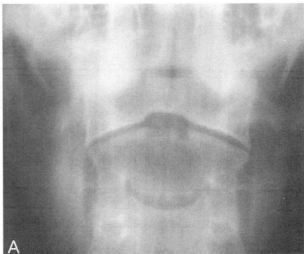

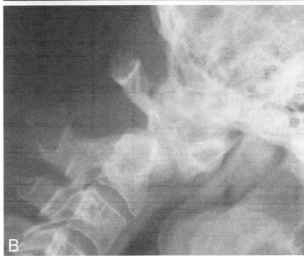

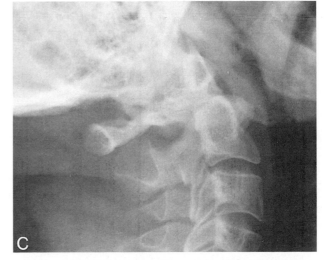

Figure 3.21.   AGENESIS OF THE ODONTOID PROCESS WITH INSTABILITY. A. AP Tomogram. Observe the complete lack of an osseous shadow of the odontoid. **B. Flexion, Lateral Cervical. C. Extension, Lateral Cervical.** There is no odontoid process allowing significant translation of the atlas in flexion and extension. COMMENT: Patients with this degree of instability and who manifest neurologic symptoms are destined for surgical arthrodesis. (Courtesy of Bryan Hartley, MD, Melbourne, Australia)

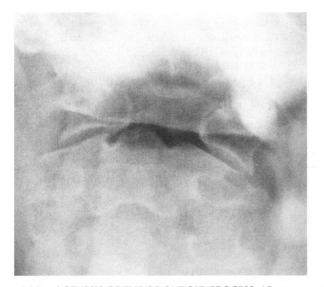

Figure 3.20.   AGENESIS OF THE ODONTOID PROCESS. AP open mouth. Observe the abbreviated peg of the odontoid process, with the remainder of its substance lacking. The lateral shift of C1 upon C2 indicates instability. (Courtesy of Klaus W Weber, MD, Fort Wayne, Indiana)

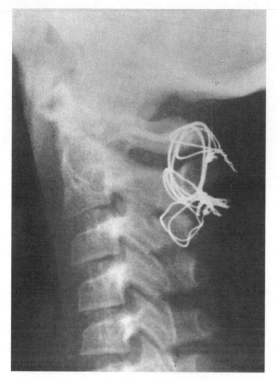

Figure 3.22.   SURGICAL ARTHRODESIS FOR AGENESIS OF THE ODON-TOID PROCESS. Coned Lateral Cervical. Posterior interspinous wiring of C1, C2, and C3 as treatment for agenesis of the odontoid process.

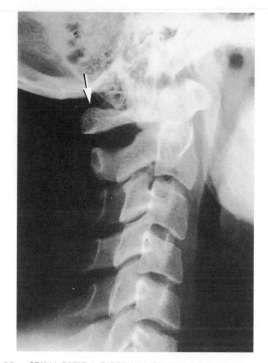

Figure 3.23.   SPINA BIFIDA OCCULTA OF THE ATLAS AND AXIS. Coned Lateral Cervical. Observe the absence of a C1 posterior cervical line (arrow) that indicates the presence of spondyloschisis at C1. Also note the hypoplastic appearance of the posterior arch of the axis. (Courtesy of John C. Slizeski, DC, Denver, Colorado)

MEDICOLEGAL IMPLICATIONS
Hypoplastic and Agenetic Odontoid Process

- Head trauma resulted in a delayed-onset, posterior circulation stroke in a 5-year-old boy who also had odontoid aplasia. (2)

- These odontoid anomalies may be found in patients with Hurler's and Morquio's syndromes. (3)

- Also, see Medicolegal Implications for os odontoideum.

SPINA BIFIDA OCCULTA

See description in "Anomalies of the Thoracic and Lumbar Spine." (Figs. 3.23, 3.24A and B)

ANOMALIES OF C3 THROUGH C7
BLOCK VERTEBRA

Description. When two adjacent vertebrae are osseously fused from birth, this joined unit is called a congenital block vertebra. Embryologically, this is the result of failure of the normal segmentation process of the somites during the period of differentiation at 3 to 8 fetal weeks. (1)

The block vertebra by itself is clinically insignificant. As there is no motion allowed at the fused level, there is no potential for degenerative disease of the disc or posterior apophyseal joints. The foramina at the blocked level may be smaller than normal, normally sized, or enlarged, but have not been shown to cause nerve compression. However, because of the lack of a motion segment the free articulations above and below the block segment are stressed and usually result in premature degenerative discogenic spondylosis and arthrosis at the fully articulated levels, especially below the fusion site. (Fig. 3.25A and B) Fusions are partial (i.e., do not completely involve the anterior and posterior spinal units) and may result in abnormal spinal curvature, usually scoliosis, because of a unilateral bar. Block vertebrae are most commonly found at C5-C6, C2-C3, T12-L1, and L4-L5 in decreasing order of incidence. (1,2)

A recent report suggests that long-standing congenital or acquired fusion of upper cervical vertebrae may lead to stretching and laxity of the ligaments between the occiput and the atlas, resulting in excessive motion and brainstem or cord compression. (2)

Radiologic Features. A typical congenital block vertebra will demonstrate the following roentgen signs: (a) a diminished AP diameter of the vertebral body; (b) a hypoplastic or rudimentary disc space that may show faint calcification; (c) possible fusion of the apophyseal joints (50% of cases); and (d) possible malformation or fusion of the spinous processes. (Figs. 3.26 A–C, 3.27)

The anterior margins of the involved vertebrae form a concave surface, because of the decreased AP diameter at the fusion that is visible on plain film and MRI. (Fig. 3.28A–C) This "*wasp waist*" (3) or "C" shape can serve as a mnemonic device, to indicate that this fusion is "congenital." (Fig. 3.29A–C) Another helpful sign of this congenital anomaly is osseous fusion of the neural arches,

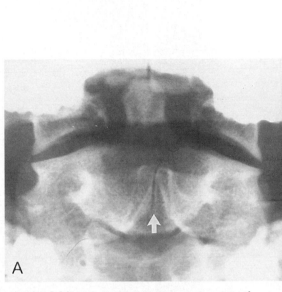

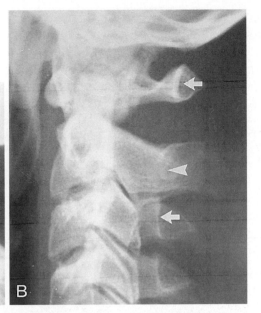

Figure 3.24.   SPINA BIFIDA OCCULTA OF THE AXIS. A. AP Open Mouth. Observe the midline radiolucent cleft of the spinous process of C2 (arrow). **B. Coned Lateral Cervical.** The cortical white line created by the junction of the lamina and spinous process is clearly noted at C1 and C3 (arrows). The white line represents the spinolaminar junction line or the posterior cervical line (PCL) and is a line drawn to connect the spinolaminar lines of the cervical vertebrae. The lack of a spinolaminar junction line at C2 (arrowhead) signifies spina bifida occulta. (Courtesy of Kenneth E. Yochum, DC, St. Louis, Missouri)

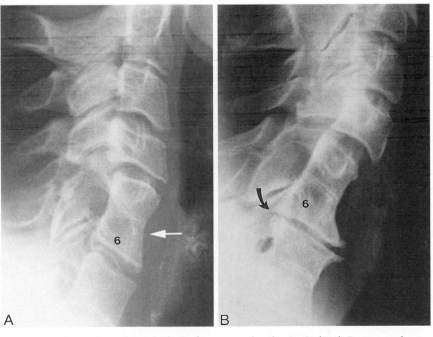

Figure 3.25.   CERVICAL BLOCK VERTEBRAE. A. Lateral Cervical: Single Block Vertebra. Observe the block vertebra present at the C5-C6 level. The arrested growth of the vertebral bodies results in an anterior concavity that has been referred to as the "wasp-waist" appearance (arrow). Facet structures at C5-C6 are also fused. **B. Lateral Cervical: Multiple Block Vertebrae.** There are block vertebrae present at C5-C6 and C7-T1. Facet joint fusion is noted at the C5-C6 level. Premature degenerative discopathy with spondylosis is present at the C6 disc level. Posterior osteophyte formation affecting the C6-C7 vertebrae (arrow) may result in spinal canal stenosis. COMMENT: Fifty percent of patients with block vertebrae have associated apophyseal joint fusion, as is present in both of these cases. (Courtesy of John Nolan, DC, Wanganui, New Zealand)

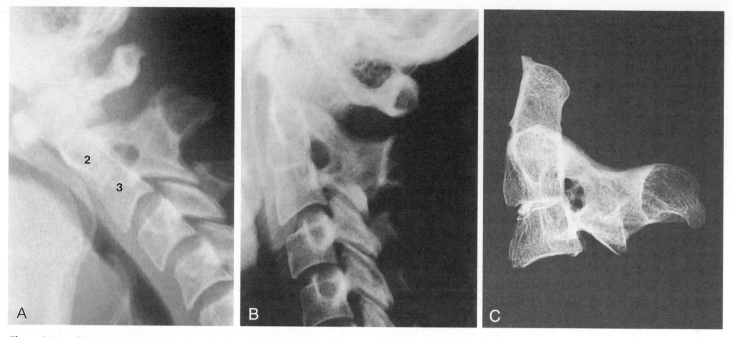

Figure 3.26. C2-C3 CERVICAL BLOCK VERTEBRAE. A. Coned Lateral Cervical Flexion and B. Coned Lateral Cervical. Observe the block vertebra present between C2-C3, with fusion of the apophyseal joints. **C. Specimen** **Radiograph.** Observe the rudimentary calcified disc at C2 in this blocked specimen. COMMENT: Block vertebrae are most commonly found at C5-C6, C2-C3, T12-L1, and L4-L5 in decreasing order of incidence.

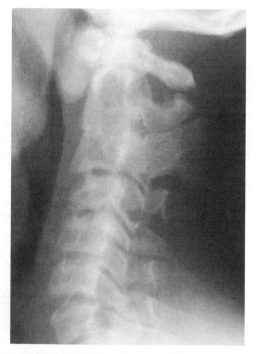

Figure 3.27. C2-C3 CERVICAL BLOCK VERTEBRA. Lateral Cervical. Observe the unusual C2-C3 block with a deformed posterior arch of C2 and C3. This abnormality resulted in increased biomechanical stress that increased the size of the anterior arch of C1. (Courtesy of James D. Abel, DC, Columbus, Nebraska)

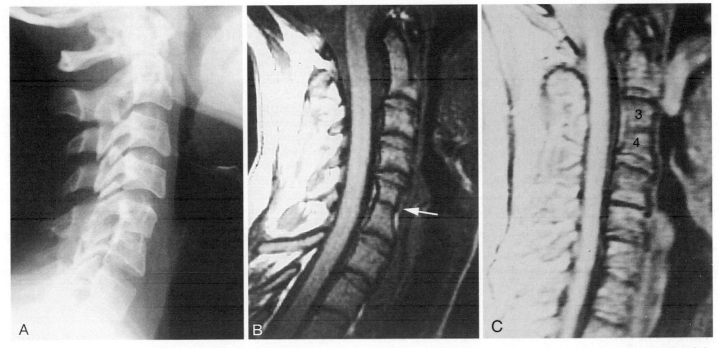

Figure 3.28.   CONGENITAL BLOCK VERTEBRAE. A. Coned Lateral Cervical. Observe the classic signs of block vertebra, including wasp-waist vertebra, "C" shape anterior margin, rudimentary disc and fusion of the posterior elements at this C5-C6 blocked segment. **B. Sagittal T1-Weighted MRI.** This is the same patient as in **A.** Recall that with T1-weighting, cortical bone has a low signal intensity. Note the characteristic "C" shape to the anterior bodies of C5-C6 (arrow). There is also a low signal intensity band that crosses, representing the endplates of the vertebrae that failed to separate. The same "C" shaping is noted at C3-C4 in **C. Sagittal T1-Weighted MRI.** This is a different patient. The congenital block is at C3-C4. In both MR images, the spinal cord is of normal intensity. (**C** Courtesy of Robert D. Thompson, DC, Buena Park, California)

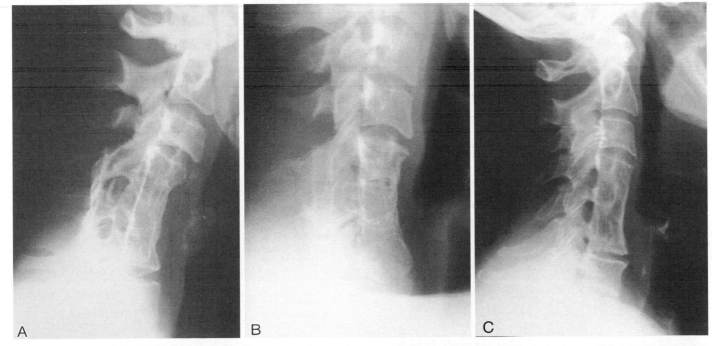

Figure 3.29.   CONGENITAL BLOCK VERTEBRAE. A-C. Coned Lateral Cervicals: Congenital. Observe the congenital block vertebrae with the characteristic "C"-shaped ("wasp-waist") deformity signifying the congenital origin of this fusion. COMMENT: Notice the coronal orientation of the intervertebral foramina within the blocked segment. This foraminal orientation occurs with an increased incidence in blocked vertebrae. (**B** Courtesy of Jon P. Carmichael, DC, Denver, Colorado, **C** Courtesy of J. Todd Knudsen, DC, DACBR, Orem, Utah)

that is almost never associated with infectious, traumatic processes or other causes of block vertebrae. (4) (Figs. 3.30 A–D, 3.31, 3.32, 3.33)

KLIPPEL-FEIL SYNDROME

Description.   In 1912 Klippel and Feil (1) described a 46-year-old man with congestion of the lungs and nephritis. They described his physical appearance as follows: The head seemed to be resting directly on the trunk, and the spine was compressed without apparent pain. This original description is typical of the patient affected with Klippel-Feil syndrome (e.g., a patient with a short, webbed neck (pterygium coli), a low hairline, and a decreased range of cervical motion) and has become known as the classic triad of this abnormality. This triad is completely expressed in only 52% of patients with the disease. (2) Men and women are equally affected. Facial asymmetry, torticollis, or webbing of the neck may be seen in 20% of patients. (3) The thoracic cage may also be deformed as a result of scoliosis or Sprengle's deformity. (Figs. 3.34A and B, 3.35)

In addition to spinal involvement, genitourinary, nervous, and cardiopulmonary systems are often affected. An alternative name for this condition, which can be found in the literature, is "*brevicollis.*" An embryologic basis for this problem has been offered that explains the association of genitourinary anomalies, a fact not completely appreciated in the Klippel and Feil case. The original patient died of complications of renal disease and uremia. (1) Duncan states: "Existing embryologic data suggest that the blastema of the cervical vertebrae, scapulae, and the genitourinary system have an intimate spatial relationship at the end of the fourth or beginning of the fifth week of fetal life. An alteration in this region can affect the cervical vertebrae and scapulae directly, and the genitourologic changes are mediated indirectly through the inductive capacity of the pronephric duct." (4)

It has been noted that the vertebral changes of Klippel-Feil syndrome resemble those of fetal alcohol syndrome; however, these are two separate entities. (5)

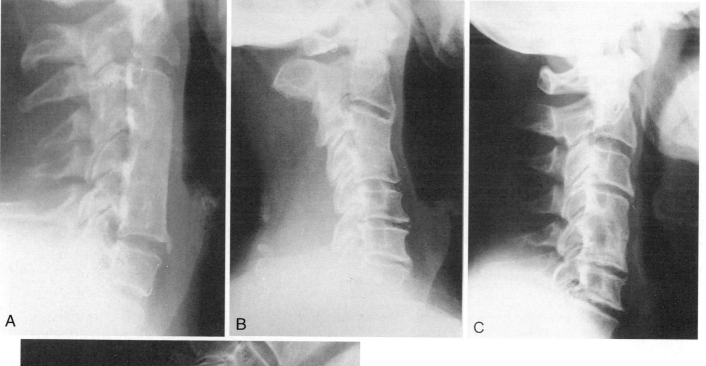

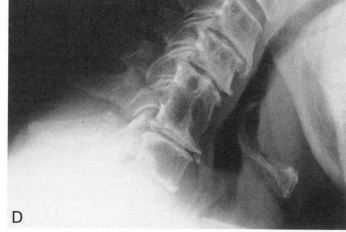

Figure 3.30.   SURGICALLY FUSED VERTEBRAE. A–D. Coned Lateral Cervicals. The lack of anterior concavity, rudimentary discs, or fusion of the apophyseal joints are all radiographic signs suggesting a surgical rather than congenital origin for these fused segments. Another clue to the surgical origin in **B** is the lack of lamina and spinous processes removed during laminectomy. (**D** Courtesy of Richard N. Garian, DC, Holliston, Massachusetts)

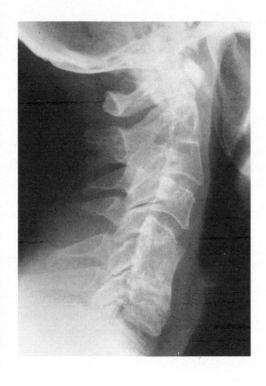

Figure 3.31.   CONGENITAL BLOCK AND SURGICALLY FUSED VERTEBRA. Coned Lateral Cervical. Note the rudimentary disc and posterior joint fusion at the congenitally blocked C2-C3 segment. These features are not present at the surgically fused C5-C6-C7 complex. (Courtesy of Paul Van Wyk, DC, Denver, Colorado)

Figure 3.32.   DEGENERATIVE FUSED VERTEBRA. Coned Lateral Cervical. Another cause of "block" vertebra is demonstrated at C4-C5. Note the opacified disc at C2-C3 (arrow), the C3-C4 facet joint sclerosis (arrowhead) and, osteophytosis at C3-C4 through C6-C7, all radiographic indicators of the degenerative process. The decrease in intervertebral disc height has allowed C4 to fuse on C5. (Courtesy of Richard L. Green, DC, Winthrop, Massachusetts)

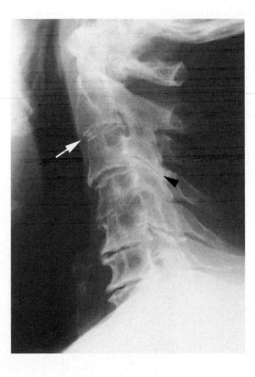

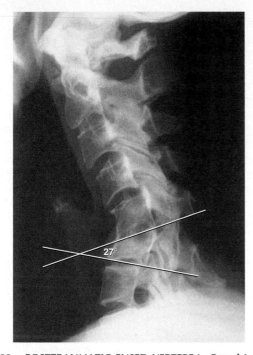

Figure 3.33. POSTTRAUMATIC FUSED VERTEBRA. Coned Lateral Cervical. Note the acute angulation of C5 upon C6 (greater than 11°), the varying interspinous distance at this level (more than 3 mm different from the adjacent segments) and uncovering of the facet joints. This was a grade 3 sprain that was unstable and ultimately fused in this position. (From White AA, Johnson RM, Panjabi MM, et al.: *Biomechanical analysis of clinical instability in the cervical spine.* Clin Orthop 109:85, 1975.)

Radiologic Features. X-ray examination of the spine will reveal multiple block vertebrae (two or more) of the cervical and upper thoracic spine. Anomalies of rib development may also be evident. (Figs. 3.34A and B, 3.35) These block vertebrae are responsible for scoliosis, the condition most commonly associated with Klippel-Feil syndrome. (2) Platybasia of the skull may be noted on the lateral cervical film. Congenital elevation of the scapula, Sprengle's deformity, is found in 25% of Klippel-Feil patients. (3) (Fig. 3.36A and B)

Magnetic resonance imaging is useful in demonstrating spinal canal stenosis, cord compression, and spinal cord abnormalities (hydromyelia and diplomyelia). (6)

MEDICOLEGAL IMPLICATIONS
Klippel-Feil Syndrome

- A patient with progressive cervical myeloradiculopathy has been reported with spinal stenosis caused by osteophyte formation at the freely articulated segment above the block vertebra. (7)
- A 16-year-old patient with Klippel-Feil syndrome and bilateral Sprengel's deformity developed transient paresthesias of both upper extremities and occasional weakness on cervical extension caused by intersegmental instability at C3-C4. (8)
- An 11-year-old patient with intermittent but progressive headaches, dizziness, nausea, vomiting, slurred speech, ataxia, and syncope has been reported. The symptoms were related to an occipital lobe infarct caused by occlusion of the vertebral arteries. (9)

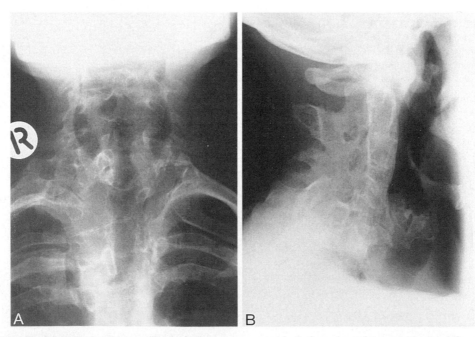

Figure 3.34. KLIPPEL-FEIL SYNDROME. A. AP Lower Cervical. There are multiple block vertebrae noted throughout the lower cervical and upper thoracic spine, as evidenced by the lack of disc spacing. Anomalous rib development is also noted. **B. Lateral Cervical**. There are multiple block vertebrae throughout the cervical spine. The zygapophyseal joints are additionally fused. Of incidental notation is posterior spondyloschisis of the atlas, as well as multiple lower cervical and upper thoracic segments.

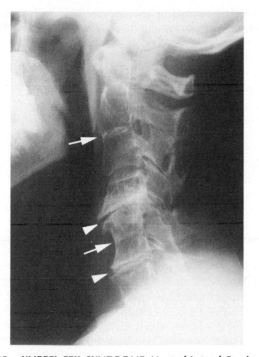

Figure 3.35.   KLIPPEL-FEIL SYNDROME. Neutral Lateral Cervical. Notice the block vertebrae at C2-C3 and C5-C6 (arrows). COMMENT: There is also significant disc degeneration noted at the C4-C5 and, to a lesser extent, the C6-C7 segments (arrowheads). This is a result of the additional stresses that these segments must withstand because of the hypomobility of the block segments. (Courtesy of Dennis V. Salisbury, DC, Chadron, Nebraska)

SPRENGLE'S DEFORMITY

Description.   Congenital elevation of the scapula, described by Sprengle in 1891, was actually first mentioned in 1863 by Eulenberg. (1) Sprengle's original report describes four children with similar scapular deformities. (2) In all four of these patients, the left scapula was elevated. Although various postulates have been advanced, the reason for this deformity remains a mystery. At the third fetal week the scapula develops in the neck, at the C4-C5 level. Under ordinary conditions the scapula migrates to its normal position by the fiftieth day of gestation. Therefore a failure to descend, rather than elevation of the scapula, is a more accurate description of the pathology. It seems likely that the problem evolves prior to the third month of skeletal development. A 2:1 female predominance has been noted. (3) The deformity can be detected at birth and is usually unilateral, but may be seen bilaterally. (3)

Examination of a patient with Sprengle's deformity will show elevation of the scapula and limited humeral abduction. Torticollis, with or without muscle spasm, may be present. The degree of fixation, as well as the quantity of malrotation and maldevelopment, should all be determined. (3)

Sprengle's deformity may present as an isolated anomaly, but it also occurs in 20 to 25% of the cases of Klippel-Feil syndrome.

Omovertebral Bone

Another frequent concomitant is the omovertebral bone, present in 30 to 40% of Sprengle's deformity cases. (4) (Fig. 3.37) It is not always bone as the name implies; it may also be composed of cartilage or fibrous tissue. The omovertebral bone usually runs from the C5 or C6 spinous process, lamina, or transverse process to the superior angle of the scapula. The earliest description of the omovertebral bone is attributed to Willett and Walsham in 1880. (5)

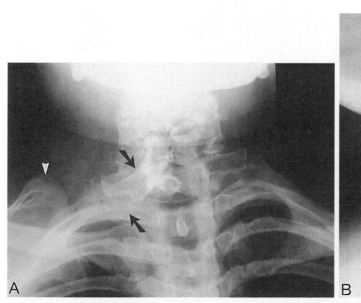

Figure 3.36.   KLIPPEL-FEIL SYNDROME WITH OMOVERTEBRAL BONE.
A. AP Lower Cervical. Observe the omovertebral bone projecting from the lamina of C7 toward the superior angle of the scapula (arrows). There is associated congenital failure of descent of the scapula (Sprengle's deformity) (arrowhead). **B. Lateral Cervical.** There are multiple congenital block vertebrae. (Courtesy of James R. Brandt, DC, FACO, Coon Rapids, Minnesota) COMMENT: Sprengle's deformity is found in 25% of patients with Klippel-Feil syndrome.

Concerning Sprengle's deformity, Lovell and Winter state: "The treatment of choice is surgery. The deformity does not progress, but it does not spontaneously improve without surgery. Conservative treatment does not result in any improvement. Physical therapy also is not helpful." Surgery is best considered between the ages of 4 and 7 years. (3)

Radiologic Features. The scapula is hypoplastic, shortened vertically, and is broad on x-ray examination. It is rotated so that the glenoid process is directed inferiorly. The inferior angle rests above the normal T7 level. The amount of elevation may be from

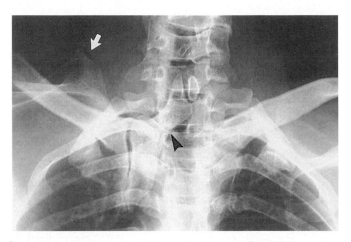

Figure 3.37. SPRENGLE'S DEFORMITY WITH OMOVERTEBRAL BONE. AP Cervicodorsal Spot. Observe the congenital failure of descent of the scapula (arrow), denoting a Sprengle's deformity. There is a large, bony bar projecting from the lamina and spinous process of C7 to the vertebral border of the scapula, representing an omovertebral bone (arrowhead). COMMENT: Thirty to 40% of the cases of Sprengle's deformity will have an associated omovertebral bone.

2 to 10 cm. Two-thirds of patients presenting with these features demonstrate associated scoliosis, hemivertebrae, block vertebrae, spina bifida occulta, or cervical ribs. (6)

CERVICAL SPONDYLOLISTHESIS

Description. The original reference to this rare anomaly is credited to Perlman and Hawes in 1951. (1) There is absence of the pedicles bilaterally with dysplasia of the articular processes, and spina bifida occulta is a constant feature. The sixth cervical vertebra is most commonly involved, but other cervical levels, particularly C2, have been described. (2–6) Males are more commonly affected. The patient may have no complaints or may report symptoms that include occipital headache, nuchal rigidity, torticollis, dysphagia, depressed deep tendon reflexes, and radicular arm pain. (2,7)

Radiologic Features. Abnormalities will be seen on anteroposterior, lateral, and oblique radiographs of the cervical spine. The lateral film will show dysplasia of the neural arch, and sometimes slight anterolisthesis of the involved level. (Fig. 3.38A and B) The anteroposterior radiograph will reveal a spina bifida occulta. (Fig. 3.39A–D) Spina bifida occulta at C6 is a rare, isolated anomaly and is a highly suggestive sign of cervical spondylolisthesis. Enlarged foramina will be present bilaterally because of the absent pedicles. Flexion and extension radiographs may demonstrate intersegmental instability. (See Chapter 5.)

Computed tomography is useful to demonstrate the bilateral defects with their smooth cortical margins. This finding clearly distinguishes the congenital anomaly from an acute fracture. (8) (Fig. 3.40A)

When a history of significant trauma is involved, magnetic resonance imaging is useful in ruling out acute injury to the discs or spinal cord. (Fig. 3.40B) The lack of edema on MRI scans confirms the nontraumatic nature of the defect.

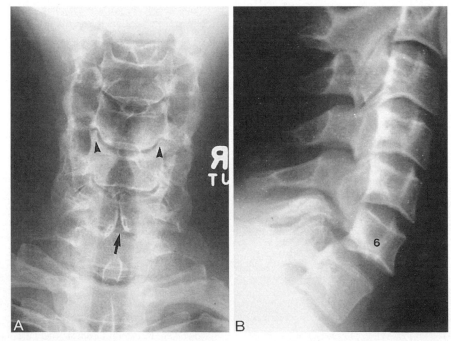

Figure 3.38. CERVICAL SPONDYLOLISTHESIS: C6. A. AP Lower Cervical. There is a spina bifida occulta present at C6 (arrow). Considerable joint of von Luschka arthrosis is present bilaterally at the C4-C5 levels (arrowheads). **B. Coned Lateral Cervical.** Note the marked dysplasia of the pedicles and articular pillars of C6. There is anterior translation of the vertebral body of C6 upon C7. COMMENT: The spinolaminar line, which is usually the most reliable indicator of translation of a vertebral segment, cannot be used in this case because of the spinal bifida occulta.

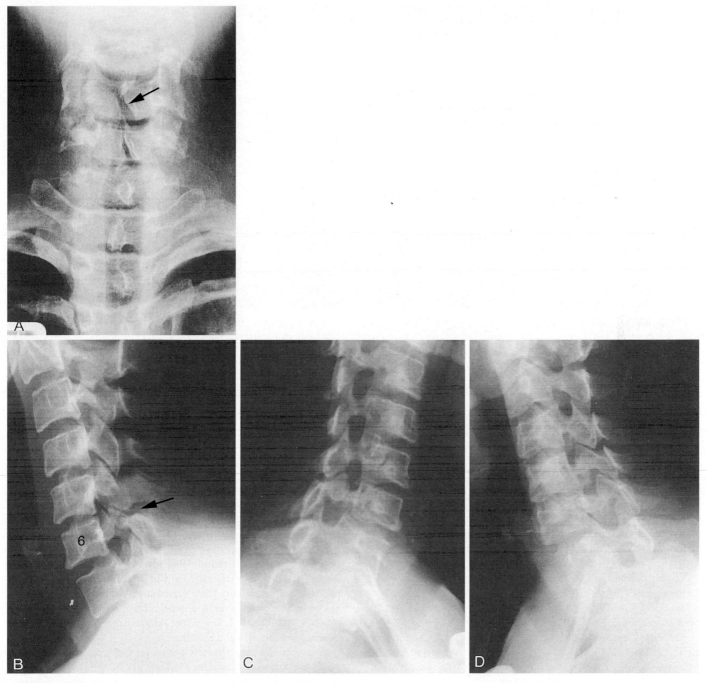

Figure 3.39.   CERVICAL SPONDYLOLISTHESIS: C5 and C6. A. AP Lower Cervical. Note the oblique lucency in the midline of both C5 and C6 representing spina bifida occulta at both segments (arrow). Incidentally and unrelated is elongation of the C7 transverse process (arrowhead). **B. Neutral Lateral Cervical.** There is a break in the posterior vertebral line (George's line) with an anterolisthesis of C6 on C7 (arrow). There are also abnormally shaped articular pillars at C6. **C and D. Cervical Obliques.** The oblique views demonstrate defects in the pedicles of C6 and dysplasia of the C6 articular processes. (Courtesy of Marc Moramarco, DC, Woburn, Massachusetts)

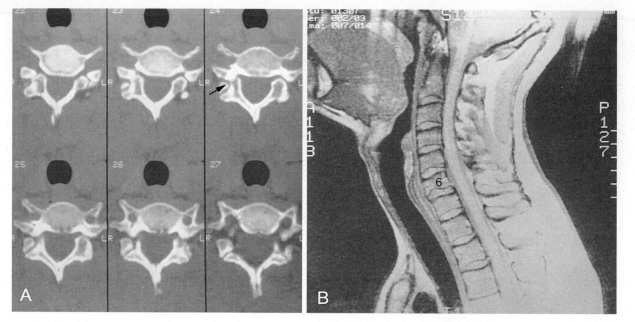

Figure 3.40.   CERVICAL SPONDYLOLISTHESIS. A. This CT bone window clearly demonstrates the bilateral defects in the C6 posterior arch (arrow). Note how the osseous margins of the defects are smoothly corticated. **B.** This sagittal T1-weighted MRI image of the same patient shows no evidence of disc herniation, bulge or spinal cord defect. (Courtesy of Jeffrey J. Pfeifer, DC, Alton, Illinois)

ABSENT PEDICLE OF THE CERVICAL SPINE

Description.   In 1946 Hadley (1) is credited with the first report of the congenital absence of a cervical pedicle. As of 1990 the literature had reported 55 cases. The cartilage anlage of the cervical vertebra develops from six centers—one for each side of the vertebral body, one in each costal process, and one for each neural arch—that then become the pedicle, articular process, transverse process, and lamina. It is a failure of development of the latter that results in this vertebral anomaly. The most common levels in the cervical spine to be affected are C6 (44%), C5 (31%), C4 (12.5%), and C7 (12.5%). (2) Each side is equally affected but is always unilateral. (3)

Dissection has demonstrated one common dural pouch with two nerve roots inside and a fibrous band at the site of the missing pedicle. (3) Clinically, symptoms of paraesthesia or pain in the upper extremity, head, or neck may be found. It is important to recognize this entity as a developmental anomaly and differentiate it from tumor destruction of the pedicle, as seen in neurofibromatosis, dural ectasia, tortuous or aneurysmal vertebral artery, or metastasis.

Radiologic Features.   Oblique projections will demonstrate an enlarged intervertebral foramen at the level of the missing pedicle. (Fig. 3.41A–C) At the same level both the transverse process and the superior aspect of the articular process may be dysplastic. This malformed articular process appears to be universally dorsally displaced. The articular dysplasia is seen on lateral views, but is best visualized on pillar projections. Hypertrophy of the contralateral pedicle may also be present and should be considered a hallmark of this congenital dysplasia. This radiographic sign of a sclerotic contralateral pedicle is far more commonly seen with agenesis of a lumbar pedicle as a result of greater weight bearing in this area. The vertebral body is unaffected, in distinction to the posterior scalloping of the body that is seen with neurofibromas (dumbbell tumors) at the intervertebral foramen.

Conservative, nonoperative therapy for patients with an absent cervical pillar has been recommended. (3–5)

CERVICAL RIB

Description.   A cervical rib is a separate piece of bone that articulates with the transverse process of one or more cervical vertebrae. It is most common at the C7, C6, and C5 levels, in descending order of occurrence. These ribs may be differentiated from elongation of a cervical transverse process (apophysomegaly or transverse mega-apophysis), that would demonstrate no costovertebral articulation. They may be differentiated from rudimentary first thoracic ribs via the orientation of the transverse processes with which they articulate. Cervical transverse processes are caudally oriented, while thoracic transverse processes project cephalically. If the orientation is equivocal, it may be necessary to count all thoracic ribs.

Cervical ribs are present in 0.5% of the population and are twice as common in females. (1) They are bilateral in 66% of cases. (1) If these ribs cause symptoms, it is usually after middle age when the shoulders begin to droop, resulting in neurovascular compression. Typically, the subclavian vessels and brachial plexus pass superior to a cervical rib, but in some instances the brachial plexus may be split by a cervical rib. (2)

Radiologic Features.   The radiographic diagnosis is made when the anomalous rib is seen to form a joint with a transverse process that is oriented in a caudal direction (thoracic transverse processes normally point cephalically, while cervical transverse processes are directed caudally). The length of the cervical rib is quite variable, from a rudimentary stump to a fully developed rib that may also articulate with the sternoclavicular junction. (Fig. 3.42A and B) Sutton considers cervical ribs to be a common anomaly. (3) Cervical ribs may be differentiated from elongation or enlargement of the transverse process. An enlarged transverse process extends laterally beyond the transverse pro-

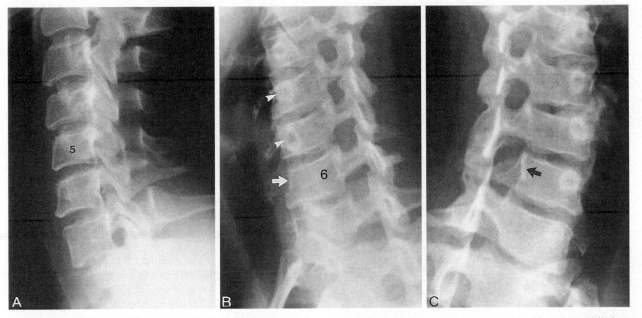

Figure 3.41. ABSENT PEDICLE OF THE CERVICAL SPINE. A. Lateral Cervical. Observe the altered appearance of the articular pillar of C6. **B. Oblique Cervical.** There is no pedicle shadow present on C6 (arrow). Observe the normal pedicle shadow on C4, C5 (arrowheads). **C. Oblique Cervical.** The failure of pedicle development has resulted in an abnormally large intervertebral foramen (arrow). (Courtesy of Gary M. Guebert, DC, DACBR, St. Louis, Missouri)

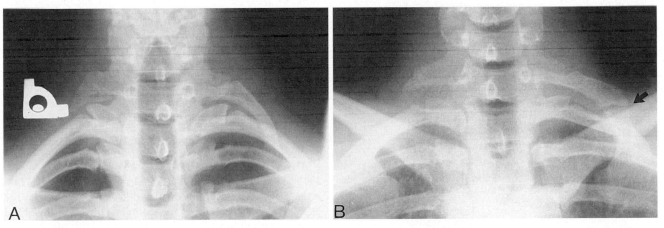

Figure 3.42. CERVICAL RIBS. A. AP Lower Cervical. There is a complete cervical rib present at C7 on the right side. An attenuated cervical rib is present at C7 on the left side. **B. AP Lower Cervical.** There is a cervical rib with an accessory articulation (arrow). A small cervical rib is also noted on the opposite side. (Courtesy of Donald E. Freuden, DC, FACO, Denver, Colorado)

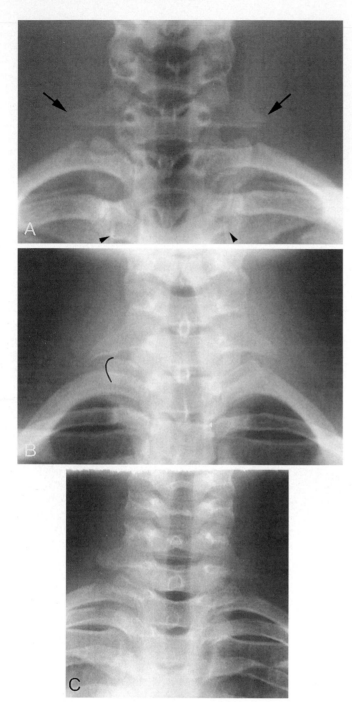

Figure 3.43. ELONGATED TRANSVERSE PROCESSES: C7. A. Coned AP Lower Cervical. Observe the bilateral elongation of the transverse processes of C7 in this 22-year-old patient (arrows). Also note the open physeal lines in the medial aspects of the clavicles (arrowheads). These growth centers appear around the age of 17 years and close around 25 years of age. **B. Coned AP Lower Cervical.** Again note the bilateral elongation of these transverse processes. The transverse process of T1 is outlined as a reference point, with the elongated transverse process of C7 beyond the distal tip of the first thoracic transverse process. **C. Coned AP Lower Cervical.** Note this finding is evident even on a patient 8 years of age. COMMENT: This finding may mimic a cervical rib with potential for thoracic outlet syndrome (TOS).

cess of the first thoracic vertebra and does not reveal a joint. (Fig. 3.43A–C)

MEDICOLEGAL IMPLICATIONS
Cervical Rib

- A case of primary or effort (exertional) thrombosis has been reported in a patient with cervical ribs. These patients present with peripheral edema, prominent superficial veins, and neurologic symptoms of pain and paresthesias. (4)
- A rare case of a cervical rib causing an aneurysm of the subclavian artery has been reported. (5)

"Cervical ribs vary greatly in size and shape, and clinical symptoms bear little relation to the radiographic abnormality." (3) One should be aware that a fibrous band may extend from the end of a small cervical rib and be the actual source of neural or vascular compression. Unfortunately, this band is unappreciated on plain film radiographs. Contrast radiographic examination demonstrating vascular occlusion would be necessary to make a preoperative diagnosis of a fibrous band creating a thoracic outlet syndrome.

ANOMALIES OF THE THORACIC AND LUMBAR SPINE

VERTEBRAL BODY ANOMALIES

BLOCK VERTEBRA

See description in the section "Anomalies of the Cervical Spine." (Figs. 3.44A–C, 3.45A and B, 3.46, 3.47A and B)

BUTTERFLY VERTEBRA

Description. The embryologic explanation for this radiologically distinctive entity has been variously described as failure of regression of the chorda dorsalis, persistence of the ventrodorsal extension of the perichordal sheath, or failure of the lateral ossification centers to unite. (1,2) Tanaka and Uhthoff (3), regarding coronal cleft vertebrae, show conclusive histopathologic correlation of lack of involvement of the notochord in development of this anomaly and attribute the defect to the placement of the intraosseous blood vessels. The opinion directly disputes the theories of Schmorl and Junghans (1) and is corroborated by the work of Emery. (4) The initial description of butterfly vertebra, attributed to von Rokitansky (5), in 1844, is where the two halves of the vertebra assume the appearance of a butterfly's wings when viewing the vertebral body from the front.

Radiologic Features. The x-ray appearance on an AP radiograph has been likened to the wings of a butterfly. It is created by indentation of the endplate cortices toward the central body, creating an hourglass central lucency that anatomically represents continuous disc material from the adjacent disc spaces above and below. The pedicles may appear slightly enlarged, and the interpediculate distance may be minimally increased. (6) (Fig. 3.48)

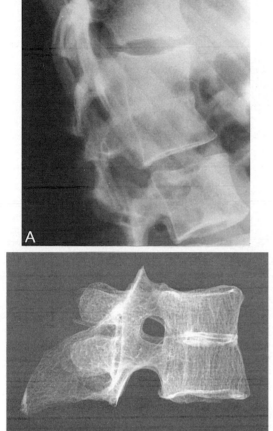

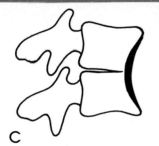

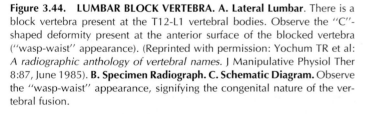

Figure 3.44. LUMBAR BLOCK VERTEBRA. A. Lateral Lumbar. There is a block vertebra present at the T12-L1 vertebral bodies. Observe the "C"-shaped deformity present at the anterior surface of the blocked vertebra ("wasp-waist" appearance). (Reprinted with permission: Yochum TR et al: *A radiographic anthology of vertebral names.* J Manipulative Physiol Ther 8:87, June 1985). **B. Specimen Radiograph. C. Schematic Diagram.** Observe the "wasp-waist" appearance, signifying the congenital nature of the vertebral fusion.

The most common areas to be affected are the thoracic and lumbar spine. (6) It is usually clinically insignificant if occurring as an isolated anomaly. The development of the ununited lateral body halves is generally symmetrical; therefore scoliosis or kyphoscoliosis are not associated. (Fig. 3.49A and B) Dysraphic spinal conditions such as meningocele, myelomeningocele, or diastematomyelia may have multiple butterfly vertebrae present. (6)

HEMIVERTEBRAE

Description. The vertebral body normally develops from two lateral ossification centers. When one of these centers fails to grow, the resultant triangular deformity of the body is called a lateral hemivertebra. Lateral hemivertebra is the most common type of presentation. As a rule, a hemivertebra does not exist singularly, and there are usually other coexistent vertebral anomalies. (1) Rarely, a dorsal hemivertebra occurs that is characterized by absence of the anterior portion of the vertebral body. (1) Even more rare is a ventral hemivertebra, where the posterior portion of the body is absent. (Fig. 3.50) The most commonly affected areas of the spine are the upper lumbar and lower thoracic regions. (1)

An isolated hemivertebra will cause a structural scoliosis with an angular lateral curvature, the hemivertebra occurring at the apex of the scoliosis. There is no hope of reducing this type of scoliosis without surgical intervention; however, if two hemivertebrae are balanced by their wedges being based on opposite sides, they produce little or no visible deformity. (2) The interposed discs at the affected level are normally developed. (3)

Hemivertebrae constitute approximately 6% of anomalies associated with congenital spinal deformities. (4) Lateral hemivertebrae have been shown to occur with other vertebral anomalies such as block vertebrae, diastematomyelia, Klippel-Feil syndrome, meningocele, multiple enchondromatosis (Ollier's disease), and spondylothoracic dysplasia. (1,3) Dorsal hemivertebrae may be seen with achondroplasia, cretinism, chondrodystrophy, Morquio's disease, and gargoylism. (3)

Radiologic Features. The laterally wedged hemivertebra is easily diagnosed from plain anteroposterior radiographs. The vertebral body will be triangular, with the endplates tapering to a point. (Fig. 3.51) Although adjacent discs are of normal height, the endplates of adjacent vertebrae are slightly deformed, giving those vertebral bodies a trapezoid shape. An isolated laterally wedged hemivertebra results in an angular scoliosis; but usually there are multiple congenital anomalies involved. (Fig. 3.52) Multiple hemivertebrae, in conjunction with block vertebrae, distort the spine and result in what has been called the *scrambled spine.* (5,6) A dorsal hemivertebra is pointed toward the anterior and results in a gibbus deformity. This is best visualized on lateral radiographs. (Fig. 3.53)

SCHMORL'S NODES

Description. Schmorl's nodes occur when the nucleus pulposus herniates through the vertebral endplate. (Fig. 3.54A and B) These defects have also been called cartilaginous nodes and intraspongy nuclear herniations. (1) There may be an inherent developmental weakness of the endplate, as occurs with regression of the chorda dorsalis or penetrating blood vessels (2), allowing for disc protrusion; or there may be pathologic weakening of the bone, as is seen in osteoporosis or osteomalacia, that permits the cartilaginous endplate and softened subchondral bone to yield to the pressure of the fluid and noncompressible nucleus pulposus. The incidence of cartilaginous nodes varies from 2% to 76%, depending on the method of assessment. (3,4)

A few cases have been reported where a Schmorl's node appears to be the cause of a patient's pain. (5–7)

Radiologic Features. A Schmorl's node looks like a squared-off, sharp, rectangular rim of sclerosis protruding above (or be-

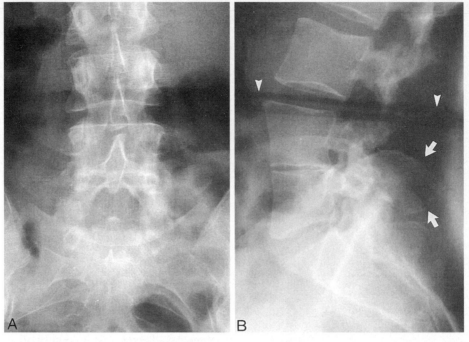

Figure 3.45.   LUMBAR BLOCK VERTEBRA. A. AP Lumbar Spine. Observe the single, large, common spinous process at the L4-L5 level. **B. Lateral Lumbar**. There is a remnant disc present between the L4-L5 block vertebra. Underdevelopment of the anterior surface of the vertebral bodies of L4-L5 has created the "wasp-waist" appearance. A single common spinous process for L4-L5 is noted (arrows). A radiolucent band (arrowheads) represents a fat-fold artifact. (Courtesy of Douglas B. Hart, DC, Carina, Queensland, Australia)

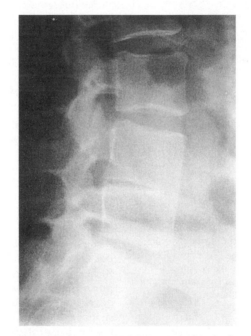

Figure 3.46.   LUMBAR BLOCK VERTEBRA. Coned Lateral Lumbar. Note the decrease in disc height and lack of endplate distinction at the L4-L5 level. The characteristic "wasp-waist" abnormality is not present in this example. (Courtesy of Gordon A. Kuether, DC, Blair, Nebraska)

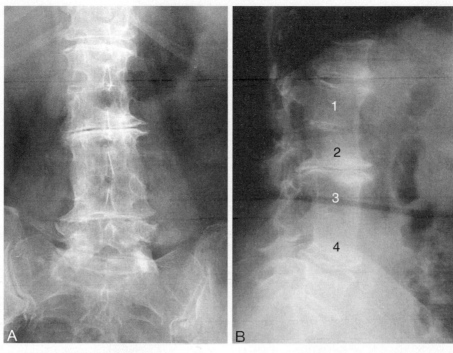

Figure 3.47.   MULTIPLE LUMBAR BLOCK VERTEBRAE. A. AP Lumbar Spine. B. Lateral Lumbar Spine. There are multiple block vertebrae throughout the lumbar spine. There is significant degenerative change noted at the freely articulated, unfused levels. (Courtesy of James F. Winterstein, DC, DACBR, Chicago, Illinois)

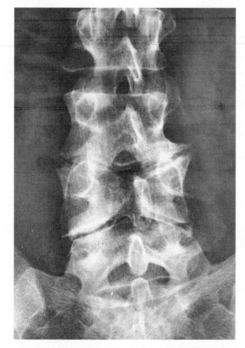

Figure 3.48.   BUTTERFLY VERTEBRA. AP Lumbar Spine. There is a butterfly vertebra present at L4. Note the widened interpediculate distance. (Reprinted with permission: Yochum TR et al: *A radiographic anthology of vertebral names.* J Manipulative Physiol Ther 8:87, June 1985) (Courtesy of Robert J. Hooke, BAppSc (Chiro), Cootamundra, New South Wales, Australia)

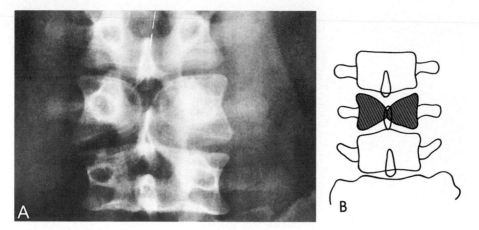

Figure 3.49.   BUTTERFLY VERTEBRA. A. AP Lumbar Spine. There is a symmetrically formed butterfly vertebra present at L3. **B. Schematic Diagram: Butterfly Vertebra**.

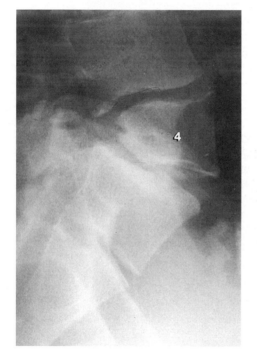

Figure 3.50.   VENTRAL HEMIVERTEBRA: LUMBAR SPINE. Lateral L5-S1 Spot. Observe the anterior hemivertebra present at the L4 lumbar level.

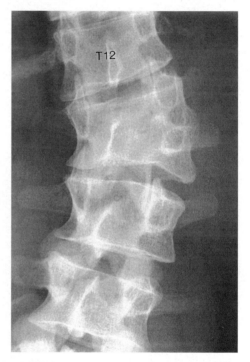

Figure 3.51.   LATERAL HEMIVERTEBRA: LUMBAR SPINE. AP Thoracolumbar Spot. Observe the duplicated pedicles and transverse processes on the L1 vertebra. There is a lateral wedging of the vertebral body consistent with a lateral hemivertebra.

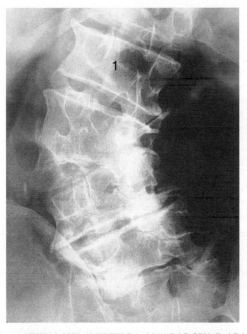

Figure 3.52. LATERAL HEMIVERTEBRA: LUMBAR SPINE. AP Lumbar. An isolated hemivertebra at L2-L3 is present. This congenital deformity has created a significant structural scoliosis throughout the lumbar spine. Observe the resultant advanced degenerative spondylophyte formation and substantial disc space narrowing present on the concave margins of this scoliotic spine. (Courtesy of Donald E. Freuden, DC, FACO, Denver, Colorado)

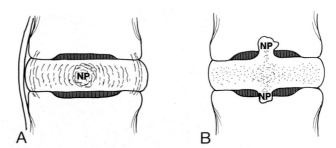

Figure 3.54. DEVELOPMENT OF SCHMORL'S NODES. A. Schematic Diagram: Normal Disc. Observe the normal location of the nucleus pulposus (*NP*). **B. Schematic Diagram: Schmorl's Node.** Observe the herniated nucleus pulposus (*NP*) through the cartilaginous endplate.

low) the endplate into the body of the vertebra. It looks as though the eraser end of a pencil had been pushed through the endplate. (Fig. 3.55A–C) The lesion may appear to be central or peripherally located. Small Schmorl's nodes are difficult to detect on plain radiographs. (5)

Giant Schmorl's nodes present a unique triad of features: anterosuperior placement, reduced supradjacent disc space, and increased anteroposterior vertebral body diameter. (6) (Figs. 3.56, 3.57A and B, 3.58) The enlarged squared-off appearance of giant Schmorl's nodes has been called the Schmorl's node phenomenon. (7) These nodes, best seen on lateral radiographs, are most common in the thoracic and lumbar spine. (Fig. 3.59) Occasionally, a narrowing of the adjacent disc space may be noted, particularly if the herniation is large, with a significant loss of nuclear material.

Nuclear Impression. Schmorl's nodes must be differentiated from nuclear impressions (notochordal persistence). These variants of development also cause irregularity of the endplates, but there is a smooth, undulating cortical surface that involves almost the entire endplate. (Fig. 3.60A–C) On a lateral radiograph of nuclear impression there is an indentation of the inferior endplate, while on an anteroposterior radiograph a *"double hump"* will be noted and has been referred to as the *"Cupid's bow contour."* (8) (Fig. 3.61A–E) A named appearance has been described because of the characteristic computed tomographic presentation of this anomaly. The *"owl's eyes"* appearance is present when paired, well-corticated radiolucencies are noted in the vertebral endplate, and the central area has the CT value of disc material. This finding has been described in the typical inferior endplate location and also in superior vertebral endplates. (9–13) (Fig. 3.61F)

VATER SYNDROME

Description. The VATER syndrome (vertebral anomalies, anal atresia, tracheo-esophageal fistula with esophageal atresia, and renal and radial dysplasia) was first proposed by Quan and Smith (1), when they described seven patients with the association of vertebral maldevelopment and multiple visceral anomalies. The reason proposed for this constellation of defects is a nonrandom association of congenital anomalies of mesodermal structures that must occur before the seventh fetal week of development, which is a tendency of concurrence and not an absolute interrelationship. The vertebral anomalies are usually hypoplastic or aplastic. (3) The "V" may also apply to vascular defects, since ventricular septal defects and a single umbilical

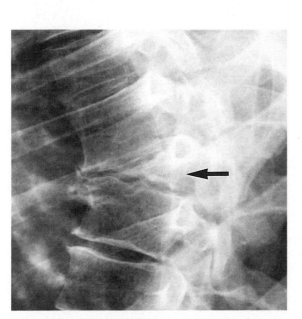

Figure 3.53. DORSAL HEMIVERTEBRA: THORACIC SPINE. Lateral Mid Dorsal Spot. Observe the dorsal hemivertebra present in the midthoracic spine (arrow). This congenital abnormality has created an increased thoracic kyphosis.

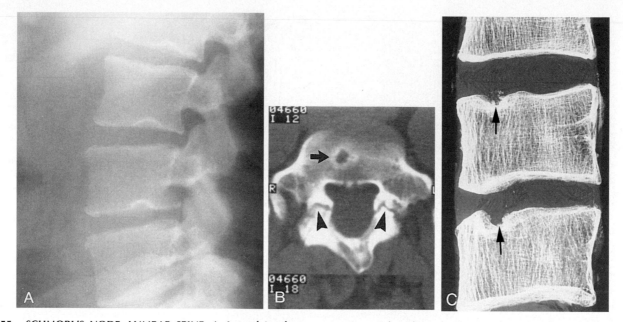

Figure 3.55.   SCHMORL'S NODE: LUMBAR SPINE. A. Lateral Lumbar Spine. The short, sharply defined defects involving the vertebral endplates on multiple lumbar levels represent Schmorl's nodes. **B. Computed Tomographic Appearance of a Schmorl's node.** (Not the same patient as in **A**) Observe the clearly defined defect present within the vertebral body, rep-resenting a Schmorl's node) (arrow). This patient has, additionally, bilateral pars defects (arrowheads). **C. Lateral Specimen Radiograph**. This demonstrates the abrupt margin and relatively shallow depth within which the herniation occurs (arrows). (Courtesy of Donald Resnick, MD, San Diego, California)

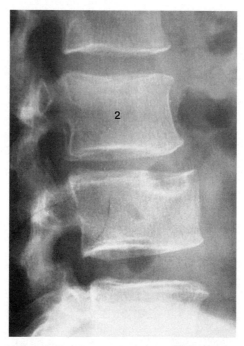

Figure 3.56.   SCHMORL'S NODE PHENOMENON: LUMBAR SPINE. Lateral L2 Spot. There is a giant Schmorl's node present on the anterosuperior corner of the third lumbar vertebra. Associated disc space narrowing is present at the L2–L3 level. Observe the increase in the anteroposterior diameter of the L3 vertebral body. This constellation of changes represents the Schmorl's node phenomenon.

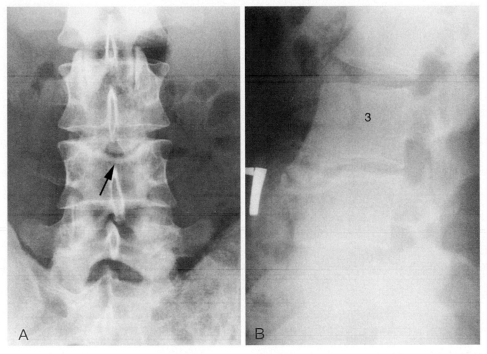

Figure 3.57.   GIANT SCHMORL'S NODE. A. Coned AP Lumbar Spine. Observe the depressed superior cortical endplate of the L4 vertebral body (arrow). Note the apparent facet asymmetry at L4-L5. **B. Coned Lateral Lumbar Spine**. Note the extension of the L3 vertebral body into the defect created by the Schmorl's node. (Courtesy of Carr Chiropractic Clinic, Huron, South Dakota)

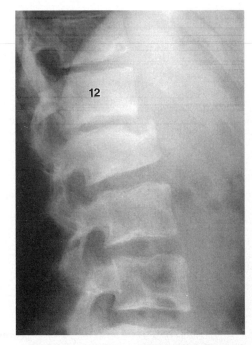

Figure 3.58.   GIANT SCHMORL'S NODE. Lateral Thoracolumbar Spot. There is a large, anteriorly placed, giant Schmorl's node present on the superior endplate of L1. Significant disc space narrowing is present at the T12-L1 level, associated with the giant Schmorl's node formation. Smaller Schmorl's node formations are present at the anteroinferior corner of T11 and at the vertebral endplates of L2 and L3. COMMENT: Multiple giant Schmorl's nodes have been previously misdiagnosed as representing Scheuermann's disease.

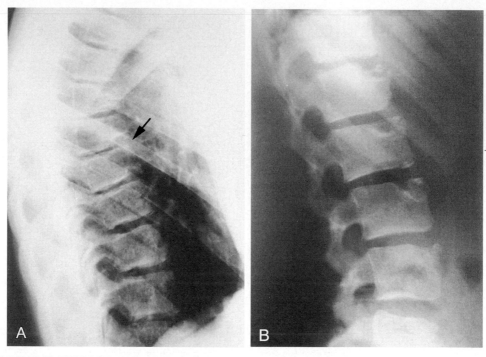

Figure 3.59.　SCHMORL'S NODES: THORACIC AND LUMBAR SPINE. A. Lateral Thoracic Spine. Observe the multiple Schmorl's nodes present in the thoracic spine (arrow). **B. Lateral Lumbar Spine.** This is the same patient as in **A**. Again note the multiple, giant Schmorl's nodes present at nearly every lumbar vertebra. COMMENT: This patient was a champion swimmer and was misdiagnosed with Scheuermann's disease. (Courtesy of Jeanne M. DesRoche, DC, Englewood, Colorado)

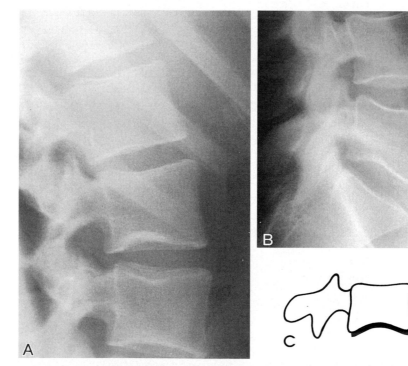

Figure 3.60.　NUCLEAR IMPRESSIONS: LUMBAR SPINE. A. Lateral Lumbar Spine. There are multiple nuclear impressions affecting the vertebral endplates of the midlumbar spine. **B. Lateral Lumbosacral Spine.** Observe the broad-based nuclear impression affecting the inferior endplate of the L5 vertebra. **C. Schematic Diagram: Nuclear Impression.** Observe the smooth and long depression of the inferior endplate found associated with nuclear impression.

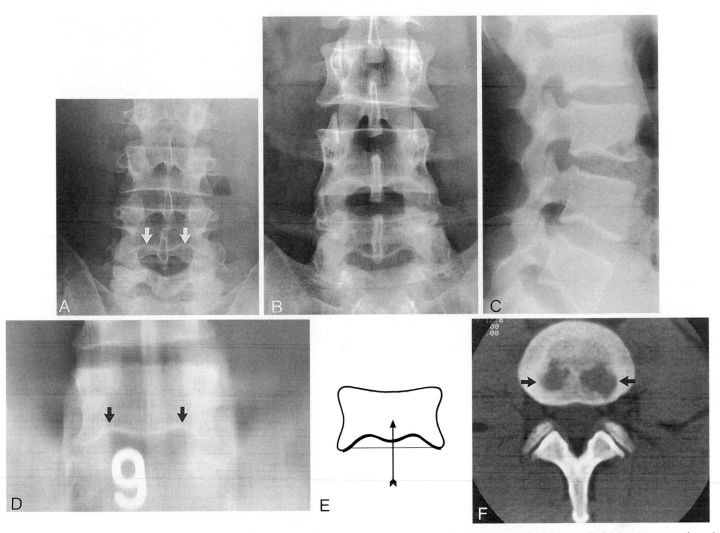

Figure 3.61. "CUPID'S BOW" CONTOUR: LUMBAR SPINE. A and B. AP Lumbar Spine. Observe the paired parasagittal concavities affecting the inferior endplate of the L4 vertebra (arrows) in these two separate examples. **C. Lateral Lumbar Spine.** Note the multiple nuclear impressions affecting the inferior endplates of L2 through L5. **D. AP Tomogram: L5 Vertebra.** Observe the "cupid's bow" contour affecting the inferior endplate of the L5 vertebra (arrows). **E. Schematic Diagram: "Cupid's Bow" Contour. F. Computed Tomogram: "Owl's Eyes" Appearance.** The computed tomographic features of nuclear impression with the "Cupid's bow" contour is that of paired, well-corticated, round areas of intervertebral disc density within the vertebral bodies. ("Owl's eyes" appearance) (arrows). COMMENT: The "Cupid's bow" contour is associated with nuclear impression deformities usually of the inferior vertebral endplates. They commonly affect the L4 and L5 vertebrae. The bilateral smooth indentations help differentiate this from a vertebral endplate fracture.

artery are frequently associated with the syndrome. (3) Karyotyping with advanced banding techniques is recommended in the diagnosis of this disorder to determine if any chromosome deletion abnormalities coexist. (4)

This rather rare entity is included as a reminder that anomalies of the spine do not always occur as isolated incidents and may be associated with other defects that may have great clinical significance in the management of the patient. It would be wise to search for and rule out additional anomalies when one appears on a radiograph.

POSTERIOR ARCH ANOMALIES

AGENESIS OF A LUMBAR PEDICLE

See discussion under "Absent Pedicle of the Cervical Spine." (1,2) (Figs. 3.62A–C, 3.63)

SPINA BIFIDA OCCULTA

The laminae meet and close posteriorly to form the spinous process. A small defect in this area will result in a cleft spinous. When this defect is mild, with only a small void in the osseous development, it is known as "spina bifida occulta (SBO)." This is not known to cause back pain and is considered to be of no clinical significance. (1) Spina bifida occulta does not predispose to low back pain, nor does it influence the chronicity of low back pain. (2) Spina bifida occulta occurs more commonly in males at the L5 and S1 levels in a 9:1 ratio. (2) Magora and Schwartz convincingly state, "All pre-employment surveys of candidates for any type of work should disregard this [SBO] finding." (2) As there is no spinous process at C1, the most correct term to describe this anomaly is spondyloschisis.

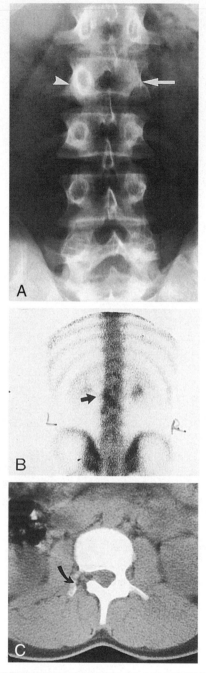

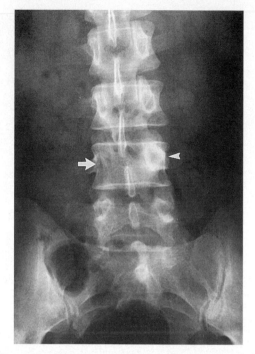

Figure 3.63. CONGENITAL ABSENCE OF A LUMBAR PEDICLE. AP Lumbar. There is agenesis of the pedicle of L4 (arrow) with contralateral reactive sclerosis and hypertrophy of the opposite pedicle (arrowhead). COMMENT: The absence of a vertebral pedicle should be considered the result of metastatic carcinoma unless the contralateral pedicle demonstrates hypertrophy and reactive sclerosis, indicating a long-standing congenital lesion with stress response.

Figure 3.62. CONGENITAL AGENESIS OF A LUMBAR PEDICLE. A. AP Lumbar Spine. Agenesis of the L2 pedicle (arrow) has created instability in the neural arch, allowing for stress to be placed upon the opposite pedicle and neural arch, producing significant reactive sclerosis (arrowhead). **B. Bone Scan: Lumbar Spine.** There is an area of increased radionuclide uptake present in the area of stress hypertrophy opposite the agenetic pedicle (arrow). **C. Computed Tomogram.** Computed tomography clearly demonstrates the agenesis of the pedicle (arrow). (Reprinted with permission from Albers VL: *Congenital absence of the lumbar pedicle, with sclerosis and hypertrophy of the contralateral pedicle.* ACA J Chiro, Radiology Case Report, April 1984)

SPINA BIFIDA VERA

This defect may be considerably larger than that found in spina bifida occulta, with no protection of the spinal cord by a bony shield, and is known as spina bifida vera or spina bifida manifesta. This void in the neural arch may allow protrusion of the meninges and/or spinal cord. There is no simple genetic explanation, but it appears that inheritance is polygenic and that 60% are genetic in origin. (3)

Spina bifida vera may be diagnosed in utero through analysis of the amniotic fluid, looking for an elevated level of alpha fetoprotein. The postpartum diagnosis of spina bifida manifesta can be suspected when on physical examination there is discovered the cutaneous signature in the form of a hair patch, lipoma, or dimple. The clinical effects of spina bifida manifesta are related to the extent of local cord and nerve root deficit, plus the delayed effects of hydrocephalus and infection of the cord.

Radiologic Features

Spina Bifida Occulta. This defect is well seen on anteroposterior radiographs of the spine. A lucent cleft is noted between the laminae, and the spinous process at that level is diminutive or absent. (Fig. 3.64A–E) A lateral view of the cervical spine may suggest the presence of a spina bifida occulta by absence of the posterior cervical line (spinolaminar junction line) and is found most commonly at C1. (Fig. 3.10B)

Spina Bifida Vera. This defect will be seen on anteroposterior and lateral views of the spine as a result of the wide defect in the posterior neural arch structures at multiple levels. A soft tissue

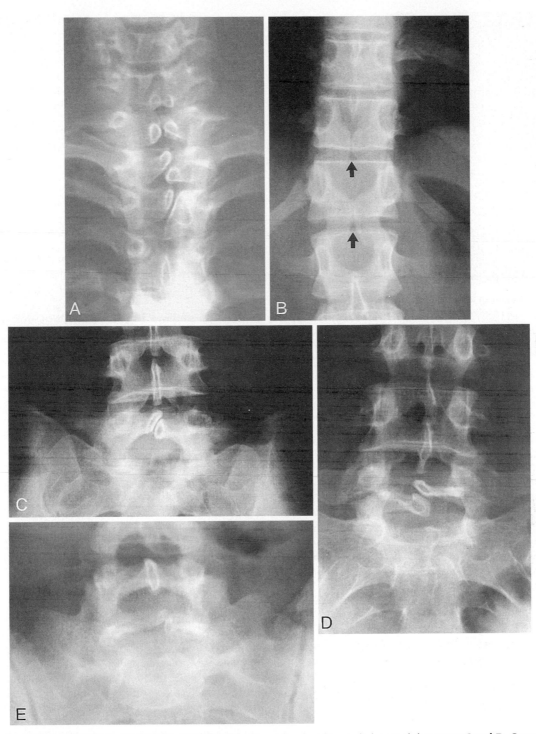

Figure 3.64. SPINA BIFIDA OCCULTA: MULTIPLE LOCATIONS. A. Coned AP Thoracic. There are multiple spina bifidae affecting C6, C7, T1, and T2. **B. Coned Lower Thoracic**. Failure of formation of the spinous processes of the eleventh and twelfth thoracic vertebrae have left a clearly de-fined midline radiolucent cleft (arrows) **C and D. Coned AP Lumbar.** Spina bifida occulta is present at the fifth lumbar vertebrae. **E. AP L5-S1 Tilt-Up.** Spina bifida occulta is present at the first sacral tubercle.

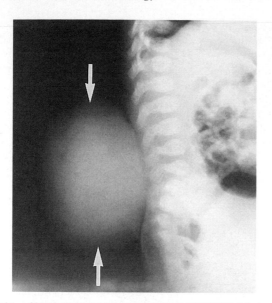

Figure 3.65. SPINA BIFIDA VERA: MYELOMENINGOCELE. Lateral Lumbar Spine. There is a large myelomeningocele posterior to the lower lumbar spine and upper sacral area in this infant (arrows).

mass posterior to the spine may also be present, representing the meningocele or myelomeningocele. (Fig. 3.65)

MENINGOCELE AND MYELOMENINGOCELE

Description. If a defect of the neural arch of a vertebra or vertebrae allows protrusion of the protective coverings of the spinal cord (the leptomeninges) or allows herniation of the spinal cord itself into the meningeal diverticulum, then there exists a meningocele or myelomeningocele. (1,2) Failure of fusion of the neural arch halves, resulting in a spina bifida vera, must take place during the twenty-first to twenty-ninth fetal day for a posterior myelomeningocele to result. (2)

At about the eighteenth fetal week spinal canal closure defects can be diagnosed via assay of alpha fetoprotein from maternal serum or from amniotic fluid aspirate. (3) All meningoceles do not protrude to the posterior. Commonly, in the upper thoracic spine a lateral herniation of the meninges through the intervertebral foramen may be seen as a water-density mass on thoracic or chest radiographs in association with neurofibromatosis. (4) Meningoceles have also been reported to occur anteriorly through the sacrum, creating a curvilinear erosion on the anterior aspect of the sacral canal. When viewed laterally on a radiograph, it creates a distinctive appearance known as the *scimitar sacrum*, since the sacrum resembles the shape of a curved Turkish sword. (5,6)

There are related problems seen with myelomeningocele, but differentiation based on clinical findings may not be possible. These problems include skin manifestations such as a hairy or pigmented patch, malformed fibrous tissue and blood vessels, and fatty tumors (lipomas). In patients with severe manifestations the protruding sac will be evident at birth, along with bilateral clubbed feet and paralysis, depending on the level of involvement. With mild expression, the child may not begin to show motor disturbances in gait until age 5 or 6.

Radiologic Features. The roentgenographic findings demonstrate spina bifida vera at one or more vertebral levels. The interpediculate distance will usually be increased at the site of involvement. Rarely, there is erosion of the vertebral body. The presence of a water-density mass may be seen, representing the sac filled with cerebrospinal fluid. Myelography, MRI, or ultrasonography is necessary to determine if the sac contains spinal cord elements. When myelography is performed water-soluble contrast media is preferred over oil-based contrast, as the communication of subarachnoid space and meningocele may be quite small. (7)

DIASTEMATOMYELIA

Description. The term "diastematomyelia" was first coined by Ollivier in 1837. (1) It represents a rare form of spinal dysraphism wherein an osseous, cartilaginous, or fibrous bar partially or completely divides the spinal cord or cauda equina and fixes it in the midline, effectively tethering the cord. (2) The thoracolumbar area is most commonly affected; less commonly affected is the cervical spine. (3) Prenatal diagnosis is possible (4), and symptoms usually lead to a diagnosis in early childhood; however, a patient may be an adult before diagnosis is made. (5–7)

Physical findings in patients with diastematomyelia include anal dimple, hairy lumbar patch, asymmetrical size of the lower extremities and lipoma. (2)

Radiologic Features. If an osseous bar is present, it may be demonstrable on plain film radiographs; a fibrous septum will not be seen. There is usually widening of the interpediculate distance at the level of the abnormality. Vertebral body deformities such as spina bifida occulta, hemivertebrae, and congenital bar and scoliosis are present in 50% of cases. (8) (Fig. 3.66A and B)

TRANSITIONAL VERTEBRAE

At the cervicothoracic, thoracolumbar, and lumbosacral junctions the morphologic characteristics of the vertebrae normally change markedly from one area to the next. It is here that transitional vertebrae occur, demonstrating features of both adjacent spinal segments. The lumbosacral junction is the most common site for transitional vertebrae to occur. Here the lowest lumbar vertebra may have some or all of the anatomic characteristics of the first sacral segment, so-called *sacralization*. Conversely, the first sacral segment may have the radiographic appearance of a lumbar vertebra, known as *lumbarization*. These changes are found in 4 to 8% of the general population. (1)

Description. Much time and effort has been spent determining the appropriate name for these affected segments such as "sacralization of the fifth lumbar vertebra," where the segment has more characteristics of the sacrum, or "lumbarization of the first sacral segment," which has more characteristics of a lumbar vertebra. The term *transitional segment* is less descriptive but encompasses both lumbarization and sacralization. The name found in a radiology report is considerably less important than the biomechanical or clinical significance.

If the transitional segment is partially or completely fused to the adjacent segment, then a motion segment is lost. The clinical significance of transitional vertebrae, especially at the lumbosacral junction, is still being debated and researched. The exhaustive study of Tini, Wieser, and Zinn (2) examined the radiographs of 4000 Swiss workers and concluded that " . . . carriers of a lumbosacral transitional vertebra do not have more backache than controls." These findings corroborate the work of Nachemson (3); however, Castellvi and coworkers (4) found that there is a significant incidence of herniation of the nucleus pulposus at the

19 mm (Castellvi type IA and IB, respectively). (4) (Fig. 3.67A–B) The L5 transverse process may, unilaterally or bilaterally, fuse with the sacrum (Castellvi type IIIA and type IIIB, respectively) (Figs. 3.68A and B, 3.69A and B) or may form an accessory joint with the sacrum (Castellvi type IIA and type IIB, respectively). When the development of the transitional segment is asymmetric and long-standing, it is not uncommon to see signs of degenerative joint disease at this accessory articulation in the form of subchondral sclerosis and marginal osteophytes. However, the presence of degenerative change at this accessory articulation does not necessarily correlate with the site of pain. (1) The body of L5 is usually normal in size and shape, but the interposed disc is generally hypoplastic or vestigial and decreased in its vertical dimension. (7)

FACET TROPISM

Description. The joint formed between articulating processes in the lumbar spine is not planar but is curved. Biomechanically, bilaterally symmetric sagittal joints at each level should allow equal ranges of motion, but these circumstances also limit flexion and rotation of the lumbar spine. (1)

In some individuals the planes of articulations at a single level are asymmetric. When this condition exists, the term *tropism* (literally meaning "turning") is applied. The significance of this anomaly has not been clearly delineated and remains an area of clinical controversy. (2,3) Recent studies have demonstrated no correlation between facet tropism and the genesis of lumbar disc degeneration. (4–7)

Radiologic Features. Facet tropism may be seen on the anteroposterior projection of the lumbar spine. In the normal lumbar spine the facet joints are visible as linear radiolucent regions between each superior and inferior articular process. Tropism at any level will manifest as nonvisualization of the facet joint space on one side, while being clearly seen on the contralateral side. (Fig. 3.70) This is most frequently encountered at the lumbosacral joint, but may be seen at any lumbar level. Tropism may be simulated by facets that are no longer oriented tangentially to the x-ray beam, as in scoliosis or intersegmental rotation. Computed tomography will most clearly demonstrate the true plane of the asymmetric facets. (8)

Facet asymmetry has been reported as a cause for excessive sclerosis of a pedicle. (9)

CLASP KNIFE SYNDROME

Description. This syndrome is named for the painful effect created upon extension of the lumbar spine in a patient who has a spina bifida of the first sacral segment and an associated caudal enlargement of the fifth lumbar spinous process. The earliest description of this finding appears to be by Ferguson in 1934. (1) In 1935 Bellerose termed the condition the long spinous process. (2) The elongation of the spinous process may be the result of inclusion of the first sacral tubercle with the ossification center for the spinous process of the fifth lumbar. DeAnguin (3) reported 15 patients with this defect and surmised that, because of the absence of the sacral tubercle, the L5 vertebra demonstrated an increased range of motion and, further, that low back pain may be caused by pressure on the laminar stumps at S1 or by pressure on a membrane that covers the sacral defect. Gill and White reported that in their experience conservative treatment, including a "flexion jacket" and postural exercises, gives relief in most instances. If this approach is unsuccessful, surgical removal of the

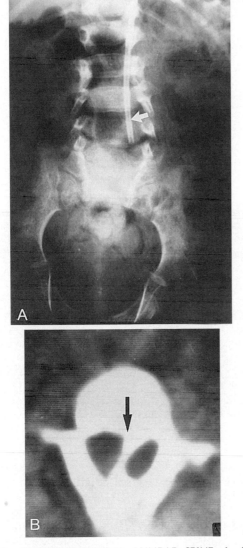

Figure 3.66. DIASTEMATOMYELIA: LUMBAR SPINE. A. AP Lumbar Spine. Observe the widened interpediculate spaces present throughout the lumbar spine. Observe an osseous bar dividing the spinal canal (arrow). **B. Computed Tomogram.** Note the osseous bar dividing the spinal canal (arrow).

next disc level above some lumbosacral transitional vertebra. They feel this may be caused by abnormal mechanical forces placed on the superior disc that may lead to premature degeneration of the disc. The disc between transitional segments is usually rudimentary in nature, but it has been shown that there is a potential for nuclear herniation with certain classifications of transitional vertebrae. (4) It is known that the accessory joints that develop between the enlarged lumbar transverse processes and the sacral alae may eventually degenerate because of the asymmetric forces of movement and that they are therefore a potential source of low back pain. (5) The combination of transitional vertebrae causing scoliosis and sciatica is known as Bertolotti's syndrome. (6)

Radiologic Features. The radiographic appearance of transitional lumbosacral vertebrae may vary greatly. The L5 vertebra may be considered transitional if the vertical dimension of one or both of its transverse processes measures greater than or equal to

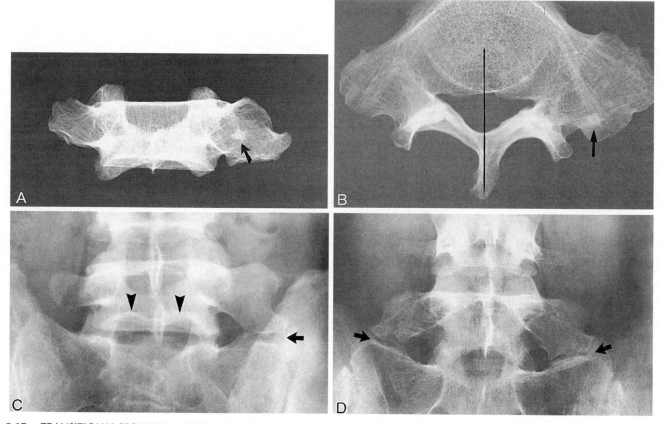

Figure 3.67.   TRANSITIONAL SEGMENT: LUMBOSACRAL JUNCTION. A. Specimen Radiograph. The large, spatulated transverse process of the fifth lumbar vertebra is noted in this transitional anatomic specimen. Of incidental notation is a benign bone island within the spatulated transverse process of L5 (arrow). **B. Specimen Radiograph**. An axial projection of the specimen demonstrates the large, spatulated transverse process of the transitional seg- ment. A benign bone island is noted (arrow). **C. AP Lumbosacral Junction.** A unilateral transitional segment is noted, with an accessory articulation (arrow). Of incidental notation is a "Cupid's bow" contour on the inferior endplate of L5 (arrowheads), resulting from nuclear impression. **D. AP Lum- bosacral Junction.** Observe the bilateral transitional segment present at the lumbosacral junction with bilateral accessory joints (arrows).

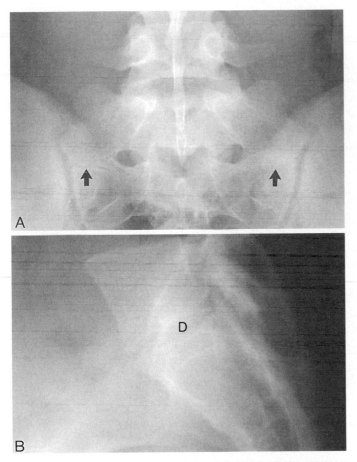

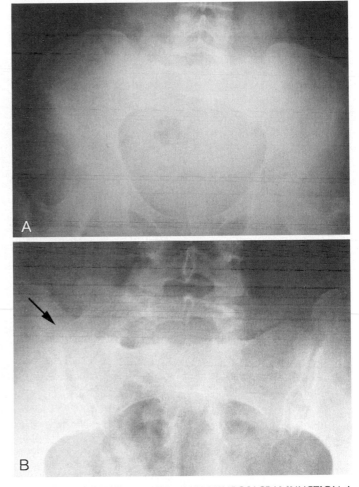

Figure 3.68.   TRANSITIONAL SEGMENT: LUMBOSACRAL JUNCTION. A. AP Lumbosacral Junction. There is a bilateral, nearly completely fused transitional segment (arrows) present at the lumbosacral junction. **B. Lateral Lumbosacral View.** Observe the hypoplastic disc (*D*) between the transitional segment and the sacral base.

Figure 3.69.   TRANSITIONAL SEGMENT: LUMBOSACRAL JUNCTION. A. Coned AP Lumbopelvic. Note the difficulty in determining the precise anatomic structures at the L5-S1 junction in this commonly utilized view. This is because the L5-S1 disc angle is not coincident with the central ray. **B. AP L5-S1 Tilt-Up.** With this view the transitional segment is clearly seen to be fused with the sacrum unilaterally (arrow). (Courtesy of Paul Van Wyk, DC, Denver, Colorado)

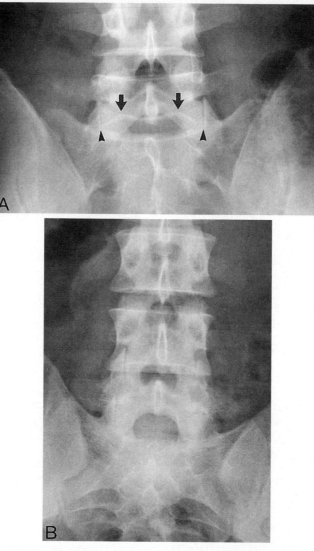

**Figure 3.70.   ABNORMALITIES OF FACET ORIENTATION: LUMBOSA-
CRAL JUNCTION. A. AP Lumbosacral View**. There are bilateral sagittal facet
facings present at the lumbosacral junction (arrowheads). Asymmetric facet
facings (tropism), are noted at the L4-L5 level. A "Cupid's bow" deformity
is present, affecting the inferior endplate of L5 (arrows). **B. AP Lumbosacral
View.** There is facet asymmetry present at the lumbosacral junction (tropism). COMMENT: Computed tomography has clearly demonstrated that
patients with plain film radiographic demonstration of bilateral sagittal facet
facings at the lumbosacral junction in fact have "cupped" facet facings
rather than purely sagittal joints in many instances.

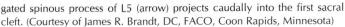

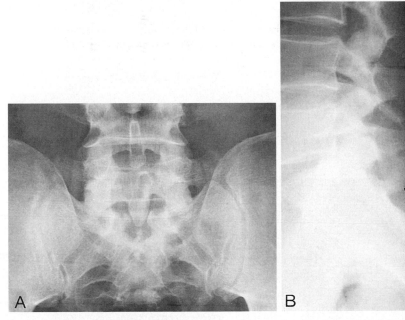

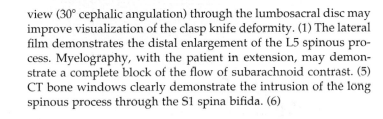

Figure 3.71. **"CLASP KNIFE" DEFORMITY. A. AP Lumbosacral View.** Observe the large spinous process of L5, which projects into a spina bifida affecting the first sacral segment. **B. Lateral Lumbosacral View.** The elongated spinous process of L5 (arrow) projects caudally into the first sacral cleft. (Courtesy of James R. Brandt, DC, FACO, Coon Rapids, Minnesota)

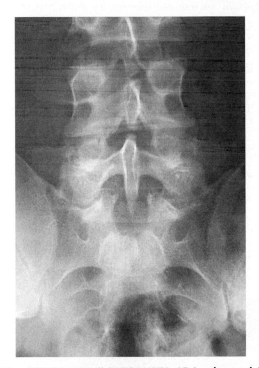

Figure 3.72. **"CLASP KNIFE" DEFORMITY. AP Lumbosacral Spot.** Observe the large spina bifida present in the first sacral segment, which allows the elongated spinous process of L5 to enter this defect.

long spinous process and rudiments of the sacral tubercle will give relief. (4)

Radiologic Features. AP roentgenograms will reveal a spina bifida occulta of the S1 level and an increased vertical dimension of the L5 spinous process. (Figs. 3.71A and B, 3.72) The tilt-up view (30° cephalic angulation) through the lumbosacral disc may improve visualization of the clasp knife deformity. (1) The lateral film demonstrates the distal enlargement of the L5 spinous process. Myelography, with the patient in extension, may demonstrate a complete block of the flow of subarachnoid contrast. (5) CT bone windows clearly demonstrate the intrusion of the long spinous process through the S1 spina bifida. (6)

ANOMALIES OF THE THORAX

RIB ANOMALIES

CONGENITAL PSEUDOARTHROSIS OF THE FIRST RIB

Occasionally, the first rib does not completely ossify in its midportion. Typically, this area is painless. Radiographically, the rib is slightly expanded and the site of the pseudoarthrosis demonstrates smooth and sclerotic cortical margins. (Fig. 3.73) This finding must be distinguished from a stress fracture of the first rib that is classically found in patients who carry heavy items using a shoulder strap.

SRB'S ANOMALY

Description. Srb's anomaly is involution of one or both first ribs as a result of diminished length and incomplete fusion of the first and second ribs to form a solid bony plate. (1)

Radiologic Features. Views taken for the chest or ribs will demonstrate this anomaly. The normal rib interspace between the first and second ribs is absent. (Fig. 3.74A and B) A pseudoarthrosis may be seen in the midportion of the fused rib.

LUSCHKA'S BIFURCATED RIB

Occasionally, the anterior aspect of an upper thoracic rib may be split or bifurcated. It is clinically insignificant, but must not be mistaken for a cavity within the lung. (1) (Fig. 3.75A–C).

RIB FORAMEN

Anomalous foraminal development in a rib may rarely be noted and is of no clinical significance. (Fig. 3.76)

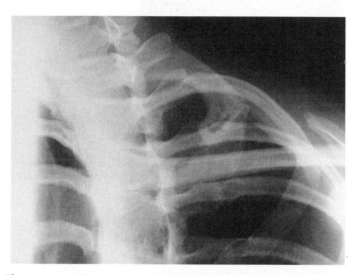

Figure 3.73. CONGENITAL PSEUDOARTHROSIS, FIRST RIB. This PA (with cephalic angulation) view of the first rib shows a developmental defect in its midportion. This finding must be differentiated diagnosed from all causes of stress fracture of the first rib. Typically, there is no local pain in patients with such a congenital pseudoarthrosis.

INTRATHORACIC RIB

Occasionally, an anomalous rib is present that protrudes through instead of around the thoracic cavity. (Fig. 3.77)

CHEST ANOMALIES

PECTUS EXCAVATUM

This is the most common deformity of the chest wall. It is also known as funnel chest, because of the midline depression of the sternum that is seen on physical examination. A lateral radiograph of the chest will confirm the physical examination finding of the posterior displacement of the sternum and a decreased retrosternal clear space. (Fig. 3.78A and B)

PECTUS CARINATUM

This deformity is produced by an anterior displacement of the sternum. An alternate name for this condition is pigeon breast. It has been found associated with Morquio's syndrome. A lateral chest film will demonstrate a prominent sternum with an increased retrosternal clear space.

STRAIGHT BACK SYNDROME

Description. A reduced thoracic kyphosis causes the anteroposterior diameter of the chest to be reduced. The lack of kyphosis has been called the cobbler's chest. (1) This change causes the heart and mediastinal structures to be compressed between the thoracic spine and the sternum. The result is a ''pancake'' heart, a shift of the heart shadow to the left, a prominent upper left heart border, and altered hemodynamics creating an ejection systolic murmur. This murmur is probably functional and typically decreases when the patient sits up or inspires. (2)

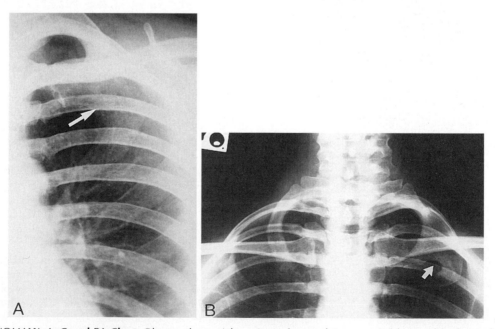

Figure 3.74. SRB'S ANOMALY. A. Coned PA Chest. Observe the partial congenital synostosis of the first and second ribs (arrow). **B. AP Ribs**. There is nearly complete congenital fusion of the first and second ribs on the right side (arrow).

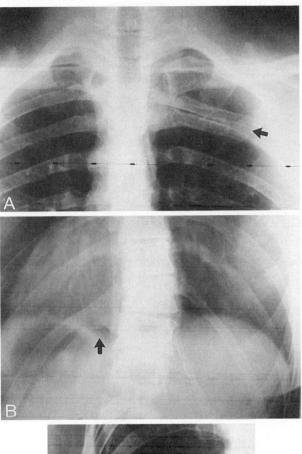

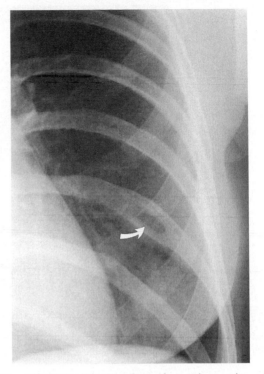

Figure 3.76.   RIB FORAMEN. Coned PA Chest. Observe the radiolucent foramen present within the posterolateral aspect of the eighth left rib (arrow). (Courtesy of Kenneth E. Yochum, DC, St. Louis, Missouri)

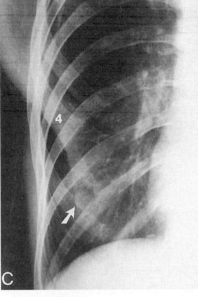

Figure 3.75.   LUSCHKA'S BIFURCATED RIB. A. PA Ribs. Observe the congenital fusion of the posterolateral surface of the third and fourth rib on the right side (arrow). The black transverse line though the lower half of the radiograph represents the perforated crease of a folding film. **B. PA Ribs.** There is congenital synostosis of the posterior surface of the 11th and 12th ribs on the left side (arrow). **C. PA Ribs.** A focal bifurcation of the anterior surface of the right fourth rib is present. The circular, radiopaque density present over the right lower lung field represents a nipple shadow (arrow). COMMENT: Luschka's bifurcated rib is clinically insignificant, but must not be mistaken for a cavity within the lung.

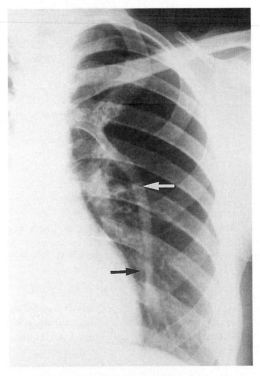

Figure 3.77.   INTRATHORACIC RIB. Coned PA Chest. Observe the accessory intrathoracic rib (arrows). This is a rare congenital anomaly. (Courtesy of Bryan Hartley, MD, Melbourne, Australia)

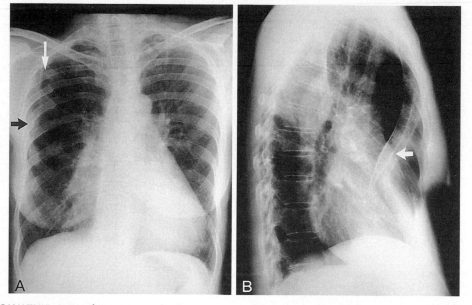

Figure 3.78.   PECTUS EXCAVATUM. A. PA Chest. As a result of posterior protrusion of the sternum, the right atrial heart border cannot be visualized on this PA radiograph. There is excessive caudal angulation of the ribs anteriorly. Of incidental notation are old healed fractures present on the right at ribs 4, 5, 6, and 7 (arrows). **B. Lateral Chest**. Observe the posterior protrusion of the sternum (arrow), which has displaced the heart so that the cardiac shadow overlaps the lower thoracic spine.

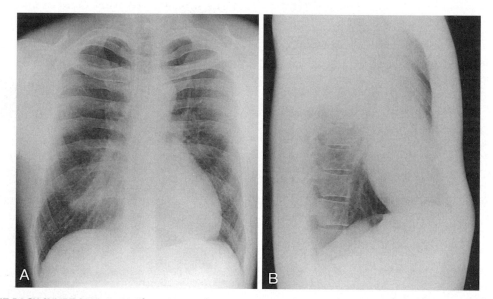

Figure 3.79.   STRAIGHT BACK SYNDROME. A. PA Chest. Notice there is no portion of the heart shadow visible to the right of the spine. Also see how the ribs angle excessively, inferiorly. **B. Lateral Chest**. The sternum is minimally depressed, as in pectus excavatum, but the thoracic kyphosis is markedly reduced, thus compressing the heart and shifting it toward the left. (Courtesy of Jay D. Fullinwider, DC, Littleton, Colorado)

It is significant that there is an increased incidence of mitral valve prolapse in patients with straight back syndrome. Therefore straight back syndrome should no longer be considered a form of pseudoheart disease, and patients should be investigated for associated mitral valve prolapse and their relatives screened. (3)

Straight back syndrome has been suggested to be inherited as an autosomal dominant with the antigenic determinants located on chromosome 6. (3)

Radiologic Features.   The PA chest view demonstrates an unusual downward angulation of the anterior rib ends. The heart shadow is displaced toward the left with no border of the heart visualized on the right side of the lower thoracic spine. The lateral chest view demonstrates a diminished kyphosis or straight thoracic spine. (Fig. 3.79A and B) A pectus excavatum is variably present.

Measurement for straight back syndrome is performed by dividing the AP diameter of the chest by the transthoracic ratio. (4)

Another method of measuring for this syndrome can be performed on the lateral chest radiograph. The distance from the middle of the anterior border of T8 to a vertical line connecting

T4 and T12 was found to be significantly reduced compared with controls, and an absolute value less than 1.2 cm indicates a straight back. Of 58 subjects with this syndrome 67% had clinical and/or echocardiographic evidence of mitral valve prolapse, while respiratory function testing revealed no significant abnormality. (3)

MEDICOLEGAL IMPLICATIONS
Straight Back Syndrome

- Three patients with Ehlers-Danlos syndrome had this syndrome. (5)
- Complaint of palpitations on swallowing. Electrocardiogram revealed supraventricular ectopics each time the patient swallowed. (6)
- A patient with a complaint of high fever following dental treatment has been reported. He had a straight thoracic spine with absence of physiologic kyphosis. Blood culture was positive for *Streptococcus sanguis I*. Echocardiography revealed mitral valve regurgitation with some vegetation at the ruptured chordae tendinae of the posterior leaflet. (7)
- Patients with straight back syndrome have a significant incidence of echocardiographically proven mitral valve prolapse. Isolated nonejection systolic click(s) were the major cardiac auscultatory finding, while 60% showed pansystolic prolapse on echocardiography. (8)
- A case of complete absence of the left pericardium coexisting with straight back syndrome in a 30-year-old female has been reported. Echocardiography showed paradoxical movement of the ventricle septum, hyperkinetic movement of the free wall of the left ventricle, and enlargement of the right ventricle. Computed tomography and magnetic resonance imaging with an artificial pneumomediastinum clearly showed rotation of the heart into the left hemithorax, prominence of the pulmonary trunk, and pneumopericardium. (9)

ANOMALIES OF THE HIP AND PELVIS

CONGENITAL HIP DYSPLASIA

Description. Congenital hip dysplasia includes deformities of the acetabulum, as well as dislocation of the femur from a malformed acetabulum. If congenital hip dislocation is suspected at birth, Ortolani's and Barlow's tests may aid in the diagnosis. The main reason for the dislocation is inversion of the fibrocartilaginous limbus and capsular contraction, which makes reduction of the dislocation difficult or impossible. (1)

Radiologic Features. The description of congenital hip dislocation by Putti in 1929 remains accurate today. The combination of an absent or small proximal femoral epiphysis, lateral displacement of the femur, and increased inclination of the acetabular roof is known as *Putti's triad*. (2) (Fig. 3.80) With long-standing dislocations and attempted weight bearing the proximally and posteriorly luxated femoral head may create a shallow pseudoacetabulum superior to the deformed primary acetabulum. (Fig. 3.81A–C)

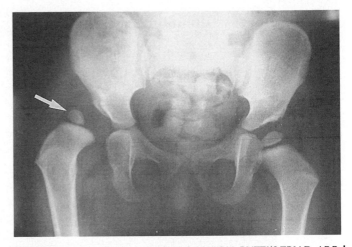

Figure 3.80.   CONGENITAL HIP DISLOCATION: PUTTI'S TRIAD. AP Pelvis. There is lateral displacement of the affected proximal femur, with underdevelopment of the femoral capital epiphysis (arrow). Additionally, a shallow acetabulum is associated.

SACRAL DYSPLASIA
SACRAL AGENESIS

Description. Congenital absence of the distal portion of the spinal column, also known as caudal regression syndrome, was first reported by Hohl in 1850. (1) Lack of development of the caudal spine has been reported as high as the 10th thoracic level. (2) An extensive study of 853 British infants (3) demonstrated that the incidence of all congenital malformations occurs at a rate three times higher than normal when it is shown that the mother had diabetes mellitus. The association of maternal diabetes with sacral agenesis has been well documented. (4)

The diagnosis is usually apparent at birth. The child has a flat or depressed sacral area with deficient musculature of the lower extremities. Associated problems include spinopelvic instability, scoliosis (most common), myelomeningocele, hip dislocation or contracture, knee contracture, and foot deformity. Renshaw has described four types based on the variable sacral/vertebral development seen radiographically. (4)

There is evidence that this condition is teratogenically induced or is a spontaneous genetic mutation. This evidence includes (a) the association with maternal diabetes mellitus; (b) the relationship of insulin-dependent diabetes mellitus with the major histocompatibility system; and (c) demonstration of a defect at a locus or loci on the sixth chromosome. This site codes for the major histocompatibility system of cell surface antigens. (4)

Radiologic Features. Radiographs will demonstrate absence of the sacrum and possibly some of the caudal lumbar segments. If the patient ever assumes a weight-bearing posture, abnormal biomechanics will cause typical degenerative joint changes to occur where the two ilia articulate. (Figs. 3.82, 3.83A and B)

COXA VARA AND COXA VALGA

Description. The noun *coxa* loosely refers to the hip, while the terms *varus* and *valgus* are adjectives that describe angulation of a part toward or away from the midline, respectively. The normal angle of incidence of the proximal femur is 120 to 130°

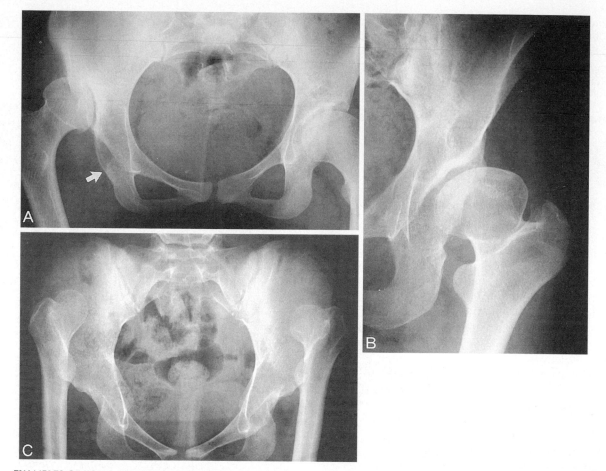

Figure 3.81.   EXAMPLES OF LONG-STANDING CONGENITAL HIP DYS-PLASIA. A. AP Pelvis. Observe the shallowness of the original acetabulum (arrow), as compared with the accessory acetabulum, which has formed on the lateral edge of the ilium. **B. AP Hip.** There is deformity and flattening of the femoral head. The acetabulum is shallow. **C. AP Pelvis.** There is complete bilateral dislocation of the femoral heads from the acetabuli, both of which are shallow. (Courtesy of Lynton G.F. Giles, MSc, DC, PhD, Townsville, Queensland, Australia)

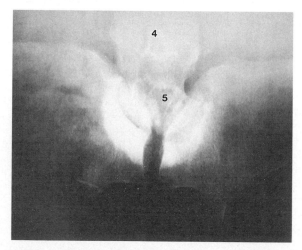

Figure 3.82.   CAUDAL REGRESSION SYNDROME. AP Lumbosacral Spot. Failure of formation of the sacrum creates close proximity of the posterior iliac surfaces. Degenerative reactive sclerosis is present on approximated iliac surfaces. (Courtesy of Appa L. Anderson, DC, DACBR, Fellow, ACCR, Portland, Oregon)

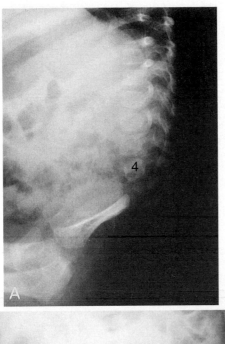

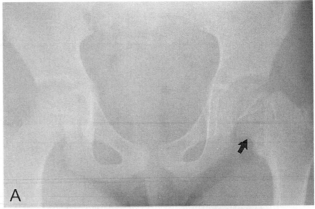

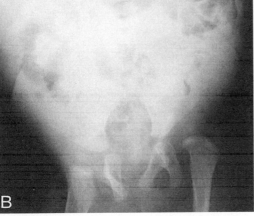

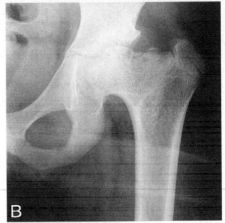

Figure 3.83.   CAUDAL REGRESSION SYNDROME. A. Lateral Lumbar Spine. Note the absence of the sacrum and L5 in this lateral film. The lowest lumbar vertebra present is L4 and it is dysplastic. **B. AP Pelvis**. The sacrum is not present and the approximation of the ilia can be noted. COMMENT: Caudal regression syndrome occurs at a much higher rate in children of mothers with diabetes mellitus. (Courtesy The Children's Hospital, Dept. of Radiology, Denver, Colorado)

Figure 3.84.   COXA VARA. A. AP Pelvis. There is a decreased femoral angle, with an inverted radiolucent "V" in the proximal metaphysis of the femur (arrow). This is a characteristic appearance for infantile coxa vara. An associated widening of the metaphysis is related to the deformity. There is no evidence of degenerative joint changes at this time. (Courtesy of C.H. Quay, MD, Melbourne, Australia) **B. AP Hip**. There is significant reduction of the femoral angle, with broadening of the metaphysis. A characteristic enlargement of the greater trochanter is noted. Associated deformity and osteophyte formation is present, affecting the lateral edge of the acetabulum.

(Mikulicz's angle). If this angle measures less than 120°, coxa vara exists. An angle greater than 130° indicates coxa valga. (See Chapter 2)

Coxa Vara. This femoral deformity is the result of eccentric cessation of growth of the medial aspect of the growth plate between the proximal femoral epiphysis and the femoral neck. It may occur in isolation or accompany proximal femoral focal deficiency, osteogenesis imperfecta, rickets, fibrous dysplasia, (2) and cleidocranial dysplasia. (3) The sex incidence is equal, and it is unilateral in 75% of cases. Acquired coxa vara may also complicate proximal femoral fractures.

Coxa Valga. This deformity appears to be the result of muscular imbalance of the abductor mechanism of the hip. (1) This imbalance, in turn, reduces the traction effect on the physis at the base of the greater trochanter. Histologic studies show that this growth plate is continuous (along the lateral aspect of the femoral neck)

with the growth plate of the proximal femoral epiphysis. Therefore this region of growth has great influence on the developing angulation of the femoral neck/shaft.

Radiologic Features.

Coxa Vara. Patients with coxa vara will have a decreased femoral angle, an inverted radiolucent "V" in the proximal metaphysis of the femur, an enlarged greater trochanter, and, depending on the length of existence, some deformity of the acetabulum may be present. (Fig. 3.84A and B) Degenerative joint changes may be superimposed findings in long-standing cases.

Coxa Valga. Patients with coxa valga will demonstrate an increased femoral angle (greater than 130°). Partial lateral dislocation of the femoral head out of the acetabular cavity is frequently found. Coxa valga is common with lesions that predispose to atrophy or disease of the structures contiguous to the hip such as chronic injuries to the lower extremities.

ANOMALIES OF THE EXTREMITIES

PATELLAR ANOMALIES

BIPARTITE, TRIPARTITE, AND MULTIPARTITE PATELLAE

Description. The patella is a sesamoid bone that normally develops from a single ossification center about the fifth or sixth year of life. Occasionally, this ossification center may be fragmented and may fail to unite osseously, although there is usually a fibrous bridge. The result is a mature patella made up of two or more separate pieces of bone. The most common presentation of this anomaly is a *bipartite patella*: two separate pieces of bone. Of these 80% are bilateral. (1) A *tripartite patella* has three pieces. More than three pieces is called a *multipartite* or *segmented patella*. These patellar anomalies affect 2 to 3% of the population with an equal sex incidence. (1) Although clinically insignificant, these anomalies must be differentiated from fractures.

It should be noted that there have been reports of pain associated with bipartite patellae. The pain appears to be the result of traumatic loosening of the fibrous connection and is localized to the area of the osseous defect, is exacerbated with activity, and does not abate with conservative treatment. The most effective treatment seems to be surgical excision of the accessory portion of the patella. (1–3)

Radiologic Features. Anteroposterior, lateral, and axial views of the knee are most helpful for diagnosing patellar anomalies and differentiating them from fractures. The ununited segment is usually in the *superolateral* aspect of the patella, although bone fragments have been demonstrated in various quadrants. (4) (Figs. 3.85, 3.86) Particular attention should be directed to the margins of the separated bone. The bone edges should be smooth,

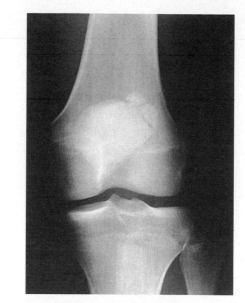

Figure 3.86. OSSIFICATION ABNORMALITIES OF THE PATELLA: TRIPARTITE PATELLA. AP Knee. (Courtesy of Kenneth E. Yochum, DC, St. Louis, Missouri)

rounded, and well corticated. Soft tissue swelling is unrelated to bipartite patellae.

FONG'S SYNDROME

Description. Also known as iliac horn syndrome and possibly associated with the nail-patella syndrome, hereditary onycho-osteo dysplasia, this hereditary syndrome is transmitted as an autosomal dominant. The patient demonstrates abnormalities of the nails of the hands and feet, renal dysplasia, and bone deformities. (1,2)

Radiologic Features. The patellae are hypoplastic and laterally placed. Exostoses from the posterior aspect of the ilia are noted (iliac horns). The articulations of the elbow are malformed. (For further discussion, see Chapter 8.)

TARSAL AND FOOT ANOMALIES

TARSAL COALITION (TARSAL BARS)

Description. Tarsal coalition consists of a fibrous union or a bony bar between two or more tarsal bones. Some coalitions are acquired posttraumatically or are the sequellae of inflammatory arthritic conditions. The majority of tarsal coalitions seen in clinical practice are present from birth. (1,2) Symptoms appear after the first decade. The majority of symptoms are secondary to biomechanically induced osteoarthritis. It affects 1 to 2% of the population. (3)

The patient may complain of pain, which may be severe, in the tarsal area. Limited subtalar or midtarsal joint motion, a rigid or semirigid flatfoot deformity, and prominence of the peroneal tendons may be noted. (4) Peroneal prominence may be present with or without spasm. (5) Tarsal coalition can be a cause of chronic inversion injuries to the ankle and should be looked for in patients with such histories, since it may be corrected surgically, reestablishing normal, subtalar-joint weight bearing.

Tarsal coalitions are known to be present in phocomelia, hemimelia, and other gross limb anomalies. (6) An extensive and au-

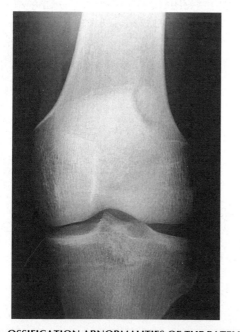

Figure 3.85   OSSIFICATION ABNORMALITIES OF THE PATELLA: BIPARTITE PATELLA. AP Knee. COMMENT: Bipartite and tripartite patellae almost always occur on the superolateral margin of the patella. They should not be confused with patellar fracture, since fractures usually occur through the waist of the patella. (Courtesy of Kenneth E. Yochum, DC, St. Louis, Missouri)

thoritative account of tarsal coalition by Jacobs et al. (3) should be consulted. A talar beak may be associated. (3)

Radiologic Features. The diagnosis of tarsal coalition can usually be made on plain film radiographs by performing dorsoplantar, lateral, and medial oblique views of the foot and an axial view of the calcaneus to visualize the subtalar joints. When an expected normal joint is obliterated by a bony bar that is continuous with the normally articulated adjacent bones, the diagnosis is certain. (Fig. 3.87A and B) The two most common sites for tarsal coalition are the talocalcaneal and calcaneonavicular articulations. (3) The demonstration of fusion of bones by syndesmoses, synchondroses, or synostoses may require tomography or CT evaluation.

VERTICAL TALUS

Description. Congenital vertical talus is a developmental anomaly consisting of primary dislocation of the talonavicular joint. The more vertical orientation of the talus appears to be the result of a short Achilles tendon. (1) The characteristic foot deformity is known as "rocker bottom" foot because of the rounded prominence on the medial plantar surface. It is often associated with spina bifida manifesta, myelomeningocele, and Down's syn-

drome. The sex ratio is equal, and it is bilateral in 50% of patients. (2)

Radiologic Features. On the dorsoplantar film a calcaneus valgus is present, along with metatarsus adductus. The lateral film will show plantar flexion of the calcaneus and an increased plantar inclination of the talus. (Fig. 3.88A and B) The navicular then articulates with the dorsal aspect of the talus. The altered plane of articulations for the talus predisposes these patients to development of degenerative joint disease later in life.

MORTON'S SYNDROME

Description. Morton's syndrome, named after Dudley Morton, (1) occurs in the presence of an abnormally short first metatarsal, and a second metatarsal that is unusually broad based. The patient complains of pain on activity at the plantar surface of the foot, in the vicinity of the second cuneiform-metatarsal joint. On observation a significant callus may be present under the second and third metatarsal heads. Morton suggested the term "*metatarsus atavicus,*" (1) but the condition is more commonly known as *Morton's foot or first ray insufficiency syndrome.*

Radiologic Features. A dorsoplantar view of the affected foot will reveal the first metatarsal bone to be significantly shorter than the second metatarsal. There is a varus deformity of the first

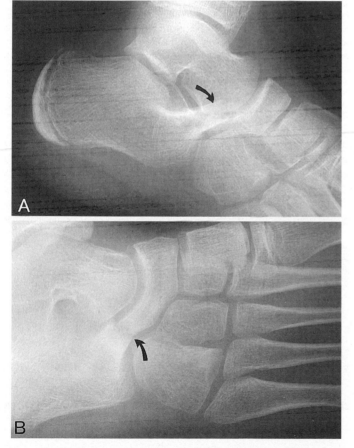

Figure 3.87.   TARSAL COALITION. A. Lateral Calcaneus. There is a large bony bar projecting from the anterior process of the calcaneus (arrow). **B. Oblique Foot**. An accessory articulation (arrow) has formed between the anterior calcaneal bar and the tarsal navicular. This coalition is fibrous in nature. COMMENT: Tarsal coalition often goes unrecognized and may be the underlying etiology in patients with chronic inversion injuries of the ankle.

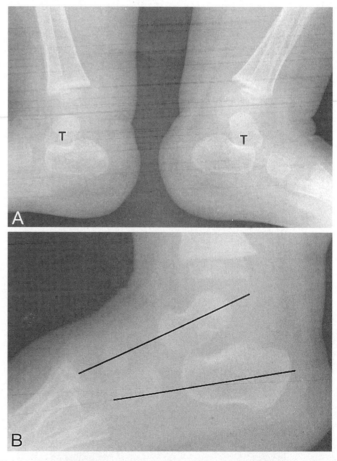

Figure 3.88.   VERTICAL TALUS. A. Bilateral Lateral Ankles. The talus (*T*) has assumed a vertical position bilaterally. (Courtesy of David M. Walker, DPM, Melbourne, Australia). **B. Coned Lateral Foot: Normal Axial Relationships**. The enhanced lines demonstrate the normal axial relationships of the talus with the remainder of the forefoot and the calcaneus with the talus.

metatarsal. Because of the increased biomechanical forces placed on the second metatarsal bone, its shaft and base will be increased in transverse diameter through periosteal bone deposition. The tibial and fibular sesamoids are proximally displaced. Stress fractures of the second and third metatarsals may complicate this condition. (2)

POLYDACTYLY

See discussion under "Finger Anomalies." (Fig. 3.89)

ELBOW ANOMALIES

SUPRACONDYLAR PROCESS OF THE HUMERUS

Description. A rudimentary exostosis of bone seen in man and lower animals may be present on the anteromedial aspect of the distal humeral metaphysis and is known as a supracondylar process. It can be differentiated from an osteochondroma by the fact that the supracondylar process grows toward the adjacent joint, whereas an osteochondroma grows away from the joint. It may occur in approximately 3% of the population and is slightly more common in Europe. (1) It has been variously called "supracondyloid," "supraepitrochlear," or "epicondylic process." (2)

The presence of a supracondylar process may have clinical significance in two instances: First, it is bone and is therefore subject to fracture. Second, it may compress the median nerve and the brachial, radial, or median arteries if they happen to travel in the course of the median nerve. (2) Rarely, compression of the median nerve may create a median nerve neuralgia; however, most remain asymptomatic. (2,3) Anatomically, a fibrous or fibroosseous ligament may extend from the end of the process to the medial epicondyle of the humerus and is known as Struther's ligament. (4)

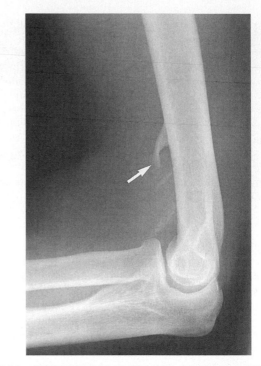

Figure 3.90.   SUPRACONDYLAR PROCESS: DISTAL HUMERUS. Lateral Elbow. A slender bony spur projects from the anterior distal diaphyseal surface of the humerus (arrow). The supracondylar process projects toward the joint, a helpful differential point from an osteochondroma, which projects away from the point. COMMENT: The supracondylar process is usually asymptomatic; however, it may be complicated with fracture or, if large, may compress the median nerve, creating a median nerve palsy.

Radiologic Features. Radiographically, a supracondylar process is composed of cortical and trabeculated bone, forming a beaklike bony spur at the anterior and medial portions of the distal humeral metaphysis. This excrescence of bone is angled toward the elbow joint and is usually not larger than 2 cm in length. (Fig. 3.90) It is not well seen on frontal radiographs but is clearly defined in lateral or oblique projections.

MEDICOLEGAL IMPLICATIONS
Supracondylar Process of the Humerus

- Possible fracture
- Median nerve compression
- Supracondylar process of the humerus may also be found in patients with the rare disease Cornelia de Lange syndrome. (5)

RADIOULNAR SYNOSTOSIS

Description. When there is a failure of longitudinal segmentation of the proximal radius and ulna, a bone fusion results. This defect is transmitted as an autosomal dominant, with an equal sex incidence. It may be seen unilaterally, but 80% of the time it is bilateral. (1) The length of the fusion may extend from 3 to 6 cm and may be osseous or fibrous. From a clinical standpoint,

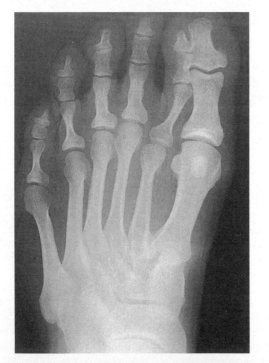

Figure 3.89.   POLYSYNDACTYLY: FOOT. DP Foot. Duplication and hypoplasia of the second ray with soft tissue fusion to the great toe is noted. (Courtesy of Bryan Hartley, MD, Melbourne, Australia)

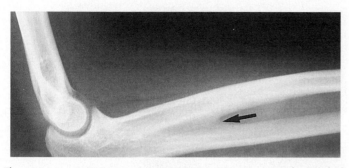

Figure 3.91. RADIOULNAR SYNOSTOSIS: ELBOW. Coned Lateral Elbow. There is congenital fusion of the proximal interosseous space between the radius and ulna (arrow). This usually occurs as an isolated congenital anomaly.

pronation and supination may be limited to nonexistent, depending on the degree and type of fusion. The defect may be diagnosed at birth, but diagnosis is delayed in most instances until childhood. Surgery may result in a more normal position for hand function. (2) Associated conditions include congenital dislocated hip, clubfoot, Madelung's deformity, and syndactyly or polydactyly. (3)

Radiologic Features.   This diagnosis can be made on anteroposterior and lateral views of the elbow. These will demonstrate bone in the area between the proximal radius and ulna, usually occupied by the interosseous membrane for a distance of up to 6 cm. (Fig. 3.91)

WRIST ANOMALIES
MADELUNG'S DEFORMITY

Introduction.   This entity was first defined in 1878 by a German surgeon, Madelung (1), who described a young woman with a deformity of her wrist. He also reported that this deformity had been described as early as 1834, but it is his name that has persisted as the eponym of this congenital anomaly. It now seems that Madelung's deformity of the wrist may exist alone or as part of a more generalized condition known as dyschondrosteosis.

Description.   The problem is passed on as an autosomal dominant trait and is usually more manifest in females. The deformity is twice as common in bilateral form. The diagnosis is usually made in early adolescence, during periods of rapid growth, when associated wrist pain develops. This pain will usually subside after the growth period; therefore observation of the patient is recommended until closure of the growth plate before any operation is considered. (2,3)

The fundamental abnormality is retarded growth of the medial portion of the distal radial epiphysis, resulting in asymmetric growth. This results in ulnar deviation of the hand and a dorsal prominence of the ulnar styloid process caused by posterior subluxation of the distal ulna. Manual reduction of the subluxation may be attempted, but is only a temporary measure. The physical appearance of the resulting wrist deformity has been called the "*bayonette*" appearance. (4)

Radiologic Features.   On a posterior to anterior film of the wrist the x-ray appearance shows a triangular shape to the distal radial epiphysis, with retarded growth of its medial aspect, resulting in an ulnar slant to the distal radial articulating surface. The radius is shortened, and a lucent defect is noted along its medial metaphysis. The distal radioulnar joint is widened. The carpal angle is decreased (less than 117°). A lateral film usually

shows a volar tilt of the distal radial articular surface greater than the normal 5° and dorsal subluxation of the ulna. The carpal alignment is altered to accommodate the radial changes, with the lunate being at the proximal apex of the carpal deformity. (Fig. 3.92A and B)

NEGATIVE ULNAR VARIANCE

Description.   This is a condition where the ulna is unusually shorter than the distal radial articular surface. (Fig. 3.93A) It is also known as the ulnar minus variant. It has also been shown that the triangular fibrocartilage complex at the distal ulna is thicker in patients with negative ulnar variance. (1)

Ulnar variance changes with wrist and forearm position. Supination increases the measurement of negative ulnar variance, and pronation decreases the measurement of negative ulnar variance. Wrist deviation and alterations of the x-ray beam in the longitudinal plane also influence this measurement. Standardized wrist positioning has been advocated to allow accurate and reproducible measurements of ulnar variance. (2)

In 1928 Hulten indicated that this developmental anomaly created an increased potential for Kienböck's disease, an avascular necrosis of the carpal lunate. (3) (See Chapter 13.) (Fig. 3.93B) However, there is controversy over this association. (4–9)

Posttraumatic Scapholunate Dissociations.   The results showed a significantly greater amount of negative ulnar variance in patients with scapholunate dissociations than in normal controls. Again, there is controversy over this association. (10–13)

Treatment.   The association of a negative ulnar variance in patients with Kienböck's disease provides the rationale for a radial shortening osteotomy. This osteotomy, to realign the radiocarpal joint and shorten the radius, attempts to lessen the presumed increased compressive forces on the lunate. By "unloading" the lunate through this procedure, the possibility for revascularization exists. (14) Radial shortening has been shown to be an effective treatment for Kienböck's disease in wrists that do not have degenerative changes in adjacent carpal joints. (15)

CARPAL COALITION

Description.   Carpal coalition is the fusion of two or more carpal bones. It may occur as an isolated anomaly or as part of more widespread anomalous developments. The cause of congenital fusion of the carpal bones is lack of segmentation and cavitation in the cartilage template for the affected bones. Carpal coalition is twice as common in females and slightly more common in blacks. (1) Bridging between the lunate and triquetral bones is the most common fusion in the wrist. (2) Some of the associated conditions include Madelung's deformity, Holt-Oram syndrome, Turner's syndrome, and Ellis-van Creveld syndrome. (1,2) Generally, isolated fusions affect the bones in one row of the wrist, (1) whereas fusions that cross from one row to the other tend to be associated with congenital syndromes. (2) The greatest clinical risk associated with carpal coalition is fracture.

Radiologic Features.   Because of the incomplete fusion in some examples, plain film demonstration of the osseous bridge may be difficult and require multiple views of the affected wrist. The diagnosis can be made when continuity of cortical and trabecular bone between adjacent carpal bones is demonstrated. (Figs. 3.94, 3.95) Diagnosis will be delayed until ossification is radiographically evident. Fusions secondary to acquired disease, such as psoriatic arthritis, rheumatoid arthritis, or septic arthritis, may be differentiated through historical and clinical data.

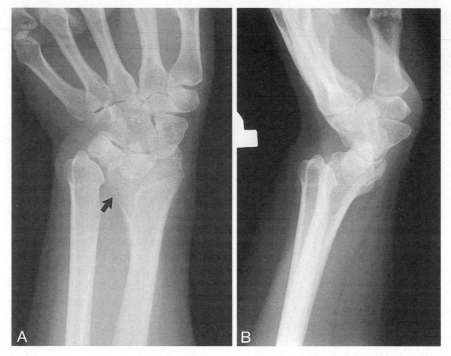

Figure 3.92.   MADELUNG'S DEFORMITY: WRIST. A. PA Wrist. Premature closure of the medial portion of the distal radial physis (growth plate) has created an ulnar slant to the distal articulating surface of the radius. A characteristic "V"-shaped deformity is present on the ulnar side of the distal radius (arrow). There is a widening of the radioulnar articulation and disorientation of the radiocarpal articulation. This has created a decreased carpal angle. **B. Lateral Wrist**. There is characteristic posterior subluxation in the ulna, which has been referred to in Madelung's deformity as the "bayonette" appearance.

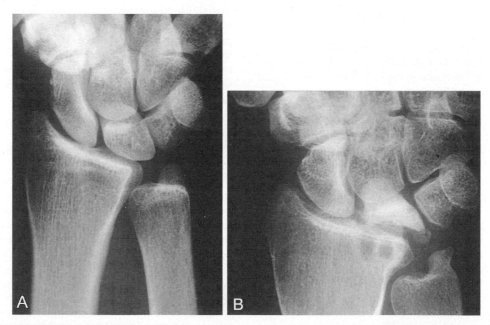

Figure 3.93.   NEGATIVE ULNAR VARIANCE: WRIST. A. PA Wrist. Notice that the distal end of the ulna is shorter than the distal articulating surface of the radius. **B. PA Wrist.** Another patient also has negative ulnar variance and an advanced stage of avascular necrosis of the lunate (Kienböck's disease). The long-standing collapsed lunate has resulted in mild narrowing of the radiocarpal joint and degenerative subchondral cysts in the subarticular radius.

FINGER ANOMALIES

POLYDACTYLY

Description.   Polydactyly is an increased number of fingers or toes. There is a predominance for this condition in black patients. The significance of polydactyly depends on whether the extra digit is on the radial (preaxial) or ulnar (postaxial) side of the hand. Preaxial polydactyly is seen in Apert's syndrome, Fanconi's syndrome, and Holt-Oram syndrome. Postaxial polydac-

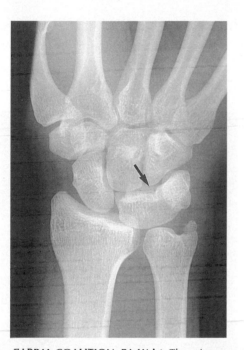

Figure 3.94.   CARPAL COALITION. PA Wrist. There is congenital synostosis affecting the lunate and triquetrum. The arrow indicates where the normal articulation should have occurred. Of incidental notation is nonunion of the ulnar styloid tip.

tyly is associated with Ellis-van Creveld syndrome and Laurence-Moon-Biedl syndrome. (1)

Radiologic Features.   The diagnosis of polydactyly is evident clinically. The role of x-ray is to determine the nature of osseous development within the extra finger, as well as any additional bony maldevelopment associated with coexisting syndromes.

SYNDACTYLY

Description.   Syndactyly is the most common developmental anomaly of the hand, but it may also affect the foot and is manifest in the form of fusion of the skin between the digits (syndactyly) or fusion of the osseous phalanges of adjacent digits (synostosis). The incidence is thought to be one in 2500 births, (1) with a distinct male predominance, (2) and is more common in whites than blacks in a 10:1 ratio. (3) It may be considered partial when the fusion involves the proximal segments, or complete if the fusion extends to the distal aspect. If the fusion is distal, with the proximal segments free, the appropriate name is acrosyndactyly. It is not a bone or cartilage disease but a defect of mesenchymal organization during the fifth fetal week, resulting in failure of an interphalangeal joint to develop. (4)

Five types of syndactyly have been described: (a) zygodactyly (most common type), involving the third and fourth fingers and/or the second and third toes; (b) synpolydactyly of the third and fourth fingers, with partial or complete reduplication of fingers three and four in the web (or may be toes four and five); (c) ring and little finger syndactyly, where the middle phalanx of the fifth finger is rudimentary or absent; (d) complete syndactyly, involving all fingers; and (e) syndactyly associated with metacarpal and/or metatarsal synostosis. (5) It more commonly affects the medial side of the hand. (6)

Syndactyly may be associated with other syndromes, including Poland, Apert, Saethre, and Pfeiffer syndromes. (5)

Radiologic Features.   X-ray examination of the affected extremity will show soft tissue fusion between the fingers or toes and any osseous anomalies of development. In some instances fusion of the phalanges of the same finger or toe may be present; in other cases fusion of the phalanges between adjacent digits may be noted. (Fig. 3.96)

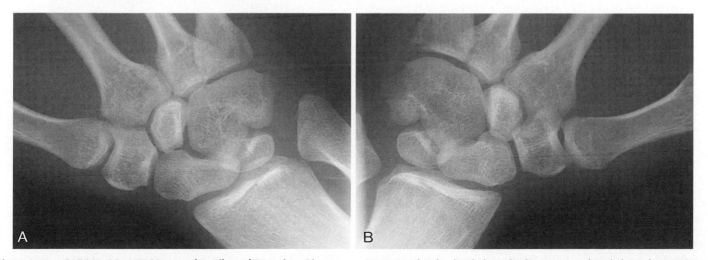

A

B

Figure 3.95.   CARPAL COALITION. A and B. Bilateral PA wrists. Observe the union of the pisiform, capitate, and hamate in this patient who also has only four fingers on each hand. It appears the triquetra are agenetic. It is also interesting that the distal ulnae display an unusual medial angulation. (Courtesy of James R. Brandt, DC, FACO, Coon Rapids, Minnesota)

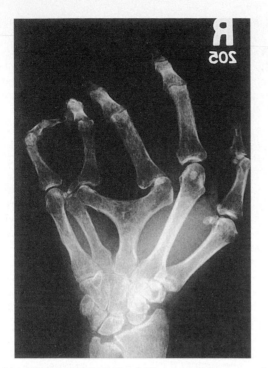

Figure 3.96.   SYNDACTYLY. PA Hand. Observe the bifurcation of the third metacarpal. Note that there are still only 5 digits because of the hypoplasia of the fourth ray phalanges. (Courtesy of John Chomyn, MD, Denver, Colorado)

KIRNER'S DEFORMITY

Description.   Kirner's deformity, a type of curvature of the fifth finger, is also known as dystelephalangy. (1) It occurs sporadically or is transmitted as an autosomal dominant trait. This abnormality usually affects the fifth fingers bilaterally. (2) Physical examination will show a palmar curvature of the distal phalanx in a patient beyond 5 years of age. Before this age, the deformity is usually unnoticeable. Soft tissue swelling may precede the bone deformity. (3)

Radiologic Features.   Radiographically, there is volar curvature of the fifth digits, with separation (widening) of the growth plate and deformity of the epiphysis. There is no apparent clinical significance of this deformity.

AN ATLAS OF NORMAL SKELETAL VARIANTS

INTRODUCTION

To properly interpret skeletal radiographs, a thorough understanding of normal radiographic anatomy and its skeletal variations is essential. Often, the skeletal variations from normal may simulate various disease processes. The authors therefore offer the following pictorial atlas of *"skeletal variants"* to familiarize the reader with the more common variations from normal.

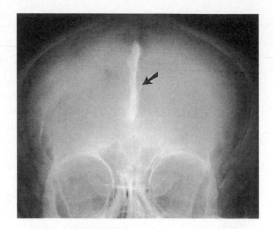

Figure 3.97.   FALX CALCIFICATION. There is calcification of the falx cerebri (arrow), which is of no clinical significance.

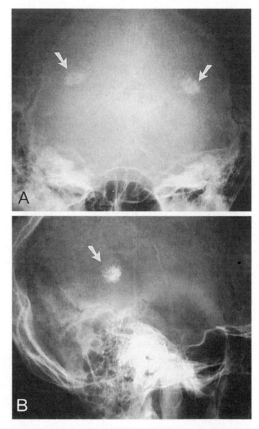

Figure 3.98.   CHOROID PLEXUS CALCIFICATION. A and B. There are calcifications noted in the choroid plexuses (arrows), which are of no clinical significance.

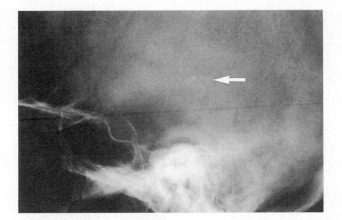

Figure 3.99. PINEAL GLAND CALCIFICATION. There Is calcification present within the pineal gland (arrow), which is of no clinical significance. (Courtesy of Kenneth E. Yochum, DC, St. Louis, Missouri)

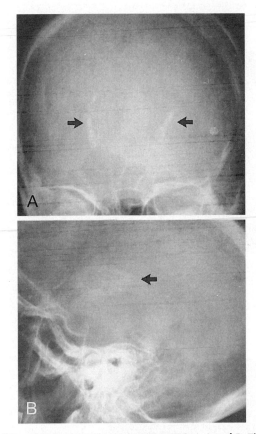

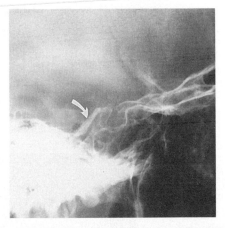

Figure 3.100. BASAL GANGLIA CALCIFICATION. A and B. There is calcification noted within the basal ganglia (arrows). COMMENT: Calcification of the basal ganglia may occur as a normal variant or can be associated with pseudohypoparathyroidism and pseudopseudohypoparathyroidism.

Figure 3.101. PETROCLINOID LIGAMENT CALCIFICATION. Calcification of the petroclinoid ligament is present (arrow), which is a normal variant.

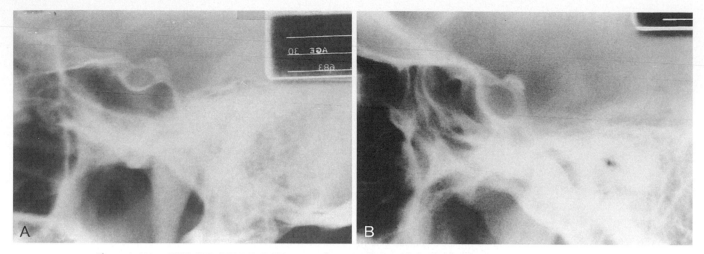

Figure 3.102. BRIDGED SELLA TURCICA. A and B. Coned Lateral Skull. Note the thin osseous "bridge" covering the superior portion of the sella turcica. (**B** Courtesy of James M. Kolodziej, DC, Denver, Colorado)

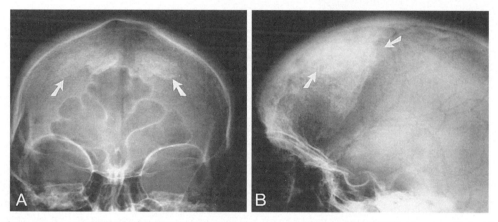

Figure 3.103. HYPEROSTOSIS FRONTALIS INTERNA. A and B (arrows). COMMENT: Hyperostosis in this area must be differentiated from meningioma.

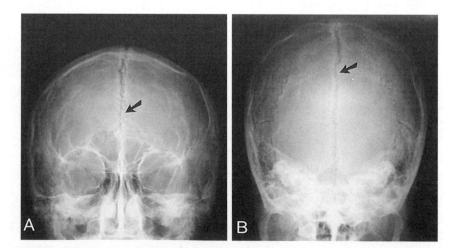

Figure 3.104. PERSISTANT METOPIC SUTURE. A and B. There is persistence of the metopic suture (arrows). COMMENT: This suture may persist throughout life and be mistaken for a fracture. It is also found associated with cleidocranial dysplasia.

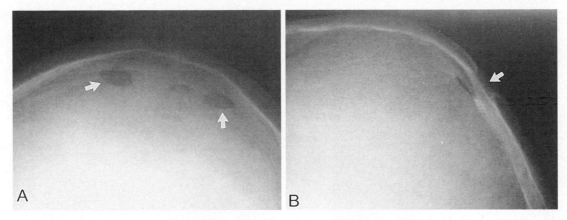

Figure 3.105.   PARIETAL FORAMINA. A and B. Observe the parietal foramina, which serve as a conduit for the emissary veins of Santorini (arrows).

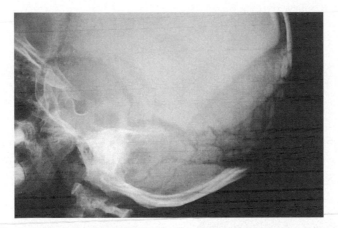

Figure 3.106.   WORMIAN BONES. There are multiple wormian bones present at the lambdoidal suture. COMMENT: Wormian bones represent isolated intrasutural bones occurring along the course of the cranial sutures. They may be seen as a normal variant or can occur with cleidocranial dysplasia, osteogenesis imperfecta, and other congenital anomalies. (Courtesy of C.H. Quay, MD, Melbourne, Australia)

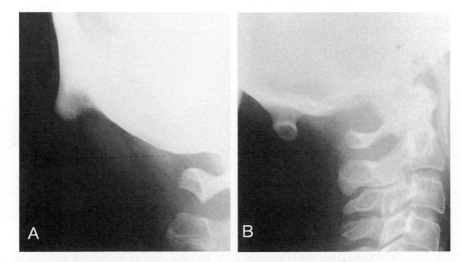

Figure 3.107.   PROMINENT EXTERNAL OCCIPITAL PROTUBERANCE. A and B. There is a prominent external occipital protuberance, which is considered a variation of normal.

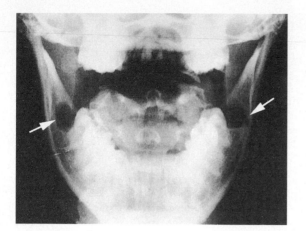

Figure 3.108.   BILATERAL RADIOLUCENCIES FROM WISDOM TOOTH EXTRACTIONS. AP Open Mouth. This patient had wisdom teeth removed a short time prior to this radiograph being taken (arrows). The smooth margin and short zone of transition should suggest a benign process and not an aggressive infectious or neoplastic lesion. (Courtesy of Leslie Pepper, DC, Denver, Colorado)

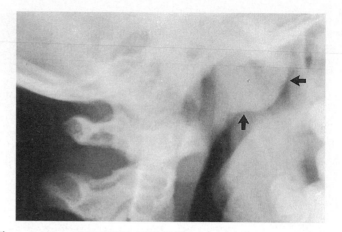

Figure 3.109.   ADENOIDAL TISSUE. There is an indentation on the posterior surface of the nasopharyngeal air space from slight enlargement of adenoidal tissue (arrows).

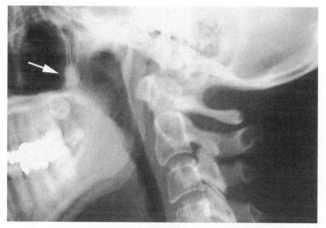

Figure 3.110.   PSEUDOTUMOR: NASAL CAVITY. Coned Neutral Lateral Cervical. A rounded soft tissue density (arrow) is superimposed on the dorsal wall of the maxillary sinus and represents the normal inferior turbinates and the superimposed mandibular coronoid processes. This finding should not be confused with an intranasal neoplasm or maxillary polyp. (Courtesy of Ronald D. Myhra, DC, Denver, Colorado) (From Sistrom CL, Keats TE, Johnson CM: *The anatomic basis of the pseudotumor of the nasal cavity.* AJR 147:782, 1986.)

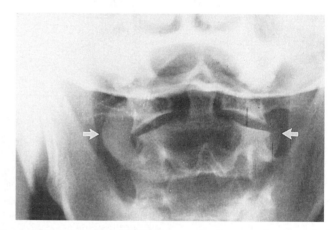

Figure 3.111.   TONGUE. The radiopaque density seen adjacent to the lateral mass and articular pillars of C2 (arrows) represents the water density of the tongue and not an ossific or calcific abnormality.

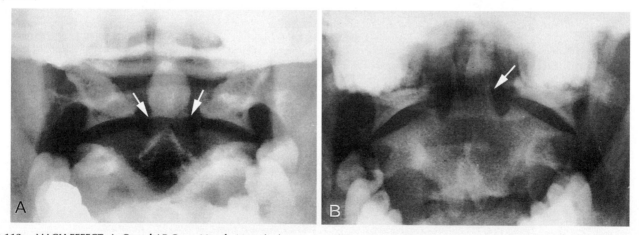

Figure 3.112.   MACH EFFECT. A. Coned AP Open Mouth. Note the lucent pseudofracture (arrows) created at the base of the dens by a Mach effect. This simulates a type II odontoid fracture, but is differentiated by following the arc of the posterior arch of the atlas and seeing where it crosses the odontoid. **B. Coned AP Open Mouth**. Again note where the posterior arch of the atlas overlies the base of the dens (arrow). Also observe the bilateral paraodontoid notches that are a normal variant (see also Fig. 3.174). COMMENT: A Mach effect is created whenever two osseous densities overlie one another. It is a lucent line at their junction that is a physiologic optical illusion.

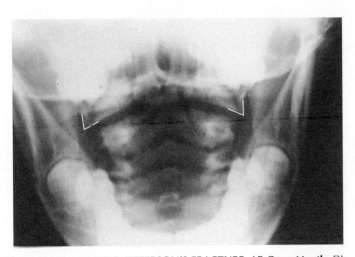

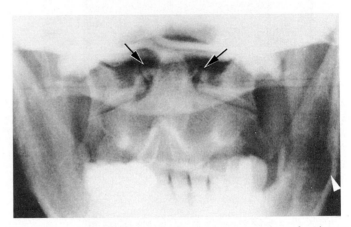

Figure 3.113.   PSEUDO-JEFFERSON'S FRACTURE. AP Open Mouth. Observe the overhanging edges of the C1 lateral masses (artist-enhanced lines) bilaterally in this 10-year-old male. COMMENT: In an adult this finding would suggest a Jefferson's fracture; however, in a child, this represents the differential ossification rate between C1 and C2. (Courtesy of Appa L. Anderson, DC, DACBR, Fellow, ACCR, Portland, Oregon)

Figure 3.114.   VIKING HELMET SIGN. Coned AP Open Mouth. Observe the "horns" (arrows) protruding from the sides of the dens. This is a rare morphological variation of the dens. Also seen in the right lower jaw is a lucent area left by a recent tooth extraction (arrowhead). (Courtesy of William E. Litterer, DC, DACBR, Fellow, ACCR, Elizabeth, New Jersey)

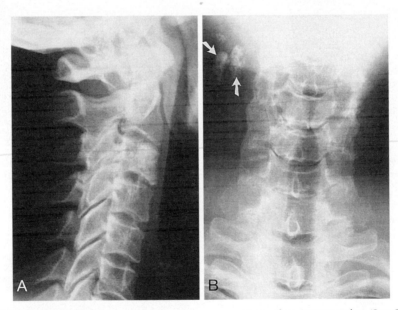

Figure 3.115.   CALCIFIED CERVICAL LYMPH NODES. A and B. Calcification of the cervical lymph nodes (arrows) are noted lateral to the cervical spine. COMMENT: The superimposition of the calcified cervical lymph nodes over the cervical vertebrae on the lateral projection may mimic the appearance of an ivory vertebra (See C-3). This emphasizes the point of having two views at 90° to each other as a minimum radiologic investigation. (Courtesy of Allan J. Warrener, DC, Melbourne, Australia)

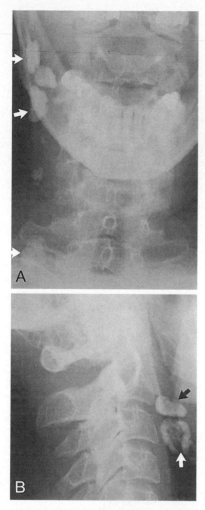

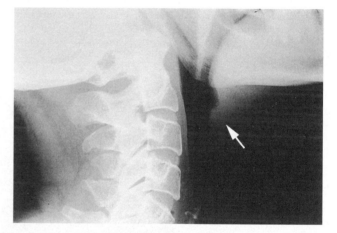

Figure 3.116.   CALCIFIED CERVICAL LYMPH NODES. A and B. There is unilateral calcification of the cervical chain of lymph nodes (arrows). COMMENT: Calcifications of this degree frequently follow prior inflammatory disease of the lymph nodes, but are otherwise of no clinical significance.

Figure 3.117.   SUBLINGUAL THYROID. Coned Neutral Lateral Cervical. Note the rounded, soft tissue mass at the base of the tongue (arrow) that represents ectopic thyroid tissue that failed to descend into its normal position. (Courtesy of Michael A. Fox, MD, Memphis, Tennessee)

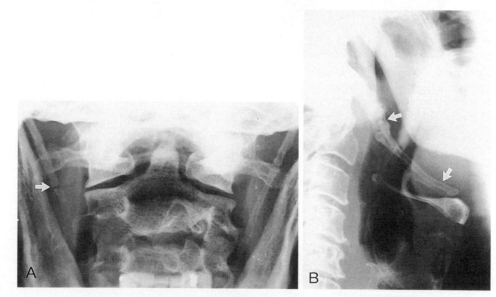

Figure 3.118.   CALCIFIED STYLOHYOID LIGAMENT. A and B. There is bilateral calcification of the stylohyoideus ligament (arrows).

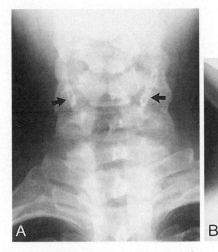

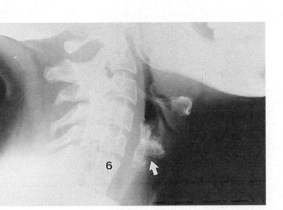

Figure 3.119.   THYROID CARTILAGE CALCIFICATION. A and B. Calcification of the wings of the thyroid cartilage simulates vertebral artery calcification (arrows). Note the oblique orientation is wrong for vertebral artery calcification (which is very rare and seldom seen on x-rays). There is a congenital block vertebra present between C6 and C7.

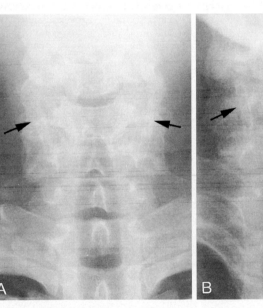

Figure 3.120.   THYROID CARTILAGE CALCIFICATION. A. AP Lower Cervical. Note the bilateral calcifications (arrows) of the wings of the thyroid cartilage at the levels of C5-C6-C7. **B. AP Lower Cervical.** Note the bilaterally calcified thyroid cartilage (arrows) extending obliquely from C6, cephalad. COMMENT: This calcification is commonly mistaken for atherosclerosis in the vertebral artery. Recall that the vertebral artery passes through the transversarium foramen and would run vertically.

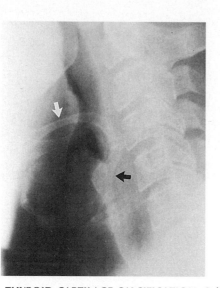

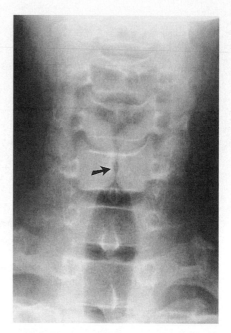

Figure 3.121.   THYROID CARTILAGE CALCIFICATION. Calcification of the superior cornua of the thyroid cartilage is noted (arrows).

Figure 3.122.   LARYNGEAL SHADOW. The thin area of radiolucency superimposed on the C6 vertebral body represents the contracted larynx (arrow). This should not be confused with a spina bifida occulta or a vertical fracture line.

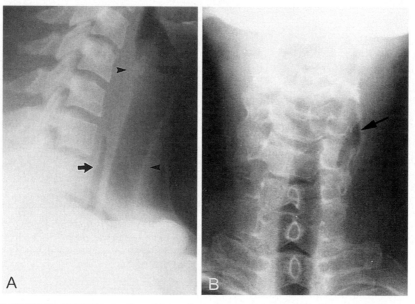

Figure 3.123.   AIR-TRAPPED IN CERVICAL REGION. A. Coned Lateral Cervical. Observe the air present in the esophagus (arrow). The normal air density of the pharynx and trachea are identified (arrowheads). **B. Coned AP** **Lower Cervical.** Note the air trapped in the vallecula of the larynx adjacent to C4-C5 (arrow). (**B** Courtesy of Michael J. Nehring, DC, Boulder, Colorado)

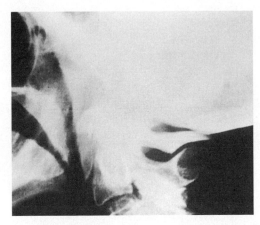

Figure 3.124.   C1 POSTERIOR ARCH DEFORMITY. Observe the peculiar knifelike configuration to the posterior arch and tubercle of the atlas.

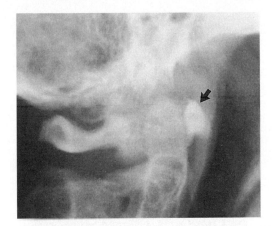

Figure 3.126.   SCLEROTIC ANTERIOR TUBERCLE. The area of increased density in the anterior tubercle of the atlas is considered a variation of normal (arrow). COMMENT: If the anterior tubercle of the atlas appears radiopaque and enlarged, it signifies compensatory stress hypertrophy. The lack of enlargement signifies a variation of normal.

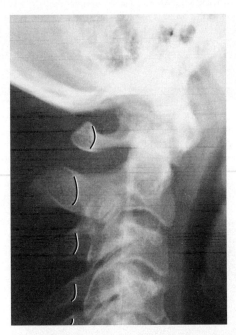

Figure 3.125.   SHORT POSTERIOR ARCH OF C1. Coned Lateral Cervical. Note the break in the spinolaminar line (posterior cervical line) with the anteriorly placed C1 spinolaminar line. This was asymptomatic in this patient but, if it doesn't measure 16 mm in the sagittal dimension, stenosis may be present. COMMENT: A reduced sagittal diameter of the C1 spinal canal could be due to subluxation secondary to rheumatoid arthritis or ankylosing spondylitis. However, there would be an increased atlantodental interspace not present in this case. (Courtesy of Ron D. Myhra, DC, Denver, Colorado)

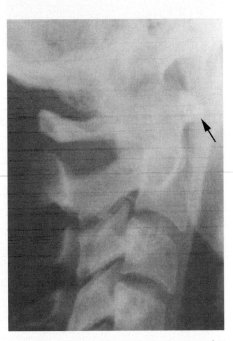

Figure 3.127.   SMALL ANTERIOR TUBERCLE: C1. Coned Neutral Lateral Cervical. Note how small the anterior tubercle of the atlas is (arrow). This is a normal variant.

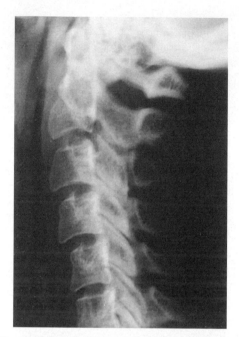

Figure 3.128.   LARGE POSTERIOR TUBERCLE: C1. Coned Neutral Lateral Cervical. Observe the large posterior tubercle at C1. This anomalous size of the posterior tubercle facilitates the articulation with the C2 spinous process. (Courtesy of Dennis P. Nikitow, DC, Denver, Colorado)

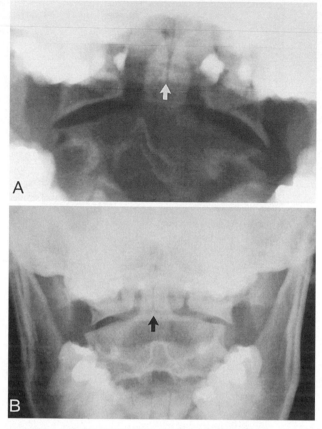

Figure 3.130.   CENTRAL INCISOR GAP. A and B. Observe the vertical radiolucent line that appears to split the odontoid process (arrows). This represents the space between the central incisors. COMMENT: This may appear to simulate a vertical fracture of the odontoid process; however, these have not been reported.

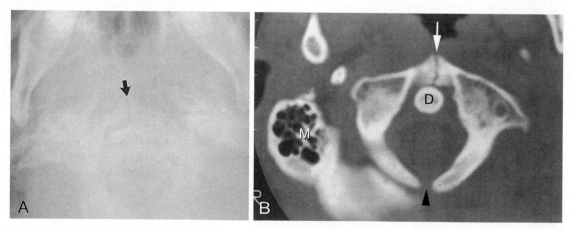

Figure 3.129.   ANTERIOR C1 SPONDYLOSCHISIS. A. Coned Base Vertex. There is a cleft in the anterior arch of the atlas (arrow). **B. Computed Axial Tomography**. Note the failure of fusion of both the anterior (arrow) and posterior arch (arrowhead) of the atlas. Also identified in this study are the dens (*D*) and mastoid air cells (*M*). (Courtesy of William E. Litterer, DC, DACBR, Fellow, ACCR, Elizabeth, New Jersey)

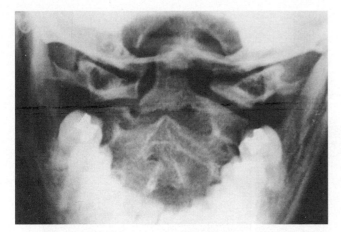

Figure 3.131.   ODONTOID PROCESS CLEFT. Odontoid View. A congenital horizontal cleft at the base of the odontoid process creates a pseudofracture appearance (arrow). Incidentally, note the Mach effect created by the base of the occiput overlying the dens. This is commonly mistaken for a fracture. (Courtesy of Bruce Kniegge, DC, Honduras)

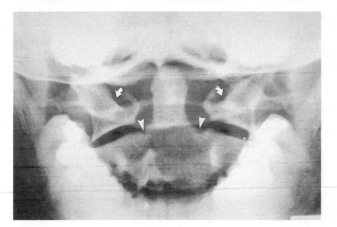

Figure 3.132.   NORMAL C1 SUPERIOR ARTICULATING SURFACES. Observe the symmetric normal, radiolucent appearance of the concave medial surfaces of the lateral masses of the atlas (arrows). Observe also the normal paraodontoid notches (arrowheads) near the base of the odontoid process.

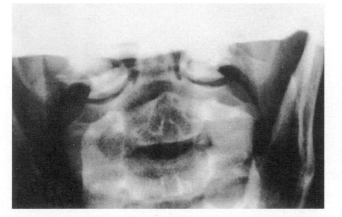

Figure 3.133.   ATLANTOAXIAL ARTICULATION: NORMAL VARIANT. Coned AP Open Mouth. Note the "ball-and-socket" articular variant at the atlantoaxial junction bilaterally. The normal atlantoaxial articulations are more flattened than in this anomalous example. Also note the paraodontoid notches (see also Fig. 3.132) and the Mach effect creating a lucent pseudolesion across the base of the dens. (Courtesy of Tyrone Wei, DC, DACBR, Portland, Oregon)

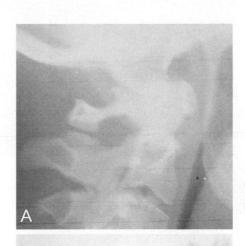
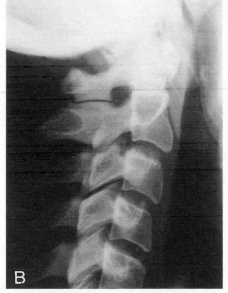

Figure 3.134.   C1-C2 ACCESSORY JOINT. A and B. Coned Lateral Cervicals. These are two examples of accessory joints noted at the inferior aspect of the posterior tubercle/posterior arch of the atlas and the superior surface of the lamina of the axis. This anomaly effectively limits flexion and extension at C1-C2. (Courtesy of John C. Slizeski, DC, Denver, Colorado)

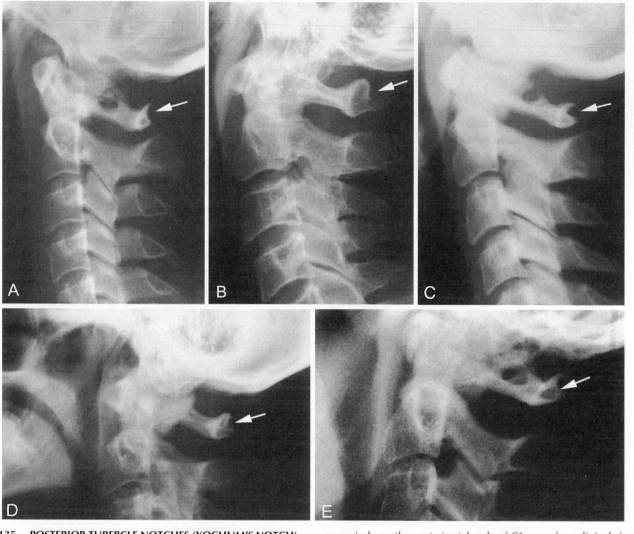

Figure 3.135.   POSTERIOR TUBERCLE NOTCHES (YOCHUM'S NOTCH). A–E. Coned Lateral Cervicals. These developmental notches, seen poster- osuperiorly on the posterior tubercle of C1, are of no clinical significance (arrows).

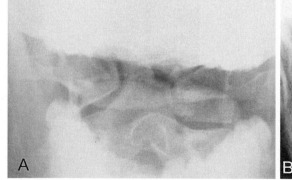

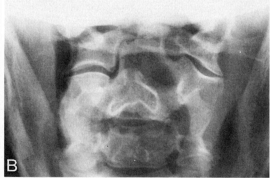

Figure 3.136.   PERSISTENT INFANTILE ODONTOID PROCESS. A and B. These are two examples of anomalous development of the base of the odontoid process and a right angle formation of the lateral mass of C1 and the superior facet of the axis on one side. (Courtesy of Donald E. Freuden, DC, FACO, Denver, Colorado) (From McClellan R, El Gammal T, Willing S, et al: *Persistent infantile odontoid process: A variant of abnormal atlantoaxial segmentation*. AJR; 158:1305, 1992)

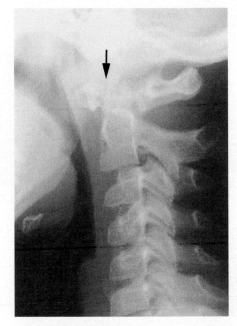

Figure 3.137. "V"-SHAPED ATLANTODENTAL INTERSPACE. Coned Neutral Lateral Cervical. Observe how the normal ADI in children (arrow) can appear shaped as the letter "V." This 10-year-old boy had neck trauma justifying this radiograph. The maximum ADI in children is 5 mm, just larger than the 3 mm normally allowed in adults. This measurement should be obtained halfway from the top to the bottom of the articulation.

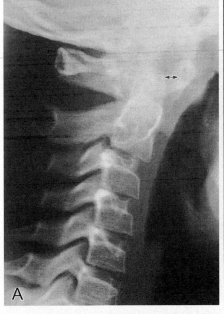

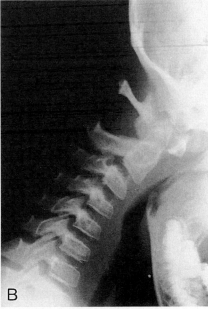

Figure 3.138.   PSEUDOSUBLUXATION OF C2. A. Coned Neutral Lateral Cervical. There is a pseudosubluxation of C2 upon C3 as a result of hypermobility in this area in children, that is frequently misinterpreted as a pathologic instability. Note the trapezoid appearance of the cervical vertebral bodies, which is normal in a child of this age (10 years old). Observe the normal appearance of the atlantodental interspace (ADI) (double-headed arrow). This measured 5 mm, representing the upper limit of normal in a pediatric patient. **B. Flexion Lateral Cervical.** Another child demonstrating pseudosubluxation of C2 on C3. Also note the unusual but normal gapping between the neural arches of C1 and C2 that in an adult would represent a grade 2 ligamentous sprain. In the pediatric patient this is within normal limits. This range of motion at C1-C2 has created a "V"-shaped atlantodental interspace. (**B** Courtesy of Donald E. Freuden, DC, FACO, Denver, Colorado)

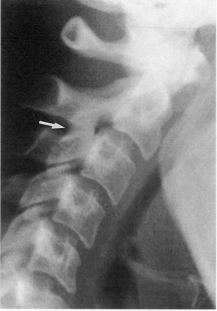

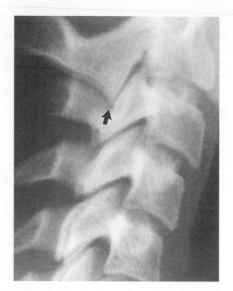

Figure 3.139.   NORMAL C2-C3 FACET JOINTS. There is an apparent an-kylosis of the C2-C3 zygapophyseal joints demonstrated on this flexion lat-eral radiograph (arrow). This is a pseudofusion, since the zygapophyseal joint spaces at C2-C3 are seldom seen clearly on the neutral lateral cervical spine because of their oblique anatomic orientation.

Figure 3.140.   FACET NOTCH. Observe the normal notching of the apoph-yseal joint surface of the C3 vertebra (arrow). This should not be mistaken for erosion or fracture.

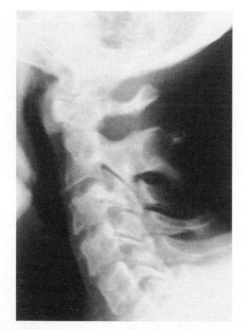

Figure 3.141.   FORKED SPINOUS PROCESS: C2. Although C2 is an atyp-ical cervical vertebra, the spinous process can bifurcate. This bifurcation is typically in transverse orientation, while in this normal variant it is a pre-dominantly sagittal bifurcation. (Courtesy of George E. Springer, DC, Clear-water, Florida)

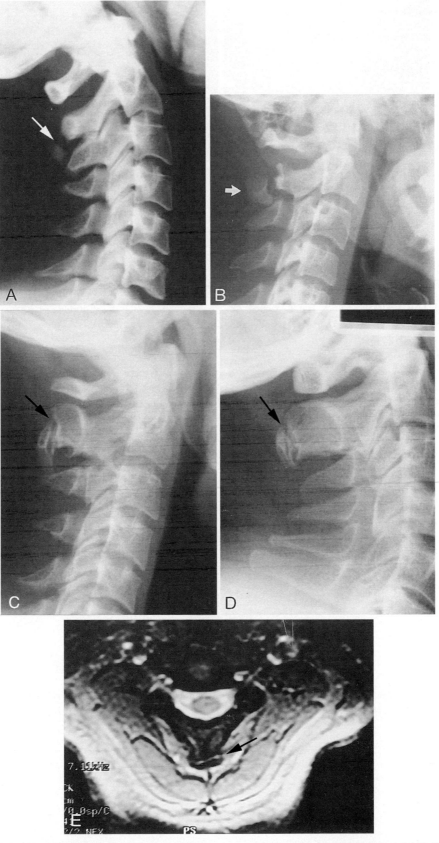

Figure 3.142.   NONUNION OF SPINOUS PROCESS: C2. A, B, C, and D. Coned Lateral Cervicals. There is nonunion of the spinous process (arrows) to the lamina of C2 in all images. When a fracture occurs at the tip of a spinous process, the fracture fragment displaces caudally. This and the sclerotic margins help differentiate this anomaly from a recent fracture. **C** was initially called a fracture avulsion because of the apparent caudal displacement of the "avulsed" fragment. **E. Axial T2-Weighted MRI**. This is an axial slice through the C2 spinous process shown in **D**. The gap in the spinous process (arrow) is noted and there is no edema as there would be with an acute avulsion fracture. It was then determined that **D** was also nonunion of the growth center. (**C** Courtesy of Ralph E. Brewer, DC, Denver, Colorado)

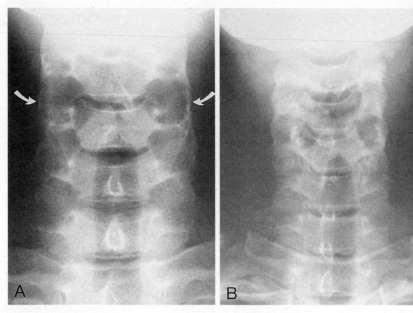

Figure 3.143.   CERVICAL PSEUDOLESIONS: C5. A and B. Coned AP Lower Cervicals. Notice the paired radiolucencies (arrows) which are a normal variant. **B**. (Courtesy of Richard N. Garian, DC, Holliston, Massachusetts)

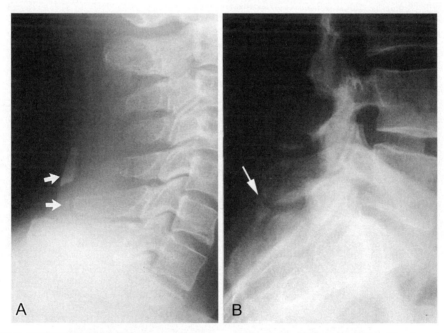

Figure 3.144.   SUPRASPINOUS LIGAMENT OSSIFICATION. A. Lateral Cervical. Note the calcification in the ligamentum nuchae, creating "nuchal bones" (arrows). **B. Coned Lateral Lumbar**. Accessory ossification within the supraspinous ligament at L5-S1 (arrow).

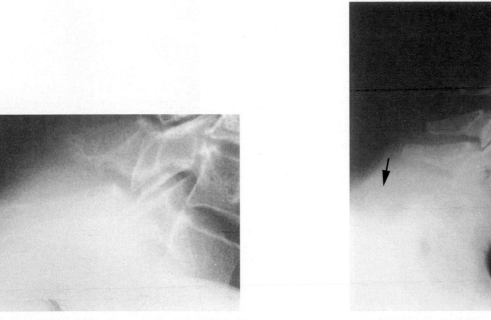

Figure 3.145. NONUNION: SECONDARY GROWTH CENTER. Lateral Cervicodorsal Spot. Nonunion of the secondary growth center for the spinous process is present at C7 (arrow). COMMENT: This must be differentiated from a "clay shoveler's" avulsion fracture. This is accomplished by the demonstration of the sclerotic margins between the bony segments and the lack of caudal displacement of the distal portion of the spinous process, which is usually present in avulsion fractures.

Figure 3.146. BENT SPINOUS PROCESS: T1. Coned Neutral Lateral Cervical. Observe the caudal angulation displayed by the dorsal half of the spinous process of T1 (arrow). This deformity is more closely associated with midthoracic spinous processes instead of transitional vertebrae. This patient reported no history of trauma.

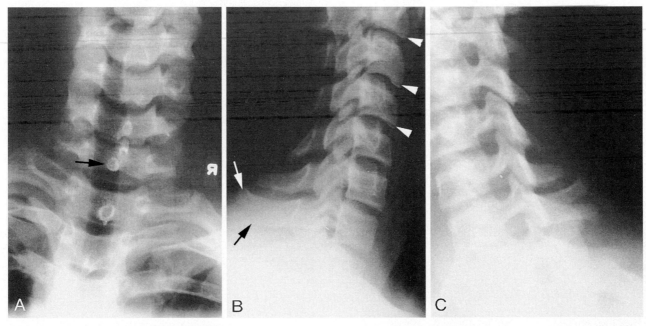

Figure 3.147. CONGENITAL BIFID SPINOUS PROCESS: C7. A. Coned AP Lower Cervical. This radiograph was taken of a 14-year-old boy because of cervical trauma, and a cervical spinal fracture was considered in the differential diagnosis. Note the two circular densities indicating the bifid spinous process at C7 (arrow). **B. Coned Neutral Lateral Cervical**. Note the twin tips to the bifurcated spinous process of the C7 vertebra (arrows). With the soft tissue overlap of the shoulder, a fracture of one of the spinous processes is difficult to rule out. Incidentally noted are the normal, ununited secondary growth centers for the vertebral bodies (ring apophysis) at C2, C3, and C4 (arrowheads). **C. Coned Posterior Cervical Oblique.** On this oblique view, with 15° cephalad tube angulation, we are better able to separate the spinous processes from the surrounding soft tissue. COMMENT: As described in Figure 3.145, a "clay-shoveler's" fracture typically involves caudal displacement of the fractured fragment, that is not displayed here. (Courtesy of Donald E. Freuden, DC, FACO, Denver, Colorado)

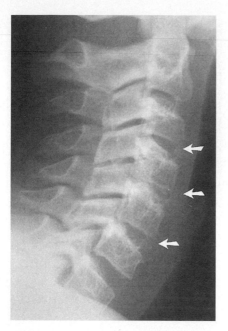

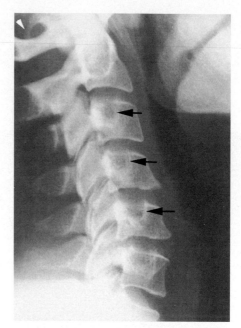

Figure 3.148.   ELONGATED CERVICAL TRANSVERSE PROCESSES. Observe the bony densities superimposed on the intervertebral discs, representing elongated transverse processes of the midcervical spine (arrows).

Figure 3.149.   PSEUDOTUMOR: TRANSVERSE PROCESSES AT C3, C4, AND C5. A. Coned Neutral Lateral Cervical. Observe the circular radiolucencies at C3, C4, and especially C5 that are the normal appearance of the transverse processes when viewed on end (arrows). The radiolucency is especially prominent at C5 because of the overlap and obliteration of its superior cortical endplate. Incidentally noted is calcification of the posterior atlantooccipital ligament creating a posterior ponticle at C1 (arrowhead) (also see Figs. 3.13, 3.14). COMMENT: The sclerotic "U" shaping and relative symmetry in three adjacent vertebral segments help to distinguish them from a neoplastic or infectious lytic process. (Courtesy of Carr Chiropractic Clinic, Huron, South Dakota)

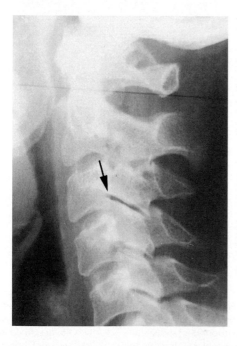

Figure 3.150.   PSEUDOFRACTURE: MILD ROTATION CAUSING POSTERIOR BODY LUCENCY. Coned Neutral Lateral Cervical. There is a lucency extending through the posterior vertebral body margin of C3 (arrow). This lucency is caused by a slight cervical curvature with spinal rotation that projects the normal lucency of the well-maintained zygapophyseal joint anteriorly over the vertebral body. This finding is enhanced by the facet plane at C3-C4 being coincident with (parallel to) the primary x-ray beam. (Courtesy of Scott A. Sole, DC, Denver, Colorado)

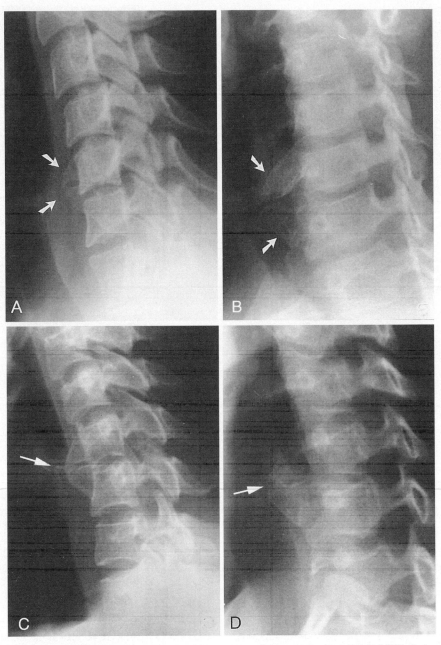

Figure 3.151.   ENLARGED CERVICAL TRANSVERSE PROCESSES, ANTERIOR TUBERCLE: C5-C6. A. Coned Lateral Cervical and B. Coned Posterior Cervical Oblique. Anomalous articulation between the transverse processes of C5 and C6 has occurred due to elongation of the anterior tubercles (arrows). **C. Coned Lateral Cervical and D. Coned Posterior Cervical Oblique.** The anomalous articulation is again demonstrated (arrows). (**A** and **B** Courtesy of Gary M. Guebert, DC, DACBR, St. Louis, Missouri. **C** and **D** Courtesy of William E. Litterer, DC, DACBR, Fellow, ACCR, Elizabeth, NJ) (From Applebaum Y, Gerald P, Bryk D: *Elongation of the anterior tubercle of a cervical vertebral transverse process: An unusual variant.* Skeletal Radiol 10:265, 1983.)

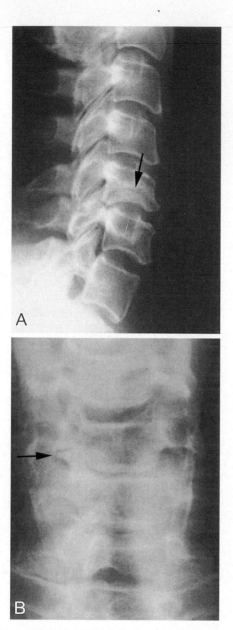

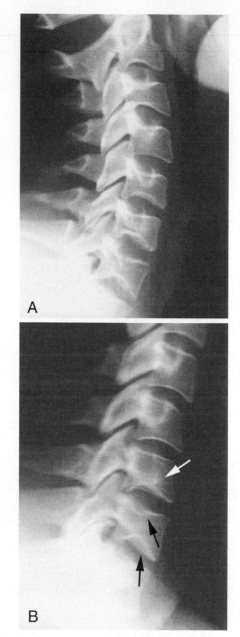

Figure 3.152.   PSEUDOFRACTURE: C5. A. Coned Neutral Lateral Cervical. Observe the arcing radiolucency overlying the body of C5 (arrow). **B. Coned AP Lower Cervical**. Note the advanced degenerative hypertrophy of the uncovertebral joint and how the osteophytes have created a horizontal cleft (arrow). COMMENT: This pseudofracture is caused by advanced degenerative joint disease of the uncovertebral joint. With this degree of degeneration there is probably significant foraminal stenosis also present at this level.

Figure 3.153.   CERVICAL NUCLEAR IMPRESSIONS (NOTOCHORDAL PERSISTENCY). A. Coned Neutral Lateral Cervical. There are multiple smooth indentations affecting the superior and inferior endplates throughout the cervical spine. These represent nuclear impressions and are a variant of normal. **B. Coned Neutral Lateral Cervical**. Nuclear impressions are again noted in the inferior endplate of C6 and both endplates of C7 (arrows). (Courtesy of Wendy Neale, DC, Portland, Maine)

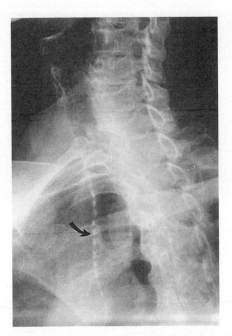

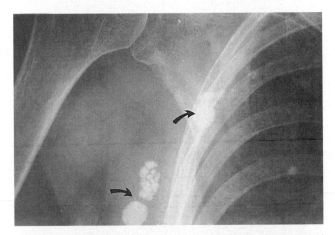

Figure 3.154.   TRACHEAL CARTILAGE CALCIFICATION. Clinically insignificant calcification of the tracheal cartilages is present (arrow). (Courtesy of Kenneth E. Yochum, DC, St. Louis, Missouri)

Figure 3.156.   CALCIFIED AXILLARY LYMPH NODES. There is calcification in multiple axillary lymph nodes (arrows). These should not be confused with blastic bone lesions or pulmonary nodules when they overlie these anatomic structures. It is unusual for the axillary lymph nodes to calcify. (Courtesy of Kenneth E. Yochum, DC, St. Louis, Missouri)

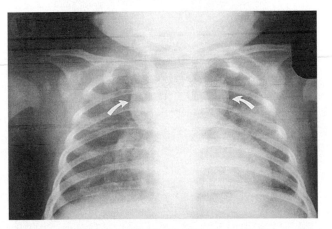

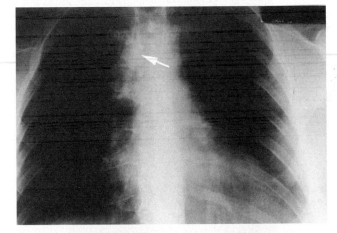

Figure 3.155.   NORMAL THYMUS GLAND. The radiopaque paraspinal density just above the heart (arrows) represents the normal infant thymus gland.

Figure 3.157.   CALCIFIED LYMPH NODE: MEDIASTINAL. Coned AP Thoracic. Note the large, irregular calcification present in the right paratracheal lymph node (arrow) at the T5 level. These structures may rarely cause compression of the adjacent trachea or bronchus or rarely may erode through the bronchial wall to become a broncholith. (Courtesy of Douglas L. Forsstrom, DC, Denver, Colorado)

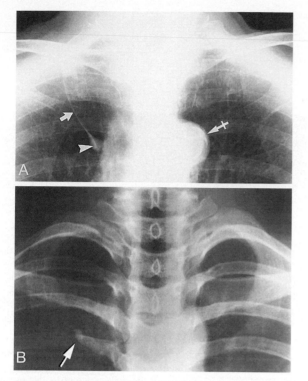

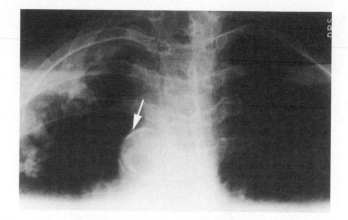

Figure 3.160.   THUMBNAIL SIGN: AORTIC ARCH. Coned AP Thoracic. Observe the fine radiopaque margins at the superior edge of the aortic arch (arrow). This is atherosclerotic plaquing within the aortic arch and is called the "thumbnail sign." Also note the patchy calcification and fibrosis in the left lung apex, the result of prior tuberculosis. (Courtesy of Scott A. Sole, DC, Denver, Colorado)

Figure 3.158.   AZYGOS FISSURE, AZYGOS VEIN, AZYGOS LOBE. A. Coned AP Chest. Observe the fine radiopaque line present in the right upper lung apex, representing the azygos fissure (arrow). The radiopaque density at the base of this fissure represents the azygos vein (arrowhead). Extensive atherosclerotic plaquing is present within the aortic knob, demonstrating a "thumbnail" sign (crossed arrow). **B. AP Thoracic.** This same finding in a bone film with a grid (instead of the previous chest technique) makes the finding more subtle (arrow). COMMENT: The azygos fissure creates an accessory lobe, referred to as the azygos lobe. This is of no clinical significance.

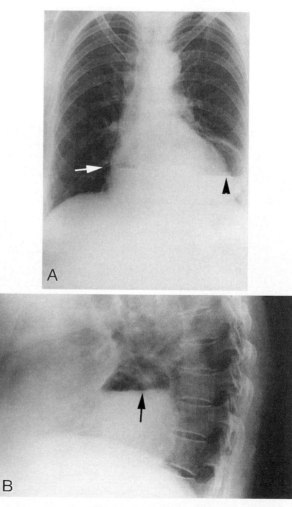

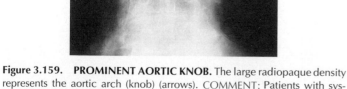

Figure 3.159.   PROMINENT AORTIC KNOB. The large radiopaque density represents the aortic arch (knob) (arrows). COMMENT: Patients with systemic hypertension often will have significant prominence of the aortic arch.

Figure 3.161.   HIATAL HERNIA. A. PA Chest. Note the air-fluid level that extends from near the right border of the heart (right atrium) (arrow) across midline to the left lateral wall of the thoracic cage (arrowhead). These air-fluid levels represent gas in the fundus of the stomach after herniation through the diaphragm. **B. Coned Lateral Chest.** Note the air-fluid level (arrow) above the level of the diaphragm in the retrocardiac space.

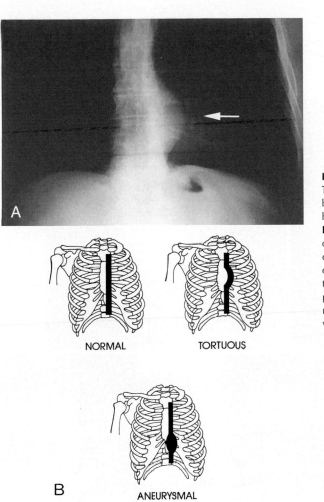

Figure 3.162. TORTUOUS DESCENDING THORACIC AORTA. A. Coned AP Thoracic. Observe the convex density lying to the left of the lower thoracic verte-brae (arrow). This represents tortuosity of the descending thoracic aorta. The aorta becomes tortuous (elongates) in elderly and hypertensive patients. **B. Schematic Diagram.** The normal descending thoracic aorta maintains a uniform caliber and overlies the left half of the thoracic spine. The tortuous aorta also has a uniform caliber but buckles away from the spine. The medial border is difficult to visualize on radiographs. The aneurysmal descending thoracic aorta also has a lateral margin that buckles away from the spine; however, this section of the aorta has lost its parallel walls. The caliber of the aneurysmal section becomes dilated. Unfortu-nately, the medial portion of the aneurysm overlies the spine and is difficult to visualize on radiographs.

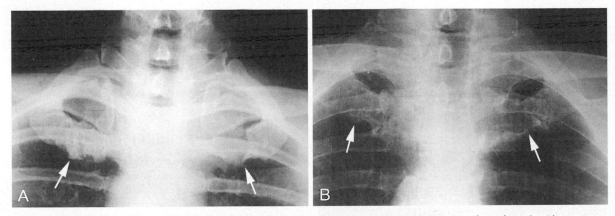

Figure 3.163. IDIOPATHIC COSTOCHONDRAL JOINT IRREGULARITY. A and B. Coned AP Thoracic. Ob-serve the irregularity and prominence of the calcified first costochondral junctions (arrows).

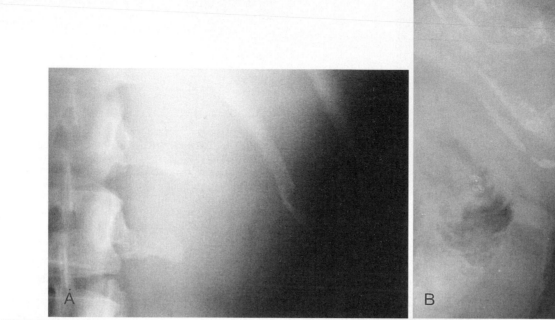

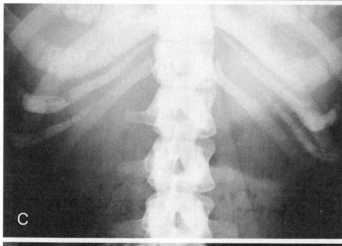

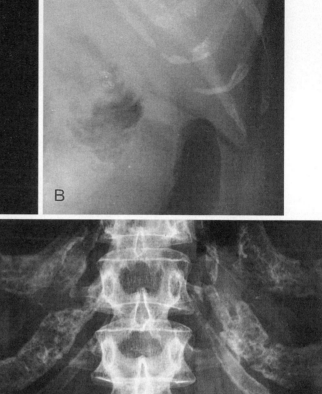

**Figure 3.164.   IDIOPATHIC COSTOCHONDRAL CARTILAGE CALCIFI-
CATION. A–E. View.** Observe the varying amounts of costochondral calcification involving the lower ribs (arrow). These may appear very dense, symmetric, and homogeneous; however, they have no pathologic significance.
Costochondral calcification may occur in children, as well as in adults, and
is a variation of normal. (**A** Courtesy of Daniel L. Perkins, DC, Denver, Colorado) COMMENT: An increased incidence of costal cartilage calcification
in children with hyperthyroidism has been reported. (From Senac MO, Lee
FA, Gilsnaz V: *Early costochondral calcification in adolescent hyperthyroidism.* Radiology 156:375, 1985)

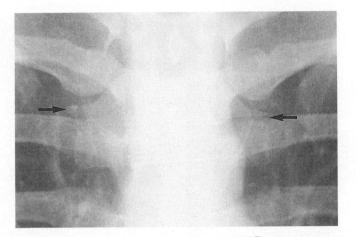

Figure 3.165.   NONUNION: SECONDARY GROWTH CENTERS: MA-NUBRIUM. There is nonunion of the secondary growth centers for the ma-nubrium (arrows).

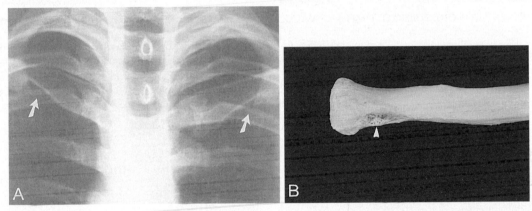

Figure 3.166.   RHOMBOID FOSSAE. A and B. There are bilateral rhomboid fossae present on the inferior surface of the medial aspect of the clavicles (arrows). A photograph of an anatomic specimen clearly defines the inden-tation of the rhomboid fossae (arrowhead). COMMENT: The rhomboid fossa represents a developmental variation at the insertion of the rhomboid liga-ment, which is of no clinical significance.

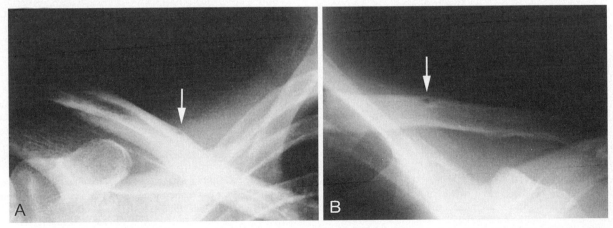

Figure 3.167.   SUPRACLAVICULAR FORAMEN. A. PA Clavicle. Observe the pseudolesion created by a foramen in the middle clavicle (arrow). **B. PA Clavicle.** Observe the small, circular radiolucency along the superior aspect of the medial one-third of the clavicle (arrow). This represents a foramen that may transmit the supraclavicular nerve.

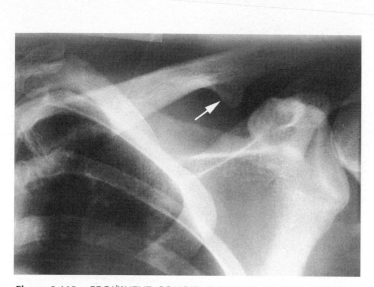

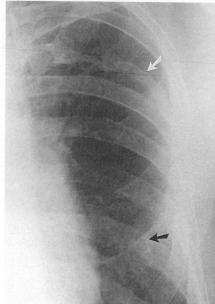

Figure 3.168. PROMINENT CONOID TUBERCLE OF THE CLAVICLE. Coned PA Clavicle. The osseous density extending from the clavicle inferiorly represents an enlarged conoid tubercle (arrow) and must be differentiated from ossification of the coracoclavicular ligaments. The lack of a trauma history and the smooth, corticated margin point to a congenital origin for this anomaly. (Courtesy of James J. Holland, DC, FACO, Carmichael, California)

Figure 3.170. POSTSURGICAL RIB REGROWTH. Reformation and growth of a previously resected rib is present (arrows). This is a common occurrence following rib resection if residual periosteum is left behind. COMMENT: The patient's history of previous surgery is very helpful, since the radiographic appearance may simulate a destructive rib lesion.

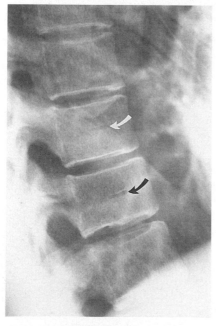

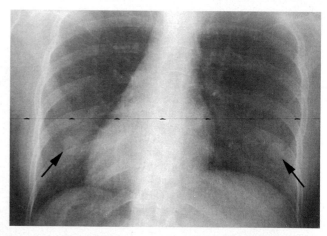

Figure 3.169. HAHN'S VENOUS CLEFTS. Hahn's venous clefts (arrows) are seen throughout the central portion of the thoracic vertebral bodies. COMMENT: These venous grooves are most frequently seen in the lower thoracic spine and should not be confused with any pathologic process.

Figure 3.171. NIPPLE SHADOWS. Coned AP Full Spine. Observe the two circular opacities overlying the chest in the region where the nipples are normally located. This finding is sometimes confused with a true pulmonary nodule (also see Fig. 3.75). COMMENT: The dark line traversing the film in midline is the perforation for the film-fold of a 14″ by 36″ film. (Courtesy of George E. Springer, DC, Clearwater, Florida)

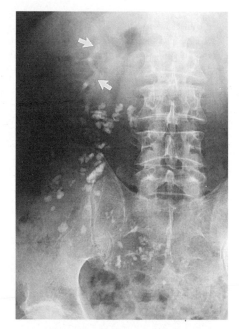

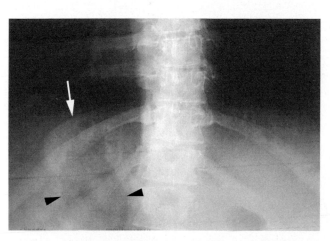

Figure 3.172.   FLUID IN FUNDUS OF STOMACH: PSEUDOTUMOR APPEARANCE. Coned AP Lumbar. Note the circular water density present just under the left hemidiaphragm (arrow). This density is caused by fluid in the fundus of the stomach with a superimposed air density in the body of the stomach extending inferiorly off the photograph (arrowheads).

Figure 3.174.   CALCIFIED MESENTERIC LYMPH NODES. There are multiple, scattered, irregular areas of calcification present in the right lower abdomen, representing mesenteric lymph nodes. Contrast media is noted within the collecting system of the kidney (arrows). (Courtesy of Kenneth E. Yochum, DC, St. Louis, Missouri)

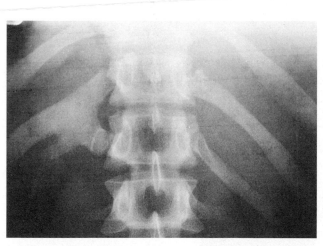

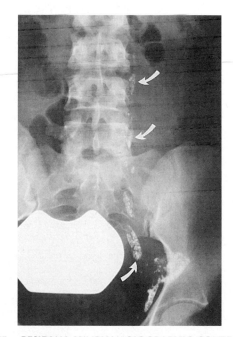

Figure 3.173.   RIB SYNOSTOSIS. Coned AP Thoracic. There is a congenital fusion of the eleventh and twelfth ribs on the left just lateral to T11-T12. (Courtesy of Ron D. Myhra, DC, Denver, Colorado)

Figure 3.175.   RESIDUAL LYMPHANGIOGRAPHIC CONTRAST MEDIA. The radiopaque material present adjacent to the lumbar spine and extending into the pelvic basin (arrows) represents residual contrast media from a previous lymphangiogram. Note the ovarian shield superimposed upon the pelvic inlet.

Figure 3.176.   ILIOLUMBAR LIGAMENT OSSIFICATION.
A. Coned AP Lumbar. There is early ossification of the iliolumbar ligament (arrow). **B–E. AP L5-S1 Spot.** Note the unilateral ossification of the iliolumbar ligament (arrows). Also
note the clarity with which you can visualize the L5-S1 intervertebral joint space, the L5 pedicles, and the sacroiliac
joints using the AP L5-S1 spot. This is also called the "Ferguson's" or "tilt-up" view. **F. AP L5-S1 Spot.** Observe bilateral ossification of the iliolumbar ligaments (arrows) and
contrast media present within the subarachnoid space above
the first sacral level (arrowhead) as a result of previous myelographic investigation. (**B** Courtesy of William E. Litterer,
DC, DACBR, Fellow, ACCR, Elizabeth, New Jersey; **C** Courtesy of David J. Byrnes, DC, Coffs Harbor, New South Wales,
Australia, **D** and **E** Courtesy of Max L. Denton, DC, Marlon,
Ohio)

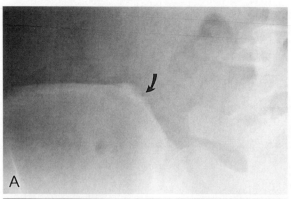

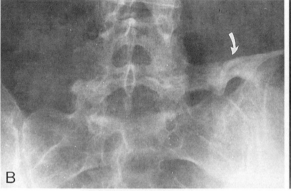

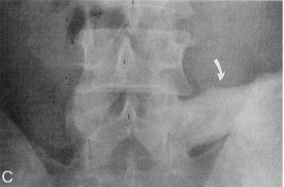

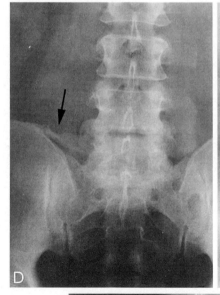

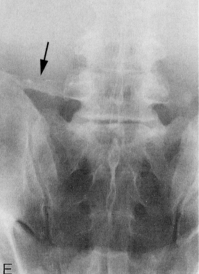

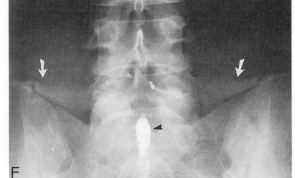

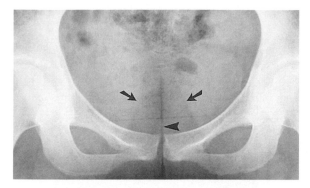

Figure 3.177. GLUTEAL FASCIAL PLANES. The radiolucent shadows above the pubic rami (arrows) represent the fascial planes within the gluteus maximus muscles. The clear, sharply demarcated radiolucent linear line (arrowhead) represents the fold between the buttocks.

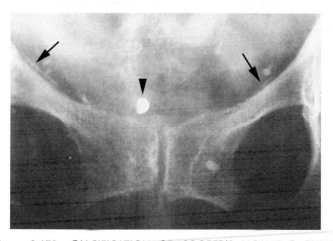

Figure 3.178. CALCIFICATION OF COOPER'S LIGAMENT: PUBIS. Coned AP Pelvis. Observe the fine radiopaque lines paralleling the superior aspect of the pubic bones (arrows). This is reported to be an aging phenomena. The opaque density (arrowhead) is retained barium contrast in a rectal diverticulum. (Courtesy of Harry R. Shepard, DC, Marion, Indiana) (From Steinfeld, JR. et al: *Calcification in Cooper's ligament.* AJR; 121:107, 1974)

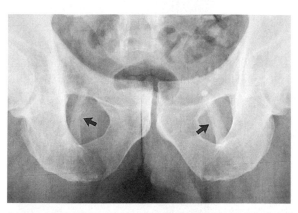

Figure 3.179. CALCIFIED SACROTUBEROUS LIGAMENTS. Calcification of the sacrotuberous ligaments is noted (arrows). COMMENT: Calcification of the sacrotuberous ligaments is more commonly found in diffuse idiopathic skeletal hyperostosis (DISH) and fluorosis. It may, however, occur as an isolated variant, as was the case in this patient.

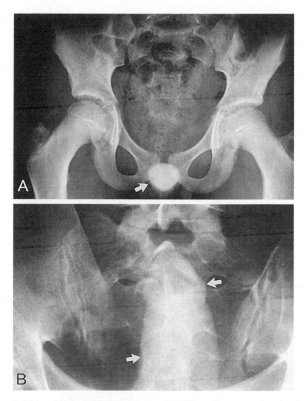

Figure 3.180. PENILE SHADOW. A and B. The radiopaque circular density present in the area of the pubic articulation in **A** represents the penis seen *en face* (arrow). The elongated radiopacity seen superimposed on the sacrum (arrows) in **B** represents the water density of the penis.

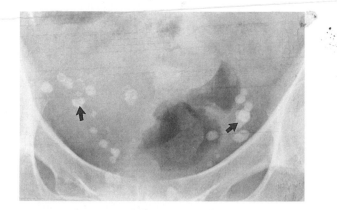

Figure 3.181. PELVIC PHLEBOLITHS. The multiple radiopacities above the superior pubic rami represent phleboliths. The radiolucent center (arrows) is typical of phleboliths, which are located within the pelvic veins. COMMENT: Phleboliths in this location are of no clinical significance to the patient.

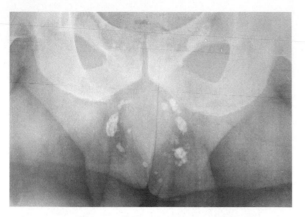

Figure 3.182. CALCIFIED SCROTAL LYMPH NODES. The irregular calcifications seen below the pubic rami bilaterally represent calcified scrotal lymph nodes. COMMENT: Calcification of the scrotal lymph nodes are of no clinical significance.

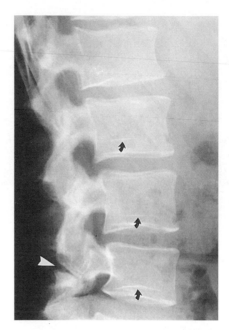

Figure 3.184. LUMBAR HARRIS' GROWTH ARREST LINES. There are Harris' growth arrest lines that parallel the endplates of the lumbar vertebrae (arrows). A defect in the pars interarticularis is noted at a single lumbar vertebra (arrowhead). No evidence of spondylolisthesis is present. COMMENT: Harris' growth arrest lines are seldom seen within the spine and should not be interpreted as lead lines or associated with any other metabolic abnormality or bone-sclerosing dysplasia.

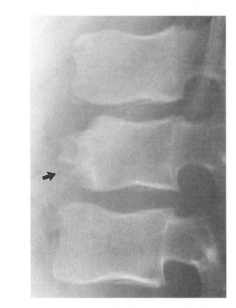

Figure 3.183. NORMAL LUMBAR VERTEBRAL OSSIFICATION. Observe the normal "step" defect (arrow) present on the anterior surface of this juvenile lumbar vertebra. This is a developmental variation of normal and will disappear with ossification of the ring apophysis.

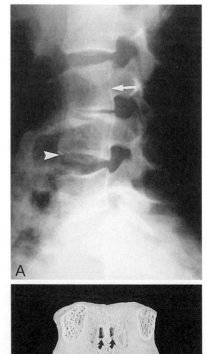

Figure 3.185. LUMBAR BLOCK VERTEBRA. A and B. There is a partial congenital block vertebra present at L3-L4. A posterior venous cleft is present at the L3 vertebra (arrow). Observe the persistent secondary growth center at the anteroinferior aspect of L4 (arrowhead). The posterior venous cleft is clearly demonstrated in the photograph of the anatomic specimen (arrows) and represents a growth variant. The neural arch has been removed at the pedicles.

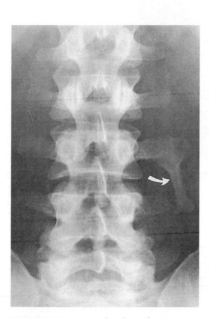

Figure 3.186.   LUMBAR RIB. A rare lumbar rib is present, projecting from the inferior aspect of the third lumbar transverse process (arrow). (Courtesy of Gary M. Guebert, DC, DACBR, St. Louis, Missouri)

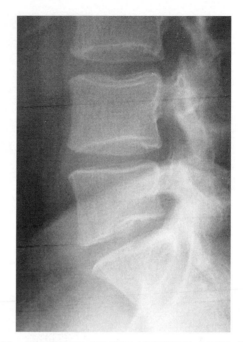

Figure 3.188.   TRAPEZOID LUMBAR VERTEBRAL BODY. Observe the trapezoidal shape of the L5 vertebral body. This is a developmental variation of normal and should not be confused with a compression fracture.

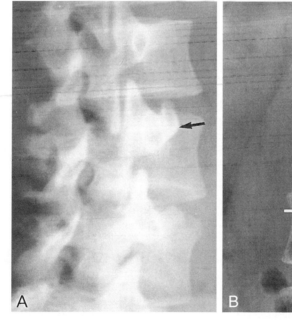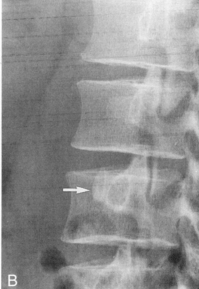

Figure 3.187.   PIG SNOUT VERTEBRA. A and B. An anomalous malformation of the transverse process (arrows) of a lumbar vertebra creates the ''pig snout'' appearance of the Scotty dog. (**A**, Reprinted with permission: Keats, TE: *Atlas of Normal Roentgen Variants That May Simulate Disease,* ed. 3. Chicago Year Book Medical Publishers, 1984) (Courtesy of William E. Litterer, DC, DACBR, Fellow, ACCR, Elizabeth, New Jersey)

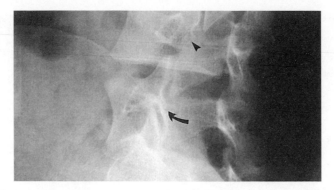

Figure 3.189.   THIN L5 PARS INTERARTICULARIS. The pars interarticularis of the L5 vertebra is congenitally thin (arrow) in comparison to the normal width present at the L4 vertebra (arrowhead). COMMENT: Patients born with a thin pars interarticularis may be predisposed to spondylolysis.

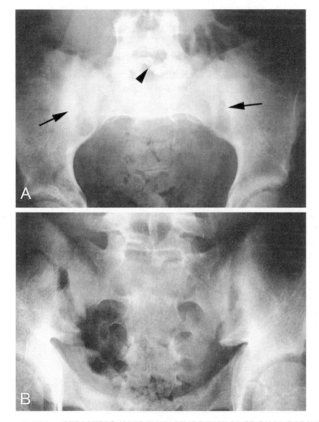

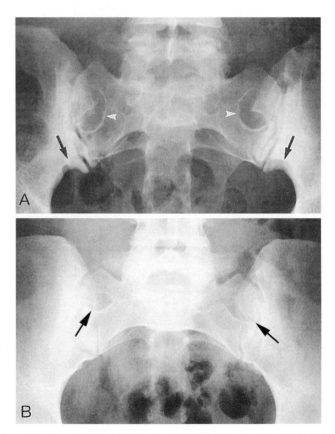

Figure 3.190.   PEDIATRIC "WIDENING" OF THE SACROILIAC JOINTS. A. Coned AP Pelvis. The sacroiliac joints in pediatric patients may appear ill defined, with the joints being wide (arrows). This is a normal appearance in younger patients, like this 13 year old. Also note the spina bifida occulta of S1 (arrowhead). **B. AP L5-S1 Tilt-Up.** This is a much better radiographic view to visualize the normal widening of these pediatric sacroiliac joints. (Courtesy of John C. Slizeski, DC, Denver, Colorado)

Figure 3.191.   ACCESSORY SACRAL FORAMINA. A. Coned AP Pelvis. There are bilateral accessory sacral foramina noted (arrowheads). Bilateral paraglenoid sulci are present (arrows). **B. Coned AP Pelvis.** Another example of bilateral accessory sacral foramina (arrows). (**B** Courtesy of John H. Phillips, DC, Carbondale, Colorado)

Figure 3.192.   ILIAC FOSSA. A. AP L5–S1 Tilt-Up. Observe the fossa present in the upper ilium (arrow), creating the appearance of a sacroiliac erosion. **B and C. Coned AP Pelvis.** Again note the bilateral fossae present on the lower portions of the ilia altering the appearance of the normal sacroiliac joints (arrows). (**C** Courtesy of Richard L. Green, DC, Winthrop, Massachusetts)

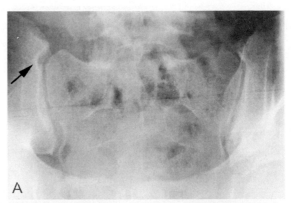

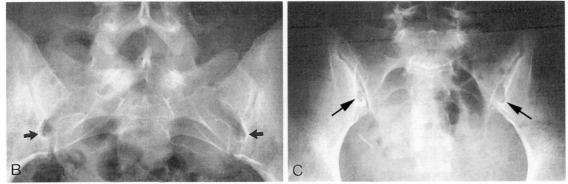

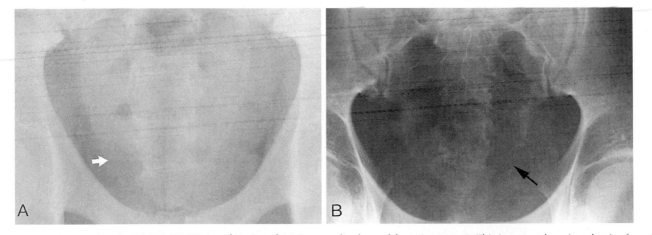

Figure 3.193.   SACRAL OSSIFICATION DEFECT. A and B. Coned AP Sacral Views. Observe the failure of ossification of the lateral margin of the distal sacral foramina (arrow). This is a growth variant that is of no clinical significance and should not be interpreted as a destructive lesion.

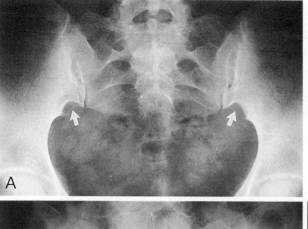

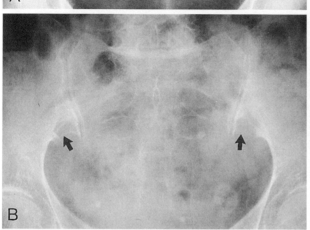

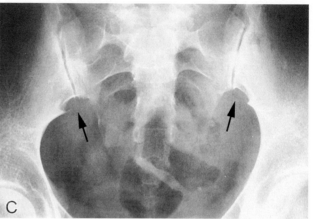

Figure 3.194.   PARAGLENOID SULCI. A–C. Observe the deep paraglenoid sulci (arrows) affecting the iliac portion of the lower aspect of the sacroiliac joint. COMMENT: This sulcus transmits the superior branch of the gluteal artery and supplies insertion for a portion of the sacroiliac ligament. It is a characteristic of the female pelvis, since it is rarely found in the male pelvis. It is occasionally unilateral but is most often found bilaterally, although asymmetrical in its presentation. It has also been referred to as the "preauricular" sulcus.

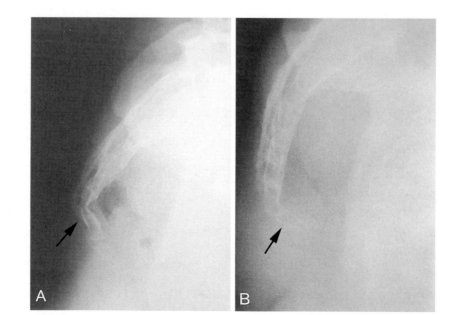

Figure 3.195.   SACRAL AND COCCYX VARIATIONS. A and B. Coned Lateral Sacrum. Note the angular variation in the sacrococcygeal region (arrows). This angulation may represent healed trauma and/or normal anatomic variation; however, it may also represent a problem site for the delivery of a child.

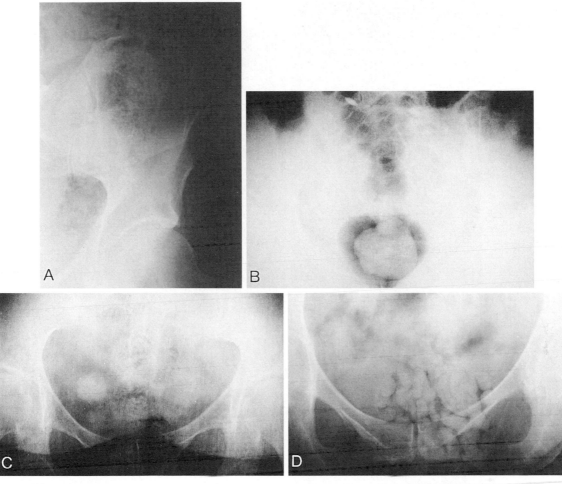

Figure 3.196.   GAS/FECAL MATERIAL. A–D. Coned AP Lumbar. This is a common pseudolesion of the ilium and pelvis. It is caused by a mixture of gas and fecal material in the descending colon, sigmoid colon, and/or rectum. When you scrutinize these "lesions", look for extension of the "lesion" beyond the edges of the underlying bone and bony trabeculae through the gas shadow. This is more commonly present on the patient's right side. (**C** Courtesy of Scott H. Smith, DC, Greeley, Colorado)

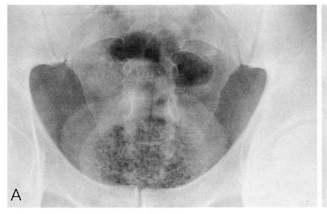

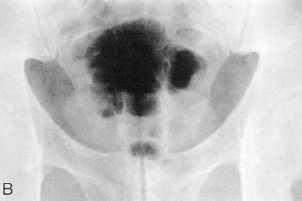

Figure 3.197.   GAS/FECAL MATERIAL: EVACUATION. A and B. Coned AP Sacrum. In **A** the distal sacrum and coccyx are obscured by a mottled mass of superimposed feces. **B** is the same patient, the same day, in a postevac-uation film. COMMENT: Considering any sacral or coccygeal films, it would improve visualization of those structures to order an enema for the patient before the exam. (Courtesy of Wesley E. Wilvert, DC, Parker, Colorado)

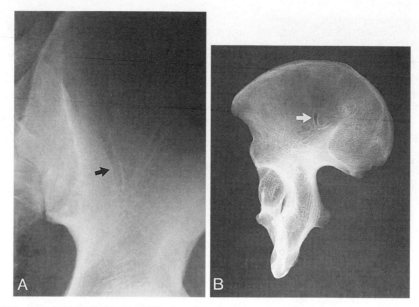

Figure 3.198.   ILIAC VASCULAR GROOVE. A and B. The "V"- and "Y"-shaped grooves (arrows) represent the passageway for the nutrient arteries of the ilium.

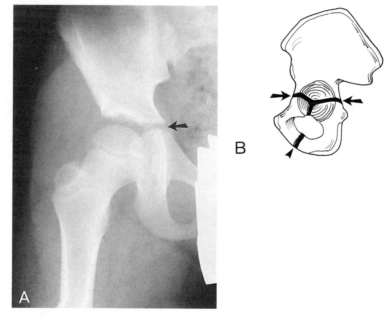

Figure 3.199.   TRIRADIATE CARTILAGE. A. AP Hip. The radiolucent defect present on the medial surface of the acetabulum represents the normal triradiate cartilage (arrow). **B. Schematic Diagram**. This represents a lateral perspective of the ilium, demonstrating the triradiate cartilage (arrows) and the ischiopubic synchondrosis (arrowhead).

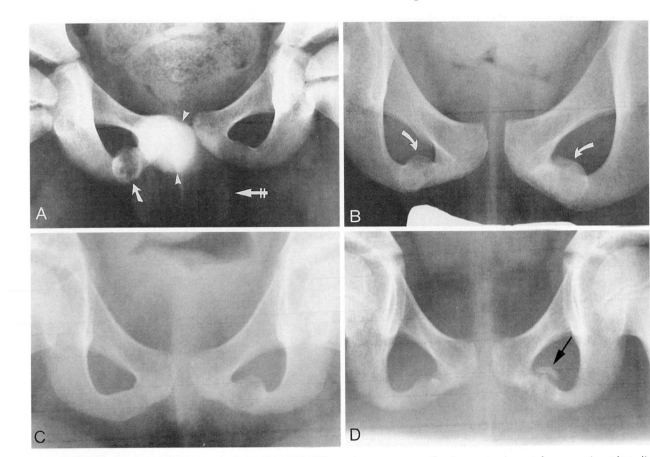

Figure 3.200.   ISCHIOPUBIC SYNCHONDROSIS GROWTH VARIANT. Coned AP Pelvis. A. The area of radiolucency and bulbous deformity of the ischiopubic synchondrosis (arrow) denotes a developmental growth variant. The adjacent radiopacity (arrowheads) represents the penis. The linear radiopaque margin (crossed arrow) represents the lateral edge of the scrotum. **B.** There are bilateral areas of bony expansion at the junction of the ischiopubic synchondrosis (arrows). These represent a growth abnormality. **C.** This normal variant finding is also seen unilaterally in this female child. **D.** Here is a separate ossification center (arrow) for a prominent but clinically unimportant ischiopubic synchondrosis. COMMENT: The growth irregularity occurring at the ischiopubic synchondrosis often creates an expansile abnormality at the junction of the growth center or the previous site of same. This should not be referred to as an area of ischemic necrosis, as had been described by van Neck. (Courtesy of The Children's Hospital, Department of Radiology, Denver, Colorado)

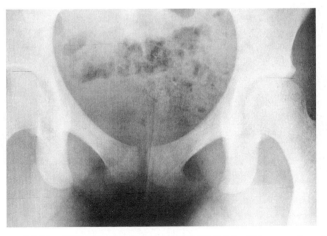

Figure 3.201.   ISCHIAL AGENESIS. Coned AP Pelvis. This asymptomatic 24-year-old patient presented with bilateral failure of ossification of the ischium. The fusion of the ischium with the pubis should have occurred by eight years of age. (Courtesy of Mark T. Clark, DC, Denver, Colorado)

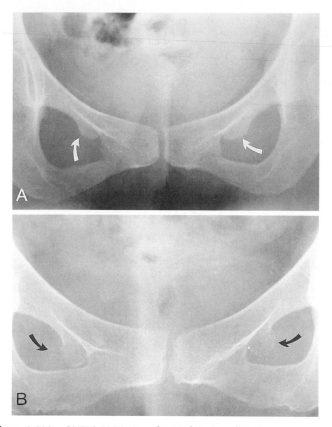

Figure 3.202.   PUBIC EARS. Coned AP Pelvis. A and B. There are congenital protuberances noted projecting toward the obturator foramen (arrows), representing a variation of normal referred to as "pubic ears."

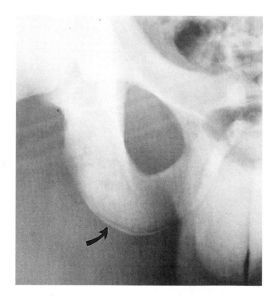

Figure 3.203.   NORMAL ISCHIAL GROWTH CENTER. Coned AP Hip. Observe the fine linear area of radiopacity below the ischial tuberosity, representing the ischial apophysis (arrow).

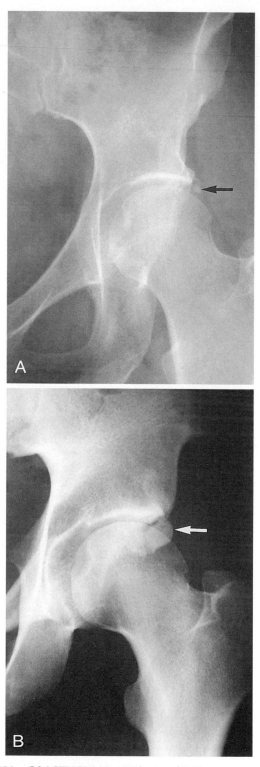

Figure 3.204.   OS ACETABULAE. AP Hip. A and B. These are two examples of os acetabulae (arrows), accessory bones. (Courtesy of Kenneth E. Yochum, DC, St. Louis, Missouri)

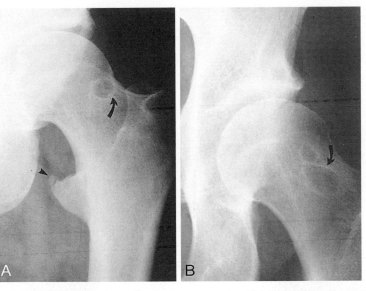

Figure 3.205. FEMORAL HERNIATION PITS. A and B. The well-corticated, geographic areas of radiolucency present within the femoral neck (arrows) represent herniation pits (also Pitt's pits), a bone reaction to an irregular capsular surface. They should not be confused with smaller linear defects on the superior and lateral border of the femoral neck caused by penetrating blood vessels known as perforation grooves. Previously, herniation pits have erroneously been called benign fibrocystic conversion defects. Note on **A** the small osteophyte formation on the lesser trochanter at the insertion of the psoas muscle (arrowhead).

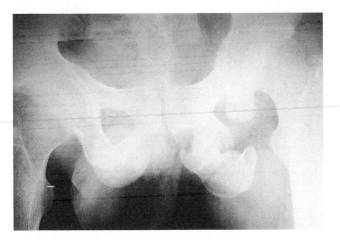

Figure 3.206. ACCESSORY ACETABULUM: THIRD LEG SYNDROME. Coned AP Pelvis. Observe the supernumerary and rudimentary "third leg," which articulates with the inferior pubic ramus creating an accessory acetabulum. Additionally, there is incomplete development of the ischium. (Courtesy of Robert L. Lile, MD, Denver, Colorado)

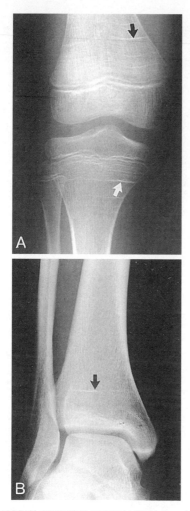

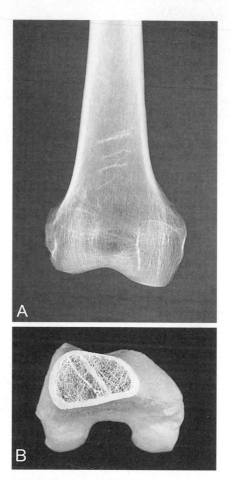

Figure 3.207.   HARRIS' GROWTH ARREST LINES. A and B. There are Harris' growth arrest lines present in the distal metaphysis of the femur, proximal metaphysis of the tibia, and distal metaphysis of the tibia (arrows). COMMENT: These radiopaque transverse bands should not be confused with heavy metal intoxication, bone-sclerosing dysplasia, or any metabolic underlying abnormalities.

Figure 3.208.   BONE BARS. A and B. The radiopaque densities present through the metaphysis of the distal femur represent confluent trabeculae known as "bone bars." This appearance on the radiograph is a variation of normal.

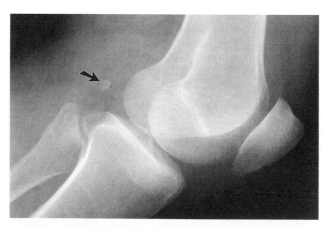

Figure 3.209.   FABELLA. The small spherical radiopacity present in the popliteal fossa (arrow) represents a fabella. COMMENT: A fabella represents a normal sesamoid bone within the lateral gastrocnemius tendon. This should not be confused with an osteochondral fragment within the joint capsule, as found in patients with osteochondritis dissecans.

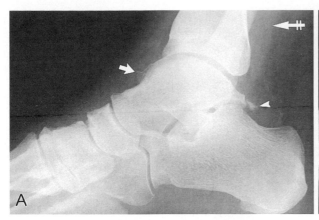

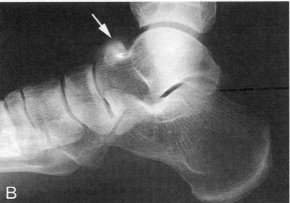

Figure 3.210.   TALAR BEAK, A and B. Views. There is a talar beak present on the anterior surface of the talus in both images (arrows). In addition, **A** also displays an os trigonum in the area of the posterior aspect of the talus (arrowhead) and calcification of the posterior tibial artery (crossed arrow) of the Monckeberg medial sclerosis variety in this diabetic patient. COMMENT:

The talar beak is a developmental variant that should not be confused with hypertrophic spurring seen adjacent to the talonavicular joint. It may be associated with tarsal coalition. The os trigonum is a variation of normal and should not be mistaken for a fracture of the posterior process of the talus.

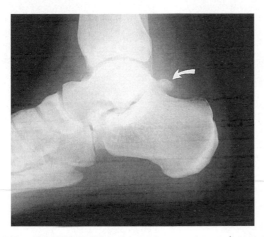

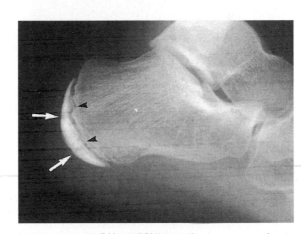

Figure 3.211.   OS TRIGONUM. An os trigonum is noted posterior to the talus (arrow). COMMENT: The os trigonum represents an accessory ossicle and should not be mistaken for a fracture of the posterior process of the talus.

Figure 3.212.   CALCANEAL APOPHYSIS. The increase in density in the secondary ossification center for the calcaneal apophysis (arrows) is a normal manifestation of the growing pediatric calcaneus. The multiserrated margins to the parent calcaneus (arrowheads) additionally represent a normal manifestation of growth before complete closure of the calcaneal growth center occurs. COMMENT: Young patients with pain in the calcaneus should always have the opposite calcaneus radiographed for comparison. The normal increased radiopacity of the calcaneal apophysis has often been erroneously referred to as "avascular necrosis" (Sever's disease).

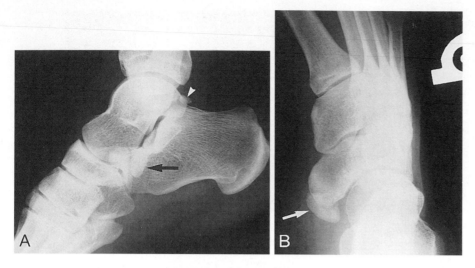

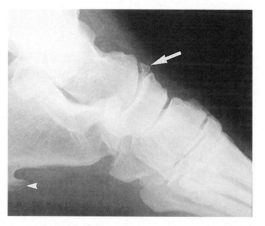

Figure 3.213. OS TIBIALE EXTERNUM. A and B. An accessory ossicle is noted medial to the tarsal navicular bone (arrows), representing an os tibiale externum. An os trigonum is also noted (arrowhead).

Figure 3.214. OS SUPRANAVICULARE. An os supranaviculare, an accessory ossicle, is noted (arrow). A large plantar calcaneal exostosis is also seen (arrowhead). COMMENT: The os supranaviculare should not be mistaken for an avulsion fracture. The os supranaviculare has been referred to as "Pirie's bone."

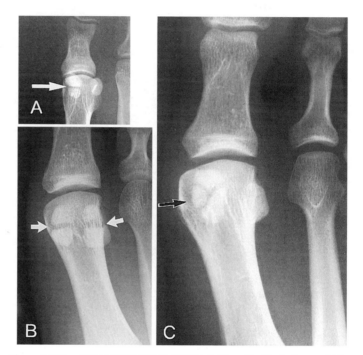

Figure 3.216. SESAMOID BONE: FOOT. A. Bipartite Single Sesamoid (arrow). B. Bipartite Double Sesamoid (arrows). C. Tripartite Single Sesamoid (arrow). COMMENT: The sesamoids outlined here are found in the flexor hallucis brevis tendons. These sesamoid bones lie below the first metatarsophalangeal articulation and are occasionally subject to stress fracture.

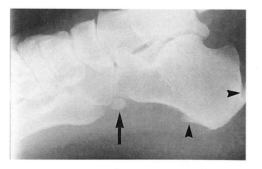

Figure 3.215. OS PERONEUM. There is an accessory ossicle present near the cuboid (arrow). This is referred to as an "os peroneum." There are large calcaneal spurs projecting from the Achilles and plantar surfaces of the calcaneus (arrowheads).

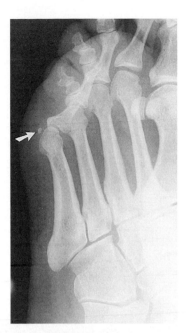

Figure 3.217.   SESAMOID BONE: FOOT. There is a small sesamoid bone noted adjacent to the fifth metatarsophalangeal articulation (arrow).

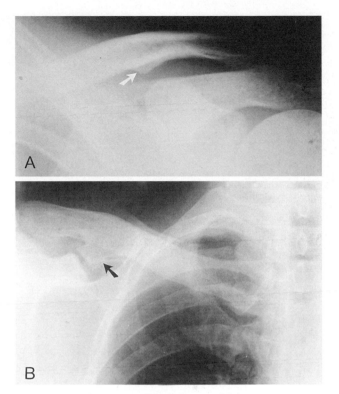

Figure 3.219.   CONOID TUBERCLE. A. A small bony process projecting from the inferior surface of the clavicle (arrow) represents the conoid tubercle and should not be confused with any underlying pathology. **B.** There is an enlarged conoid tubercle projecting as an exostosis and forming an accessory articulation with the coracoid process of the scapula (arrow).

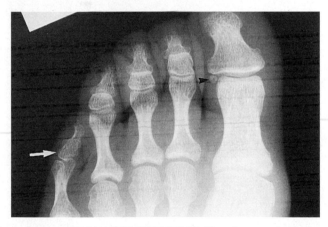

Figure 3.218.   PHALANGEAL SYNOSTOSIS. There is congenital synostosis of the mid and distal phalanges of the fifth toe (arrow). This is a frequent congenital variation of normal and should not be confused with any underlying pathology. A small accessory ossicle is noted adjacent to the distal interphalangeal articulation of the great toe (arrowhead).

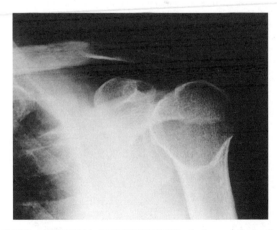

Figure 3.220.   HUMERAL PSEUDOTUMOR. A ''pseudotumor'' appearance is noted in the humeral head. This is created with internal rotation and represents the ball-shaped articular surface of the humeral head, along with superimposition of the tuberosities. This appearance is frequently seen on PA chest radiographs and should be regarded as a variation of normal.

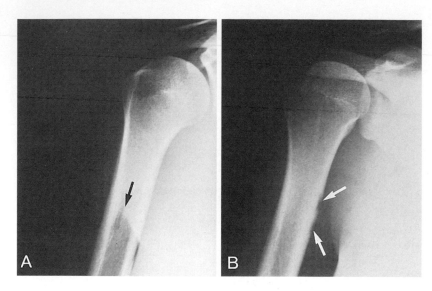

Figure 3.221. PECTORALIS MAJOR: HUMERAL INSERTION. A and B. The radiolucencies noted in the humeral cortex (arrows) are produced by the insertion of the pectoralis major muscle.

Figure 3.222. PECTORALIS MAJOR: HUMERAL INSERTION. A and B. The radiolucent defect in the area of the humeral cortex represents the area of insertion of the pectoralis major muscle (arrows). The slight cortical bump on the lateral surface of the humerus represents the normal deltoid tuberosity (arrowheads).

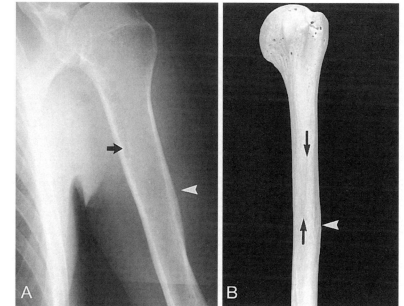

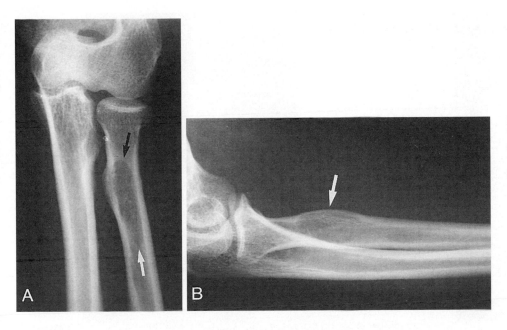

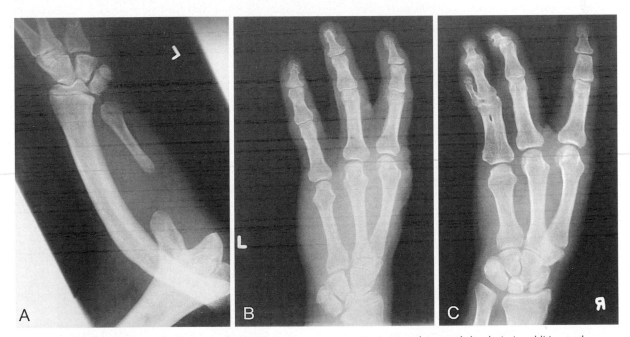

Figure 3.223. RADIAL PSEUDOTUMOR. There is a "pseudotumor" appearance noted in the proximal metaphysis of the radius (arrows). This is created by an unusually large radial tuberosity. (Courtesy of Gary M. Guebert, DC, DACBR, St. Louis, Missouri)

Figure 3.224. CONGENITAL ABSENCE OF ULNA. A. AP Forearm. Even though the distal aspect of the ulna is present, there is extreme negative ulnar variance in the wrist. Observe the lateral bowing of the radius due to increased stress from the lack of an intact ulna. Also note the malformation and dislocation of the elbow. **B. PA Left Hand.** This is the left hand from the patient in **A**. Note the carpal dysplasia in addition to the presence of only three digits. **C. PA Right Hand.** The opposite hand of this patient also displays carpal dysplasia and three digits although the third digit demonstrates synostosis. (Courtesy of Richard Edmonds, BAppSc (Chiro), Port Macquarie, New South Wales, Australia)

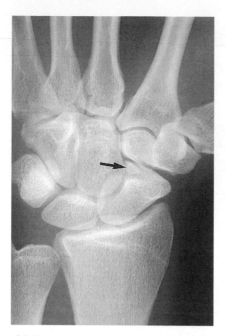

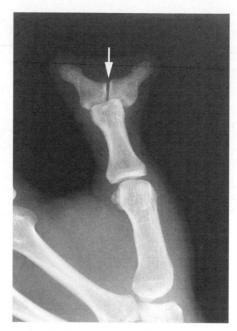

Figure 3.225.   OS CENTRALE. An os centrale is present on the dorsum of the carpus (arrow), lying among the scaphoid, trapezoid, and capitate.

Figure 3.226.   POLYDACTYLY. AP Thumb. Observe the twin distal phalanges on the thumb. Note that these phalanges have an articulation between themselves (arrow), as well as an articulation with the proximal phalanx.

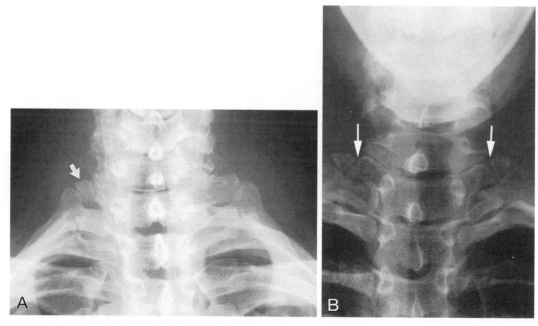

Figure 3.227.   NONUNION OF THE SECONDARY GROWTH CENTER OF T1 TRANSVERSE PROCESSES. A. Coned AP Lower Cervical. Nonunion of the secondary growth center is noted (arrow). **B. Coned AP Lower Cervical**. Observe the radiolucent lines (arrows) separating the distal aspects of both transverse processes of T1. COMMENT: This must be differentiated from a fracture, done by noting its smooth margins and sclerotic borders.

Fractures of the transverse processes of the lower cervical and upper thoracic spine are rare and, when present, are found associated with severe trauma and other fractures. Note that the transverse processes of the thoracic vertebrae angle superiorly, while those of the cervical vertebrae angle inferiorly. This allows distinction between the normal thoracic ribs and the anomalous cervical ribs. See also Figure 3.229 for a similar process in the lumbar spine.

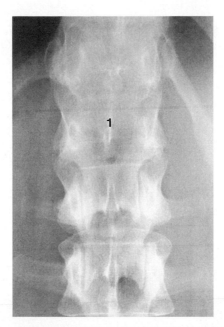

Figure 3.228.   AGENETIC LUMBAR TRANSVERSE PROCESSES. There is agenesis of the transverse processes of L1 bilaterally. This is a rare anomaly. (Courtesy of Kenneth E. Yochum, DC, St. Louis, Missouri)

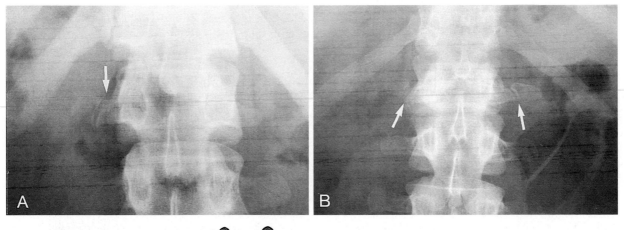

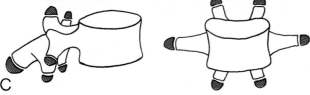

Figure 3.229.   UNUNITED SECONDARY OSSIFICATION CENTERS. Lumbar Spine. A. Unilateral nonunion of the ossification center for the transverse process (arrow). **B.** Bilateral nonunion (arrows). **C.** This schematic diagram demonstrates the normal secondary growth centers for the spine.

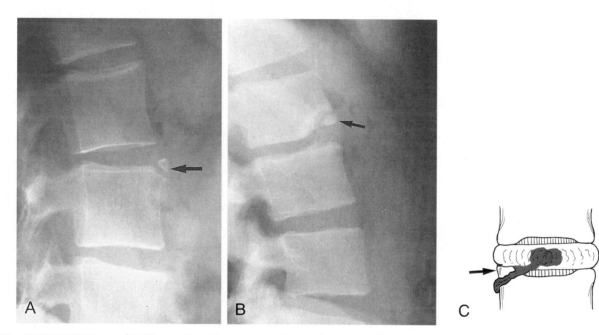

Figure 3.230.   LIMBUS BONE. A and B. The small ossicles present at the anterior corners of the vertebral bodies (arrows) represent limbus bones. **C.** This schematic diagram demonstrates herniation of nuclear material as the basis for the production of the limbus bone (arrow). COMMENT: The limbus bone is produced as a result of migration and herniation of nuclear material through the secondary growth center for the corner of the vertebral body. This nuclear migration results in nonunion of the secondary growth center.

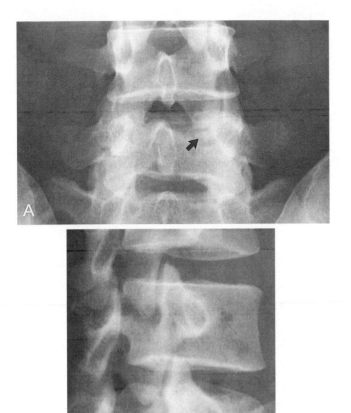

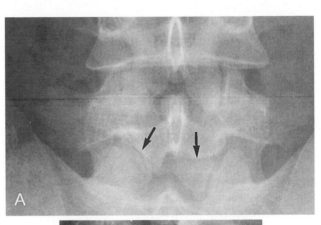

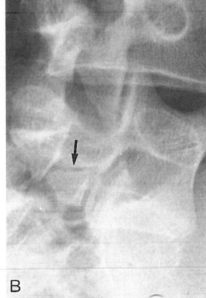

Figure 3.231.   UNUNITED SECONDARY OSSIFICATION CENTERS. Lumbar Spine. A. Frontal View. B. Oblique View. There is nonunion of the secondary ossification center for the end of the inferior articulating process of L4 (arrows), which may be mistaken for a fracture.

Figure 3.232.   UNUNITED SECONDARY OSSIFICATION CENTERS. Lumbar Spine. A and B. Bilateral failure of union of the ossification centers for the inferior articulating processes of L5 is identified (arrows). COMMENT: This has been referred to as "Oppenheimer's ossicles."

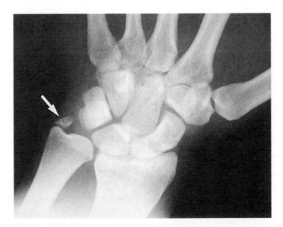

Figure 3.233.   UNUNITED SECONDARY OSSIFICATION CENTER. Ulna.
Observe the nonunion of the ulnar styloid process (arrow). COMMENT: This should not be mistaken for a fracture and is differentiated from same by its smooth sclerotic margins and lack of displacement.

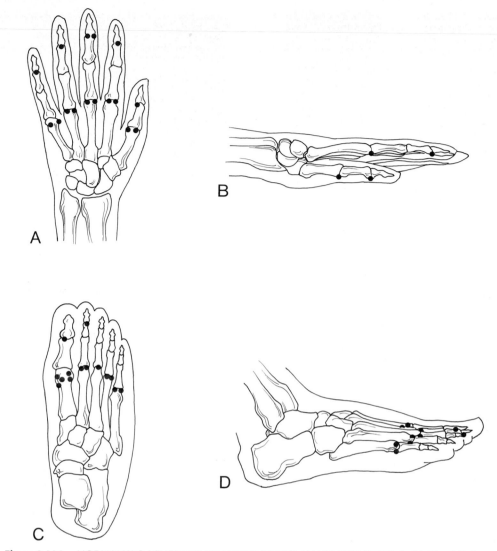

**Figure 3.234.   NORMALLY OCCURRING SESAMOID BONES: HAND AND FOOT. A. PA Hand. B. Lateral
Hand. C. Dorsoplantar Foot. D. Lateral Foot.**

REFERENCES

ANOMALIES OF THE CRANIOVERTEBRAL REGION

Occipitalization of the Atlas

1. **Macalister A:** *Notes on the development and variations at the atlas.* J Anat Physiol 27:519, 1893.
2. **Dunsker SB, Brown O, Thompson N:** *Craniovertebral anomalies.* Clin Neurosurg 27:430, 1980.
3. **Harcourt BT, Mitchell TC:** *Occipitalization of the atlas.* J Manipulative Physiol Ther 13:532, 1990.
4. **Bassi P, Corona C, Contri P, et al:** *Congenital basilar impression: Correlated neurological syndromes.* Eur Neurol 32:238, 1992.
5. **Aragaki Y, Takatsu A, Shigeta A:** *Unusual mechanism of lethal cervical spinal cord injury in a case of atlanto-axial diastasis.* Int J Legal Med 106:41, 1993.
6. **Tokuda K, Miyasaka K, Abe H, et al:** *Anomalous atlantoaxial portions of vertebral and posterior inferior cerebellar arteries.* Neuroradiology 27:410, 1985.
7. **Bernal Sprekelsen M, Hormann K, Weh L:** *Sudden hearing loss and the craniocervical junction.* An Otorrinolaringol Ibero Am 17:353, 1990.

Occipital Vertebrae

1. **Hadley LA:** *Atlanto-occipital fusion, ossiculum terminale and occipital vertebra as related to basilar impression with neurological symptoms.* AJR 59:511, 1948.
2. **Lombardi G:** *The occipital vertebra.* AJR 86:260, 1961.
3. **Tulsi RS:** *Some specific anatomical features of the atlas and axis: Dens, epitransverse process and articular facets.* Aust NZ J Surg 48:570, 1978.
4. **Bertini G, Celenza M, Orsi R, et al:** *Osseous anomalies of the craniovertebral junction: A case report.* Ital J Orthop Traumatol 17:135, 1991.

5. **Gross A:** *Traumatic basal subarachnoid hemorrhages: Autopsy material analysis.* Forensic Sci Int 45:53, 1990.
6. **Schumacher S:** *Ein Beitrag zur Manifestation des Okcipitalwirbels.* Anat Anz 31:145, 1907.
7. **Fischer E:** *Akzessorische freie Knochenelemente in der Umgebung des Foramen occipitale magnum.* Fortschr Geb Rontgenstrahlen Nuklearmedizin 91:638, 1959.

Platybasia/Basilar Invagination

1. **Chamberlain WE:** *Basilar impression (platybasia).* Yale J Biol Med 11:487, 1939.
2. **Rothman RH, Simeone FA:** *The Spine,* ed 2. Philadelphia, WB Saunders, 1982.
3. **Bernal Sprekelsen M, Hormann K, Weh L:** *Sudden hearing loss and the craniocervical junction.* An Otorrinolaringol Ibero Am 17:353, 1990.
4. **Keats TE, Lusted LB:** *Atlas of Roentgenographic Measurement,* ed 5. Chicago, Year Book Medical Publishers, 1985.
5. **Kaden B, Cedzich C, Schultheiss R, et al:** *Disappearance of syringomyelia following resection of extramedullary lesion. A contribution to the aetiological enigma of syringomyelia.* Acta Neurochir (Wien) 123:211, 1993.
6. **Aragaki Y, Takatsu A, Shigeta A:** *Unusual mechanism of lethal cervical spinal cord injury in a case of atlanto-axial diastasis.* Int J Legal Med 106:41, 1993.

Arnold-Chiari Malformation

1. **Chiari H:** *Uber veranderungen des kleinhirns infolge von hydrocephalie des grosshirns.* Dtsch Med Wochenschr 17:1172, 1881.
2. **Elster AD, Chen MYM:** *Chiari I malformations: Clinical and radiologic reappraisal.* Radiology 183:347, 1992.
3. **Susman J, Jones C, Wheatley D:** *Arnold-Chiari malformation: A diagnostic challenge.* Am Fam Physician 39:207, 1989.
4. **DaSilva JA:** *Basilar impression and Arnold-Chiari malformation. Surgical findings in 209 cases.* Neurochirurgia (Stuttg) 35:189, 1992.

5. **Hida K, Iwasaki Y, Imamura H, et al:** *Birth injury as a causative factor of syringomyelia with Chiari I deformity.* J Neurol Neurosurg Psychiatry 57:373, 1994.
6. **Aronson DD, Kahn RH, Canady A, et al:** *Instability of the cervical spine after decompression in patients who have Arnold-Chiari malformation.* J Bone Joint Surg (Am) 73:898, 1991.
7. **Yochum TR, Barry MS, Gould SJ, et al:** *Wrong-sided scoliosis: When left isn't right.* J Neuromuscoskeletal Sys 2:195, 1994.

ANOMALIES OF THE CERVICAL SPINE

Agenesis of the Posterior Arch of the Atlas

1. **Gehweiler JA, Daffner RH, Roberts, L:** *Malformations of the atlas simulating the Jefferson fracture.* AJR 140:1083, 1983.
2. **Page GT, Yock DH:** *Total aplasia of the posterior arch of the atlas.* Minn Med 64:666, 1981.

Posterior Ponticle of the Atlas

1. **Kimmerly:** Roentgenpraxis 2:479, 1930. Cited by Dugdale LM: *The ponticulus posterior of the atlas.* Australas Radiol 25:237, 1981.
2. **Lamberty BGH, Zivanovic S:** *The retro-articular vertebral artery ring of the atlas and its significance.* Acta Anat 85:113, 1973.
3. **Limousin CA:** *Foramen arcuale and syndrome of Barre-Lieou: Its surgical treatment.* Int Orthop 4:19, 1980.
4. **Buna M, Coghlan W, deGruchy M, et al:** *Ponticles of the atlas: A review and clinical perspective.* J Manipulative Physiol Ther 7:261, 1984.
5. **Gatterman MI:** *Contraindications and complications of spinal manipulative technique.* ACA J Chiro 15:75, 1981.
6. **Gross A:** *Traumatic basal subarachnoid hemorrhages: Autopsy material analysis.* Forensic Sci Int 45:53, 1990.

Agenesis of the Anterior Arch of the Atlas

1. **Dwight T:** *Account of two spines with cervical ribs, one of which had a vertebra suppressed, and absence of the anterior arch of the atlas.* J Anat Physiol 21:539, 1886.
2. **Carella A:** *Slight anomalies of the atlas: Their pathogenetic meaning.* Neuroradiology 3:224, 1972.
3. **Mace SE, Holliday R:** *Congenital absence of the C1 vertebral arch.* Am J Emerg Med 4:326, 1986.
4. **Verjaal A, Harder NC:** *Backward luxation of the atlas: Report of a case.* Acta Radiol 3:173, 1965.
5. **Chapman S, Goldin JH, Hendel RG, et al:** *The median cleft face syndrome with associated cleft mandible, bifid odontoid peg and agenesis of the anterior arch of atlas.* Br J Oral Maxillofac Surg 29:279, 1991.
6. **Gamble JG, Rinsky LA:** *Combined occipitoatlantoaxial hypermobility with anterior and posterior arch defects of the atlas in Pierre-Robin syndrome.* J Pediatr Orthop 5:475, 1985.

Down's Syndrome

1. **Greenfield GB:** *Radiology of Bone Diseases,* ed 3. Philadelphia, JB Lippincott, 1980.
2. **Diamond LS, Lynne D, Sigman B:** *Orthopedic disorders in patients with Down's syndrome.* Orthop Clin North Am 12:57, 1981.
3. **Martel W, Tischerler JM:** *Observation on the spine in Mongoloidism.* AJR 97:630, 1966.
4. **Ozonoff MB:** *Pediatric Orthopedic Radiology,* Philadelphia, WB Saunders, 1979.
5. **La France ME:** *A chiropractic perspective on atlantoaxial instability in Down's syndrome.* J Manipulative Physiol Ther 13:157, 1990.
6. **Martich V, Tamar BA, Yousefzadeh DK, et al:** *Hypoplastic posterior arch of C-1 in children with Down syndrome: A double jeopardy.* Radiology 183:125, 1992.
7. **Yochum TR:** *Mongolism.* Euro J Chiro 30:158, 1982.
8. **Weinberg B, Maldjiian, Kass EG, et al:** *The prominent conoid process of the clavicle: A new radiographic sign in Down's syndrome.* AJR 160:591, 1993.
9. **Special Olympics Committee.** Special Olympics news release: Participation by individuals with Down syndrome who suffer from the atlanto-axial subluxation condition. Washington, D.C.: Special Olympics, March 31, 1983.
10. **Rosenbaum DM, Blumhagen JD, King HA:** *Atlantooccipital instability in Down syndrome.* AJR 146:1269, 1986.
11. **El-Khoury GY, Clark CR, Dietz FR, et al:** *Posterior atlantooccipital subluxation in Down syndrome.* Radiology 159:507, 1986.
12. **Tredwell SJ, Newman DE, Lockitch G:** *Instability of the upper cervical spine in Down syndrome.* J Pediatr Orthop 10:602, 1990.
13. **Segal LS, Drummond DS, Zanotti RM, et al:** *Complications of posterior arthrodesis of the cervical spine in patients who have Down syndrome.* J Bone Joint Surg (Am) 73:1547, 1991.
14. **Olive PM, Whitecloud TS III, Bennett JT:** *Lower cervical spondylosis and myelopathy in adults with Down's syndrome.* Spine 13:781, 1988.

Ossiculum Terminale Persistens of Bergman

1. **Rothman RH, Simeone FA:** *The Spine,* vol 1. Philadelphia, WB Saunders, 1982.

Os Odontoideum

1. **Minderhound JM, Braakman R, Penning L:** *Os odontoideum: Clinical, radiological, and therapeutic aspects.* J Neurol Sci 8:521, 1969.
2. **Rothman RH, Simeone FA:** *The Spine,* ed 2. Philadelphia, WB Saunders, 1982.
3. **Fielding JW, Hensiger RN, Hawkins RJ:** *Os odontoideum.* J Bone Joint Surg (Am) 62:376, 1980.
4. **Hukuda S, Ota H, Okabe N, et al:** *Traumatic atlantoaxial dislocation causing os odontoideum in infants.* Spine 5:207, 1980.

5. **Fielding JW, Griffin PP:** *Os odontoideum: An acquired lesion.* J Bone Joint Surg (Am) 56:187, 1974.
6. **Woolin DG:** *The os odontoideum.* J Bone Joint Surg (Am) 45:1459, 1963.
7. **Stevens JM, Chong WK, Barber C, et al:** *A new appraisal of abnormalities of the odontoid process associated with atlanto-axial subluxation and neurological disability.* Brain 117:133, 1994.
8. **Morgan MK, Onofrio BM, Bender CE:** *Familial os odontoideum. Case report.* J Neurosurg 70:636, 1989.
9. **Kirlew KA, Hathout GM, Reiter SD, et al:** *Os odontoideum in identical twins: Perspectives on etiology.* Skeletal Radiol 22:525, 1993.
10. **Takakuwa T, Hiroi S, Hasegawa H, et al:** *Os odontoideum with vertebral artery occlusion.* Spine 19:460, 1994.
11. **McGoldrick JM, Marx JA:** *Traumatic central cord syndrome in a patient with os odontoideum.* Ann Emerg Med 18:1358, 1989.
12. **Dempster AG, Heap SW:** *Fatal high cervical spinal cord injury in an automobile accident complicating os odontoideum.* Am J Forensic Med Pathol 11:252, 1990.
13. **Epstein BS:** *The Spine-A Radiological Text and Atlas,* ed 4. Philadelphia, Lea & Febiger, 1976.
14. **Holt RG, Helms CA, Munk PL, et al:** *Hypertrophy of C-1 anterior arch: Useful sign to distinguish os odontoideum from acute dens fracture.* Radiology 173:207, 1989.
15. **Yamashita Y, Takahashi M, Sakamoto Y, et al:** *Atlantoaxial subluxation. Radiography and magnetic resonance imaging correlated to myelopathy.* Acta Radiol 30:135, 1989.
16. **Moser EA, Harbough RE, Cromwell L, et al:** *Os odontoideum and posterior circulation stroke in childhood.* J Neuromuscoskel Sys 1:170, 1993.
17. **Bhatnagar M, Sponseller PD, Carroll C IV, et al:** *Pediatric atlantoaxial instability presenting as cerebral and cerebellar infarcts.* J Pediatr Orthop 11:103, 1991.

Hypoplastic and Agenetic Odontoid Process

1. **McRae DL:** *The significance of abnormalities of the cervical spine.* AJR 84:3, 1960.
2. **Phillips PC, Lorentsen KJ, Shropshire LC, et al:** *Congenital odontoid aplasia and posterior circulation stroke in childhood.* Ann Neurol 23:410, 1988.
3. **Thomas SL, Childress MH, Quinton B:** *Hypoplasia of the odontoid with atlanto-axial subluxations in Hurler's syndrome.* Pediatr Radiol 15:353, 1985.

Block Vertebra

1. **Lovell WW, Winter RB:** *Pediatric Orthopedics,* Philadelphia, JB Lippincott, 1978.
2. **Wiesel SW, Rothman RH:** *Occipitoatlantal hypermobility.* Spine 4:187, 1979.
3. **Meschan I:** *Analysis of Roentgen Signs,* Philadelphia, WB Saunders, 1973.
4. **Sutton D:** *A Textbook of Radiology and Imaging,* ed 3. New York, Churchill Livingstone, 1980.

Klippel-Feil Syndrome

1. **Klippel M, Feil A:** *Un cas d'absence des vertebres cervicales. Avec cage thoracique remontant jusqu'a la base du crane (cage thoracique cervicale).* Nouv Iconog Salpetriere 25:223, 1912.
2. **Hensinger RN, Lang JE, MacEwen GD:** *Klippel-Feil syndrome. A constellation of associated anomalies.* J Bone Joint Surg (Am) 56:1246, 1974.
3. **Duncan PA:** *Embryologic pathogenesis of renal agenesis associated with cervical vertebral anomalies (Klippel-Feil phenotype).* Birth Defects 13:91, 1977.
4. **Lovell WW, Winter RB:** *Pediatric Orthopedics,* Philadelphia, JB Lippincott, 1978.
5. **Tredwell SJ, Smith DF, Macleod PJ, et al:** *Cervical spine anomalies in fetal alcohol syndrome.* Spine 7:331, 1982.
6. **Ritterbusch JF, McGinty LD, Spar J, et al:** *Magnetic resonance imaging for stenosis and subluxation in Klippel-Feil syndrome.* Spine 16:S539, 1991.
7. **Ducker TB:** *Cervical myeloradiculopathy: Klippel-Feil deformity.* J Spinal Disorders 3:439, 1990.
8. **Hall JE, Simmons ED, Danylchuk K, et al:** *Instability of the cervical spine and neurological involvement in Klippel-Feil syndrome.* J Bone Joint Surg (Am) 72:460, 1990.
9. **Born CT, Petrik M, Freed M, et al:** *Cerebrovascular accident complicating Klippel-Feil syndrome.* J Bone Joint Surg (Am) 70:1412, 1988.

Sprengel's Deformity

1. **Eulenberg M:** *Casuistis Mittheilungen aus dem Begiete der Orthopadie.* Arch Klin Chir 4:301, 1863.
2. **Sprengle OGK:** *Die angeborene Verschiebung des Schulterblattes nach oben.* Arch Klin Chir 42:545, 1891.
3. **Lovell WW, Winter RB:** *Pediatric Orthopedics,* Philadelphia, JB Lippincott, 1978.
4. **Ogden JA, Conlogue AB, Phillips SB, et al:** *Sprengel's deformity. Radiology of the pathologic deformation.* Skeletal Radiol 4:204, 1979.
5. **Willett A, Walsham WJ:** *An account of the dissection of the parts removed after death from the body of a woman the subject of congenital malformation of the spinal column, bony thorax, and left scapular arch. With remarks on the probable nature of the defects in development producing the deformities.* Med Chir Trans 63:257, 1880.
6. **Jenkinson SG:** *Undescended scapula associated with omovertebral bone: Sprengel's deformity.* J La State Med Soc 129:13, 1977.

Cervical Spondylolisthesis

1. **Perlman R, Hawes LE:** *Cervical spondylolisthesis.* J Bone Joint Surg (Am) 33: 1012, 1951.
2. **Niemeyer T, Penning L:** *Functional roentgenographic examination in a case of cervical spondylolisthesis.* J Bone Joint Surg (Am) 45:1671, 1963.
3. **Rowe L, Steiman I:** *Anterolisthesis in the cervical spine-spondylolysis.* J Manipulative Physiol Ther 10:11, 1987.

4. **Jeanneret B, Magerl F:** *Congenital fusion C0-C2 associated with spondylolysis of C2.* J Spinal Disorders 3:413, 1990.
5. **Hanson EC, Shook JE, Wiesseman GJ, et al:** *Congenital pedicle defects of the axis vertebra.* Spine 15:236, 1990.
6. **Riebel GD, Bayley JC:** *A congenital defect resembling the hangman's fracture.* Spine 16:1240, 1991.
7. **Barnes DA, Borns P, Pizzutillo PD:** *Cervical spondylolisthesis associated with multiple nevoid basal cell carcinoma syndrome.* Clin Orthop 162:26, 1982.
8. **Black KS, Gorey MT, Seidman B, et al:** *Congenital spondylolisthesis of the 6th cervical vertebra: CT findings.* J Comput Assist Tomogr 15:335, 1991.

Absent Pedicle of the Cervical Spine

1. **Hadley LA:** *Congenital absence of pedicle from cervical vertebra.* AJR 55:193, 1946.
2. **Tiyaworabun S, Beeko D, Bock WJ:** *Congenital absence of a pedicle in the cervical spine.* Acta Neurochir 61:303, 1982.
3. **van Dijk Azn R, Thijssen HOM, Merx JL, et al:** *The absent cervical pedicle syndrome.* Neuroradiology 29:69, 1987.
4. **Sakou T, Morizono Y:** *Congenital absence of a vertebral pedicle in the cervical spine. A case report.* Clin Orthop 175:51, 1983.
5. **Wiener MD, Martinez S, Forsberg DA:** *Congenital absence of a cervical spine pedicle: Clinical and radiologic findings.* AJR 155:1037, 1990.

Cervical Rib

1. **DuToit J, DeMuelenaere P:** *Isolated fracture of a cervical rib.* S Afr Med J 18:62, 1982.
2. **Kosenak LM, Knorr EJ, DeRojas JJ, et al:** *Cervical rib variant: Report of a case.* Ann Vasc Surg 6:292, 1992.
3. **Sutton D:** *A Textbook of Radiology and Imaging,* ed 3. New York, Churchill Livingstone, 1980.
4. **Nemmers DW, Thorpe PE, Knibbe MA, et al:** *Upper extremity venous thrombosis. Case report and literature review.* Orthop Rev 19:164, 1990.
5. **Engel A, Adler OB, Carmeli R:** *Subclavian artery aneurysm caused by cervical rib: Case report and review.* Cardiovasc Intervent Radiol 12:92, 1989.

ANOMALIES OF THE THORACIC AND LUMBAR SPINE

Butterfly Vertebra

1. **Schmorl G, Junghans H:** *The Human Spine in Health and Disease,* ed 2. New York, Grune & Stratton, 1971.
2. **Murray RO, Jacobson HG:** *The Radiology of Skeletal Disorders,* New York, Churchill Livingstone, 1977.
3. **Tanaka T, Uhthoff HK:** *Coronal cleft vertebrae, a variant of normal enchondral ossification.* Acta Orthop Scand 54:389, 1983.
4. **Emery JL:** *Deformities of the vertebral bodies.* Dev Med Child Neurol 24:692, 1982.
5. **von Rokitansky C:** *Handbuch du Pathologischen Anatomie,* Wien, Braumuller und Seidel, 1844.
6. **Epstein BS:** *The Spine-A Radiological Text and Atlas,* ed 4. Philadelphia, Lea & Febiger, 1976.

Hemivertebrae

1. **Epstein BS:** *The Spine-A Radiological Text and Atlas,* ed 4. Philadelphia, Lea & Febiger, 1976.
2. **Murray RO, Jacobson HG:** *The Radiology of Skeletal Disorders,* New York, Churchill Livingstone, 1977.
3. **Gjorup PA:** *Dorsal hemivertebrae.* Acta Orthop Scand 35:117, 1964.
4. **Blummel J:** *An analysis of the charts and roentgenograms of 264 patients.* Am Surg 28:501, 1962.
5. **Wilkinson RH, Strand RD:** *Congenital anomalies and normal variants.* Semin Roentgenol 1:7, 1979.
6. **Yochum TR, Hartley B, Thomas DP, et al:** *A radiographic anthology of vertebral names.* J Manipulative Physiol Ther 8:87, 1985.

Schmorl's Node

1. **Resnick D, Niwayama G:** *Intravertebral disk herniations: Cartilaginous (Schmorl's) nodes.* Radiology 126:57, 1978.
2. **Coventry MB, Ghormley RK, Kernohan JW:** *Intervertebral disc—its microscopic anatomy and pathology; changes in the intervertebral disc concomitant with age.* J Bone Joint Surg (Am) 27:233, 1945.
3. **Coventry MB, Ghormley RK, Kernohan JW:** *Intervertebral disc—its microscopic anatomy and pathology; pathologic changes in the intervertebral disc.* J Bone Joint Surg (Am) 27:460, 1945.
4. **Hilton RC, Ball J, Benn RT:** *Vertebral end-plate lesions (Schmorl's nodes) in the dorsolumbar spine.* Ann Rheum Dis 35:127, 1976.
5. **Lipson SJ, Fox DA, Sosman JL:** *Symptomatic intravertebral disc herniation (Schmorl's node) in the cervical spine.* Ann Rheum Dis 44:857, 1985.
6. **Walters G, Coumas JM, Akins CM, et al:** *Magnetic resonance imaging of acute symptomatic Schmorl's node formation.* Pediatr Emerg Care 7:294, 1991.
7. **Yochum TR, Wylie J, Green RL:** *Schmorl's node phenomenon.* J Neuromusculoskel Sys 2:19, 1994.
8. **Takahashi K, Takata Z:** *A large painful Schmorl's node: A case report.* J Spinal Disorders 7:77, 1994.
9. **Malmivaara A, Videman T, Kuosma E, et al:** *Plain radiographic, discographic, and direct observations of Schmorl's nodes in the thoracolumbar junctional region of the cadaveric spine.* Spine 12:453, 1987.
10. **Resnick D, Niwayama G:** *Diagnosis of Bone Disorders,* Philadelphia, WB Saunders, 1981.

11. **Rothman RH, Simeone FA:** *The Spine,* ed 2. Philadelphia, WB Saunders, 1982.
12. **Dietz GW, Christensen EE:** *Normal "Cupid's bow" contour of the lower lumbar vertebrae.* Radiology 121:577, 1976.
13. **Ramirez H, Navarro JE, Bennett WF:** *"Cupid's bow" contour of the lumbar vertebral endplates detected by computed tomography.* J Comput Assist Tomogr 8:121, 1984.

VATER Syndrome

1. **Quan L, Smith DW:** *The VATER association: Vertebral defects, anal atresia, tracheoesophageal fistula with esophageal atresia, radial and renal dysplasia: A spectrum of associated defects.* J Pediatr 82:104, 1973.
2. **Barne JC, Smith WL:** *The VATER Association.* Radiology 126:445, 1978.
3. **Temtamy SA, Miller JD:** *Extending the scope of the VATER association: Definition of the VATER syndrome.* J Pediatr 85:345, 1974.
4. **McNeal RM, Skoglund RR, Francke U:** *Congenital anomalies including the VATER association in a patient with a del(6)q deletion.* J Pediatr 91:957, 1977.

Agenesis of a Lumbar Pedicle

1. **Wortzman G, Steinhardt MI:** *Congenitally absent lumbar pedicle: A reappraisal.* Radiology 152:713, 1984.
2. **Sener RN, Ripeckyj GT, Jinkins JR:** *Agenesis of a lumbar pedicle: MR demonstration.* Neuroradiology 33:464, 1991.

Spina Bifida Occulta and Vera

1. **Nachemson A:** *The lumbar spine—an orthopedic challenge.* Spine 1:59, 1976.
2. **Magora A, Schwartz A:** *Relation between the low back pain syndrome and x-ray findings. III. Spina bifida occulta.* Scand J Rehabil Med 12:9, 1980.
3. **Carter CO:** *Genetics of spina bifida.* In: Proceedings of Symposium on Spina Bifida. London, Christofer Foss, 1965.

Meningocele/Myelomeningocele

1. **Epstein BS:** *The Spine-A Radiological Text and Atlas,* ed 4. Philadelphia, Lea & Febiger, 1976.
2. **Turek SL:** *Orthopedics Principles and Their Application,* ed 4. Philadelphia, JB Lippincott, 1984.
3. **Adams MJ, Windham GC, James LM, et al:** *Clinical interpretation of maternal alpha fetoprotein concentrations.* Am J Obstet Gynecol 148:241, 1984.
4. **Greenfield GB:** *Radiology of Bone Diseases,* ed 3. Philadelphia, JB Lippincott, 1980.
5. **Epstein BS:** *The Vertebral Column: An Atlas of Tumor Radiology,* Chicago, Year Book Medical Publishers, 1974.
6. **Yochum TR, Hartley B, Thomas DP, et al:** *A radiographic anthology of vertebral names.* J Manipulative Physiol Ther 8:87, 1985.
7. **Resnick D, Niwayama G:** *Diagnosis of Bone and Joint Disorders.* Philadelphia, WB Saunders, 1981.

Diastematomyelia

1. **Ollivier CP:** *Traites des maladies de la moelle epiniere,* ed 3. Paris, Mequignon-Marvis, 1837.
2. **Scatliff JH, Till K, Hoare RD:** *Incomplete, false, and true diastematolyelia.* Radiology 116, 349, 1975.
3. **Herman TE, Siegel MJ:** *Cervical and basicranial diastematomyelia.* AJR 154:806, 1990.
4. **Boulot P, Ferran JL, Charlier C, et al:** *Prenatal diagnosis of diastematomyelia.* Pediatr Radiol 23:67, 1993.
5. **Mick TJ, Tuchscherer MM:** *Diastematomyelia diagnosed in adulthood.* Top Diagn Radiol Adv Imag 1:4, 1993.
6. **Rawanduzy A, Murali R:** *Cervical spine diastematomyelia in adulthood.* Neurosurgery 28:459, 1991.
7. **Hesselink JW, Tans JT, Hoogland PH:** *Diastematomyelia presenting in two male adults with low back pain.* Clin Neurol Neurosurg 88:223, 1986.
8. **Hilal S, Marton D, Pollack E:** *Diastematomyelia in children.* Radiology 112:609, 1974.

Transitional Vertebrae

1. **Elster AD:** *Bertolotti's syndrome revisited: Transitional vertebrae of the lumbar spine.* Spine 14:1373, 1989.
2. **Tini PG, Wieser C, Zinn WM:** *The transitional vertebra of the lumbosacral spine: Its radiological classification, incidence, prevalence, and clinical significance.* Rheumatol Rehabil 16:180, 1977.
3. **Nachemson A:** *Towards a better understanding of low-back pain.* Rheumatol Rehabil 14:129, 1975.
4. **Castellvi AE, Goldstein LA, Chan DPK:** *Lumbosacral transitional vertebrae and their relationship with lumbar extradural defects.* Spine 9:493, 1984.
5. **Hadley LA:** *Anatomico-roentgenographic Studies of the Spine,* ed 2. Springfield, Charles C Thomas, 1973.
6. **Bertolotti M:** *Contributo alla conoscenza dei vizi di differenzazione regionale del rachide con speciale riquardo all assimilazione sacrale della V lombare.* Radiol Med 4:113, 1917.
7. **Nicholson AA, Roberts GM, Williams LA:** *The measured height of the lumbosacral disc in patients with and without transitional vertebrae.* Br J Radiol 61:454, 1988.

Facet Tropism

1. **Rothman RH, Simeone FA:** *The Spine,* ed 2. Philadelphia, WB Saunders, 1982.
2. **Nachemson A:** *The lumbar spine-an orthopaedic challenge.* Spine 1:59, 1976.
3. **Farfan HF, Sullivan JD:** *The relationship of facet orientation to intervertebral disc failure.* Can J Surg 10:179, 1967.

4. **Hagg O, Wallner A:** *Facet joint asymmetry and protrusion of the intervertebral disc.* Spine 15:356, 1990.
5. **Murtagh FR, Paulsen RD, Rechtine GR:** *The role and incidence of facet tropism in lumbar spine degenerative disc disease.* J Spinal Disord 4:86, 1991.
6. **Cassidy JD, Loback D, Yong-Hing K, et al:** *Lumbar facet joint asymmetry. Intervertebral disc herniation.* Spine 17:570, 1992.
7. **Vanharanta H, Floyd T, Ohnmeiss DD, et al:** *The relationship of facet tropism to degenerative disc disease.* Spine 18:1000, 1993.
8. **Cox JM, Aspegren DD, Trier KK:** *Facet tropism: Comparison of plain film and computed tomography examinations.* J Manipulative Physiol Ther 14:355, 1991.
9. **Downey EF, Nason SS, Massoud M, et al:** *Asymmetrical facet joints: Another cause for the sclerotic pedicle.* Spine 8:340, 1983.

Clasp Knife Syndrome

1. **Ferguson AB:** *The clinical and roentgenographic interpretation of lumbosacral anomalies.* Radiology 22:548, 1934.
2. **Bellerose MN:** *Low-back pain caused by lumbosacral abnormalities.* NEJM 213:177, 1935.
3. **DeAnguin CE:** *Spina bifida occulta with engagement of the fifth lumbar spinous process.* J Bone Joint Surg (Br) 41:486, 1959.
4. **Gill GG, White HL:** *Mechanisms of nerve-root compression and irritation in backache.* Clin Orthop 5:66, 1955.
5. **Stark WA:** *Spina bifida occulta and engagement of the fifth lumbar spinous process.* Clin Orthop 81:71, 1971.
6. **Goobar JE, Erickson F, Pate D, et al:** *Symptomatic clasp-knife deformity of the spinous processes.* Spine 13:953, 1988.

ANOMALIES OF THE THORAX
Srb's Anomaly/Luschka's Rib

1. **Srb:** *Med Jb kk Ges Artze,* Vienna, 1862. Cited in: Kohler A, Zimmer EA: *Borderlands of the Normal and Early Pathologic in Skeletal Radiology,* ed 3. New York, Grune & Stratton, 1968.

Straight Back Syndrome

1. **Wermut W, Rein B:** *Straight back syndrome. Case report.* Polski Tygodnik Lekarski 45:225, 1990.
2. **Datey KK, Deshmukh MM, Engineer SD, et al:** *Straight back syndrome.* Br Heart J 26:614, 1964.
3. **Davies MK, Mackintosh P, Cayton RM, et al:** *The straight back syndrome.* Q J M 49:443, 1980.
4. **Twigg HL, DeLeon A, Perloff JK, et al:** *The straight-back syndrome: Radiographic manifestations.* Radiology 88:274, 1967.
5. **Ayres JG, Pope FM, Reidy JF, et al:** *Abnormalities of the lungs and thoracic cage in the Ehlers-Danlos syndrome.* Thorax 40:300, 1985.
6. **Wander GS, Garg K, Anand IS:** *Swallowing induced supraventricular ectopics in a patient with straight back syndrome.* Jpn Heart J 30:523, 1989.
7. **Takeuchi E, Tamaki S, Watanabe T, et al:** *A case report of mitral valve regurgitation due to the infective endocarditis associated with the straight back syndrome.* J Jpn Sur Soc 91:914, 1990.
8. **Kumar UK, Sahasranam KV:** *Mitral valve prolapse syndrome and associated thoracic skeletal abnormalities.* J Assoc Physicians India 39:536, 1991.
9. **Iwafuchi Y, Okada Y, Kato T, et al:** *A case of complete absence of the left pericardium coexisting with straight back syndrome.* Respir Circ 39:1055, 1991.

ANOMALIES OF THE HIP AND PELVIS
Congenital Hip Dysplasia

1. **Resnick D, Niwayama G:** *Diagnosis of Bone Disorders.* Philadelphia, WB Saunders, 1981.
2. **Putti V:** *Early treatment of congenital dislocation of the hip.* J Bone Joint Surg (Am) 11:798, 1929.

Sacral Dysplasia

1. **Hohl AF:** *Die Geburten missgestalteter, kranker und todter Kinder.* Verlag der Buchhandlung des Waisenhauses, 1850.
2. **Friedel G:** *Defekt der Wirbelsaule vom 10. Brust an abwarts bei einem Neugeborenen.* Arch Klin Chir 93:944, 1910.
3. **Pedersen LM, Tygstrup I, Pedersen J:** *Congenital malformations in newborn infants of diabetic women.* Lancet 1:1124, 1964.
4. **Renshaw TS:** *Sacral agenesis: A classification and review of 23 cases.* J Bone Joint Surg (Am) 60:373, 1978.

Coxa Vara/Coxa Valga

1. **Katz JF, Siffert SS:** *Management of Hip Disorders in Children,* Philadelphia, JB Lippincott, 1983.
2. **Calhoun JD, Pierret G:** *Infantile coxa vara.* AJR 115:561, 1972.
3. **Sutton D:** *A Textbook of Radiology and Imaging,* ed 3. Edinburgh, Churchill Livingstone, 1980.

ANOMALIES OF THE EXTREMITIES
Bipartite, Tripartite, and Multipartite Patellae

1. **Weaver JK:** *Bipartite patellae as a cause of disability in the athlete.* Am J Sports Med 5:137, 1977.
2. **Green WT:** *Painful bipartite patellae.* Clin Orthop 110:197, 1975.

3. **Halpern AA, Hewitt O:** *Painful medial bipartite patellae.* Clin Orthop 134:180, 1978.
4. **Keats TE:** *An Atlas of Normal Roentgen Variants that May Simulate Disease,* ed 3. Chicago, Year Book Medical, 1984.

Fong's Syndrome

1. **Fong EE:** *Iliac horns (symmetrical bilateral central posterior iliac processes): Case report.* Radiology 47:517, 1946.
2. **Murray RO, Jacobson HG:** *Radiology of Skeletal Disorders,* Edinburgh, Churchill Livingstone, 1977.

Tarsal Coalition

1. **Harris BA:** *Anomalous structures in the developing human foot.* Anat Rec 121:1339, 1955.
2. **Leonard MA:** *The inheritance of tarsal coalitions and its relationship to spastic flatfoot.* J Bone Joint Surg (Br) 56:520, 1974.
3. **Jacobs AM, Sollecito V, Oloff L, et al:** *Tarsal coalitions: An instructional review.* J Foot Surg 20:214, 1981.
4. **Outland T, Murphy ID:** *Relation of tarsal anomalies in spastic rigid flatfeet.* Clin Orthop 1:217, 1953.
5. **Kaplan EG, Kaplan GS, Vaccari OA:** *Tarsal coalition: Review and preliminary conclusions.* J Foot Surg 16:136, 1977.
6. **O'Rahilly R:** *A survey of carpal and tarsal anomalies.* J Bone Joint Surg (Am) 35:626, 1953.

Vertical Talus

1. **Patterson WR, Fitz DA, Smith WS:** *The pathologic anatomy of congenital convex pes valgus.* J Bone Joint Surg (Am) 50:458, 1968.
2. **Jacobsen ST, Crawford AH:** *Congenital vertical talus.* J Pediatr Orthop 3:306, 1983.

Morton's Syndrome

1. **Morton D:** *The Human Foot,* New York, Columbia University Press, 1948.
2. **Jahss MH:** *Disorders of the Foot,* Philadelphia, WB Saunders, 1982.

Supracondylar Process of the Humerus

1. **Terry RJ:** *A study of the supracondyloid process in the living.* Am J Phys Anthropol 4:129, 1921.
2. **Laha RK, Dujovny M, DeCastro SC:** *Entrapment of median nerve by supracondylar process of the humerus.* J Neurosurg 46:252, 1977.
3. **Barnard LB, McCoy SM:** *The supracondyloid process of the humerus.* J Bone Joint Surg (Am) 28:845, 1946.
4. **Struthers J:** *On a peculiarity of the humerus and humeral anatomy.* Month J Med Sci 9:264, 1849.
5. **Curtis JA, O'Hara AE, Carpenter GG:** *Spurs of the mandible and supracondylar process of the humerus in Cornelia de Lange syndrome.* AJR 129:156, 1977.

Radioulnar Synostosis

1. **Hansen OH, Anderson NO:** *Congenital radio-ulnar synostosis. Report of 37 cases.* Acta Orthop Scand 41:225, 1970.
2. **Turek SL:** *Orthopedics Principles and Their Application,* ed 4. Philadelphia, JB Lippincott, 1984.
3. **Freyer B:** *Ungewohnliche beobachtung dobbelseitiger kongenitaler synostosen zwischen radius und ulna.* Radiologie 6:253, 1966.

Madelung's Deformity

1. **Madelung OW:** *Die spontane subluxation der hand nach vorne.* Verh Dtsch Ges Chir 7:259, 1878.
2. **Lichenstein JR, Sundaram M, Burdge R:** *Sex-influenced expression of Madelung's deformity in a family with dyschondrosteosis.* J Med Genet 17:41, 1980.
3. **Nielsen JB:** *Madelung's deformity. A follow-up study of 26 cases and a review of the literature.* Acta Orthop Scand 48:379, 1977.
4. **Kaitila II, Leisti JT, Rimoin DL:** *Mesomelic skeletal dysplasias.* Clin Orthop 114:94, 1976.

Negative Ulnar Variance

1. **Werner FW, Palmer AK, Fortino MD, et al:** *Force transmission through the distal ulna: Effect of ulnar variance, lunate fossa angulation, and radial and palmar tilt of the distal radius.* J Hand Surg (Am) 17(3):423, 1992.
2. **Epner RA, Bowers WH, Guilford WB:** *Ulnar variance—the effect of wrist positioning and roentgen filming technique.* J Hand Surg (Am) 7(3):298, 1982.
3. **Hulten O:** *Uber anatomische variationen der Hand-Gelenkknochen.* Acta Radiol 9:155, 1928.
4. **Gelberman RH, Salamon PB, Jurist JM, et al:** *Ulnar variance in Kienbock's disease.* J Bone Jt Surg (Am) 57(5):674, 1975.
5. **Chen WS, Shih CH:** *Ulnar variance and Kienbock's disease. An investigation in Taiwan.* Clin Orthop Rel Res. (255):124, 1990.
6. **Kristensen SS, Sobaile K:** *Kienbock's disease—the influence arthrosis on ulnar variance measurements.* J Hand Surg (Br) 12:301, 1987.
7. **Kristensen SS, Thomassen E, Christensen F:** *Ulnar variance in Kienbock's disease.* J Hand Surg (Br) 11:258, 1986.
8. **D'Hoore K, De Smet L, Verellen K, et al:** *Negative ulnar variance is not a risk factor for Kienbock's disease.* J Hand Surg (Am) 19:229, 1994.
9. **De Smet L:** *Ulnar variance: Facts and fiction review article.* Acta Orthop Belgica 60:1, 1994.

10. **Czitrom AA, Dobyns JH, Linscheid RL:** *Ulnar variance in carpal instability.* J Hand Surg (Am) 12:205, 1987.
11. **Larsen CF, Lindequist S, Bellstrom T:** *Lack of correlation between ulnar variance and carpal bone angles on lateral radiographs in normal wrists.* Acta Radiol 33:275, 1992.
12. **Voorhees DR, Daffner RH, Nunley JA, et al:** *Carpal ligamentous disruptions and negative ulnar variance.* Skeletal Radiol 13:257, 1985.
13. **De Smet L:** *Ulnar variance: Facts and fiction review article.* Acta Orthop Belgica 60:1, 1994.
14. **Weiss AP:** *Radial shortening.* Hand Clinics 9:475, 1993.
15. **Weiss AP, Weiland AJ, Moore JR, et al:** *Radial shortening for Kienbock's disease.* J Bone Joint Surg (Am) 73:384, 1991.

Carpal Coalition

1. **Cope JR:** *Carpal Coalition.* Clin Radiol 25:261, 1974.
2. **Poznanski AK, Holt JF:** *The carpals in congenital malformation syndromes.* AJR 112:443, 1971.

Polydactyly

1. **Poznanski AK:** *The Hand in Radiologic Diagnosis,* ed 2. WB Saunders, 1984.

Syndactyly

1. **MacCollum DW:** *Webbed fingers.* Surg Gynecol Obstet 71:782, 1940.
2. **Nylen B:** *Repair of congenital finger syndactyly.* Acta Chir Scand 113:310, 1957.
3. **Kelikian H:** *Congenital Deformities of the Hand and Forearm,* Philadelphia, WB Saunders, 1974.
4. **Castilla EE, Paz JE, Orioli-Parreiras IM:** *Syndactyly: Frequency of specific types.* Am J Med Genet 5:357, 1980.
5. **Temtamy SA, McKusick VA:** *The genetics of hand malformations.* Birth Defects 14:1, 1978.
6. **Poznanski AK:** *The Hand in Radiologic Diagnosis,* ed 2. Philadelphia, WB Saunders, 1974.

Kirner's Deformity

1. **Kirner J:** *Doppelseitige Verkrummungen des Kleinfingerendgliedes als Selbstandiges Krankheitsbild.* Fortschr Geb Rontgenstrahlen 36:804, 1927.
2. **Poznanski AK:** *The Hand in Radiologic Diagnosis,* ed 2. Philadelphia,WB Saunders, 1984.
3. **Steinback H, Gold R, Preger L:** *Roentgen Appearance of the Hand in Diffuse Disease,* Chicago, Year Book Medical, 1975.

4

Scoliosis

Lindsay J. Rowe and Terry R. Yochum

GENERAL CONSIDERATIONS

The term *scoliosis* is usually credited to Hippocrates.(1) Its derivation is from the Greek word *skolios*, meaning twisted or crooked. Within the disciplines of orthopedics and radiology, scoliosis describes any lateral deviation of the spine from the midsagittal plane. A review of past and present literature available on this subject reveals a voluminous amount of information and sophisticated research. This chapter is not intended to be an encyclopedic compilation of this data. Rather, it presents fundamental concepts, principles, and knowledge, particularly in relation to the role, evaluation, and clinical application of the radiologic examination.

CLASSIFICATION AND TERMINOLOGY

A standard vocabulary and classification system is utilized in the literature and is essential for accurate communication and description. (2,3)

CLASSIFICATION

Etiology

An etiologic classification for scoliosis is the most accepted method of categorizing lateral deviations of the spinal column. (2) (Table 4.1)

Location

Curvatures are described by the region of the spine in which the apex vertebra is located. (Fig. 4.1) (Table 4.2)

TERMINOLOGY

Numerous terms are commonly employed in the description of scoliotic deviations, vertebral abnormalities, and related findings. These have been standardized by the Terminology Committee of the Scoliosis Research Society. (3)

Scoliosis

Adolescent Scoliosis. Spinal curvature presenting at or about the onset of puberty and before maturity (10 to 25 years).

Adult Scoliosis. Spinal curvature existing after skeletal maturity.

Cervical Curve. Spinal curvature that has its apex from C1 to C6.

Cervicothoracic Curve. Spinal curvature that has its apex at C7 or T1.

Compensatory Curve. A curve above or below the primary curve, functioning as an adaptation to the primary curve and maintaining normal body alignment. It may be structural.

Congenital Scoliosis. Scoliosis due to congenitally anomalous vertebral development.

Curve Measurement. *Cobb Method:* Select the upper and lower end vertebrae; erect perpendiculars to their transverse axes. They intersect to form the angle of the curve. If the vertebral endplates are poorly visualized, a line through the bottom or top of the pedicles may be used.

Risser-Ferguson Method: The angle of a curve is formed by the intersection of two lines drawn from the center of the superior and inferior end vertebral bodies to the center of the apical vertebral body.

Double Major Scoliosis. A scoliosis with two structural curves.

Double Thoracic Curve (Scoliosis). A scoliosis with a structural upper thoracic curve, a larger, more deforming lower thoracic, and a relatively nonstructural lumbar curve.

Functional Curve. A compensatory curve that is incomplete because it returns to the erect. Its only horizontal vertebra is its caudad or cephalad one.

Table 4.1. Etiologic Classification of Scoliosis

STRUCTURAL SCOLIOSIS

I. IDIOPATHIC
  A. INFANTILE
    1. Resolving
    2. Progressive
  B. JUVENILE (3–10 years)
  C. ADOLESCENT (>10 years)
II. NEUROMUSCULAR
  A. NEUROPATHIC
    1. Upper Motor Neuron
     (a) Cerebral palsy
     (b) Spinocerebellar degeneration
      (1) Friedreich's disease
      (2) Charcot-Marie-Tooth disease
      (3) Roussy-Levy disease
     (c) Syringomyelia
     (d) Spinal cord tumor
     (e) Spinal cord trauma
     (f) Other
    2. Lower Motor Neuron
     (a) Poliomyelitis
     (b) Other viral myelitides
     (c) Traumatic
     (d) Spinal muscular atrophy
      (1) Werdnig-Hoffmann
      (2) Kugelberg-Welander
     (e) Myelomeningocele (paralytic)
    3. Dysautonomia (Riley-Day)
    4. Other
  B. MYOPATHIC
    1. Arthrogryposis
    2. Muscular Dystrophy
     (a) Duchenne (pseudohypertrophic)
     (b) Limb-girdle
     (c) Facioscapulohumeral
    3. Fiber Type Disproportion
    4. Congenital Hypotonia
    5. Myotonia Dystrophica
    6. Other
III. CONGENITAL
  A. FAILURE OF FORMATION
    1. Wedged Vertebra
    2. Hemivertebra

  B. FAILURE OF SEGMENTATION
    1. Unilateral (Unsegmented Bar)
    2. Bilateral
  C. MIXED
IV. NEUROFIBROMATOSIS
V. MESENCHYMAL DISORDERS
  A. MARFAN'S
  B. EHLERS-DANLOS
  C. OTHERS
VI. RHEUMATOID DISEASE
VII. TRAUMA
  A. FRACTURE
  B. SURGICAL
    1. Postlaminectomy
    2. Postthoracoplasty
  C. IRRADIATION
VIII. EXTRASPINAL CONTRACTURES
  A. POSTEMPYEMA
  B. POSTBURNS
IX. OSTEOCHONDRODYSTROPHIES
  A. DIASTROPHIC DWARFISM
  B. MUCOPOLYSACCHARIDOSES (e.g., Morquio's syndrome)
  C. SPONDYLOEPIPHYSEAL DYSPLASIA
  D. MULTIPLE EPIPHYSEAL DYSPLASIA
  E. OTHER
X. INFECTION OF BONE
  A. ACUTE
  B. CHRONIC
XI. METABOLIC DISORDERS
  A. RICKETS
  B. OSTEOGENESIS IMPERFECTA
  C. HOMOCYSTINURIA
  D. OTHERS
XII. RELATED TO LUMBOSACRAL JOINT
  A. SPONDYLOLYSIS AND SPONDYLOLISTHESIS
  B. CONGENITAL ANOMALIES OF LUMBOSACRAL REGION
XIII. TUMORS
  A. VERTEBRAL COLUMN
    1. Osteoid Osteoma
    2. Histiocytosis X
    3. Other
  B. SPINAL CORD (See Neuromuscular)

NONSTRUCTURAL SCOLIOSIS

I. POSTURAL SCOLIOSIS
II. HYSTERICAL SCOLIOSIS
III. NERVE ROOT IRRITATION
  A. HERNIATION OF NUCLEUS PULPOSUS
  B. TUMORS

IV. INFLAMMATORY (e.g., Appendicitis)
V. RELATED TO LEG LENGTH DISCREPANCY
VI. RELATED TO CONTRACTURES ABOUT THE HIP

Full Curve. A curve in which the only horizontal vertebra is at the apex.

Genetic Scoliosis. A structural spinal curvature inherited according to a genetic pattern.

Hysterical Scoliosis. A nonstructural deformity of the spine that develops as a manifestation of a conversion reaction.

Idiopathic Scoliosis. A structural spinal curvature for which no cause is established.

Infantile Scoliosis. Spinal curvature developing during the first 3 years of life.

Juvenile Scoliosis. Spinal curvature developing between skeletal age of 3 years and the onset of puberty (3 to 10 years).

Kyphoscoliosis. Lateral curvature of the spine associated with either increased posterior or decreased anterior angulation in the sagittal plane in excess of the accepted norm for that region. In the thoracic region, 20 to 40° of kyphosis is considered normal.

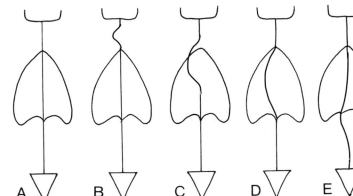

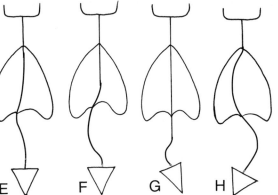

Figure 4.1. CLASSIFICATION OF SCOLIOSIS ACCORDING TO LOCA-
TION. A. Normal Spine. B. Cervical. C. Cervicothoracic. D. Mid Thoracic.

E. Thoracolumbar. F. Lumbar. G. Lumbosacral. H. Double Lumbar and
Thoracic.

Table 4.2. Classification of Scoliosis by Location	
Classification	Apex Vertebra
Cervical	C1–C6
Cervicothoracic	C7–T1
Thoracic	T2–T11
Thoracolumbar	T12–L1
Lumbar	L2–L4
Lumbosacral	L5–S1

Lordoscoliosis. Lateral curvature of the spine associated
with an increase in anterior curvature or a decrease in posterior
angulation in the sagittal plane in excess of normal for that region.
In a thoracic spine, where posterior angulation is normally present, less than 20° would constitute lordoscoliosis.

Lumbar Curve. Spinal curvature that has its apex from L1 to
L4.

Lumbosacral Curve. Spinal curvature that has its apex at L5
or below.

Major Curve. Term used to designate the larger(est) curve(s),
usually structural.

Minor Curve. Term used to refer to the smaller(est) curve(s).

Myogenic Scoliosis. Spinal curvature due to disease or
anomalies of the musculature.

Neurogenic Scoliosis. Spinal curvature due to disease or
anomalies of nerve tissue.

Nonstructural scoliosis (Functional). A curve that has no
structural component and that corrects or over corrects on recumbent side-bending radiographs.

Osteogenic Scoliosis. Spinal curvature due to abnormality of
the vertebral elements and/or adjacent ribs, acquired or
congenital.

Primary Curve. The first or earliest of several curves to appear, if identifiable.

Structural Curve. A segment of the spine with a fixed lateral
curvature. Radiographically, it is identified in supine lateral side-
bending films by the failure to correct. They may be multiple.

Thoracic Curve. Scoliosis in which the apex of the curvature
is between T2 and T11.

Thoracogenic Scoliosis. Spinal curvature attributable to disease or operative trauma in or on the thoracic cage.

Thoracolumbar Curve. Spinal curvature that has its apex at
T12 or L1.

Vertebral and Other Related Terms

Angle of Inclination. With the trunk flexed 90° at the hips,
the angle between the horizontal and a plane across the posterior
rib cage at the greatest prominence of a rib hump.

Apical Vertebra. The most rotated vertebra in a curve; the
most deviated vertebra from the vertical axis of the patient.

Body Alignment, Balance, Compensation. (a) The alignment
of the midpoint of the occiput over the sacrum in the same vertical
plane as the shoulders over hips. (b) In radiology, when the sum
of the angular deviations of the spine in one direction is equal to
that in the opposite direction.

End Vertebra. The most cephalad vertebra of a curve whose
superior surface or the most caudad one whose inferior surface
tilts maximally toward the concavity of the curve.

Gibbus. A sharply angular kyphosis.

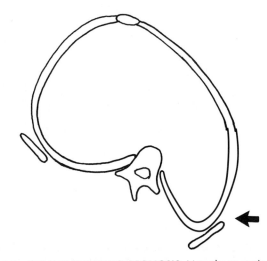

Figure 4.2. RIB HUMP DUE TO SCOLIOSIS. Note the posterior vertebral
body rotation on the side of the rib hump (arrow), which is usually most
prominent on the convex surface at the apex of the curve.

Iliac Epiphysis (Apophysis). The epiphysis along the wing of the ilium.

Iliac Epiphysis Sign (Apophysis Sign, Risser's Sign). In the anteroposterior roentgenogram of the spine, when the excursion of ossification in the iliac epiphysis (apophysis) reaches its ultimate medial migration, vertebral growth may be complete.

Kyphosis. A change in the alignment of a segment of the spine in the sagittal plane that increases the posterior convex angulation.

Pelvic Obliquity. Deviation of the pelvis from the horizontal in the frontal plane. Fixed pelvic obliquities can be attributable to contractures either above or below the pelvis.

Rib Hump. The prominence of the ribs on the convexity of a spinal curvature, usually due to vertebral rotation, best exhibited on forward bending. (Fig. 4.2)

Skeletal Age (Bone Age). The age obtained by comparing an anteroposterior roentgenogram of the left hand and wrist with the standards of the Gruelich and Pyle *Atlas.*

CLINICAL FEATURES

STRUCTURAL SCOLIOSIS

A structural scoliosis is a lateral curvature that is fixed and that fails to correct on recumbent lateral-bending radiographic studies. Many disorders are related to this type of spinal disorder. (Table 4.1)

Idiopathic Scoliosis

This is the most common form of lateral spinal deviation, accounting for up to 80% of scolioses. (4) The etiology is unknown, although many factors have been implicated. These include connective tissue disease, diet, enzymes, muscular imbalance, vestibular dysfunction, and inheritance. (5,6) Patients with scoliosis can have associated osteopenia while the intervertebral discs remain immature. (6,7)

Of all causes, an inherited genetic defect appears to play a significant role with up to 30% of patients having another family member with significant scoliosis. (8–10) A positive family history does not translate into worse curves or progressive curves. (10) The age of onset distinctively occurs within the growth period and allows for an age-based classification—infantile, juvenile, and adolescent.

Infantile Idiopathic Scoliosis. This occurs between birth and 3 years of age. The majority will disappear (resolving infantile idiopathic scoliosis), but some will occasionally progress (progressive infantile idiopathic scoliosis). (11) This progressive form is rare in the United States, is slightly more common in males, and is usually a left convex thoracic curve.

Juvenile Idiopathic Scoliosis. The onset is between 3 and 10 years of age, with an average age of 7 years. There is female gender predominance of 4 to 1. (12) As many as 30% will eventually have corrective surgery.

Adolescent Idiopathic Scoliosis. The curvature develops in the period between the age of 10 and skeletal maturity. The natural history of scoliosis has not significantly changed over the years. (13) The adolescent form remains the most common type of idiopathic scoliosis. Females are predominantly affected, with a ratio of 9 to 1 over males. (14) There is an increased incidence of coexisting pes cavus deformity. (15) The critical time period for progression, which may be rapid, is between the ages of 12 and 16. (Fig. 4.3) Once spinal growth has ceased, as indicated by

Figure 4.3. IDIOPATHIC SCOLIOSIS. A. No abnormality was observed in this 25-year-old female until 12 years of age, when her deformity was first detected. Despite bracing, her scoliosis progressed and has remained unchanged until this present radiograph. **B.** This 23-year-old female was radiographed for evaluation of midthoracic pain. Until this examination she had been unaware of her scoliotic deviation. COMMENT: Many idiopathic scolioses remain asymptomatic and may be found as an incidental finding in adulthood. Cosmetic deformity may be relatively slight despite even relatively large magnitude scoliotic curvatures.

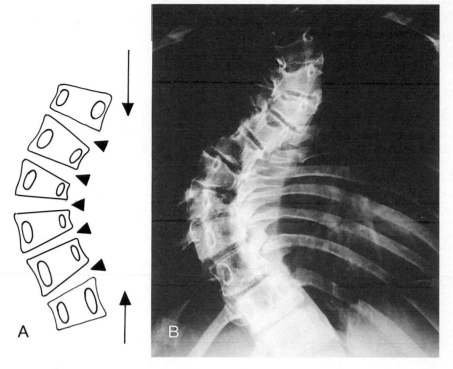

Figure 4.4. HUETER-VOLKMANN PRINCIPLE. A. Diagram. Excessive compressive axial loading at the discovertebral junction (arrowheads) due to scoliosis during the period of bone growth may produce permanent wedge-shaped vertebral bodies. **B. Radiograph.** The four vertebral bodies at the apices of the curves are notably wedged. Also observe the pedicle migration of these segments signifying vertebral rotation. (Courtesy of Leo C. Wunsch Sr., DC, DACBR, Denver, Colorado)

fusion of the iliac apophysis, further progression is unlikely. Later in adult life, superimposed degenerative changes may allow the curvature to increase on an average of 15° (16) and occasionally create nerve entrapment syndromes. (17)

A frequent finding in a developing scoliosis is a lateral wedged deformity of the vertebral body, which will persist into adult life. This is a result of impaired growth at the discovertebral junction on the concave side of the curvature because of excessive compressive forces (Hueter-Volkmann principle) (Fig. 4.4). The most frequent curve pattern is the right convex thoracic type. Three other curves that are frequently present include a right thoracolumbar, a left lumbar, and a combined form of left lumbar and right thoracic. (4,18) The psoas shadow on frontal radiographs is often absent on the concave side of a lumbar scoliosis. (19)

There is a 10 times greater incidence of congenital heart disease than in the general population when the idiopathic curve is more than 20°. (20)

Congenital Scoliosis

Congenital scoliosis is distinguished by anomalies of the vertebrae or ribs. The most frequently observed anomalies include hemivertebrae, block vertebrae, spina bifida, bridging vertebral bars, joint deformities, fusion of ribs, and other rib malformations. (21) (Fig. 4.5) This curve is typically a short "C" curve and may be rapidly progressive in the growing years. Occasionally, anterior vertebral body defects may cause superimposed kyphosis (kyphoscoliosis). (22) There is a frequent association of congenital scoliosis with anomalies of the genitourinary system. (23)

Neuromuscular Scoliosis

A large spectrum of neuropathic and myopathic disorders may produce a progressive spinal deformity. (Refer to Table 4.1) The most common neuropathy associated with scoliosis is poliomyelitis. (24) The scoliotic pattern produced is distinctively a long

C-shaped curve, frequently extending from the sacrum to the lower cervical region. The convex side is oriented toward the unaffected muscle group. Intersegmental rotation may be severe in these curves, and rapid progression in the curvature angle frequently occurs between the ages of 12 and 16 years. Cerebral palsy produces the same type of long C-shaped curve. Other neurologic disorders associated with scoliosis include syringomyelia, spinal cord tumor, trauma, and dysautonomia.

Idiopathic scoliosis of 15° or more that occurs before the age of 11 years should be viewed with a high index of suspicion as evidence of the presence of a significant intraspinal pathology. (25) (Fig. 4.6) *Left-sided* thoracic curves similarly can more often be associated with these same abnormalities, including tumors, syringomyelia, and Arnold-Chiari malformations, which are best evaluated with magnetic resonance (MR) imaging. (26,27) (See Chapter 3 for more discussion of left-sided thoracic curves.) Myopathic scoliotic curves are relatively infrequent. The most frequent cause is muscular dystrophy of Duchenne. An increasing lordosis usually precedes the onset of the scoliotic deformity. (28) The scoliosis that forms is often rapidly progressive and severe, requiring fusion and Harrington rod implantation. Once the patient has been confined to a wheelchair, the formation of a scoliosis is almost inevitable. (29)

Neurofibromatosis

Neurofibromatosis is an inherited congenital disorder of neuroectodermal and mesodermal tissues. The first description of the relationship between the formation of nerve and skin tumors was given by von Recklinghausen in 1882. (30) Scoliosis was first associated with neurofibromatosis in 1921 by Weiss. (31) The classic triad of diagnostic findings include: (a) multiple, soft, elevated cutaneous tumors (fibroma molluscum); (b) cutaneous pigmentation (café au lait spots); and (c) neurofibromas of peripheral nerves. In addition, various skeletal lesions, including erosions, intraosseous cystic defects, deformity, pseudarthrosis, growth ab-

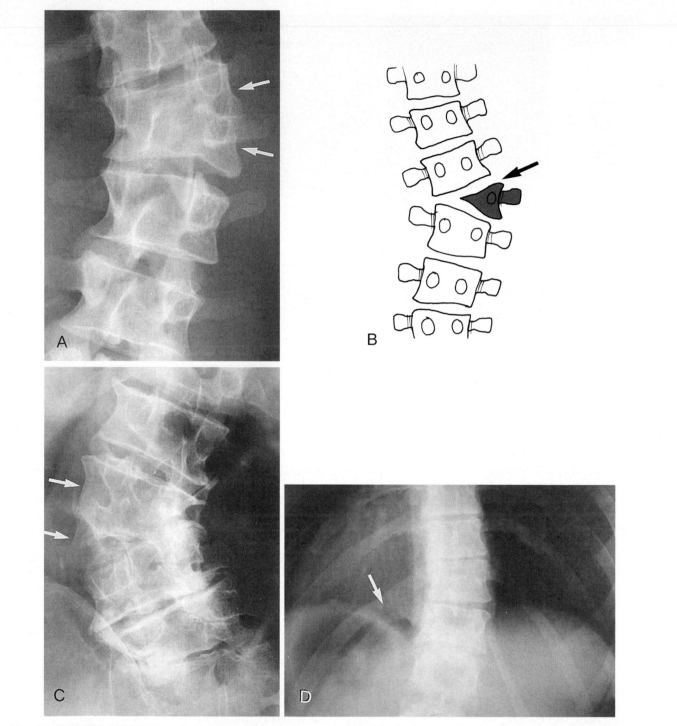

Figure 4.5. CONGENITAL SCOLIOSIS. A–C. Hemivertebrae. The presence of an additional portion of a vertebral body (arrows) produces a structural malformation, leading to the scoliotic deformity. **D. Rib Synostosis.** A localized lack of rib separation (arrow) precipitates this thoracolumbar scoliosis.

errations, and cranial abnormalities, may be present in up to 50% of these patients. (32)

Scoliosis is the most common bony abnormality and is present in approximately 10 to 50% of patients. (32–34) Varying degrees of scoliosis occur, from mild to severe, deforming angulations. (Figs. 4.7, 4.8) The most conspicuous features, when present, consist of a short, angular deformity with dysplasia of the vertebral bodies. Kyphosis is the most common superimposed deformity. Additional findings suggestive of a neurofibromatosis-induced scoliosis include enlarged foramina, posterior and lateral vertebral body scalloping, deformed ribs ("twisted ribbons"), and an adjacent smooth soft tissue mass due either to a neurofibroma or to a protruding meningocele. Notably, the scoliosis frequently progresses and requires surgical fusion and stabilization.

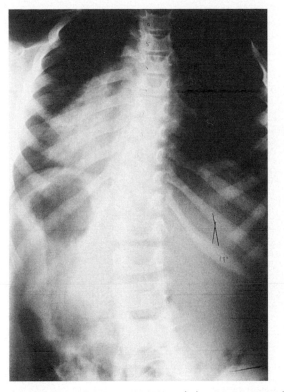

Figure 4.6. LEFT THORACIC SCOLIOSIS. Left thoracic curves under the age of 11 years may be a marker for underlying intracanal tumors, syringomyelia, and Arnold-Chiari malformations. (Courtesy of Anne P. Odenweller, DC, Baton Rouge, Louisiana)

Other Causes

Infection.   Infectious processes, such as tuberculosis, may precipitate spinal deformity due to collapse and bony destruction. (Fig. 4.9) The most distinctive deformity is a sharp, angular kyphosis (gibbus), although varying degrees of scoliosis may also occur.

Radiation.   Irradiation to the growing spine may produce vertebral abnormalities in up to 75% of patients. (35) These changes consist of growth arrest lines, endplate irregularities, altered vertebral shape, and scoliosis. The most common childhood disorders to be irradiated are Wilm's tumor and neuroblastoma. The treatment field is usually lateral to, but includes, the spine and results in one side absorbing more radiation than the other. This may produce two types of deformity: (a) a mobile flexion curve or (b) a fixed rotatory scoliosis due to unilateral shortened laminae and pedicles. (36) In both curves the convexity is away from the side of irradiation.

Trauma.   Injuries to the spine that produce fracture or dislocation may also induce a lateral spinal curvature, which may be permanent. (Fig. 4.10) Fractures of the transverse processes in the lumbar spine can be associated with a scoliosis convex to the side of the fractures. (37)

Degenerative Joint Disease.   Advanced discopathy and facet arthrosis may result in a scoliotic deviation, especially when the changes are extensive unilaterally. (Fig. 4.11) These curvatures are designated "degenerative scolioses."

Miscellaneous Disorders.   Many other conditions precipitate a structural scoliosis, including bone tumors, connective tissue diseases, and surgery. (Figs. 4.12, 4.13)

NONSTRUCTURAL SCOLIOSIS

Curvatures that have no structural alteration and that correct on recumbent lateral-bending radiographic studies are classified as nonstructural and have a number of possible etiologies. (Table 4.1) These include such conditions as leg length inequality, antalgia from discal herniations ("sciatic scoliosis"), and inflammatory bowel disease. (Figs. 4.14, 4.15)

COMPLICATIONS ASSOCIATED WITH SCOLIOSIS

Complications of a scoliotic curve are numerous. These occur with and without treatment.

Nontreatment-Related Complications

Cardiopulmonary Complications.   In more severe thoracic curvatures, restricted rib cage movement and lung volume ultimately produce pulmonary hypertension with subsequent right-(cor pulmonale) and left-sided congestive heart failure. (38) Congestive heart failure is the single most common direct cause of death in the patient with scoliosis. Altered lung ventilation also predisposes to pulmonary infection and dyspnea.

Degenerative Spinal Arthritis.   Loss of disc height, osteophytes, and intersegmental instability frequently accompany adult scoliosis and occasionally even adolescent scoliosis. (16,39,40) Distinctively, these degenerative changes are most pronounced on the concave side of the curve and extend to involve other stressed articulations, including costotransverse, sacroiliac, and hip joints. (Fig. 4.16) The most common area of secondary spinal pain from a thoracic scoliosis is the lumbar spine. (40) Secondary spatial compromise of the central and lateral spinal recesses may result in nerve root entrapment syndromes. (17)

Curvature Progression.   The most rapid and severely deforming time period for scoliosis is in the adolescent growth spurt (age 12 to 16 years), where the curve may increase at the rate of 1° per month. (39) In the adult, progression does occur but is relatively less, in the range of 10 to 15°. (16,39)

Fatigue and Joint Dysfunction Syndromes.   Altered biomechanical spinal stresses frequently produce asymmetric muscle and joint loadings. Muscular and ligamentous strain ensues, and spinal and sacroiliac joints become inflamed and altered in their normal kinematics, which all contribute to produce significant pain, discomfort, and disability. (41,42) These symptoms are frequently the most immediately debilitating feature in a patient with scoliosis. (40) Sites of pain in lumbar curves include the curve convexity (most common), the lumbosacral region, the curve concavity, and the costoiliac region with impingement of the ribs over the iliac crest (rare). (42)

Radiation Exposure.   A considerable amount of concern has focused on the long-term effects of repeated radiologic examinations. The average patient undergoing conservative therapy with bracing over 3 years has an average of 22 radiographs taken. The chance of an increased risk of malignancy in patients with scoliosis appears to be minimal in comparison with the natural incidence in the general population (0.2% for breast carcinoma; 5% for leukemia). (43–45)

Pregnancy.   The implications for pregnancy in the presence of scoliosis remain sketchy. In general, severe lumbar curves may be associated with obstetrical difficulties, while severe thoracic curves may be linked to other medical problems. (46) A higher incidence of premature delivery has been recorded. (47) Cesarean rates are not increased nor is the incidence of back pain during

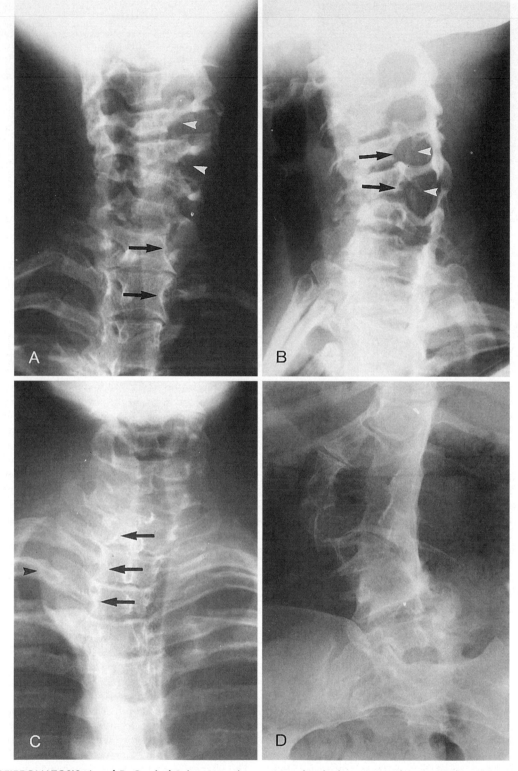

Figure 4.7.   NEUROFIBROMATOSIS. A and B. Cervical Spine. Note the lower cervical curvature, scalloped vertebral bodies (arrows), and widened foramina (arrowheads). (Courtesy of William E. Litterer, DC, DACBR, Fellow, ACCR, Elizabeth, New Jersey) **C. Upper Thoracic Spine.** Observe the upper thoracic curvature, lateral body scalloping (arrows), and the paraspinal mass (arrowhead) of an associated meningocele. (Courtesy of Clayton F. Thomsen, DC, Sydney, Australia) **D. Lumbar Spine.** A bizarre distortion of the lumbar bodies, posterior arches, and intervertebral foramina accompany the scoliosis. (Courtesy of Lawrence A. Cooperstein, MD, Pittsburgh, Pennsylvania)

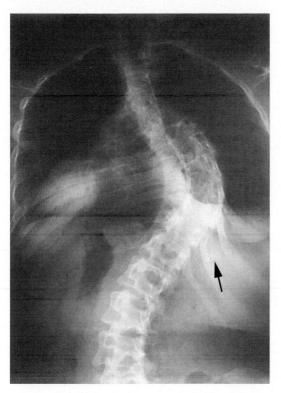

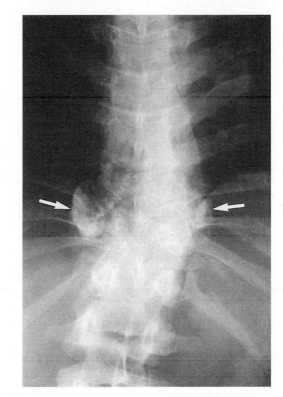

Figure 4.8.   NEUROFIBROMATOSIS. A marked right, short segment thoracic scoliosis is apparent. Note the presence of the soft tissue opacity over the left eleventh rib, denoting a cutaneous fibroma molluscum (arrow).

Figure 4.9.   TUBERCULOUS SPONDYLITIS (POTT'S DISEASE) PRODUCING A STRUCTURAL SCOLIOSIS. Tuberculous infection of the thoracolumbar vertebrae has precipitated collapse and a lateral scoliosis. The abnormal rib angulation is due to the associated gibbus deformity. Note the flocculent soft tissue calcification within the accompanying cold abscess (arrows).

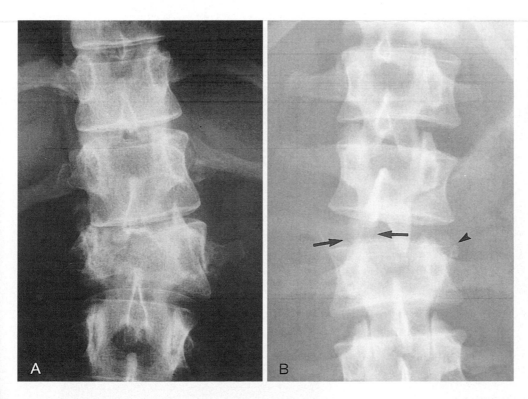

Figure 4.10.   TRAUMATIC SCOLIOSIS. A. A traumatic anterior and lateral vertebral body fracture of the first lumbar segment has created an accompanying scoliosis. **B.** A complete facet luxation at the L2-L3 interspace (arrows) has produced a minor scoliosis. Observe the superior endplate compression fracture of L3 (arrowhead).

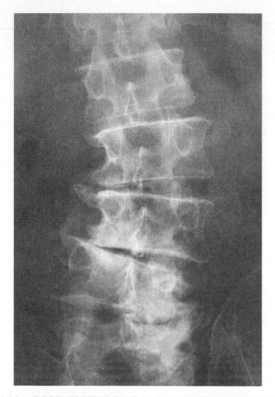

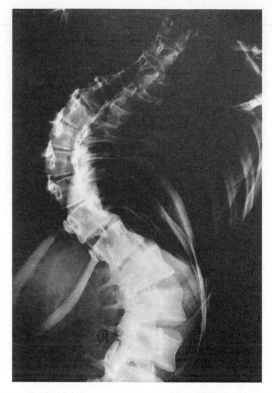

Figure 4.11.   DEGENERATIVE DISC AND APOPHYSEAL JOINT DISEASE PRODUCING SCOLIOSIS. Severe discopathic alterations at the second, third, and fourth lumbar discs with associated facet arthrosis have produced lateral listhesis and lateral flexion at these levels. These degenerative changes have resulted in a mild structural scoliosis. Such degenerative changes predispose to spinal stenosis.

Figure 4.13.   SCOLIOSIS ASSOCIATED WITH MARFAN'S SYNDROME. A severe double lumbar and thoracic curve is typical of this connective tissue defect.

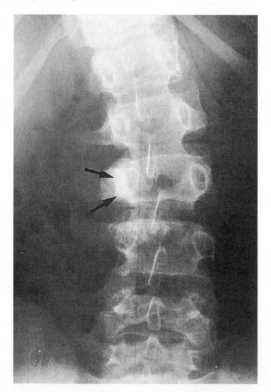

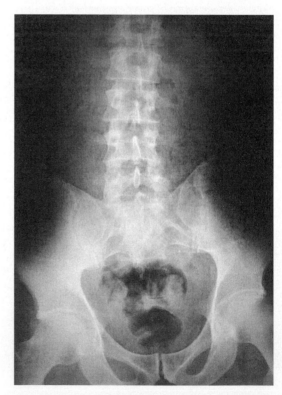

Figure 4.12.   SCOLIOSIS DUE TO OSTEOID OSTEOMA. Observe the localized sclerotic focus adjacent to the pedicle (arrows). These tumors are painful and characteristically induce a rotatory scoliosis with the lesion usually being located on the concave side. (Courtesy of Jack Edeiken, MD, Houston, Texas)

Figure 4.14.   SCOLIOSIS SECONDARY TO SHORT LEG SYNDROME. On this upright radiograph observe the pelvic unleveling and compensatory mild mid lumbar rotatory curvature convex to the low side of the pelvic unleveling.

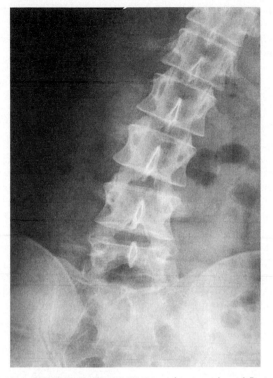

Figure 4.15. ANTALGIC SCOLIOSIS. Note the acute lateral flexion at the fourth lumbar segment and the failure of the vertebrae to rotate despite the lateral spinal deviation. This patient exhibited classic clinical signs of fourth lumbar disc protrusion.

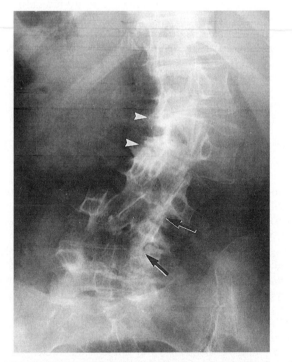

Figure 4.16. COMPLICATING DEGENERATIVE ARTHRITIS. There is severe facet arthrosis (arrows), discal degeneration, and spondylophytes (arrowheads) accompanying this idiopathic lumbar curve. These degenerative changes have occurred at the regions of maximal stress.

pregnancy, even if fusion has been performed. (48,49) Whether or not a pregnancy has a significant effect on curve progression is inconclusive. (42,50)

Treatment-Related Complications

Nonsurgical and surgical measures utilized in the treatment of scoliosis may produce a wide gamut of complications.

Nonsurgical Complications. The majority of deleterious side effects arise from the use of external braces and supports. Psychologically, the patient undergoes a good deal of mental stress. In long-term bracing, superficial skin irritations may be a persistent problem, either due to sweating or to allergy. It is rare for pressure sores to occur. Occasionally, nerve compression may occur with numbness and paresthesias, especially of the anterior femoral cutaneous nerve and, less commonly, of the brachial plexus. With curvature correction, compression of the duodenum under the superior mesenteric artery may create obstruction with nausea and vomiting (cast syndrome). (51) In the past the chin rested on Milwaukee braces frequently producing lower facial and dental abnormalities, but these are rare findings today. (52)

Surgical Complications. During the operative procedure, cardiac arrest and spinal cord injury are the most feared complications. Early postoperative problems include respiratory distress, infection, and loosening of the fixation device. Later, following release from the hospital, infection may still supervene. However, the most frequent complications are pseudarthrosis of the fusion (15% of cases) and instrumentation failure. (53)

RADIOLOGIC ASSESSMENT

The radiologic examination is the most definitive and important diagnostic tool in the assessment and management of the patient with scoliosis. (54) A number of nonradiologic methods, such as moire contourography and back contour devices, have been employed. (55) The role of the radiograph is multiple: (a) determining etiology; (b) evaluating curvature, including site, magnitude and flexibility; (c) assessing bone maturity; (d) monitoring progression or regression; and (e) aiding in the selection of appropriate treatment. A wide variety of factors are involved in the process of obtaining practical clinical information while avoiding unnecessary radiation exposure. (Table 4.3)

STANDARD RADIOGRAPHIC TECHNIQUES
Projections

Erect Anteroposterior and Lateral Projections. These projections are the absolute minimum required for accurate assessment of any scoliosis. Preferably, the anteroposterior (AP) projection should be done by a single exposure on a 14″ by 36″ cassette in order to allow for total and continuous curvature evaluation. (56) However, if such equipment is not available, sectional projections can be utilized just as effectively. The disadvantages of the single exposure full spine projection are the irradiation of unnecessary body parts, sacrifice of bone detail for pathology, and the expense of the equipment necessary to do the projections adequately. (Fig. 4.17) Wherever possible, a long focal-film distance, rare earth screens, density equaling filtration, collimation, optimal kilovoltage, and lead shielding of breasts, thyroid, and gonads should be utilized. (56) Obtaining the projection posterior-anterior also significantly reduces the dose to sensitive tissues.

Lateral-Bending Projections. These are primarily projections to evaluate curvature flexibility. The patient laterally flexes as

Table 4.3. Radiologic Examinations in Scoliosis

Projection	Indications-Information
Standard Techniques	
Erect AP	Curve analysis, contributing etiologies
Erect Lateral	Sagittal curvatures (kyphosis, lordosis)
Lateral Bending	Flexibility
Left Hand, Wrist	Skeletal age
Supplementary Technique	
Chest	Cardiopulmonary status
Contrast Studies	
Angiogram	Vascular compromise, neoplasm
Gastrointestinal	Duodenal obstruction
Genitourinary	Kidney anomalies, obstruction
Myelogram	Cord integrity, anomalies, stenosis
Derotated	Anatomy, anomalies
Erect PA	Reduction of radiation dose
Flexion, Extension	Sagittal curve flexibility
Lumbosacral Spot	
AP	Anomalies
Lateral	Spondylolisthesis
CT	Osseous detail
MRI	Spinal cord lesion
Obliques	Fusion and instrumentation status
Supine	Flexibility
Tangential	Efficacy of rib hump surgery
Tomography	Anatomy, abnormalities
Traction	Flexibility in neuromuscular disease

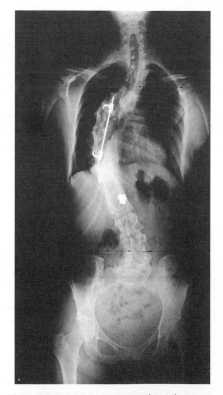

Figure 4.17. FULL SPINE RADIOGRAPH. The right primary thoracic scoliosis is stabilized with a short segment Harrington rod. COMMENT:Technical problems, especially in obtaining adequate collimation, make it difficult to reduce patient dose and exclude radiosensitive tissues such as the breast, thyroid, and gonads in obtaining a full spine projection. (Courtesy of Craig Reese, DC, Boulder, Colorado)

much as possible, and the exposure is made. This must be done both to the right and left.

Left Hand and Wrist. A spot AP radiograph is taken of the left hand and wrist in patients under 20 years of age. This is compared with the Greulich and Pyle *Atlas* to ascertain the skeletal age of the patient, which is important in planning the treatment regime. (57)

Technology

Film Identification. Films are usually viewed as if the examiner were observing the patient from the posterior, so the markers should be reversed to simplify interpretation. In addition to the traditional identification by name, age, institution, date, and file number, further information may be helpful. When lateral-bending studies are being taken, it is important to show the direction of bending and to identify the projection as a lateral-bending study. It is also vital to identify whether the projections are being taken with the patient erect or recumbent.

Equipment. In producing a quality radiograph for scoliosis mensuration, it is desirable to use a machine capable of exposures at 84 inches. A minimum capacity for such exposures would be a 125-kilovolts peak (kVp), 300-milliamperes (mA) machine. Use of high frequency generators (100 kHz) is preferable. (56) A grid ratio of no less than 10 to 1, in combination with rare earth screens, produces acceptable images while reducing the radiation dose. (52,56,57) Similarly, the use of split screens to compensate for differing body thicknesses should be avoided; balancing filtration at the collimator is preferred. (59) Technique factors will vary according to each patient, but a minimum kilovoltage of 90 is recommended. (56,60) Compression devices reduce tissue thickness and motion, which results in improved anatomic detail and diminished radiation dose. (56)

Sectional AP films should be taken when the patient's body thickness measures more than 24 cm. Gonadal protection must be applied in all instances of scoliosis evaluation, both in the AP and lateral projections. In repeated examinations the majority of the pelvis, except for the sacral base, should not be exposed. Lateral collimation on AP films should be as close as practical, without compromising necessary rib and curvature details.

SUPPLEMENTARY RADIOGRAPHIC TECHNIQUES

Projections

Numerous specialized projections are available to provide additional information. (Refer to Table 4.3)

Chest. Specific evaluations of the lungs and heart should be obtained periodically in order to establish any alteration in cardiopulmonary status, especially cor pulmonale and congestive heart failure.

Contrast Examinations. Occasionally, these studies may be employed to better evaluate certain body systems. Myelography may be employed to evaluate spinal cord integrity, congenital anomalies, and stenosis. Intravenous pyelograms are often used in congenital deformities of the spine because of the increased frequency of renal anomalies and possible obstructive uropathy. Gastrointestinal studies are used when abdominal symptoms suggest duodenal obstruction by the superior mesenteric artery as the curvature is corrected. (51) Angiograms are rarely used except when vascular compression or vascular neoplasm in the cord is suspected.

Derotated View. This view is used only in severe kyphoscoliotic curves (over 100°). By rotating the patient, the effects of segmental rotation are reduced, which allows for better evaluation for underlying anomalies. (61)

Flexion-Extension. These are analogous to the lateral flexion views for flexibility evaluation. Their main purpose is to demonstrate the degree of mobility within the curvature in the sagittal plane.

Posterior-Anterior. Various studies have shown significant reductions in radiation doses to such radiosensitive structures as the thyroid, breasts, and active bone marrow by performing the frontal film in a posterior-anterior position. (59,62-65) As an example, this projection reduces the dosage to the breast by a factor of approximately 3, from 60 mRad (0 to 60 Gy) to 20 mRad (0 to 20 Gy). However, inherent in the placement of the vertebrae farther from the film are the magnification, the loss of geometric sharpness, and a change in the measured Cobb's angle, therefore making AP comparisons of dubious value. (63,64)

Lumbosacral Spot Views. Due to technical underexposure, the details of the lumbosacral region are frequently obscured. An anterior-posterior projection with a cephalad tube tilt of 20 to 30° will show the junctional region clearly. (66) Additionally, a lateral erect projection may demonstrate a spondylolisthesis frequently seen in conjunction with scoliosis, especially if rotation is evident on the frontal radiograph. (67,68)

Magnetic Resonance Imaging. Evaluation of the spinal cord is best achieved with MR. In curves of 15° or more, in left thoracic curves, or from clinical suspicion, MR readily detects lesions, including intracanal tumors, syringomyelia and Arnold-Chiari malformation. (69)

Oblique. The object of these films is usually to assess the status of a previous bone graft or corrective instrumentation. Additional information is also obtained, such as the integrity of the pars interarticularis and paraspinal soft tissues.

Supine. When compared with erect radiographs, the effect of gravity on the curve can be observed and, once again, provide data on the curvature flexibility. An additional bonus is the improved structural detail that is obtained in this position.

Tangential ("Rib Hump" View). This view is used only when cosmetic surgery is contemplated for the posterior rib hump. The patient faces the bucky and flexes forward with the x-ray beam directed tangentially across the back. If the vertebrae are seen to be rotated under the ribs, no surgery is performed, because the patient will maintain the hump even if the ribs are removed. (65)

Tomography. The depiction of obscured anatomic details and deformity is best examined by sequential tomography. This is only utilized in selective instances.

Traction. This is only used in patients with neuromuscular disease who are unable to perform lateral-bending studies unassisted. A supine projection is taken with traction applied to the head and feet, and the projection is compared to the neutral AP film.

Technology

Segmented Field Radiography. A standard AP full spine is taken at the initial visit. (70) Transitional and end levels are located from which the Cobb angles are constructed. Subsequent examinations, which may follow with treatment, only take collimated, small field views of these same transitional and end levels, with the Cobb method applied again. This technique reduces the radiation dose considerably.

Specialized Shields and Filters. Numerous shields have been developed to reduce doses to radiosensitive organs, such as the

breast, thyroid, and gonads. (59) These are especially useful on lateral radiographs because of the higher level of exposure necessary to produce this film. Additional filtration is also instrumental in substantially decreasing the absorbed dose and obtaining a better quality image. (71)

Digital Radiography. A computerized system of acquiring radiographic images has considerable application in the assessment of scoliosis. (72) Frontal and lateral studies of adequate diagnostic quality for scoliosis evaluation can be obtained with a dose reduction of at least 50%.

SCOLIOSIS MENSURATION

The four basic spinal parameters evaluated in scoliosis are: (a) curvature, (b) rotation, (c) flexibility, and (d) skeletal maturation.

Curvature Measurement

The two most popular measuring methods are the Cobb-Lippman and Risser-Ferguson systems. The Cobb method is the most accepted standard for quantifying scoliotic deviation. (73)

Cobb-Lippman Method. This procedure was introduced by Lippman in 1935 and popularized later by Cobb. (2) (Figs. 4.18, 4.19) A line is drawn along the superior border of the cephalad end vertebra. A similar line is drawn along the inferior surface of the caudad end vertebra. If the endplates are not visible, the bottom or tops of the pedicles can be used. Perpendicular lines are then erected from each horizontal line, and the angle of their intersection measured. Seven groups are categorized according to the Cobb angle: group 1: 0 to 20°; group 2: 21 to 30°; group 3: 31 to 50°; group 4: 51 to 75°; group 5: 76 to 100°; group 6: 101 to 125°; and group 7: 126° and above.

The Cobb method gives larger measurements than the Risser technique by an average of 25%, or about 10°. (73,74) With larger curves this percentage difference increases, and some have ad-

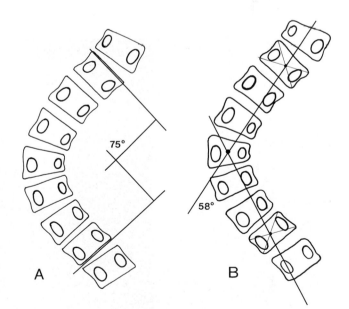

Figure 4.18. CURVATURE MENSURATION. A. Cobb Method. The end vertebrae are located, and lines are drawn on their appropriate endplates. Perpendiculars are erected to these endplate lines and the intersecting acute angle measured. **B. Risser-Ferguson Method.** A dot is placed in the center of each end vertebra as well as in the apical segment. These are then joined and their intersecting acute angle measured.

vocated using the Risser method to reduce this discrepancy, but this practice is to be discouraged. The Cobb procedure also has the distinction of being more easily applied and reproducible by different observers. (75) In double curvatures both curves should be measured.

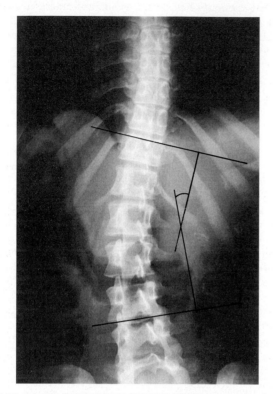

Figure 4.19.   COBB METHOD OF MENSURATION. Perpendicular lines to the endplates of the end vertebrae intersect on the concave side, where the angle is measured.

Risser-Ferguson Method.   Ferguson first introduced his methodology in the early 1920s and later published his findings along with Risser in the 1930s and 1940s. (74,76,77) (Fig. 4.18) In this procedure the centers of the end and apical vertebral bodies are identified. These points are then connected and the angle of intersection measured.

Rotation

Rotation is invariably present in scoliosis and is intimately associated with the degree of external cosmetic deformity, especially in the thoracic spine. The anterior column (vertebral body-disc) rotates more than the posterior column (neural arch). (69)

Spinous Method.   Cobb first described an evaluation based on the position of the spinous tip to the vertebral body. (2) It provides an estimate of posterior vertebral deformity. (69) Spinous processes are prone to malformation and displacement and are frequently difficult to identify. Consequently, these structures should not be used to assess rotation.

Pedicle Method.   Described by Nash and Moe in 1969, this is the most accepted method of determining rotation. (78) (Fig. 4.20) The movement of the pedicle on the convex side of the curve is graded between 0 and 4 and is a measure of anterior deformity. (69,78) CT examination of scoliotic vertebral rotation has demonstrated that the pedicle method is not entirely accurate but is the most usable available. (79) A Nash-Moe grade of 0, which is given when there is no apparent rotation present, in fact may have greater than 10° of rotation present. (79)

Flexibility

Flexibility is defined as the degree of mobility within a scoliosis. This is an important parameter to assess since it shows not only the correctability of a scoliosis, but also that it may continue to progress. To the surgeon a lack of flexibility is a contraindication to spinal fusion. The radiographic assessment of flexibility is evaluated primarily by a supine lateral-bending radiograph

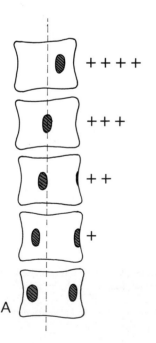

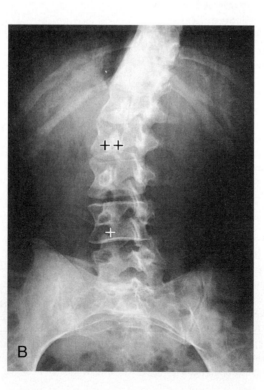

Figure 4.20. ROTATION ASSESSMENT: PEDICLE METHOD. A. Diagrammatic Representation. B. Radiographic Depiction. The maximal rotation is at the apical vertebra (+2). (Courtesy of William E. Litterer, DC, DACBR, Fellow, ACCR, Elizabeth, New Jersey)

into the convex side of the scoliosis. The Cobb method is applied, and the degree of correction induced is the measure of flexibility. (Fig. 4.21)

Skeletal Maturation

Ascertaining skeletal maturity is vital to determining treatment and prognosis. While the potential for growth remains, there is the possibility of curvature progression. Three observations are used in this determination: (a) comparing the left hand and wrist with the Greulich and Pyle *Atlas*; (b) observing the vertebral ring epiphyses; and (c) observing the iliac epiphysis.

Left Hand and Wrist. This is compared with the Greulich and Pyle *Atlas*. In general, scoliotic female individuals are more mature than normal between 11 and 12 years of age and less mature between 15 and 17. (80,81) Practically interpreted, this means that the growth period in scoliotic females is lengthened. (82) The distal radial epiphysis closes at the same time as the vertebral body epiphysis.

Vertebral Ring Epiphyses. These are normal traction epiphyses at the peripheral body margins. Although they do not contribute to vertical vertebral body growth, their fusion to the body rim very closely parallels arrest in spinal growth. (Fig. 4.22D–F) The recognition of this fusion is the most accurate indicator of completed spinal growth and can be interpreted as a strong inhibiting factor to future scoliotic progression.

Iliac Epiphysis (Risser's Sign). The recognition of the iliac crest epiphysis as an indicator of spinal maturity was first noted by Risser in 1948 (83) and later confirmed. (64,84,85)

In the majority of individuals the apophysis appears laterally near the anterior superior iliac spine and progresses medially toward the posterior superior iliac spine ("capping"). This gradual extension in excursion is graded by quarters: 1+, 25%; 2+, 50%; 3+, 75%; and 4+, 100%. When the epiphysis is fused to the ilium, it is graded 5+. (Figs. 4.22, 4.23)

The process of capping usually begins in boys at the age of 16 and in girls at the age of 14. From the time of appearance to complete excursion to the posterior superior iliac spine, a time period of 1 year has usually elapsed. It then will take 2 to 3 years for complete osseous union to occur. This pattern of formation and closure parallels the formation and progression of the scoliosis. In the preadolescent child (10 to 15 years), prior to the ap-

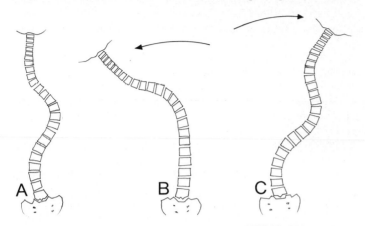

Figure 4.21. FLEXIBILITY EVALUATION BY LATERAL BENDING. A. Erect, Neutral Position. The presence of a left lumbar and right thoracic curvature is evident. **B. Left Lateral Bending.** Note the left lumbar curve disappears, indicating it to be nonstructural. **C. Right Lateral Bending.** The right thoracic curve remains unchanged, indicating it to be structural. COMMENT: When there is failure of a curvature to correct on lateral bending, the curvature can be interpreted as being irreversible and also non progressive.

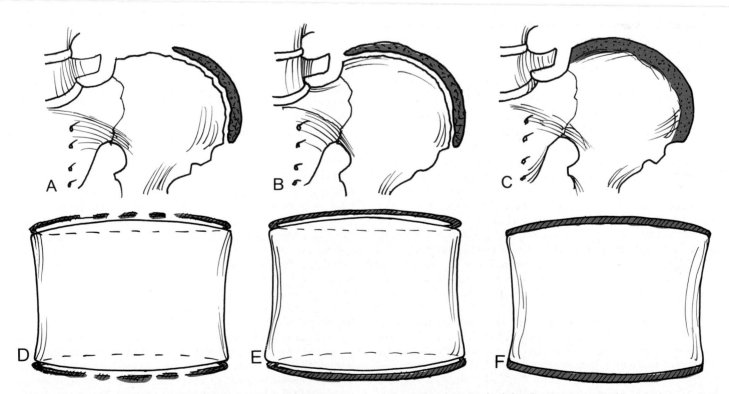

Figure 4.22. RADIOGRAPHIC DETERMINATION OF THE SPINAL MATURITY. A-C. Iliac Epiphysis. D-F. Vertebral Body Epiphysis. The two most reliable signs of maturation are the status of the iliac and vertebral body epiphyses. When they are both fused and no longer visible, spinal maturation is complete and curvature progression is less likely.

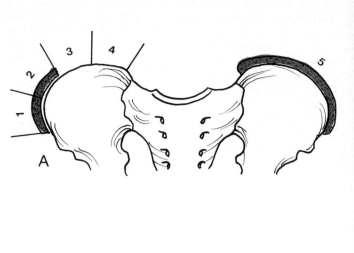

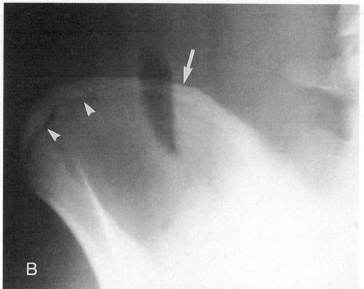

Figure 4.23.   ILIAC EPIPHYSIS: RISSER'S SIGN. A. Grading System. The epiphysis first appears at the anterior superior iliac spine and gradually progresses posteromedially before fusing to the ilium. Five grades are utilized, one for each quarter ossified, 1+, 2+, 3+, 4+, and 5+, when complete osseous fusion has occurred. **B. Radiographic Depiction.** A 4+ Risser's sign (arrow). The radiolucent line (arrowheads) represents the cartilaginous growth plate. COMMENT: The distal radial epiphysis closes at the same time as the iliac epiphysis.

pearance of the iliac epiphysis, it is usual for the curve to show the greatest rate of progression. (84) Once the epiphysis becomes visible, curve progression slows and eventually ceases when the epiphysis fuses. A Risser 4 in females and a Risser 5 in males usually signals the end of curve progression. (86)

CLINICAL RADIOLOGIC CORRELATION

Application of the radiographic information is vital to the diagnosis, treatment, and management of scoliosis. Specific applications include selection of therapy, monitoring patient response, and long-term assessment.

Therapy Selection

Therapy selection is based on combining all facts together. The major objectives in selecting a therapeutic regime hinge on curve progression and its effect on cosmetic appearance and body function. Approximately 25% of all curves will show some degree of progression. (87) Indicators of likely progression include curvature pattern, age, onset of menarche, and an absent (0) or early (1+) Risser sign. (87) Curve patterns that are at the highest risk of progression and should be braced earlier are double primary curvatures (two curves in one region) and primary lumbar with compensatory thoracic curves. (88) The lumbar component is the most likely part to progress. In addition, other factors, such as the magnitude of the curve (curves greater than 20° are three times more likely to progress), flexibility, and family history, should be considered. (87,88)

The major therapeutic decision is among three alternatives—close observation, bracing, and surgery. (89) The use of surface electrical stimulation in some studies has been as effective as the Milwaukee brace in halting progression (90), while other studies have yielded disappointing results. (91,92) In minor curves, less than 20°, there is general agreement that the patient does not require bracing (93,94); however, in view of possible rapid progression during the growth period (10 to 15 years), these patients must be frequently and carefully examined for signs of increasing

deformity. Radiographic examination every 3 months should be done as part of this monitoring process. The use of noninvasive methods as alternatives has been advocated by some researchers. (55,95) If more than a 5° increase is demonstrated, bracing should be contemplated. (93) Additionally, if rotation and a rib hump are prominent, bracing is also indicated. Exercise has not been shown to decrease scoliosis, but it does have value in improving posture, flexibility, muscular tone, and psychological awareness. Chiropractic spinal manipulation frequently decreases associated musculoskeletal symptoms.

Indications for bracing include curves that are flexible, skeletally immature, between 20 and 40°, and that are progressive in nature. (67,87,93) The most commonly utilized brace is the Milwaukee brace. (96) Its purpose is not to correct a curve but to prevent further progression. The brace functions by exerting longitudinal traction between the occiput and pelvis, with pressure pads appropriately placed to limit rotation and lateral displacement. Physiologically, the cumulative effect is to decrease the curvature and the segmental torsion. Additionally, this aids in decreasing the compressive forces on the discovertebral growth plate and helps prevent the lateral wedged deformities of the vertebral bodies. The wearing of the brace should be for 23 hours per day, until skeletal maturity, and should be combined with a specific exercise regime. (93,94) A weaning period of from 6 to 12 months is usually necessary, with gradually increased hours without the brace. Radiographs should be obtained every 3 months during this period to evaluate for stability or progression. If progression is evident, the bracing time must again be increased.

Surgical intervention may be done where an underlying abnormality can be treated, rapid progression is occurring in an immature spine, or the curve is over 40°, although these criteria are not definitive. (94,97) Occasionally, milder deformities may be surgically stabilized for cosmetic reasons. The most common surgeries performed include the insertion of Harrington rods and the Dwyer procedure of wire cable and screws. (98) (Figs. 4.24, 4.25)

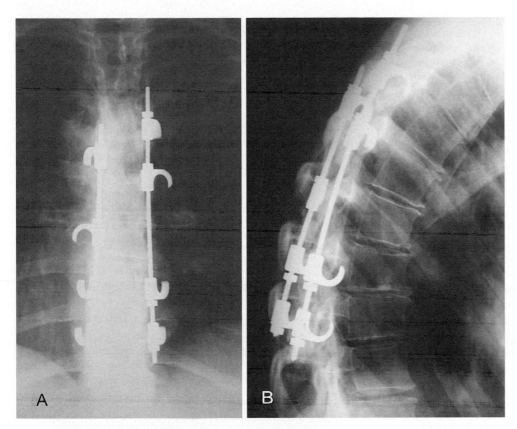

A   B

Figure 4.24. A and B. Harrington Rod Procedure. Two rods are placed on either side of the spine and anchored to the bone by hooks. These effectively fuse the spinal segments and prevent progression of the curve. (Courtesy of William E. Litterer, DC, DACBR, Fellow, ACCR, Elizabeth, New Jersey)

Response Monitoring and Long-Term Assessment

In both the braced and unbraced patient with scoliosis careful and frequent examination should be performed. A radiographic study should be done every 3 to 4 months until skeletal maturity, as demonstrated by closure of the iliac epiphysis. Once a brace has been removed, an annual examination for 5 years is suggested to observe and monitor any delayed tendency for progression. If the curve does show progression, surgical stabilization may be indicated. In surgical cases radiographs will aid in the placement of stabilizing instruments and graft material. During the postoperative period the degree of correction, the integrity of the fusion, and any complicating infection can be assessed. Postfusion radiographs show decreased Cobb angles of around 35%, but the shape of the curve and apical vertebral rotation remain unchanged. (53,99) Over an extended time period the radiographic examination can be used to evaluate superimposed degenerative changes and progressive spinal changes. Those fusions that extend below L2 have a higher incidence of discal syndromes requiring a further surgery at a later time. (100)

MEDICOLEGAL IMPLICATIONS
Scoliosis

- In all cases of scoliosis a cause must be sought. There needs to be a systematic evaluation both clinically and radiologically to identify segmentation defects, neuromuscular disorders, neurofibromatosis, spinal cord and vertebral tumors, as well as other etiologies. The diagnosis of idiopathic scoliosis is a diagnosis by exclusion.

- In idiopathic scoliosis appropriate follow-up radiologic examination must be considered at a minimum of 3 to 4 month intervals

Figure 4.25. DWYER PROCEDURE. The intervertebral discs are removed, screws are inserted, and the connecting wire is shortened to compress the vertebrae together and reduce the flexibility for progression of the curvature. (Courtesy of William E. Litterer, DC, DACBR, Fellow, ACCR, Elizabeth, New Jersey)

during the growth phase to monitor for progression. Failure to recognize progression of scoliosis during the growth phase may delay more aggressive intervention and result in more severe deformity and longer-term complications. Individuals who possess high-risk indicators of likely progression should be followed more closely (double primary or lumbar primary curvature, younger age, early menarche, low-grade Risser sign, curves greater than 20°, positive family history).

- Radiographs must be of high quality with state-of-the-art equipment (high frequency generators, rare earth screens, and so forth) to minimize radiation dose, since multiple examinations are often required during the growth period. Removal of radiosensitive tissues from the irradiated field, either by collimation, filters, or shielding, should be a priority. The frequency of radiographic examinations should be minimized as much as possible.

- The technical inadequacies for pathologic evaluation of full spine exposures should be considered. Where clinically indicated or if there is a questionable area noted on the full spine radiograph, sectional or spot films should be obtained.

- Measurements must be accurate and consistent. The method of choice remains the Cobb analysis, which hinges on the correct choice of end vertebrae, accurate placement of lines, and accurate angle measurement. It is critical to use the same landmarks and end vertebrae at subsequent examinations to provide meaningful comparison data on curvature development.

- Complications may arise and need to be recognized. These may include pulmonary hypertension and heart failure, degenerative spinal syndromes, curve progression, and joint dysfunctions. In patients with previous surgery, infection, bony fusion, or hardware failure can supervene.

- In idiopathic scoliosis, claims for reducing or arresting further progression of curvatures with conservative methods should be made with caution. These may result in unrealistic expectations and a false sense of security in light of the unpredictability of the deformity.

CAPSULE SUMMARY *Scoliosis*

GENERAL CONSIDERATIONS
- Scoliosis: from Greek word *skolios*, meaning twisted or crooked. Lateral deviation of the spinal column.

CLASSIFICATION AND TERMINOLOGY
- Scolioses are classified according to etiology (Table 4.1) and location. Specific standardized terminology is utilized in the discipline.

CLINICAL FEATURES
- Structural scoliosis is a fixed deformity that does not correct on lateral bending.
- Idiopathic scoliosis is the most common scoliosis. Three different types—infantile, juvenile, adolescent.
- Adolescent idiopathic scoliosis: 10 years of age until skeletal maturity. Females: 9 to 1, usually right thoracic, wedged vertebrae (Hueter-Volkmann principle); most rapid growth between age 12 and 16.
- Congenital scoliosis: structural anomalies, short curve, high incidence of genitourinary anomalies.
- Neuromuscular scoliosis: nerve or muscle disease, long curve convex to weak side.
- Neurofibromatosis: mesoectodermal dysplasia. Scoliosis common, often short and angular kyphosis, and with vertebral dysplasia.
- Others: infection, radiation, trauma, degenerative joint disease, neoplasm.

- Nonstructural scoliosis: deformity fully corrects on lateral bending. Etiology: leg deficiencies, antalgia.
- Complications of scoliosis: cardiopulmonary disease, degenerative arthritis, curve progression, pain, radiation-induced abnormalities, psychological disturbances, nerve palsies, infections, pseudoarthrosis, and instrumentation failure.

RADIOLOGIC ASSESSMENT
- Standard projections: erect AP and lateral full spine, right and left lateral bending, left hand and wrist.
- Supplementary projections: many. (Table 4.3)
- Technology: 84 inches TFD, compensating filtration, rare earth screens.
- Measurements: curvature-Cobb method; rotation-pedicle method; flexibility-lateral flexion; skeletal maturation—left hand and wrist, vertebral ring epiphyses, iliac epiphysis (Risser's sign).
- Therapy selection: indicators of progression include double curvatures, young age, early onset of menarche, absent or early Risser's sign.
- No treatment: less than 20°, but must be monitored carefully every 3 months. Greater than 5° increase should be braced.
- Bracing: flexible, immature, 20 to 40° curves, which are progressive; usually, Milwaukee brace. Evaluated every 3 months, until maturity, then weaned gradually.
- Surgery: abnormality, progression, more than 40°; Harrington rods, Dwyer procedure.

REFERENCES

1. **Hippocrates:** *The genuine works of Hippocrates,* London, F. Adams, 1849.
2. **Cobb JR:** *Outline for the study of scoliosis.* Am Acad Orthop Surgeons Lect 5:261, 1948.
3. **Terminology Committee, Scoliosis Research Society.** *A glossary of scoliosis terms.* Spine, 1:57, 1976.
4. **Keim HA:** *Scoliosis.* CIBA Clin Symp 30(1):1, 1978.
5. **Wynne-Davies, R:** *Genetic and environmental aspects.* J Bone Joint Surg (Br) 50:24, 1968.
6. **Worthington V, Shambaugh P:** *Systemic abnormalities in idiopathic scoliosis.* J Manipulative Physiol Ther 14:467, 1991.
7. **Cook SD, Harding AF, Morgan EL, et al:** *Trabecular bone density in idiopathic scoliosis.* J Pediatr Orthop 7:168, 1987.

8. **MacEwan DG, Cowell HR:** *Familial incidence of idiopathic scoliosis and its implication in patient treatment.* J Bone Joint Surg (Am) 52:405, 1970.
9. **Riseborough T, Wynne-Davies RA:** *Genetic survey of idiopathic scoliosis in Boston, Massachusetts.* J Bone Joint Surg (Am) 56:974, 1973.
10. **Brunnell WP:** *The natural history of idiopathic scoliosis before skeletal maturity.* Spine 11:773, 1986.
11. **Lloyd-Roberts GC, Pilcher MF:** *Structural idiopathic scoliosis in infancy. A study of the natural history of 100 patients.* J Bone Joint Surg (Br) 47:520, 1965.
12. **Mannherz RE, Betz RR, Clancy M, et al:** *Juvenile idiopathic scoliosis followed to skeletal maturity.* Spine 13:1087, 1988.
13. **Montgomery F, Willner S:** *The natural history of idiopathic scoliosis. A study of the incidence of treatment.* Spine 13:401, 1988.
14. **Hoppenfield S:** *Scoliosis. A Manual of Concept and Treatment,* Philadelphia, JB Lippincott, 1967.

15. **Carpintero P, Gonzalez I, Garcia E, et al:** *The relationship between pes cavus and idiopathic scoliosis.* Spine 19:1260, 1994.

16. **Collis DK, Ponsetti IV:** *Long term followup of patients with idiopathic scoliosis not treated surgically.* J Bone Joint Surg (Am) 51:425, 1969.

17. **Epstein JA, Epstein BS, Lavine LS:** *Surgical treatment of nerve root compression caused by scoliosis of the lumbar spine.* J Neurosurg 41:449, 1974.

18. **Ponsetti IV, Friedman B:** *Prognosis in idiopathic scoliosis.* J Bone Joint Surg (Am) 32:381, 1950.

19. **Bloom RA, Gheorghiu D, Verstandig A, et al:** *The psoas sign in normal subjects without bowel preparation: The influence of scoliosis on visualization.* Clin Radiol 41:204, 1990.

20. **Reckles LN, Peterson HA, Bianco AJ, et al:** *The association of scoliosis and congenital heart disease.* J Bone Joint Surg (Am) 57:449, 1975.

21. **Winter RB, Moe JH, Eilers VE:** *Congenital scoliosis.* J Bone Joint Surg (Am) 50:1, 1968.

22. **Winter RB, Moe JH, Wang JF:** *Congenital kyphosis.* J Bone Joint Surg (Am) 55:223, 1973.

23. **MacEwan GD, Hardy JH, Winter RB:** *Evaluation of kidney anomalies in congenital scoliosis.* J Bone Joint Surg (Am) 54:1451, 1972.

24. **Kilfoyle RM, Foley JJ, Norton PL:** *Spine and pelvic deformity in childhood and adolescent paraplegia. A study of 104 cases.* J Bone Joint Surg (Am) 47:659, 1965.

25. **Lewenowski K, King JD, Nelson MD:** *Routine use of magnetic resonance imaging in idiopathic scoliosis patients less than 11 years of age.* Spine 17:S109, 1992.

26. **Goldberg CJ, Dowling FE, Fogarty EE:** *Left thoracic scoliosis configurations. Why so different?* Spine 19:1385, 1994.

27. **Barnes PD, Brody JD, Jaramillo D, et al:** *Atypical idiopathic scoliosis: MR imaging evaluation.* Radiology 186:247, 1993.

28. **Spencer GE Jr:** *Orthopedic considerations in the management of muscular dystrophy.* Curr Pract Orthop Surg 5:279, 1973.

29. **Siegel IM:** *Scoliosis in muscular dystrophy.* Clin Orthop 93:235, 1973.

30. **von Recklinghausen FD:** *Über die multiplen Fibrome der Haut und ihre Beziehungen zu den Neuromen.* Virchow, Festschr R 1882.

31. **Weiss RS:** *Curvature of the spine in von Recklinghausen disease.* Arch Dermatol Syphilis 3:144, 1921.

32. **Hunt JC, Pugh DG:** *Skeletal lesions in neurofibromatosis.* Radiology, 76:1, 1961.

33. **Scott JC:** *Scoliosis and neurofibromatosis.* J Bone Joint Surg (Br) 47:240, 1965.

34. **Akbarnia BA, Gabriel KR, Beckman E, et al:** *Prevalence of scoliosis in neurofibromatosis.* Spine, 17:S244, 1992.

35. **Neuhauser EBD, Wittenhoy MH, Berman CF, et al:** *Irradiation effects of roentgen therapy on the growing spine.* Radiology 59:737, 1952.

36. **Rutherford H, Dodd GD:** *Complications of radiation therapy: Growing bone.* Semin Roentgenol 9:15, 1974.

37. **Gilsanz V, Miranda J, Cleveland R, et al:** *Scoliosis secondary to fractures of the transverse processes of lumbar vertebrae.* Radiology 134:627, 1980.

38. **Samuelson S:** *Cor pulmonale resulting from deformities of the chest.* Acta Med Scand 142:399, 1952.

39. **Risser JC:** *Scoliosis: Past and present.* J Bone Joint Surg (Am) 46(1):167, 1964.

40. **Grubb SA, Liscomb HJ:** *Diagnostic findings in painful adult scoliosis.* Spine 17:518, 1992.

41. **Diakow PRP:** *Pain: A forgotten aspect of idiopathic scoliosis.* J Can Chir Assoc 28(3):315, 1984.

42. **Nykoliation JW, Cassidy JD, Arthur BE, et al:** *An algorithm for the management of scoliosis.* J Manipulative Physiol Ther 9:1, 1986.

43. **Drummond D, Ranallo F, Lonstein J, et al:** *Radiation hazards in scoliosis management.* Spine 8(7):741, 1983.

44. **Rao PS, Gregg EC:** *A revised estimate of the risk of carcinogenesis from X rays to scoliosis patients.* Invest Radiol 19(1):58, 1984.

45. **Nash CL, Gregg EC, Brown RH, et al:** *Risk of exposure to X rays in patients undergoing long term treatment for scoliosis.* J Bone Joint Surg (Am) 61:371, 1979.

46. **DeCarle DW:** *Pregnancy associated with severe angular deformities of the spine.* Am J Obstet Gynecol 73:296, 1957.

47. **Visscher W, Lonstein JE, Hoffman DA, et al:** *Reproductive outcomes in scoliosis patients.* Spine 13:1096, 1988.

48. **Betz RR, Bunnell WP, Lambecht-Mulier E, et al:** *Scoliosis and pregnancy.* J Bone Joint Surg (Am) 69:90, 1987.

49. **Siegler D, Zorab PA:** *Pregnancy in thoracic scoliosis.* Br J Dis Chest 75:367, 1981.

50. **Berman AT, Cohen DL, Schwentker EP:** *The effects of pregnancy on idiopathic scoliosis: a preliminary report on eight cases and a review of the literature.* Spine 7:76, 1982.

51. **Skandalaikis JE, Akin JT, Milsap JH, et al:** *Vascular compression of the duodenum.* Contemp Surg 10:33, 1977.

52. **Alexander RG:** *The effects on tooth position and maxillofacial vertical growth during treatment of scoliosis with the Milwaukee brace.* Am J Orthod 52:161, 1966.

53. **van Dam BE, Bradford DS, Lonstein JE, et al:** *Adult idiopathic scoliosis treated by posterior spinal fusion and Harrington instrumentation.* Spine 12:32, 1987.

54. **Young LW, Oestreich AE, Goldstein LA:** *Roentgenology in scoliosis: Contribution to evaluation and management.* AJR 108:778, 1970.

55. **Pearsall DJ, Reid JG, Hedden DM:** *Comparison of three noninvasive methods for measuring scoliosis.* Phys Ther 72:648, 1992.

56. **Taylor JAM:** *Full-spine radiography: A review.* J Manipulative Physiol Ther 16:460, 1993.

57. **Greulich WW, Pyle SI:** *Radiographic Atlas of Skeletal Development of the Hand and Wrist,* ed 2. Stanford, Stanford University Press, 1959.

58. **Fearon T, Vucich J, Butler P, et al:** *Scoliosis examinations: Organ dose and image quality with rare-earth screen-film systems.* AJR 150:359, 1988.

59. **Gray JE, Hoffman AD, Peterson HA:** *Reduction of radiation exposure during radiography for scoliosis.* J Bone Joint Surg (Am) 65(1):5, 1983.

60. **Davies WG:** *Radiography in the treatment of scoliosis and in leg lengthening. Part II—Radiography in scoliosis.* Radiography 26(311):349, 1960.

61. **Archer BR, Whitmore RC, North LB, et al:** *Bone marrow dose in chest radiography: The posteroanterior vs. anteroposterior projection.* Radiology 133:211, 1979.

62. **Stagnara P:** *Examen du scoliotique. In: Deviations laterales du rachio: Scoliosis.* Paris, Encyclopedic Medicochirurgicale, 7, 1974.

63. **DeSmet AA, Fritz SL, Asher MA:** *A method for minimizing the radiation exposure from scoliosis radiographs.* J Bone Joint Surg 63:156, 1981.

64. **Schock CC, Brenton L, Agawal KK:** *The effect of PA versus AP x rays on the apparent scoliotic angle.* Orthop Trans 4:32, 1980.

65. **Lodin H:** *Transversal tomography in the examination of thoracic deformities, funnel chest and kyphoscoliosis.* Acta Radiol 57:49, 1962.

66. **Yochum TR, Guebert GM, Kettner NW:** *The tilt-up view: A closer look at the lumbosacral junction.* Appl Diagn Imag 1(6):49, 1989.

67. **Tojner H:** *Olisthetic scoliosis.* Acta Orthop Scand 33:291, 1963.

68. **Fisk JR, Moe JH, Winter RB:** *Scoliosis, spondylolysis, and spondylolisthesis. Their relationship as reviewed in 539 patients.* Spine 3(3):234, 1978.

69. **Herzenberg JE, Waanders NA, Closkey RF, et al:** *Cobb angle versus spinous process angle in adolescent scoliosis.* Spine 15:874, 1990.

70. **Daniel WW, Barnes GT, Nasca RJ, et al:** *Segmented field radiography in scoliosis.* AJR 144:325, 1985.

71. **Merkin JJ, Sportelli L:** *The effects of two new compensating filters on patient exposure in chiropractic full spine radiography.* J Manipulative Physiol Ther 5(1):25, 1982.

72. **Kling TF, Cohen MJ, Lindseth RE, et al:** *Digital radiography can reduce scoliosis x-ray exposure.* Spine 15:880, 1990.

73. **Goldstein LA, Waugh TR:** *Classification and terminology of scoliosis.* Clin Orthop Rel Res 93:10, 1973.

74. **George K, Rippstein J:** *A comparative study of the two popular methods of measuring scoliotic deformity.* J Bone Joint Surg (Am) 43(6):809, 1961.

75. **Lusskin R:** *Curves and angles. A comparison of scoliosis measurements.* Clin Orthop Rel Res 23:232, 1962.

76. **Risser JC, Ferguson AB:** *Scoliosis: Its prognosis.* J Bone Joint Surg (Am) 18:667, 1936.

77. **Ferguson AB:** *Roentgen Diagnosis of the Extremities and Spine,* ed 2. New York, PB Hoebner, 1949.

78. **Nash CL, Moe JH:** *A study of vertebral rotation.* J Bone Joint Surg (Am) 51(2):223, 1969.

79. **Ho EKW, Upadhyay SS, Ferris L, et al:** *A comparative study of computed tomographic and plain radiographic methods to measure vertebral rotation in adolescent idiopathic scoliosis.* Spine 17:771, 1992.

80. **Willner S, Nordwall A:** *A study of skeletal age and height in girls with idiopathic scoliosis.* Clin Orthop 110:6, 1975.

81. **Low WD, Mok CK, Leong AC, et al:** *The development of southern Chinese girls with adolescent idiopathic scoliosis.* Spine 3:152, 1978.

82. **Gross C, Graham J, Neuwirth M, et al:** *Scoliosis and growth. An analysis of the literature.* Clin Orthop Rel Res 175:243, 1983.

83. **Risser JC:** *Important practical facts in the treatment of scoliosis.* Am Acad Orthop Surgeons Lect 5:248, 1948.

84. **Risser JC:** *The iliac apophysis: An invaluable sign in the management of scoliosis.* Clin Orthop Rel Res 11:111, 1958.

85. **Zaoussis AL, James JIP:** *The iliac apophysis and the evaluation of curves in scoliosis.* J Bone Joint Surg (Br) 40(3):442, 1958.

86. **Suh PB, MacEwan GD:** *Idiopathic scoliosis in males. A natural history study.* Spine 13:1091, 1988.

87. **Lonstein JE, Carlson JM:** *The prediction of curve progression in untreated idiopathic scoliosis during growth.* J Bone Joint Surg (Am) 66(7):1061, 1984.

88. **Meade KP, Bunch WH, Vanderby R, et al:** *Progression of unsupported curves in adolescent idiopathic scoliosis.* Spine 12:520, 1987.

89. **Farady JA:** *Current principles in the nonoperative management of structural adolescent idiopathic scoliosis.* Phys Ther 63(4):512, 1983.

90. **Fisher DA, Rapp GF, Emkes M:** *Idiopathic scoliosis: Transcutaneous muscle stimulation versus the Milwaukee brace.* Spine 12:987, 1987.

91. **Aspegren DD, Cox JM:** *Correction of progressive idiopathic scoliosis utilizing neuromuscular stimulation and manipulation: A case report.* J Manipulative Physiol Ther 10:147, 1987.

92. **Durham JW, Moskowitz A, Whitney J:** *Surface electrical stimulation versus brace in the treatment of idiopathic scoliosis.* Spine 15:888, 1990.

93. **Keim HA:** *The Adolescent Spine,* New York, Grune & Stratton, 1976.

94. **Calliet R:** *Scoliosis: Diagnosis and Treatment,* Philadelphia, FA Davis, 1978.

95. **Denton TE, Randall FM, Deinlein DA:** *The use of instant moire photographs to reduce exposure from scoliosis radiographs.* Spine 17:509, 1992.

96. **Blount WP, Schmidt AC, Keever D, et al:** *The Milwaukee brace in the operative treatment of scoliosis.* J Bone Joint Surg (Am) 40:511, 1958.

97. **Hassan I, Bjerkreim I:** *Progression in idiopathic scoliosis after conservative treatment.* Acta Orthop Scand 54(1):88, 1983.

98. **Dwyer AF, Newton NC, Sherwood AA:** *An anterior approach to scoliosis. A preliminary report.* Clin Orthop 62:192, 1969.

99. **Stokes AF, Ronchetti PJ, Aronsson DD:** *Changes in shape of the adolescent idiopathic scoliosis curve after surgical correction.* Spine 19:1032, 1994.

100. **Paonessa KJ, Engler GL:** *Back pain and disability after Harrington rod fusion to the lumbar spine for scoliosis.* Spine 17:S249, 1992.

5

Natural History of Spondylolysis and Spondylolisthesis

Terry R. Yochum, Lindsay J. Rowe, and Michael S. Barry

DEFINITIONS

Spondylolysis is an interruption of the pars interarticularis, which may be either unilateral or bilateral. The term *spondylolysis* is derived from two Greek roots: *spondylos*, meaning vertebra, and *lysis*, meaning a dissolution or a loosing, a setting free, a releasing. (Fig. 5.1A and B)

Spondylolisthesis is traditionally defined as an anterior displacement of a vertebral body in relation to the segment immediately below. The Greek origin of this word is *spondylos*, meaning vertebra, and *listhesis*, which refers to slippage or displacement but without regard for direction. (Fig. 5.1A and B) Traditionally, and even today, the term *spondylolisthesis* in medical literature is synonymous with forward displacement. Unfortunately, this is an erroneous use of the word *spondylolisthesis*. While a more precise term for this anatomic disrelationship would be "anterolisthesis with or without spondylolysis," we will yield to convention in this chapter and use *spondylolisthesis* to mean anterior vertebral displacement, unless otherwise indicated. Spondylolisthesis (anterolisthesis) may occur with a defect in the vertebral arch (spondylolytic spondylolisthesis) or without a defect in the vertebral arch (nonspondylolytic spondylolisthesis). (1)

Prespondylolisthesis has been used to indicate the presence of spondylolysis without forward vertebral displacement. This term is misleading and should be discarded since it erroneously implies that displacement will necessarily occur.

HISTORICAL CONSIDERATIONS

Spondylolisthesis has been a focal point of academic and clinical interest for over 100 years, and still many questions remain unanswered in regard to the etiology, clinical significance, treatment, and prognosis of this common condition.

The first recorded description of spondylolisthesis was written in 1782 by a Belgian obstetrician, Herbinaux. (2) The term *spon-dylolisthesis* was introduced by Kilian (3), who concluded that these displacements occurred gradually. Herbinaux's original report was of a patient who experienced difficulty in childbirth because of displacement of the fifth lumbar vertebra relative to the first sacral segment. This condition stimulated the interest of obstetricians, who identified it as a cause of obstructed labor. It is doubtful that the spondylolisthesis had anything to do with the patient's difficulty with delivery. Wiltse has never observed difficulty with delivery, no matter how severe the displacement. (L.L. Wiltse, personal communication, 1990) In 1855 Robert (4) performed experiments on cadavers in which he removed all soft tissues around the spondylolysis at the lumbosacral junction, exposing the pars interarticularis. His studies revealed that no displacement occurred if the neural arch was intact, an observation later challenged. (5,6) In 1858 Lambl (5) demonstrated the pars interarticularis defect that is known as "spondylolysis." In 1895 Neugebauer (6) was the first to describe displacement of the L5 vertebral body upon the sacrum that occurred without pars interarticularis defects as a result of congenital elongation of the pars interarticularis (type I: Dysplastic).

PREVALENCE

Approximately 90% of all spondylolytic spondylolistheses involve the fifth lumbar vertebra. (7) The remaining 10% are found throughout the other lumbar and cervical vertebrae. (Table 5.1)

Several studies have suggested that there are variations in the prevalence of spondylolysis in different populations. There is a 5 to 7% prevalence of pars defects in the white population, with a 2 to 1 male predominance. (8) Moreton (9) found a 7.2% prevalence of spondylolysis in a preemployment study of 32,600 asymptomatic young men aged 18 to 35 years.

Stewart (10) in 1953 studied the skeletal remains of 243 Alaskan Eskimos and found a 40.3% prevalence of pars defects in the specimens. Kettelkamp and Wright (11) reviewed the radio-

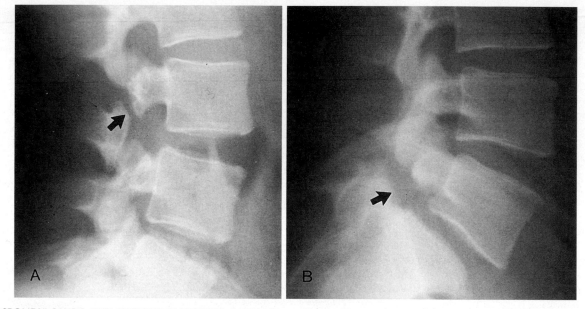

Figure 5.1.   SPONDYLOLYSIS AND SPONDYLOLISTHESIS. A. Spondy-lolysis: Third Lumbar. Observe the pars defects (arrow), but note the absence of anterolisthesis of the third lumbar body. **B. Spondylolisthesis: Fifth Lum-bar.** In this case the pars defects (arrow) are accompanied by anterolisthesis of the fifth lumbar body.

Table 5.1.   Common Sites for Spondylolysis and/or Spondylolisthesis (7)

Location	Percentage*
L5	90
L4	5
L1, 2, 3	3
C5, 6, 7	2

*Excludes degenerative

Table 5.2.   Hypothesized Mechanisms of Development of Spondylolysis and/or Spondylolisthesis (13)

Separate ossification centers
A fracture that occurs at the time of birth
An ordinary fracture at that region
A stress or fatigue fracture
Displacement secondary to an increased lumbar lordosis
Displacement secondary to a pinching mechanism of superior and
    inferior articular processes
Weakness of regional ligamentous and fascial support structures
Aseptic necrosis of the pars interarticularis
Dysplasia of the pars interarticularis
Pathologic changes of the pars interarticularis

graphs of 153 Alaskan Eskimos and noted the presence of pars defects in 28%. In addition to a much higher overall prevalence of spondylolysis compared with other groups, Alaskan Eskimos have demonstrated a proportionately higher percentage of upper lumbar involvement (L1-L3) compared with other groups. (10) We suggest that carrying infants in a cradleboard places an undue amount of premature stress on the pars interarticularis, perhaps explaining the unusually high prevalence of pars defects in the Alaskan Eskimos. This could have serious implications for the popular use of infant carriers, which maintain children in the up-right position for extended periods of time. These devices may cause premature biomechanical stress upon the pars interarticu-laris, predisposing the children to pars defects. Perhaps use of an upright walker should be discouraged until the child can walk unassisted.

Rowe and Roche (12) report an incidence of spondylolisthesis of 2.4% in the black populations of North America and South Africa. According to Wiltse (13), there is a thirteen-fold increase in the prevalence of spina bifida occulta among persons with pars defects when compared with the general population. Spina bifida occulta is not necessarily found at the level of the spondylolysis, nor are the disorders etiologically related. (13) According to Janse, (14) patients with spina bifida occulta often have hypoplastic and asymmetric facets at the spondylolisthetic segment. This may cause aberrant motion and excessive stress in the neural arch, which may then predispose that patient to develop pars defects.

ETIOLOGY

The etiology of spondylolysis is controversial, with many sug-gested mechanisms. (Table 5.2) Although much debate has arisen regarding the true nature of isthmic spondylolysis, there is little doubt that physical forces are major factors in its production.

CONGENITAL

For many years spondylolysis and spondylolisthesis have been referred to as congenital anomalies (15,16); however, exten-sive studies of cadavers have not revealed these lesions in the newborn. Batts (17) in 1939, in a study of 200 fetal spines, found no pars interarticularis defects, nor did Rowe and Roche (12) in 509 stillborn and neonatal cadavers. Fredrickson et al. (18), re-viewed the lumbar radiographs of 500 newborns in 1984 and found no evidence of spondylolysis or spondylolisthesis, thus supporting an acquired etiology. Previously, the youngest patient reported with pars defects (15) was a 4-month-old child who was born after an uneventful pregnancy and delivery. Borkow and Kleiger (15) reported that shortly after birth the parents noted a deformity in the child's lower back and brought it to the attention of their physician. Radiologic examination revealed a pars defect at the L4 vertebra and a hypoplastic L5 vertebral body. The youngest persons previously reported were 10 and 17 months of age, respectively. (19,20) (Fig. 5.2)

Some authors attempt to explain spondylolysis as being caused by the nonunion of two separate ossification centers in the pars interarticularis or as due to a defect in cartilaginous development; however, no evidence has been produced to support these theories. (13) It should be understood that the pars is typically a fully ossified structure at birth. (21,22)

Although spondylolysis is not considered to be of congenital origin, there is an increased incidence among some families (23) and certain racial groups, such as Alaskan Eskimos and other native Americans. (10) This suggests that there are some genetic factors that may predispose an individual to develop the defect. If the defect is ultimately of mechanical origin, the amount and distribution of cortical bone within the pars interarticularis must be considered important. (24) The presence of a thin pars interarticularis may be due to genetic factors. The high familial incidence of this condition may be explained by a thin pars interarticularis, causing otherwise normal physiologic forces on the neural arch to produce critical tensile stress and fatigue fracture at the pars level. Therefore, those born with a thin pars may be predisposed to but not born with spondylolysis.

STRESS FRACTURE

Presently, the most commonly proposed etiology leading to a pars interarticularis defect is that of stress fracture. (25) The most common skeletal location for stress fracture is the pars interarticularis of the fifth lumbar vertebra. (25) Wiltse et al. (25) have

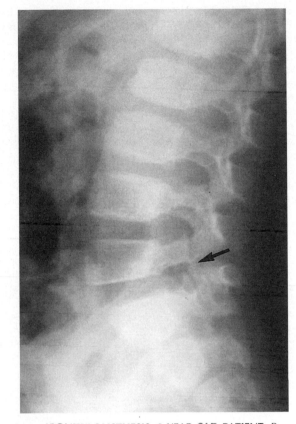

Figure 5.2. SPONDYLOLISTHESIS, 3-YEAR-OLD PATIENT. Pars defects are visible at the fifth lumbar segment (arrow), with accompanying anterolisthesis. (Courtesy of Victor Y. W. Tong, DC, DACBR, Los Angeles, California)

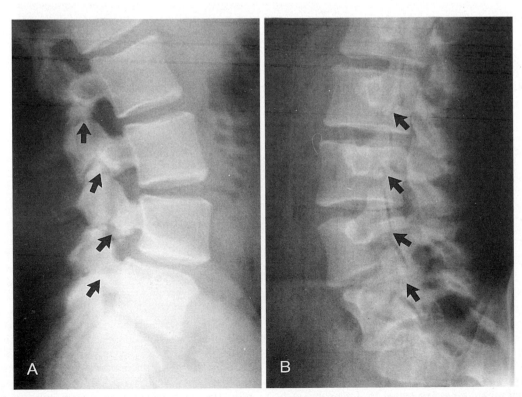

Figure 5.3. SPONDYLOLYSIS AT MULTIPLE LEVELS. A and B. A 22-year-old male power weight lifter had these films taken following an acute low back strain. Observe the multiple pars defects from the fifth to second lumbar levels (arrows). This patient totaled *eight* pars defects from L2 through L5.

proposed that spondylolysis is a fatigue fracture caused by recurrent mechanical stress. This theory is supported by an in vitro study conducted by Cyron and Hutton (26), in which they subjected 28 human lumbar spines, consisting of the lower three lumbar vertebrae and the sacrum, to repetitive mechanical stress. The lumbar vertebrae were subjected to a hyperextension loading pattern calculated to simulate walking with a heavy backpack. They found that the pars interarticularis defect of the lumbar vertebrae was related to hyperextension mechanical fatigue fracture. (Fig. 5.3A and B) Similar fatigue fractures may occur at the vertebra above a transitional segment. (Fig. 5.4A–C)

Except for a single case at C4 reported in a gorilla the defect of spondylolysis has not been reported in mammals other than humans. (27) We therefore suggest that the upright posture of humans, combined with additional repetitive hyperextension mechanical stress, would appear to be a significant etiologic factor. Rosenberg et al. (28) reviewed the radiographs of 143 lifelong nonambulatory patients. The condition underlying the nonambulatory status varied but was most commonly cerebral palsy. No case of spondylolysis or spondylolisthesis was detected in this study. These patients had the same prevalence as the general population for such other spinal anomalies as spina bifida occulta, transitional vertebrae, and structural scoliosis. These findings support the hypothesis that ambulation and upright posture, with added repetitive hyperextension mechanical stress, are intimately related to the etiology of spondylolysis.

Age of onset augments the argument for the stress fracture etiology. Spondylolysis in children can occur shortly after walk-

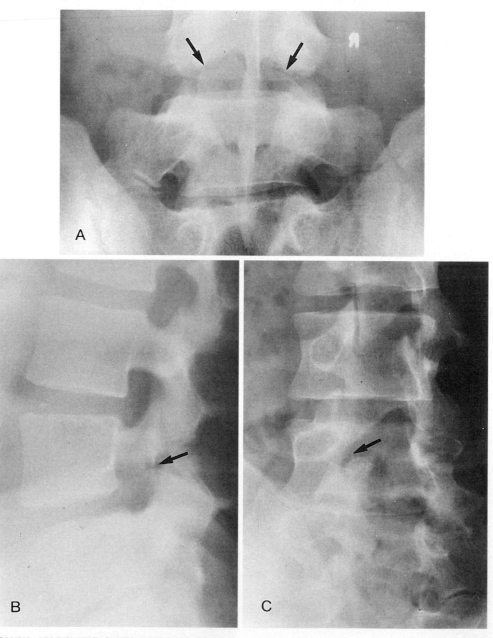

Figure 5.4. SPONDYLOLYSIS ASSOCIATED WITH A TRANSITIONAL LUMBOSACRAL SEGMENT. A. AP Angulated View. The bilateral accessory joints are identified. Note the pars defects visible on this angulated (30° cephalad) lumbosacral view (arrows). **B and C. Lateral and Oblique Views.** The pars defects (arrows) and anterolisthesis are identified.

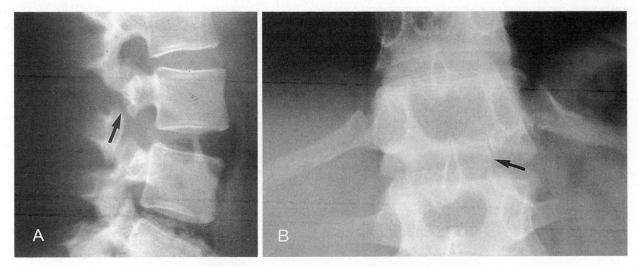

Figure 5.5. PARS INTERARTICULARIS DEFECTS AT UNUSUAL LEVELS. A. Third lumbar (arrow), male pole-vaulter.
B. Twelfth thoracic (arrow). (Courtesy of Simon Breen, BAppSc (Chiro), Adelaide, Australia)

ing begins; however, clinical and radiographic detection occurs most commonly after the age of 5 and most often between the ages of 10 and 15. (12) There appears to be a meaningful etiologic association between the onset of the pars defect, the development of the lumbar lordosis, and repeated infant falls, particularly if premature walking occurs. (29) Parents should be discouraged from prompting their child to walk before the child is prepared to do so. Repetitive lumbar hyperextension has also been implicated as a mechanism in the development of pars interarticularis defects. (20,30)

An increased prevalence of spondylolysis and spondylolisthesis has been noted in persons participating in above-average levels of physical activity, particularly when the activity involves stressful movements of the lumbar spine that are unique to certain sports. Rossi (30), in a report to the Italian Olympic Committee in 1978, reviewed 1430 lumbar spine radiographs of athletes in the 16 to 27 age range. Of these athletes, 239 (16.7%) were found to have spondylolysis and/or spondylolisthesis. Those athletic activities in which participants had the highest prevalence of spondylolysis and/or spondylolisthesis were diving and gymnastics. The prevalence among persons in those sports was higher than for the general population and supports the assertion that athletic activity resulting in greater spinal mechanical stress is related to the development of spondylolysis and spondylolisthesis. (Fig. 5.5A and B) Similarly, a high percentage of pole-vaulters develop spondylolysis. (31) Raynal et al. (32) examined the radiographs of 4619 middle-aged manual laborers involved in heavy lifting and found a 9.4% prevalence of spondylolysis and spondylolisthesis, which is similar to the prevalence among Japanese athletes, 10.9%. (33) Diving, gymnastics, weight lifting and pole-vaulting all require repetitive hyperextension of the lumbar spine, coupled with jarring, which suggests that hyperextension is a factor in the etiology of spondylolysis and spondylolisthesis. (34)

Accepting the stress fracture etiology presents a challenge. Since all other stress fractures heal with immobilization, why doesn't this one? The answer appears to be that these individuals are not immobilized at the time the spondylolysis occurs. This results in the nonunion of the stress fracture and, thereby, a spondylolysis. Micheli (35–37) has documented the healing and dis-

appearance of pars defects with the use of the Boston overlap brace (antilordotic brace).

OTHER FACTORS

Rarely, an acute traumatic fracture does occur through the pars area, creating a spondylolysis. An acute pars fracture without concomitant fracture in other parts of the vertebra (usually a compression fracture of the vertebral body) seldom occurs. (Fig. 5.6) Certain disease processes, such as osteopetrosis can weaken the bone and thereby allow spondylolysis to occur. (38) (Fig. 5.7)

WILTSE CLASSIFICATION OF SPONDYLOLISTHESIS

The most widely used classification of spondylolisthesis is that described by Wiltse, Newman, and Macnab, in which five distinct types have been identified. (39)

Type I: Dysplastic: This type includes those spondylolistheses with a congenital abnormality in the upper sacrum or the neural arch of L5 that allows displacement to occur. (Fig. 5.8)

Type II: Isthmic: This type has three subtypes that involve alteration to the pars interarticularis as follows:
A. A lytic or stress (fatigue) fracture of the pars, or
B. An elongated but intact pars, or
C. An acute fracture of the pars (rare and seldom affects the pars only).

Type III: Degenerative (Pseudospondylolisthesis): This type is secondary to long-standing degenerative arthrosis of the lumbar zygapophyseal joints and discovertebral articulations, without a pars separation.

Type IV: Traumatic: This type is secondary to a fracture of part of the neural arch other than the pars interarticularis.

Type V: Pathologic: This type occurs in conjunction with generalized or localized bone disease (e.g., Paget's disease, metastatic bone disease, osteopetrosis, etc.).

TYPE I: DYSPLASTIC

This type of spondylolisthesis involves a congenital malformation of the upper sacrum and/or the neural arch of the L5

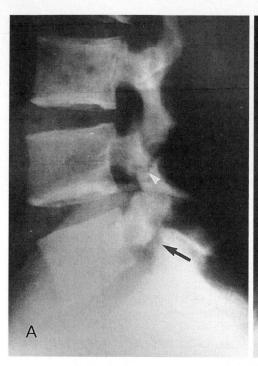

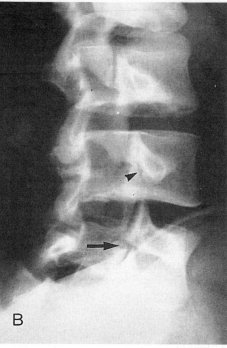

Figure 5.6. SPONDYLOLYSIS: FIFTH LUMBAR SEGMENT, WITH ACUTE UNILATERAL PARS FRACTURE AT THE FOURTH LUMBAR SEGMENT. 16-year-old male football player was "clipped" from behind. **A. Lateral View.** Note the defect at the fifth lumbar pars (arrow), with no anterolisthesis. The fractured fourth lumbar pars is also identified (arrowhead). **B. Oblique View.** The difference between the defects is apparent—smooth and more horizontal at the fifth (arrow) and irregular and more vertical at the fourth (arrowhead). COMMENT: Despite the considerable force required to fracture the fourth lumbar pars, no anterolisthesis of the fifth segment occurred, demonstrating the usual stability of spondylolytic pars defects. (Courtesy of Barton W. Dukett, DC, Bigelow, Arkansas)

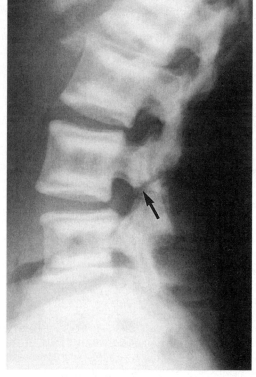

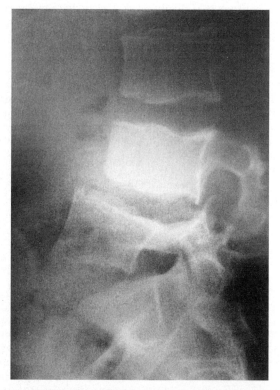

Figure 5.7. PATHOLOGIC SPONDYLOLISTHESIS: OSTEOPETROSIS. In this condition the bones are rendered brittle and prone to fracture; in this case, at the third lumbar pars interarticularis (arrow).

Figure 5.8. DYSPLASTIC SPONDYLOLISTHESIS. Observe the congenitally elongated and dysplastic pedicle and pars interarticularis of the L5 vertebral segment. This condition has allowed a significant anterolisthesis to occur without pars defect. COMMENT: This 14-year-old female patient has a dysplastic spondylolisthesis Wiltse type I. This patient also had Marfan's syndrome with spool-shaped vertebrae and scalloping of the posterior vertebral body margins. (Courtesy of Kenneth P. Stein, DC, Miles City, Montana)

vertebra. (40) There is an anterior displacement of the L5 vertebral body upon the sacrum as a result of the bony architecture being inadequate to withstand the forward vectors of thrust of the lumbar spine on the sacral promontory. (Fig. 5.8) Usually, there is an accompanying wide spina bifida occulta involving the sacrum and the L5 vertebra. This type usually progresses to a more severe grade of displacement (40) and is one of the nonspondylolytic (no pars defects) forms of spondylolisthesis. Dysplastic spondylolisthesis is much less common than the isthmic type, with a ratio of about 1:4. (40)

TYPE II: ISTHMIC

Subtype A

This subtype is caused by biomechanical stress; the mode of failure is believed to be fatigue fracture of the pars interarticularis. It is the most common type found in persons below the age of 50 and has not been noted in the newborn. (40)

Subtype B

This subtype of spondylolisthesis results from elongation of the pars interarticularis without separation. It is fundamentally the same lesion as subtype A; however, it is thought to be secondary to repeated, minor trabecular stress fractures of the pars. Healing of these fractures occurs, but the pars is elongated as the vertebral body of L5 is displaced anteriorly. Eventually, the pars may separate as displacement progresses, making differentiation from subtype A difficult. (40)

Subtype C

These spondylolistheses, rarely seen, result from acute pars fractures. The most common mechanism of injury is lower lumbar hyperextension. Displacement seldom occurs. (39)

TYPE III: DEGENERATIVE

Degenerative spondylolisthesis (type III), with an intact neural arch, has been referred to by Junghans (27) as "pseudospondylolisthesis" to differentiate it from those with a neural arch defect. (27) Macnab (41) prefers the phrase "spondylolisthesis with an intact neural arch," which is a more accurate description. Thus, degenerative spondylolisthesis is another type of nonspondylolytic spondylolisthesis. Degenerative spondylolisthesis is approximately 10 times more common at L4 than at the L3 or L5 vertebra, and no greater than 25% anterior displacement of the L4 vertebral body occurs, with the majority involving only 10 to 15% displacement. (42) (Fig. 5.9A and B) Distribution of degenerative spondylolisthesis varies among populations. It is 6 times more common in females 60 years of age or older, compared with males of the same age (42), and is rare in persons under 50 years of age. (34) Degenerative spondylolisthesis is 3 times more common in blacks than in whites, with no adequate explanations for these sexual and racial disparities. (42) Finally, degenerative spondylolisthesis is 4 times more likely to be found in association with a sacralized fifth lumbar vertebra. (42) (Table 5.3)

The mechanisms of displacement are thought to involve a combination of zygapophyseal joint arthrosis, disc degeneration, and remodeling of the articular processes and pars. (41) An in-

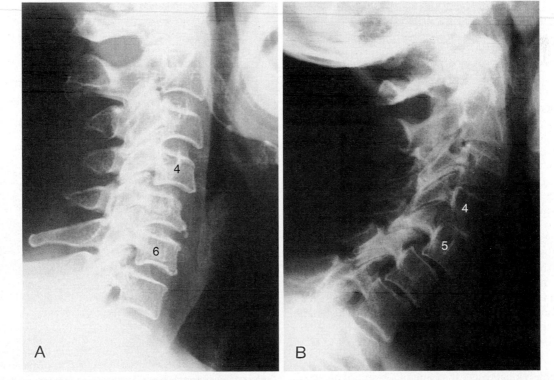

Figure 5.9. DOUBLE DEGENERATIVE SPONDYLOLISTHESES—A CERVICAL SPINE LOCATION. A. Lateral Cervical View. There is a C4 and C6 double degenerative spondylolisthesis. Extensive facet arthrosis has allowed this degenerative spondylolisthesis to occur. (Courtesy of Kevin J. La Londe, DC, Duxbury, Massachusetts) **B. Lateral Cervical View.** There is a congenital block vertebra present at the C4-C5 level with a remnant calcified disc. A significant anterolisthesis of C5 upon C6 and, to a lesser extent, C6 upon C7 has occurred as a result of extensive discogenic spondylosis and posterior facet joint arthrosis. This patient has significant spinal stenosis. (Courtesy of Jan A. Roberts, DC, Farmington, Maine)

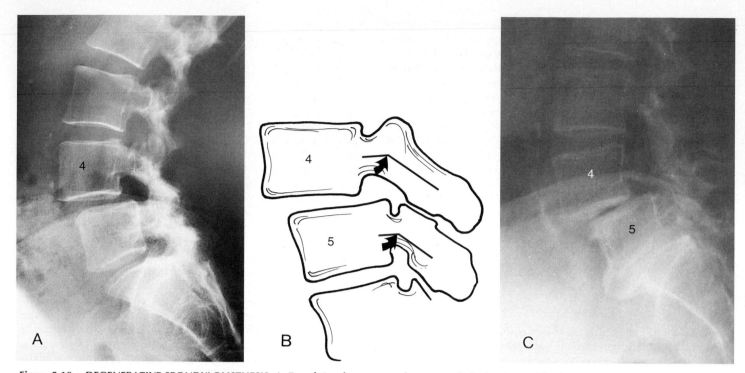

Figure 5.10. DEGENERATIVE SPONDYLOLISTHESIS. A. Fourth Lumbar. A typical anterior displacement has occurred secondary to facet arthrosis at the fourth and fifth lumbar zygapophyseal joints. Also note the altered pedicle-facet angle at this level. **B. Pedicle-Facet Angle.** A widening of this angle (arrows), due to remodeling from facet arthrosis, enhances the tendency to produce anterolisthesis. **C.** Double degenerative spondylolisthesis at the fourth and fifth lumbar vertebrae. Observe the vacuum phenomenon at the L4 disc level and extensive atherosclerosis of the abdominal aorta. (Courtesy of Daniel L. Fouts, DC, Tulsa, Oklahoma)

Table 5.3.	The Three F's of Degenerative Spondylolisthesis
	Female
	Four (L4)
	Above **F**orty years

crease of the "pedicle-facet angle" has been noted in the degenerative type of spondylolisthesis. (1) This angle, formed by the long axis of the pedicle (or vertebral root) at its intersection with the long axis of the articular pillar, indicates the more horizontal alignment of the degenerative zygapophyseal joints, as seen on the lateral radiograph, and demonstrates the overriding of the articular surfaces. (1) (Fig. 5.10)

Several explanations have been proposed for degenerative spondylolisthesis occurring with such great frequency at the L4 level. Allbrook (43) has stated that the greater mobility of L4 due to the sagittal orientation of the facets at the L4-L5 level may explain the unusual frequency of degenerative spondylolisthesis at the L4 level. Additionally, the firmly attached, normal lumbosacral joint may place increased stress on the L4-L5 intervertebral joints, ultimately leading to hypermobility and degeneration of the articular triad. (42)

TYPE IV: TRAUMATIC

Traumatic spondylolisthesis can occur as a result of an acute, severe injury that creates a fracture of a portion of the neural arch other than the pars interarticularis. (Fig. 5.6) These fractures generally heal when appropriately immobilized. (40) It is common at C2 and is referred to as a Hangman's (actually Hangee's) fracture. (Fig. 5.11)

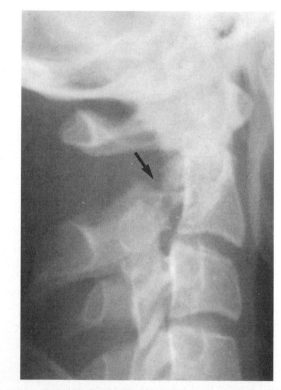

Figure 5.11. TRAUMATIC SPONDYLOLISTHESIS: AXIS (HANGMAN'S FRACTURE). Note the anterolisthesis of the axis body and fractures through the pedicles of the C2 vertebra (arrow).

TYPE V: PATHOLOGIC

Generalized or systemic disorders of bone may affect the neural arch of the spine and allow spondylolysis to develop. Metastatic carcinoma, osteopetrosis (23,38), and Paget's disease are some of the more common disorders which may contribute to the formation of spondylolysis. (Fig. 5.7)

A *sixth* type may be offered, which is called *"postsurgical"* or *"iatrogenic spondylolisthesis."* This includes two different types of lesions. The first is a stress fracture of the pars at a level immediately above or below a spinal fusion (spondylolisthesis acquisita). (1) (Fig. 5.12) Many of these patients have had previous anterior interbody fusion for spondylolisthesis. This creates abnormal stress above or below the fusion site. With the advent of posterolateral fusions for spondylolisthesis, this entity is disappearing.

The second disorder in this group is caused by removing too much bone in posterior decompression laminectomies, usually for a herniated nucleus pulposus. This unilateral decompression creates spinal instability and abnormal stress upon the neural arch opposite the surgical defect. This abnormal stress may lead to a sclerotic hypertrophied pedicle and lamina or spondylolysis (see discussion and images under Unilateral Spondylolysis).

CLINICAL FEATURES

PAIN

In addition to their controversial etiology, spondylolysis and spondylolisthesis present a challenging clinical picture. Spondy-

lolysis and/or spondylolisthesis may be found in symptomatic or asymptomatic individuals. Patients with severe displacement may experience only minimal back pain, and there is no correlation between the degree of anterior displacement and the severity of symptoms. (16,46) Of those patients with back pain related to their spondylolisthesis, 25% have a recent history of antecedent trauma. (7) These patients have a deep-seated, dull, aching pain, which is localized to the area of spondylolysis or spondylolisthesis. In most cases the lesion has been present since the age of 5 or 6 years. (18) Studies indicate that approximately one-half of patients with radiologic signs of spondylolisthesis never develop symptoms. (29,39,44,45) Nachemson (40) believes that spondylolysis does not contribute to the cause of pain at all, and according to Schmorl and Junghans (27), pain specifically related to spondylolysis and/or spondylolisthesis does not exist. Additionally, Fredrickson and colleagues (18), in their extensive prospective study, found that the development of spondylolysis, with or without spondylolisthesis, does not cause pain in most patients. We feel that back pain may often be present with patients developing spondylolysis, but its presence goes unrecognized because of the young age (2 to 10 years) of the patient and the failure of the parents to acknowledge the child's complaints, which may be simply disregarded as "growing pains." The development of spondylolysis in a teenage athlete or young adult is usually painful (30,31); therefore, why shouldn't it be in the young child? The use of single-photon emission computed tomography (SPECT) scans may allow the clinician to see increased radiotracer uptake in the area of the pars which is usually indicative of a symptomatic pars. (47)

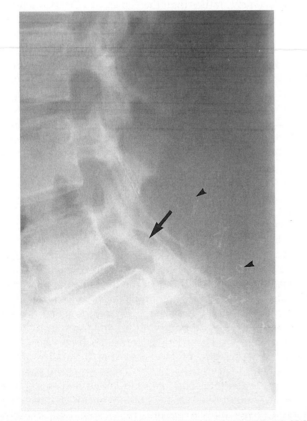

Figure 5.12. SPONDYLOLISTHESIS ACQUISITA (IATROGENIC SPONDYLOLISTHESIS). Following a decompressive laminectomy and posterior arthrodesis at the fourth and fifth lumbar vertebrae, pars defects developed at the fourth lumbar vertebra (arrow), which allowed for a grade 1 spondylolisthesis to occur. Of incidental notation are surgical metallic sutures in the soft tissues of the lumbosacral region (arrowheads).

PHYSICAL EXAMINATION FINDINGS

Examination of the patient with spondylolisthesis often reveals distinct postural changes consistent with the degree of anterolisthesis. The buttocks are often prominent, assuming a heart-shaped appearance when viewed from the posterior. A hyperlordosis of the lumbar spine and anterior shift of the gravitational weight-bearing line is often noted. Patients with advanced displacement may demonstrate bilateral transverse skin furrows, which can be seen above the iliac crest. An associated spina bifida occulta may be signaled by localized hypertrichosis. Lower lumbar spine palpation of a patient with a spondylolytic spondylolisthesis reveals prominence of the spinous process at the affected vertebral level. (Fig. 5.13A) Conversely, in a patient with a nonspondylolytic spondylolisthesis, the spinous process of the affected level will be palpated as a depression ("step defect"). (Fig. 5.13B) A clicking sensation at the level of the involved segment may be felt or heard during active trunk flexion or on straight-leg raising. This may be referred to as the *"spinal rattle"* of spondylolysis or spondylolisthesis. Demonstration of this crepitation on clinical examination mandates radiographic assessment to rule out spondylolysis or spondylolisthesis. Hamstring tightness has long been thought to be associated with spondylolisthesis, yet its cause is not known. Decreased anterior trunk flexion and reduced straight-leg raising may be manifestations of tight hamstring muscles and not evidence of an anterolisthesis. No statistically significant correlation is found between hamstring tightness, low back pain, and the radiographic evidence of pars defects or spondylolisthesis. (48) Tight hamstrings may be found in patients with spondylolysis or any grade of spondylolisthesis. In children with spondylolisthesis, tight hamstrings cause a peculiar gait that is

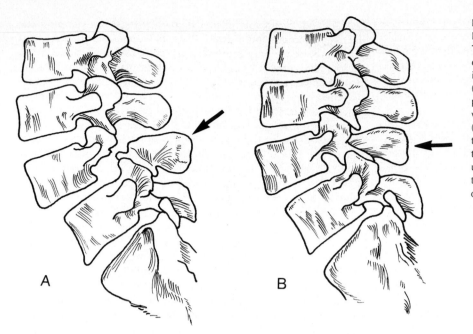

A   B

Figure 5.13.   SPONDYLOLYTIC VERSUS NONSPONDYLOLYTIC SPONDYLOLISTHESIS: LUMBAR PALPATION. A. Spondylolytic Spondylolisthesis. Bilateral pars defects at the L4 vertebra allow anterior displacement of its body and pedicles. The intact upper lumbar segments (L1-L3) move in unison with the displaced L4 body and pedicles, leaving the rest of the L4 neural arch behind, which will be palpated as the prominent spinous process (arrow). **B. Nonspondylolytic Spondylolisthesis.** Observe the anterior displacement of the intact L4 on L5. Since there are no pars defects, the neural arch of L4 must naturally accompany the anterior displacement of the vertebral body. This results in a palpable depression ("step defect") as the spinous process is drawn forward (arrow).

nearly pathognomonic for this condition. The excessively tight hamstrings tilt the inferior pelvis backward and restrict flexion of the hip. Subsequently, these patients have a stiff-legged and short-strided gait, and the pelvis rotates with each step. This gait has been referred to as a *"pelvic waddle."* Also, the child may prefer to jog or run rather than walk, or to walk on the toes with the knees bent.

Neurologic evaluation of the lower extremities is usually unremarkable. However, if leg pain is present, it may be nondermatomal and will likely be a referred-pain phenomenon following sclerotomal patterns from irritation of the mesodermal structures, such as the ligaments and muscles. (49) Disc herniations are generally not associated with spondylolisthesis, but spondylolisthesis may give a "pseudodisc" appearance on CT or MR axial imaging. (18)

DISPLACEMENT

There has been debate in the literature concerning the progression of anterior displacement in spondylolisthesis. Only 2 to 3% of patients with spondylolisthesis show progressive displacement. (18) The majority of these occur due to underlying degenerative changes. (27) The presence of a spina bifida occulta has been shown to be associated with an increased risk of anterior displacement. (50)

Progression of the anterior displacement in spondylolisthesis occurs primarily between the ages of 5 and 10, although some may continue to displace between the ages of 10 and 15. (18) Maximum anterior displacement is usually seen within 18 months to 2 years following the development of spondylolysis, which is usually below 10 years of age. (18) Very few cases demonstrate further anterolisthesis beyond the age of 18. (18,39) (Fig. 5.14A and B) It is rare for greater than 15% anterior displacement to occur in the adult patient with degenerative spondylolisthesis, unless it is associated with zygapophyseal joint instability secondary to severe arthrosis. If marked disc space narrowing occurs, some minor slip may take place. (51)

Taillard (8) has suggested that two anatomic factors are important in the development of a displacement of isthmic spon-

dylolisthesis: the *"trapezoidal"* shape of the fifth lumbar vertebra and the *"doming"* deformity of the anterior sacral promontory. Fredrickson et al. (18) found that a change in the shape of the fifth lumbar vertebra and sacrum occurred at the same time or soon after the displacement was noted. We concur with their opinion that these changes in the shape of the vertebrae are the result of the displacement, rather than the cause. (18) Occasionally, a buttressing of new bone will occur at the anterior margin of the sacrum as a protective measure to resist further anterior displacement of the L5 vertebral body and is a good prognostic sign, as progression of the anterior displacement is unlikely. (8) Turek (52) states that severe anterior displacement (grades 3 and 4) is twice as common in young females and that the most rapid displacement occurs between the ages of 9 and 15. Schmorl and Junghans (27) state that they have not found a case described in the literature that suggests that trauma induced displacement in a known preexisting spondylolysis. Although the anteriorly placed weight gain that occurs during pregnancy would seem to predispose to displacement, such is not the case. No further displacement of spondylolisthesis or fetal risk has been found to be associated with pregnancy, and most patients have no difficulty during parturition, unless the child is presented breech. (18)

The information presented concerning the signs and symptoms of patients with spondylolisthesis demonstrates the lack of direct correlation with back pain. Therefore, the clinician must look past the spondylolisthesis in the total evaluation of patients with both back pain and spondylolisthesis to identify any other causes. Medical authorities who attest to a direct correlation between the presence of spondylolysis and/or spondylolisthesis and back pain have based their conclusions on cases that also included the presence of biomechanical instability and longstanding neurologic deficits. (29,39) These represent such a small percentage of the total patients with spondylolisthesis that this conclusion is questioned by the authors of this chapter, since we feel this does not apply to the majority of spondylolisthesis cases. We concur with Fredrickson et al. (18) that a child over 10 years of age with spondylolysis or spondylolisthesis should be permitted to enjoy normal activities during childhood and adolescence without fear of progressive displacement or disabling pain. When

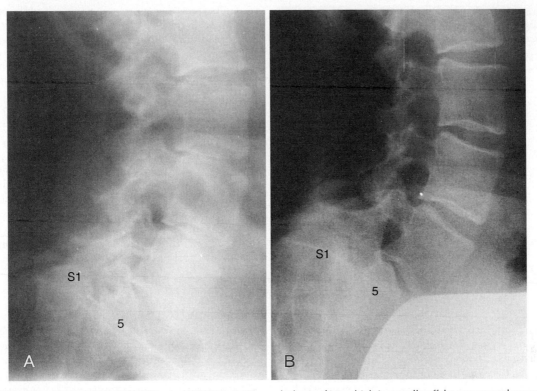

Figure 5.14. ADVANCED SPONDYLOLISTHESIS: A UNIQUE CASE STUDY WITH SERIAL FILMS. A. Lateral Lumbar View. B. Lateral Lumbar View 10 Years after Figure A. COMMENT: This young female patient presented with lower lumbar pain (**A**) and was treated successfully by a chiropractor. Ten years later (**B**) there has been no progression of this antero- listhesis of L5, which is actually off the sacrum and represents grade V spondylolisthesis (spondyloptosis). This patient has had two uneventful pregnancies without cesarean section. (Courtesy of William J. Ladson, DC, Swan Hill, Victoria, Australia)

spondylolisthesis has been detected before the age of 10, we recommend limitation of gymnastic and sports activities until serial flexion and extension upright lateral lumbar radiographic studies, taken 6 months apart, demonstrate no evidence of progressive displacement of the involved segment.

ATHLETIC ACTIVITY

There has been a trend in the clinical management of athletes with spondylolisthesis to curb or restrict their athletic activities. This in effect creates a *"spondylo-athletic invalid,"* even though only an uncomplicated bilateral pars defect with spondylolisthesis may exist. The current literature does not support this approach to the clinical management of patients with spondylolisthesis. (18,30,54) Fredrickson and colleagues (18) do not restrict children's activity in any way, and they allow full participation in sports.

Semon and Spengler (53) reviewed the records of 506 college football players from the University of Washington, spanning an 8-year period. The medical records of the football players included documentation of practices and games missed because of injury. Of the players, 135 (27%) had low back pain following their games. Because of persistent low back symptoms of pain and stiffness, 58 players had roentgenograms of the lumbosacral spine. In 12 of the 58 (20.7%) players with back pain that were radiographed, defects of the lumbar pars interarticularis were observed. We consider the significant finding in this study to be that those players with low back pain and lumbar spondylolysis had no greater time lost from games and practices than players with low back pain without spondylolysis. Ferguson (54) reported a 50% prevalence of pars defects (6 out of 12) in interior linemen on the University of Pittsburgh football team. These players were also performing their football tasks quite adequately, and it may well be the same for many others with spondylolysis and spondylolisthesis playing rigorous sports.

Many coaches and physicians have discouraged individuals with lumbar spondylolysis and/or spondylolisthesis from participating in rigorous sports, despite recent studies that do not support this approach; therefore, it is in the best interest of the patient for the clinician to reconsider seriously the management of these athletes. Semon and Spengler (53) concluded that skeletally mature football players with lumbar spondylolysis and/or spondylolisthesis are able to engage in college and professional football without problems. It seems that the presence of lumbar spondylolysis and/or spondylolisthesis is of modest clinical significance during the 4-year period of active participation in football. (53) However, those patients with spondylolysis and/or spondylolisthesis who demonstrate biomechanical instability, a positive SPECT bone scan, along with persistent symptoms, warrant further clinical consideration.

PROBLEM-BASED CLINICAL CLASSIFICATION OF SPONDYLOLISTHESIS

Hyland has recently offered a problem-based classification for spondylolisthesis. (55,56) His spondylolisthesis classification is based on four problem-based clinical presentations. (See Table 5.4.)

Table 5.4. Problem-Based Clinical Classification of Spondylolisthesis*

	Age	Additional Imaging	Management
Recent Spondylolytic	5–18	SPECT bone scan	immobilization/ restrictions
Preexisting Spondylolytic— Stable	>20	none	active treatment
Preexisting Spondylolytic— Unstable	>20	dynamic views compression/ traction views	possible surgical stabilization
Degenerative	>50	dynamic views compression/ traction views	active treatment
		MRI and CT (stenosis)	possible surgical stabilization

*From Hyland J: *Clinical Classification of Spondylolisthesis*. ACA J Chiro, August 1993.

1. **Recent Spondylolytic Spondylolisthesis (RSS)**. This is due to a recent traumatic or stress fracture and is usually painful and frequently debilitating. It is most commonly seen in adolescents who are physically active, especially in sports requiring repetitive hyperextension of the lumbar spine. These activities include, but are not limited to, diving, gymnastics, and pole-vaulting, as well as sports exerting heavy stress to the lower back such as weight lifting, football, and basketball. RSS has also been linked to inherited weakness (24) and biomechanical factors such as high sacral base angle (57) and increased disc angles, (58) which appear to predispose a child to develop a defect in the pars interarticularis.

2. **Preexisting Spondylolytic Spondylolisthesis—Stable (PSS-S)**. This is the end result of recent spondylolytic spondylolisthesis (RSS) that has gone on to nonunion and a permanent fibrous defect in the area of the pars interarticularis. Further progression of slippage is not expected after the age of 18, and most recent studies show no increase in frequency of low back pain or disability. (55,56) When spinal symptoms are present, a thorough search beyond the spondylolisthesis for altered biomechanics and alternate sources of pain is required. PSS-S is the most common type of spondylolisthesis seen in chiropractic clinical practice, and often shows excellent response to conservative chiropractic care. It is recommended that one *look past* spondylolisthesis for the true cause of back pain in these patients.

3. **Preexisting Spondylolytic Spondylolisthesis—Unstable (PSS-U)**. This is a variant of PSS-S that demonstrates incomplete fibrous union with resulting hypermobility and biomechanical instability at the spondylolisthetic level. It is uncommon, although no study has yet provided a good estimate of true incidence. This type may be the cause of recurrent episodes of back pain and prolonged disability in an adult and progressive slippage in the adolescent. Instability is best determined radiographically (see Instability Evaluation later in the chapter). SPECT bone scans may be of assistance in determining instability.

4. **Degenerative Spondylolisthesis (DS)**. This is found primarily in patients beyond the age of 40 and is much more common in women. It is estimated that 25% of spondylolisthesis cases are due to degenerative spondylolisthesis (pseudospondylolisthesis). As the population over 50 increases, this proportion will also increase.

Unlike the other types, which are spondylolytic and frequently affect L5, degenerative spondylolisthesis does not have a pars defect and occurs much more frequently at L4. (59) The forward displacement occurs secondary to disc degeneration and facet joint arthrosis and often develops later in life. The predisposing factor is believed to be a straight and stable lumbosacral joint that sits higher than normal between the ilia. This arrangement, which may include sacralization of L5, puts increased stress on the L4-L5 intervertebral joint. This can lead to segmental hypermobility, ligament laxity, disc degeneration, and multiple small microfractures of the inferior articular processes of L4.

The amount of slippage that occurs in degenerative spondylolisthesis cases seldom exceeds 25%, and is usually in the range of 10 to 15%. Foraminal compromise and/or lateral recess stenosis that results in neurologic signs and symptoms is possible due to degenerative facet arthropathy. This may lead to the lateral recess or lateral nerve root entrapment syndrome, with patients having intermittent neurogenic claudication.

RADIOLOGIC FEATURES

Radiologic evaluation is the definitive method of confirming the presence of spondylolysis and spondylolisthesis. A complete series of the lumbar spine and sacrum is recommended. It should include weight-bearing anteroposterior (AP) and lateral projections and an AP angulated (tilt-up) view. It also requires bilateral 45° anterior oblique projections, which may be taken weight-bearing or recumbent. The likelihood of not identifying pars defects increases significantly when oblique projections are not included in the radiologic evaluation. If the radiograph is taken lying down, many cases that we would call spondylolysis alone (no slip) will show slippage with erect spinal films. The most definitive imaging modality to demonstrate the pars defects is computed tomography (CT scan).

ANTEROPOSTERIOR NONANGULATED VIEW

Anteroposterior views of the lumbar spine generally do not yield sufficient information for the radiologic evaluation of the pars interarticularis. The pars interarticularis on the AP view projects immediately inferior and slightly medial to the pedicle outline. A pars defect will sometimes be visible as an irregular, linear radiolucency approximately paralleling the inferior cortex of the adjacent pedicle. Normally, the L5 pars interarticularis is not easily discernible with this view because of projectional distortion produced by the presence of the lordotic lumbosacral angle. However, when there is significant anterior displacement of the L5 segment, the vertebral body and transverse processes will become superimposed over the sacral base and alae. The subsequent superimposition of densities at the lumbosacral junction creates an appearance termed the "*inverted Napoleon's Hat*" sign or the "*Gendarme's Cap*." (60) The inferior border of this density corresponds to the anterior aspect of the L5 vertebral body with the attached transverse processes and has been referred to as the "*Bowline of Brailsford*." (60) (Fig. 5.15A and B)

According to Ravichandran (61), a useful radiologic sign in detection of spondylolisthesis is the appearance of the rotated spinous process of a single lumbar vertebra. This is found in a vertebral segment not demonstrating lateral flexion of the vertebral body and without scoliosis and is appreciated in the AP lumbar spine film by drawing a line joining the spinous processes of the lumbar vertebrae. When singular rotation is noted, it may suggest an area of spondylolysis or spondylolisthesis. (61)

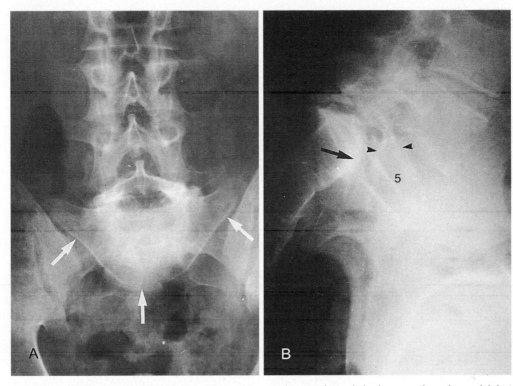

Figure 5.15. SPONDYLOPTOSIS, FIFTH LUMBAR. A 22-year-old Australian Rules football player with acute back pain. **A. AP View.** Note the "inverted Napoleon's hat" sign and the "bowline of Brailsford" (arrows). **B. Lateral View.** The fifth lumbar body has completely slipped over the sacrum. The sacral promontory is dome-shaped (arrow), and the fifth lumbar body is trapezoidal (arrowhead), which is characteristic of grades 3, 4, and 5 types of spondylolisthesis. (Reprinted with permission: Yochum TR, et al: *Reactive sclerosis of a pedicle due to unilateral spondylolysis—A case study.* ACA J Chiro, Radiology Corner, September 1980) COMMENT: Despite the severity of this spondylolisthesis, the patient quickly responded to conservative care and continued to participate in football without recurrence of back pain. He has been pain free for the past 12 years. (Courtesy of Bruce F. Walker, DC, and C. Alison Hogg, MD, Melbourne, Australia)

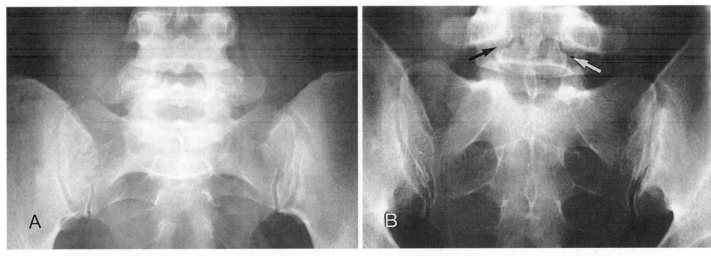

Figure 5.16. ANTEROPOSTERIOR DETECTION OF PARS DEFECTS. A. Normal AP Film. No defects are visible. **B. Angulated AP Film.** The bilateral defects now become visible (30° cephalad tube-tilt) (arrows). (Courtesy of Donald E. Freuden, DC, FACO, Denver, Colorado)

ANTEROPOSTERIOR ANGULATED VIEW

In the evaluation of spondylolisthesis the AP angulated view (also called the tilt-up or Ferguson's view) can be used to more adequately visualize the L5 pars interarticularis. (62) In Canada, this view has been referred to as the Hibbs' projection (Hibbs was a radiologist associated with Albert Ferguson). (63) The tube is angled 25 to 30° cephalad so that the central ray passes through the lumbosacral disc directed about midway between the pubic symphysis and umbilicus or at the level of the anterosuperior iliac spine (ASIS). The AP angulated view eliminates difficulties in patient positioning for oblique lumbar radiographs. Often the pars defect is not tangential to the beam at 45°, and defects, particularly at the L5 level, may not be identified on routine lumbar spine oblique films. Defects in the pars interarticularis may be identified as focal areas of radiolucency below the pedicle outline. (Fig. 5.16A and B, Fig. 5.17A–D)

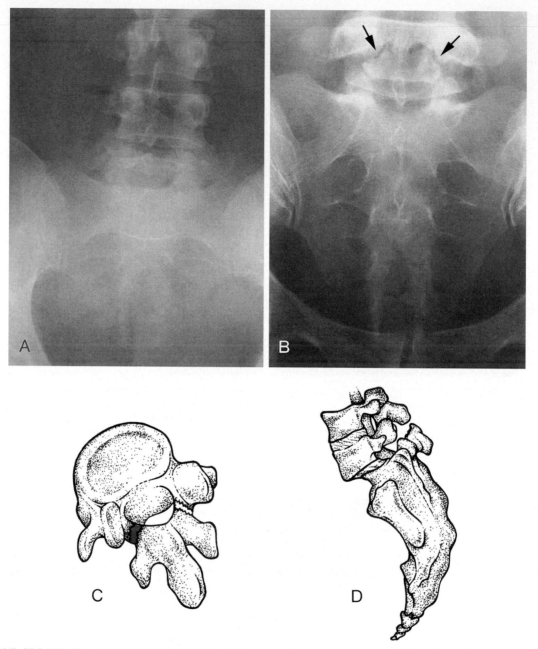

Figure 5.17. TILT-UP PROJECTION OF THE LUMBOSACRAL JUNCTION. A. Normal AP View. No pars defects are visible at the L5 level. **B. Tilt-Up View.** The bilateral pars defects now become visible (25° cephalic tube tilt) (arrows). **C and D. Schematic Demonstration of L5 Pars Defects.** COMMENT: The tilt-up projection of the lumbosacral junction is a great aid in the determination of bilateral pars defects at L5. Often the patients are not positioned tangential to the beam, and defects at the L5 level can be present and not seen on normally positioned oblique lumbar radiographs. It is strongly recommended that the tilt-up projection be added to the evaluation of all patients for lower back pain.

LATERAL VIEW

The lateral view is the most helpful projection for depicting vertebral body anterolisthesis (spondylolisthesis). Comparison of the alignment of the posterior vertebral body margins (George's line) will reveal a distinct misalignment between the involved segments. Also, a line drawn perpendicular to the sacral base from the sacral promontory (Ullmann's line) will show the anteroinferior margin of the L5 vertebral body to touch or to be anterior to this line. (Fig. 5.18) Often a slight change in position of the anterolisthesis may occur when recumbent and upright lateral lumbar films are compared, with the greatest degree of displacement found in the upright radiograph.

The degree of spondylolisthesis has been described by Meyerding. (64) The sacral base length is divided into four equal quarters, and the posterior aspect of the displaced vertebra is compared to this division and "graded" accordingly (Fig. 5.19A–F, 5.20A–D); that is, a grade 1 spondylolisthesis is present when the posterior aspect of the vertebral body lies between the posterior aspect of the sacrum and the first of the four divisions. A grade 2 corresponds to the posterior vertebral body margin positioned

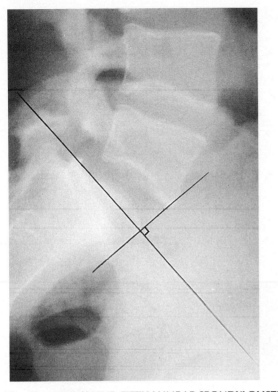

Figure 5.18.   ULLMANN'S LINE, FIFTH LUMBAR SPONDYLOLISTHESIS. A line drawn perpendicular to the sacral base line from the sacral promontory is shown intercepting the fifth lumbar body, indicating a spondylolisthesis.

OBLIQUE VIEW

This is the best view for diagnosing pars abnormalities above L5 and must be performed bilaterally. This projection can be performed in either the anterior or posterior oblique position and can be done upright or recumbent. If performed in the standing position, the anterior oblique position should be used. This allows the divergent x-ray beam to project into the lordosis, rather than against it. Occasionally, the pars defect may be difficult to see as a result of improper positioning of the patient, superimposed structures such as the iliac crest and abdominal contents, and asymmetry of the pars defects. The use of a 30° cephalic tube tilt in patients who are obliquely positioned (left anterior oblique [LAO] or right anterior oblique [RAO]) for lumbar radiography may elongate the pars and allow more adequate visualization of subtle pars defects. (Fig. 5.24A and B)

Lachapelle (60) describes the appearance of the neural arch and its processes on the oblique film as looking like a "Scotty Dog." The anatomic counterparts of the Scotty Dog are outlined in Table 5.5. (66) (Fig. 5.23B) A pars defect will appear as an irregular linear radiolucency which has often been called the "collar" or "broken neck" of the Scotty Dog. (1) The bony margin of the defect may be sclerotic, with an irregular margin at the opposing surface of the nonunion. (Fig. 5.23B and D)

An additional feature that may be noted on the oblique film is referred to as the "stepladder sign" (67) which is produced by a misalignment of the zygapophyseal joints at the involved level. The stepladder sign is demonstrated by drawing lines through the plane of each zygapophyseal joint, and it is considered positive if any line passes through the joint space below it or lies anterior to it. In such cases a stepladder pattern is formed by the lines. (Fig. 5.23C) This sign may not be present in some patients with the degenerative type of spondylolisthesis (type III).

INSTABILITY EVALUATION

Instability is defined as excessive mobility of the spondylolisthetic segment. In the context of this discussion the term does not imply altered biomechanical function at other motion segments.

In order to evaluate the stability of the spondylolisthetic segment, lateral lumbar flexion and extension erect stress radiographs should be performed. (Fig. 5.25A–C) Although conflicting views exist among clinical authorities on the definition of motion segment instability, either additional displacement of the spondylolisthetic segment of 4 mm or a difference in angular motion of two adjacent motion segments greater than 11° in response to spinal flexion and extension (68) is considered to have a poor prognosis with conservative treatment. (69) The 4 mm displacement may occur either anteriorly or posteriorly from the position seen on the erect neutral lateral lumbar film. When vertebral movement of *4-mm or more in either direction is present, the segment may be considered unstable and likely to be symptomatic.*

Limitation of physical activity in the growing child under the age of 10 with spondylolysis and/or spondylolisthesis is appropriate. However, back pain that begins several years after the development of a spondylolisthesis is more likely to be due to other causes. Segmental translatory instability has been examined with a new method in which lateral spot radiographs of the lumbosacral spine are taken (instead of flexion/extension stress lateral radiographs) during axial traction and compression. (70–73) To produce traction, the patient is positioned to hang by the

between the first and second divisions, and a grade 3, between the third and fourth divisions. Next is a grade 4, in which the posterior surface of the L5 vertebral body lies between the anterior sacral promontory and the third division. A patient may reach beyond a grade 4 spondylolisthesis and have complete anterior displacement beyond the sacral promontory; this has been referred to as "*spondyloptosis*" (29) or a grade 5 spondylolisthesis, and is rare. (29) (Fig. 5.15) A percentage of displacement may alternatively be used to grade the degree of anterolisthesis and is considered more accurate than the Meyerding method. Specific millimetric mensuration may also be used as a more accurate alternative than the Meyerding classification.

In the developing child with a grade 3 or 4 spondylolisthesis of L5, a trapezoidal posterior narrowing or wedging of the L5 vertebral body is often seen. Occasionally, a thick, bony protruding buttress may also be seen extending forward from the sacral promontory. (8) (See Fig. 5.15) This radiographic sign (buttressing) represents a stress response secondary to significant anterolisthesis and usually denotes stability of the spondylolisthetic segment. (8) (Figs. 5.21A and B, Fig. 5.22A–C)

Flexion and extension lateral radiographs will provide better visualization of the defect. The pars defect is typically seen just below the pedicle in an oblique plane as a linear radiolucency extending through the junction of the superior and inferior articular processes. The greater the vertebral body anterolisthesis, the easier it is to visualize the pars defects.

In lateral films of the upper lumbar spine, superimposition of the transverse processes over the pars region may simulate pars defects. (65) (Fig. 5.23A)

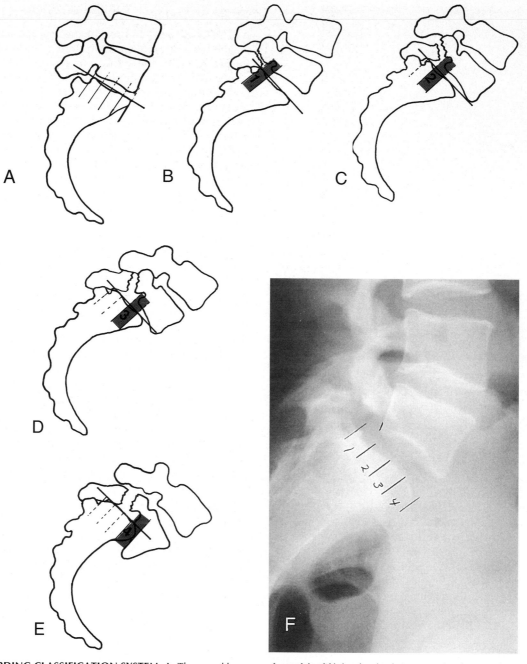

Figure 5.19. MEYERDING CLASSIFICATION SYSTEM. A. The sacral base is divided into four equal segments, and the alignment of the posterior surface of the fifth lumbar body is ascertained. **B.** grade 1. **C.** Grade 2. **D.** Grade 3. **E.** Grade 4. **F.** An example of a grade 1 spondylolisthesis.

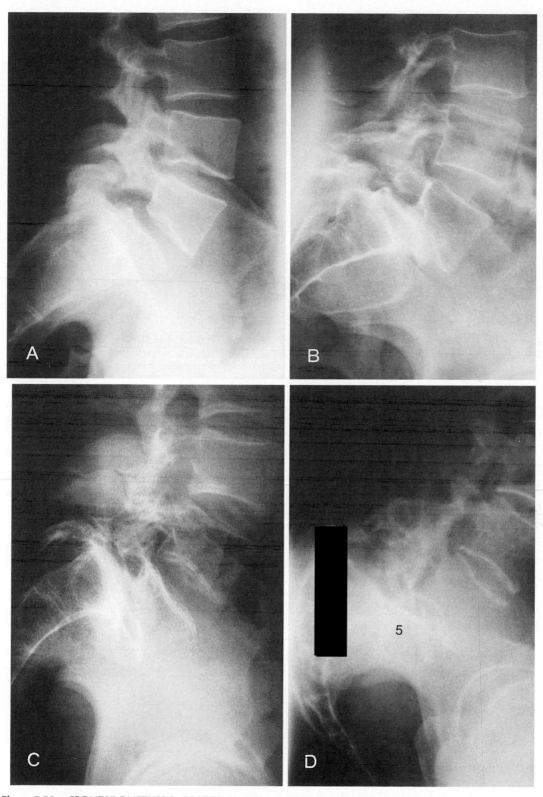

Figure 5.20.   SPONDYLOLISTHESIS: GRADED BY THE MEYERDING METHOD. A. Grade 1. **B.** Grade 2. **C.** Grade 3. **D.** Grade 4, almost a grade 5.

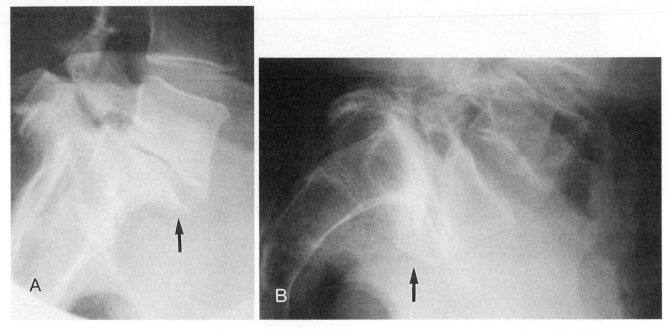

Figure 5.21.   SPONDYLOLISTHESIS: BUTTRESSING PHENOMENOM OF THE SACRUM. A. Small anterior buttressing bone formation of the sacrum (arrow). **B.** Larger anterior sacral buttress (arrow).

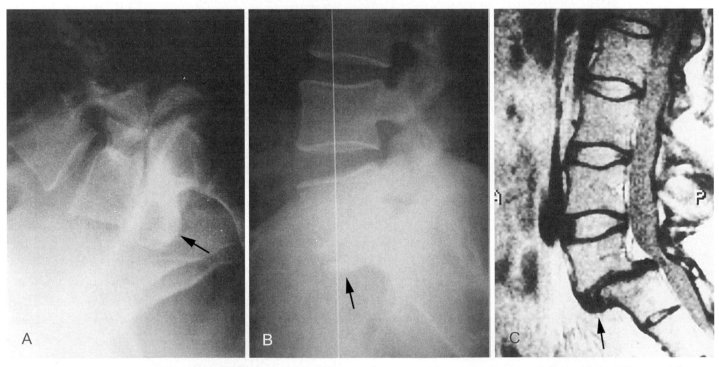

**Figure 5.22.   SPONDYLOLISTHESIS: HUGE BUTTRESS PHENOMENON
OF THE SACRUM. A.** There is a very large spondylophyte formation present
at the anterior aspect of the sacral base (arrow). (Courtesy of John Nolan,
DC, Wanganui, New Zealand) **B and C.** Observe the large anterior buttress

formation of the sacrum (arrow) and the correlative MR scan of the same
patient with low signal intensity (black appearance of the spur) at the anterior
aspect of the sacrum (arrow).

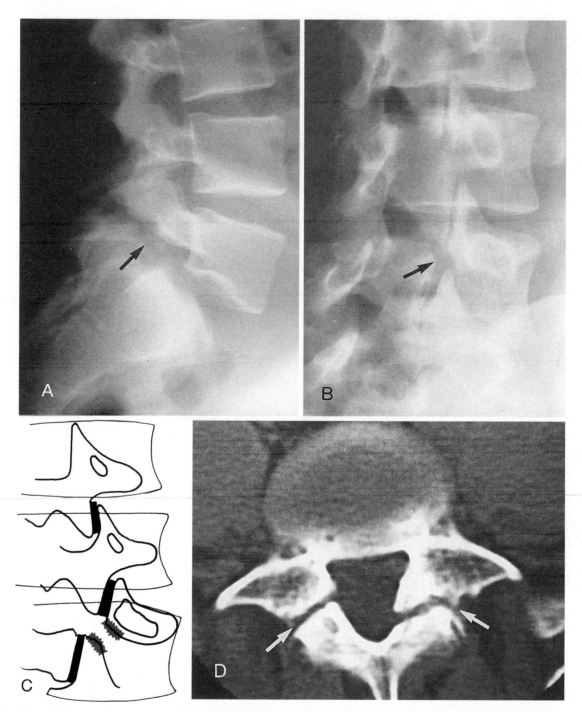

Figure 5.23.   CLASSIC SIGNS OF SPONDYLOLISTHESIS. A. Lateral View. Note the pars defects (arrow) and anterior displacement of the L5 vertebra. **B. Oblique View.** The lucent ''collar'' is clearly visible (arrow). **C. Stepladder Sign.** On an oblique film the alignment of the facet joints changes abruptly at the level of slippage. **D. CT Scan.** The pars defects are readily identified (arrows). Observe the asymmetry of the defects, which is usually present in spondylolysis and may explain why some pars defects are hard to demonstrate on symmetrically positioned 45° oblique lumbar radiographs.

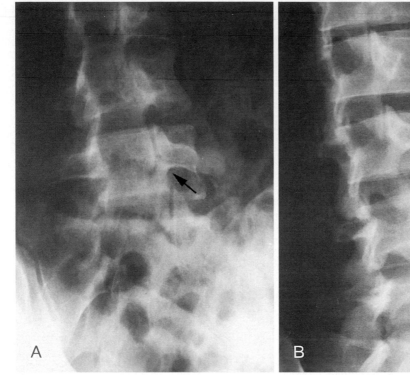

A

B

Figure 5.24. OBLIQUE LUMBAR RADIOGRAPH WITH TUBE TILT—AID IN THE DETECTION OF PARS DEFECTS. A. Oblique Lumbar Radiograph with Tube Tilt. A 30° cephalic tube tilt may be used to augment visualization of the pars at the L4 or L5 level (arrow). **B. Lumbar Radiograph—No Tube Tilt.** The pars of L4 and L5 are visible (arrow). COMMENT: The lumbar radiographs in **A** and **B** represent the same patient, with **A** using a 30° cephalic tube tilt and **B** showing no tube tilt. The L5 pars is much easier to see when it has been somewhat elongated with the cephalic tube tilt projection. However, the tilt-up projection of the lumbosacral junction (AP angulated projection) is a far more practical means to eliminate the degree of obliquity inherent to the pars defect and the problem in positioning the patient at that exact angle when doing oblique lumbar radiography. (Courtesy of Connie Jones, RT(R), Denver, Colorado)

Table 5.5.	Anatomic Counterparts of the Scotty Dog
Eye	Pedicle
Nose	Transverse Process
Ear	Superior Articular Process
Foreleg	Inferior Articular Process
Neck	Pars Interarticularis
Body	Lamina

hands from a horizontal bar perpendicular to the film plane. Thus the lumbar spine is subjected to gravitational traction of the weight of the lower extremities and the pelvis, which represents approximately 40% of total body weight. During radiography, the hips slightly contact the film cassette holder to prevent swaying and to keep the distances between the x-ray tube, the spine, and the film constant. (Fig. 5.26A–D) Then axial compression of the spine is brought about by positioning the patient to stand erect with an additional load of a rucksack filled with 20 kg of sand. (Fig. 5.27)

Kalebo and colleagues (71) have published the opinion that translatory movements (calculated as the resultant difference between compression and traction views) of greater than 3.6% (1.6 mm) may be regarded as pathologic and indicative of segmental instability. We feel the 1.6 mm figure is too low and should be 4 mm.

It appears that the axial compression/traction technique is superior to lateral lumbar flexion/extension stress radiographs in the assessment of instability in patients with spondylolysis and/or spondylolisthesis. The poor detectability of lower lumbar segmental instability using the flexion/extension method compared with the compression/traction technique might be explained by altered tension in the muscles of the spine and trunk. These muscles may limit translatory movements in the spondylolytic segment. (71) This fact does not, however, exclude the value of using lateral lumbar flexion/extension radiographs when examining spinal mobility (rotation in the sagittal plane) or instability of upper lumbar segments. (71)

Since back pain can become a major limiting factor in an athlete's continued participation in rigorous sports, clinical management should not be based on the mere presence of spondylolysis and/or spondylolisthesis alone. (53) No evidence presently exists to support the theory that cessation of sports activity will prevent the development of more serious complications of spondylolisthesis; therefore, the management of athletes should be based on their clinical symptoms rather than the presence of spondylolysis or spondylolisthesis. (74) Athletes with spondylolisthesis should be allowed to continue to participate in sports, since there is no evidence that they are any more susceptible to back injuries than athletes without spondylolisthesis and since cessation of sports may needlessly create a *"spondylo-athletic invalid."* (74)

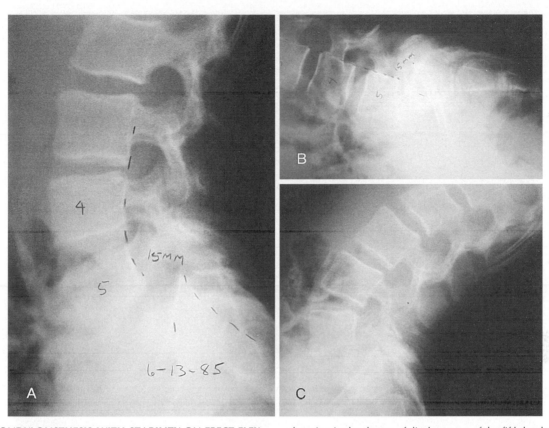

Figure 5.25.   SPONDYLOLISTHESIS WITH STABILITY ON ERECT FLEXION AND EXTENSION RADIOGRAPHS. A 9-year-old female gymnast who fell was radiographed and found to have a preexisting spondylolisthesis. **A. Lateral View.** A 15-mm displacement is evident at the fifth lumbar vertebra. **B and C. Flexion (B) and Extension (C) Views.** These views fail to show any alteration in the degree of displacement of the fifth lumbar vertebra. COMMENT: This case demonstrates the unlikelihood of further progression, based on the stability exhibited even after trauma. (Courtesy of Richard Krauss, DC, FACO, Phoenix, Arizona)

SINGLE-PHOTON EMISSION COMPUTED TOMOGRAPHY

Radionuclide skeletal scintigraphy plays a major role in the identification and evaluation of early lesions by providing correlative activity in radiographically hidden lesions. Because of its limited resolution, planar bone scintigraphy (PBS) is frequently incapable of displaying specific anatomic involvement and may altogether miss less active sites of increased uptake. Single-photon emission computed tomography (SPECT) provides sectional and multiplanar imaging and is sensitive for localizing bony remodeling in such complex areas as the spine. (Fig. 5.28)

Sports-related injuries to the spine are seen with increasing frequency among young persons who engage in a wide variety of professional or amateur sports activities. Radiology plays an important role in the differential diagnosis and follow-up of these patients. Among the imaging methods, bone scintigraphy has proved useful in the detection of active bone pathology, sometimes in the presence of normal radiographs. A pars defect may be an incidental radiographic finding. The actual cause of the low back pain may instead be such diverse entities as a herniated nucleus pulposus, nerve root compression, spinal stenosis, osteomyelitis, osteoarthritis, disc space infection, bone metastases, or muscular strain. Hence, there is a need for a test that can confirm spondylolysis or spondylolisthesis as the true cause of pain. Because planar bone scintigraphy (PBS) is often incapable of distinguishing between increased metabolic activity in the posterior neural arch and that in the underlying vertebral body, its value is somewhat limited as a means of differentiating between the various causes of low back pain. Therefore, correlation between the sites of increased metabolic activity and radiographic findings are often inaccurate. With the advent of SPECT, more accurate scintigraphic localization is possible. (Fig 5.29A–D)

TECHNIQUE

The major advantage of the SPECT technique over planar imaging is that the SPECT approach is a three-dimensional imaging technique, as compared to the two-dimensional planar technique. The SPECT technique, therefore, has an improved ability to separate adjacent structures tomographically. In addition, image contrast is significantly increased with SPECT, as it is with all tomographic techniques. Implementation of the SPECT technique requires a more uniform and stable camera system than does planar imaging. Such systems are now readily available. The time required to perform a single detector SPECT study is approximately 20 to 30 minutes, with patient imaging approximately 10 to 20 minutes for reconstruction and photography. The imaging time is proportionately decreased with new multidetector systems.

The bone SPECT technique has been applied successfully to the temporomandibular joints, hips, knees, and spine. In spite of

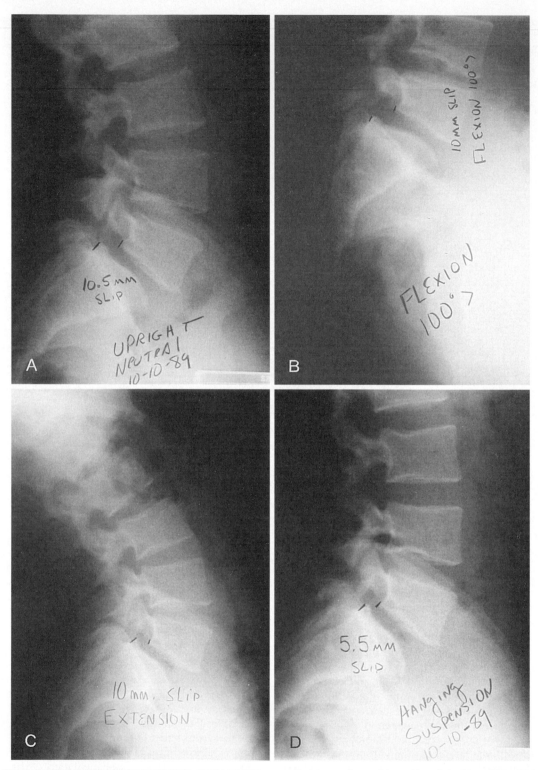

Figure 5.26.   TRACTION LUMBAR SPINE RADIOGRAPHY: INSTABILITY EVALUATION. A. An Upright Neutral Lateral Lumbar. B. Flexion. C. Extension. D. Hanging Traction Suspension Radiograph. COMMENT: This 33-year-old male runner has been unresponsive to conservative chiropractic care. The traction hanging radiographs demonstrate 5-mm translation that was not seen in the routine flexion/extension weight-bearing lateral lumbar radiographs. This represents an excessive amount of translation and indicates underlying radiographic and/or clinical instability. This patient had a successful surgical fusion, which stopped the patient's long-standing lower lumbar spine pain. The superiority of traction and/or compression radiography over flexion/extension stress radiographs of the lumbar spine for demonstrating instability is very obvious in this case study. (Reprinted with permission: Cox JM, Trier K: *Chiropractic adjustment results correlated with spondylolisthesis instability.* J Manual Med 6:67-72, 1991)

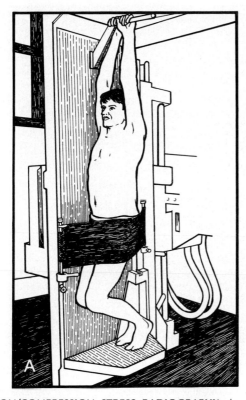
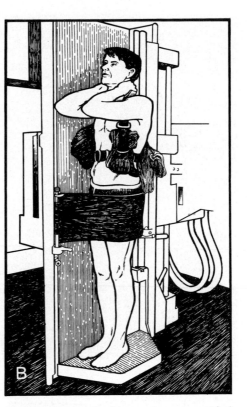

Figure 5.27. TRACTION/COMPRESSION STRESS RADIOGRAPHY. A. Traction Stress—the Patient Hangs by Hands from a Horizontal Bar. To prevent swaying, the toes slightly touch the ground. **B. Compression Stress—the Patient Stands with a 20-kg Rucksack on the Shoulders.** During traction and compression, the hips are in contact with the cassette holder to keep the distance between the lumbar spine and film constant. COMMENT: Traction/compression stress radiography appears to be the most accurate means of assessing radiographic instability of the spondylolisthetic segment.

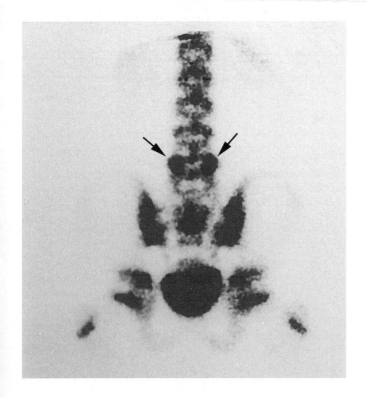

Figure 5.28. SPECT BONE SCAN. Observe the intense bilateral isotope tracer uptake (arrows) at the L4 segment, with the remaining pars throughout the lumbar spine being normal. COMMENT: SPECT is the most sensitive and accurate means to determine physiologic activity in the pars interarticularis. (Courtesy of Deborah M. Pate, DC, DACBR, San Diego, California)

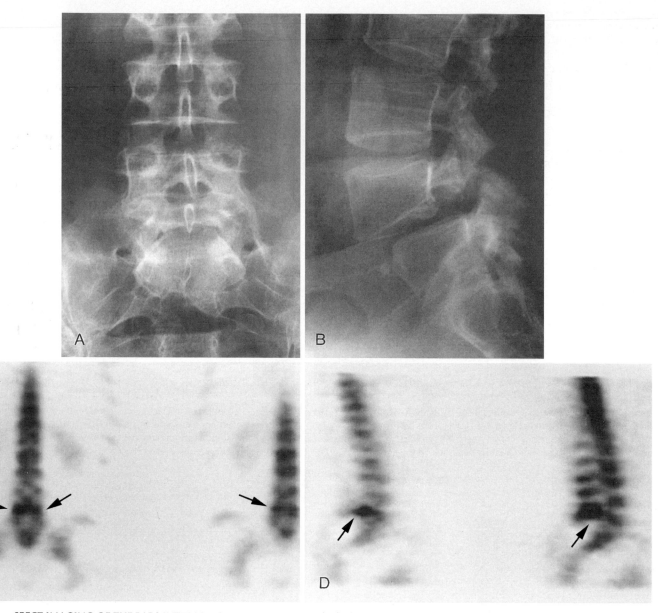

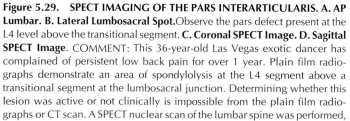

Figure 5.29.   SPECT IMAGING OF THE PARS INTERARTICULARIS. A. AP Lumbar. B. Lateral Lumbosacral Spot. Observe the pars defect present at the L4 level above the transitional segment. **C. Coronal SPECT Image. D. Sagittal SPECT Image**. COMMENT: This 36-year-old Las Vegas exotic dancer has complained of persistent low back pain for over 1 year. Plain film radiographs demonstrate an area of spondylolysis at the L4 segment above a transitional segment at the lumbosacral junction. Determining whether this lesion was active or not clinically is impossible from the plain film radiographs or CT scan. A SPECT nuclear scan of the lumbar spine was performed, which demonstrated bilateral intense uptake (arrows) at the pars interarticularis. This strongly suggests that this patient's back pain is associated with the pars defect and that this lesion has been recently acquired and is clinically active. The SPECT scan provides a truly *physiologic* investigation of the area of the pars, which tells the clinician the current nature of the defect (chronic or acute). Patients with positive SPECT images must reduce their physical activity and often are placed into a Boston overlap brace. (Courtesy of Vasanti Deuskar, MD, and Alan M. Lesselroth, MD, Mountain Diagnostics, Las Vegas, Nevada)

the advances in skeletal MR imaging, bone SPECT imaging, especially in the spine, continues to be a very valuable diagnostic tool. It is capable of providing clinical evaluation for a variety of disorders, particularly in the determination of spondylolysis with or without positive radiographs.

SPONDYLOLYSIS AND SPONDYLOLISTHESIS AND THE SPECT SCAN

Spondylolysis and spondylolisthesis are frequent findings in patients with lower back pain. Frequently, the question arises as to whether or not the radiographic abnormalities actually account for the patient's pain. Lowe et al. (75), in a study of 53 young military personnel with spondylolysis on planar bone scans, reported positive results in 10 of 23 individuals with acute or recent onset of low back pain, in 3 of 23 individuals with a long history of low back pain, and none with painless spondylolysis. Collier (76) applied planar and SPECT bone scintigraphy to 19 adults with radiographic evidence of spondylolysis or spondylolisthesis; 13 of these patients were categorized as being symptomatic due to their bony abnormalities, and the other 6 patients were asymptomatic. The sensitivity for detection of "*painful*" spondylolysis or spondylolisthesis was 85% with the SPECT technique and 62% with the planar technique in the 13 symptomatic patients. Collier (76) has cautioned that increased activity in the regions of the pars is not always specific for injury, since the activity may be secondary to osteoarthritis or malignant metastatic bone disease. These results, however, suggest that SPECT studies are more sensitive than planar imaging in the detection of stress-induced injuries, particularly spondylolysis of the lower lumbar spine. (Fig. 5.30A–D)

SPECT SCAN DRIVES PATIENT MANAGEMENT

Far too often the clinical conclusions that determine whether an athlete participates in sports are based on the radiographic presence of spondylolysis and ongoing lower back pain. Since plain film radiographs and CT scans will only show the anatomic morphology of the spondylolytic defect, they are of little use in predicting the patient's true cause of pain. A functional examination, such as SPECT scintigraphy, provides an active physiologic examination that predicts whether the spondylolytic defect is likely to be a source of specific pain. (36,37,77) Athletes with low back pain who perform repetitive lumbar hyperextension activities but who have normal plain radiographs should also be considered for SPECT scanning. If these patients do not respond to conservative management as expected, they may be in the *preradiographic phase* of developing pars defects. The SPECT scan may demonstrate a significant increase in uptake in the area of the pars, even though plain film bone radiographs are normal. (78,79) Such patients should have their activities reduced, allowing enough time to reverse the stress reaction within the pars and cease or retard the development of pars defects. Patients with a hot SPECT bone scan, with or without pars defects, should be placed into an antilordotic orthosis, such as the Boston overlap brace developed by Micheli. (35) With the use of a SPECT bone scan, information is provided indicating when a young athlete can return to competition. After an appropriate time of bracing, a SPECT scan can be repeated, and once it is normal, activity can be gradually resumed to competitive levels. The use of serial examinations following early therapeutic intervention to demonstrate resolution of the scintigraphic abnormalities can be very helpful. It is recommended that skeletal SPECT be performed on any patient with persistent symptoms suggestive of injury to the

pars interarticularis, even if results of general radiography and planar bone scanning are normal. (36,37,77–79)

SPECT SCANNING FOR THE SURGICAL SPINE

In 1987 Slizofski and co-workers (80) reported on 26 patients who had undergone lumbar spine fusion 6 months earlier; 15 patients were symptomatic, and 11 patients were asymptomatic. Focal areas of increased uptake within the fusion mass were considered positive for pseudoarthrosis. In the 15 symptomatic patients the SPECT scans demonstrated a 78% sensitivity and an 83% specificity, compared to 43% and 50%, respectively, for the planar bone scans. SPECT provided information not available on PBS in 14 of the 26 patients studied.

Lusins et al. (81) reported on 25 patients with persistent low back pain following lumbar surgery. The patients were divided into three groups: single-level laminectomies, multilevel laminectomies, and multilevel laminectomies with fusion. In the single-level laminectomy group, only 2 of 11 patients had increased activity on the SPECT scans, limited to the laminectomy site. Of the 14 remaining patients 12 demonstrated increased activity, with 10 of the sites of increased activity corresponding to the lumbar facet joints. The SPECT scan was considered to be very helpful in localizing the abnormality to the facet joints. Chronic facet joint instability (which has been previously proposed as a cause for the persistent back pain following spine surgery) can be difficult to diagnose otherwise. In two patients the focal increased activity involved the site of fusion mass. In these latter two patients CT examination demonstrated poor bony incorporation at the level of the fusion.

SPECT imaging can also be used as a means of identifying those patients who should have spinal fusion. According to Raby and coworkers (82), SPECT scanning appears to be more accurate than lumbar immobilization in predicting those patients who will benefit from a spinal fusion. Lumbar immobilization (lumbar jacket test) is uncomfortable for the patient, causes difficulties in bathing and wearing normal clothes, and delays management decisions for at least 2 months. These problems do not occur with SPECT scanning. The long-term effect of lumbar immobilization by use of the lumbar jacket on the activity of the pars defect has not been assessed in this study. Patients in whom fusion is being considered should first be evaluated with a SPECT bone scan. Raby (82) has shown that the addition of SPECT scanning seems at least as accurate as lumbar immobilization in identifying patients who obtain greater pain relief and fewer complications from spinal fusion. The presence of a positive SPECT scan in this circumstance suggests that spinal fusion may be of benefit to the patient.

CLASSIFICATION OF PROBLEMATIC PATIENTS

It is possible to identify four distinct groups of patients with spondylolysis or spondylolisthesis. (83) Classification of patients into one of the following groups through clinical examination and imaging, including scintigraphy, may be very helpful in the overall management of the patients.

1. *Patients with unilateral or bilateral focal scintigraphic abnormalities but who have not yet developed evidence of spondylolysis on radiographs.* These patients are in the *preradiographic phase* of spondylolysis, and early immobilization of these patients may halt the development of an active spondylolytic defect. In view of the high sensitivity but low specificity of scintigraphy, caution must be

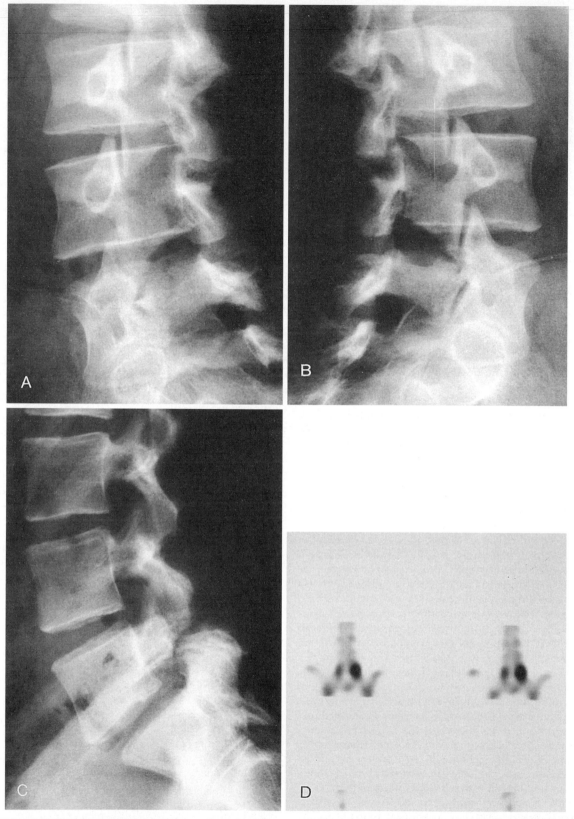

Figure 5.30. SPONDYLOLISTHESIS AND BACK PAIN: THE REAL PICTURE. A and B. Bilateral Lumbar Oblique Radiographs. C. Lateral Lumbar. D. SPECT Scan of the Lower Lumbar Spine. COMMENT: This 18-year-old male football player presents with recent onset of lower back pain following trauma in a scrimmage. Bilateral pars defects are seen at the L5 level on the plain film radiographs, and a 10% anterolisthesis (spondylolisthesis) of L5 upon the sacrum is noted. Since this patient failed to respond to conservative treatment and there was worry about continued participation in football, a SPECT bone scan was performed, which showed intense uptake in both pars at L-5. The SPECT scan in this patient tells the clinician that these pars defects are active and that this patient must not participate in football for a short period of time until this area of the pars interarticularis becomes clinically silent and is cold on SPECT scanning. (Courtesy of Gary D. Konstant, DC, Watertown, South Dakota)

exercised before rendering a definitive diagnosis of acute spondylolysis since other abnormalities, such as osteoid osteoma or other benign bone tumors of the neural arch, could create such a focal uptake.

2. *Patients in whom spondylolysis is seen on radiographs and who have increased uptake on the scintigram.* Healing is still progressing, and there is a possibility of bony union with immobilization using an antilordotic Boston overlap brace. These patients should not be participating in sports activities. Serial SPECT scans can help monitor the conservative management of these athletes by informing the clinician as to when the patients can return to competitive sports (when the SPECT scan returns to normal).

3. *Patients with unilateral spondylolysis and enhanced radiotracer uptake on the contralateral side (Wilkinson's syndrome).* These patients are at imminent risk of developing bilateral spondylolysis. Appropriate immobilization in an antilordotic brace (Boston overlap) should be considered.

4. *Patients with radiographically confirmed spondylolysis but no focal accumulation on scintigraphy.* In these patients, there is an established nonunion of the previous stress fracture, which is unlikely to heal with immobilization. This may have medicolegal implications in patients examined within 1 year of an accident alleged to be the cause of a spondylolysis.

We believe that the identification of this varied patient population clarifies the role of scintigraphy in the management of spondylolysis. Although not firmly documented in a prospective study, there is very strong empirical evidence that by determining whether there is active healing in the area of the pars, SPECT scintigraphy assists in the choice between conservative and operative management in patients with persistent symptoms secondary to spondylolysis or spondylolisthesis.

A PROBLEMATIC CIRCUMSTANCE

A distinct challenge to the clinician occurs when a patient presents with lumbosacral pain following a traumatic event. Often there is no history of back pain prior to the most recent injury. Radiographic examination reveals an L4 or L5 isthmic type IIA spondylolisthesis (bilateral pars defects), which is smooth and well corticated. The clinical dilemma is to determine whether the current trauma is related to the presence of spondylolysis or spondylolisthesis or is unrelated, and whether the current lumbosacral pain is associated with any pain-producing activity at the level of the pars defect. In most instances, patients with bilateral, well corticated, smooth pars defects have had these lesions prior to any recent traumatic episode. This conclusion is derived from the bilateral, symmetric nature of the lesion and well-corticated bone margins. Acute fractures of the pars are seldom bilateral and symmetrical. The clinical question often arises in patients with localized back pain whether the recent trauma has aggravated the preexisting pars defect, causing further separation or injury to the defect. This is a very valid question that requires further diagnostic imaging. It is recommended that flexion/extension or traction/compression (see discussion under Instability Evaluation) lateral lumbar stress radiographs be performed to determine if segmental instability is present. The presence of instability suggests that the recent traumatic episode may be implicated as an etiologic factor in the production of the patient's current lower back pain. Additional special imaging to include SPECT will prove very helpful in searching for increased physiologic activity of the subchondral bone at the level of the pars defect. A positive SPECT scan will confirm a direct cause

and effect relationship between the trauma and the patient's existing lumbosacral pain. A negative SPECT scan, coupled with negative stress radiographs, forces the clinician to look elsewhere, past the spondylolisthesis, for a biomechanical or organic cause for the patient's lumbosacral pain.

MAGNETIC RESONANCE IMAGING

The recognition of isthmic spondylolysis with surface coil MR imaging of the lumbar spine has received little attention in the literature. (84–86) Spondylolysis is a relatively common finding in the lumbar spine, occurring most often at the L5 level (90% of cases). While the plain radiographic, scintigraphic, and CT criteria for this entity (as well as those for spondylolisthesis) have been well established, corresponding findings with high-resolution surface coil MR imaging are less well known. This technique requires detailed knowledge of the normal sagittal and axial anatomy of the posterior vertebral arch.

The interruption of the cortical margins of the pars interarticularis is the primary sign of spondylolysis on MR images. Sagittal T1- and proton density-weighted images are the most accurate for demonstrating this interruption because they permit better differentiation between cortical and medullary bone. An abnormal high signal within the area of the defect, or within the pars region without a defect on T2-weighted images, suggests *bone marrow edema.* This bone marrow edema may be the precursor of the development of spondylolysis and may be seen as a low signal intensity on the T1-weighted images in the axial or parasagittal plane.

Traditionally, parasagittal images have been used to evaluate the intervertebral foramen, the position of nerve roots to surrounding anatomy, and the presence of foraminal encroachment. However, close inspection of the area of the pars may reveal bone marrow edema on both T1- and T2-weighted sequences. This finding confirms the presence of active stress in the pars and represents a precursor to the development of spondylolysis, even though the plain film radiographs are normal.

Occasionally, patients with suspected spondylolysis may present to clinicians with normal plain films, normal planar bone scans, and an MR imaging scan that may be interpreted as normal for disc herniation or stenosis. This may occur if the radiologist is not specifically looking for bone marrow edema on the parasagittal or axial images.

The author (TRY) has had experience with such a case, the MR imaging scans were read as normal when, in fact, retrospective analysis of the left and right parasagittal T2-weighted images and axial T1-weighted images revealed bone marrow edema in the area of the L4 pars in a highly active 18-year-old boy who was performing repetitive hyperextension activities as a football player. His plain film radiographs and planar bone scan were normal, and it was not until a SPECT scan was performed that the true location of his back pain was revealed. (Fig. 5.31A–F) On the basis of this experience, the authors suggest that all low back MR imaging studies, particularly in active athletes, include parasagittal T2-weighted images and axial T1- and T2-weighted images through the area of the pedicle/pars junction in order to rule out the possibility of bone marrow edema in patients with active spondylolysis.

MR imaging, in conjunction with SPECT imaging, may play a role in confirming the presence of active bone marrow edema and assist in managing complicated cases of athletic or work-related injuries to the lumbar spine.

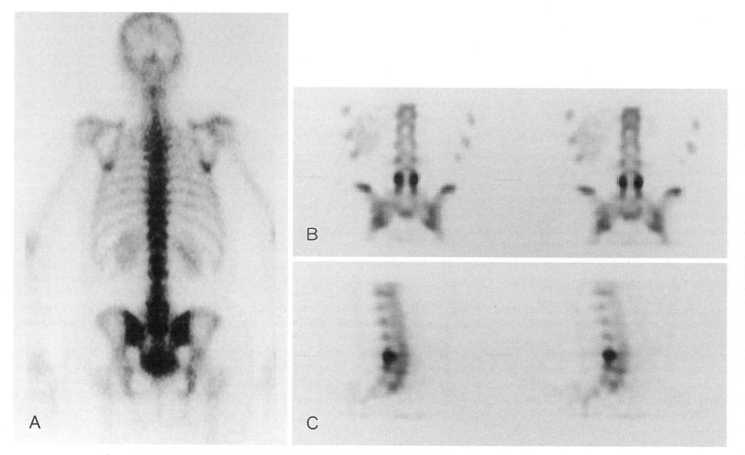

Figure 5.31A–C.   PERSISTENT LUMBAR SPINE PAIN: A MISDIAGNOSIS. A. Planar Bone Scan. Normal study. **B. Coronal SPECT Bone Scan.** Positive tracer uptake bilaterally at L4. **C. Sagittal SPECT Bone Scan.** Positive intense uptake of tracer at the L4 pars.

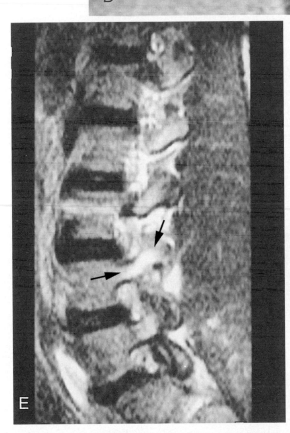

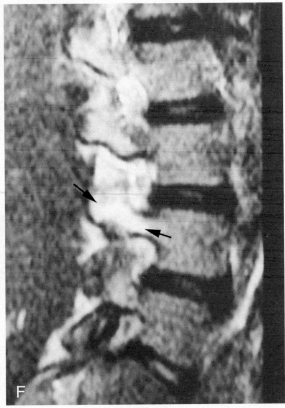

Figure 5.31D–F.   D. T1-Weighted Axial MR Imaging Scan at the Pars Pedicle Junction. Bilateral low signal intensity (arrows) in the area of the L4 pedicle pars region is indicative of bone marrow edema. **E and F. Right and Left Parasagittal MR Imaging Projections of the Lumbar Spine.** Observe the increased signal intensity consistent with bone marrow edema in the pars pedicle region of L4 (arrows). COMMENT: This 16-year-old football quarterback is the son of an orthopedic surgeon, who has failed to respond to his father's treatment for persistent lower lumbar spine pain. He hurt his back while running sprints and scrimmaging in football and has had ongoing back pain for over 3 months. Plain film radiographs performed by his father were normal, as was his planar bone scan. Two MR imaging scans were performed, which were read as normal with no evidence of disc herniation. Close retrospective inspection of the parasagittal foraminal images on both the right and left side showed bone marrow edema in the area of the pars interarticularis bilaterally at the L4 segment. This was confirmed on axial T1-weighted scans showing bilateral low signal intensity with bone marrow edema at L4. There was no evidence of pars defects seen on either MR imaging scan. Failure to respond to traditional medical treatment stimulated the orthopedic surgeon to take his son to a chiropractor. The chiropractor performed an examination and a series of manipulations, which were not successful in eliminating the pain, and at the recommendation of the chiropractor a SPECT bone scan was performed. This SPECT bone scan was intensely hot, which confirmed that this patient was in the *preradiographic phase* of active spondylolysis. This patient was placed into an antilordotic Boston overlap brace in near zero lordosis. Within 2 weeks of being placed into the brace, the back pain was totally gone. In less than 2 months, with adaptation to the brace allowing greater lateral flexion, the patient was able to run and participate in competitive contact sports. The high sensitivity of bone marrow edema detection on MR imaging scans provides one additional piece of information in the area of the lumbar spine for imaging patients with lower back pain. All interpreters of MR imaging scans are encouraged to inspect the pars interarticularis on the parasagittal views and the axial projections to determine whether there are signal alterations consistent with bone marrow edema, which may indicate that the patient is in the process of developing bilateral pars defects. (Courtesy of Richard L. Green, DC, Winthrop, Massachusetts)

UNILATERAL SPONDYLOLYSIS

Spondylolysis may involve only one pars interarticularis of a single vertebra, allowing a 5 to 10% anterolisthesis. (Fig. 5.32A and B) In this circumstance, compensatory stress hypertrophy of the contralateral pedicle can occur, creating a "sclerotic pedicle." (87,88) (Fig. 5.33A–D) This compensatory hypertrophy is manifested radiographically by a dense, sclerotic, enlarged pedicle and pars region. (Fig. 5.34) This appearance can mimic osteoid osteoma, osteoblastoma, or osteoblastic metastatic disease, which are common at this site. Agenesis of the pedicle may also show the same stress hypertrophy of the contralateral pedicle and pars region. (Fig. 5.35A–C, 5.36A and B) The key differential sign is the presence of a unilateral pars defect. Regression of the compensatory bone changes may occur, should a stress fracture develop on the same side as the dense pedicle. Bilateral spondylolysis equalizes the weight bearing and reduces the stress within the involved spinal motion segment. (45) (Fig. 5.37A–G)

The appearance of a sclerotic pedicle at any level of the vertebral column constitutes a diagnostic challenge to both the clinician and the radiologist. The numerous etiologies of this entity (Table 5.6) include a broad gamut of bone diseases. Unilateral spondylolysis with contralateral sclerosis of the pedicle has been called "Wilkinson's syndrome" (88) and is the most common cause of a sclerotic pedicle. This is most frequently seen in the mid to lower lumbar spine in highly motivated young athletes who are continually performing repetitive hyperextension activities involving the lower lumbar spine. There is often increased uptake on the scintigraphic bone scan, helping to localize and confirm physiologic activity as it relates to the sclerotic pedicle and the unilateral pars defect. Athletes with such abnormalities should be

put into an antilordotic brace (Boston overlap brace), and their activities should be severely restricted for a minimum of 3 months, or until the SPECT bone scan returns to normal. Often clinicians will miss the early changes of a sclerotic pedicle, since only the peripheral edge of the cortex of the pedicle may show the signs of increased radiodensity. In slightly underexposed radiographs of less than optimal quality, this faintly sclerotic pedicle may be easily overlooked. Oblique radiographs, along with a tilt-up view of the lumbosacral junction, may be very helpful in providing a complete assessment of the density of the pedicles and the integrity of the opposite pars.

Table 5.6.   Causes of the Sclerotic Pedicle

A. Congenital
   Agenetic/hypoplastic pedicle (contralateral side)
   Agenetic/hypoplastic facet (contralateral side)
   Asymmetric facets (contralateral side)
   Spina bifida occulta
B. Unilateral spondylolysis with contralateral stress sclerosis
C. Tumors
   Benign (bone island, osteoid osteoma, osteoblastoma)
   Malignant (blastic metastasis, lymphoma, myeloma, Ewing's sarcoma)
D. Tumorlike conditions
   Paget's disease, fibrous dysplasia, sarcoidosis, tuberous sclerosis
E. Infection
F. Iatrogenic
   Laminectomy (contralateral)
   Spinal arthrodesis
G. Idiopathic

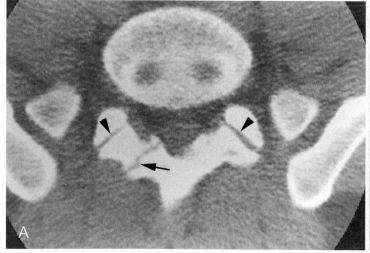
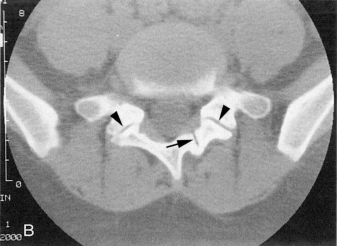

Figure 5.32.   CT DEMONSTRATION OF UNILATERAL PARS DEFECTS. A. Axial CT Scan of the L5 Level. Observe the unilateral pars defect (arrow). This should not be confused with the normal facet structures (arrowheads). The radiolucencies seen in the inferior surface of the vertebral body of L5 has been called the "owl's eye" appearance of notochordal persistency or nuclear impression. (Courtesy of W. Michael Spurlock, DC, Moorehead, Kentucky) **B. Axial CT Scan of the L5 Level.** Observe the unilateral pars defect (arrow). The facet structures (arrowheads) should not be confused with pars defect.

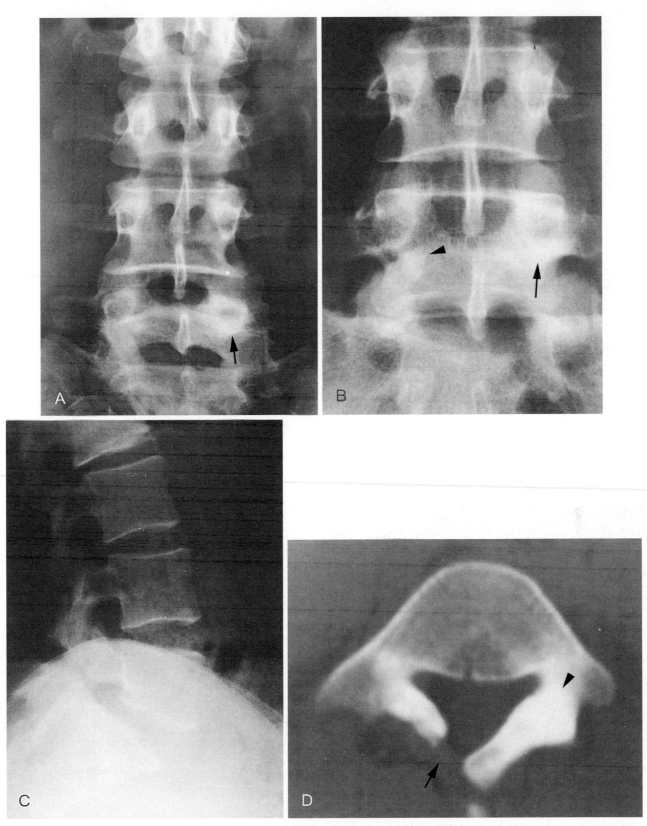

Figure 5.33.   SCLEROTIC PEDICLE: FIFTH LUMBAR VERTEBRA. A. AP Nonangulated Projection. Note the sclerotic pedicle at L5 (arrow) and no apparent pars defect. **B. AP Tilt-Up View.** Observe the sclerotic pedicle at L5 (arrow) and the contralateral unilateral pars defect on the opposite side (arrowhead). **C. Lateral Lumbar.** There has been a slight anterolisthesis of L5 upon the sacrum, 10 to 15% anterior displacement of the vertebral body can occur with unilateral pars defects. **D. CT Scan.** Demonstrates a unilateral pars defect (arrow) and contralateral sclerosis of the pedicle and pars interarticularis (arrowhead). COMMENT: The tilt-up projection is an optimum view to demonstrate unilateral or bilateral pars defects, as is nicely demonstrated in this case. Unilateral pars defects with contralateral sclerosis of the opposite pedicle (Wilkinson's syndrome) is the most common cause of a sclerotic pedicle. (Courtesy of David E. Friedman, DC, Denver, Colorado)

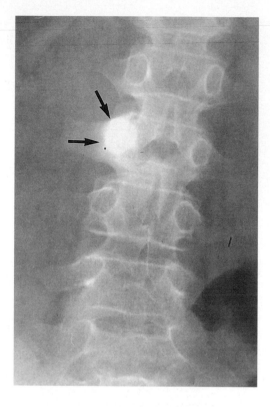

Figure 5.34.   OSTEOID OSTEOMA: PEDICLE. Observe the unilateral dense pedicle due to the benign tumor (arrows), osteoid osteoma. (Reprinted with permission: Yochum TR: *Osteoid osteoma of the thumb.* ACA Council Roent, Roentgen Brief, November 1979) (Courtesy of John E. MacRae, DC, DACBR, Toronto, Canada)

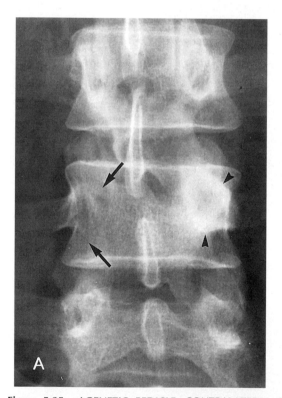

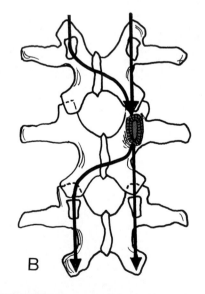

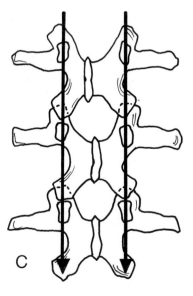

Figure 5.35.   AGENETIC PEDICLE: CONTRALATERAL SCLEROSIS. A. Note the absence of the pedicle outline (arrows) and the prominence of the contralateral pedicle (arrowheads). **B.** Diagrammatic representation of the redistribution of mechanical forces due to pedicle agenesis. The increased pedicle density and cortical thickness is a stress-induced compensatory change. **C.** Distribution of mechanical forces when the posterior arches are normal. Any disruption in the ring of the neural arch will alter this distribution.

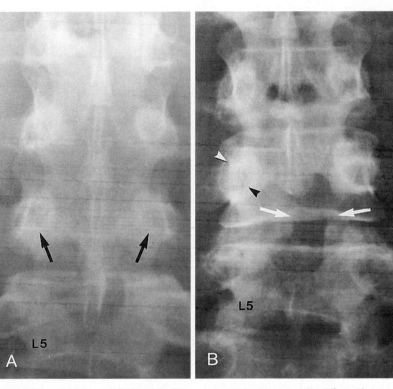

Figure 5.36.   PEDICLE STRESS HYPERTROPHY FROM CONTRALATERAL LAMINECTOMY. A. Preoperative Film. Note the symmetrically uniform density of both pedicles of the fourth lumbar vertebra (arrows).

B. 1-Year Postoperative Film. Observe the lamina defect (arrows) and the contralateral sclerotic pedicle (arrowheads). (Courtesy of Tyrone Wei, DC, DACBR, Portland, Oregon)

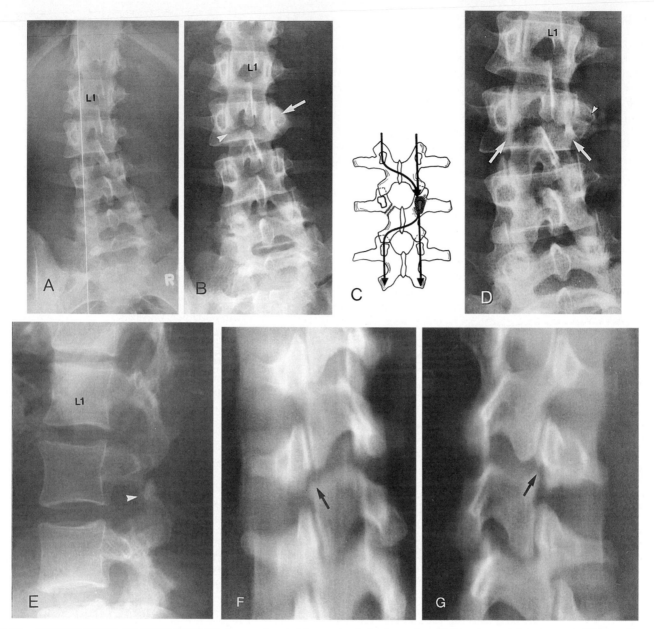

Figure 5.37.   SPONDYLOLYSIS: ITS PATHOGENESIS. A young female followed over a 4-year period. **A. Initial Film.** A left rotatory scoliosis is visible, with the second lumbar vertebra showing no pars defects or pedicle abnormalities. **B. 2 Years Later.** The scoliosis remains. Observe the second lumbar sclerotic pedicle (arrow) and the left pars interarticularis defect (arrowhead). **C. Diagrammatic Representation.** The mechanism operating to produce the sclerotic pedicle is demonstrated. The hypertrophy is due to the additional stress placed upon the pedicle by the contralateral pars defect. **D. 4 Years Later.** The scoliosis persists, but note the resolution of the sclerotic pedicle due to the formation of bilateral pars defects (arrows). Also note the retained hypertrophy of the previously sclerotic pedicle (arrowhead). **E. Lateral Film.** Shows the defect (arrowhead) and no anterolisthesis. **F and G. Oblique Tomograms.** Confirms the bilateral defects (arrows). (Courtesy of Rae Batten, BAppSc (Chiro), Perth, Western Australia) COMMENT: This case demonstrates the important role of stress in the production of pars defects. (Reprinted with permission: Yochum TR, et al: *Reactive sclerosis of a pedicle due to unilateral spondylolysis.* ACA J Chiro, Radiology Corner, September 1980)

CERVICAL SPONDYLOLISTHESIS

Isolated spondylolisthesis in the cervical spine is a rare and unusual disorder. (89) The majority of these cases are discovered accidentally during radiographic studies initiated as a result of antecedent trauma. Cervical spondylolisthesis is most commonly found at the C6 vertebral segment but has also been noted at the C2, C5, and C7 segments. (89) There are only 31 patients with cervical spondylolisthesis reported in the literature. (89) The majority of these cases of cervical spondylolisthesis have occurred in males, suggesting a sex-linked genetic disorder. (90) The most likely etiology for cervical spondylolisthesis is that of congenital dysplasia (89), which may be manifested radiographically as bilateral hypoplasia of the articular pillars and the pedicles. Some patients may also present with unilateral agenesis of the pedicle, which will allow anterolisthesis of the involved cervical segment to occur. (89) (Fig. 5.38A and B)

It is noteworthy that 50% of patients with cervical spondylolisthesis have an associated spina bifida occulta of that particular vertebra. Since spina bifida occulta of the C6 segment is uncommon as an isolated anomaly, its presence should raise high clinical suspicion for associated cervical spondylolisthesis. Flexion and extension radiographs of the cervical spine are recommended to evaluate for motion segment instability. (91) (Table 5.7)

The clinical significance of cervical spondylolysis is not well defined, leading to a spectrum of treatment regimes ranging from benign neglect to prophylactic fusion. (92) The majority of reported cases were only mildly symptomatic and responded well to conservative measures. Indications for surgical management include severe symptoms, presence of instability, and prophylaxis against possible dislocation should additional trauma occur.

Table 5.7. Cervical Spondylolisthesis
C6 level anterolisthesis (most common site)
C6 spina bifida occulta
Hypoplastic pillars, pedicles, etc.

(92) Both anterior interbody fusion and posterior fusion have been performed; both methods lead to resolution of symptoms.

Dysplasia is thought to be the most common cause of cervical spondylolisthesis; there are, however, other conditions that may predispose to anterolisthesis of a cervical body. (89) These include acute fracture, pedicle agenesis, degenerative arthritis, inflammatory arthritides (rheumatoid arthritis, ankylosing spondylitis, Reiter's syndrome, psoriatic arthropathy), and pathologic bone diseases (infection, neoplasm, and others). (89) It is, therefore, important to establish the etiology of the anterolisthesis in every patient. (93) (Fig. 5.39A and B)

TREATMENT AND PROGNOSIS
CONSERVATIVE MANAGEMENT

Considerable controversy exists concerning the treatment and management of patients with spondylolisthesis. The conservative medical approach to treatment includes the following: restriction of physical activity, strengthening exercises to abdominal and back muscles, bed rest, low back bracing, and nonnarcotic analgesics. (53)

An additional conservative approach that has proved beneficial for the treatment and management of patients with symptom-

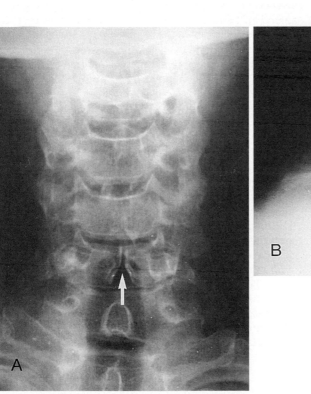

Figure 5.38. CERVICAL SPONDYLOLISTHESIS: SIXTH CERVICAL VERTEBRA. A. AP View. Note the spina bifida occulta at the sixth cervical segment (arrow). **B. Lateral View.** Almost total agenesis of the sixth articular pillar is apparent (arrowheads), with minimal anterolisthesis of the associated vertebral body. (Courtesy of James F. Winterstein, DC, DACBR, Chicago, Illinois)

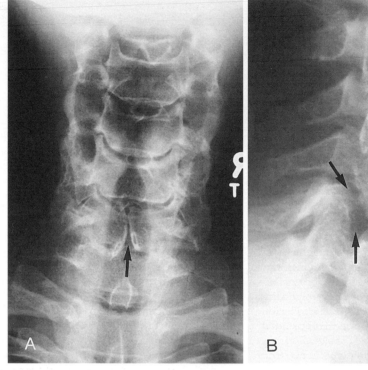
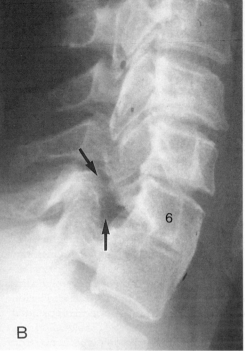

Figure 5.39.   CERVICAL SPONDYLOLISTHESIS: MISDIAGNOSIS. A 45-year-old female had radiographs following a motor vehicle accident. A diagnosis of fracture and dislocation at the sixth cervical level was made, and a surgical fusion was performed. **A. AP View.** Note the spina bifida occulta at the sixth cervical segment (arrow). **B. Lateral View.** There is partial agen- esis of the sixth cervical articular pillar (arrows). A complete interbody fusion has been performed between the sixth and seventh cervical segments. COMMENT: The findings of a spina bifida and absence of the pillar suggest a congenital rather than a posttraumatic deformity. (Courtesy of Dennis M. Richards, DC, Tweed Heads, New South Wales, Australia)

atic spondylolisthesis is chiropractic spinal manipulative therapy. (49) Since a large majority of patients with spondylolisthesis have an associated hyperlordosis, facet syndrome and/or sacroiliac fixation, these conditions are often the cause of symptoms rather than the presence of spondylolisthesis. (49,94)

According to Illi (95), restoration of normal sacroiliac joint mobility may decrease the strain on the lower lumbar spine, thereby giving patients relief from lower back pain (which he thought was an indirect effect of the lumbar spondylolisthesis). Cassidy, Potter, and Kirkaldy-Willis (49) performed chiropractic spinal manipulative therapy on patients who had varying degrees of spondylolisthesis. They found that 80% of these patients responded favorably to specific manipulation of the sacroiliac joint or the lumbar zygapophyseal joints above the segment with the pars defects, thus avoiding manipulation directly over the area of spondylolisthesis. (49) Prone recoil manipulation directly over the area of spondylolisthesis is contraindicated. (96) They concluded that spinal manipulation offers rapid symptomatic relief to many patients with back pain who coincidentally have spondylolisthesis.

Taylor (58) also found that the motion segment above spondylolisthesis, usually L4-L5, is the segment of highest biomechanical load and thus often the site of clinical subluxation and/or pain. Comparing 60 patients with spondylolisthesis with 60 patients without, Taylor found significantly higher intersegmental hyperextension at the segment above the spondylolytic defect than those without spondylolisthesis. This intersegmental hyperextension has been associated with mechanical facet pain by other researchers. (97,98)

The successful resolution of back pain in spondylolisthesis of-ten occurs only if the level above, usually L4-L5, is evaluated with regard to biomechanical load. (99) Clinical examination should delineate the nature of the biomechanical lesion involved and dictate the appropriate manipulative treatment. (99) Occasionally, it is stated that manipulation may be contraindicated in spondylolisthesis. This opinion, however, is unfounded, and Mierau et al. (96) suggest that those with spondylolisthesis may in fact respond to manipulation more quickly than those without. Comparing 25 patients with spondylolisthesis and low back pain to 260 patients with low back pain alone, Mierau et al. (96) obtained good results with manipulation in 80% with spondylolisthesis versus only 70% of those without. The number of treatments required for a good result were 6.9 and 7.5, respectively, for the two groups.

The question often arises as to the relative safety of participation in contact sports for persons with spondylolisthesis. (99) The often-used hypothesis has been that the segment is unstable and, therefore, the individual is at an increased risk of cord or nerve root damage. (99) This is probably only true in segments with grades III or IV displacement and significant disc degeneration. Lower grades are probably quite stable (100), and these individuals may even be afforded some protection from the usual low back neurogenic syndromes because of the increase in sagittal dimensions of the spinal canal at the spondylolisthetic segment.

Use of the Boston Overlap Brace in Acute Spondylolysis

Sports-related injuries to the spine are seen with increasing frequency in such varied sports as gridiron football, gymnastics, weight lifting, diving, and pole-vaulting. Since school screening programs for scoliosis and other structural deformities of the spine have improved the early detection of spinal deformities in young adolescents, a spinal brace that would maintain adequate immobilization and positioning of the spine yet allow continued participation in normal adolescent activities has become necessary. (35) Although use of exercises in conjunction with the traditional Milwaukee brace system has been repeatedly emphasized, this brace, with its metal superstructure and leather outriggers, makes vigorous athletic participation difficult, particularly in contact sports. The Boston brace system is a modification of the Milwaukee brace system. The initial Boston brace module consisted of an outer shell of polypropylene with an inner lining and padding system of foam polyethylene that could be adapted to most body builds. One of the basic objectives in orthopedic management of low back pain of varied etiologies is attainment of an antilordotic posture. (35) Traditional Williams flexion exercises are designed to decrease the lordosis of the low back and increase flexibility. A number of braces and pelvic supports have been designed to aid in this management approach by compressing the abdominal contents, thereby decreasing the mechanical load upon the spine. (35) However, none are truly effective in decreasing the lumbar lordosis. When antilordotic capabilities of the pelvic modules were fully understood, use of the brace system in the management of certain back pain problems in adolescent patients seemed appropriate. (35) Immobilization of the spine could be maintained with full activities, including athletic participation, with the appropriate bracing procedure.

Use of a new, semirigid lumbosacral orthosis that directly decreases the lumbar lordosis and lessens axial loading of the spine by increasing intraabdominal pressure to limit the pelvic torsion of the trunk seems promising on both theoretical and clinical grounds. (35) (Fig. 5.40A and B) When used full time for 3 to 6 months in conjunction with a flexibility and muscle-strengthening exercise program, this new brace has been shown to be successful in managing the back pain produced by various etiologies in over 80% of these young patients. (35) According to Micheli, use of the Boston overlap antilordotic brace in the treatment of 67 persons with symptomatic spondylolysis and spondylolisthesis yielded an excellent or good result with no pain and return to full activities in 52 (78%) of the patients. (101) The original Boston brace was designed to open posteriorly in order to facilitate scoliotic correction. The modified antilordotic brace (Boston overlap

brace) opens in the front for convenient application and removal. Heavy-duty fittings are used to decrease the incidence of brace failure. Modules can also be made with either a polypropylene or a less rigid polyethylene outer shell. The different materials are used to allow varying degrees of patient flexibility and brace rigidity. Thus, a football linebacker might be fitted with a more rigid polypropylene brace with liner, while a supple young female gymnast might be treated with a more flexible polyethylene outer shell with no liner. (35)

To allow greater freedom of movement, the braces are trimmed according to the activity performed. The lower lateral margins are cut 1 in above the greater trochanter to enhance lateral mobility and prevent impingement of the trochanters. (35) The superior lateral trim lines can be cut down to well below the rib margins and this area filled with a lateral web of heavy-duty elastic nylon. This has been particularly important in lateral bending sports such as gymnastics, and tennis, and for the football positions of linebacker and safety. (35,101)

The combination of spinal protection and immobilization, along with decreased lumbar lordosis provided by these new orthoses has been helpful in the treatment of back injuries in young athletes, particularly those with active spondylolysis and positive SPECT scans. In this situation the brace functions as both a therapeutic apparatus and protective device. Patients with active acute spondylolysis with positive SPECT scans should be placed in an antilordotic position in the Boston overlap brace for a minimum of 6 to 8 weeks. During this time repeat bone scans should be performed, guiding the patient's return to physical activity as the SPECT bone scans become less active or "cold." (35,101)

For information concerning the Boston overlap brace, contact Boston Brace International, 20 Ledin Drive, Avon, Massachusetts, 02322, phone (508)588-6060.

Spondylolisthesis and Foot Pronation

It is imperative that the complete clinical assessment of the patient with lower back pain and preexisting spondylolytic spondylolisthesis-stable include evaluation of the longitudinal arch of the foot for pronation. One of the most common lower extremity disorders implicated in chronic structural biomechanical dysfunction is hyperpronation of the longitudinal arch. This reduces the foot's ability to properly balance body weight and cushion the force of heel-strike shock. (102) Patients with spondylolisthe-

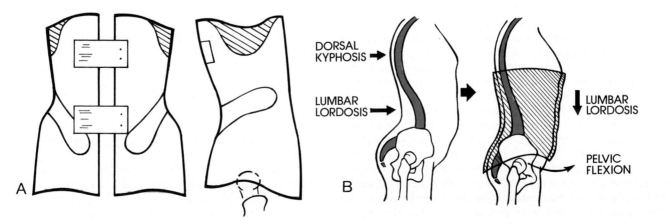

Figure 5.40. BOSTON OVERLAP BRACE. A. Schematic of the Brace. B. Schematic of the Postural Effects of the Brace on the Lumbar Lordosis.

(Adapted from Micheli LJ, Hall JE, Miller ME: *Use of modified Boston brace for back injuries in athletes.* Am J Sports Med 8 (5), 1980)

sis often have a swayback postural fault with an anterior pelvic tilt. Pronation of the longitudinal arch accentuates this. (103) Excessive pronation can progress as a serial distortion, creating a functional leg length inequality with presenting symptoms of sciatic pain, unilateral hip symptoms, and lower back pain. (104) Leg length inequality puts stress on the pelvic structures, causing an inward hip rotation and/or torquing of the pelvis, often resulting in chronic myofascial back pain, which is very common among people with spondylolisthesis. (105) Research on spondylolisthesis patients revealed a greater reduction in pain scores when orthotic therapy was combined with spinal manipulation. (55,56) Flexible orthotics enhance the biomechanics of the lower extremity by modifying minor deficits that inhibit the integrity of the pedal foundation. (106) Flexible orthotics have also been shown to decrease heel-strike shock, significantly reduce pronation, and reduce pronation velocity. (107–110) To prescribe the most effective support, use of a weight-bearing casting method to obtain quantifiable information on the extent of pedal imbalance is recommended. Casting the feet in a position of function gives real-life information on which corrections can be based. (111) This method also results in a more accurate fit, since the true length and width of the foot during the closed-chain stance are thoroughly assessed.

Orthotic therapy coupled with spinal manipulation represents a cost-effective, preventative, and integrated approach to case management of the spondylolisthetic patient.

SURGICAL MANAGEMENT

There are two main indications for surgery in the patient with spondylolisthesis: the relief of back pain in the unstable patient (as defined previously) and the elimination of neurocompressive radiculopathy. Diffuse nonradicular back pain generally requires fusion of the unstable segment but not decompression. Radicular pain often requires decompression and nearly always an added fusion. If decompressive surgery is indicated, it is critical to know, preoperatively, the precise location of stenosis in order to avoid destabilizing the segment unnecessarily.

A small percentage of patients with spondylolisthesis will demonstrate biomechanical instability (as defined previously) on erect posture radiologic stress studies. These patients may require surgical arthrodesis. Bilateral vertebral body or transverse process fusions are the most current and widely accepted surgical approaches. (16,112) Surgical intervention should be used only when conservative management has proved unsuccessful or when the patient shows signs of associated biomechanical instability and/or progressive neurologic deficits. Within these specific guidelines, arthrodesis is usually successful in the reduction of the patient's complaint.

Some patients who have undergone successful spinal fusion for spondylolisthesis may develop severe back pain months or years after the spinal surgery. The pain may be secondary to development of a stress (fatigue) fracture of the pars at a neighboring mobile vertebra as the result of increased stress placed upon these structures. (1) This condition is referred to as "spondylolisthesis acquisita." (1) Diagnosis requires flexion and extension lumbar radiographs and occasionally tomography. This fracture may heal with prolonged immobilization, but it is best treated by extending the fusion mass to include the affected vertebra. (1) SPECT imaging may also be helpful to rule out pseudoarthrosis and a failed spinal fusion.

It should be emphasized that a very small percentage of young patients will not limit their physical activities, may be unresponsive to spinal manipulative therapy or other conservative measures, and may require surgical stabilization. However, Wiltse (113) has stated that "to operate on a child simply because he has spondylolisthesis, without other reasons, would be wrong," and we applaud his view.

There is no guaranteed reduction of symptoms as a result of spinal fusion; therefore, the physician and patient should have exhausted all conservative measures prior to surgical intervention. (114) The detailed surgical treatment and management of spondylolisthesis is beyond the scope of this work, and the reader is referred to the following references: 1, 13, 18, 40, 52, 113, 115–117.

The treatment of advanced spondylolisthesis (grades III and IV) is controversial. The surgical options include decompressive laminectomy, fusion in situ, decompression followed by spinal fusion, or reduction followed by spinal fusion. (115–117) Reduction of the deformity before fusion carries the risk of neurologic deterioration, whereas fusion in situ is thought to be a more reliable option. Decompressive laminectomy is also said to be a safe procedure. Maurice and Morley (116) reported four cases in which cauda equina lesions developed after posterior spinal fusion for severe advanced spondylolisthesis-three after intertransverse fusion in situ and one after decompression laminectomy. These patients were 16, 15 (two patients), and 10 years old. All had in situ fusion and subsequently developed cauda equina signs, including bladder dysfunction, lax anal tone, and altered perineal sensations. Partial recovery was noted in two of the four patients. These findings highlight the possible dangers of surgery in patients with spondylolisthesis. The risk of neurologic damage is well recognized if reduction is attempted before fusion, but it should be documented that fusion in situ and decompressive laminectomy may be complicated by neurologic complications, even in the hands of experienced spinal surgeons. (116) It is important that all patients be counseled, before surgery, about the risks of neurologic damage following surgical fusion for spondylolisthesis.

An algorithmic approach to imaging and treatment of patients with and without spondylolysis and/or spondylolisthesis is offered. See Figures 5.41, 5.42, and 5.43.

DEGENERATIVE SPONDYLOLISTHESIS

The persistently symptomatic patient with spondylolisthesis usually has a degenerative type (type III) rather than the more common isthmic variety [type II-(a)]. Most of these patients also have lateral recess spinal stenosis of a degenerative nature, which may respond quite readily to conservative spinal manipulative therapy. If conservative treatment is unsuccessful, surgical intervention should be strongly considered. Decompressive surgery with or without fusion may provide a dramatic improvement in such patients' clinical status. (118)

PREEMPLOYMENT RADIOGRAPHIC SCREENING

In many countries, including the United States, preemployment low-back radiographs are used to screen employees for potential risk of injury in the workplace. Often, patients are denied employment or promotion because of the radiographic visualization of an asymptomatic lumbar spondylolysis and/or spondylolisthesis. (119,120) Based on the performance of the athletes in

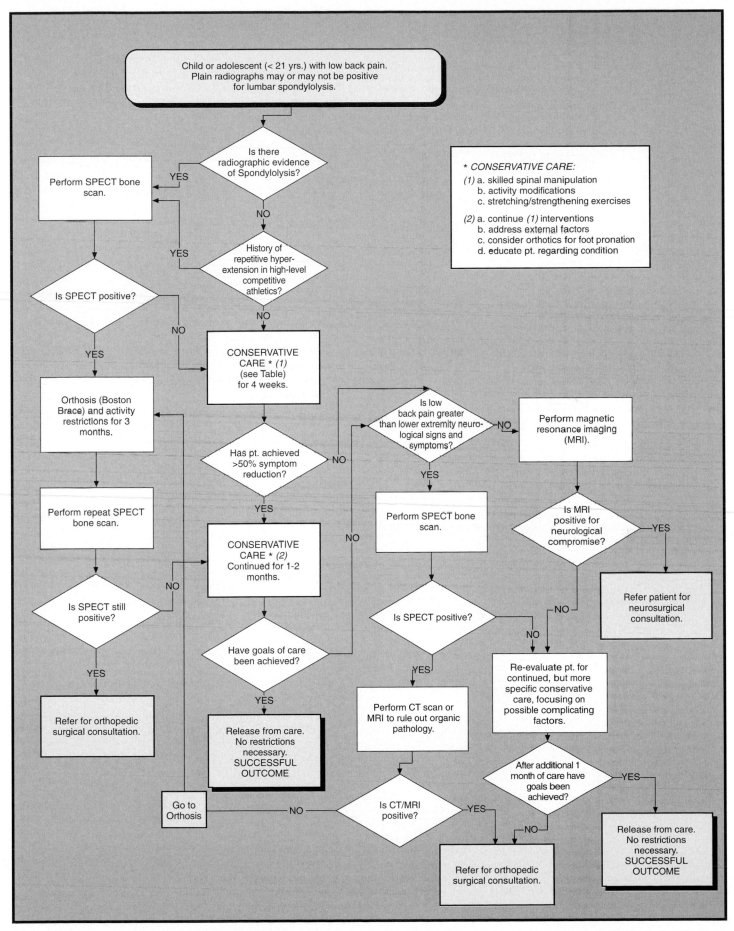

Figure 5.41.   AN ALGORITHMIC APPROACH TO SPONDYLOLYSIS AND SPONDYLOLISTHESIS. An imaging and treatment protocol for a child, ad- olescent, or young adult below the age of 21 with low back pain whose plain film radiographs may or may not be positive for lumbar spondylolysis.

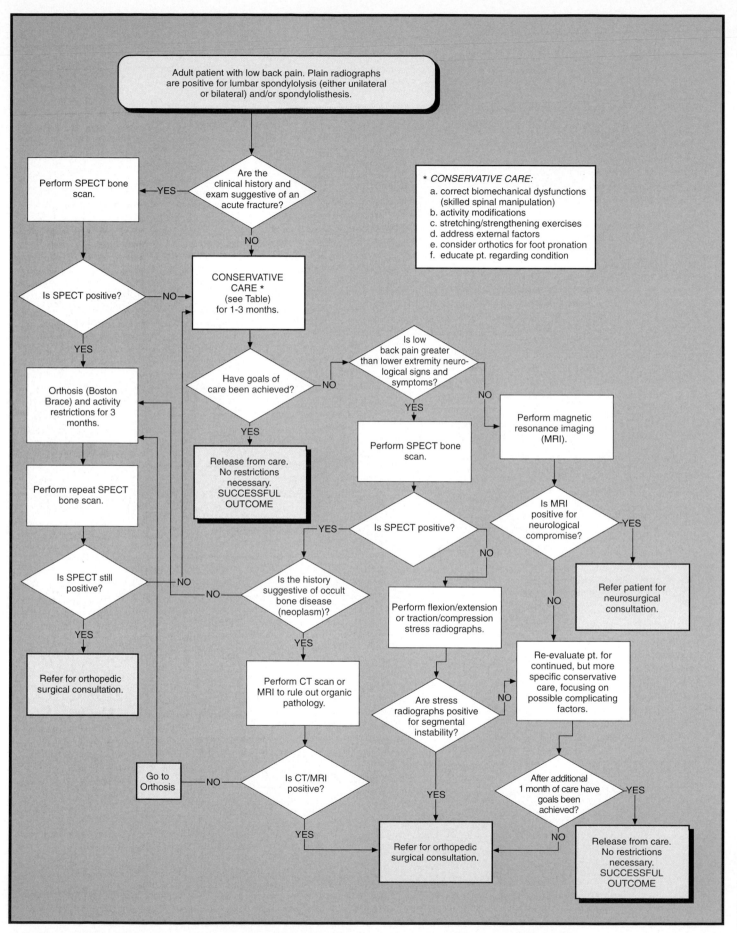

Figure 5.42. AN ALGORITHMIC APPROACH TO SPONDYLOLYSIS AND SPONDYLOLISTHESIS. An imaging and treatment protocol for an adult patient with low back pain whose plain film radiographs are positive for spondylolysis (either unilateral or bilateral) with or without spondylolisthesis.

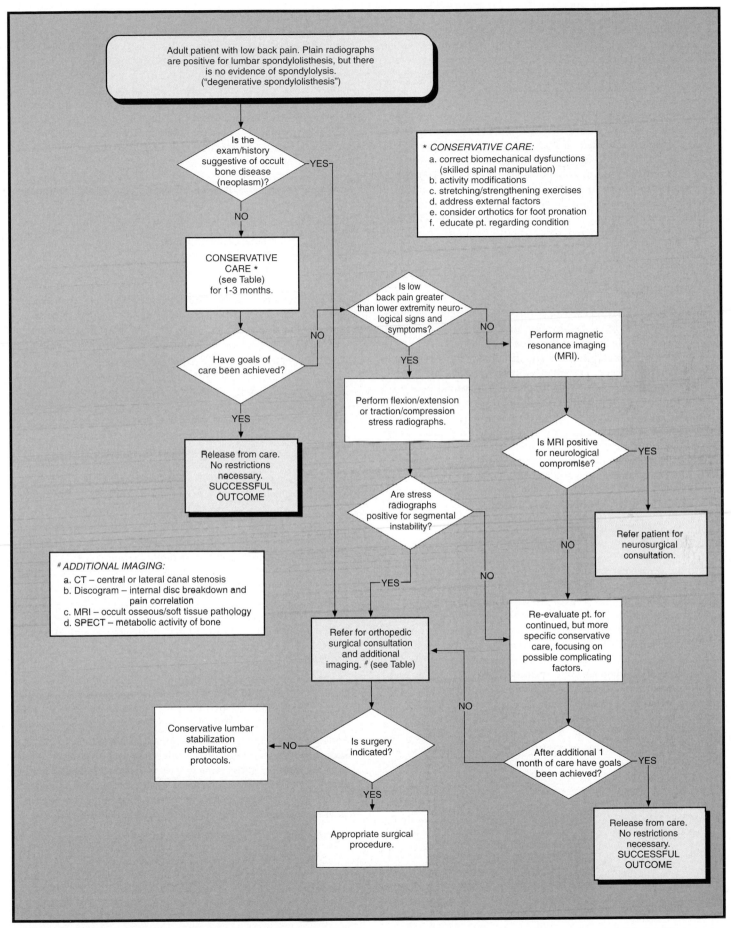

Figure 5.43.   AN ALGORITHMIC APPROACH TO SPONDYLOLYSIS AND SPONDYLOLISTHESIS. An imaging and treatment protocol for an adult patient with low back pain whose plain film radiographs are positive for spondylolisthesis, without evidence of spondylolysis (degenerative spondylolisthesis).

the previously cited studies, this attitude may not be justified. (30,33,53,54) We found no studies that demonstrate that workers with spondylolysis or spondylolisthesis involved in the heavy-labor sector of industry are at any greater risk from back injuries or have any greater loss of work time than those employees without spondylolysis or spondylolisthesis. A plethora of personal opinions exist to the contrary; these opinions, however, cannot be supported by documented clinical case studies or research data. It is our opinion that refusal of employment based on the existence of spondylolysis and/or spondylolisthesis is as antiquated as the procedure of preemployment radiographic screening itself, which is now receiving considerably less emphasis. (119,120)

Until the true etiology of low back pain in patients with these lesions is definitively proved, there should be no discrimination against workers with coincidental asymptomatic spondylolysis and/or spondylolisthesis.

IMPAIRMENT RATING

In a recent issue (June 1993) of *Guides to the Evaluation of Permanent Impairment,* published by the American Medical Association (68), spondylolisthesis (in those patients who have not been operated on for spondylolysis or spondylolisthesis) is dealt with in the following fashion. For spondylolysis or grade I or II (up to 50% slippage) spondylolisthesis, that is accompanied by a medically documented injury that is stable and medically documented pain and rigidity, with or without muscle spasm, a 7% impairment of the whole person is rendered. Spondylolisthesis of grade III and grade IV (up to 100% of anterior displacement) that is accompanied by a medically documented injury that is stable and medically documented pain and rigidity, with or without muscle spasm is rated at 9% impairment of the whole person. These numbers are far more realistic than what had been cited in earlier editions of these guidelines.

SUMMARY

Although the true etiology of spondylolysis and/or spondylolisthesis has been unclear for many years, stress fracture has emerged as the most likely cause for isthmic type IIA. Some populations demonstrate an apparent genetic predisposition to spondylolysis. The relationship between spondylolisthesis and back pain appears to encompass an unclearly defined primary cause for the pain. A small percentage of patients may have instability or spinal stenosis (degenerative spondylolisthesis), which eventually may require surgical intervention. Most, however, will respond to conservative care.

Many athletes with spondylolisthesis compete in rigorous sports without any reduction in their performance or any greater prevalence of back pain, as compared with controls. (53,74) Therefore, participation in sports should not be discouraged unless biomechanical instability, spinal stenosis, or neurologic deficit is present. The use of preemployment low back radiographs as a screening measure to detect spondylolisthesis for industry is antiquated. There is no evidence to support the premise that a patient (over the age of 18 years) with a spondylolysis and/or

spondylolisthesis is unable to perform heavy manual labor or is at greater risk of injury. Until data become available to contradict this premise, these individuals should not be discriminated against when seeking employment. Additionally, the *Guides to the Evaluation of Permanent Impairment, 4th Edition* published by the American Medical Association (68), has recently changed. In June of 1993 an updated whole-person impairment (7 and 9%) was established and is much more realistic than the earlier inflated rates.

MEDICOLEGAL IMPLICATIONS
Spondylolysis and/or Spondylolisthesis

- It is important to document the presence of unilateral or bilateral pars defects as it may relate to the degree of displacement or potential for displacement. Complete radiographic assessment to adequately demonstrate this information is considered essential.

- The importance of flexion/extension or traction/compression radiography along with SPECT bone scans is essential in the overall assessment of patients with unstable spondylolisthesis. Often patients may have a history of significant trauma that has precipitated symptoms of lower back pain. Plain film radiography and CT don't provide physiologic information concerning the pars defect. SPECT may assist in determining whether this defect is a source of pain and whether the recent trauma has produced symptoms, aggravating the preexisting spondylolysis and/or spondylolisthesis.

- It is important to establish the etiology of anterolisthesis in the cervical spine in every patient. In the presence of cervical spondylolisthesis, associated dysplasia of the neural arch frequently tips off the clinician to the underlying congenital etiology. Fifty percent of patients with cervical spondylolisthesis have an associated spina bifida occulta deformity. This is an important radiographic sign that should alert the clinician that this is not a fracture-dislocation and that under no circumstance should such a patient receive spinal fusion for the misdiagnosis of fracture. Cervical spondylolisthesis is rarely unstable upon flexion/extension radiography.

- Inappropriate spinal manipulation, which may worsen the patient's symptoms, is contraindicated in patients with spondylolisthesis. An example of such inappropriate manipulation is prone recoil adjustments directly over the spondylolisthesis.

- Patients who demonstrate radiographic instability of lumbar spondylolisthesis by means of upright flexion/extension or compression/traction stress radiographs and positive SPECT scans should be referred for orthopedic or neurologic consultation as part of the overall management of the unstable spondylolisthetic segment.

CAPSULE SUMMARY   *Spondylolysis and Spondylolisthesis*

DEFINITIONS

- *Spondylolysis* is an interruption of the pars interarticularis; this may be either unilateral or bilateral. The term *spondylolysis* is derived from two Greek roots, *spondylos*, meaning vertebra, and *lysis*, meaning a dissolution or a loosing, setting free, releasing.
- *Spondylolisthesis* is defined as an anterior displacement of a vertebral body in relationship to the segment immediately below (an incorrect use of the term- -see text for complete explanation). The Greek origin of this word is *spondylos*, meaning vertebra, and *olisthesis*, referring to displacement. Spondylolisthesis may be associated with defects in the pars interarticularis (spondylolytic spondylolisthesis) but may occur without them (nonspondylolytic spondylolisthesis).
- *Prespondylolisthesis* is defined as the presence of spondylolysis without forward vertebral displacement. This term is misleading and should be discarded since it implies that displacement will necessarily occur.

GENERAL CONSIDERATIONS

- The first recorded article relating to spondylolisthesis was in 1782 by a Belgian obstetrician, Herbinaux.
- A historical overview as well as a new perspective of spondylolysis and/or spondylolisthesis are offered.

INCIDENCE

- A prevalence of 5 to 7% is found in the white population, with a much higher figure being noted in highly active individuals and athletes.
- An explanation regarding the true reason for a 40% prevalence in Stewart's studies of the Alaskan Eskimo is still not available. We offer a hypothesis related to the early upright posture in the infant.

ETIOLOGY

- The etiology of this peculiar disorder is now clearly classified by Wiltse and Micheli, with the majority of these lesions being acquired stress fractures (type II(a)—isthmic).
- Presence of a thin pars at birth may be a predisposing factor to the development of spondylolysis.
- A small percentage of cases are dysplastic in origin (type I).
- Since this lesion has been reported only in humans (except for one gorilla), upright posture, coupled with inappropriate stresses, would appear to be a strong etiologic factor.

WILTSE CLASSIFICATION

- *Type I: Dysplastic*: A congenital abnormality in the upper sacrum or the neural arch of L5, allowing displacement to occur
- *Type II: Isthmic:* (a) a lytic or fatigue fracture of the pars, (b) elongated but intact pars, (c) acute fracture of the pars
- *Type III: Degenerative:* Secondary to long-standing degenerative arthrosis of the zygapophyseal joints and discovertebral articulation
- *Type IV: Traumatic:* Secondary to fractures in the area of the neural arch other than the pars interarticularis
- *Type V: Pathologic:* In conjunction with generalized or localized bone disease (e.g., Paget's disease, metastatic bone disease, osteopetrosis, etc.)

CLINICAL FEATURES

- A very large percentage (estimated at 50%) of the patients with spondylolysis and/or spondylolisthesis never develop back pain.
- Those patients who suffer back pain usually have a separate biomechanical or pathologic cause for their symptoms.
- Progression of displacement seldom occurs after the age of 18. It is thought by many that by the age of 10 the greatest degree of displacement has been obtained.
- Physical examination findings in patients with spondylolisthesis often reveal prominent, heart-shaped buttocks, hyperlordosis of the lumbar spine, and a palpable "step defect" in nonspondylolytic spondylolisthesis. Patients with advanced displacement often demonstrate a symmetric transverse skin furrow, which may be seen above the iliac crests. Associated spina bifida occulta may be signaled by localized hypertrichosis. A clicking sensation at the level of the involved segment may be felt or heard during active trunk flexion or on straight leg raising ("spinal rattle"). Unexplained hamstring tightness is frequently associated with spondylolisthesis. The resultant stiff-legged and short-strided gait creates a characteristic "pelvic waddle."
- Many athletes with spondylolisthesis compete in vigorous sports without any reduction in their performance or any greater prevalence of back pain, as compared with controls. Participation in sports should not be discouraged unless biomechanical instability, spinal stenosis, or neurologic deficit is present.
- Hyland has offered a problem-based clinical classification of spondylolisthesis: (a) recent spondylolytic spondylolisthesis (RSS); (b) Preexisting spondylolytic spondylolisthesis—stable (PSS-S); (c) Pre-existing spondylolytic spondylolisthesis—unstable (PSS-U); and (d) Degenerative spondylolisthesis (DS).

RADIOLOGIC FEATURES

- A bowline of Brailsford and an inverted Napoleon's hat sign, or the Gendarme's cap, are radiographic features of an advanced grade 3 or grade 4 spondylolisthesis as seen on the AP radiograph.
- Meyerding's method for determining the degree of spondylolisthesis (grades 1, 2, 3, and 4) is offered. A trapezoidal posterior narrowing of the L5 body, creating a doming of the anterior surface of the sacrum, is found with advanced spondylolisthesis.
- A radiolucent defect in the pars interarticularis is visualized optimally on oblique lumbar radiographs and referred to as the "collar" or "broken neck" of the "Scotty Dog." Equivocal defects at the L5 level may be better visualized by using a 30° cephalic tube tilt with the patient in the routine anterior oblique position. This may elongate the pars and allow more adequate visualization of subtle pars defects. The angulated AP projection (tilt-up or Ferguson's view) of the lumbosacral junction is a positive alternative to oblique views to identify spondylolysis at L5. This view eliminates the degree of obliquity in patient positioning, allowing a more accurate evaluation of equivocal lesions on other films.
- The stepladder sign is produced by malalignment of the zygapophyseal joints at the involved level of spondylolisthesis.
- AP translatory motion of greater than 4 mm or a difference in angular motion of greater than 11° in two adjacent motion segments during spinal flexion and extension has been reported as diagnostic of instability. More recently Friberg and others have documented that axial compression/traction is superior to lateral lumbar flexion/extension stress radiography in the assessment of instability in patients with spondylolysis and/or spondylolisthesis.
- SPECT is a tomographic method to obtain sectional and multiplanar images, which allows a more accurate means than

planar bone scans to determine increased radiotracer uptake in lumbar spondylolysis. It is the most sensitive tool to localize bone remodeling in an area of complex spinal anatomy. The SPECT scan plays a significant role in evaluating increased physiologic activity in the area of the pars in patients who are symptomatic, and it can dictate patient management (i.e., reducing physical activity and athletic participation in various sporting activities). Patients with positive SPECT bone scans, with or without pars defects, should be placed in an antilordotic position, such as with the Boston overlap brace.

- An additional application of SPECT imaging is the evaluation of the postsurgical spine for pseudoarthrosis. Focal areas of increased uptake within the fusion mass are considered positive for a pseudoarthrosis. SPECT scanning provides more accurate information not available on planar bone scans.
- MR imaging of spondylolysis has recently been documented in the literature. Careful evaluation of the neural arch in patients exhibiting the appropriate clinical features of developing spondylolysis may reveal bone marrow edema in the preradiographic phase. This finding is seen as an area of high signal in the pars on T2-weighted axial and parasagittal images of the lumbar spine. A unique case study with MR imaging of the pars is offered.

UNILATERAL SPONDYLOLYSIS

- Unilateral spondylolysis often creates compensatory stress hypertrophy of the contralateral pars and pedicle region (Wilkinson's syndrome).
- This finding (sclerotic pedicle) may simulate neoplastic disorders, such as osteoid osteoma, osteoblastoma, or a focus of osteoblastic metastasis.
- A key differential clue is to search for the unilateral pars defect opposite the sclerotic pedicle.

CERVICAL SPONDYLOLISTHESIS

- This is a rare and unusual disorder.
- The majority of these lesions are asymptomatic.
- It is most commonly found at the C6 vertebral segment; however, it has been noted at C2, C5, and C7.

- The defect is nearly always bilateral and is most frequently found in males.
- The most likely etiology is congenital agenesis or dysplasia of the pedicle.
- Approximately 50% of the patients with cervical spondylolysis have an associated spina bifida occulta of the involved vertebra.
- This lesion should not be misinterpreted as a fracture, and the presence of spina bifida occulta at C6 confirms its congenital etiology.

TREATMENT AND PROGNOSIS

- Medical management is conservative initially, although surgical fusion is still being recommended by many orthopedic surgeons. Maurice and Morley reported four cases in which cauda equina lesions occurred after posterior spinal fusion for severe advanced spondylolisthesis.
- Caution is advised to those patients who consider surgery without exhausting all conservative measures first. A more conservative approach, including chiropractic spinal manipulative therapy, has been found beneficial in managing patients' low back pain with the presence of spondylolysis or spondylolisthesis. The use of the Boston (antilordotic) overlap brace in patients with symptomatic spondylolysis in the preradiographic or radiographic phase is thoroughly discussed. SPECT imaging plays an important role in determining when an antilordotic brace or surgical intervention is used in patient management.
- Some innovative thoughts are presented concerning the ability of patients with spondylolisthesis to continue to participate in rigorous sports and function in a work place requiring heavy manual labor.

With the most recent issue (1993) of *Guides to the Evaluation of Permanent Impairment,* published by the American Medical Association, a 7% impairment of whole person is rendered in patients with grade I or grade II spondylolisthesis with ongoing back pain. A 9% impairment of whole person has been assigned to patients with grade III or grade IV spondylolisthesis with accompanying persistent lower back pain. These numbers are far more realistic than the inflated percentages cited in earlier editions of the guidelines.

REFERENCES

1. **Gehweiler JA, Osborne R, Becker, RF:** *The Radiology of Vertebral Trauma,* Philadelphia, WB Saunders, 1980.
2. **Herbinaux G:** *Traite sur divers laborieux, et sur les polypes de la matrice,* Bruxelles: JL DeBoubers, 1782.
3. **Kilian HF:** *Spondylolysteses gravissimae causa nuper detecta.* In: *Commentatio anatomica obstetricia.* Bonnae Lit. C. Geirgii, 1854. Cited in Clin Radiol 20:315, 1969.
4. **Robert H:** Monatsschrift fur Geburtskunde und Frauenkrankheiten, 5:81, 1855.
5. **Lambl W:** *Beitr ge zur Geburskunde und Gynackologie,* von FWV Scanzoni, 1858.
6. **Neugebauer FL:** *Neuer Beitrag zur Aetiologie und Causistik der Spondylolisthesis.* Arch Gynaekol 1895: 25:182. Translated in part in Clin Orthop 117:4, 1976.
7. **McKee BM, Alexander WJ, Dunbar JS:** *Spondylolysis and spondylolisthesis in children: A review.* J Can Assoc Radiol 22:100, 1971.
8. **Taillard WF:** *Etiology of spondylolisthesis.* Clin Orthop 117:30, 1976.
9. **Moreton RD:** *Spondylolysis.* JAMA 195:671, 1966.
10. **Stewart TD:** *The age incidence of neural arch defects in Alaskan natives, considered from the standpoint of etiology.* J Bone Joint Surg (Am) 35:937, 1953.
11. **Kettlekamp DB, Wright DG:** *Spondylolysis in the Alaskan Eskimo.* J Bone Joint Surg (Am) 53:563, 1971.
12. **Rowe GG, Roche MB:** *The etiology of separate neural arch.* J Bone Joint Surg (Am) 35:102, 1953.
13. **Wiltse LL:** *The etiology of spondylolisthesis.* J Bone Joint Surg (Am) 44:539, 1962.
14. **Janse J:** In: Hildebrant RW, ed, *Principles and practice of chiropractic. An anthology.* Lombard, IL: National College of Chiropractic, 1976.
15. **Borkow SE, Kleiger B:** *Spondylolisthesis in the newborn: A case report.* Clin Orthop 81:73, 1971.
16. **Turner RH, Bianco AJ:** *Spondylolysis and spondylolisthesis in children and teenagers.* J Bone Joint Surg (Am) 53:1298, 1971.
17. **Batts M Jr:** *The etiology of spondylolisthesis.* J Bone Joint Surg (Am) 21:879, 1939.
18. **Fredrickson BE, Baker D, McHollick WJ, et al:** *The natural history of spondylolysis and spondylolisthesis.* J Bone Joint Surg (Am) 66:699, 1984.
19. **Kleinberg S:** *Spondylolisthesis in an infant.* J Bone Joint Surg (Am) 16:441, 1934.
20. **Laurent L, Emola S:** *Spondylolisthesis in children and adolescents.* Acta Orthop Scand 31:45, 1961.
21. **McCarville B, Sundaram M, Gabriel K:** *Spondylolysis in a two-year-old girl.* Orthopedics 16:10, 1993.
22. **Hensinger RN:** *Current concepts review: Spondylolysis and spondylolisthesis in children and adolescents.* J Bone Joint Surg (Am) 71:1098, 1989.
23. **Saha MM, Bhardwaj OP, Srivastava G, et al:** *Osteopetrosis with spondylolysis: Four cases in one family.* Br Radiol 43:738, 1970.
24. **Cyron BM, Hutton WC:** *Variations in the amount and distribution of cortical bone across the partes interarticularis of L5-a predisposing factor in spondylolysis?* Spine 4:2, 1979.
25. **Wiltse LL, Widell EH, Jackson DW:** *Fatigue fracture: The basic lesion in isthmic spondylolisthesis.* J Bone Joint Surg (Am) 57:17, 1975.
26. **Cyron BM, Hutton WC:** *The fatigue strength of the lumbar neural arch in spondylolysis.* J Bone Joint Surg (Br) 60:462, 1978.

27. **Schmorl G, Junghans H:** *The Human Spine in Health and Disease,* ed 2. New York, Grune & Stratton, 1971.
28. **Rosenberg NJ, Bargar WL, Friedman B:** *The incidence of spondylolysis and spondylolisthesis in nonambulatory patients.* Spine 6:35, 1981.
29. **Newman PH, Stone KH:** *The etiology of spondylolisthesis.* J Bone Joint Surg (Br) 45:39, 1963.
30. **Rossi F:** *Spondylolysis, spondylolisthesis and sports.* Sports Med 18:317, 1978.
31. **Gainor BJ, Hagen RJ, Allen WC:** *Biomechanics of the spine in the pole-vaulter as related to spondylolysis.* Am J Sports Med 11:53, 1983.
32. **Raynal L, Coaard M, Elbanna S:** *Contribution a l'etude de la spondylolyse traumatique.* Acta Orthop Belg 43:653, 1977.
33. **Kono S, Hayashi M, Kashahara T:** *A study on the etiology of spondylolysis with reference to athletic activities (Japanese).* J Jpn Orthop Assoc 49:125, 1975.
34. **Schulitz KP, Niethard FU:** *Strain on the interarticular stress distribution—measurements regarding the development of spondylolysis.* Arch Orthop Trauma Surg 96:197, 1980.
35. **Micheli LJ, Hall JE, Miller ME:** *Use of modified Boston brace for back injuries in athletes.* Am J Sports Med 8:5, 1980.
36. **Bellah RD, Summerville DA, Micheli LJ, et al:** *Low back pain in adolescent athletes: Detection of stress injury to the pars interarticularis with SPECT.* Radiology 180:509, 1991.
37. **Papanicolaou N, Wilkinson RH, Micheli LJ, et al:** *Bone scintigraphy and radiography in young athletes with low back pain.* AJR 145:1039, 1985.
38. **Szappanos L, Szepesi K, Thomazy V:** *Spondylolysis in osteopetrosis.* J Bone Joint Surg (Br) 70(3):426, 1988.
39. **Wiltse LL, Newman PH, Macnab I:** *Classification of spondylolysis and spondylolisthesis.* Clin Orthop 117:23, 1976.
40. **Moe JH, Winter RB, Bradford DS, Lonstein JE:** *Scoliosis and Other Spinal Deformities,* Philadelphia, WB Saunders, 1978.
41. **Macnab I:** *Spondylolisthesis with an intact neural arch-so-called pseudospondylolisthesis.* J Bone Joint Surg (Br) 32:325, 1950.
42. **Rosenberg MJ:** *Degenerative spondylolisthesis.* Clin Orthop 117:112, 1976.
43. **Allbrook B:** *Movements of the lumbar spine column.* J Bone Joint Surg (Br) 39:339, 1957.
44. **Pease CN, Najat H:** *Spondylolisthesis in children.* Clin Orthop 52:187, 1967.
45. **Yochum TR, et al:** *Reactive sclerosis of a pedicle due to unilateral spondylolysis—a case study.* ACA J Chiro, Radiology Corner, September 1980.
46. **Friberg S:** *Studies on spondylolisthesis.* Acta Chir Scand 82(Suppl): 55, 1939.
47. **Bodner RJ, Heyman S, Drummond DS, et al:** *The use of single-photon emission computed tomography (SPECT) in the diagnosis of low back pain in young patients.* Spine 13:10, 1988.
48. **Albanese M, Pizzutillo PD:** *Family study of spondylolysis and spondylolisthesis.* J Pediatr Orthop 2:496, 1982.
49. **Cassidy JD, Potter GE, Kirkaldy-Willis WH:** *Manipulative management of back pain in patients with spondylolisthesis.* J Can Chirop Assoc 22:15, 1978.
50. **Blackburne JS, Velikas EP:** *Spondylolisthesis in children and adults.* Royal Soc Med 70:421, 1977.
51. **Monticelli G, Ascani E:** *Spondylolysis and spondylolisthesis.* Acta Orthop Scand 46:498, 1975.
52. **Turek SL:** *Orthopedic Principals and Their Application,* ed 4. Philadelphia, JB Lippincott, 1984.
53. **Semon RL, Spengler D:** *Significance of lumbar spondylolysis in college football players.* Spine 6:172, 1981.
54. **Ferguson RJ, McMasters JH, Stanitski CL:** *Low back pain in college football linemen.* Am J Sports Med 2:63, 1974.
55. **Hyland J:** *Spondylolisthesis.* Foot Levelers Practical Research Studies 3:6, 1993.
56. **Hyland J:** *Clinical classification of spondylolisthesis.* ACA J Chiro, August 1993.
57. **Saward L:** *Spondylolysis and the sacral-horizontal angle in athletes.* Acta Radiol 30:359, 1989.
58. **Taylor DB:** *Foraminal encroachment syndrome in true lumbosacral spondylolisthesis.* J Manipulative Physiol Ther 10:253, 1987.
59. **Cox JM:** *Degenerative spondylolisthesis of C7 and L4 in the same patient.* J Manipulative Physiol Ther 11:195, 1988.
60. **Zatkin HR:** *The Roentgen Diagnosis of Trauma,* Chicago, Year Book Medical Publishers, 1965.
61. **Ravichandran G:** *A radiological sign in spondylolisthesis.* AJR 134:113, 1980.
62. **Libson E, Bloom RA:** *Anteroposterior angulated view—A new radiographic technique for the evaluation of spondylolysis.* Radiology 149:315, 1983.
63. **Hibbs RA, Swift WE:** *Developmental abnormalities at the lumbo-sacral juncture causing pain and disability: A report of 147 patients treated by the spine fusion operation.* Surg Gynec Obst 48:604, 1929.
64. **Meyerding HW:** *Low backache and sciatic pain associated with spondylolisthesis and protruded intervertebral disc.* J Bone Joint Surg (Am) 23:461, 1941.
65. **El-Khoury GY, Yousefzadeh DK, Kathol MH, et al:** *Normal roentgen variant: Pseudospondylolysis.* Radiology 139:72, 1981.
66. **Kohler A:** In: EA Zimmer, ed. *Borderlands of the Normal and Early Pathologic in Skeletal Roentgenology,* ed 3. New York, Grune & Stratton, 1968.
67. **Edeiken J, Hodes PJ:** *Roentgen Diagnosis of Diseases of Bone,* Baltimore, Williams & Wilkins, 1973.
68. **American Medical Association:** *Guides to the evaluation of permanent impairment,* ed 4. Chicago: The Association, 1993.
69. **Nachemson A:** *Lumbar spine instability—A critical update and symposium summary.* Spine 10:290, 1985.
70. **Friberg O:** *Lumbar instability: A dynamic approach by traction-compression radiography.* Spine 12:2, 1987.
71. **Kalebo P, Kadziolka R, Saward L, et al:** *Stress views in the comparative assessment of spondylolytic spondylolisthesis.* Skeletal Radiol 17:570, 1989.
72. **Kalebo P, Kadziolka R, Saward L:** *Compression-traction radiography of lumbar segmental instability.* Spine 15:5, 1990.
73. **Cox JM, Trier K:** *Chiropractic adjustment results correlated with spondylolisthesis instability.* J Manual Med 6:67, 1991.
74. **Knight NA, Burleson RJ, Higginbotham JA:** *Spondylolysis of the L2 vertebra-in the female gymnast—A case report.* J Med Assoc Alabama December 23, 1977.
75. **Lowe J, Schachner E, Hirschberg E, et al:** *Significance of bone scintigraphy in symptomatic spondylolysis.* Spine 6:653, 1984.
76. **Collier BD, Johnson RP, Carrera GF, et al:** *Painful spondylolysis or spondylolisthesis studied by radiography and single-photon emission computed tomography.* Radiology 154:207, 1985.
77. **Ryan PJ, Evans BA, Gibson T, et al:** *Chronic low back pain: Comparison of bone SPECT with radiography and CT.* Radiology 182:849, 1992.
78. **Pennell RG, Maurer AH, Bonakdarpour A:** *Stress injuries of the pars interarticularis: Radiological classification and classifications for scintigraphy.* AJR 145:763, 1985.
79. **Read MTF;** *Single-photon emission computed tomography (SPECT) scanning for adolescent back pain: A sine qua non?* Br J Sports Med 28(1):94, 1994.
80. **Slizofski WJ, Collier BD, Flatley TJ, et al:** *Painful pseudoarthrosis following lumbar spine fusion: Detection by combined SPECT and planar bone scintigraphy.* Skeletal Radiol 16:136, 1987.
81. **Lusins JO, Danielski EF, Goldsmith SJ:** *Bone SPECT in patients with persistent back pain after lumbar spine surgery.* J Nucl Med 30:490, 1989.
82. **Raby N, Mathews S:** *Symptomatic spondylolysis: Correlation of CT and SPECT with clinical outcome.* Clin Radiol 48:97, 1993.
83. **Oever M, Merrick MV, Scott JHS:** *Bone scintigraphy in symptomatic spondylolysis.* J Bone Joint Surg (Br) 69:3, 1987.
84. **Jinkins JR, Matthes JC, Sener RN, et al:** *Spondylolysis, spondylolisthesis, and associated nerve root entrapment in the lumbosacral spine: MR evaluation.* AJR 159:799, 1992.
85. **Johnson DW, Farnum GN, Latchaw RE, et al:** *MR imaging of the pars interarticularis.* AJR 152:327, 1989.
86. **Grenier N, Kressel HY, Schiebler ML, et al:** *Isthmic spondylolysis of the lumbar spine: MR imaging at 1.5 T.* Radiology 170:489, 1989.
87. **Wilkinson RH, Hall JE:** *The sclerotic pedicle: Tumor or pseudotumor?* Radiology 111:683, 1974.
88. **Yochum TR, Sellers LT, Oppenheimer DA, et al:** *The sclerotic pedicle—how many causes are there?* Skeletal Radiol 19:411, 1990.
89. **Schwartz AM, Wechsler RJ, Landy MD, et al:** *Posterior arch defects of the cervical spine.* Skeletal Radiol 8:135, 1982.
90. **Bellamy R, Lieber A, Smith SD:** *Congenital spondylolisthesis of the sixth cervical vertebra.* J Bone Joint Surg (Am) 56:22, 1974.
91. **Niemeyer T, Penning L:** *Functional roentgenographic examination in a case of cervical spondylolisthesis.* J Bone Joint Surg (Am) 45:1671, 1973.
92. **Faure BT, Taylor W, Greenberg BJ:** *Cervical spondylolysis.* Orthopedics 13:2, 1990.
93. **Quint DJ:** *CT of bilateral cervical spondylolysis Letter to the editor.* AJR 156:24, 1991.
94. **Mooney V, Robertson J:** *The facet syndrome.* Clin Orthop 115:157, 1976.
95. **Illi FW:** *The Vertebral Column: Lifeline of the Body,* Chicago: National College of Chiropractic, 1951.
96. **Mierau D, Cassidy JD, McGregor M, et al:** *Comparison of the effectiveness of spinal manipulative therapy for low back pain patients with and without spondylolisthesis.* J Manipulative Physiol Ther 10:49, 1987.
97. **Banks SD:** *The use of spinographic parameters in the differential diagnosis of lumbar facet and disc syndromes.* J Manipulative Physiol Ther 6:113, 1983.
98. **Banks SD:** *Lumbar facet syndrome: Spinographic assessment of treatment by spinal manipulation.* J Manipulative Physiol Ther 6:175, 1983.
99. **Banks SD:** *Athletic low back pain originating from the neural arch.* Chiro Sports Med 1988; 2:2.
100. **Pearcy M, Shepherd J:** *Is there instability in spondylolisthesis?* Spine 10:175, 1985.
101. **Steiner ME, Micheli LJ:** *Treatment of symptomatic spondylolysis and spondylolisthesis with the modified Boston brace.* Spine 10:937, 1985.
102. **Root ML:** *Clinical Biomechanics II: Normal and Abnormal Function of the Foot.* Los Angeles: Clinical Biomechanics Corp, 1977.
103. **Foster A:** *Spondylolisthesis in chiropractic: Case report.* J Chiro 2711:73, 1990.
104. **Hlavac HF:** *The Foot Book Advice for Athletes.* Mountain View, CA: World Publications, 1977.
105. **Yochum TR, Barry MS:** *The Short Leg Syndrome.* Foot Levelers Practical Research Studies 4(5), 1994.
106. **Gross ML, Davlin LB, Evanski PL:** *Effectiveness of orthotic shoe inserts in the long-distance runner.* Am J Sports Med 19(4):409, 1991.
107. **McPoil TG, Cornwall MW:** *Use of soft orthoses in prevention of injuries.* JAPMA 81(12):638, 1991.
108. **Schwellnus MP, Jordaan G, Noakes TD:** *Prevention of common overuse injuries by the use of shock absorbing insoles.* Am J Sports Med 18(6):636, 1990.
109. **Clarke TE, Frederick EC, Hlavac HF:** *Effects of a soft orthotic device on rearfoot movement in running.* Pod Sports 1:20, 1983.
110. **Smith LS, Clarke TE, Hamill CL, et al:** *The effects of soft and semirigid orthoses upon rearfoot movement in running.* JAPMA 76:227, 1986.
111. **Wu KK:** *Foot orthoses. Principles and Clinical Applications.* Baltimore, William & Wilkins, 1990.
112. **Wiltse LL:** *Etiology of spondylolisthesis.* Clin Orthop 10:48, 1957.

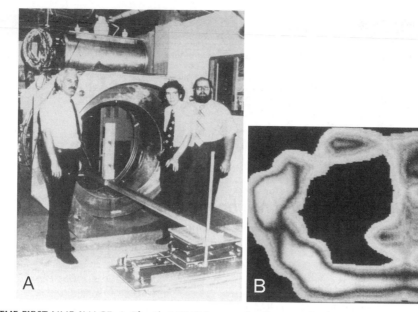

Figure 6.1.   THE FIRST NMR IMAGE. A. The First NMR Scanner for Humans. Left-to-right, R. Damadian, L. Minkhoff, M. Goldsmith. **B. The First NMR Image of a Human.** This is an axial image through the chest at the level of T8. The heart (arrow) is noted centrally within the chest cavity. This image was obtained in 1977 with the scanner depicted in **A**. COMMENT: This historic, crude image began the cascade of events that soon followed and led to the development of magnetic resonance technology. (**A** Courtesy of Partain CL, Price RR, Patton JA, et al (eds): Magnetic Resonance Imaging, WB Saunders, 1988)

Gradually, the name of this new technology was forced to change because of the negative connotation associated with the term *nuclear*. By the mid 1980s, nuclear magnetic resonance imaging became magnetic resonance imaging (MRI). MRI has rapidly gained favor with physicians and patients alike because of its noninvasive nature and lack of ionizing radiation or other harmful biologic effects.

The discovery and development of MRI is the most significant milestone in medical imaging since Roentgen's discovery of x-ray in 1895. MRI, like CT, is capable of providing an axial demonstration of human anatomy, but *without* ionizing radiation. The soft tissue contrast and spatial resolution also exceed that which is provided by computed tomography. MRI also has multiplanar capabilities, enabling anatomic information to be extracted in virtually any orientation without altering the patient's position within the scanner. Like nuclear scintigraphy, MRI is capable of obtaining physiologic data, but without the radiation dose associated with radiopharmaceutical use. Because of the aforementioned attributes, MRI has quickly gained worldwide acceptance in the medical imaging community.

Originally, MRI was used to image the central nervous system. Its clinical applications in the extremities were not initially envisioned but have been realized. Numerous applications now exist for the evaluation of disorders outside of these regions, including vascular analysis using magnetic resonance angiography (MRA) and the imaging of disorders of the chest and abdomen. In 1982 approximately a dozen MR scanners were in use worldwide. This number has increased rapidly, and it is predicted that by the turn of the century there will be at least one MR unit per 100,000 persons in the United States, Japan, and European communities. (9) The following text will briefly discuss the physics of image production, contraindications for use, and common musculoskeletal applications of MRI.

Glossary of Terms

Cardiac gating: the method used to diminish the artifact produced by pulsatile vascular flow. The pulse sequence used to obtain the MR image is synchronized with the patient's heart rate and images are continually obtained through only the diastole phase of the cardiac cycle.

Echo time (TE): the time interval from the 90° RF pulse and echo detection (measured in milliseconds).

Fast spin-echo (FSE): a pulse sequence that uses multiple echoes per repetition time (TR) to obtain the data necessary for image formation. In contrast, conventional spin-echo sequences use only a single echo per TR. The benefits of this newer, fast MR technique include reduced examination time, increased spatial resolution, and versatility in neuroimaging; in particular, superb myelographic images of the spine may be obtained. (10)

Fat suppression: an imaging technique that suppresses the signal derived from fat, thereby making small areas of pathologic change (which are often seen as areas of high signal because of their fluid content) more evident and increasing the overall sensitivity of the examination. This is usually accomplished through the use of inversion recovery techniques such as STIR (*Short T1 Inversion Recovery*) or chemical saturation (*fat sat*) sequences.

Field of view (FOV): this represents the size of the image and plays an integral part in determining the overall spatial resolution of the final image. Generally, the smaller the field of view, the greater the spatial resolution.

Flip angle: the angular deflection a hydrogen proton experiences when the RF pulse is applied. Spin-echo techniques displace the nuclear axis of rotation 90° from its equilibrium orientation (parallel or antiparallel) within the magnetic field.

Free induction decay: the loss of energy experienced by an excited proton after a 90° RF pulse. (11) The proton decays to its equilibrium (low-energy) state in an exponential fashion.

Gradient-echo pulsed sequences: this is a generic term used to describe fast MR imaging using short TR and short TE parameters. This technique differs from T1-weighted spin-echo sequences in that the RF pulses (flip angles) are less than 90°. This essentially provides a T2-weighted image in less time. Major disadvantages include the susceptibility to arti facts and the poor demonstration of bone marrow. Acronyms used to describe this type of imaging vary according to the manufacturer and include T2*-weighted, GRE (gradient recalled echo), GRASS (gradient recalled acquisition in the steady state), FLASH (fast low-angle shot), FISP (fast imaging with steady-state procession), MPGR (multiplanar GRASS), and SPGR (spoiled GRASS).

Hyperintense: relatively increased signal intensity. Areas of hyperintense (high) signal intensity are bright on MR images.

Hypointense: relatively decreased signal intensity. Areas of hypointense (low) signal intensity are dark gray or black on MR images.

Isointense: relatively equal in signal intensity.

Larmor frequency: the frequency of precession for a given proton. This frequency varies with the applied magnetic field, but is unique for each different type of proton within a given field (i.e., all hydrogen ions in a given magnetic field precess at roughly the same Larmor frequency).

Precession: the rotational motion a given proton experiences as it wobbles about the axis of an external magnetic field. This phenomenon is similar to the motion displayed by a spinning gyroscope or top, relative to the earth's rotational motion.

Proton density–weighted: a long TR and short TE MR imaging technique. The resultant image is unique in that it provides good anatomic detail and has mixed properties of both T1 and T2 relaxation times. This pulse sequence derives its information based on the relative concentrations of water (hydrogen) in the tissue.

Radiofrequency (RF) pulse: an applied radiofrequency that is used to change the orientation of the magnetic axes of the hydrogen protons from an equilibrium state to an excited state. The RF is specific for each proton species within a given magnetic field, as defined by the Larmor equation (i.e., Larmor frequency). These pulses are generally described in terms of 90° or 180° pulses.

Relaxation time: following an RF pulse, the excited hydrogen protons return to their equilibrium (preexcitation) state within the magnetic field. The time interval that is necessary for this process is known as the relaxation time and incorporates two different relaxation methods that occur simultaneously.

T1 (spin-lattice) relaxation time: the time interval required for 63% of the hydrogen protons to reestablish their equilibrium through transfer of energy to the environment (lattice).

T2 (spin-spin) relaxation time: the time interval required for 63% of the hydrogen protons to reestablish their equilibrium by energy transfer between protons precessing at slightly different frequencies.

Repetition time (TR): the time between 90° radiofrequency (RF) pulses (measured in milliseconds).

Signal: the information obtained from a tissue sample is often described in terms of its signal or signal intensity. The signal of a given tissue is a function of the hydrogen proton characteristics and type of pulse sequence chosen. Low signal tissues are hypointense and high signal tissues are hyperintense.

Signal-to-noise ratio (SNR): the amount of usable signal received compared with the noise present within the system at a given voltage. Generally, increased signal-to-noise ratios are achieved with higher-strength magnets and through the use of surface coils. The higher the signal-to-noise ratio, the greater the overall image resolution.

Signal void: the lack of signal originating from a structure or component of a structure. This has a black appearance on MR images.

Spin-echo sequences:

T1-weighted: this pulse sequence uses short TR and short TE parameters to produce a pulse sequence that emphasizes T1 relaxation effects and provides superior anatomic detail. This imaging technique produces essentially a *fat image* in which structures containing fat (i.e., bone marrow, subcutaneous fat) appear bright and structures containing water (i.e., edema, neoplasm, inflammation, CSF, sclerosis, large amounts of iron) appear dark. The substances that appear bright on the T1-weighted image shorten the T1 relaxation effects, while those that appear dark on T1-weighted images lengthen the T1 relaxation effects.

T2-weighted first echo: this is also known as a proton density–weighted image.

T2-weighted second echo: this pulse sequence utilizes long TR and long TE parameters creating a *water image.* When this imaging sequence is utilized, substances that contain predominantly free or loosely bound water molecules (i.e., neoplasms, edema, inflammation, healthy nucleus pulposus, CSF) appear bright, while substances with tightly bound water (i.e., ligaments, menisci, tendons, calcification, sclerosis) or large amounts of iron appear dark (hypointense). The hyperintensity of the CSF relative to the spinal cord and nerve roots is known as the *myelographic effect.* Fat is also relatively hyperintense on T2-weighted sequences, but is not as bright as water.

Surface coils: small coils designed to image a small region of interest (field of view). A smaller field of view provides greater contrast resolution. There is an inverse relationship between the coil diameter and the signal-to-noise ratio. (12) Numerous types of surface coils exist, varying with the size and shape of the body part to be imaged and the manufacturer.

T2* relaxation time: the time interval necessary for free induction decay to occur. This results from protons within the tissue sample precessing incoherently because of magnetic field inhomogeneity. (11)

Three-dimensional (3-D) images: these images are obtained from a volume of data acquired through a specific anatomic area and can be manipulated (reformatted) into any imaging plane. Coupled with this technique's ability to produce contiguous thin slices (1 mm or less), 3-D MR images are ideal for imaging small structures of the knee, wrist, and ankle.

TECHNICAL CONSIDERATIONS
EQUIPMENT

The largest and most costly component of the MRI system is the magnet. Three types of magnets exist: resistive (electromagnetic), permanent, and superconductive. The most frequently employed system today utilizes superconducting magnets. These magnets are comprised of metallic alloys that are maintained at a temperature near absolute zero through the use of liquid cryogens (helium and nitrogen). (11) This process is known as *supercooling* and the supercooled electromagnets are known as *superconducting* magnets.

Magnetic strength is measured in tesla (T) or gauss (one tesla equals 10,000 gauss). The magnetic strength of a 1.5 T (15,000 gauss) magnet is approximately 25,000 times greater than the earth's magnetic pull. (13) Five general categories of magnetic field strength are commercially available. The ultra high-field systems operate at greater than 2 tesla. High-field systems range from 1.5 to 2 tesla; medium-field magnets range from 0.5 to 1 tesla; low-field magnets operate between 0.1 and 0.5 tesla; and ultralow-field magnets are generally below 0.1 tesla. Mobile MRI scanners use trucks to transport their systems to rural communities and are limited in the size of the magnet they can contain. Most trucks can only accommodate magnet sizes up to 0.5 T.

The larger the strength of the magnet, the greater the signal-to-noise capabilities. When MR imaging was in its infancy, this translated into a better image. Currently, with updated software and the advent of surface and quadrature coils, some less powerful magnets are capable of producing excellent image quality. In fact, many 0.5 T systems with newer software packages that optimize the available signal-to-noise ratio yield better images than 1.5 T systems with outdated (inefficient) software.

The magnet is housed in the gantry. (Fig. 6.2) Patients are placed on the couch and moved longitudinally in and out of the magnet for spinal exams. Once inside the magnet, the couch (and patient) are stationary during the entire exam. When surface coils are employed, the patient usually remains outside the gantry.

IMAGE GENERATION
PRINCIPLES OF SIGNAL PRODUCTION

The MR image is the end product of an extremely complex process that revolves around the interaction of hydrogen protons with an external magnetic field. A brief overview of this process is provided in the following paragraphs. An in-depth discussion of the physics behind MRI is beyond the scope of this text.

The abundance and paramagnetic properties of the hydrogen proton make it the ideal substance for magnetic resonance imaging of living tissue. Only those atomic nuclei with odd numbers of protons or neutrons have the potential to be manipulated (imaged) with MRI. The solitary proton in the hydrogen nucleus causes this atom to have an intrinsic charge. Combined with the inherent spinning movement (*angular momentum*) of the atom, this charge provides the paramagnetic properties necessary for MR imaging. Charge and spin cause the hydrogen proton to behave as a magnetic dipole, with positively (north) and negatively (south) charged poles.

Normally, protons in the human body are in random orientation. When an external magnetic field is applied, the protons align themselves in either a parallel or antiparallel orientation relative to the magnetic field. This produces a very small net magnetization because a slight majority of the protons align with the applied magnetic field (parallel orientation). These protons, however, are not arranged in a static orientation, but are in constant motion. Each proton spins along its vertical axis. As it is spinning, it also wobbles slightly around the axis of the external magnetic field. (Fig. 6.3) This motion is analogous to a gyroscope or spinning top in relation to the earth's axis of rotation and is known

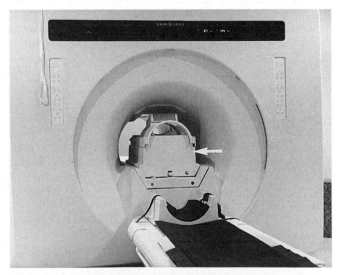

Figure 6.2.   GANTRY OF A MAGNETIC RESONANCE SCANNER. This device resembles a CT gantry, but is much longer. The bore (center) of the gantry is usually smaller than that of a CT scanner. Note the device within the center of the gantry (arrow), which is used to image the head and neck. The couch is similar to a CT scanner couch in that it moves longitudinally into and out of the center of the gantry. The couch and patient, however, are stationary during the entire examination.

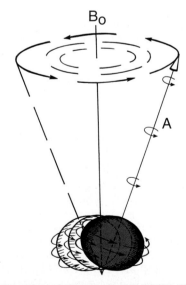

Figure 6.3.   PRECESSION: SCHEMATIC DIAGRAM. This illustration depicts the dynamic nature of a proton under the influence of an external magnetic field. The orientation of the external magnetic field (B_0) is noted. The proton continually spins about its axis (A) as it wobbles, or precesses, around the axis of the magnetic field (B_0). This creates a magnetic moment that parallels the orientation of the proton's axis. COMMENT: This motion is analogous to the spinning of a top relative to the earth's constant rotation.

as *precession*. Precession is very specific for each atomic species in a given magnetic field and occurs at a frequency known as the Larmor frequency. It results from the inherent electromagnetic characteristics of the examined proton sample and the strength of the magnetic field.

The magnetic field of an MR scanner is generally oriented longitudinally with respect to the position the patient will assume (i.e., the patient will lie in the north-south axis of the field). When

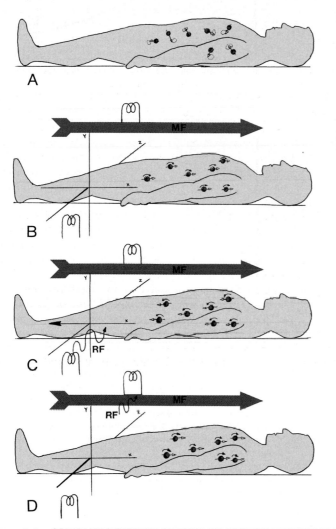

a patient is placed in the magnetic field, the spinning hydrogen protons in the patient's tissue will align their magnetic axes in either a parallel (*north* magnetic pole of proton toward *north* magnetic pole of scanner) or antiparallel (*north* of proton toward *south* of scanner) orientation. Slightly more protons will assume the parallel state, since this is a lower energy state. As the protons orient themselves about this longitudinal axis, they simultaneously spin about their own magnetic axis while precessing about the longitudinal axis of the magnetic field. When a pulse of radiofrequency energy (*RF pulse*) that matches the Larmor frequency of the protons is applied at a 90° angle to the magnetic field, the hydrogen protons *resonate* and absorb the energy of the RF pulse. This causes the protons to become misaligned relative to the magnetic field of the scanner. By carefully controlling the RF pulse, the proton orientation can be made to assume a specific angle of misalignment, usually 90° or 180°. When the RF signal is turned off, the protons re-align themselves with the longitudinal axis. (Fig. 6.4) Energy is released during this process and is expressed as an RF signal. In a uniform magnetic field, all atoms of a given species will produce a signal of similar frequency. The MR scanner, however, generates a *gradient* magnetic field, which causes the RF signal from the protons to be specifically altered according to their location within the field. (12) This proton-generated RF signal that is slightly different for each area within the scanner, is received and processed by computer to generate the actual MR image.

In spin-echo sequences, the RF pulses are repeated several times. First, a 90° pulse is applied, followed by a 180° pulse. The same process is then repeated, starting with a new 90° pulse. The interval between the two 90° pulses is called the repetition time (TR). The time between the pulse and the detection of the MR signal is known as the echo time (TE). (Fig. 6.5) It is the manipulation of these two parameters that is responsible for producing the image characteristics.

When the TR and TE are properly selected, the MR image will display contrast related to differences in proton density, T1 and T2 relaxation times. T1 (spin-lattice) and T2 (spin-spin) relaxation occur simultaneously, and the contributions of each of these parameters can be customized to offer predominantly T1 relaxation (T1-weighted image) or T2 relaxation (T2-weighted image). If the

Figure 6.4.   SCHEMATIC REPRESENTATION OF PROTON DEFLECTION IN MAGNETIC RESONANCE IMAGING. A. Random Proton Alignment. Without the influence of an external magnetic field, the randomly aligned protons are in constant motion, precessing around their individual axes of rotation. **B. Proton Alignment Under the Influence of a Strong Magnetic Field**. The electromagnet housed within the MRI gantry exerts an external magnetic force causing alignment of the precessing hydrogen protons into parallel and antiparallel positions. A net magnetic moment is created by this alignment. **C. Angular Deflection of the Hydrogen Proton**. When a radiofrequency (*RF*) pulse is generated at the appropriate Larmor frequency, the atoms are excited to a higher energy state by altering their orientation relative to the external magnetic field. The angular deflection varies based on the type of image being produced (e.g., spin-echo, gradient-echo). **D. Proton Reorientation**. When the RF pulse is removed, the coil "listens" for the energy transferred from the realignment of protons to their equilibrium position (parallel or antiparallel). The signal received by the transmitter from the reorientation of the proton is what produces the MR image. COMMENT: The above schematic is a very simplistic explanation of a complicated series of events that are necessary to produce an MR image.

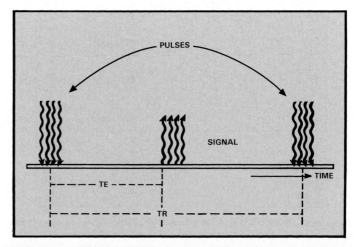

Figure 6.5.   MRI PULSE CYCLE. The diagram illustrates the simplified MRI pulse cycle. The interval between radiofrequency pulses is the repetition time or TR. Note, there is also a radiofrequency signal that echoes from the patient. The time interval from the initial RF pulse to the signal generated from proton realignment is the echo time or TE.

TR and TE are selected so that the effects of both the T1 and T2 relaxation are minimized, the resulting pulse sequence is known as a *proton density-weighted* image.

T1-weighted images utilize short repetition and echo times and provide excellent anatomic information. The resultant image is also known as the *fat image*. Fat is hyperintense (bright) and water (edema, intervertebral discs, CSF) is hypointense (dark) with this pulse sequence. The T2-weighted image (long TR and long TE) is known as the *water image* since tissues containing mobile hydrogen protons (intervertebral discs, CSF and areas of edema) are hyperintense or bright. Proton density-weighted images (long TR and short TE) provide characteristics of both T1-weighted and T2-weighted sequences.

Following the initial 90° excitation pulse, the hydrogen protons rapidly decay from an excited (high-energy) state to equilibrium (low-energy state). This process is known as free induction decay (FID) and occurs in a sinusoidal fashion. (Fig. 6.6) The time necessary for this process is the T2* relaxation time and is a function of the inhomogeneous magnetic field effect on the hydrogen protons in a given tissue sample. (11,14)

The effectiveness of a given MR examination is highly dependent on the imaging parameters selected. (Fig. 6.7) This is a complex decision, and knowledge of MR physics is necessary to choose the appropriate pulse sequences. Most imaging protocols for common disorders of the musculoskeletal system have been well documented in the radiologic literature. However, readers are encouraged to discuss the established protocols used by a particular facility prior to patient referral.

Numerous fast spin-echo and gradient-echo sequences have been developed. The acronyms used to describe these techniques are numerous, and an individual discussion of each one is beyond the scope of this text. Essentially, these techniques acquire imaging information with a reduced scan time. Three-dimensional (3-D) volume acquisitions are useful in providing a thin-section evaluation of an anatomic area. This is particularly valuable when assessing minute structures in areas such as the knee, ankle, and wrist. Compared with conventional 2-D image acquisitions, which typically employ a 3 to 5 mm slice thickness, 3-D acquisitions are capable of producing a slice thickness as small as 1 mm or less.

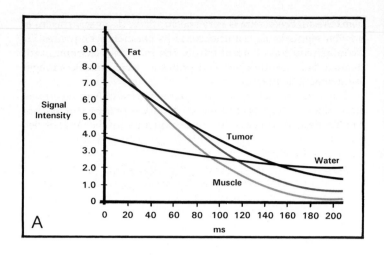

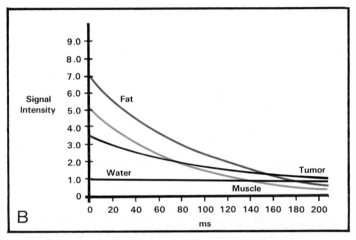

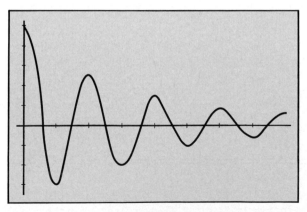

Figure 6.6. FREE INDUCTION DECAY. This schematic diagram depicts the proton decay following a 90° RF pulse. The high energy proton oscillates in a sinosoidal fashion and decreases in amplitude with time. This loss of energy (signal) occurs as the high energy protons interact with incoherently spinning protons produced by the inhomogeneous magnetic field. COMMENT: The rate at which free induction decay occurs is designated the T2* relaxation time.

Figure 6.7. MRI CONTRAST FORMATION. These two diagrams illustrate the impact of TR (time of repetition) and TE (time of echo) on tissue contrast. **A.** Note the difference in tissue contrast as a function of this 2000 ms TR. There are marked contrast differences between tumor, muscle, and fat near the TE of 100 ms. The combination of long TR and TE defines a T2-weighted image. This "weighting" emphasizes the relaxation characteristics between tumor and its surrounding tissues. **B.** Note the maximum difference in signal intensity as a function of this 500 ms TR. The shorter TE of 20 ms provides large differences in the signal intensity of tissues such as water and tumor. COMMENT: Both T1 and T2 relaxation occur simultaneously and are necessary for the complete evaluation of tumors and other pathology.

KINEMATIC MRI

Multiple MR images can be obtained at various defined points of joint movement and are displayed in rapid succession to produce a kinematic display that simulates joint motion. (14) These slices can be added to a video loop and displayed in *real time*. These techniques are particularly useful in the cervical spine, knee, wrist, shoulder, and temporomandibular joint.

PARAMAGNETIC AND FERROMAGNETIC SUBSTANCES

It is important to note that a large number of substances are influenced to a variable degree by the magnetic field. The degree to which substances are affected is based on the composition and location of the material in question as well as the strength of the magnetic field. Paramagnetic substances are weakly attracted toward the strongest region of the magnetic field and appear bright on T1-weighted images. Because of its paramagnetic properties, hydrogen is a fundamental part of MR imaging. Gadolinium is a paramagnetic ion that is often used as part of a contrast-enhancing agent. It is attached to a chelating agent (DTPA–diethylene triamine pentaacetic acid) and is administered intravenously to aid in the detection or further evaluation of numerous pathologic conditions. GD-DTPA is the most frequently used contrast agent for MR imaging. Its uses include the detection of occult central nervous system lesions; the evaluation of the vascularity, dimensions, and tissue characteristics of a known lesion; and the assessment of symptomatic postsurgical disc patients for recurrent disc herniation or scar formation. Unlike the iodinated contrast used with myelographic and CT examinations, this contrast agent has few reported adverse reactions.

Ferromagnetic substances are strongly attracted toward the strongest region of the magnetic field. Most contraindications to MR imaging are related to the ferromagnetic properties of a foreign material. The ferromagnetic properties of a given substance are dependent to a great degree on the magnetic field strength. A list of ferromagnetic materials that are relative contraindications to MR imaging may be found in the following section.

CONTRAINDICATIONS TO MRI

Contraindications to obtaining an MRI examination are based on several factors, and each individual circumstance should be evaluated prior to the denial of such an examination.

Large patients (in excess of 300 pounds) are often too large to fit into the bore of most scanners. Rectangular and open-architecture magnets permit scanning of larger individuals. Claustrophobic patients may find that lying within the small gantry for 30 to 60 minutes can be a very difficult experience. There is an approximate 5% rejection rate because of claustrophobia. Music transmitted through nonferromagnetic headphones, prism glasses, and open-architecture magnets may reduce the effects of claustrophobia. Medications (such as Valium and Xanax) are sometimes used to sedate such individuals and may also be necessary to image infants and small children.

Contraindications to an MRI examination because of the ferromagnetism of a certain device depend upon the magnet strength and the anatomic location of the device. Aneurysm clips (especially those near the circle of Willis), intraocular foreign bodies (commonly seen in welders), subcutaneous metal shards (found in sheet metal workers), and some shrapnel are frequent contraindications to an MRI examination. In addition, cardiac pacemakers or defibrillators, implanted neurostimulators (TENS units), some prosthetic heart valves (especially mitral), cochlear implants or other hearing aids, tattooed eyeliner and certain other makeup, life-support equipment, and early (first trimester) pregnancy are also contraindications. (Fig. 6.8) Most surgical clips, including those from vasectomy, tubal ligation, vagotomy, lymph node resection, splenectomy, cholecystectomy, and sympathectomy, are not ferromagnetic and do not prevent MR examination. Individual patient rejection criteria have been established by each MRI facility and should be stringently enforced.

Joint prostheses, Harrington rods, and most other orthopedic appliances are not contraindications for an MRI. With MRI, these

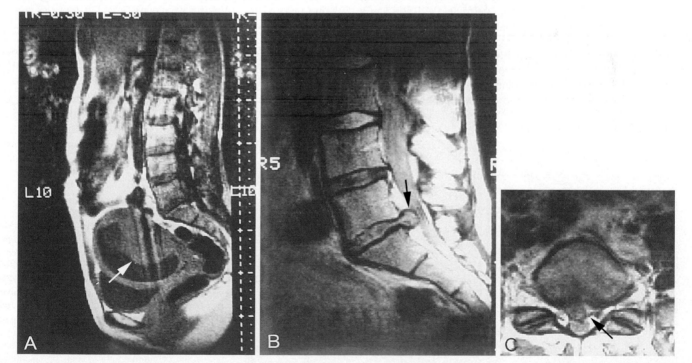

Figure 6.8. HERNIATED NUCLEUS PULPOSUS: PREGNANCY. This 31-year-old gravid female presented with severe low back pain, intractable sciatica with leg atrophy and loss of the Achilles reflex. This patient failed chiropractic treatment, and an MRI was performed in the fourteenth week of pregnancy. **A. MRI, T1-Weighted Sagittal Lumbar.** Observe the fetus in utero (arrow). The vertical striping through the gravid uterus is an artifact. **B. MRI, T2-Weighted Sagittal Lumbar. C. MRI, T2-Weighted Axial Lumbar.** Observe the large right paracentral disc herniation and posterior compres-sion of the thecal sac (arrow). The patient underwent a successful discectomy during her fourth month of pregnancy. The child was born healthy and eight years after birth showed normal development. COMMENT: MRI during pregnancy is indicated only if alternative diagnostic modalities are inadequate or potentially harmful by virtue of ionizing radiation and the host's life is threatened! It is recommended that pregnant patients provide written informed consent prior to examination. (Courtesy of Marsha J. Carry, MS, DC, Manhattan Beach, California)

devices produce a tolerable signal void rather than the offending metallic artifact produced with computed tomography.

MEDICOLEGAL IMPLICATIONS
Magnetic Resonance Imaging

- All ferromagnetic devices and metallic objects must be removed from the patient prior to examination since they may become projectile hazards.

- MRI is contraindicated in patients with any of the following electronic and/or metallic implants: cardiac pacemakers, aneurysm clips, intraocular metal fragments, cochlear implants, and implanted drug infusion devices. Some other vascular implants and devices such as prosthetic heart valves and penile implants may contraindicate the use of MRI. Patients should be assessed on an individual basis since the ferromagnetic properties of the implanted device and the strength of the magnetic field determine which materials should not be in or around the scanner.

- The only direct indication to perform an MRI scan during pregnancy is if the host's life is at risk.

THE SPINE

INDICATIONS FOR MRI

The current list of indications for magnetic resonance imaging (MRI) of the spine is long and continues to expand. Magnetic resonance technology provides contrast and spatial resolution superior to computed tomography (CT) and allows optimal visualization of the spinal cord, intervertebral discs, paravertebral musculature, ligaments, and vertebral marrow. The multiplanar capability of MR, provided by standard spin-echo and three-dimensional volume techniques, produces incomparable image quality over the axial and reformatted images of computed tomography. In addition, MRI is noninvasive and delivers no ionizing radiation to the patient.

MRI has replaced CT as the *gold standard* in the evaluation of cervical, thoracic, and lumbar disc disease. No other imaging modality defines the anatomic relationship of the intervertebral disc and the contents of the spinal canal as accurately as MRI. MRI is frequently employed in the evaluation of patients who have sustained trauma to the vertebral column or spinal cord. In particular, unparalleled evaluation of cord injury can be achieved with MRI, clearly depicting the exact location and extent of cord involvement. Other indications for MRI of the spine are congenital disorders, such as Arnold-Chiari malformation and syrinx. Evidence of early tumor infiltration of bone marrow may be observed with MRI much sooner than with CT or even bone scan. Additionally, the late stages of metastasis and many primary bone neoplasms of the spine (benign and malignant) are better evaluated with MRI. Enhancement of cord tumor neovascularity with gadolinium further increases the rate of accurate, early detection. MRI, coupled with intravenous contrast, is also beneficial in the assessment of failed back syndrome, allowing differentiation of recurrent disc herniation from postsurgical epidural scar formation.

IMAGING PROTOCOLS FOR THE SPINE
MRI Techniques for Spinal Imaging

Generally, most MRI facilities have established specific protocols for routine spinal examinations. MRI has the capability of being tailored to optimally image pathologic processes as they relate to specific spinal tissues. All spine sequences should be performed using a surface coil to reduce the field of view. *Phased array* surface coils with a 48-cm field of view allow long segments (multiple regions) of the spine to be imaged simultaneously. (1,2)

Standard spin-echo (T1- and T2-weighted) sagittal images are often employed in the cervical region. (Fig. 6.9) In addition, gra-

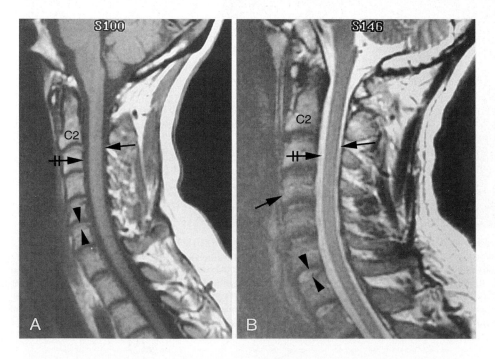

Figure 6.9. NORMAL MRI: CERVICAL SPINE, SPIN-ECHO SEQUENCES. A. MRI, T1-Weighted Sagittal. Note the high signal originating from the vertebral bodies and spinal cord (arrow) secondary to their fatty composition. The intervertebral discs are of intermediate signal intensity (arrowheads), and the cerebrospinal fluid (CSF) (arrows) is hypointense. **B. MRI, T2-Weighted Sagittal.** Note the relatively hypointense signal of the vertebral bodies and spinal cord (arrows). The intervertebral discs (arrowheads) are of intermediate to high signal intensity, and the CSF is very hyperintense (crossed arrow).

dient-echo axial and sagittal pulse sequences are frequently used. The T2-weighted second echo (long TR/long TE) sequences are susceptible to flow artifact, but provide a more accurate representation of tissue characteristics than gradient-echo images. The gradient-echo sequences employ short TR/short TE factors and flip angles of 10 to 30° to provide a *myelographic* appearance of the thecal sac and spinal cord with shorter scan times. (Fig. 6.10) This pulse sequence, however, is susceptible to overestimating the dimensions of the osseous structures and does not optimally display subtle marrow changes.

Standard cervical spine imaging sequences employ 3 to 5 mm

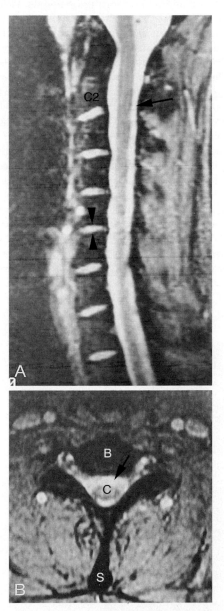

Figure 6.10. NORMAL MRI: CERVICAL SPINE, GRADIENT-ECHO SE-QUENCES. A. MRI, Gradient-Echo Sagittal. B. MRI, Gradient-Echo Axial. The marrow-containing structures are low in signal intensity. The cerebrospinal fluid (arrows) and intervertebral discs (arrowheads) are very hyperintense because of their water content. *C*, spinal cord; *B*, vertebral body; *S*, spinous process. COMMENT: The hyperintense signal of the CSF contrasts the intermediate signal intensity of the spinal cord creating the *myelographic effect.* This soft tissue contrast enables disc lesions and other extradural pathology to be accurately defined.

slice thickness. 3-D gradient-echo volume acquisitions may be used to provide thin-section and image reorientation capability (helpful in evaluating the obliquely oriented intervertebral foramina).

MRI protocols for the thoracic region typically involve the use of T1- and T2-weighted sagittal images. (Fig. 6.11) Axial slices increase the sensitivity for visualizing disc lesions.

Commonly employed pulse sequences used in MR imaging of the lumbar spine include T1- and T2-weighted and gradient-echo sagittal images. (Fig. 6.12) Parasagittal images are useful in demonstrating abnormalities of the exiting nerve roots, relative to the lateral recess and intervertebral foramen. (Fig. 6.13) Axial T1- and/or T2-weighted second echo images are also routinely performed to improve spatial localization. (Fig. 6.14) Fast spin-echo techniques may be employed to reduce the overall scan time. This technique sacrifices imaging of the marrow fat within the vertebral bodies; however, the *myelographic effect* of the spinal cord and thecal sac is enhanced.

Artifacts and Antiartifact Techniques

The quality of a given MR image of the spine can be degraded because of motion artifact originating from CSF pulsations, swallowing, peristalsis, and cardiac and respiratory motions. Therefore it is necessary to add antiartifact techniques to MR imaging protocols. When the thoracic spine is examined, for example, the use of presaturation pulses within the field of view suppress ar-

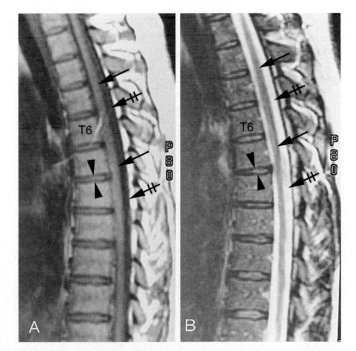

Figure 6.11. NORMAL MRI: THORACIC SPINE. A. MRI, T1-Weighted Sagittal. The intermediate to hyperintense signal of the vertebral bodies and spinal cord (arrows) occurs because of their fat content. The intervertebral discs (arrowheads) are of slightly lower signal intensity, while the cerebrospinal fluid (crossed arrows) is hypointense. The linear, high signal intensity area extending through the spinal cord and posterior vertebral margin of the T6 vertebral body is artifactual in nature. **B. MRI, T2-Weighted Sagittal.** The intervertebral discs (arrowheads) are relatively hyperintense compared to the low signal intensity vertebral bodies. The spinal cord (arrows) is intermediate in signal intensity, while the surrounding CSF (crossed arrows) is very hyperintense.

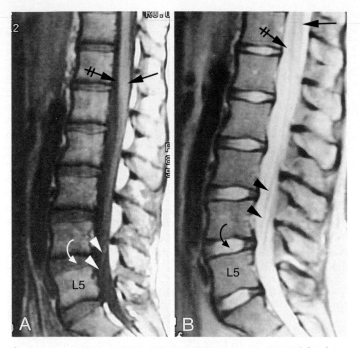

Figure 6.12.   NORMAL MRI: LUMBAR SPINE. A. MRI, T1-Weighted Sagittal. B. MRI, T2-Weighted Sagittal. The conus medullaris (arrow) is seen on the T1-weighted image as a hyperintense structure and becomes lower in signal with T2-weighting. Similar signal changes are seen in the traversing nerve roots of the cauda equina (arrowheads). The CSF (crossed arrows) is dark or hypointense on T1-weighted images and is very hyperintense with T2-weighting. Well-hydrated intervertebral discs (curved arrows) are of intermediate to low signal intensity on T1-weighted images and become hyperintense with T2-weighting. Fatty marrow is high in signal on T1-weighted images and is of intermediate to low signal intensity with T2-weighting.

tifacts originating from the heart, diaphragm, and abdominal structures. (3) Identical saturation techniques can be employed to minimize or eliminate the signal from flowing blood in major vessels adjacent to the spine. Pulsation artifacts produced by cerebral spinal fluid (CSF) can also affect the image quality. To diminish the effects CSF pulsations have on the overall image quality, cardiac gating or gradient moment nulling techniques should be used. (4,5,6)

Limited MRI Scan: A New Concept

MRI provides a unique means for evaluation of injury to the vertebral column and its supporting ligaments. Often, evidence of bone contusion, fracture, or ligamentous injury is not appreciated on the plain film examination. An abbreviated MR scan tailored to image subtle areas of edema may be helpful in assessing acute trauma that may otherwise be dismissed as insignificant. Two clinical circumstances where this would be particularly valuable are in the evaluation of a patient who has sustained significant hyperflexion/extension spinal trauma (whiplash) and in the differentiation between an old or new vertebral compression deformity (fracture). (Fig. 6.15)

MRI is clearly the modality of choice in evaluating injury to the soft tissues and in demonstrating bone marrow edema. However, it is neither practical nor cost-effective to assess each patient suspected of having subtle osteoligamentous injury with a *complete* MRI scan. The authors recommend the use of an *abbreviated* scan designed to demonstrate subtle areas of edema (in bone and soft tissue). A limited MRI scan using only sagittal T2-weighted images with or without fat-suppression techniques would accomplish this task and could be made available to a select patient population at a reduced fee.

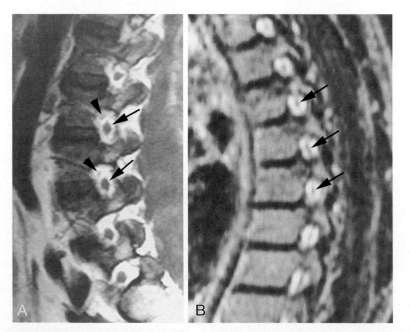

Figure 6.13.   NORMAL MRI: PARASAGITTAL IMAGES. A. MRI, T1-Weighted Far Lateral Lumbar. Note the low signal intensity dorsal root ganglia (arrows) and radicular veins (arrowheads). The surrounding hyperintense fat provides the contrast necessary to delineate these structures and assess intraforaminal pathology. **B. MRI, T1-Weighted Far Lateral Thoracic.** The dorsal root ganglia (arrows) are seen as low signal intensity structures within the hyperintense intraforaminal fat.

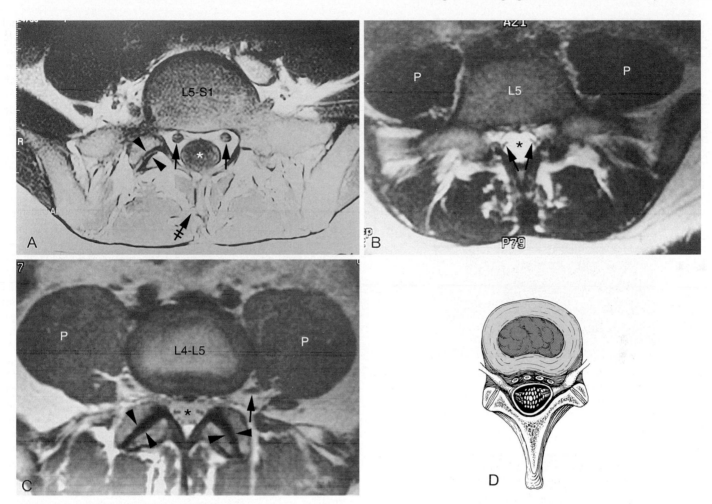

Figure 6.14. NORMAL MRI: LUMBAR SPINE. Axial slices at varying levels using different pulse sequences are demonstrated. **A. MRI, T1-Weighted Axial, L5-S1 Level.** The S1 nerve root sheaths (arrows) contain CSF and therefore parallel the signal changes of the CSF within the thecal sac (*). The right L5-S1 facet joint is also noted (arrowheads). The spinous process (crossed arrow) is seen dorsally. **B. MRI, T2-Weighted Axial.** The CSF (*) is very hyperintense and provides the necessary contrast to visualize the rootlets of the cauda equina (arrows). The psoas muscles (P) are seen lateral to the vertebral body. **C. MRI, Proton Density-Weighted Axial.** The CSF (*) is intermediate in signal and contrasts the low signal intensity of the cauda equina. The extraforaminal portion of the left L4 nerve root is observed (arrow). The psoas muscles (P) and facet joints (arrowheads) are also well visualized on this image. **D. Schematic Diagram: L4-L5 Level.**

CONGENITAL DISORDERS

Tethered Cord Syndrome

The conus medullaris usually reaches the normal adult level of L1-L2 by approximately 2 months of age. In general, after 12 years of age the tip of the conus should not extend below the L2 level. (7) The tethered cord is defined as an abnormally low position of the conus tip, below the level of the L2 vertebral body in adults. Lipomas and thickening of the filum terminale may be seen in conjunction with a tethered cord. (8) (Fig. 6.16) These focal collections of fat and connective tissue must be differentiated from epidural lipomatosis. Epidural lipomatosis may be seen in obese individuals, but is most frequently seen in those patients receiving exogenous corticosteroids. (9) (Fig. 6.17)

The clinical symptoms in tethered cord syndrome are thought to be related to mechanical factors and chronic repetitive cord ischemia. (10) Often, a mass or dural adhesions may be implicated as the cause of the restricted cord ascent. This results in stretching of the distal cord and subsequent ischemia. The onset of symptoms usually occurs between the ages of 3 and 35. Most patients experience symptoms for the first time during the adolescent growth spurt (11), supporting the hypothesis that the onset of symptoms is related to the development of the lumbar lordosis and stretching of the distal cord. The most common complaint is gait difficulty, ranging from a sensation of leg stiffness to true weakness with hyperreflexia. Frequent findings include bladder dysfunction, sensory abnormalities, back pain, focal hypertrichosis, and congenital foot deformities. Occult tethered cord syndrome presents a diagnostic challenge since symptoms appear much later in life.

MRI Findings. T1-weighted axial images are the best means to evaluate the tethered cord syndrome. (12,13) Axial imaging allows for differentiation of the centrally positioned conus and filum terminale from the laterally arrayed nerve roots of the cauda equina. The sagittal images assist in locating the cauda equina and the tip of the conus medullaris. Lipomas are frequently seen in the caudal aspect of the thecal sac, attached to the

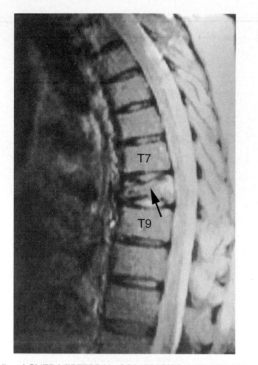

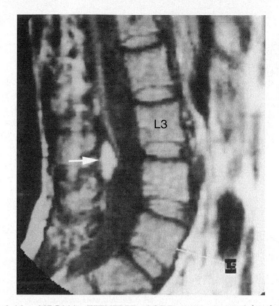

Figure 6.15.   ACUTE VERTEBRAL COMPRESSION FRACTURE. MRI, T2-Weighted Sagittal Thoracic. Note the biconcave deformity of the T8 vertebral endplates. The increased marrow signal intensity adjacent to the T8 superior endplate (arrow) represents edema. These changes are consistent with an acute injury.

Figure 6.16.   LIPOMA: TETHERED CORD. MRI, T1-Weighted Sagittal Lumbar. Notice the high signal intensity mass (arrow) with ventral deflection of a low terminating conus medullaris. These findings indicate a lipoma with an associated tethered cord. COMMENT: The conus medullaris normally terminates at the L1-L2 level. (Courtesy of Kenneth B. Reynard, MD, Denver, Colorado)

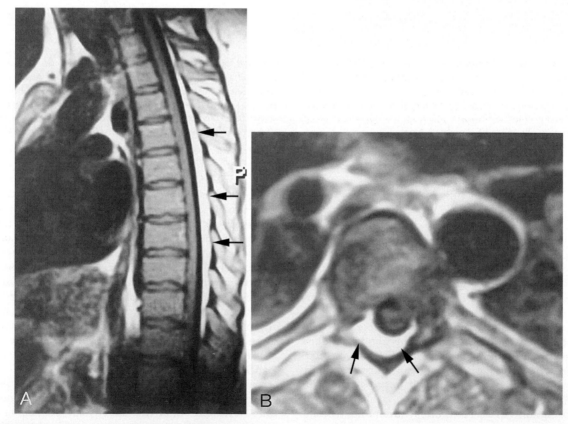

Figure 6.17.   EPIDURAL LIPOMATOSIS: THORACIC SPINE. A. MRI, T1-Weighted Sagittal Thoracic. B. MRI, T1-Weighted Axial Thoracic. There is an increased amount of high signal intensity fat within the posterior epidural space. Note the anterolateral displacement of the spinal cord and thecal sac.

COMMENT: Epidural lipomatosis is usually idiopathic or the sequelae of prolonged corticosteroid use causing redistribution of fat reserves. (Courtesy of William P. Yapp, DC, Green Cove Springs, Florida)

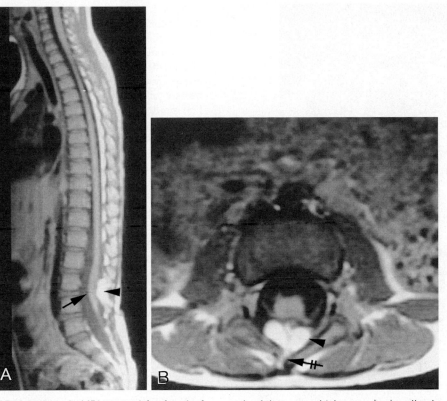

Figure 6.18.   TETHERED CORD: LIPOMA. A. MRI, T1-Weighted Sagittal Lumbar. B. MRI, T1-Weighted Axial Lumbar. Observe the low-lying position (L4) of the enlarged conus medullaris (arrow) in an ectatic thecal sac. The region of high signal intensity posterior to the conus (arrowhead) is an ex-tradural lipoma, which extends dorsally through a neural arch defect (crossed arrow). COMMENT: The conus medullaris is normally located at the L1-L2 level.

filum. (Fig. 6.18) These fatty collections are best seen on T1-weighted axial and sagittal images. The key advantage of MR over myelography and CT myelography in the evaluation of teth-ered cord syndrome is its noninvasive nature and multiplanar capabilities, as well as its ability to positively identify the cause of the cord tethering in most cases.

Diastematomyelia

Diastematomyelia is a sagittal separation of the spinal cord into two hemicords. (Fig. 6.19) These hemicords are frequently separated by a fibrous or osseous bar that may progressively stretch the cord as the patient grows, producing neurologic symp-toms in adolescent and adult patients. Sagittal MR images are better than CT at demonstrating congenital anomalies of the cord (e.g., tethered cord, lipoma, Arnold-Chiari malformation, syrinx, cyst).

Scoliosis

The majority of scolioses are idiopathic in nature, and respond favorably to conservative management. However, intraspinal ab-normalities occur in approximately 5 to 20% of the scolioses seen in children, providing an organic cause for the scoliosis and/or its progression. (14,15) These intraspinal abnormalities include Arnold-Chiari malformation, hemivertebra (structural scoliosis), hydrocephalus, syringomyelia and hydromyelia, spinal cord tu-mor, myelomeningocele, tethered cord syndrome, and diaste-matomyelia. (16)

Scolioses may be asymptomatic or may result in symptoms ranging from mild back pain to severe back pain with loss of bladder function and lower extremity neurologic deficit. A com-prehensive discussion on imaging and treatment of scoliosis is beyond the scope of this chapter, but a brief description of the features and clinical importance of *left-sided* scoliosis is provided.

Most idiopathic spinal curvatures are convex to the right. The finding of a *left-sided* scoliosis is worrisome and must be further evaluated, particularly if the curve is large or if rapid progression is observed. (Fig. 6.20) Coonrad (17) reported that of 550 consec-utive scoliosis patients 1.6% (27 patients) had left curves of the thoracic or lumbar regions. Nine of those 27 patients had evidence of neurologic dysfunction. Of those, two patients had occult sy-ringomyelia. Another recent study evaluated 18 patients with left thoracic or thoracolumbar scoliosis. Eight of these patients had abnormal MRI findings, and six exhibited nonneoplastic syrinx formation. (18) Yochum et al. (19) reported two challenging cases that exemplify the vast contrast that may be observed in different patients with the same underlying abnormality. Both patients had a progressive left scoliosis secondary to syrinx formation. One case demonstrated neurologic deterioration, and the other was asymptomatic except for the progressive left curve and minimal back pain.

MRI is helpful in detecting syrinx formation and surgical plan-ning, as well as in postsurgical follow-up. Longitudinal evalua-tion of the spinal cord and base of the skull with MRI is critical in the assessment of a rapidly progressing scoliosis (whether it be *left-* or *right-sided*) in a child or adolescent patient. Even when a *left-sided* scoliosis is asymptomatic, MR evaluation should be considered. Certainly, MRI is indicated for all individuals pre-

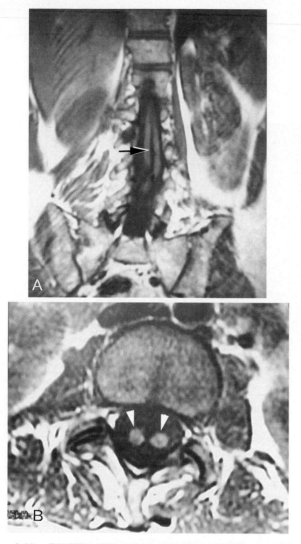

Figure 6.19. DIASTEMATOMYELIA: LUMBAR SPINE. A. MRI, T1-Weighted Coronal Lumbar. B. MRI, T1-Weighted Axial Lumbar. Observe the fibrous or osseous septum extending longitudinally through the tethered spinal cord (arrow). This septum divides the spinal cord into two symmetric hemicords (arrowheads). COMMENT: A fibrous or osseous spur increases cord tension and exacerbates the signs and symptoms of tethering. (Courtesy of Stephen J. Mattaga, DC, Burlington Township, New Jersey)

senting with severe or rapidly progressive scoliosis (especially a *left-sided* curve), or for those with neurologic symptoms. A timely and accurate diagnosis is of utmost importance in preventing permanent cosmetic disfigurement and/or neurologic impairment. Beware of the frequently sinister nature of *left-sided* curves and ensure that a complete evaluation of these patients is performed, including consideration for an MRI scan of the cervical and thoracic regions of the spinal cord. A list of indications for performing an MRI in patients with scoliosis is provided. (Table 6.1)

Arnold-Chiari Malformation

Arnold-Chiari malformation is characterized by a caudal herniation of the cerebellar tonsils through the foramen magnum and is often associated with various other abnormal neurologic and skeletal findings. Four types have been described:

Type I. The type I malformation is defined as a herniation of the cerebellar tonsils greater than 5 mm beyond the most caudal aspect of the foramen magnum. (20,21) (Fig. 6.21) This type of malformation is associated with hydrosyringomyelia (60 to 70% of patients), hydrocephalus (20 to 25% of patients), and segmentation anomalies of the craniovertebral junction (24%), including basilar impression, upper cervical assimilation, and Klippel-Feil syndrome. (22) Chiari I malformations are often clinically asymptomatic (31%), but may present in adulthood with subtle symptoms. Radiographs are important in that they may reveal vertebral anomalies, suggesting an underlying spinal cord abnormality.

Type II. The most commonly occurring Chiari malformation (representing approximately 40% of all Chiari malformations) is the type II variety. (20) This type also involves caudal displacement of the cerebellar tonsils. In addition, deformity of the calvarium and displacement of the fourth ventricle and brain stem are seen. Midline cleft defects in the cervical neural arches and myelomeningocele are often associated with this type of malformation.

Types III and IV. Type III and IV Chiari malformations are rare and exhibit a combination of those findings demonstrated in the type I and type II varieties. All types of Chiari malformations may be associated with syrinx, progressive hydrocephalus, and scoliosis. (20) A more complete discussion of Arnold-Chiari malformation is presented in Chapter 3.

Syrinx

The term *syrinx* encompasses syringomyelia, hydromyelia, and syringohydromyelia and is utilized if the exact location of the cavity within the spinal cord is unknown. Syringomyelia is defined as an eccentrically placed cavity within the parenchyma of the spinal cord. This cavity is lined with altered glial elements and contains cerebral spinal fluid (CSF). These cavities may be unilocular or septated. Pressure on the medial nuclei innervating the trunk musculature has been suggested as a mechanism for

Table 6.1.   Indications for MRI in Scoliosis Patients

Young patient (less than 11 years of age)
Severe or rapidly progressing thoracic/thoracolumbar scoliosis
  (particularly left-sided)
No family history of scoliosis
Unusually rigid scoliosis in a young patient
Scoliosis associated with pain that is unresponsive to conservative
  treatment
Abnormal radiographic findings
  Segmentation defects
  Platybasia
  Basilar impression
  Increased spinal canal diameter
  Posterior vertebral body scalloping
  Pedicle widening
Abnormal neurologic findings
  Muscular weakness and/or atrophy
  Sensory loss (particularly pain and temperature)
  Bladder/bowel dysfunction
  Unexplained/painless swollen joint (Charcot's joint)
  Abnormal superficial abdominal wall reflex
  Abnormal deep tendon reflexes (increased or decreased)
  Cranial nerve abnormality

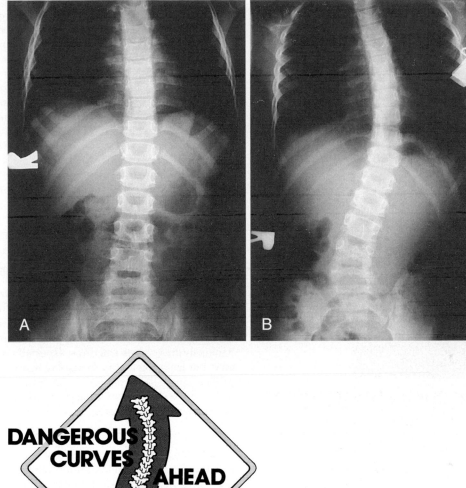

Figure 6.20.   LEFT-SIDED SCOLIOSIS: A WARNING TO BE OBSERVED BY ALL. This 4-year-old girl presented with a 10° scoliosis that progressed to 34° in one year. Note that this is a left-sided scoliosis, the opposite of what is usually expected in classic "idiopathic" scoliosis. **A. AP Thoracic: 10° Left-Sided Scoliosis. B. AP Thoracic 1 Year Later: 34° Left-Sided Scoliosis. C. Schematic Diagram Illustrating the Importance of Recognizing the Sinister Nature of the "Left-Sided" Curve.** COMMENT: Patients presenting with left-sided scolioses (especially when rapidly progressive) should be thoroughly evaluated to exclude an underlying cause for the unusual curvature. The presented case revealed an Arnold-Chiari type I malformation with syrinx. A posterior fossa decompression with installation of a syringoperitoneal shunt was performed, which allowed for decompression of the syrinx. The patient was then placed in a Boston brace, and the scoliosis was reduced to 24°. The curvature has remained stable for three years following surgery. (Reprinted with permission of Yochum TR, Barry MS, Gould SJ, et al: *Wrong Sided Scoliosis: When Left Isn't Right.* JNMS 2:195, 1994)

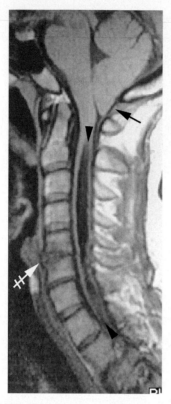

Figure 6.21.   ARNOLD-CHIARI I MALFORMATION: WITH SYRINX. MRI, T1-Weighted Sagittal Cervical. Observe the ectopic cerebellar tonsils projecting caudally to the C1 level (arrow) and the uniformly low signal intensity syrinx that enlarges the entire cervical spinal cord (arrowheads). The borders of the syrinx are well defined. Also note the unrelated changes of degenerative spondylosis at C5-C6 (crossed arrow). COMMENT: MRI is the most sensitive imaging modality to determine the presence of Arnold-Chiari malformations with or without syrinx. It provides a noninvasive means of obtaining this diagnosis.

the association of scoliosis with syrinx formation. (23) In a recent study by Elster and Chen (22) syringomyelia was detected in 40% of patients with Chiari I malformations.

MRI is the definitive imaging modality for detecting a syrinx and is recommended for young adults and adolescents with rapidly progressive scoliosis or for evaluation of any progressive *left-sided* spinal curve. Syringes are best demonstrated on axial and sagittal T1-weighted images, where the low signal intensity CSF creates a *black column* relative to the surrounding high signal intensity spinal cord parenchyma. (Fig. 6.22)

Perineural Sacral (Tarlov's) Cyst

The terminology used in describing these meningeal cyst-like structures is quite confusing. The terms used include *meningeal cyst, perineural sacral (Tarlov's) cyst, spinal nerve root perineural cyst, meningeal diverticula,* or *occult intrasacral meningocele.* (24) These lesions probably represent various forms of congenital diverticula and are distinct from classic meningocele or myelomeningocele and should not be confused with dural ectasia. (Fig. 6.23)

Diverticula of the spinal nerve root sleeves (including Tarlov's cysts and spinal nerve root diverticula) can be quite large and may be multiple. They usually involve the dorsal nerve roots and may occur at any level, although they are most frequently observed in the sacral region. Nerve fibers lie within the cyst wall

or centrally within the cyst, surrounded by CSF. These cysts are usually asymptomatic, even when quite large. Rarely, neurologic symptoms result, requiring surgical excision. (24)

MRI Findings.   Cystic masses in the spinal canal or the neural foramina that exhibit low signal intensity on T1-weighted images and high signal intensity on T2-weighted images (paralleling the CSF signal changes) are consistent with spinal meningeal cysts (Tarlov's cysts). (Fig. 6.24) Bone erosion may occur and is evidenced radiographically by canal widening, pedicle erosion, foraminal enlargement, or scalloping of the posterior vertebral bodies or sacrum. (Fig. 6.25) Parasagittal MR images may demonstrate enlargement of the nerve root sleeve, which must be differentiated from a neural tumor. (Fig. 6.26) It is important to recognize the nature of this lesion to avoid unnecessary biopsy.

TRAUMA

Spinal fractures and their complexities have traditionally been imaged by plain film radiography, bone scan, and computed tomography. These modalities, however, are terribly deficient in their ability to demonstrate damage to the various supporting ligaments (short of complete dislocation) and spinal cord contusion. (Figs. 6.27, 6.28)

Magnetic resonance imaging has revolutionized the evaluation of trauma to the spine. Computed tomography is superior in demonstrating subtle fractures, especially in the posterior neural arch, but lacks the ability to display ligamentous tears, bone contusions, spinal hematomas, and/or spinal cord contusions. (25,26) (Fig. 6.29) MRI is the only imaging modality to assess these traumatic sequelae accurately.

Fractures

Both CT and MRI are capable of evaluating retropulsed fracture fragments and their position relative to the spinal cord and nerve roots. (Fig. 6.30) CT is better at identifying small bone fragments within the spinal canal. When injury to the spinal cord (Fig. 6.31) or nerve root is suspected, however, MRI should also be employed because of its superior spatial and contrast resolution. In the acute and subacute stages, hemorrhage or bone marrow edema within the vertebral body will demonstrate a low signal intensity area within the marrow on T1-weighted images that becomes hyperintense with T2-weighting. (Fig. 6.32) This signal pattern is consistent with bone marrow edema and suggests that the vertebral fracture is recent (less than 6 weeks in duration). A chronic or long-standing fracture does not demonstrate increased signal intensity on any pulse sequence. (27)

Limited MRI Scan: A New Concept

MRI provides a unique imaging modality to differentiate old versus new compression fractures. Plain film radiographs are helpful; however, step defects and radiodense bands of trabecular condensation are unreliable signs of determining the age of a fracture. (Fig. 6.33) Vertebral wedging is found in both old and new fractures, and reinstatement in height of the vertebral body, even in healed fractures, does not occur. The authors suggest that a limited T2-weighted or STIR sagittal scan be performed to assess the compressed vertebra for high signal intensity bone marrow edema. (Fig. 6.34) This examination can be performed in 15 minutes and will unequivocally determine the presence or absence of bone marrow edema in the vertebral body. This limited scan can be performed at a reduced fee, making it more cost-effective than bone scan or CT, while rendering no radiation dose to the patient.

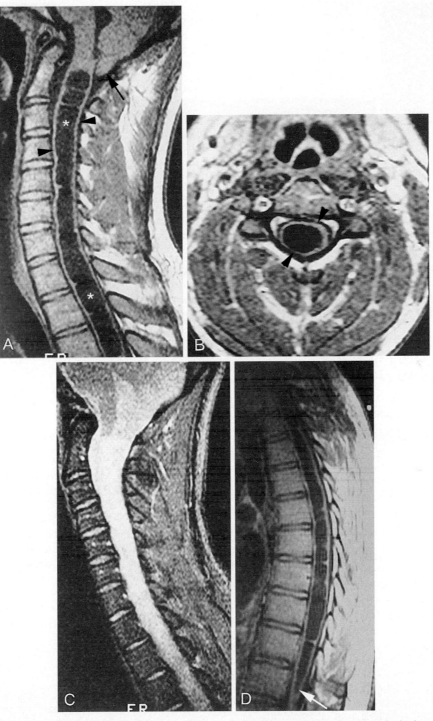

Figure 6.22.   ARNOLD-CHIARI TYPE I MALFORMATION WITH A HOL-OCORD SYRINX. This 25-year-old male patient presented with cervical spine pain in extension. A thorough neurologic examination revealed a uni-lateral decreased pinwheel sensation on the right in a shawl-like distribution. **A. MRI, T1-Weighted Sagittal Cervical. B. MRI, T1-Weighted Axial Cervical**. There is caudal displacement of the cerebellar tonsils several millimeters below the foramen magnum (arrow). Observe the large size of the spinal cord (arrowheads) secondary to the huge central canal (*). Note the low signal intensity of the central canal which contains CSF. The cephalad por-tion of the syrinx extends to the C1-C2 level. **C. MRI, Gradient-Echo Sagittal Cervical.** The low signal intensity cerebrospinal fluid (CSF) becomes hyper-intense on this pulse sequence. The thin margins of the spinal cord are ob-scured by the large amount of CSF within the syrinx. **D. MRI, T1-Weighted Sagittal Thoracic.** The caudal extent of the syrinx terminates in the conus medullaris (arrow). (Courtesy of Mark L. Taylor, DC, Las Vegas, Nevada)

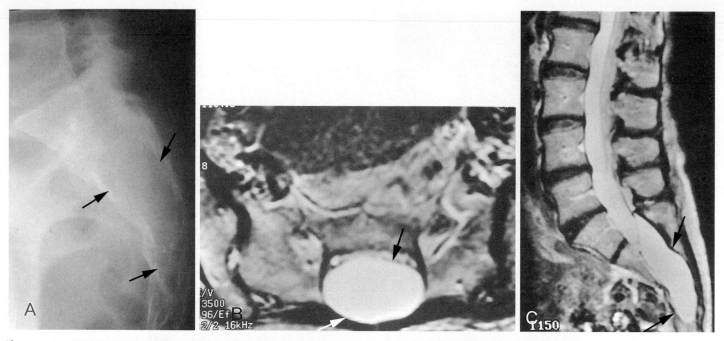

Figure 6.23.   DURAL ECTASIA: IDIOPATHIC. A. Lateral Sacrum. Observe the erosion of the posterior sacral body and neural arch (arrows) resulting in enlargement of the sacral spinal canal. The eroded margins are smooth, suggesting an indolent process. **B. MRI, T2-Weighted Axial Lumbar. C. MRI,**

T2-Weighted Sagittal Lumbar. Note the high signal intensity cerebrospinal fluid (CSF) within the ectatic thecal sac (arrows) and sacral canal enlargement. (Courtesy of Patricia A. Youmans, DC, Colorado Springs, Colorado)

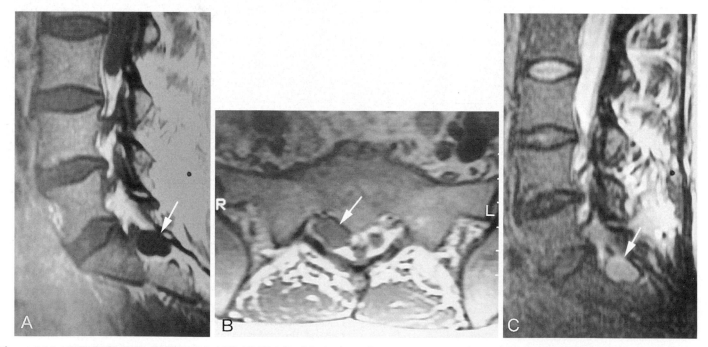

Figure 6.24.   TARLOV'S CYST: SACRUM. A. MRI, T1-Weighted Sagittal Lumbar. B. MRI, T1-Weighted Axial Sacrum. There is a large, well-defined, low signal intensity cyst adjacent to the S1 level (arrow). This cyst occupies the right lateral aspect of the sacral canal and produces minimal erosion of

the posterior margin of S1. **C. MRI, T2-Weighted Sagittal Lumbar.** The sacral cyst (arrow) becomes hyperintense with T2-weighting, paralleling the signal intensity changes of the CSF. COMMENT: Most Tarlov's cysts are asymptomatic and incidental lesions.

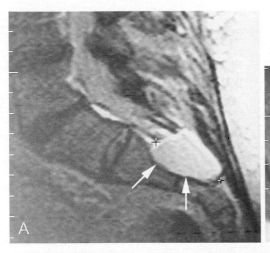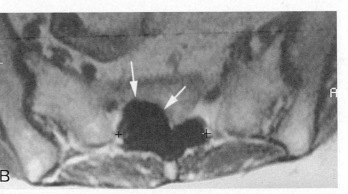

Figure 6.25.   GIANT TARLOV'S CYST. A. MRI, T2-Weighted Sagittal Lumbar. B. MRI, T1-Weighted Axial Lumbar. Note the large, well-defined mass within the neural canal, adjacent to the S1-S2 segment. This mass is hypointense on T1-weighted images and hyperintense with T2-weighting. These changes are consistent with a benign cystic mass containing CSF. Note the pressure erosion of the posterior sacral margin (arrows). (Courtesy of Frank E. Seidelmann, DO; Kingsley A. Orraca-Tetteh, MD; and Matthew M. Brown, RT(R), Advanced MRImaging, Richmond Heights, Ohio)

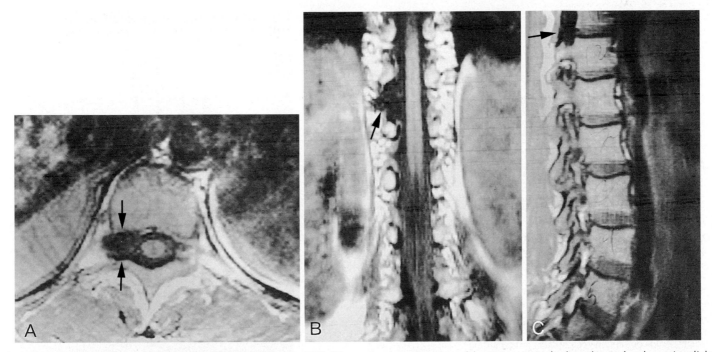

Figure 6.26.   THORACIC NERVE ROOT DIVERTICULUM. A. MRI, T1-Weighted Axial Thoracic. B. MRI, T1-Weighted Coronal Thoracic. C. MRI, T1-Weighted Sagittal Thoracic. Observe the marked low signal intensity of the nerve root diverticulum (arrows), which is isointense with the CSF. There is minimal erosion of the T11 posterior body and neural arch causing slight enlargement of the corresponding intervertebral foramen. COMMENT: Nerve root diverticula are typically asymptomatic and of no clinical concern.

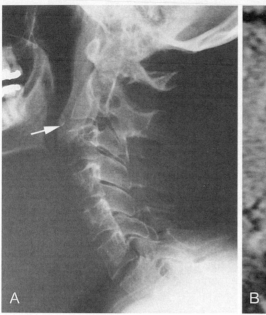

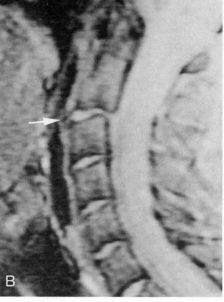

Figure 6.27. EXTENSION TEARDROP FRACTURE OF C2. This 40-year-old male suffered a cervical hypertextension injury. **A. Lateral Cervical.** Note the small fracture fragment (arrow) avulsed from the anteroinferior aspect of the C2 vertebral body. There is also a posterior subluxation of C2 on C3. The focal enlargement of the retropharyngeal tissues is secondary to edema and hemorrhage. **B. MRI, Gradient-Echo Sagittal Cervical.** Observe the interruption and increased signal intensity in the anterior longitudinal ligament (ALL) (arrowhead). The low signal intensity, avulsed fragment (arrow) is seen adjacent to the anteroinferior margin of the C2 vertebral body. (Courtesy of R.E. Marchand, DC, Calgary, Alberta, Canada)

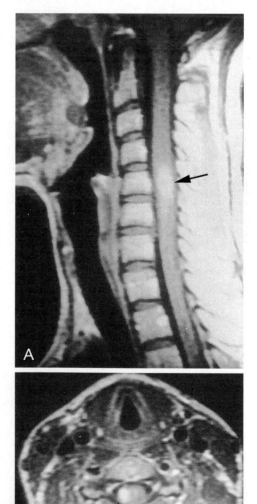

Figure 6.28. SPINAL CORD CONTUSION: CERVICAL SPINE. This young female sustained an injury to her cervical spine, resulting in progressive neurologic deficits in the upper and lower extremities. **A. MRI, T1-Weighted Contrast-Enhanced Sagittal Cervical. B. MRI, T1-Weighted Contrast-Enhanced Axial Cervical.** There is a well-defined region of increased signal intensity involving the right lateral aspect of the spinal cord (arrows) at the C5 level. Note the minimal increase in the sagittal dimensions of the cord at this level. COMMENT: Focally increased signal intensity and expansion of the cord suggest a differential diagnosis that ranges from neoplasm to multiple sclerosis. MRI is the only imaging modality that accurately detects spinal cord contusion.

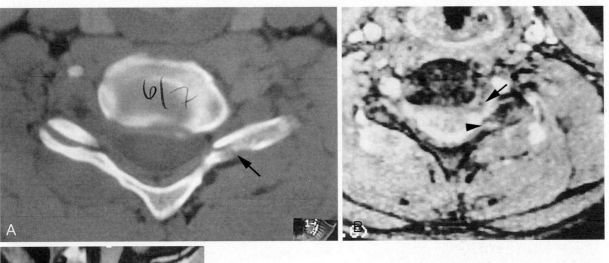

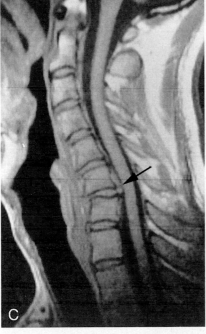

Figure 6.29.   FRACTURE OF THE NEURAL ARCH WITH ASSOCIATED C6-C7 HERNIATED NUCLEUS PULPOSUS (HNP). This patient developed acute neck pain following a motor vehicle accident. **A. CT, Bone Window Axial Cervical.** Note the laminar fracture adjacent to the articular pillar (arrow). **B. MRI, Gradient-Echo Axial Cervical.** Observe the large, left lateral disc herniation (arrow) resulting in foraminal stenosis. This finding is not seen on the CT scan. Note the hyperintense area of edema associated with the acute laminar fracture (arrowhead). **C. MRI, T1-Weighted Sagittal Cervical.** Observe the acute kyphotic angulation and anterior subluxation of C6 on C7 accompanying the large disc herniation (arrow). COMMENT: The CT scan showed no HNP, and the acute nature of the laminar fracture could not be confirmed. The axial MRI demonstrates a lateral HNP plus edema within the laminar fracture site, securing the diagnosis of a recent (less than 6 weeks) injury.

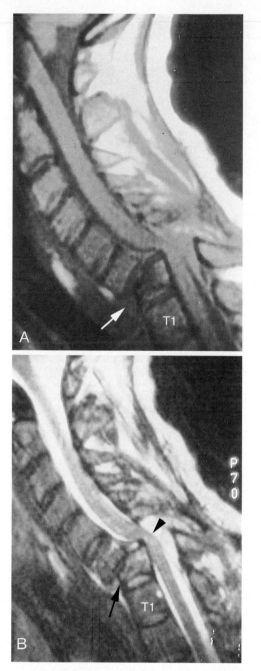

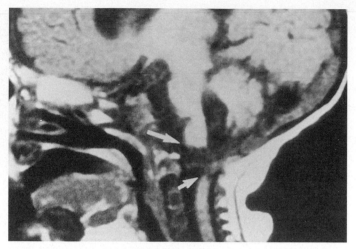

Figure 6.31.   CORD TRANSECTION: CERVICAL CORD. This child was struck by an automobile. **MRI, T1-Weighted Sagittal Cervical.** Observe the sharply delineated interruption of the spinal cord (arrows) indicating complete cord transection from C2 to the foramen magnum. This condition is incompatible with life. COMMENT: MRI may provide the physician with valuable information that limits further invasive investigation.

Figure 6.30.   FRACTURE/DISLOCATION: C6-C7. This patient was involved in a motor vehicle accident that resulted in quadriplegia. **A. MRI, T1-Weighted Sagittal Cervical.** Note the anterior dislocation of C6 on C7. Observe the compression fracture and decreased signal intensity of the C7 vertebral body (arrow) representing bone marrow edema. The dislocation has markedly narrowed the spinal canal. **B. MRI, T2-Weighted Sagittal Cervical.** The subtle, high signal intensity bone marrow edema (arrow) indicates the acute nature of the fracture. The *myelographic effect* of the T2-weighted image better demonstrates the canal narrowing with compression and angulation of the spinal cord (arrowhead). In addition, there is a small, hyperintense area within the spinal cord, representing a contusion. (Courtesy of Steven R. Nokes, MD, Baptist MRI, Little Rock, Arkansas)

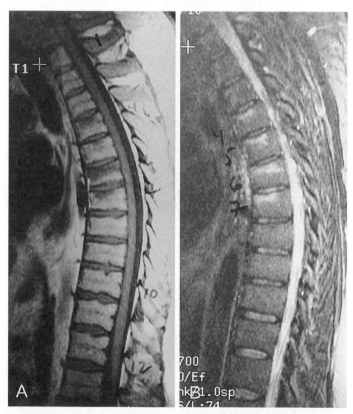

Figure 6.32.   ACUTE COMPRESSION FRACTURE: MULTIPLE LEVELS. A. MRI, T1-Weighted Sagittal Thoracic. B. MRI, T2-Weighted Sagittal Thoracic. Note the ill-defined hypointense signal intensity area within the marrow adjacent to the T4 through T7 superior vertebral endplates on the T1-weighted image. This hypointense signal becomes hyperintense with T2-weighting, consistent with bone marrow edema. Observe the slight anterior wedging of the T6 and T7 vertebral bodies. (Courtesy of Alan M. Lesselroth, MD, Mountain Diagnostics, Las Vegas, Nevada)

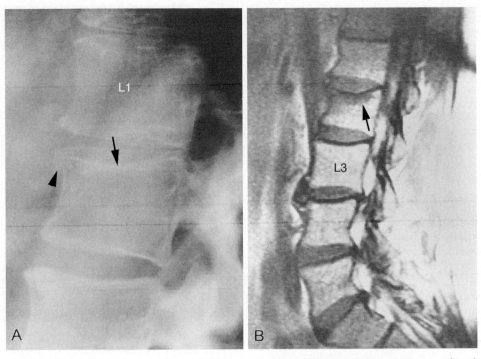

Figure 6.33.   OLD FRACTURE VERSUS NEW? A COMMON PROBLEM. This patient presents with a complicated history of multiple traumas. The clinical challenge is to differentiate an acute or recent injury acute from an old vertebral fracture. **A. Lateral Lumbar.** A mild concave deformity (arrow) and a step defect (arrowhead) of the L2 superior endplate suggest an acute etiology. How can one be certain? **B. MRI, T1-Weighted Sagittal Lumbar.** Observe the compression deformity and associated low signal intensity bone marrow edema (arrow). These findings confirm the acute nature of the compression fracture. Also, note the anterior disc herniation at L3-L4 and posterior bulging of the L5-S1 disc. COMMENT: An abbreviated sagittal MRI scan (15 minutes) is a cost-effective method of defining old versus new compression fractures. The presence of bone marrow edema denotes an injury of 6 weeks or less In duration.

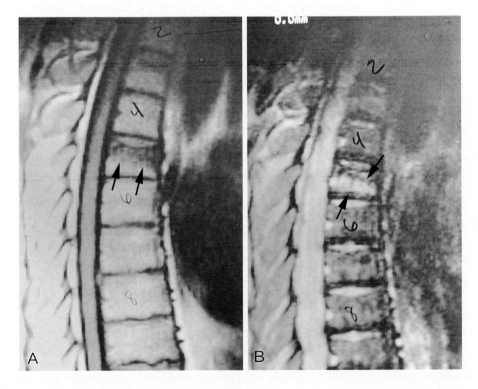

Figure 6.34.   ACUTE VERTEBRAL COMPRESSION FRACTURE: T5. A. MRI, T1-Weighted Sagittal Thoracic. Note the concave deformity of the T5 superior vertebral endplate resulting from a flexion injury of the thorax 3 weeks prior. The low signal intensity within the T5 vertebral body represents bone marrow edema (arrow). **B. MRI, T2-Weighted Sagittal Thoracic.** Observe the hyperintense bone marrow edema within the T5 vertebral body. These findings are consistent with an acute compression fracture. COMMENT: MR is the definitive imaging modality to differentiate recent versus old compression fracture.

Benign Versus Malignant Compression Fracture

Yuh (28) has suggested that MRI may be helpful in the evaluation of benign versus malignant compression fractures. Benign osteoporotic compression fractures render a low signal intensity band that is often parallel with the endplates on T1-weighted images. If the fracture represents a recent injury, this band becomes hyperintense with T2-weighting. Gadolinium scans can help characterize the fracture etiology by enhancing areas of neoplastic replacement. Often however, benign compression fractures cannot be differentiated from malignancy without biopsy.

Posttraumatic Syrinx

A significant complication associated with spinal trauma is the development of a posttraumatic syrinx. This entity should be considered in patients who sustain significant injury to the spine and in the postsurgical patient. (Fig. 6.35) The pathogenesis of posttraumatic syrinx is not well understood, but the diagnosis, using standard spin-echo sequences, is usually straightforward. If the syrinx is small, however, it may be mistaken for a focal area of myelomalacia. Differentiation usually can be made using T2-weighting. Myelomalacia has intermediate to high signal intensity on the first echo or proton density image, whereas the CSF filled syrinx has a low signal intensity on this pulse sequence.

Epidural Hematoma

Spinal epidural hematoma may arise from traumatic injury or from spontaneous bleeding, as might be seen in individuals with bleeding disorders or adjacent to neoplasms, vascular malformations or in areas of previous spinal puncture. (29) The signal characteristics of epidural hematomas vary with the age of the lesion (30) and may have a similar appearance to extruded disc material. (31) Axial images are needed to accurately assess the location of the lesion (epidural versus intradural). (Fig. 6.36) Epidural hematomas are biconcave and produce extrinsic cord compression, while subdural hematomas are located within the dural confines and conform to the borders of the thecal sac (i.e., crescent shaped). (27) Intraspinal epidural hematomas arise from venous bleeding and are much more common than subdural hematomas, but are still rare. Gundry and Heithoff (31) have suggested that these lesions arise from tearing of the fragile epidural veins.

Miscellaneous Traumatic Lesions

Schmorl's nodes may be posttraumatic in nature and associated with vertebral compression fractures. Massive herniation of the nucleus through a deformed and fractured endplate can occur and may be a disabling injury. MRI displays the full extent of the nuclear migration and is far more anatomically specific and sensitive than plain film imaging. (Fig. 6.37) Acute Schmorl's nodes may be observed on T2-weighted images as a focal intrabody herniation of disc material surrounded by adjacent high signal intensity edema.

MRI provides a unique anatomic visualization of the spinal ligaments, including the anterior longitudinal ligament, posterior longitudinal ligament, interspinous ligaments, and capsular ligaments. Disruption of these ligaments and associated hemor-

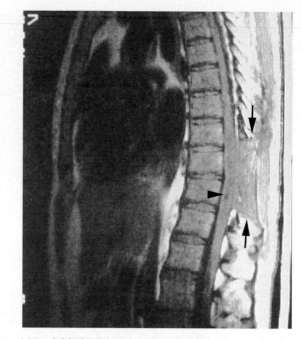

Figure 6.35. POSTOPERATIVE SYRINX: THORACIC SPINE. This patient had a history of a multilevel thoracic laminectomy and developed persistent pain near the surgical site. **MRI, T1-Weighted Sagittal Thoracic.** Observe the laminectomy defect (arrows) and focal area of decreased signal within the spinal cord, representing a syrinx (arrowhead). (Courtesy of Thomas E. Hyde, DC, DACBSP, North Miami, Florida)

rhagic edema may be demonstrated with MRI and indicates severe injury. These findings may be observed in traumatized patients when there is no plain film evidence of fracture or dislocation.

Spinal Cord Contusion

Injury to the spinal cord may result in ischemia, secondary to direct mechanical compression. This may be caused by displaced bone fragments or articular dislocation. (Fig. 6.38) In addition, during a hyperextension cervical spine injury, congenital spinal stenosis, ligamentum flavum buckling, posterior spondylosis and herniated nucleus pulposus (Fig. 6.39), may trap the cord, resulting in significant cord injury. Cord damage may also occur as a result of vascular injury, especially when the terminal perforating arteries are involved. (32)

Cord damage assumes *four* major clinical patterns: anterior cord syndrome, central cord syndrome, Brown-Sequard syndrome, and complete transection. (32) A host of varying neurologic deficits occur, depending on the type of spinal cord injury. Any of the spinal cord syndromes that are incomplete have the potential for recovery. Neurologic assessment after 48 hours usually provides a good indication of the eventual prognosis for recovery of function. (32) If there is no return of sensation or motor function within 48 hours, some degree of permanent damage is likely. The development of MR criteria for assessing cord damage may, in the future, modify the current methods of prognostication. (32)

MRI Findings.   Acute cord insult on T1-weighted scans may demonstrate isointense focal cord swelling at the site of injury. (33) On T2-weighted scans, cord contusions usually exhibit a focal area of hyperintense signal resulting from the associated edema

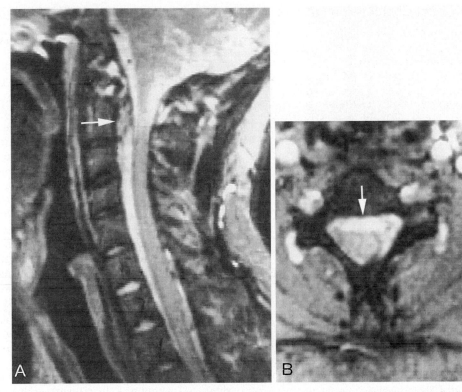

Figure 6.36.   EPIDURAL HEMATOMA: CERVICAL SPINE. This patient presented following a severe motor vehicle accident. **A. MRI, Gradient-Echo Sagittal Cervical. B. MRI, Gradient-Echo Axial Cervical**. A well-defined collection of high signal intensity is noted ventrally within the epidural space (arrows). This produces slight posterior displacement and deformity of the spinal cord. (Courtesy of Robert A. Seigel, MD, St. Anthony Hospital, Denver, Colorado)

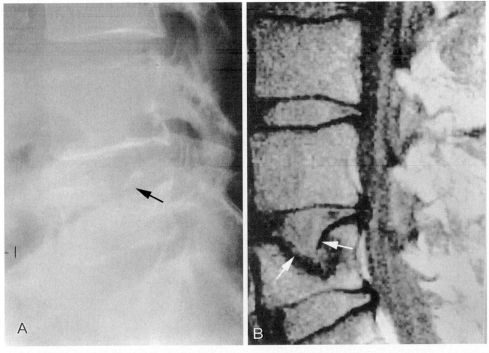

Figure 6.37.   TRAUMATIC SCHMORL'S NODE/COMPRESSION FRACTURE: LUMBAR SPINE. This patient was disabled in an automobile accident. **A. Lateral Lumbar**. The plain film exam underestimates the extent of the injury. Observe the fractured and depressed L5 superior endplate (arrow). **B. MRI, Proton Density-Weighted Sagittal Lumbar**. The cortical endplate is interrupted in its midportion with intermediate signal intensity nuclear material extending into the mid body of L5 (arrows). The lack of high signal intensity bone marrow edema surrounding the Schmorl's node suggests an old injury. COMMENT: The superior contrast resolution of MRI accurately identified the extent of this patient's injury.

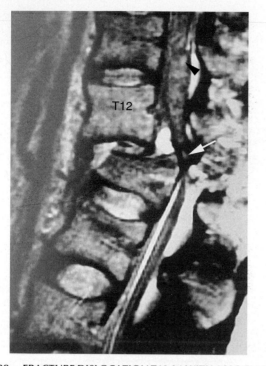

Figure 6.38.   FRACTURE DISLOCATION T12-L1 WITH ASSOCIATED SPINAL CORD HEMORRHAGE. This 29-year-old male was struck by a boat trailer. **MRI, T2-Weighted Sagittal Thoracolumbar.** Observe the compression fracture of the L1 vertebral body. There is disruption of the T12-L1 disc and anterior longitudinal ligament with a 50% anterior luxation of T12 on L1. Note the marked compression of the spinal cord (arrow) with a small area of hyperintense signal, consistent with spinal cord hemorrhage (arrowhead). COMMENT: The presence of cord hemorrhage negatively impacts the prognosis of patients with spinal cord injuries. (Courtesy of Steven R. Nokes, MD, Baptist MRI, Little Rock, Arkansas)

and hemorrhage. Acute spinal cord damage assumes one of two general patterns: *hemorrhagic* or *non-hemorrhagic*. (33) The non-hemorrhagic pattern is characterized by normal signal intensity on T1-weighted images in conjunction with abnormal high signal intensity on the T2-weighted image. This high signal can usually be seen extending inferiorly and superiorly from the injury epicenter. Gradual dissipation of this hyperintense region within the cord occurs over a period of 7 to 21 days. (33) This abnormal pattern can be seen in patients who are neurologically normal.

The second major pattern of cord damage represents intramedullary hemorrhage. This is an ominous finding representing significant, and often permanent, cord damage. The MR appearance of intramedullary hemorrhage is similar to that of intracranial hemorrhage and therefore depends on its age. The signal characteristics change according to the phase of deoxyhemoglobin degradation at the time of the examination. Initially, low signal intensity may be demonstrated within the cord on T2-weighted images and may be accentuated on gradient-echo images. (32,33) The late stage of cord hemorrhage is seen as an area of residual intramedullary hemosiderin deposition. When sufficient methemoglobin has accumulated, hemorrhage has high signal intensity on both T1- and T2-weighted images. (Fig. 6.40)

Magnetic resonance imaging has become the *gold standard* in the evaluation of the traumatized spine, particularly when cord contusion is suspected. MRI should be recommended for patients reporting a history of spinal trauma and displaying neurologic signs and symptoms. In patients with preexisting disc herniations, or herniations occurring at the time of injury, there may be a direct mechanical cause for cord contusion. Even if the herniation predates the accident, it may be implicated when injury to the spinal cord is sustained during hyperextension-rotatory cervical spine trauma.

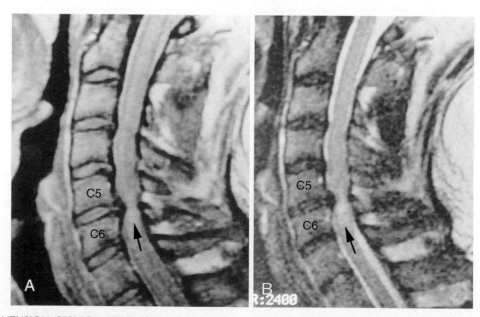

Figure 6.39.   CORD CONTUSION: CERVICAL SPINE. This patient was involved in a motor vehicle accident and subsequently complained of tingling in the upper and lower extremities. Treatment consisted of high-dose corticosteroids and bed rest. The symptoms resolved after treatment. **A. MRI, Proton Density-Weighted Sagittal Cervical. B. MRI, T2-Weighted Sagittal**

Cervical. Herniation of the nucleus pulposus is noted at C5-C6, resulting in central compression of the thecal sac. The increased signal intensity within the spinal cord adjacent to the site of herniation (arrow) represents a spinal cord contusion. (Courtesy of Kenneth B. Reynard, MD, Center for MRI, Ltd., Denver, Colorado)

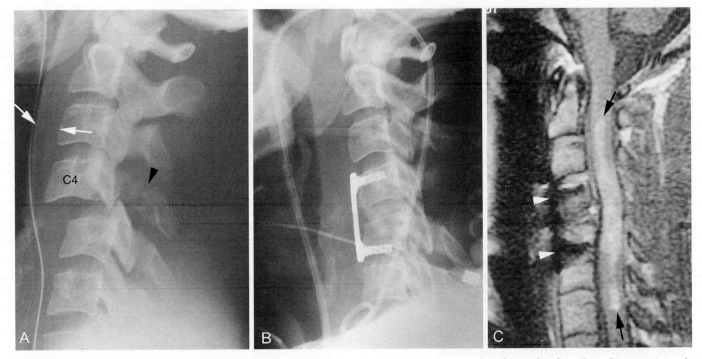

Figure 6.40. BILATERAL C4-C5 FACET DISLOCATION WITH CORD CONTUSION. This 30-year-old male was in a motor vehicle accident. **A. Lateral Cervical.** Note the bilateral anterior dislocation of C4 on C5 with locked facets. There is thickening of the retropharyngeal interval secondary to edema (arrows). Additionally, a fracture of the C4 lamina is present (arrowhead). **B. Lateral Cervical, Postsurgery.** Note the C4-C5 arthrodesis. There was no improvement in the patient's neurologic status. **C. MRI, T1-Weighted Sagittal Cervical.** One month later, the MRI revealed high signal intensity within the spinal cord extending from C2 to C7 (arrows), consistent with hemorrhage. Note the signal void produced by the anteriorly placed fixation device (arrowheads). COMMENT: MRI was helpful in limiting more invasive imaging in this patient who suffered permanent disability following this injury. No other imaging modality provides direct visualization of the integrity of the spinal cord. (Courtesy of Ted D'Amico, DC, Calgary, Alberta, Canada)

INFECTION

Infectious Spondylitis

Infections of the spine usually involve the vertebral body (osteomyelitis) and the disc space (discitis) and can be collectively referred to as infectious spondylitis. (32) In general, suppurative spondylitis progresses more rapidly than the nonsuppurative (tuberculous) variety. With suppurative spondylitis, clinical symptoms generally occur within weeks of the infection and vary greatly with the type of organism, location of the lesion, and extent of involvement. The most common organism is *Staphylococcus aureus*, with streptococci and gram-negative organisms being less commonly involved. Pain is usually present, but may be either intermittent or constant and varies widely in severity. The patient may be febrile. The *radiographic latent period* (the time necessary for radiographically demonstrable changes) may be as long as 21 days. Symptoms associated with tuberculous spondylitis are similar to suppurative spondylitis; however, they usually are more insidious in nature, with a slower rate of progression. Active pulmonary tuberculosis may or may not be present at the time of diagnosis.

The initial infectious focus in the spine often begins at the subchondral vertebral endplate and spreads by imbibition into the disc. The early stages of plain film radiographic findings are disc space narrowing and endplate destruction. Late changes include marked disc space thinning and vertebral body destruction. Tuberculous spondylitis more commonly demonstrates anterior gouge defects of the vertebral body, a structural flexion deformity of the vertebral column (gibbus deformity), and formation of an abscess, which has a strong tendency to eventually calcify along the psoas muscle. (Fig. 6.41) Suppurative spondylitis generally involves one level, while tuberculous spondylitis may track underneath the anterior longitudinal ligament, eventually affecting multiple contiguous segments. (Fig. 6.42) The reader is referred to Chapter 12 for a detailed discussion on the pathophysiologic mechanism and plain film radiographic findings of infectious spondylitis.

MRI Findings. Both suppurative and nonsuppurative spondylitis demonstrate similar changes with MRI. On the T1-weighted images, a confluent decreased signal intensity may be seen within the affected vertebral bodies and adjacent disc. This altered signal is caused by the increased water content of the exudative polymorphonuclear leukocyte response and local ischemia replacing the normal high signal fatty marrow. (34,35) With T2-weighting, the infected disc may appear normal, abnormally hyperintense, (36) or hypointense. (32) The normally clear demarcation between the disc and vertebral body is frequently distorted. Additionally, the signal abnormalities that affect the adjacent marrow can extend deep within the vertebral bodies. (Fig. 6.43) The early changes of infection versus those of tumor are readily apparent with MRI before there is any visible evidence of abnormality with plain film or CT. Neoplasms rarely involve or cross a disc space, whereas infections invariably infiltrate and destroy the disc and adjacent vertebral endplates. (34,35)

Other forms of inflammatory or infectious disorders of the spine, such as spinal cord infections (transverse myelitis), lepto-

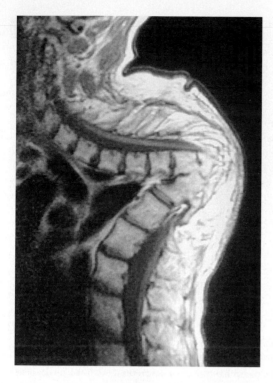

Figure 6.41.   TUBERCULOUS SPONDYLITIS: GIBBUS DEFORMITY. This patient had a history of pulmonary tuberculosis with spinal involvement. **MRI, T1-Weighted Sagittal Thoracic.** There is collapse and marked deformity with ankylosis of several midthoracic vertebrae. A pronounced kyphosis or gibbus deformity is present resulting in sharp angulation and stretching of the spinal cord. The contents of the thoracic cage are severely compromised by the spinal deformity. COMMENT: Tuberculosis of the spine results in disc destruction and vertebral body involvement that progresses to multiple levels. Since the posterior elements of the vertebral segment are typically spared, body destruction results in a sharp angulation (gibbus) across the affected segments. MRI is highly sensitive and specific, allowing for accurate evaluation of the acute and chronic phases of infectious spondylitis.

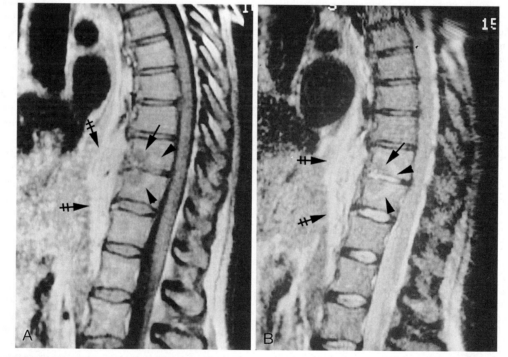

Figure 6.42.   SPONDYLODISCITIS: SEVERE THORACIC SPINE PAIN. A. MRI, Proton Density-Weighted Sagittal Thoracic. B. MRI, T2-Weighted Sagittal Thoracic. Observe the hypointense signal within the subchondral bone of T7 and T8 (arrows). This decreased signal intensity is surrounded by a hyperintense rim (arrowhead). In addition, the T7-T8 disc is abnormally hyperintense and is surrounded by irregular endplates. Note the large prevertebral abscess (crossed arrows). COMMENT: MRI is highly sensitive and specific for the diagnosis of vertebral osteomyelitis and disc infection. (Courtesy of David A. Oppenheimer, MD, Boulder, Colorado)

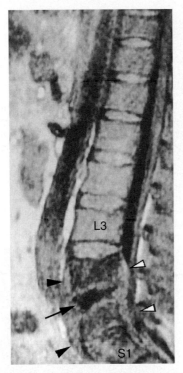

Figure 6.43.   SPONDYLODISCITIS: L4-L5. MRI, T2-WEIGHTED SAGITTAL LUMBAR. There is a marked loss of the signal originating from the L4-L5 disc, consistent with exudative material (arrow). Decreased signal intensity is also noted in the L4 and L5 vertebral segments. In addition, observe the loss of cortical definition and irregularity of the opposing L4-L5 endplates. A low to intermediate signal intensity mass is present anterior to the vertebral bodies and within the epidural space (arrowheads), representing an abscess. (Courtesy of Craig P. Church, DC, DACBR, Toledo, Ohio)

meningeal infections, cysticercosis, and blastomycosis (Fig. 6.44) are recognized to cause changes demonstrable on MRI; however, an individual discussion on each of these entities is beyond the scope of this text.

Epidural Abscess

Spinal epidural abscess is an infectious process of the epidural space that may consist of pus or granulation tissue. (37) The most common primary focus of the infection is in the thoracic spine (approximately 50%). (38) Epidural abscesses are most frequently iatrogenic, usually the result of invasive procedures such as discectomy/vertebral fusion, epidural steroid injections, and myelography. On MRI, abscesses are usually well defined and exhibit signal changes that are similar to neural tissue on T1-weighted images, becoming bright with T2-weighting. (30) Gradient-echo and STIR images should be employed if an epidural abscess is suspected clinically. Gadolinium-enhanced images are helpful in delineating the margins of the lesion on otherwise equivocal scans.

OSSEOUS TUMORS OF THE VERTEBRAL COLUMN

Introduction

Primary and metastatic tumors of the vertebral column will be presented in a limited fashion with an emphasis on their MRI manifestations. A more complete discussion of all primary benign

and malignant bone tumors, along with an extensive discussion of the pathophysiology of tumor metastasis, is presented in Chapter 11.

Metastasis

Metastatic disease of the vertebral column is difficult to image in its earliest stages. Most metastatic lesions (80%) are osteolytic in nature and require approximately 50% loss of bone density before the earliest signs of destruction can be detected with plain film spinal radiographs. Computed tomography is able to demonstrate these bony changes earlier than plain films. Bone scans are far superior to plain film radiography and CT, requiring only 3 to 5% of bone destruction before abnormal radiopharmaceutical activity is apparent. The most sensitive imaging modality in the detection of osseous metastatic disease in the spine is MRI. Its disadvantage in comparison with nuclear medicine scans is that it does not image the full skeleton, limiting its ability to a regional evaluation of the disease.

The earliest MR findings usually detect vertebral metastasis in the marrow adjacent to the posterior cortical margin. (39) (Fig. 6.45) The remaining portions of the vertebral body, pedicles, and other sections of the neural arch may be involved secondarily as the neoplastic process spreads throughout the intravertebral venous system. (Fig. 6.46) Replacement of the normal fatty marrow within the vertebral body is often seen with MRI in the absence of gross morphologic alterations. (Fig. 6.47) This provides valuable information that is not readily attainable with plain film radiography or CT. The high cellular activity (high water and low fat content) of the metastatic process appears as a low signal intensity area on the T1-weighted image. With T2-weighting this area becomes hyperintense. (Fig. 6.48) Osteoblastic metastasis is observed as low signal intensity on both the T1- and T2-weighted spin-echo pulse sequences.

MRI provides anatomic information concerning tumor extension into the paravertebral and epidural soft tissues. This information is of prognostic value and also assists in treatment planning.

Multiple Myeloma

Multiple myeloma is the most common primary malignant tumor of bone. It represents a proliferation of plasma cells, usually within bone marrow. The spine is frequently a primary site, and localized lesions may spread throughout the body in later stages. The typical appearance of untreated multiple myeloma on MR images is similar to that of other malignant lesions that replace fatty bone marrow. Well-circumscribed areas of marrow replacement are observed diffusely involving multiple vertebral bodies. (32) These areas appear hypointense on T1-weighted images and hyperintense with T2-weighting. (32) Multiple myeloma should be considered, along with metastatic disease, in the differential diagnosis for patients between the ages of 50 and 70 with insidious back pain of a nonmechanical nature.

Other Primary Malignant Bone Tumors

Other primary malignant tumors of bone such as Ewing's sarcoma, osteosarcoma, chondrosarcoma, and chordoma (Fig. 6.49) cause similar marrow replacement with no definitive MRI findings to assist in the determination of the tumor's histologic composition. The histologic diagnosis of these and other primary malignant bone tumors is usually determined by biopsy. The role of MRI in the evaluation of primary bone tumors is to display the *extent* of the neoplastic processes within the marrow cavity and

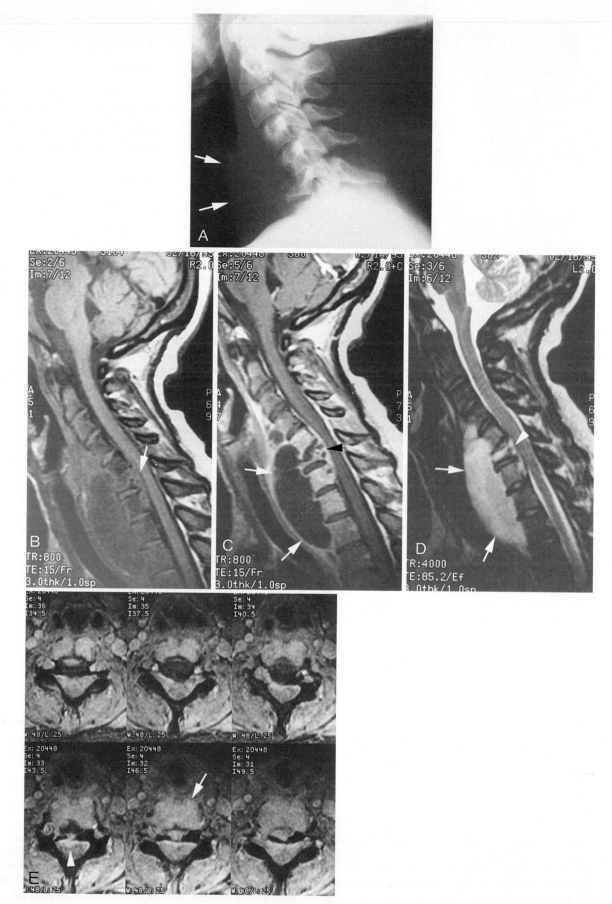

Figure 6.44.

Figure 6.44. BLASTOMYCOSIS WITH A LARGE PARAVERTEBRAL ABSCESS: CERVICAL SPINE. This 22-year-old black female presents with neck pain three months following a motor vehicle accident. **A. Lateral Cervical.** There is gross destruction of the anterior C5 and C6 vertebral bodies with marked narrowing of the interposed disc. Osteopenia is also present at the anterior aspect of the C4 vertebral body. Note the enlarged prevertebral soft tissues (arrows), suggesting an underlying mass. **B. MRI, T1-Weighted Noncontrast Sagittal Cervical.** Observe the large, intermediate to low signal intensity, prevertebral soft tissue mass with extension into the C5-C7 vertebral bodies and epidural space (arrow). **C. MRI, T1-Weighted Contrast-Enhanced Sagittal Cervical.** Peripheral rim enhancement of the large mass is seen. Note the lack of central contrast uptake. These findings are character-

istic, but not definitive, of an infectious process. **D. MRI, T2-Weighted Sagittal Cervical. E. MRI, Gradient-Echo Axial Cervical.** Note the large, soft tissue mass within the prevertebral space extending from C4 to T3 (arrows). The central portion of this mass is very hyperintense on this pulse sequence, consistent with a fluid-filled or exudative internal composition. Note the epidural extension of the abscess, posterior to the C5-C7 levels (arrowheads), which produces compression on the ventral portion of the thecal sac and spinal cord. COMMENT: Aspiration of 40 cc of fluid from the prevertebral mass and culture revealed *Blastomyces dermatitidis* as the causative organism for this large abscess (blastomycosis). (Courtesy of Steven R. Nokes, MD, Baptist MRI, and Ronald G. Kelemen, DC, Little Rock, Arkansas)

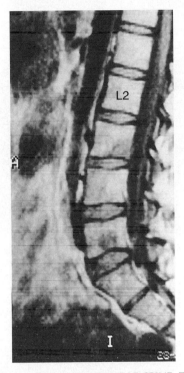

Figure 6.45. SPINAL METASTASIS: LUMBAR SPINE. This patient's plain film radiographs (not shown) were normal. Her unresponsiveness to conservative management prompted this examination. **MRI, T1-Weighted Lumbar Sagittal.** Two low signal intensity foci are seen posteriorly, adjacent to the inferior endplates of L3 and L5 and represent marrow replacement from breast metastasis. No visible cortical disruption or local soft tissue invasion is evident. COMMENT: Plain film radiographs require 30 to 50% bone destruction before radiographic findings are readily visible. MRI is the MOST SENSITIVE imaging modality in the detection of spinal metastasis.

to detect adjacent soft tissue invasion. This information is not attainable with any other imaging modality and is valuable in determining the type of treatment to be initiated, establishing a more accurate prognosis, and monitoring treatment results. These data become very crucial when chemotherapy, radiation therapy, and limb salvage procedures are being considered. (40) Following treatment with chemotherapy and/or radiation therapy, MRI can be utilized to monitor tumor cell response.

Hemangioma

Hemangioma is the most common benign tumor of the vertebral column. It is most frequently found in the lower thoracic and upper lumbar vertebral bodies. These lesions consist of cavernous, capillary, and venous vascular channels intermixed with

thickened osseous trabeculae. (32) Cystic, blood-filled spaces may be contained within the tumor. The trabeculae form characteristic vertical striations, which are commonly noted on plain film radiographs. This *corduroy cloth* or *striated vertebrae* appearance is a characteristic radiographic finding. Most lesions are limited to the vertebral body; however, 10 to 15% may extend into the posterior arch and, if expansion occurs, can produce spinal stenosis with resultant cord compression. If hemangiomas reach a large size, the soft tissue mass can expand beyond the bony margins, requiring surgical decompression. (41) Most hemangiomas are asymptomatic and seldom cause pathologic fracture.

These tumors range in size from a small, round focus within the vertebral body to involvement of the entire vertebral body and neural arch. (Fig. 6.50) The high fat content of hemangiomas produces hyperintense signal within the vertebral body on T1-weighted images. On the second echo of the T2-weighted sequence, the fat signal is diminished and appears iso- or slightly hyperintense. (Fig. 6.51) In the rare instances of cord compression the soft tissue mass extending beyond the confines of the vertebral body is clearly shown on T1-weighted axial scans.

SPINAL CORD TUMORS
Introduction

Before magnetic resonance imaging, myelography and CT myelography were the gold standard in the evaluation of spinal cord tumors. Magnetic resonance imaging has replaced these modalities in most clinical situations. However, in locations where access to MRI is restricted or unavailable, these invasive modalities are still routinely utilized.

Tumors of the spinal cord are pathologically similar to, but less common than, brain tumors (1:6 ratio). (42) They may arise from the neural tissue, meninges, surrounding bone and soft tissues, embryonal rests or as metastases from primary intracranial neoplasms (drop metastases) or other primary neoplasms located elsewhere in the body. Spinal cord tumors have classically been divided into three anatomic categories: *intradural extramedullary*, *intradural intramedullary*, and *extradural*. In the adult, intradural extramedullary tumors represent approximately 60% of all spinal cord tumors. Intradural intramedullary and extradural tumors represent 15% and 25% of cord tumors, respectively. (42) Rasmussen et al. (43) reported the following distribution of spinal cord tumors: cervical, 18%; thoracic, 54%; lumbar, 21%; sacral, 7%; and multiple regions, 1%.

Although spinal cord tumors may occur at any age, they are more common between the third and sixth decades, with no apparent sex predilection. There are a number of significant differences between spinal cord tumors in childhood and in adults. First, the anatomic distribution differs, with a greater concentra-

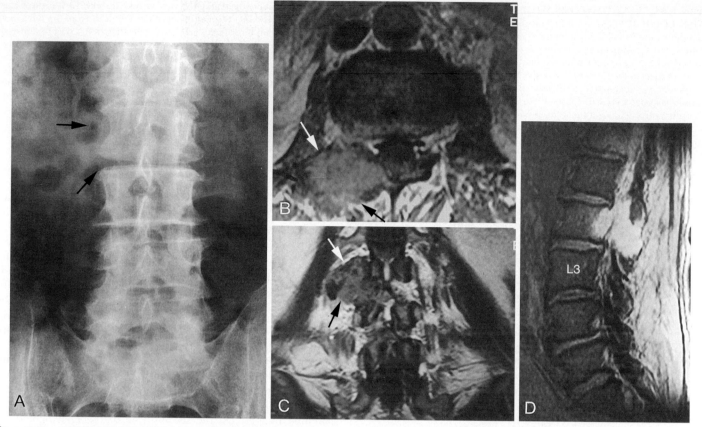

Figure 6.46.   CHRONIC LOW BACK PAIN: METASTASIS. A. AP Lumbar. Observe the missing right pedicle and poorly defined right neural arch of L2 (arrows). **B. MRI, T1-Weighted Axial Lumbar. C. MRI, T1-Weighted Coronal Lumbar.** Note the intermediate signal intensity mass that has destroyed the right lamina-pedicle region of L2, extending into the adjacent soft tissues (arrows). There is minimal displacement of the right lateral thecal sac. **D. MRI, Gradient-Echo Sagittal Lumbar.** Note the hyperintense mass involving the right neural arch and posterior one-third of the L2 vertebral body. (Courtesy of Alan M. Lesselroth, MD, Mountain Diagnostics, Las Vegas, Nevada)

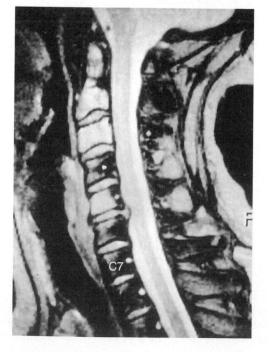

Figure 6.47.   OCCULT BREAST METASTASIS: CERVICAL SPINE. This 48-year-old female complained of neck and arm pain. The plain film and bone scan examinations (not shown) were negative. An MRI was performed to rule out a herniated disc. **MRI, Gradient-Echo Sagittal Cervical.** An unexpected finding was the increased signal intensity foci within numerous cervical vertebrae. The marrow infiltrate is hyperintense relative to the normally low signal fatty marrow. These findings were proven to be metastatic carcinoma from a primary breast carcinoma. Also note the contained disc herniation at C5-C6. (Courtesy of James E. Carter, DC, DACBR, Danville, California)

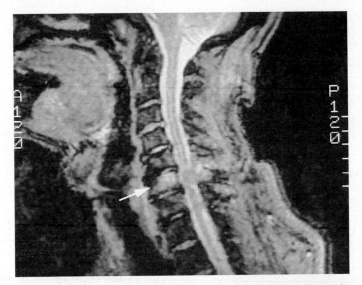

Figure 6.48. VERTEBRAL NEOPLASM: MARROW REPLACEMENT. This 55-year-old long-standing smoker complained of increasing neck pain and upper extremity paresthesia. **MRI, Gradient-Echo Sagittal Cervical.** Note the increased signal intensity area replacing the normally low signal vertebral marrow (arrow) at C6. There is also posterior extension of the malignant tissue into the spinal canal and neural arch. COMMENT: MRI, like radionuclide scintigraphy, is a highly sensitive imaging modality for the evaluation of occult neoplasms of the vertebral column. (Courtesy of The Deaconess West Hospital, Department of Radiology, St. Louis, Missouri)

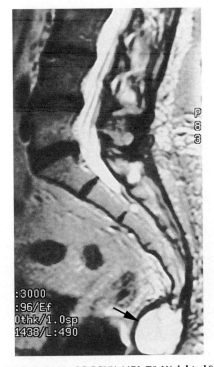

Figure 6.49. CHORDOMA: COCCYX. MRI, T2-Weighted Sagittal Sacrum. Chordomas present as isointense or hypointense masses on T1-weighted images. Note the well-defined homogeneously hyperintense mass surrounded by a thin band of low signal intensity cortex at the level of the coccyx (arrow) on this T2-weighted image. COMMENT: Fifty percent of chordomas occur in the sacrum and coccyx, 30% in the clivus, and the remaining 20% in the vertebral column; C2 has the highest predilection. (Courtesy of The University Hospital, Department of Radiology, Denver, Colorado)

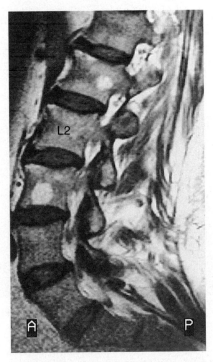

Figure 6.50. HEMANGIOMAS: AN INCIDENTAL FINDING. MRI, T1-Weighted Sagittal Lumbar. Two well-defined high signal intensity foci are noted within the L1 and L3 vertebral bodies. COMMENT: Intraosseous hemangiomas are the most common benign tumor of the vertebral column. The fatty nature of these neoplasms produces hyperintense signal on both T1- and T2-weighted images. Occasionally, a variable pattern of signal intensity may be seen.

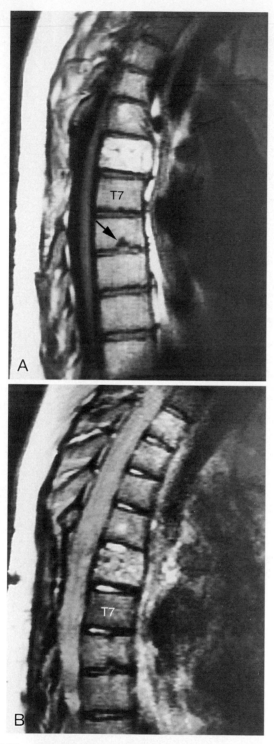

tion in the cervical, lumbar, and sacral regions in childhood, largely as a result of the increased frequency of congenital lesions in these areas. Second, intramedullary and extradural tumors occur with greater frequency and intradural extramedullary tumors with considerably less frequency in childhood. Finally, the relative incidence of the various pathologic types of spinal cord tumors differs considerably. Gliomas and congenital tumors are more common in children, whereas meningiomas and neurofibromas are usually found in adults. Ependymomas and astrocytomas constitute approximately one-third of the acquired tumors in children. (42) These tumors are occasionally quite bulky and may extend from the foramen magnum to the lumbar region. These so-called *giant tumors* of the spinal cord are often associated with progressive scoliosis. (42)

Magnetic resonance imaging has greatly enhanced the ability to detect and characterize lesions of the spinal cord. Short TR/TE (T1-weighted) sagittal sequences generally demonstrate excellent morphologic detail and assist in defining the cord width. Cystic cavities may occur within or adjacent to the tumor and are usually disclosed with MRI. However, some proteinaceous cysts may be isointense with the cord and difficult to appreciate on T1-weighted images. (44) T2-weighted sagittal images demonstrate high signal within the substance of the cord, consistent with either tumor or surrounding edema. Because of MRI's sensitivity to hemorrhage, areas of bleeding are easily detected. The MR appearance of hemorrhage depends on the acute, subacute, or chronic nature of the bleed. This is caused by hemoglobin break-

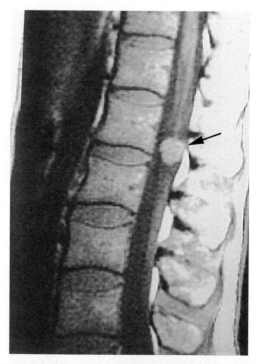

Figure 6.51. HEMANGIOMA: MULTIPLE SITES. A. MRI, T1-Weighted Sagittal Thoracic. B. MRI, T2-Weighted Sagittal Thoracic. Observe the uniform expansion of the T6 vertebral body with bulging of the anterior cortex. The signal originating from the vertebral marrow at this level is markedly increased on the T1-weighted image. In addition, similar high signal intensity areas are present within the marrow of the T4 and T5 vertebral bodies. These represent smaller hemangiomas. With T2-weighting, the high signal intensity hemangiomas become intermediate in signal. A Schmorl's node is incidentally noted affecting the T8 inferior endplate (arrow).

Figure 6.52. EPENDYMOMA: 8 YEARS OF LOW BACK PAIN. This 38-year-old male presented with cauda equina symptoms (coughing causing urination, dyspareunia, and premature ejaculation). **MRI, T1-Weighted Sagittal Lumbar.** There is a well-defined, round, hyperintense lesion within the spinal cord at the L1-L2 level (arrow). This lesion was not proven by biopsy, but was thought to be an ependymoma. A CT was obtained 3 years prior and was normal. COMMENT: Usually, routine CT examinations include only axial slices from L3 to S1. Symptoms suggesting conus medullaris pathology are best evaluated with MRI since it provides direct visualization of this structure. (Courtesy of Kevin J. Loughlin, DC, Boston, Massachusetts)

down and the evolution of blood into its various by-products. Hemosiderin deposition, which is often observed in hemorrhagic cord tumors, appears as a peripheral, markedly hypointense area on spin-echo sequences.

Contrast-enhanced (gadolinium) MRI scans can help in the early detection and characterization of cord lesions. (45,46) Enhancement with gadolinium is most useful in cases of focal, poorly defined masses, especially metastases. (47) These lesions tend to be fairly well circumscribed, but are obscured by the extensive surrounding edema that often extends far beyond the region of the actual tumor. Gadolinium can be very effective in pinpointing the exact location of the lesion. (47) Although the area of cord enlargement can be extensive, the actual lesion may be small (less than one vertebral body in height). Meningiomas are common primary neoplasms in the adult and often require gadolinium enhancement to define their borders.

Intradural Intramedullary Tumors

These neoplasms are predominantly gliomas. Subgroups in this category include ependymoma, astrocytoma, oligodendroglioma, glioblastoma multiforme, and medulloblastoma.

Ependymoma. By far the most common glioma of the spinal cord is the ependymoma, representing 65% of all intraspinal gliomas. (42) (Fig. 6.52) Ependymomas usually occur in the third to fifth decade of life and are most commonly located in the lumbar region, especially at the conus and filum. In the filum terminale it may appear as a fusiform swelling or as one or more fairly well encapsulated nodules. Ependymomas of the conus and filum are frequently large, bulky lesions extending over a considerable distance, often filling the entire circumference of the spinal canal without visible radiographic changes. (Fig. 6.53) These large lesions, however, occasionally produce thinning and erosion of pedicles, with scalloping of the posterior vertebral body. The scalloping of the vertebra may occur at a single level or over several vertebral segments. Small encapsulated ependymomas may not give rise to any detectable bone lesions.

On the T1-weighted images homogeneous or heterogeneous areas of low signal intensity are seen within the cord and may represent tumor, cystic degeneration within the tumor, or tumor with adjacent syrinx formation. With T2-weighting intramedullary ependymomas demonstrate increased signal intensity relative to the cord. This area of high signal is well circumscribed with smaller ependymomas. Contrast-enhanced, T1-weighted

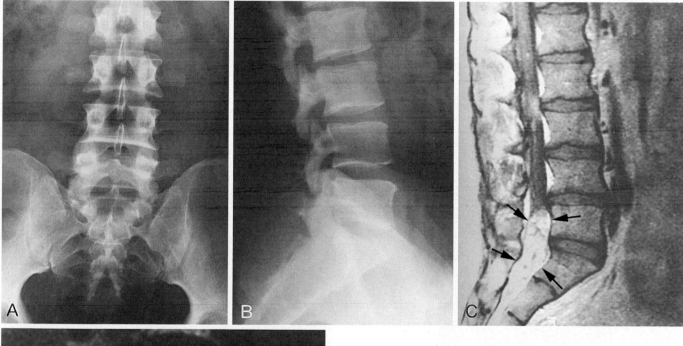

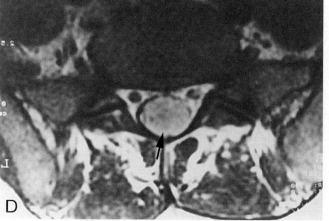

Figure 6.53. EPENDYMOMA: LUMBOSACRAL JUNCTION. This 29-year-old male presented with low back and leg pain of 2 years' duration. **A. AP Lumbar. B. Lateral Lumbar.** The plain films are normal. **C. MRI, T1-Weighted Contrast-Enhanced Sagittal Lumbar**. There is a large intramedullary lesion occupying the lumbosacral canal (arrows). **D. MRI, T2-Weighted Axial L5-S1.** The entire volume of the thecal sac (arrow) is replaced by this tumor. The tumor was surgically removed. COMMENT: Ependymoma is the most common intramedullary tumor of the lumbar spine. They commonly arise from the conus medullaris and filum terminale. Because of their slow growth characteristics, they may enlarge the spinal canal. It is often difficult to differentiate ependymomas from other intramedullary tumors such as astrocytoma. (Courtesy of Craig F. Morrow, DC, Bloomington, Indiana)

MR scans are superior to T2-weighted scans in detecting and defining the margins of ependymomas due to the permeability of the blood-brain barrier. Surgical removal is the treatment of choice for ependymomas and may be curative.

Astrocytoma. The second most common glioma is the astrocytoma, which constitutes approximately 30% of intraspinal gliomas. Generally, astrocytomas in the cord are of a lower histologic grade than those in the brain. The distribution of astrocytomas is fairly uniform in the spinal cord, regardless of tumor grade. (48) Approximately 75% of lesions occur at the thoracic and cervical levels, 20% occur in the distal cord, and 5% occur in the filum terminale. (32) (Fig. 6.54) Most patients with spinal cord astrocytomas present in the fourth or fifth decade; there is a slight tendency for the more aggressive lesions to become symptomatic earlier. (48) The usual clinical presentation in most patients is pain in the neck, back or lower extremity. Spasticity and stiffness in the lower extremity is the presenting sign in 20 to 30% of these patients and, in higher-grade tumors, occurs more frequently than pain. Sensory changes (numbness and tingling), constipation, and urinary incontinence may also exist.

Astrocytomas of the spinal cord are typically large and involve multiple levels. (Fig. 6.55) The tumor is hypointense relative to the spinal cord on T1-weighted images. The degree of heterogeneity depends on the size of the tumor and the amount of associated hemorrhage. Edema is difficult to distinguish from tumor on unenhanced spin-echo images because both demonstrate low signal on T1-weighted images and high signal intensity on T2-weighted images. Early diagnosis is hastened by the use of intravenous contrast (gadolinium).

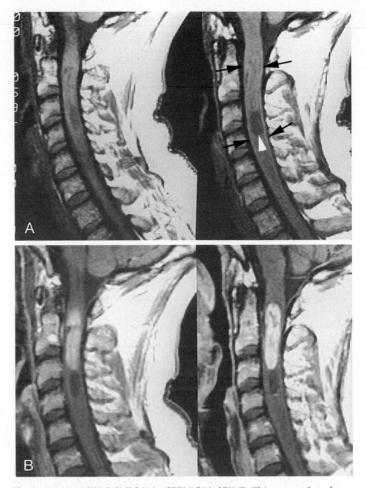

Figure 6.55. ASTROCYTOMA: CERVICAL SPINE. This young female patient presents with progressive neck and arm pain with unexplained weakness in the lower extremities. **A & B. MRI, T1-Weighted Sagittal Cervical Without Contrast.** There is diffuse enlargement of the spinal cord extending from C2 to C4 (arrows). Several poorly defined areas of low signal intensity and a sharply delineated hypointense cyst are present (arrowhead). The cyst is nearly isointense to cerebrospinal fluid and may represent cystic necrosis or a small syrinx. **C & D. MRI, T1-Weighted Contrast-Enhanced Sagittal Cervical.** Observe the marked enhancement of the tumor following intravenous injection of contrast (gadolinium). COMMENT: MRI, even with contrast, cannot definitively confirm the histologic diagnosis of intramedullary tumors. (Courtesy of Mr. Bruce D. Bowen, MR Imaging of Lehigh Valley, Allentown, Pennsylvania)

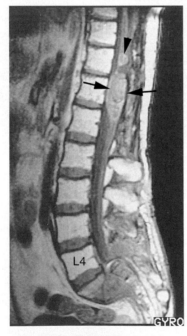

Figure 6.54. ASTROCYTOMA: DUAL LESIONS. This patient reported progressive weakness of the lower extremities and urinary incontinence. **MRI, T1-Weighted Contrast-Enhanced Sagittal Lumbar.** Note the fusiform expansion and increased signal intensity of the conus medullaris (arrows). A satellite lesion (arrowhead) is also seen superior to the larger lesion. Additionally, observe the grade V spondylolisthesis of L5 exhibiting the typical trapezoidal shape and remodeling (doming) of the sacral base. COMMENT: Differentiation between most intramedullary tumors is difficult, even with the use of gadolinium contrast infusion. The two most common intramedullary tumors are ependymoma and astrocytoma.

An important differential consideration in a cord lesion with mass effect and abnormal signal intensity is multiple sclerosis (MS), which may be indistinguishable from tumor. (32) MS lesions may show focal enlargement of the cord and can become extensive enough to enlarge the entire cervical cord. MS plaques are usually more homogeneous in signal intensity than astrocytomas (even in large lesions) and may involve the cord asymmetrically. Comparatively, cord tumors tend to be more symmetric and diffuse. MS lesions often show resolution of the mass effect in 3 to 6 months, whereas the high signal intensity region on T2-weighted images persists beyond 6 months in astrocytomas. An acute MS plaque can enhance on postcontrast scans.

The survival period for patients with spinal cord astrocytomas is variable and depends primarily on the histologic grade of the tumor (I to IV). Patients with low-grade tumors (I and II) tend to

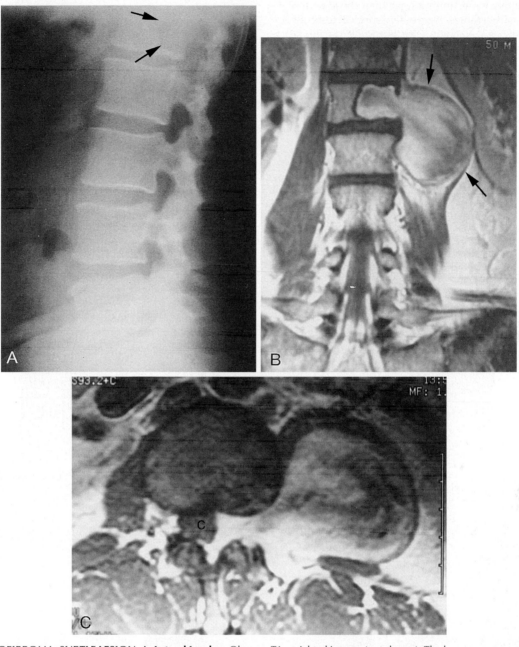

Figure 6.56.   NEUROFIBROMA: SUBTLE LESION. A. Lateral Lumbar. Observe the subtle curvilinear erosion of the posterior L1 vertebral body (arrows) in this 50-year-old male with chronic thoracolumbar pain. **B. MRI, T1-Weighted Coronal Contrast-Enhanced Lumbar.** Note the erosion of the L1 vertebral body by a huge heterogeneous paraspinal mass (arrows). There is minimal enhancement of this lesion when compared with the unenhanced T1-weighted images (not shown). The larger component of the mass projects outside the spinal canal through the enlarged IVF. **C. MRI, T2-Weighted Axial Lumbar Without Contrast.** There is displacement of the spinal cord (C) by the intraforaminal component of this tumor. These findings are consistent with a neurofibroma. (Courtesy of Richard L. Riley, DC, FACO, and Steven R. Nokes, MD, Baptist MRI, Little Rock, Arkansas)

survive approximately eight times longer than those with high-grade (III and IV) astrocytomas. Aggressive surgical resection appears to improve survival statistics with astrocytomas, but necessitates early diagnosis and accurate tumor localization. MR imaging provides important information for early diagnosis (especially when intravenous contrast is utilized) and successful treatment.

Miscellaneous Gliomas

Less common gliomas include glioblastoma multiforme, oligodendroglioma, and medulloblastoma. Other uncommon intramedullary tumors include dermoid cyst, melanoma, sarcoma, and hemangioblastoma. Discussion of these uncommon intraspinal tumors is beyond the scope of this text.

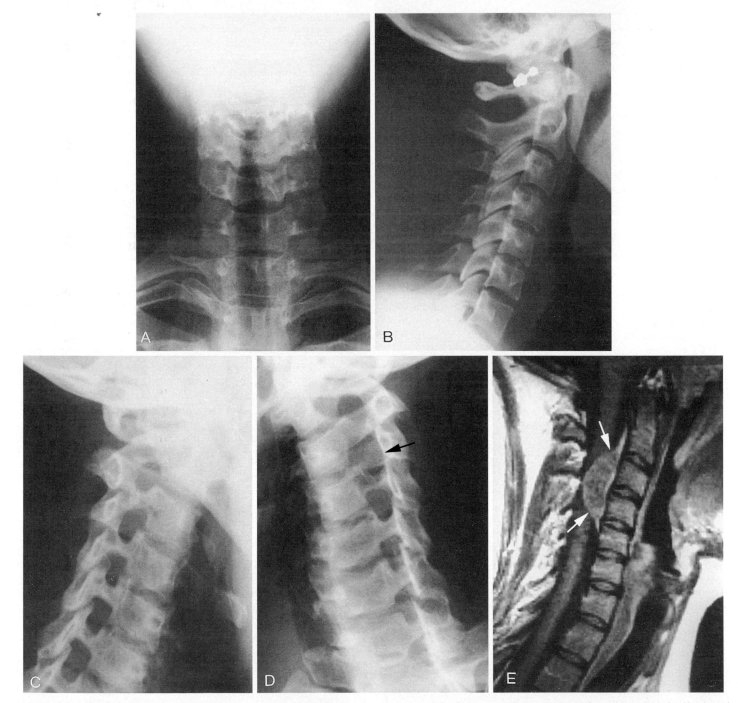

Figure 6.57.   NEUROFIBROMA: NECK AND SHOULDER PAIN. This 19-year-old female complained of neck and shoulder pain. **A. AP Lower Cervical. B. Lateral Cervical. C. Left Posterior Oblique Cervical**. These radiographs are normal. **D. Right Posterior Oblique Cervical**. Note the enlarged C3-C4 intervertebral foramen (arrow). **E. MRI, T1-Weighted Sagittal Cervical. F. MRI, T1-Weighted Axial Cervical.** Observe the heterogeneous, intermediate signal intensity tumor (arrows) resulting in marked, right lateral,

spinal cord displacement and compression. The posterior vertebral body and the left pedicle are eroded by the intraforaminal, "dumbbell-shaped" tumor causing foraminal enlargement (arrowheads). **G. Lateral Cervical Postoperative**. There is a multilevel laminectomy from C2 through C4 with reversal of the cervical lordosis, creating a "goose-neck" deformity. This patient experienced an otherwise uncomplicated recovery. (Courtesy of Philip N. Hardinger, DC, Denver, Colorado)

Intradural Extramedullary Tumors

This group represents the largest number of spinal cord tumors, mostly benign, and is composed primarily of meningiomas and nerve sheath tumors (neurofibromas), which occur with equal frequency.

Meningiomas. Spinal meningiomas originate from cells covering the arachnoidal villi. These tumors are most commonly found in the thoracic spine (approximately 80%) and are usually solitary, but may be multiple in neurofibromatosis. (49) They have a definite predilection for females (4:1 ratio) in this location. (49) The cervical spine is the second most common site of involvement, with a 15% incidence. Meningioma is the most common extramedullary intradural tumor in the region of the foramen magnum. (48) When they occur in this area, they usually arise high in the cervical cord and may extend into the posterior fossa. These tumors vary in size from a small nodule to a large, lobulated mass. Microscopic psammomatous calcification is a common histologic feature for meningiomas, but dense, grossly visible calcification is uncommon in spinal meningiomas (reported in only 1 to 5 % of cases). (48–50) These calcifications are poorly visualized with MRI. Most meningiomas are histologically benign, slow growing, and compress, but do not directly invade, the spinal nerves or cord. Malignant meningiomas are rare and tend to invade neural tissue.

The clinical signs of intraspinal meningioma depend on the location of the lesion and include focal sensory and motor disturbances, transverse myelitis, paralysis, and loss of sphincter control. The symptoms result from slow, progressive nerve root and cord compression and may be present from 6 months to 2 years before the patient seeks medical attention.

MRI Findings. Meningiomas appear as discrete masses with signal intensity similar to the spinal cord on T1- and T2-weighted images. With gadolinium these lesions appear as sharply defined hyperintense masses. Cord compression can be clearly seen on sagittal and axial images.

Nerve Sheath Tumors. Unfortunately, these tumors have been designated by a variety of names: neurofibroma, neurinoma, perineural fibroblastoma, neurilemoma, and schwannoma. Presently, it is thought that these tumors arise from the cells of Schwann in the nerve sheath. Consequently, they are more properly termed neurofibromas or schwannomas. In contrast to meningiomas, neurofibromas tend to occur somewhat earlier in life with the average age of onset at approximately 38 years. (42) According to Bull (51), in a series of 163 neurofibromas 43% were found in the thoracic spine, 33% in the lumbar spine, 22% in the cervical spine, 1% in the sacrum, and less than 1% at multiple levels. These tumors are quite variable in size and shape, and tend to be larger than meningiomas. The average neurofibroma is a smooth, soft, often cystic, lesion attached to the dorsal nerve root. Unlike meningiomas, neurofibromas are rarely adherent to the dura. Large lesions may be lobulated with occasional internal hemorrhage and cyst formation. Intraspinal neurofibromas are usually located in the subdural space of the thecal sac, but may also extend through the neural foramina, resulting in *hourglass-* or *dumbbell-*shaped lesions. Occasionally, these lesions may produce large masses outside the spinal canal with considerable erosion of the adjacent neural foramina. (Fig. 6.56)

Multiple neurofibromas occur in association with neurofibromatosis (von Recklinghausen's disease). Neurofibromatosis is frequently associated with intracranial acoustic nerve lesions, multiple spinal meningiomas, and gliomas.

MRI Findings. On T1-weighted images, neurofibromas appear as discrete masses with isointense or hypointense signal intensity relative to the spinal cord. Cord compression is often seen on both the sagittal and axial images. Intradural neurofibromas deviate the cord with widening of the adjacent subarachnoid space. Extension into the neural foramen is frequent and is best seen on the axial images, appearing as an intermediate signal intensity mass replacing the normal high signal intensity fat on T1-weighted images. (Fig. 6.57) The main differential diagnosis, from an imaging perspective, is meningioma. Both of these le-

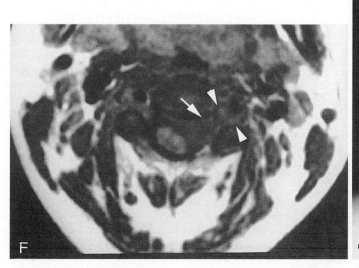
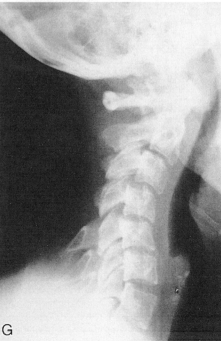

Figure 6.57F and G.

sions have similar signal intensity on T1- and T2-weighted images and enhance with gadolinium.

All neurofibromas originate as histologically benign lesions, but peripheral lesions may occasionally undergo malignant transformation. Intraspinal lesions usually remain benign. (49) The treatment of choice for all nerve sheath tumors is surgical excision and, if removed early, one can expect a complete surgical cure.

Extradural Tumors. Approximately 25 to 30% of all spinal cord tumors are extradural in location. The greatest number of these tumors, particularly in the older age group, are malignant. The high incidence of malignant tumors and low incidence of benign tumors in the extradural space contrasts sharply with the tumor incidence in the subdural space, where most extramedullary tumors are benign. The most common cause of extradural tumor is metastasis from breast or lung carcinoma. (42) (Fig. 6.58) Hodgkin's lymphoma and multiple myeloma are other malignant neoplasms that may produce spinal cord compression. The benign extradural tumors include neurofibroma (most common), meningioma (often malignant in the extradural space), lipoma, and dermoid and epidermoid tumors.

PATHOLOGY OF THE INTERVERTEBRAL DISC

Historical Perspectives

The intervertebral disc was first described by Vesalius in 1555 in his classic monograph "De Humani Corporis Fabrica." (52) In 1857 Virchow elaborated on the anatomy of the intervertebral

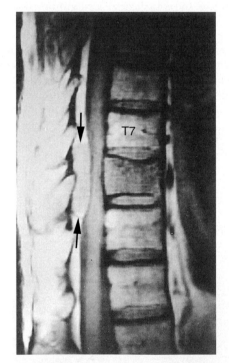

Figure 6.58. EXTRADURAL METASTASIS: THORACIC SPINE. This 55-year-old female had a history of treated breast cancer and had recently developed progressive lower extremity weakness. **MRI, T1-Weighted Sagittal Thoracic.** Observe the high signal intensity, soft tissue mass (arrows) compressing the dorsal aspect of the spinal cord. The tumor has slightly lower signal intensity than the adjacent epidural fat. Note the low signal intensity of the T8 vertebral body and mild compression deformity of the superior endplate. This finding is consistent with marrow replacement from tumor metastasis. (Courtesy of Reed B. Phillips, DC, DACBR, PhD, Los Angeles, California)

disc, (53) and in 1858 von Luschka published a more detailed anatomic description of the disc and discussed its embryology. (54)

The earliest known report on the traumatic rupture of an intervertebral disc was made by Kocher in 1896. (55) He described a posterior L1-L2 herniation at postmortem in a man who landed upright after a fall of 100 feet. In 1911 Middleton and Teacher (56) reported on a young man who developed pain and flaccid paralysis of the lower extremities after lifting a heavy weight. Sixteen days after the injury the patient died and necroscopy disclosed a posterior disc herniation at the T12-L1 segment. The same year Goldthwait (57) reported and diagrammatically illustrated the role of trauma in a typical posterior L5-S1 herniation of the nucleus pulposus. In 1913 Elsberg (58) described a benign extradural spine "tumor," which he termed a *chondroma*. This lesion actually represented a disc herniation; however, an increasing number of intraspinal "chondromas" and "enchondromas" were reported by various surgeons, some of whom appreciated the discogenic origin of these lesions. In 1918 Sicard (59) pointed out the role of irritation of the intraspinal sciatic nerve roots in the production of sciatica. Interestingly enough, the clinical syndrome of sciatica had been described by an Italian, Dominico Cotunio, approximately a century and a half before Sicard's description (1764). (60)

The most exhaustive contribution to the literature on the anatomy and pathology of the intervertebral disc was made by Schmorl, whose incomparable postmortem studies of the spine appeared between 1927 and 1932. (61) In 1929 Dandy (62) reported two cases of nerve root compression caused by extruded cartilaginous fragments of the intervertebral disc. However, it remained for Mixter and Barr in 1934 (63) to report the first removal of herniated disc material, which they initially thought was tumor. Theirs was the first description of sciatica caused by nerve root compression from disc herniation. While quite accurate, this mechanical model was unfortunately accepted for decades as the sole mechanism for discogenic back pain and nerve root irritation. Recent studies by Franson et al. (64), as well as other investigators, have shown that other important mechanisms also play a role in the production of radicular and discovertebral pain.

ANATOMY OF THE INTERVERTEBRAL DISC

The Normal Intervertebral Disc

The adult intervertebral disc consists of three parts: the articular endplates, nucleus pulposus, and annulus fibrosus.

Articular Endplate. In the growing spine the cartilaginous articular plates overlap the anterior and lateral margins of each vertebral body, forming the *epiphyseal ring*. When full growth is attained, enchondral bone formation stops, and there is fusion between the epiphyseal ring and the vertebral body. The fibers of the annulus fibrosus (Sharpey's fibers) are firmly attached to the compact bony ring. The residual central portion of the articular surface of the vertebral body consists of spongy bone that abuts the cartilaginous endplate. This spongy surface is subject to invasion by nuclear tissue and subsequent erosion from nuclear migration (*Schmorl's node formation*).

Nucleus Pulposus. The demarcation between the nucleus pulposus and the annulus fibrosus is not sharply defined. The nucleus pulposus varies in size, but usually occupies a position posterior to the center of the disc. This position varies slightly in different segments of the spine, being somewhat more anterior in the upper thoracic region.

The nucleus pulposus consists of remnant notochordal cells and a network of type II collagen fibrils, similar to those found in articular hyaline cartilage. These fibrils are embedded in a proteoglycan substance that binds water, giving the normal nucleus the consistency of a semiliquid gel, which offers resistance to compressive forces. Proteoglycans are composed of polypeptides with side chains consisting of mucopolysaccharides such as chondroitin sulfate, keratin sulfate, and a small amount of hyaluronic acid. Grossly, the fibrocartilaginous nucleus has a semigelatinous, white, glistening appearance. The turgor of the nucleus depends on its water content, which diminishes with age.

In infancy, the nucleus pulposus contains approximately 90% water. The decrease in fluid content of the nucleus normally begins in the third and fourth decades and usually progresses slowly. The factors responsible for age-related changes within the disc are related, in part, to its biomechanical constituents and are accelerated by any condition that produces disc degeneration (e.g., trauma or inflammatory disorders).

The discs are avascular and nourished by a diffusion process that provides a metabolic exchange via the vessels supplying the vertebral bodies. The fluid exchange takes place through the perforated cartilaginous endplates that separate the disc and the adjacent vertebral spongiosa. (42) This physiologic transfer of nutrients is substantiated by the fairly rapid disappearance of aqueous contrast material from the nucleus pulposus after discography.

The biomechanical behavior of the intervertebral disc is related to its hydration status. (65) Generally, a well-hydrated disc is able to withstand the compressive forces of weight-bearing better than a dehydrated disc. The fluid of the nucleus pulposus acts not only to resist compression, but also to distribute forces in a radial fashion through the annulus fibrosus. As the disc's water-binding capacity decreases, it becomes fibrous and rigid, ultimately resulting in a functionally impaired disc that exhibits altered load distribution through its individual components (nucleus pulposus and annulus fibrosus). Even repetitive normal forces initiated by the activities of daily living produce cartilage fibrillation and annular fissuring. These tears provide the means through which the nucleus pulposus may progressively migrate toward the perimeter of the annulus fibrosus and provoke pain. When fissures extend to the outer margin of the annulus, herniation of the nucleus pulposus may follow. A variety of factors, including the magnitude of weight-bearing loads, rapidity of degeneration, annular fissuring, and healing determine the extent of the herniation. (66)

Annulus Fibrosus. The annulus fibrosus is the strongest portion of the intervertebral disc and firmly binds the vertebrae together. It also determines the size and configuration of the disc. There is no clear anatomic distinction between the nucleus pulposus and the annulus in the adult, although in children the nucleus and annulus are more distinct. The normal annulus fibrosus is made up of 12 to 15 concentric lamellae surrounding the nucleus. Joining these concentric lamellae are obliquely oriented fibers that extend between the lamellae. Together, these structures form a dense gelatinous network of fibers. The inner annular fibers, consisting mainly of type II collagen, are similar to those in the nucleus and also help in resisting compressive forces. The outer one-third of the annulus of the disc has a documented nerve supply, which is provided from the recurrent meningeal nerve of von Luschka. (67)

DISC LESIONS: AN ATTEMPT TO STANDARDIZE THE CONFUSING TERMINOLOGY

Numerous overlapping terms have been used to describe disc lesions. Great confusion exists among clinicians when communicating about the many types of disc pathology. Post (68) suggests a clear and succinct classification. (Table 6.2) Three basic types are offered (Fig. 6.59):

1. *Bulging disc* (bulging annulus, disc bulge, ballooning disc). This is a circumferential, symmetric bulge of the annular fibers. It may be likened to letting half the air out of an inner tube and applying pressure to create a larger outer circumference. Disc bulges represent a part of the natural aging process associated with disc degeneration.
2. *Contained disc* (disc herniation, HNP, protrusion, slipped disc). This represents focal migration of nuclear material that is contained by the outer fibers of the annulus fibrosus.
3. *Noncontained disc* (ruptured disc, prolapse, free-fragment, sequestered disc, extruded disc, floating disc, migrated disc, wrapped disc [a disc herniation engulfed by reparative granulation tissue]). This represents nuclear disc material that is not contained by the outer fibers of the annulus fibrosus. Noncontained discs usually migrate either in a cephalad or caudad direction, relative to the parent disc.

The terms *hard disc* and *soft disc* have been used to describe disc lesions. Hard discs are those bulges or herniations that are comprised of disc material with adjacent marginal osteophytes. This finding suggests a chronic disc lesion. Soft discs are not surrounded by adjacent osteophytes. These lesions may be acute, subacute, or chronic in nature.

Uniformity in describing these disc lesions is necessary for chiropractors, general practitioners, orthopedic surgeons, radiologists, and neurosurgeons so that decisions concerning patient management can be effectively conveyed.

Table 6.2. Classification of Disc Lesions*

Bulging Disc

Bulging annulus
Disc bulge
Ballooning disc

Contained Disc

Protrusion
Herniated disc
Herniated nucleus pulposus (HNP)
Slipped disc (term often used by the lay public)
Subligamentous disc herniation

Noncontained Disc

Prolapse
Extruded disc
Sequestered disc
Fragmented disc
Floating disc
Free-fragment
Ruptured disc
Amputated disc
Wrapped disc (discal fragment wrapped in postsurgical adhesions)
Migrated disc

*From Post MJD: *Computed Tomography of the Spine.* Baltimore, Williams & Wilkins, 1984.

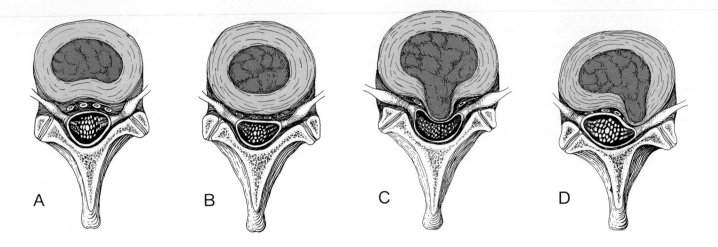

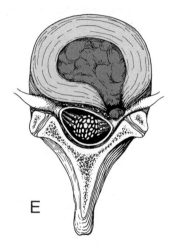

Figure 6.59.   DISC ABNORMALITIES: THEIR MANY APPEARANCES. A. Normal: Schematic Diagram. Note the normal concave configuration of the posterior border of the disc. **B. Bulging Disc: Schematic Diagram.** Observe the circumferential symmetric bulging of the disc creating a convex posterior discal border, slightly compressing the epidural veins. **C. Contained Central Disc Herniation (HNP): Schematic Diagram. D. Contained Paracentral Disc Herniation (HNP): Schematic Diagram. E. Noncontained or Sequestered Disc (Free Fragment): Schematic Diagram.**

Figure 6.60.   BULGING DISC: LUMBAR SPINE. A. MRI, T2-Weighted Sagittal Lumbar, L5-S1. B. MRI, T1-Weighted Axial Lumbar, L5-S1. Observe the circumferential disc bulge (arrows). Note the slight ventral efface-ment of the thecal sac. The high signal intensity area within the posterior vertebral body of L1 represents an intraosseous hemangioma (arrowhead).

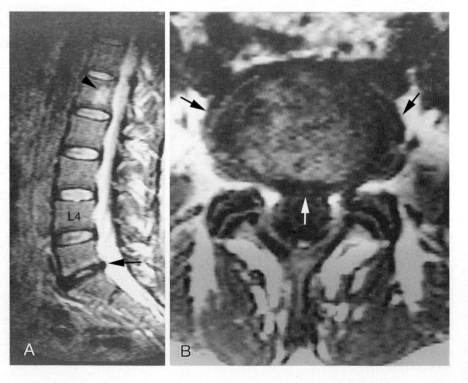

MRI Findings

Bulging Disc. Disc bulges become more prevelant with age and are often associated with degenerative discs. (69) The annulus fibrosis becomes stretched, allowing diffuse concentric bulging of the disc beyond the margins of the adjacent vertebral bodies. (Fig. 6.60) This probably occurs as a result of tearing of the collagen bridges between the annular fibers. (70) Typically, disc bulges are symmetric and maximal in the midline, but the degree of disc extension may be greater on one side. (71)

Contained Disc. Disc herniations that produce myelopathy are usually large and maintain a significant midline component coupled with a congenitally narrowed canal or ligamentous hypertrophy; even small herniations may produce *front-to-back stenosis*.

The MR appearance of cervical, thoracic, and lumbar disc herniations is essentially similar and will be discussed in a combined fashion. (Figs. 6.61–6.64) Most disc herniations (contained discs) are easy to detect on T1- or T2-weighted scans. (72) They are paramidline in location, making them readily detectable on both

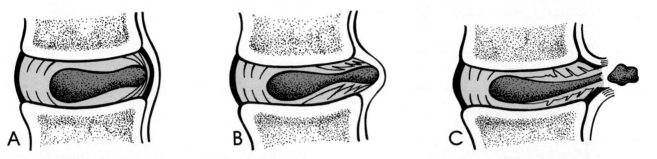

Figure 6.61. PATTERNS OF DISC DERANGEMENT: A SAGITTAL PERSPECTIVE. A. Disc Bulge. This diagram illustrates posterior migration of the nucleus pulposus. The annulus is intact posteriorly, but demonstrates a convex contour. **B. Contained Disc Herniation**. There is posterior extension of the nucleus pulposus through annular tears and fissures. This focal protrusion

elevates the posterior longitudinal ligament and increases the convex deformation of the posterior disc margin. **C. Non-Contained (Sequestered) Disc.** A *noncontained* nuclear fragment is detached from the herniation and is extruded into the epidural space. A free disc fragment usually migrates cranially or caudally within the spinal canal.

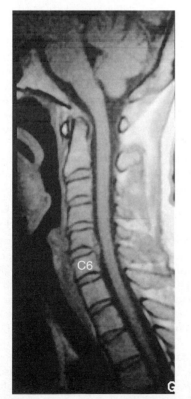

Figure 6.62. HERNIATED NUCLEUS PULPOSUS: SEVERE NECK PAIN. This patient noted exacerbation of his upper extremity pain on neck extension. **MRI, T1-Weighted Sagittal Cervical**. There is a focal midline herniation of the C5-C6 intervertebral disc with compression of the subarachnoid space. COMMENT: MRI represents the *gold standard* for imaging disc herniations.

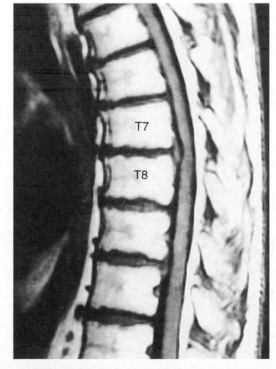
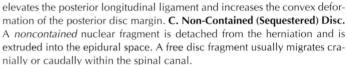

Figure 6.63. HERNIATED DISC: THORACIC SPINE. This 30-year-old male complained of acute onset of severe interscapular pain. **MRI, T1-Weighted Sagittal Thoracic.** Observe the curvilinear focal herniation arising from the posterior T7-T8 disc space. Mild extradural effacement of the ventral spinal cord is present.

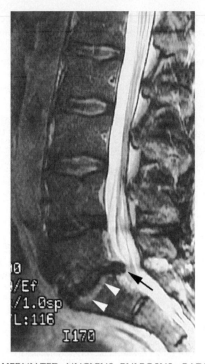

Figure 6.64. HERNIATED NUCLEUS PULPOSUS: RADICULITIS. This 44-year-old male experienced radiating leg pain and numbness of his posterior thigh. **MRI, T2-Weighted Fast Spin-Echo Sagittal Lumbar.** Note the large contained posterior herniation of the L5-S1 disc (arrow). There is decreased signal intensity in both the L4-L5 and L5-S1 discs. The increased signal intensity of the S1 endplate is consistent with the Modic type I pattern of marrow degeneration (arrowheads). With T1-weighting, these type I changes become low in signal due to fibrovascular conversion of the fatty bone marrow.

sagittal and axial images. (Figs. 6.65, 6.66) The *far-out lesions* (foraminal and extraforaminal herniations) are best appreciated in the axial plane.

On T1-weighted images, disc herniations appear as focal areas of intermediate signal intensity extending beyond the posterior vertebral margin into the epidural space. The nuclear material has a mildly hyperintense signal relative to the adjacent CSF. Herniated discs are visualized on T1-weighted images because of displaced epidural fat and deformity of the dural sac and nerve root sleeves. On T2-weighted and gradient-echo pulse sequences, epidural fat is not as hyperintense and often does not provide sufficient contrast for the detection of subtle disc lesions. Therefore the diagnosis is dependent on the signal of the disc contrasting with the high-signal CSF. (Fig. 6.67)

The appearance of a disc herniation on MRI does not provide reliable information regarding the chronicity of the lesion. When significant inflammatory tissue surrounds the herniation, it may be seen on T2-weighted images as an area of abnormal hyperintense signal surrounding the disc. However, these findings are often unreliable. Peripheral gadolinium enhancement of the granulation tissues surrounding the disc suggests active repair of a relatively recent lesion. Focal enhancement within the annulus fibrosis related to tearing has been reported. (73) Beltran et al. (74) suggest that this finding is caused by the ingrowth of vascular granulation tissue into a relatively acute tear.

Far-Out Lesions. Contained and noncontained disc lesions may be lateral to the intervertebral foramina at the pedicle, often

making detection difficult. Both axial and parasagittal T1-weighted scans are best at demonstrating these far-out disc herniations because of the resulting asymmetry and displacement of the epidural fat near the dorsal root ganglion. (Fig. 6.68) T2-weighted second echo images are not as helpful in assessing these lesions.

Non-Contained Disc (Free Fragment). A non-contained disc lesion, or sequestered *free fragment,* is best detected on sagittal scans that show fragment migration from the native disc space along the dorsal surface of the adjacent vertebral bodies. (Fig. 6.69) These free fragments are also seen on axial scans, but their separation from the disc is best appreciated on the sagittal images. (Fig. 6.70) The free disc material often is still hydrated and thus can show relatively high signal intensity on T2-weighted images. Schelinger et al. (75) reported that there is no consensus on preferred direction of free fragment disc migration. Historically, free fragments have been thought to more commonly migrate in a superior direction; however, Williams et al. (76) recently reported a higher prevalence of inferior migration.

Clinical Features of Disc Disease

The symptoms suggestive of disc disease can be mimicked by other disease entities. It is therefore important for an imaging study of the lumbar spine to include examination of the cauda equina and the conus medullaris. This is the analog to the conus view that was a standard part of lumbar myelography. In addition, numerous pelvic disorders, including neoplastic and inflammatory diseases, as well as osteonecrosis of the hip, may mimic lumbar radiculopathy. Awareness of all potential nerve root compressors and their clinical correlates is useful in making MRI interpretations more meaningful.

All disc lesions must be correlated with the patient's clinical symptoms and physical examination findings. Without clinical correlation, the value of the MR findings diminishes. It is important to note that myelograms, discograms, computed tomographic scans, and magnetic resonance images reveal abnormal disc findings in 20 to 30% of subjects who have no history of pain. (77,78) In the horizontal (supine) scanning position, existing pathologic conditions might relax into a *decompressed* state. Anatomic derangements are affected by weight-bearing positions, and if an upright scanning posture were used, altered anatomic relationships might be more obvious.

ARE DISC LESIONS A SOURCE OF PAIN?

Discogenic pain at any spinal level can occur as a result of *tearing of the pain sensitive outer annular fibers of the disc.* Two mechanisms are commonly offered to explain why disc herniations cause radiculopathy: *mechanical compression* of the nerve root and *secondary inflammatory changes* following nuclear extrusion. The inflammatory response has been shown to cause sensitization of the adjacent neurologic structures, including the exiting nerve roots. (64)

As mentioned previously, MRI offers physiologic information concerning disc hydration. The appearance of discal abnormality may or may not correlate with the patient's symptoms. Aprill and Bogduk (79) suggested that, when a zone of hyperintense signal is observed within the annulus fibrosus on T2-weighted images, severe tearing of these fibers has occurred and these discs are symptomatic. This sign was seen in less than one-third of the patients they studied, but was highly specific. Often, however, additional testing such as discography and neurophysiologic

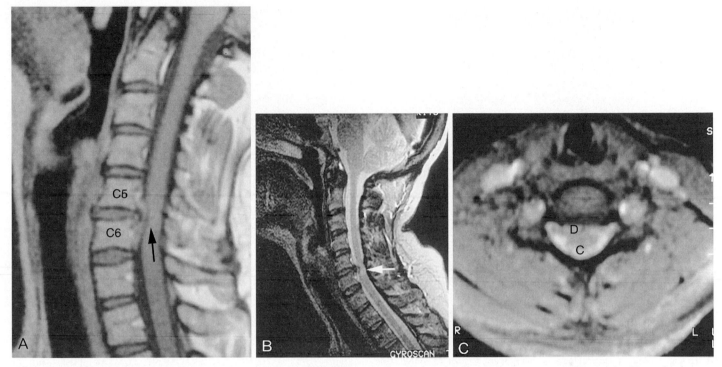

Figure 6.65. HERNIATED NUCLEUS PULPOSUS: SPINAL CORD CON-TUSION. A. MRI, T1-Weighted Contrast-Enhanced Sagittal Cervical. Observe the focal disc herniation at C5-C6 that compresses the ventral aspect of the spinal cord. There is a subtle hyperintense signal intensity within the adjacent spinal cord (arrow) representing a cord contusion. **B. MRI, T2-Weighted Sagittal Cervical.** The herniation has obliterated the ventral CSF column. The subtle hyperintense area on the T1-weighted image has become more hyperintense on this T2-weighted image (arrow). **C. MRI, Gradient-Echo Axial Cervical.** Note the large, right paracentral disc herniation (*D*) at C5-C6 producing ventral compression of the spinal cord (*C*). COMMENT: MRI is the only imaging modality capable of detecting spinal cord contusions.

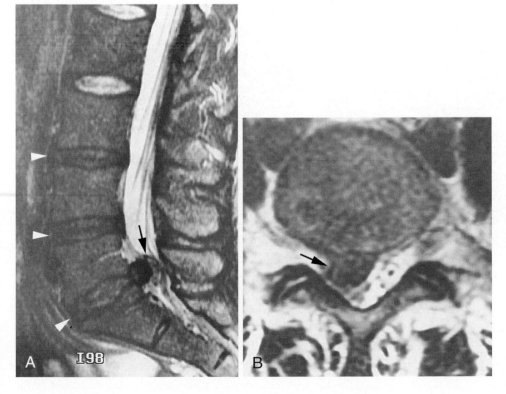

Figure 6.66. HERNIATED NUCLEUS PULPOSUS AND DESICCATION: LUMBAR SPINE. A. MRI, T2-Weighted Sagittal Lumbar. B. MRI, T2-Weighted Axial Lumbar. Note the large, contained, right paracentral disc herniation at L5-S1 (arrow) that nearly fills the entire spinal canal and displaces the adjacent nerve roots. In addition, the L3-L4, L4-L5, and L5-S1 discs are low in signal intensity, indicating desiccation (arrowheads). (Courtesy of Alan M. Lesselroth, MD, Mountain Diagnostics, Las Vegas, Nevada)

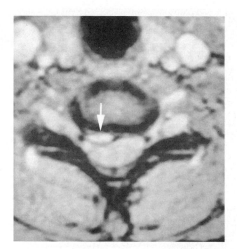

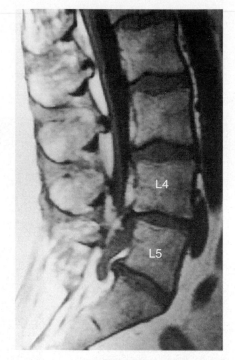

Figure 6.67.   HERNIATED NUCLEUS PULPOSUS: CERVICAL SPINE. This patient experienced neck pain related to a work injury. **MRI, Gradient-Echo Axial Cervical.** Note the right paracentral disc herniation (arrow) compressing the ventral aspect of the spinal cord. COMMENT: MRI provides a highly sensitive means for assessing disc herniation and spinal cord compression.

Figure 6.69.   A HUGE DISC FRAGMENT: LUMBAR SPINE. MRI, T1-Weighted Sagittal Lumbar. An extraordinarily large intermediate signal intensity nuclear fragment has been extruded from the L4-L5 disc and extends caudally to S1. In addition, there is a contained L5-S1 disc herniation. (Courtesy of Robin R. Canterbury, DC, DACBR, Davenport, Iowa)

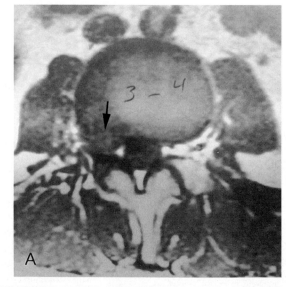

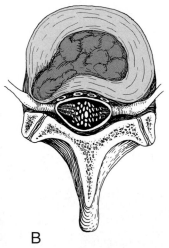

Figure 6.68.   FAR LATERAL DISC HERNIATION: LUMBAR SPINE. A. MRI, T1-Weighted Axial Lumbar, L3-L4. B. Schematic Diagram, L3-L4. Observe the far lateral disc herniation at L3-L4 (arrow). The normal epidural fat has been displaced by the disc material, obscuring the far lateral recess. COMMENT: This patient would have had a normal myelogram because of the "far lateral" or "far-out" position of the disc herniation.

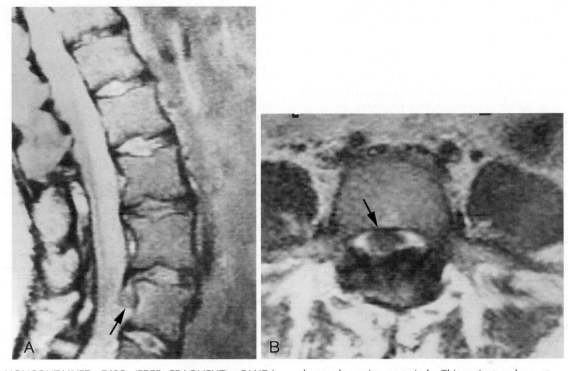

Figure 6.70. NONCONTAINED DISC (FREE FRAGMENT): CAUDA EQUINA SYNDROME. A. MRI, T2-Weighted Sagittal Lumbar. Observe the noncontained L5-S1 disc (sequestered free fragment) that has migrated caudally (arrow). **B. MRI, T1-Weighted Axial Lumbar**. Note the very large, intermediate signal intensity disc fragment (arrow) compressing and displacing the cauda equina posteriorly. This patient underwent emergency surgical decompression. COMMENT: The symptoms of bowel and bladder incontinence, sensory disturbance, and motor weakness in the lower extremities suggest the presence of *cauda equina syndrome* and warrant immediate neurosurgical referral.

tests (e.g., somatosensory evoked potentials, nerve conduction velocity) are necessary to conclude whether a given disc lesion is symptomatic.

Radiculitis

In human experiments, it has been shown that compression and traction can elicit radicular pain only when the nerve root is inflamed. (80,81) Since myelograms, discograms, CT, and MRI frequently reveal abnormal findings in asymptomatic patients, (77,78) it would appear that the true cause of pain production is more complex than traction or compression of the nerve root. Some secondary changes have been assumed to be critical factors in radicular pain.

Anatomic Considerations of Spinal Nerve Roots

Spinal nerve roots connect the peripheral nervous system to the spinal cord. They can be defined anatomically as the proximal part of the spinal nerve, bathed in cerebral spinal fluid (CSF). A key structure of the nerve root as it relates to low back pain and radicular pain is the dorsal root ganglion (DRG). The position of the DRG is not constant. It can be located in the spinal canal, intervertebral foramina, or outside the foramen, depending on the specific segmental level and patient variation. The dura mater and its root sleeve are fixed to the surrounding ligamentous structures in the lumbar spine. Variation in these ligamentous checkreins can be related to pain production. (80) The nerve root is covered only by a thin membranous structure, or root sheath, which is permeable to the CSF. The epineurium of the peripheral nerve is continuous with the dura mater, and the endoneurium also continues from the peripheral nerve to the nerve root.

An hypothesis for the pathomechanism of radicular pain involves mechanical compression of the DRG. These changes are observed by monitoring the circulatory dynamics, which are altered because of the mechanical and vascular vulnerability of the nerve root. This mechanical compression may produce local nerve root ischemia, inducing symptoms of *intermittent neurogenic claudication*. The production of radicular pain by compression has been well documented in the literature, but the pathophysiologic mechanism is still poorly understood. Hasue and Saal have suggested the possibility of a *chemical radiculitis* from inflammatory mediators generated by either degenerated facets and discs or by an autoimmune reaction that occurs in response to disc herniation. (64,82) Disturbed CSF flow due to compression or fibrosis may compound local circulatory and inflammatory changes, resulting in malnutrition of the nerve root. (82) The debris associated with discal injury may create blockage of axonal flow and cause electrophysiologic changes such as ectopic discharges and interneural crosstalk. (82) Pharmacologic changes, including disturbed transit or altered synthesis of neuropeptides, have also been reported in association with disc herniation. Any manipulative technique that can alter this chemical radiculitis may be one hypothesis to explain the reduction of symptoms that can occur in disc lesions.

The Cauda Equina Syndrome

Occasionally, a large midline disc herniation may compress several roots of the cauda equina. Raff (83) reported an incidence of 2% of 624 patients with protruded discs who developed symptoms of cauda equina syndrome. A higher incidence of cauda equina syndrome is associated with noncontained disc (free) fragments in the upper lumbar spine. If a disc lesion becomes large, it may mimic an intraspinal tumor, particularly if it has been slowly progressing.

When compromised, the centrally placed sacral fibers to the lower abdominal viscera produce symptoms that characterize *cauda equina* compression. Perianal numbness and loss of the anal or bulbocavernosus reflex characterize an advanced cauda equina syndrome. Sensory deficit is common and frequently is manifested superior to the involved motor level. Often, back pain or perianal anesthesia will predominate and leg symptoms may be masked. Difficulty with urination, consisting of frequency or overflow incontinence, may develop relatively early. In males, recent impotence may be included in the history. Leg pain may occur and progress to numbness of the feet and difficulty in walking.

Haldeman and Rubinstein (84) have reported ten cases of cauda equina syndrome that developed in patients following manipulation. They concluded that patients who present with bowel or bladder disturbance, leg weakness, or rectal or genital sensory changes after manipulation should be referred immediately for treatment of *cauda equina syndrome*.

The presenting lesion frequently may still be evolving, resulting in changing signs and symptoms. Initial examination may indicate an isolated radiculopathy or show nonspecific neurologic findings. It is imperative that the clinician be alert to promptly recognize the signs and symptoms of cauda equina syndrome. Immediate surgical intervention is necessary, since spontaneous neurologic recovery has not been observed. If incontinence is present, only prompt surgery can lessen the potential for per-

manent urinary drainage complications. Similarly, sudden severe paraplegia requires immediate decompression. When symptoms are extensive, a careful preoperative MRI is indicated for level identification. Contrast-enhanced MRI scans have replaced myelography in the assessment of patients with cauda equina syndrome, as might be expected.

DEGENERATIVE JOINT DISEASE
General Considerations

Degeneration of the intervertebral disc complex begins early in life and is a consequence of a variety of environmental factors, as well as of normal aging. The precise pathophysiology of disc degeneration is not known. The most common factor that results in disc degeneration is acute or chronic repetitive trauma. Repeated minimal vertebral trauma probably causes disruption of nutrient flow across the osteocartilaginous endplate. Immunologic, metabolic, and genetic factors may also play a role in degenerative disc disease. For example, ochronosis, a rare hereditary disorder of amino acid metabolism, causes severe disc degeneration at virtually all intervertebral disc levels in affected juvenile patients.

As the disc degenerates, it loses water and accumulates fibrous tissue. During this process, the proteoglycan loss results in weakening and stretching of the annular fibers. This causes generalized bulging or ballooning of the disc. At the same time, radial tears develop through the annulus fibrosus and some of the Sharpey's fibers are torn from their attachments. This causes an inflamma-

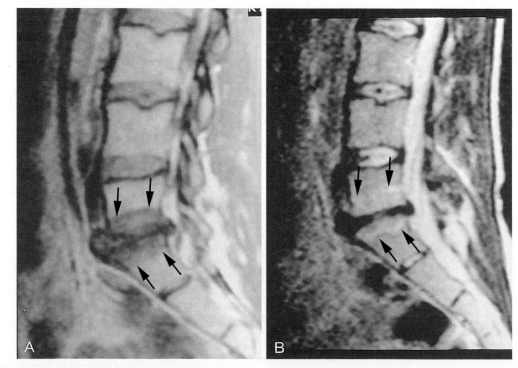

Figure 6.71. DEGENERATIVE ENDPLATE: MODIC TYPE I. A. MRI, T1-Weighted Sagittal Lumbar. Note the low signal intensity within the marrow adjacent to the opposing endplates of L5-S1 (arrows). Also note the large anterior and smaller posterior disc herniations, as well as the marked disc space narrowing, at this level. **B. MRI, T2-Weighted Sagittal Lumbar**. The L5-S1 endplate changes increase in signal intensity with T2-weighting (ar-

rows). These findings represent vertebral endplate disruption with fibrovascular marrow replacement. COMMENT: The low signal intensity on the T2-weighted image confirms the degeneration of the L5-S1 disc. Compare this with the normal signal intensity originating from the disc above. In addition, observe the high contrast provided by the bright cerebrospinal fluid. This is the *myelographic effect* of the T2-weighted image.

tory and reparative response leading to osteophyte formation and other sequelae of degenerative disease.

A more complete and penetrating discussion of degenerative disc disease from an anatomic, pathophysiologic, and clinical perspective is offered in Chapter 10 of this text.

MRI Findings. MRI provides an accurate method of investigating diseases of the spine and spinal cord not previously accessible with other imaging techniques. For this reason, some long-held diagnostic criteria must be modified. MRI certainly has a greater sensitivity to disc abnormalities than any other imaging modality and has now assumed its rightful place as the *gold standard* in imaging the various pathologic lesions of all intervertebral disc disorders.

Healthy intervertebral discs are intermediate in signal on T1-weighted images and become hyperintense centrally with T2-weighting. The desiccated (degenerated) disc demonstrates partial or complete loss of this hyperintense signal. In addition, decreased disc height and annular fiber bulging are often associated. Modic et al. (85) have described signal changes in the marrow of vertebral bodies adjacent to degenerated discs:

Modic Type I

Type I changes demonstrate a decreased signal intensity on T1-weighted images and an increased signal intensity on T2-weighted images. (Fig. 6.71) These changes have been identified in approximately 4% of patients undergoing MR imaging for lumbar disc disease. Histopathologic sections of type I changes demonstrate disruption and fissuring of the endplate by vascularized fibrous tissues that invade the adjacent marrow. This produces prolongation of the T1 and T2 relaxation times.

Modic Type II

Type II changes are represented by an increased signal intensity on T1-weighted images and an isointense or slightly hyperintense area with T2-weighting. (Fig. 6.72) In both type I and type II changes there is evidence of associated degenerative disc disease at the level of involvement. Histologically, type II changes demonstrate endplate disruption with fatty marrow replacement in the adjacent vertebral body. In addition to a degenerative etiology, type II changes are also seen in approximately 30% of chymopapain-treated discs, which may be viewed as a model of acute disc degeneration.

Modic Type III

Type III changes are represented by decreased signal intensity on both T1- and T2-weighted images. (Fig. 6.73) This may or may not correlate with bone sclerosis on plain radiographs. Modic type I and II changes show no radiographic alterations, which is not surprising when one considers the histology. Advanced sclerosis on plain radiographs is a reflection of dense, woven bone within the vertebral body, which replaces the marrow elements. The lack of signal in Modic type III reflects the relative absence of marrow in areas of fibrous or compact bone deposition.

Future Needs

Modic offers a unique MRI classification of marrow changes associated with degenerative intervertebral disc disease. There appears to be a relationship between these changes because type I changes have been observed to convert to type II, while type II

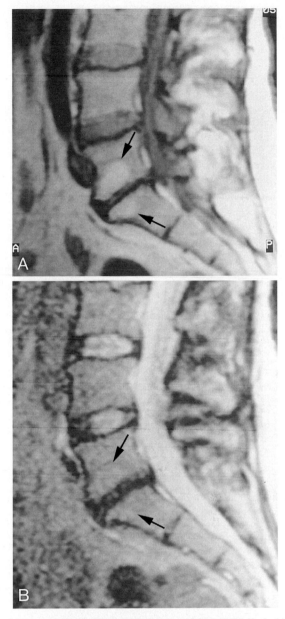

Figure 6.72. DEGENERATIVE ENDPLATE: MODIC TYPE II. A. MRI, T1-Weighted Sagittal Lumbar. Observe the marked narrowing and diminished signal intensity of the L5-S1 disc. The marrow adjacent to the L5-S1 disc space demonstrates abnormally increased signal intensity (arrows). **B. MRI, T2-Weighted Sagittal Lumbar.** The marrow signal adjacent to the L5-S1 disc is slightly hyperintense (arrows). COMMENT: These findings suggest long-standing degenerative disc disease with resultant fatty marrow conversion.

changes seem to remain stable. To date, no biomechanical or clinical significance has been offered in relation to these histologic changes. Modic's concluding thoughts in his landmark article suggest that, while much is known about the structure and biochemistry of the intervertebral disc, little has been offered to impact the patient's overall clinical picture. (85) It is imperative that we improve our understanding of the anatomic and biochemical basis for MR signal intensity changes so that this information can be applied to longitudinal studies of both symptomatic and asymptomatic animal models and humans. (85) Only through this process will we be able to modify the debilitating sequelae of degenerative disc disease. (85)

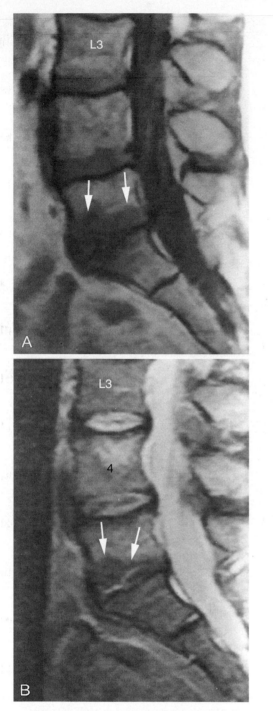

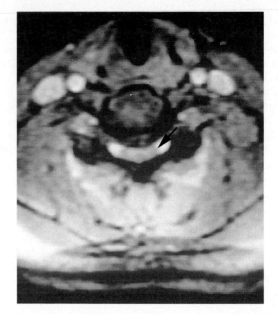

Figure 6.74.   CONGENITAL STENOSIS: A PREDISPOSING FACTOR TO NECK PAIN. MRI, Gradient-Echo Axial Cervical. The anteroposterior diameter of the spinal canal is narrowed, producing compression of the spinal cord (arrow). COMMENT: This condition arises as a result of congenitally short pedicles that reduce the dimensions of the spinal canal. The diminished osseous dimensions of the central canal predispose the spinal cord to injury, even with trivial trauma.

Figure 6.73.   DEGENERATIVE ENDPLATE: MODIC TYPE III. A. MRI, T1-Weighted Sagittal Lumbar. There is decreased signal intensity along the opposing vertebral endplates of L5-S1 (arrows). **B. MRI, T2-Weighted Sagittal Lumbar.** The previously identified marrow signal adjacent to the L5-S1 disc is unchanged (arrows). These findings are consistent with vertebral fibrosis and sclerosis. Incidentally, there is a hemangioma within the L4 vertebral body.

Spinal Stenosis

The term *spinal stenosis* refers to any narrowing of the spinal canal. This can occur as a result of congenitally short pedicles, (Fig. 6.74) or it can occur from a long list of acquired causes (see Chapter 10 for a complete list), which are beyond the scope of this chapter. This discussion will be limited to some general com-

ments concerning MR features of proliferation or thickening of the ligamentum flavum, bony proliferation creating the lateral recess syndrome, synovial cysts as a complication of facet joint disease, and degenerative spondylolisthesis.

Ligamentum Flavum Hypertrophy

The ligamentum flavum (ligamenta subflava) connects the lamina of the adjacent vertebrae from C2 to the first sacral segment. Each ligament consists of two lateral portions that commence on either side of the roots of the articular processes, and extend dorsally to the spinolaminar junction. Each consists of elastic tissue, thus the term *yellow ligaments* of the spine. In the cervical region, the ligaments are thin, but broad and long; they are thicker in the thoracic region and thickest in the lumbar region. These ligaments may undergo stress hypertrophy as a result of weight-bearing and degenerative processes on the facet structures. Patients with extensive facet arthrosis and joint instability may have a greater degree of ligamentum flavum hypertrophy. Flaval hypertrophy, if advanced, may produce posterior compression on the spinal cord or cauda equina, leading to localized or referred pain. Kirkaldy-Willis et al. (86) have succinctly described the stenosis associated with thickening of the ligamentum flavum in the posterior aspect of the spinal canal and discal or bony proliferation in the anterior aspect of the spinal canal, which they refer to as *front-to-back* stenosis. This may produce an hourglass indentation on the spinal cord or cauda equina and lead to significant neurologic symptoms.

While traditionally CT and CTM have been used in the evaluation of bony stenosis, MRI is felt by many (the authors included) to provide more useful information concerning the impact of the stenosis as it relates to the adjacent neurologic structures. The clinical relevance of demonstrating bony stenosis, ligamentum flavum hypertrophy, or facet joint arthrosis (creating lateral recess spinal stenosis) lies in determining what effect enlargement of these structures has on the surrounding soft tissue anatomy. MRI provides a precise evaluation of the dorsal root ganglion, exiting nerve roots, and cauda equina.

Synovial Cyst Formation

Synovial cysts are degenerative in nature and can occur in or adjacent to degenerative facet joints. (87,88) They may reach considerable size and cause localized back pain. On T1-weighted images, synovial cysts may be seen as low signal intensity masses in the posterior spinal canal. They may be better delineated with T2-weighting, as their fluid contents become hyperintense. (32) The key to the diagnosis is their location and the proximity of the cyst to the synovial joint. (Fig. 6.75) Although an unusual finding, gas-filled synovial cysts have been reported. This degenerative vacuum phenomenon may be present in the apophyseal joints, and the continuity of cysts with the synovial joint can allow gas to become entrapped within the cyst.

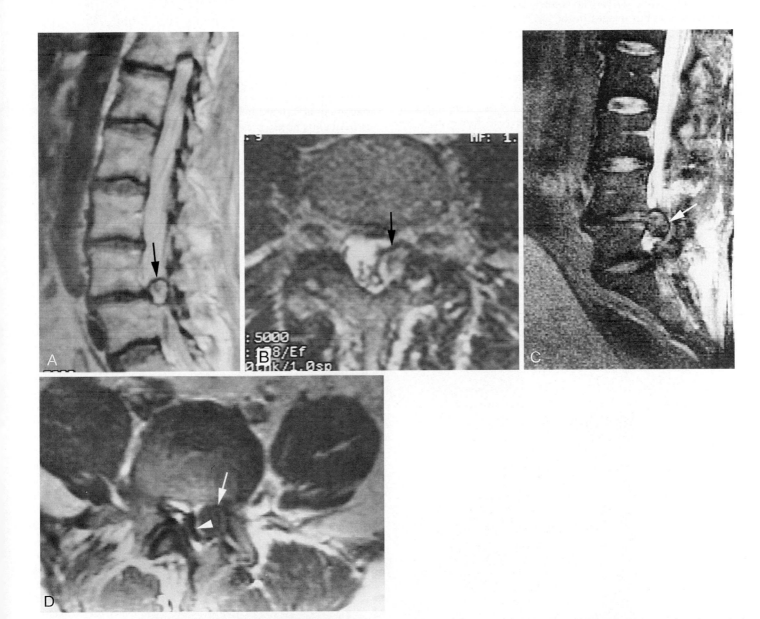

Figure 6.75.   SYNOVIAL CYST: LUMBAR SPINE. A. MRI, Proton Density-Weighted Sagittal Lumbar. There is an anterolisthesis of L4 on L5 associated with narrowing and decreased signal intensity within the disc. Note the well-defined, high signal intensity fluid collection (arrow) within the neural canal, posterior to the L4-L5 disc. **B. MRI, T2-Weighted Axial Lumbar.** The thin, low signal intensity margin of the cyst (arrow) surrounds the intermediate signal intensity joint fluid. This cyst is adjacent and contiguous with the apophyseal joint capsule. **C. MRI, T2-Weighted Sagittal Lumbar.** There is a large mass extending into the neural canal which appears contiguous with the L4-L5 disc (arrow). This finding is highly suggestive of a large disc her-

niation. **D. MRI, T1-Weighted Axial Lumbar.** The mass noted on the sagittal images is actually adjacent to and contiguous with the left apophyseal joint (arrow). Note the marked deformity of the left lateral thecal sac (arrowhead). COMMENT: A synovial cyst usually arises secondary to the capsular laxity and instability of the apophyseal joint. The enlarged capsule accumulates joint fluid, often resulting in a space-occupying mass within the spinal canal. Symptoms of compression may occur and occasionally necessitate aspiration of the cyst. (**C** and **D**, Courtesy of Robert A. Seigel, MD, St. Anthony Hospital, Denver, Colorado)

Ossification of the Posterior Longitudinal Ligament

Ossification of the posterior longitudinal ligament (OPLL) is a special subcategory of degenerative disease that can cause severe cervical spine and, sometimes, thoracic or lumbar spine stenosis. (89,90) It is characterized by marked multilevel hypertrophy and calcification (ossification) of the posterior longitudinal ligament, which may be seen on plain films when prominent. This disease is more common in Japanese patients, but its etiology is unknown. It may occur as an isolated entity in the cervical spine, or it may be associated with diffuse idiopathic skeletal hyperostosis (DISH). The diagnosis can be made on sagittal T1- and T2-weighted scans, but images in the axial plane are required for accurate detection of central canal compromise. (Fig. 6.76) The pattern of calcification and ossification can be quite irregular and often has a bizarre serpentine appearance. The most severe involvement usually occurs at the C4 to C6 levels and is seen as an irregular, low signal intensity area on T1-and T2-weighted images. Computed tomography yields the most accurate image of the ossified posterior longitudinal ligament. MRI, however, better demonstrates the impact of the ossification as it relates to the spinal cord and nerve roots.

Degenerative Spondylolisthesis

Degenerative spondylolisthesis is a forward displacement of a vertebral body secondary to extensive superior and inferior facet arthrosis. This is frequently associated with degenerative disc disease and is most commonly found at the L-Four segment in Females over the age of Forty (*the three F's of degenerative spondylolisthesis*). The absence of a pars defect (which would increase the sagittal dimensions of the central canal) results in narrowing of the anteroposterior diameter of the spinal canal, causing central spinal stenosis, in addition to lateral recess and neuroforaminal stenosis. The contours of the thecal sac have an hourglass or constricted outline. Because the vertebral body projects anterior and inferior in relation to the disc below, a *pseudodisc* appearance can be created on the CT or MR images. (91)

THE POSTOPERATIVE SPINE

Recurrent Disc Herniation Versus Epidural Scar: An Imaging Dilemma

The failed postoperative back syndrome is a diagnostic challenge to treating physicians, radiologists, and surgeons. Clinical assessment is difficult because the physical signs and symptoms are frequently nonspecific. Conventional radiography of the spine displays only the bony changes at laminectomy sites and the ossified fusion masses. CT myelography is an invasive procedure that may show certain conditions such as dural tears with cyst formation and arachnoiditis at the surgical site (92); however, it does not provide adequate information for the differentiation of epidural fibrotic scar from recurrent disc herniation. Today, mag-

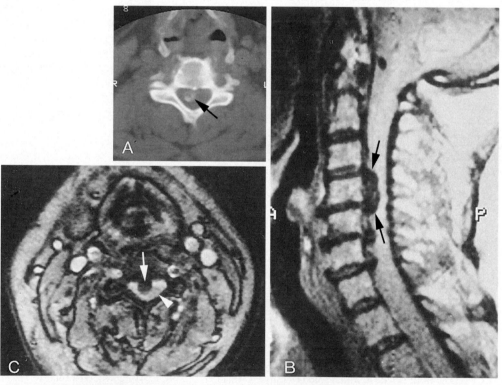

Figure 6.76.   OSSIFICATION OF THE POSTERIOR LONGITUDINAL LIGAMENT (OPLL). This 57-year-old male presented with transient motor weakness in the lower extremities. Movement of the head produced upper extremity motor weakness and an occasional shocklike pain into the upper extremities (Lhermitte's sign). **A. CT, Bone Window Axial Cervical** . Note the dense ossification immediately posterior to the vertebral body (arrow) within the posterior longitudinal ligament (PLL). The ossified ligament occupies a large portion of the neural canal, producing central spinal stenosis. **B. MRI, Proton Density-Weighted Sagittal Cervical. C. MRI, Gradient-Echo**

Axial Cervical. The lobulated, low signal intensity, ossified PLL (arrows) is situated in the ventral spinal canal and produces high grade extradural cord compression at multiple levels. Note the compressed and posteriorly displaced spinal cord (arrowhead). COMMENT: MRI provides optimal visualization of the spinal canal contents. There are numerous etiologies of spinal stenosis ranging from degenerative to neoplastic. The superior contrast resolution of magnetic resonance imaging makes it the ideal modality for differential diagnosis of these entities. (Courtesy of The Wood River Memorial Township Hospital, Department of Radiology, Wood River, Illinois)

netic resonance imaging has established itself as the modality of choice for imaging the postoperative spine. (93) The multiplanar imaging capability, superior soft tissue contrast resolution, and excellent tissue characterization are its major advantages. In addition, MR images of postoperative patients with orthopedic hardware (e.g., pedicle screws, Harrington rods, etc.) are superior to CT images. The signal void produced by these structures on MRI does not distort or obscure adjacent tissues. In contrast, an offensive metallic artifact that obscures adjacent structures is observed with CT. Most recently, gadolinium-DTPA–enhanced MRI of the spine has shown unparalleled sensitivity and accuracy in differentiating recurrent disc herniation from epidural scar tissue. (94)

What is Gadolinium's Role?

An epidural low signal intensity mass on T1-weighted images, with or without nerve root or spinal cord displacement, is the characteristic MR feature of disc herniation. The appearance is similar in the nonsurgical and postsurgical back. Surgical procedures often cause scar tissue to accumulate within the epidural space, adjacent to the nerve roots and posterior vertebral margin, often mimicking disc herniation. Differentiation between recurrent herniated nucleus pulposus and postsurgical scar is crucial because recurrent disc lesions may benefit from surgical intervention following failed conservative care, whereas epidural scar formation should not be treated surgically. Therefore Gadolinium-enhanced MR plays a key role in selecting the appropriate management for the postsurgical back pain patient. (Fig. 6.77)

Early imaging helps to differentiate these two entities. Following gadolinium injection there is limited, if any, enhancement of the herniated disc on early (6- to 10-minute) postinjection T1-weighted images, but enhancement appears on delayed (30- to 45-minute) images. (94) Conversely, scar tissue is relatively well vascularized and enhances soon after contrast administration.

The lack of early enhancement of the intervertebral disc is attributed to its relative avascularity. Its late enhancement is presumed to be caused by diffusion of contrast into the disc from surrounding vascular tissues. The criteria used to identify postoperative epidural scar are the same as for disc: morphology, location, presence or absence of mass effect, and gadolinium-enhancement characteristics.

MRI Findings. Morphologically, postoperative scar usually presents as an irregularly configured extradural mass with unsharp margination and is not typically contiguous with the disc. It is located along the surgical pathway and presumably arises as a result of tissue insult. The MR signal intensity characteristics of nonenhanced scar tissue depend on many factors, including scar morphology, fat content, chronicity, vascularity, specific location, inflammation (or absence thereof), and other various technical factors. A *young* scar, or scar in the immediate postoperative period, consists of budding granulation tissue that has high signal intensity on T2-weighted images. As the scar *ages*, fibrous elements predominate and the signal characteristics become hypointense on both T1- and T2-weighted images. Scar morphology and volume also seem to affect its signal intensity. When scar appears mostly in strands of tissue, it tends to have low signal intensity on both T1- and T2-weighted images. However, mass or bandlike scars more often demonstrate intermediate signal intensity. Some investigators have stated that the location of the scar influences its signal characteristics. (95) A difference between scars located anteriorly and posteriorly within the spinal canal has been reported. Laterally placed scar has a signal intensity somewhere between the two. Differentiation of epidural fibrosis from herniated disc material is crucial since reoperation on epidural scar often leads to a poor surgical outcome. Occasionally, recurrent

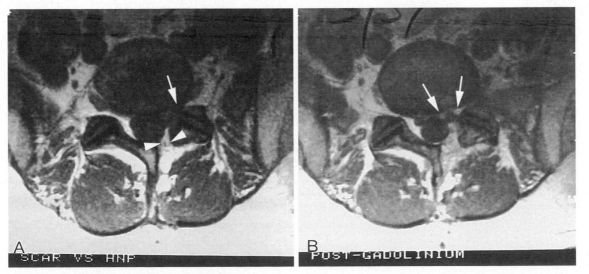

Figure 6.77.   CONTRAST-ENHANCED MRI: SCAR VERSUS DISC. This 47-year-old male underwent unilaminectomy 2 years ago for the diagnosis of acute HNP. Two years after surgery, his back pain returned and progressively worsened. His clinical differential diagnosis included recurrent herniation versus post-surgical scar. **A. MRI, T1-Weighted Axial Lumbar Without Contrast.** Note the large area of low signal intensity posterior to the disc (arrow). Is this scar or recurrent disc material? Observe the laminectomy defect with fat graft (arrowheads). **B. MRI, T1-Weighted Contrast-Enhanced Axial Lumbar.** There is mild enhancement of the mass in the ventral epidural space (arrows), consistent with scar tissue. COMMENT: Postoperative scar tissue is typically present in the anterior epidural space and may be confused with recurrent disc herniation or free fragment. The use of gadolinium is often necessary to differentiate scar from disc. Disc material is avascular and may enhance peripherally on postcontrast images because of the vascularity of the surrounding granulation tissue. Postsurgical scar tissue enhances throughout because of its extensive neovascularity. (Courtesy of Merritt L. Armstrong, DC, Freeport, Maine)

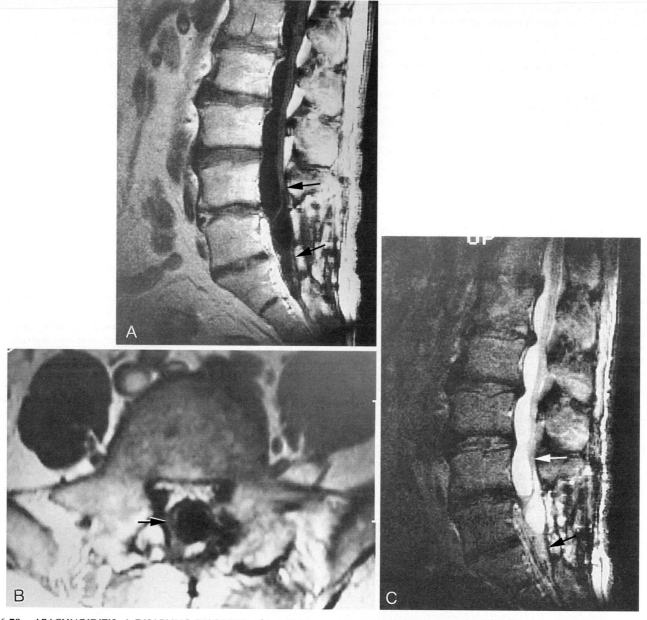

Figure 6.78.   ARACHNOIDITIS: A DISABLING DISORDER. This patient experienced five surgical procedures for low back pain and now complains of severe left lower extremity radiculopathy. **A. MRI, T1-Weighted Contrast-Enhanced Sagittal Lumbar. B. MRI, T1-Weighted Contrast-Enhanced Axial Lumbar.** The intermediate signal intensity rootlets of the cauda equina are adherent to the posterolateral aspect of the thecal sac (arrows). The central and lateral rootlets do not enhance and are not easily discernible. This finding is known as the *empty thecal sac sign* of arachnoiditis. Also note the

presence of a disc herniation at L1-L2 and posterior bulging of the L2-L3 disc. **C. MRI, T2-Weighted Sagittal Lumbar.** The high signal intensity CSF highlights the abnormal position of the cauda equina (arrows). COMMENT: Arachnoiditis occurs most frequently in the lumbar spine. Its etiologies include surgery, Pantopaque myelography complicated by hemorrhage, chymopapain injection, epidural steroid injection, and meningeal infection. Arachnoiditis results in severe and often unrelenting spinal pain. (Courtesy of Robert A. Seigel, MD, St. Anthony Hospital, Denver, Colorado)

disc herniation may be sequestered and wrapped in epidural scar tissue creating what has been referred to as the *wrapped* noncontained (sequestered) disc or *wrapped disc*. (74)

ARACHNOIDITIS

Arachnoiditis can result from several etiologies, including myelography, surgery, infection, and trauma. Symptoms include chronic intractable pain radiating into the extremities. No matter

what the etiology, arachnoiditis has a similar morphologic appearance on MR, myelography, and CT myelography. Clumping and irregular separation of nerve roots are characteristic of arachnoiditis and may obscure the demarcation of the conus medullaris from the cauda equina. (96) T1- and T2-weighted axial images optimally display the distortion of the thecal sac and nerve roots. Gadolinium enhancement increases the diagnostic yield in the evaluation of these patients. Often, central clumping of the nerve roots is visible as asymmetric rounded areas of intermediate signal intensity located centrally within the thecal sac. Adhesion of the nerve roots to the wall of the thecal sac may also be seen and has been termed the *empty thecal sac sign*. (96) (Fig. 6.78) Arachnoiditis may also affect the peripheral roots. If severe arachnoiditis is present, there may be complete obliteration of normal CSF signal by a soft tissue mass extending below the conus. Contrast-enhanced MRI is helpful in detecting arachnoiditis in its moderate to advanced stages or when standard spin-echo images are inconclusive.

MULTIPLE SCLEROSIS
CLINICAL CONSIDERATIONS

The diagnosis of multiple sclerosis (MS) is made on the basis of clinical symptoms, confirmatory paraclinical tests, imaging findings, and the exclusion of other neurologic diseases. (1) This common neurologic disorder most frequently affects young adults of northern European extraction. Pathologically, the disease is characterized by the cyclical appearance of *plaque-like* inflammation and demyelination of scattered areas throughout the central nervous system (CNS) white matter. The cause of the disease is unknown, but susceptibility is determined predominantly by multiple genetic variants.

Clinically, most patients have periodic remissions followed by relapses, with increasing neurologic deficit following each relapse. (2) After years, this clinical pattern becomes chronic and progressive. Less often the clinical course may be gradually or rapidly progressive from the onset. (3) The remarkably broad spectrum of clinical symptoms and signs has been well described in many clinical reviews. (4–9) Despite the dramatic advances in the laboratory evaluation of MS, the diagnosis still rests primarily on the clinical findings. Schumacher (10) has defined specific clinical criteria for the diagnosis of MS, requiring the demonstration of clinical abnormalities that implicate at least two noncontiguous CNS white matter sites and at least two relapses into gradual progression over 6 months. Patients must be evaluated by an experienced neurologist, and the symptoms expressed must be best explained by MS. This judgment is based mainly on the clinical demonstration of the multiplicity of neurologic events, separated by time and/or anatomic location, and partly on the knowledge of certain CNS sites that are involved more frequently with MS. (10)

LHERMITTE'S SIGN

Lhermitte's sign is classically defined as a rapid, *lightninglike, pins-and-needles* sensation into the upper and lower extremities on flexion of the head and neck. This sensation was first described by Marie and Chatelin in 1917. (11) During the next 25 years Lhermitte studied and discussed this sign (which came to bear his name) and arrived at the conclusion that it resulted from lesions in the posterior and lateral columns of the cervical spinal cord. (12) He believed the lesion was specifically linked to demyelination in the presence of axonal continuity and that it occurred commonly in patients with multiple sclerosis. (12) One-third of MS patients will experience Lhermitte's sign during their illness and this may be the presenting symptom of MS in more than 15% of patients. (13–15) In addition to MS, Lhermitte's sign may also be present in patients with cervical cord neoplasms, cervical spondylosis, radiation myelopathy, subacute combined degeneration, and head and neck trauma. (16)

MRI FINDINGS

MR imaging is the first and only imaging modality that allows direct visualization of the CNS plaques that characterize MS. Recently, the use of contrast (gadolinium) has made it possible to identify *acute* inflammation and *fresh* plaques in areas of chronic involvement. (17) Nesbit et al. (1) demonstrated excellent correlation between contrast enhancement and the histologic activity of lesions; all 29 histologically active lesions they studied showed enhancement, whereas no enhancement was observed in the four inactive lesions they evaluated. Because gadolinium enhances lesions that disrupt the blood-brain barrier, these observations substantiate the hypothesis that breakdown of this barrier in MS may be related to macrophage migration and infiltration, a relatively early histologic finding. In most instances the duration of clinical symptoms in patients with enhancing lesions range from 5 to 12 weeks. Persistence of enhancement beyond 12 weeks is unusual but has been documented. (18)

These features should lead to a better understanding of the natural history of this unpredictable disorder. Already, surprising results have been reported, with considerable disease activity occurring in patients without clinical evidence of relapse. (19) Serial MR imaging, with and without contrast enhancement, will also contribute greatly in monitoring the progress of the disease in clinical trials. MRI has already made it possible to virtually eliminate the use of other imaging techniques, such as CT and myelography, in excluding other diagnoses. In addition, MRI may eliminate certain paraclinical tests and prove complimentary to others in the diagnosis, management and clinical study of this disabling disorder.

Standard spin-echo and gradient-echo pulse sequences are often adequate in demonstrating suspected MS lesions. (Fig. 6.79) T1-weighted images provide anatomic localization of affected areas and may be performed before and after contrast to evaluate the integrity of the blood-brain barrier. T2-weighted dual echo images allow optimal assessment of the hyperintense plaques relative to the CSF and cerebral parenchyma. (Fig. 6.80) Unfortunately, there is a long list of disorders that exhibit similar imaging characteristics. The classic appearance of MS is one of multiple periventricular lesions with prolongation of the T1 and T2 relaxation times, appearing as low signal intensity foci on T1-weighted images that become high in signal intensity with T2-weighting. (20) These irregularly bordered lesions are usually less than 2.5 cm and have a *lumpy bumpy* appearance. (21) (Fig. 6.81) They may be homogeneous, or may have a thin rim of relative T2 hypointensity or T1 hyperintensity. (1) Infratentorial white matter lesions are common. Some of the MS lesions are ovoid and perpendicular to the long axis of the brain and lateral ventricles, a finding that appears to be quite specific for MS. (22)

Most patients with clinical symptoms of MS will have a positive MR head scan; however, 15% of affected individuals have lesions in the spinal cord with a negative MRI of the brain. (23) MS frequently targets the cervical cord, with the thoracic and lumbar regions of the cord involved in decreasing order of incidence. (16) In postmortem examinations posterior column plaques have been found in two thirds of MS patients. (24) The spinal cord plaques have the same imaging appearance as the cerebral plaques and can resemble spinal cord contusion. (25,26) (Fig. 6.82)

Patients who are suspected of having multiple sclerosis should

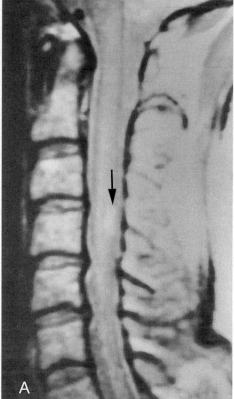

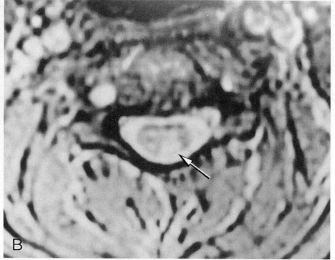

Figure 6.79. MULTIPLE SCLEROSIS PLAQUE: CERVICAL CORD. A. MRI, T1-Weighted Sagittal Cervical. B. MRI, Gradient-Echo Axial Cervical. Note the high signal intensity lesion in the spinal cord at the C4 level (arrows), consistent with a multiple sclerosis plaque.

Figure 6.80. MULTIPLE SCLEROSIS: INTRA-CRANIAL AND SPINAL CORD LESIONS. A. MRI, Proton Density-Weighted Sagittal Brain. Observe the multiple, high signal intensity lesions within the corpus callosum (arrows). These focal sites of myelin destruction and glial reaction represent the plaques of multiple sclerosis. **B. MRI, T2-Weighted Sagittal Cervical.** There is a solitary, high signal intensity plaque extending to the ventral margin of the cervical cord (arrow). COMMENT: MRI provides an accurate and non-invasive means for evaluation of multiple sclerosis in the brain and spinal cord. These plaques, however, may mimic cord injury or neoplasm. Focal hyperintense lesions of the brain or spinal cord must be correlated with other clinical or paraclinical (e.g., spinal tap, nerve conduction velocity) testing for the definitive diagnosis.

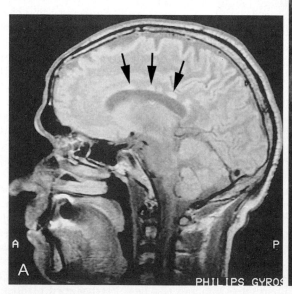

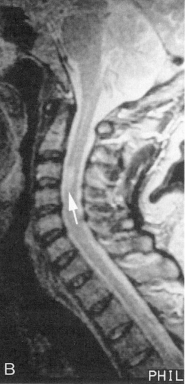

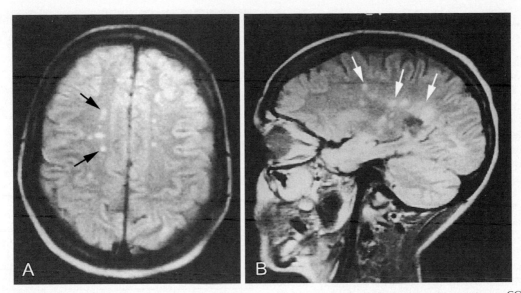

Figure 6.81.   MULTIPLE SCLEROSIS: BRAIN PLAQUES. This 34-year-old female presented with ataxia and complained of periodic tingling in the upper and lower extremities. **A. MRI, Proton Density-Weighted Axial Brain. B. MRI, Proton Density-Weighted Sagittal Brain.** Observe the multiple, discrete, round and oval lesions scattered bilaterally throughout the cerebral white matter (arrows). The lesions are hyperintense relative to the normal white matter. The increased signal intensity results from an initial inflammatory response and gliosis within the MS plaque. COMMENT: The clinical course of multiple sclerosis includes neurologic deficits that usually exhibit periodic exacerbations and remissions. The lesions of multiple sclerosis may be present in the brain and/or spinal cord. Contrast enhancement is of assistance in determining the acute versus chronic nature of the lesions and monitoring treatment. (Courtesy of George E. Springer DC, Clearwater, Florida and Kenneth B. Reynard, MD, Denver, Colorado)

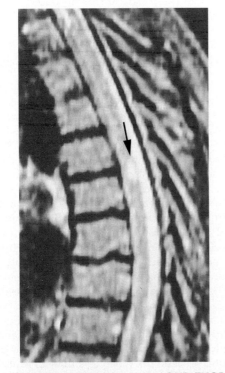

Figure 6.82.   MULTIPLE SCLEROSIS (MS) PLAQUE: THORACIC CORD. MRI, T2-Weighted Sagittal Thoracic. Note the high signal intensity lesion within the thoracic spinal cord (arrow). This appearance is consistent with an MS plaque. COMMENT: Fifteen to twenty percent of multiple sclerosis patients have a normal MR head scan with concurrent plaques in the spinal cord. The cervical, thoracic, and lumbar regions of the spinal cord should be imaged when clinically indicated to exclude MS plaques in the spinal cord.

have an MRI scan of the head performed before any other imaging modality. If the head scan is normal, a cervical, thoracic, or lumbar spine MRI scan should be performed to rule out MS plaques of the spinal cord. A negative brain MRI cannot be considered definitive in ruling out MS, since lesions of the spinal cord may exist. Additionally, an MRI scan of the head may be normal in patients with early clinical evidence of MS.

DIFFERENTIAL DIAGNOSIS

The differential diagnosis of multiple cerebral white matter lesions on MRI is extensive and includes vascular and inflammatory conditions of the CNS such as white matter ischemia/infarction, normal aging, vasculitis, radiation injury, moyamoya disease, acute disseminated encephalomyelitis, subacute sclerosing panencephalitis, brucellosis, viral encephalitis, AIDS, granulomatous diseases such as sarcoidosis and tuberculosis, and autoimmune diseases (systemic lupus erythematosus and others). (18,23,27–32)

The most common differential considerations are multiple white matter lesions from normal aging and/or white matter ischemic changes. They appear on T2-weighted images as small foci of increased signal within the white matter of the brain. Small ischemic foci are frequently noted in healthy patients more than 50 years of age, but they are relatively rare in healthy young people. These ischemic lesions have been referred to as *unidentified bright objects (UBOs)* and are associated with the vascular changes of normal aging. Notably, UBOs are randomly oriented; a key observation that often allows their differentiation from MS plaques, which are usually in a characteristic supraventricular or periventricular anatomic distribution.

THE HIP

INTRODUCTION

The large muscles of the thigh and pelvis, as well as the ball-and-socket nature of the articulation contribute to the exceptional stability of the hip. Common pathologies of this joint such as fracture (including stress fracture), arthritis, osteonecrosis, infection, reflex sympathetic dystrophy syndrome, dysplasia, and tumor can be demonstrated on magnetic resonance (MR) images. MRI is indicated when information obtained from conventional radiographs is inconclusive or equivocal. For example, soft tissue inflammatory processes (bursitis, capsulitis, tendinitis, myositis), muscular atrophy, hematomas, and neoplasms are well demonstrated with MRI. Because of the large size of the hip, MR examinations must be performed with a surface coil large enough to cover the entire joint. For comparison purposes it is recommended that both hip joints be imaged simultaneously in the axial and coronal planes. Sagittal images are not routinely performed but may be obtained to supplement the standard images. The use of intravenous contrast may be helpful in detecting certain subtle pathologies such as infection, arthritis, and tumor.

High-resolution MR images clearly display the normal, hyperintense bone marrow of the adult femoral head and neck, surrounded by the hypointense cortex. It should be noted that the signal intensity of the bone marrow varies with age. The hematopoietic (red) marrow is low in signal intensity compared with the bright, fatty (yellow) marrow. In children and young adults the femoral neck, because of its red marrow content, often contains hypointense areas, compared with the hyperintense, fatty epiphyseal region. The conversion from hematopoietic to fatty marrow occurs in a symmetric fashion from the distal end of the long bone to the proximal portion. Marrow reconversion may occur when the demand on the body's hematopoietic system is increased and it becomes necessary to enhance hematopoiesis by converting the ends of the long bones from fatty marrow back to red marrow. This process occurs in some trained marathon runners (sports anemia) (1) and in hematologic disorders. (2)

OSTEONECROSIS OF THE HIP

This disorder is also referred to as avascular necrosis (AVN) or ischemic necrosis of bone. Osteonecrosis or in situ death of a segment of bone is still a challenge for radiologists, pathologists, and clinicians alike. This discussion is confined to adult onset osteonecrosis, which can occur in association with a myriad of clinical disorders. A long list of causes of unilateral and bilateral femoral head osteonecrosis is offered. (Table 6.3)

Medullary bone infarcts represent a form of osteonecrosis that is usually clinically silent; affecting only the marrow cavity and its trabecular architecture. Only when both the medullary bone and surrounding cortex are involved, is the process termed osteonecrosis. (2,3)

Magnetic resonance imaging is the most sensitive imaging modality for detection of osteonecrosis, especially at the early stages of the disease. It is more sensitive than nuclear bone scans. Osteonecrosis occurs most frequently in the immediate subchondral regions of the proximal femur, distal femur, and the proximal humerus. (2,3) Early osteonecrotic lesions are seen as focal, subchondral areas of abnormal signal intensity. (Fig. 6.83) Typically, these lesions are surrounded by a rim of low signal intensity on

Table 6.3. Conditions Associated with Avascular Necrosis of the Femoral Head	
Unilateral	**Bilateral**
Common	
Spontaneous (idiopathic)	Alcoholism
Surgery	Corticosteroid therapy
Trauma (fracture, dislocation)	Spontaneous (idiopathic)
Uncommon	
Gout	Arteriosclerosis
Hemophilia	Caisson disease
Infection	Cushing's disease
	Gaucher's disease
	Hemoglobinopathy
	Lupus erythematosus
	Pancreatitis
	Pheochromocytoma
	Rheumatoid arthritis
	Sickle cell anemia

T1-weighted images, creating a ringlike appearance. This *double line* or *ring* pattern is comprised of a low signal intensity band surrounding a central high signal intensity area. (Fig. 6.84) These signs are seen on both T1- and T2-weighted images and are pathognomonic of early osteonecrosis. At a later stage the necrotic lesion becomes hypointense on both T1- and T2-weighted images. Other late signs include deformity, collapse, and sclerosis of the femoral head. (4–8) These signs are readily observed on plain film radiographs and carry a poor prognosis.

CORE DECOMPRESSION FOR HIP OSTEONECROSIS: A CONTROVERSIAL TREATMENT MODALITY

Since osteonecrosis of the hip is relentless in its progression, it behooves the clinician to establish the diagnosis early and seek treatment modalities that are aimed at arresting the progression of this disease. Steinberg (9) has reported uninhibited progression of osteonecrosis to arthroplasty in 80% of patients, regardless of the stage at clinical presentation. Progression of the disease is inevitable in all patients who present with evidence of femoral head collapse. (9)

Core decompression is a relatively new surgical procedure that has met with some degree of success in the treatment of early femoral head osteonecrosis. Supporters claim this procedure alleviates the elevated intraosseous pressure, permitting neovascularization and restoration of the vascular supply. (10) If the osteonecrosis is diagnosed early, core decompression may save the femoral head from collapse and obviate the need for hip arthroplasty. (Fig. 6.85)

Beltran et al. (10) have described a method of assessing the risk of femoral head collapse following core decompression by preoperatively evaluating the extent of femoral head involvement by the necrotic process. (3) When less than 25% of the weight-bearing surface of the femoral head is involved, femoral head collapse is unlikely. With 25 to 50% involvement, femoral head collapse occurred in 43% of the patients. With greater than 50% involvement, femoral head collapse occurred in 80% of the hips examined. The time interval from surgical procedure to collapse was typically 6½ months. It is important for the clinician to realize that if a significant area of the femoral head is involved (indicated

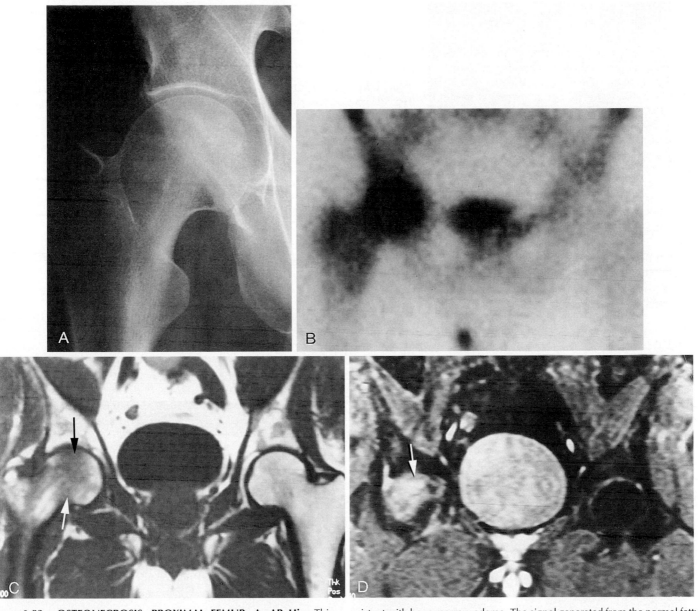

Figure 6.83. OSTEONECROSIS: PROXIMAL FEMUR. A. AP Hip. This exam is normal. **B. Bone Scan, Anterior Pelvis.** There is marked tracer uptake within the right femoral head and neck. **C. MRI, T1-Weighted Coronal Pelvis.** Observe the diffuse low signal intensity within the right femoral head (arrows) consistent with bone marrow edema and suggestive of osteonecrosis. **D. MRI, Short T1 Inversion Recovery (STIR) Coronal Pelvis.** The large area of hyperintense signal within the right proximal femur (arrow) is con-

sistent with bone marrow edema. The signal generated from the normal fatty marrow within the opposite hip is suppressed, appearing very low in signal (black). COMMENT: STIR sequences can be of great value in imaging the musculoskeletal system since it suppresses the signal of fat while enhancing the signal intensity generated by subtle fluid accumulation. (Courtesy of Patrick J. Russmano, DC, Easton, Pennsylvania)

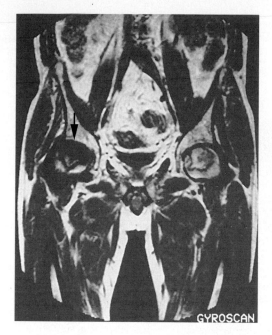

Figure 6.84. BILATERAL HIP PAIN: OSTEONECROSIS. MRI, T1-Weighted Coronal Hip. The central hyperintense signal within both femoral heads is surrounded by a low signal intensity margin. This represents the *double line sign* of osteonecrosis. The central area of hyperintense signal represents reparative granulation tissue and marrow edema, while the hypointense signal has been described as either reactive sclerosis and/or fibrosis. The right femoral head also demonstrates a diffuse, low signal intensity area within the subchondral bone and flattening of the femoral head (arrow). These findings are consistent with necrotic bone and reactive sclerosis. (Courtesy of Frank E. Seidelmann, DO; Kingsley A. Orraca-Tetteh, MD; and Matthew M. Brown, RT(R), Advanced MRImaging, Richmond Heights, Ohio)

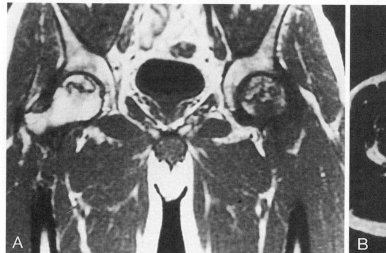

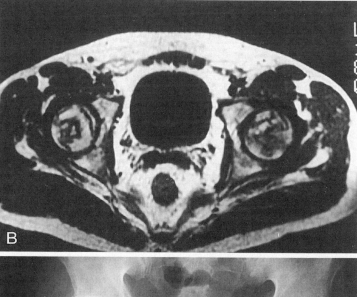

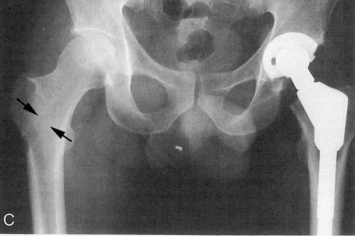

Figure 6.85. IDIOPATHIC OSTEONECROSIS: BILATERAL HIP. This 38-year-old male presented with bilateral hip pain of increasing severity. There was no history of steroid use or trauma. **A. MRI, T1-Weighted Coronal Bilateral Hip. B. MRI, T1-Weighted Axial Bilateral Hip.** Both hips are affected by the disease process, but the larger area of mixed signal intensity is seen on the left. Both femoral heads display a central high signal intensity area and a surrounding hypointense halo, consistent with the *double line sign* of osteonecrosis. This halo of low signal intensity represents fibrous tissue or sclerosis surrounding the central area of active granulation tissue. **C. Bilateral AP Hip.** A core decompression with residual tracking artifact is noted within the right proximal femur (arrows). This patient underwent a left total hip arthroplasty. COMMENT: Approximately 3 years following core decompression there is no evidence of disease progression.

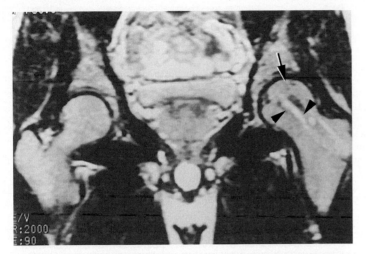

Figure 6.86.   PAINFUL HIP: NEGATIVE RADIOGRAPHS. This 40-year-old patient was involved in a motor vehicle accident and sustained trauma to his left hip. His hip pain persisted, but radiographs of the area were unremarkable. A core decompression was performed based on the initial MRI (not shown), which suggested early osteonecrosis. **MRI, T2-Weighted Coronal Pelvis.** Note the subtle heterogeneous signal intensity within the left femoral head (arrow). A core decompression artifact is noted tracking through the proximal femur to the subchondral bone of the femoral head (arrowheads). This patient's hip pain resolved and a 2-year follow-up MRI (not shown) demonstrated no evidence of osteonecrosis or femoral head deformity. COMMENT:Core decompression is a controversial surgical technique used to alleviate the elevated intraosseous pressure, permitting the revascularization of necrotic bone and often halting the osteonecrotic process.

by volumetric evaluation of the ischemic changes), subchondral collapse may occur following core decompression, despite the initial absence of subchondral fracture on conventional plain film radiographs. (10)

The key to this clinical decision is early diagnosis; therefore MR imaging should be performed as early as possible in any patient with risk factors for osteonecrosis and persistent hip pain. The core decompression procedure may provide a window of opportunity to halt the progression of the osteonecrosis in patients with early disease. (Fig. 6.86) Even though the procedure may fail in these patients, the risk may be worth taking since most are destined for total hip replacement, regardless of the treatment employed.

BONE MARROW EDEMA OF THE HIP

This poorly understood abnormality has been described in the literature as a nonspecific, yet distinct, entity and as a precursor to osteonecrosis. (11) In addition, it has been reported in association with other conditions such as transient osteoporosis of the hip (TOH) (12–18), osteomyelitis (19), infiltrative neoplasms (20), and posttraumatic bone bruise. (21)

MR imaging characteristics of bone marrow edema (BME) include a diffuse, heterogeneous pattern of decreased signal intensity on T1-weighted images. This area becomes hyperintense with T2-weighting and involves most of the femoral head, often extending into the femoral neck and intertrochanteric region. The increased signal intensity seen on the T2-weighted images is consistent with increased free water or edema within the normal fatty marrow. (6,22–24) Vande Berg et al. (25) emphasize the importance of high-resolution T2-weighted images in distinguishing

between osteonecrosis and other conditions associated with bone marrow edema. With BME, there is typically no evidence of an underlying, focal subchondral defect, a finding that is usually suggestive of osteonecrosis. (25)

THE OCCULT HIP FRACTURE: A NEW ASSESSMENT PROTOCOL

One of the most difficult orthopedic challenges is the demonstration of occult fractures of the hip in the elderly patient. Often, plain film x-rays are inadequate or equivocal. Bone scan and CT deliver a significant radiation dose to the patient and may not render a definitive answer.

Mink and Deutsch (21) have suggested the use of coronal T1-weighted MR images to demonstrate bone marrow edema associated with occult fractures of the hip. MRI provides a magnificent imaging modality to identify these occult fractures because of its ability to detect areas of abnormal marrow signal (bone marrow edema).

In a cost-conscious health care environment, the authors suggest that an abbreviated MRI examination of the hip using T1-weighted coronal images be considered for the detection of hidden fractures in patients with the appropriate clinical manifestations and equivocal plain films. (Fig. 6.87) The overall scan time for this examination is diminished (no more than 15 minutes), allowing a significantly reduced fee. We recommend that the clinician forgo the needless radiation and expense of a bone scan or CT and go directly to a *limited* MRI scan of the hip.

TRANSIENT OSTEOPOROSIS OF THE HIP

This condition was first reported in 1959 by Curtis and Kincaid (26) as a rare disorder that was seen primarily in the third trimester of pregnancy. Currently, it is more frequently described in young and middle-aged persons and has a male predominance. (27) The clinical presentation consists of the spontaneous onset of hip pain that is progressive over several weeks. A history of minor trauma may or may not be reported. (27–29) In the early stage, conventional plain films may be normal. Usually within 3 to 6 weeks there is severe osteoporosis of the subchondral bone and loss of the subchondral cortex adjacent to the femoral head and neck. The acetabulum may be affected in some cases, but the joint space is unaffected. (18) In some patients similar lesions may develop in the opposite hip or in other joints (regional migratory osteoporosis). (29) Bone scintigraphy demonstrates homogeneously increased uptake in the femoral head, with lesser involvement of the neck. These findings are seen prior to radiographic changes.

Transient osteoporosis of the hip (TOH) may progress to osteonecrosis. Conversely, complete resolution of the clinical and imaging manifestations of TOH usually occurs without specific treatment in 2 to 6 months. The exact cause of transient osteoporosis of the hip is uncertain, but its mechanism may be similar to that of reflex sympathetic dystrophy syndrome, suggesting a neurogenic origin. Minor trauma, neurovascular dysfunction, synovitis, and transient ischemia (also called *reversible* osteonecrosis) have been reported in association with TOH. (27,29)

The MRI signal changes in TOH are related to an increased amount of free water (edema). The T1-weighted images demonstrate diffuse, hypointense bone marrow edema involving the femoral head, neck, and intertrochanteric area. (Fig. 6.88) With T2-weighting, the lesion has a hyperintense signal that may also

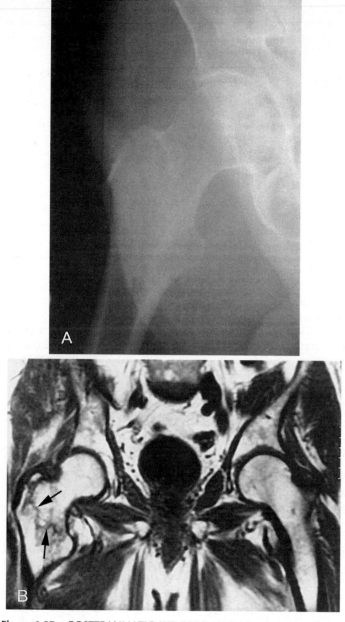

Figure 6.87. POSTTRAUMATIC HIP PAIN: LIMITED MRI SCAN. A. AP Hip. The plain films were normal. **B. MRI, T1-Weighted Coronal Pelvis**. Note the spiderlike, low signal intensity pattern and surrounding marrow edema within the intertrochanteric region of the right femur (arrows). These findings are consistent with an occult fracture of the proximal femur. COMMENT: The superior contrast resolution of MRI increases the likelihood of detecting occult fractures and their complications. A limited MR scan, using only coronal slices, can provide valuable information in patients suspected of having an occult hip fracture. This examination can be performed without the expense of a complete MRI exam or the use of bone scan or CT. (Courtesy of Steven R. Nokes, MD, Baptist MRI, Little Rock, Arkansas)

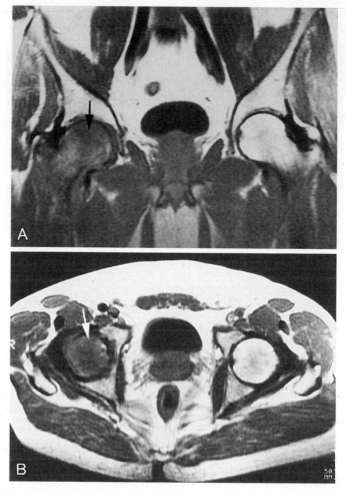

Figure 6.88. TRANSIENT OSTEOPOROSIS OF THE HIP: A CLINICAL ENIGMA. The radiographs of this patient (not shown) revealed osteopenia of the right hip. **A. MRI, T1-Weighted Coronal Hip. B. MRI, T1-Weighted Axial Hip.** Note the diffuse loss of signal intensity in the right femoral head and neck (arrows). On T2-weighted images (not shown) this low signal intensity area became hyperintense, consistent with transient osteoporosis. COMMENT: Transient osteoporosis of the hip is a controversial and poorly understood disorder. The clinical presentation is variable and MRI plays an important role in establishing the differential diagnosis and excluding other pathology such as osteonecrosis. Patients with this disorder usually recover with conservative management.

STRESS FRACTURE OF THE HIP

This type of injury often occurs as a result of overload and is frequently diagnosed in the femoral neck of long-distance runners (particularly in marathoners). The osteoporotic female population is also at risk for developing stress fractures of the hip. These are actually *insufficiency fractures* and may occur with trivial trauma or normal activity. Often these injuries are not visible on conventional plain radiographs. On MR images the fracture line appears hypointense on both T1- and T2-weighted images. It is usually surrounded by a broad, ill-defined, hypointense area of edema on T1-weighted images that becomes hyperintense with T2-weighting. (4) (Fig. 6.89) Other pathologies such as osteomyelitis and arthritis may also have the same MR characteristics.

involve the acetabulum. These changes are often ill-defined and heterogeneous, especially on long TR/TE images. Minimal to moderate joint effusions may be detected. (16,18) As with scintigraphy, MRI is positive before the changes are demonstrated on plain radiographs. When this condition is suspected clinically, the MR images should be obtained first.

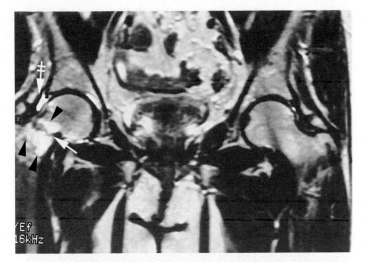

Figure 6.89.   STRESS FRACTURE: FEMORAL NECK. MRI, T2-Weighted Coronal Pelvis. Observe the low signal intensity fracture line traversing the right femoral neck (arrow). In addition, there is a region of hyperintense signal adjacent to the fracture, representing bone marrow edema (arrowheads). Minimal intracapsular edema is evident (crossed arrow). COMMENT: Stress fractures characteristically present as a linear decrease in signal intensity on T1-weighted images and remain low in signal with T2-weighting. The edema associated with the fracture is also hypointense on T1-weighted images, but brightens with T2-weighting.

MISCELLANEOUS BONE AND SOFT TISSUE MASSES OF THE THIGH

Numerous bone and soft tissue lesions may occur about the hip and proximal femur. Characterization of these lesions often is not possible without biopsy. However, if some basic principles of MR image interpretation are observed and correlated with the patient's clinical history and paraclinical examination findings, the differential diagnosis can be narrowed.

Iliopsoas Bursitis

As the psoas tendon crosses over the iliopectineal eminence of the pubis, it may cause inflammation of the iliopsoas bursa. Clinically, the patient may experience pain and a "snapping" sensation with internal and external rotation activities. (30) The MRI appearance of these lesions is characteristic of similar cystic soft tissue masses. On T1-weighted images the lesion appears isointense or slightly hypointense to the surrounding musculature and brightens with T2-weighting. (Fig. 6.90)

Malignant Fibrous Histiocytoma

Malignant fibrous histiocytoma is the most common soft tissue sarcoma occurring in late adult life. (30,31) These lesions generally occur in the lower extremities of patients greater than 50

Figure 6.90.   AN INGUINAL MASS: HISTORY OF RIGHT HIP PAIN. This patient's history includes an inguinal hernia and the recent onset of right hip pain. At examination a slightly pulsatile soft tissue mass was noted on deep palpation. **A. CT, Soft Tissue Window Axial Pelvis.** Note the cystic, low-attenuation mass immediately anterior to the right femoral head (arrow). **B. MRI, Proton Density-Weighted Axial Pelvis.** The previously noted area of decreased attenuation on the CT displays a homogenous low signal intensity (arrow). **C. MRI, T2-Weighted Axial Pelvis.** Observe the homogeneous hyperintense signal intensity in this localized fluid collection (arrow). These findings are representative of iliopsoas bursitis.

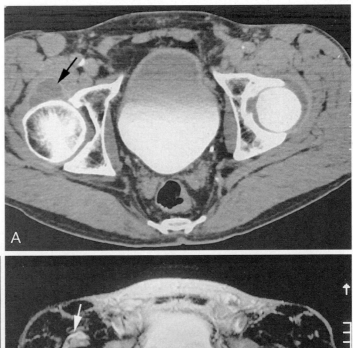

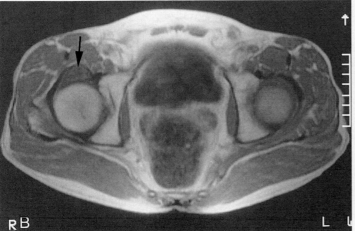

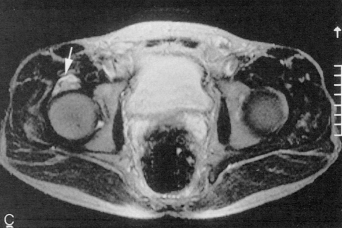

years of age. Radiographic changes include the presence of a large soft tissue mass that may calcify. (31) These lesions are frequently 5 to 10 cm at the time of diagnosis and can cause adjacent cortical erosion or periostitis. (31)

The MRI features of malignant fibrous histiocytoma are non-specific. Typically, a multinodular, well circumscribed mass that demonstrates inhomogeneous signal on conventional spin-echo images is observed. Low to intermediate signal intensity areas are seen on T1-weighted images, and areas of hyperintense signal are seen with T2-weighting. This mixed signal pattern has been described as the *bowl of fruit* appearance (32) and is a reflection of the variable distribution of hemorrhage, necrosis, and calcification. A variable pattern of contrast enhancement is usually observed. (Fig. 6.91)

Aneurysmal Bone Cyst

Aneurysmal bone cyst (ABC) is a benign neoplastic-like lesion that most commonly affects the axial and proximal appendicular skeleton, but may occur in any bone. These lesions generally occur in younger patients (10 to 30 years of age) and are usually primary, but may be seen in association with numerous other benign and malignant preexisting neoplasms (i.e., giant cell tumor, fibrous dysplasia, osteosarcoma, and chondromyxoid fibroma). (30,33) Those lesions that affect the long bones occur most frequently in the metaphysis. Radiographically, ABCs are eccentric, expansile lesions that frequently exhibit a *soap bubble* appearance.

Aneurysmal bone cysts contain varying amounts of blood,

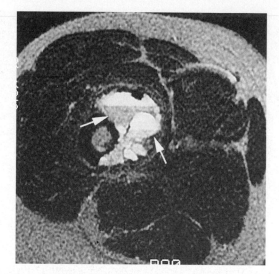

Figure 6.92. ANEURYSMAL BONE CYST: FLUID-FLUID LEVEL. MRI, T2-Weighted Axial Thigh. Observe the expansile nature of the eccentrically positioned aneurysmal bone cyst that destroys the outer two-thirds of the femoral cortex, but does not extend into the medullary cavity. The thin cortical rim seen on plain films (not shown) is not well demonstrated on these images. A characteristic fluid-fluid level is present. No soft tissue invasion is seen, consistent with the benign nature of this lesion. COMMENT: The fluid-fluid level arises from the settling of blood products to the dependent portion of the lesion (arrows), similar to the plasma red-blood-cell interface of centrifuged blood. The hyperintense proteinaceous fluid is less dense and rises to the less dependent portion of the lesion. This finding is highly suggestive, of, but not exclusive to, aneurysmal bone cyst. (Courtesy of Ronald N. Baxter, MD, Denver, Colorado)

fluid, and fibrous tissue. (30) These factors and their relative prevalence within the lesion are responsible for its heterogeneous MR appearance. Generally, ABCs have areas of internal septation with areas of bright signal on both T1- and T2-weighted or gradient-echo images, depending on the chronicity of the associated hemorrhage (34). *Fluid-fluid* levels may be present and probably represent layering of uncoagulated blood and blood products (specifically, methemoglobin). (30) (Fig. 6.92) Fluid-fluid levels are most commonly seen with aneurysmal bone cysts; however, the differential diagnosis also should include giant cell tumor, chondroblastoma, hemangioma, fibrous dysplasia, simple bone cyst, osteosarcoma, synovial sarcoma, and even metastasis. (32,33)

Chondrosarcoma

Chondrosarcoma represents the third most common primary malignant neoplasm. These lesions most frequently affect individuals in the fourth to sixth decade of life. Chondrosarcomas may be primary (arising de novo) or secondary (arising in existing benign cartilaginous lesions undergoing malignant degeneration) and characteristically involve the axial or proximal appendicular skeleton.

On standard spin-echo and gradient-echo images these lesions are large and heterogeneously low in signal, relative to the normal fatty marrow. (Fig. 6.93) A significant soft tissue component is often present. Higher-grade, more cellular lesions are generally more heterogeneous. (35) T2*-weighted images are sensitive to low signal intensity calcifications that are frequently present within the otherwise hyperintense tumor. (30)

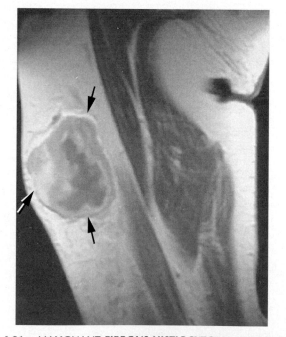

Figure 6.91. MALIGNANT FIBROUS HISTIOCYTOMA: ELDERLY MALE WITH A PAINFUL THIGH MASS. MRI, T1-Weighted Contrast-Enhanced Sagittal Thigh. There is a sharply defined mass (arrows) with inhomogeneous signal intensity located in the musculature of the anterior thigh. The central lower signal intensity is surrounded by moderately increased signal intensity. Minimal contrast enhancement is noted when compared with the noncontrast images (not shown). COMMENT: Malignant fibrous histiocytoma is the most common soft tissue sarcoma occurring in the adult and is most frequently located in the thigh.

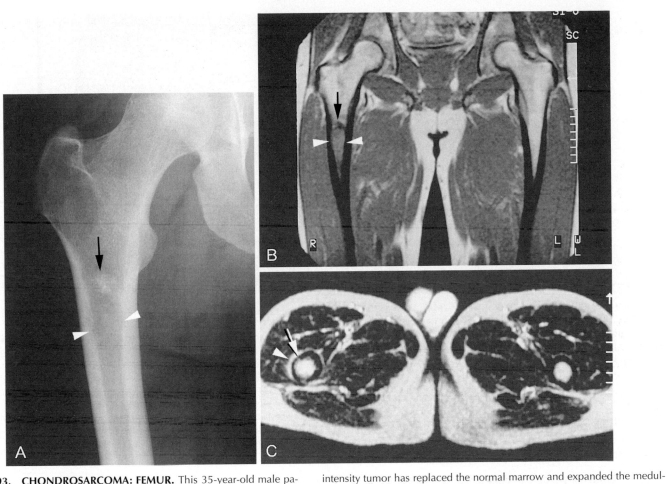

Figure 6.93. CHONDROSARCOMA: FEMUR. This 35-year-old male patient presented with a deep ache in his right hip. **A. AP Spot Hip.** Observe the intramedullary, stippled calcification (arrow) in the right femoral diaphysis. There is a subtle radiolucency with early endosteal erosion of the femur (arrowheads). **B. MRI, T1-Weighted Coronal Pelvis.** Observe the low signal intensity intramedullary calcification (arrow). The intermediate signal intensity tumor has replaced the normal marrow and expanded the medullary space (arrowheads). The contralateral side is normal. **C. MRI, T2-Weighted Bilateral Axial Femur.** Tumor infiltration has caused endosteal erosion (arrow). The high signal intensity region along the cortical perimeter represents edema (arrowhead). No cortical fracture or soft tissue tumor invasion is identified.

THE KNEE

Magnetic resonance imaging is now recognized as the *gold standard* in imaging of the knee. With the use of a dedicated extremity coil, high-resolution images can be obtained with detailed information concerning the bone marrow, cortex, cartilage, menisci, ligaments, tendons, and surrounding synovium. (Fig. 6.94) MR evaluation of the knee can be performed in sagittal, axial, and coronal planes, with 3 to 4 mm slice thickness. With three-dimensional (3-D) volume acquisitions, thinner slices can be acquired (1 mm or less). In contrast to arthrography, MRI can obtain information in multiple planes without movement of the knee (which is an integral part of the arthrographic examination). This section briefly describes the conditions of the knee that are best imaged by MRI, and is not intended to be an all-inclusive list.

MEDIAL MENISCUS

The medial meniscus is asymmetric in the sagittal plane with the posterior horn being longer, taller, and wider than the anterior horn. Viewed axially, the medial meniscus has a *banana*-shaped appearance with a wider radius of curvature than its lateral counterpart. (1) Because of its fibrocartilage content, it appears on all pulse sequences as an area of homogeneously low signal intensity.

Meniscal lesions are seen as areas of increased intrameniscal signal that may or may not extend to the articular surface. Frank tears more commonly affect the posterior horn of the medial meniscus because of its steeper concavity and firm ligamentous attachments. Conversely, horizontal degenerative tears are more common laterally. (2–7) The posterior medial meniscal body is the most common site for myxoid degenerative change. This appears as a thin, relatively hyperintense (gray) line on a proton density- or T1-weighted image with a *V shape* that often communicates with the peripheral capsular surface. Meniscal cysts are far less common on the medial side than the lateral side, but when they occur medially, they are often giant and painless and may extend posteriorly (rarely anteriorly). (1)

LATERAL MENISCUS

The lateral meniscus is seen as a symmetric *bow tie* signal void in the sagittal plane on at least one or two slices. When visualized in the axial plane, it has a *C shape* with its radius of curvature being smaller than the medial meniscus. The more medial sections demonstrate two triangular horns (anterior and posterior)

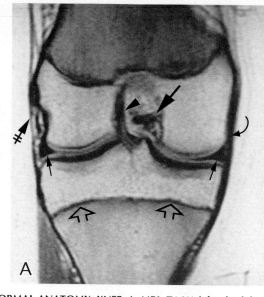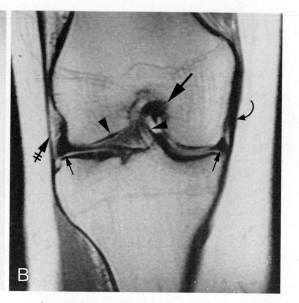

Figure 6.94. NORMAL ANATOMY: KNEE. A. MRI, T1-Weighted Adolescent Knee. B. MRI, T1-Weighted Coronal Adult Knee. The adult knee is a slightly more anterior slice, which explains the differing appearance of the cruciate ligaments. The posterior cruciate ligament (large arrows) is always seen as a homogeneous low signal intensity structure that attaches at the lateral aspect of the medial femoral condyle. This ligament runs in a caudal direction from its insertion on the femur to its tibial insertion. The anterior cruciate ligament (arrowheads) is of either low or intermediate signal intensity with interspersed areas of hyperintense signal. Striations are often visualized. Anteriorly, this ligament has a "*fanlike*" insertion on the lateral aspect of the tibial spines and narrows as it extends in a cephalad direction along the medial aspect of the lateral femoral condyle. The menisci (small arrows)

are homogeneous areas of triangular low signal. The lateral collateral ligament (crossed arrows) is seen as a homogeneous linear area of low signal extending from the lateral femoral condyle to the fibular head. The thicker, more firmly attached medial collateral ligament (curved arrows) is seen extending from the medial epicondyle of the femur to the proximal tibial metaphysis, several centimeters inferior to the tibial plateau. This low signal intensity structure is poorly differentiated from the signal void originating from the adjacent bony cortex. Observe the distinct margin delineating the fatty marrow within the epiphysis from the red marrow in the metaphyses in the adolescent patient (open arrows). A residual physeal scar is seen in a similar location in the adult patient.

that appear as symmetric triangles. The anterior horn of the lateral meniscus is quite variable in its height and overall length. Hypoplasia of this horn is not uncommon. Volume averaging of the anterolateral meniscal recess, its interface with the anterolateral horn, and the transverse ligament of Winslow may create the false impression of a horizontal meniscal tear. (1) Tears of the lateral meniscus are less common than medial meniscal tears. This has been attributed to its greater mobility, stemming from its looser peripheral attachments.

GRADING SYSTEM FOR MENISCAL LESIONS

Assessing the MR characteristics of meniscal abnormalities is crucial in guiding the clinician to the most effective form of treatment. (Fig. 6.95) The following grading system (Table 6.4) has been offered by Pomeranz (1) and Stoller. (6)

Grade I

A grade I meniscal abnormality represents a nonarticular, globular or focal, intrasubstance, increased signal intensity. This correlates pathologically with early mucinous degeneration. (6) This has also been referred to as myxoid or hyaline degeneration with a focal accumulation of mucopolysaccharide ground substance in stressed or strained areas of the meniscal fibrocartilage. (6) These changes usually occur in response to mechanical loading and degeneration. Grade I signal alterations may be observed in asymptomatic athletes and normal volunteers and are usually not clinically significant. (6)

Grade II

A grade II meniscal abnormality presents on MRI as a horizontal line of increased signal intensity, usually extending to the capsular periphery of the meniscus, but *not reaching either meniscal articular surface*. (6) Pathologically, the increased signal is thought to represent microscopic clefting and collagen fragmentation with areas of hypocellularity within the fibrocartilaginous matrix. (6) Patients with grade II meniscal abnormalities may or may not present with symptoms of knee pain. However, it should be noted that grade II meniscal abnormalities may be a precursor to frank (grade III) tears. This is especially common in the posterior horn of the medial meniscus, which is the most common location of grade II lesions. (6)

Grade III

Grade III meniscal tears exhibit an area of increased signal intensity that communicates or *extends to at least one articular surface*. (6) These areas of high signal represent confined intrasubstance cleavage tears. Diagnosis of these closed meniscal tears requires surgical probing during arthroscopy. These lesions might be missed altogether on arthrographic examination. (6) Grade III tears have been subdivided by Pomeranz (1) into grades IIIa and IIIb, as defined in Table 6.4. These represent complex intrameniscal cleavage tears. Grade III tears are the most symptomatic of all the meniscal abnormalities. Some may require surgical intervention, and most should at least be referred for orthopedic consultation before any rehabilitative exercises are per-

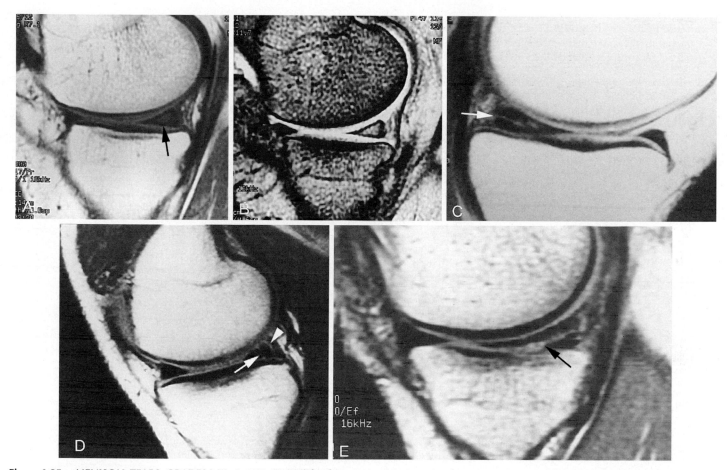

Figure 6.95.   MENISCAL TEARS: GRADES I-III. A. MRI, T1-Weighted Sagittal Knee. B. MRI, T2*-Weighted Sagittal Knee. Note the hyperintense signal within the posterior horn of the medial meniscus on the T1-weighted image (arrow). On the T2*-weighted sequence this area becomes very hyperintense. This finding is consistent with myxoid degenerative change in a grade I meniscal lesion. (Courtesy of Frank E. Seidelmann, DO; Kingsley A. Orraca-Tetteh, MD; and Matthew M. Brown, RT(R), Advanced MRImaging, Richmond Heights, Ohio) **C. MRI, T1-Weighted Sagittal Knee.** There is a linear hyperintense area horizontally positioned within the posterior horn of the medial meniscus (arrow). This finding is consistent with a *grade II* (degen-erative) meniscal tear. **D. MRI, T1-Weighted Sagittal Knee.** There is a vertical hyperintense signal extending to both the superior and inferior articulating surfaces of the posterior horn of the lateral meniscus (arrow). This finding is consistent with an *acute grade III* meniscal tear. The second vertical hyperintense signal (arrowhead) represents the meniscofemoral attachment and should not be confused with a vertical meniscal tear. **E. MRI, T2-Weighted Sagittal Knee.** There is a horizontally oriented meniscal tear extending to the inferior articulating surface of the posterior horn of the medial meniscus (arrow). This finding is consistent with a grade III tear.

Table 6.4.	Meniscal Grading Table*
Grade 0	Homogeneously black signal
Grade I	Subtle intermediate high signal that is rounded or ovoid (invariably asymptomatic)
Grade II	Linear intermediate signal with "V" shape communicating with the capsular surface of the meniscus (may be symptomatic or asymptomatic)
Grade IIIa	Linear signal alteration communicating with the articular surface of the meniscus (usually a symptomatic lesion)
Grade IIIb	Complex high-signal alterations that are intermediate and that communicate with the articular and capsular surface (usually symptomatic, often requiring surgical intervention)

*From Pomeranz SJ: *Orthopedic and Sports Medicine MRI Review Lecture Notes.* Cincinnati, OH: MRI Education Foundation, 1993; and Stoller DW: *Magnetic Resonance Imaging in Orthopaedics and Sports Medicine.* Philadelphia, JB Lippincott, 1993.

formed. Typically, the more peripheral the tear, the greater the likelihood that conservative (nonsurgical) management will be successful.

Parrot beak, horizontal cleavage, flap, and *bucket handle* tears are all different types of grade III meniscal tears. (Figs. 6.96, 6.97) Bucket handle tears occur secondary to acute injury and are severely symptomatic, usually requiring surgical intervention. Type III tears (either *a* or *b*) may assume a vertical or horizontal orientation, or they can occur in a complex multidirectional orientation, depending on the extent of injury.

Meniscocapsular separations usually involve the medial meniscus and occur peripherally at the meniscocapsular attachment. These are poorly demonstrated on conventional MR images, but are seen well with specialized radial slices through the medial compartment. (6) Because these injuries occur at the periphery, adjacent to the perimeniscal vessels, they usually heal spontaneously.

The classic *Big 3* injury to the knee, or *O'Donoghue's Unhappy Triad* (8), has been defined as follows (Fig. 6.98):

1. A grade III tear of the posterior horn of the medial meniscus.
2. A partial or complete tear of the medial collateral ligament.
3. A partial or complete tear of the anterior cruciate ligament.

Accordingly, close inspection of the anterior cruciate ligament and medial collateral ligament for injury is always advised in patients with a grade III tear of the posterior horn of the medial meniscus.

DISCOID MENISCUS

Discoid meniscus is a congenital anomaly. The lateral meniscus, which is more frequently affected, assumes a biconcave disc-like shape on the coronal and sagittal images. The midportion of the meniscus (the space between the anterior and the posterior horns), can be seen on three or more consecutive sagittal slices. (9) (Fig. 6.99) This finding should be confirmed on the coronal

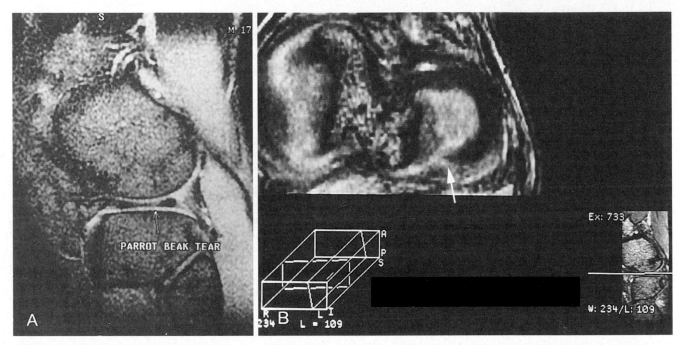

Figure 6.96.   PARROT-BEAK TEAR: POSTERIOR HORN, LATERAL MENISCUS. A. MRI, T2*-Weighted Far Lateral, Sagittal Knee. B. MRI, 3-D Volume Acquisition, Axial Knee. Note the subtle hyperintense signal within the posterior horn of the medial meniscus (arrows). (Courtesy of Frank E. Seidelmann, DO; Kingsley A. Orraca-Tetteh, MD; and Matthew M. Brown, RT(R), Advanced MRImaging, Richmond Heights, Ohio)

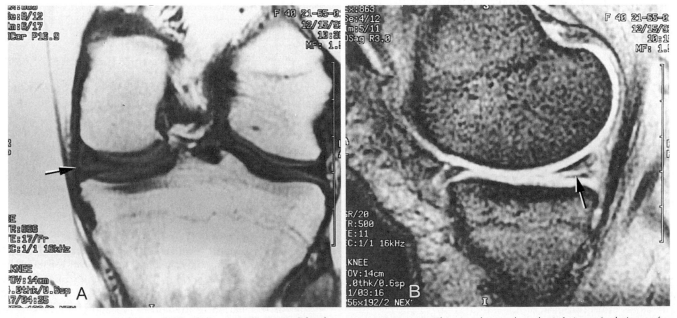

Figure 6.97.   GRADE III MENISCAL TEAR: KNEE. A. MRI, T1-Weighted Coronal Knee. B. MRI, T2*-Weighted Sagittal Knee. There is an area of horizontally oriented hyperintense signal within the posterior horn of the medial meniscus on both the T1-weighted and T2*-weighted pulse se-quences (arrows). This signal extends to the inferior articulating surface and is consistent with a horizontal cleavage tear. (Courtesy of Frank E. Seidelmann, DO; Kingsley A. Orraca-Tetteh, MD; and Matthew M. Brown, RT(R), Advanced MRImaging, Richmond Heights, Ohio)

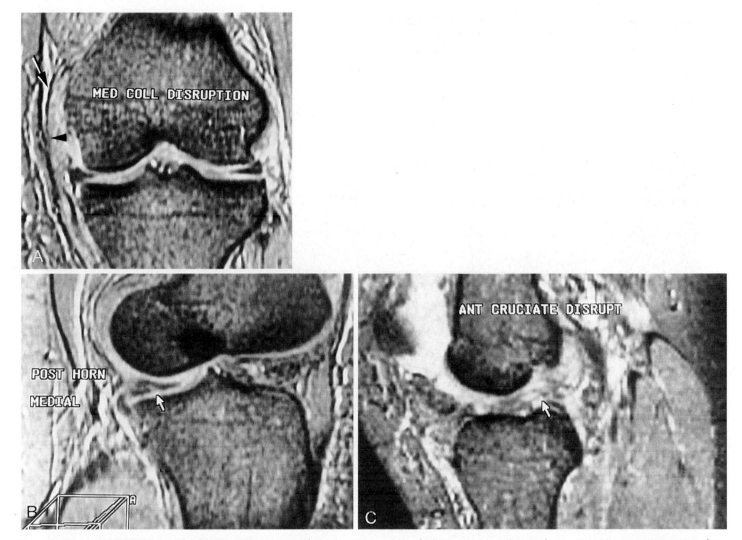

Figure 6.98.   O'DONOGHUE'S UNHAPPY TRIAD: KNEE. This 21-year-old sustained a football injury and complained of severe and persistent knee pain. **A. MRI, 3-D Volume Acquisition Coronal Knee.** The medial collateral ligament (MCL) is normally seen as a thin, low signal intensity band coursing along the medial joint space (arrow). The MCL of this individual is interrupted by a hyperintense signal (arrowhead), consistent with a tear. Also note the displacement of the ligament secondary to the adjacent effusion. **B. MRI, 3-D Volume Acquisition Sagittal-Oblique Knee.** High signal intensity interrupts the meniscus and extends to the opposing articular surfaces (ar-

row). This is consistent with a grade III meniscal tear. **C. MRI, 3-D Volume Acquisition Sagittal Knee.** The anterior cruciate ligament (ACL) is poorly seen and obscured by high signal intensity swelling and edema (arrow). These findings suggest disruption of the ACL. COMMENT: The triad of ACL, MCL, and posterior horn medial meniscus tears (O'Donoghue's Unhappy Triad) is typically a result of significant valgus forces that disrupt the medial joint compartment. (Courtesy of Kenneth B. Reynard, MD, Center for MRI, Ltd., Denver, Colorado)

images. The discoid meniscus is mostly seen in children and may manifest clinically by a *click* during flexion and extension of the knee (snapping knee syndrome). There is a higher incidence of meniscal lesions in these individuals, probably because of its abnormal thickness and anomalous tibial attachment.

MENISCAL CYST

A meniscal cyst is a collection of mucinous or synovial fluid that arises in association with some meniscal tears. This may present as a giant painless mass on the medial side, but is smaller and 10 times more common on the lateral side. (1) The cyst may extend to the joint space or more anteriorly toward the infrapatellar fat-pad. It is usually well defined and can be multiloculated. These cystic masses are best demonstrated in the axial and coronal planes and are low in signal intensity on T1-weighted im-

ages, becoming hyperintense with T2-weighting. (Fig. 6.100) The differential diagnosis includes ganglion, capsular cyst, and bursitis. (10)

ANTERIOR CRUCIATE LIGAMENT

The anterior cruciate ligament (ACL) is attached to the posteromedial aspect of the lateral femoral condyle. It extends inferiorly and medially to the anterior tibial intercondylar area, where it inserts between the anterior attachments of the menisci. (6) Its function is to prevent anterior translation of the tibia and resist posterior translation of the femur. Normally, it courses parallel to the *Blumensaat line*, a line drawn along the posterior surface of the femoral notch on the midsagittal images. (11)

The ACL is approximately 11 to 12 mm thick and, in the most frequently scanned position, appears straight and taut without

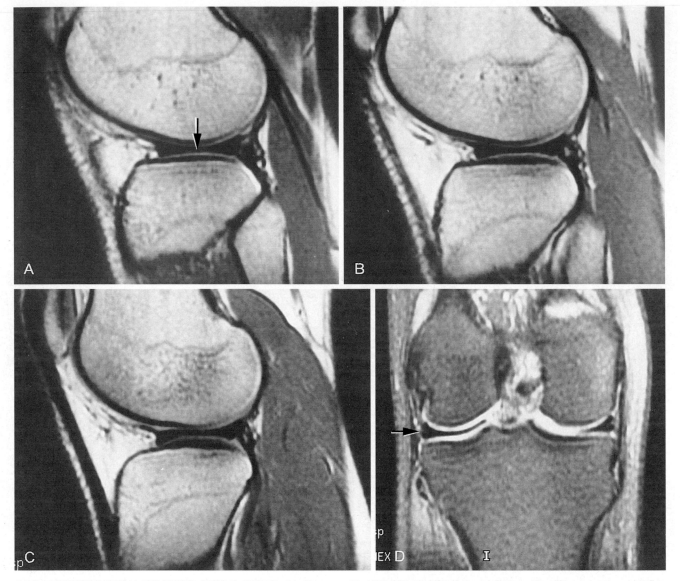

Figure 6.99.   DISCOID LATERAL MENISCUS: KNEE. A. MRI, Proton Density-Weighted Sagittal Knee. B. MRI, Proton Density-Weighted Sagittal Knee. C. MRI, Proton Density-Weighted Sagittal Knee. As the slices progress from lateral to medial (**A–C**), note the absence of separation of the low signal intensity lateral meniscus (arrow) into anterior and posterior horns.

D. MRI, T2*-Weighted Coronal Knee. The lateral meniscus is abnormally thickened (arrow). COMMENT: The discoid meniscus is a congenital anomaly that most frequently involves the lateral meniscus. This anomaly results in an increased prevalence of meniscal degeneration and tearing. (Courtesy of Kenneth B. Reynard, MD, Center for MRI, Ltd., Denver, Colorado)

angulation. (6) Its MR signal intensity is intermediate to hypointense. The tibial attachment is *fanlike* and its two separate bundles (anterolateral and posteromedial) are sometimes seen in the lateral aspect of the femoral tunnel on the coronal images. (Fig. 6.101) The intermediate signal observed along its distal tibial insertion is caused by the presence of synovial sheath thickening. (1) The ACL and its femoral attachment are best seen in the sagittal plane.

MRI Findings

Magnetic resonance can accurately demonstrate tears of the ACL. The diagnosis is based on direct and indirect signs (11,12) visualized on sagittal T1- and T2-weighted images. The *direct* signs of ACL tear include focal or diffuse intermediate signal intensity areas within the substance of the ligament on proton density–weighted images that become hyperintense with T2-weighting, a wavy contour of the ligament or lack of continuity, and the inability to visualize the structure. (11–14) (Fig. 6.102) These signs have a sensitivity of 93% and a specificity of 97%. (11) *Indirect* signs include a horizontal orientation of the ACL (11), a bone bruise or osteochondral fracture at the posterolateral aspect of the tibia and lateral femoral condyle (called *kissing contusions*) (11,12), (Fig. 6.103) anterior displacement of the tibia or *anterior drawer sign* (11), an abnormally high arc or buckling of the posterior cruciate ligament (11,15), and posterior displacement of the lateral meniscus (secondary to the anterior tibial displacement). (11,16) ACL tears are more frequently observed than PCL tears because the ACL is only half as thick as the PCL. *O'Donoghue's unhappy triad* (8) is frequently found accompanying anterior cruciate ligament tears.

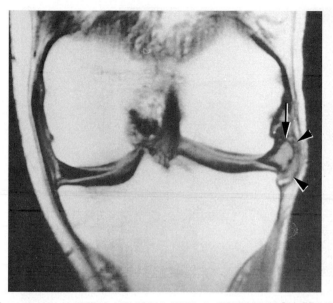

Figure 6.100. LATERAL MENISCAL CYST: A COMPLICATION OF ME-NISCAL TEAR. This patient complained of chronic lateral knee pain. **MRI, T1-Weighted Coronal Knee.** There is a horizontal tear of the lateral meniscus associated with a meniscal cyst (arrow). This cyst displaces the lateral joint capsule (arrowheads). COMMENT: Meniscal cysts are benign fluid collections that occasionally complicate meniscal tears. Initially intrameniscal, the cyst may enlarge and expand the meniscus peripherally, displacing the joint capsule. Meniscal cysts may present as a giant painless mass on the medial aspect of the joint, but are smaller and 10 times more common on the lateral side.

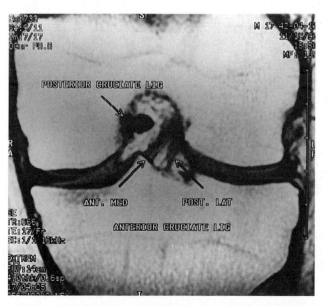

Figure 6.101. MRI OF THE KNEE: NORMAL ANATOMY REVISITED. MRI, T1-Weighted Coronal Knee. Note the circular low signal intensity of the normal posterior cruciate ligament and the fanlike insertion of the antero-medial and posterolateral fibers of the anterior cruciate ligament. (Courtesy of Frank E. Seidelmann, DO; Kingsley A. Orraca-Tetteh, MD; and Matthew M. Brown, RT(R), Advanced MRImaging, Richmond Heights, Ohio)

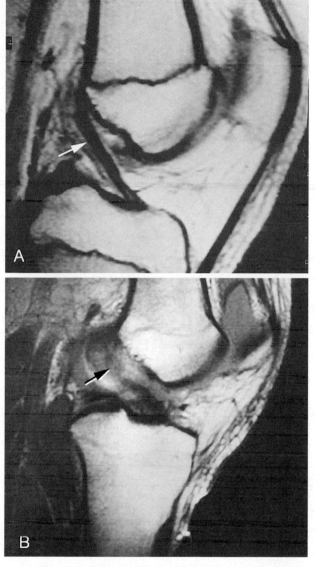

Figure 6.102. ANTERIOR CRUCIATE LIGAMENT (ACL) TEAR. A. MRI, Proton Density-Weighted Sagittal Knee. Note the normal low signal intensity ACL in this pediatric patient (arrow). The ACL originates on the lateral femoral condyle posteriorly and courses caudally in an anteroinferior direction to insert on the lateral portion of the intercondylar area of the tibia. Anterior translation of the tibia and posterior translation of the femur are limited by this ligament. **B. MRI, Proton Density-Weighted Sagittal Knee.** The ACL has been avulsed from its proximal femoral attachment (arrow). Note the retraction of the ligament and surrounding hemorrhagic edema.

POSTERIOR CRUCIATE LIGAMENT

Both the anterior and posterior cruciate ligaments are intracapsular and extrasynovial. The posterior cruciate ligament (PCL) originates at the lateral aspect of the medial femoral condyle, crosses the ACL, and attaches to the posterior intercondylar portion of the tibia. (Fig. 6.101) The PCL is viewed as a central stabilizer of the knee, resisting posterior tibial displacement on the femur when the knee is flexed. (17–19) Posterior to the PCL, the ligament of Wrisberg connects with the posterior horn of the lateral meniscus and inserts on the medial femoral condyle. (17,19) The ligament of Humphrey passes anterior to the PCL. The ligaments of Humphrey and Wrisberg are taut in flexion and exten-

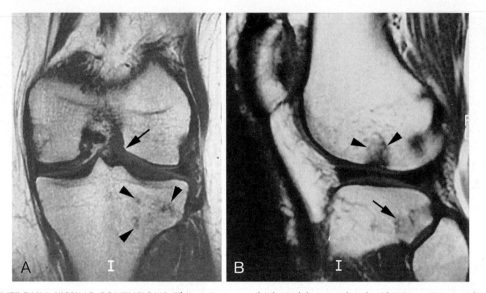

Figure 6.103.   ACUTE KNEE PAIN: KISSING CONTUSIONS. This patient sustained a twisting injury to the knee during a recent football game. A complete plain film radiographic evaluation of the knee (not shown) was normal. **A. MRI, T1-Weighted Coronal Knee.** Note the intermediate signal intensity within the distal anterior cruciate ligament (arrow), consistent with hemorrhage and edema within and around the ligament. The lack of discernible fibers within the ligament is suggestive of a complete tear. Low signal intensity areas are noted within the subcortical bone of the lateral tibial condyle (arrowheads). This is consistent with a bone contusion. **B. MRI, T1-Weighted Sagittal.** This far lateral sagittal slice demonstrates low signal intensity within the posterior aspect of the lateral tibial plateau (arrow) and lateral femoral condyle (arrowheads). These findings are consistent with bone contusions. (Courtesy of Frank E. Seidelmann, DO; Kingsley A. Orraca-Tetteh, MD; and Matthew M. Brown, RT(R), Advanced MRImaging, Richmond Heights, Ohio)

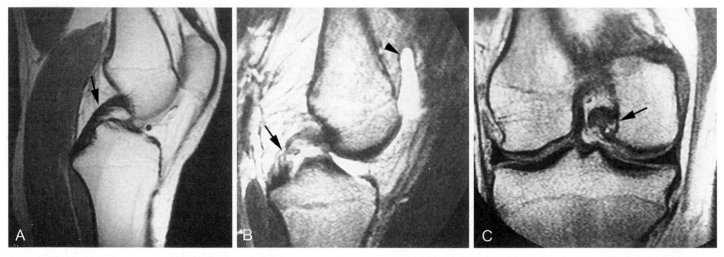

Figure 6.104.   POSTERIOR CRUCIATE LIGAMENT (PCL): NORMAL VERSUS TEAR. A. MRI, T1-Weighted Sagittal Knee. The PCL is identified in virtually every examination of the knee and is seen in its entirety on this single slice. It arises from the posterior surface of the intercondylar region of the tibia and attaches on the lateral surface of the medial femoral condyle, having an *inverted hockey stick* appearance. The PCL maintains a low signal intensity throughout and is broader and thicker than the anterior cruciate ligament (ACL). **B. MRI, T2-Weighted Sagittal Knee**. Observe the increased signal intensity with interruption and distortion of the midportion of the PCL (arrow). Note the posterior subluxation of the tibia (posterior drawer sign). Additionally, there is a large hyperintense suprapatellar effusion (arrowhead). **C. MRI, T2-Weighted Coronal Knee.** There is a heterogeneous signal intensity of the slightly enlarged PCL (arrow), consistent with a tear. COMMENT: PCL tears require significant trauma, greater than that required to tear the ACL. MRI is the only imaging modality that offers a completely noninvasive evaluation of the injured knee.

sion, respectively. The PCL is generally 15 to 20 mm thick, uniformly hypointense (black), more curved than the ACL, and assumes an *inverted hockey stick* appearance when the knee is extended on sagittal images. (19) It may appear taut with knee flexion or buckled with knee hyperextension. This buckling may be mistakenly interpreted as an indication of an ACL tear, since buckling of the PCL is one of the indirect signs of ACL laxity. The PCL is twice as strong as the ACL, with a larger cross-sectional area and higher tensile strength. These features account for the lower incidence of rupture of the PCL. (17,19) Tears of the PCL represent approximately 4 to 20% of knee ligament injuries. (17,19)

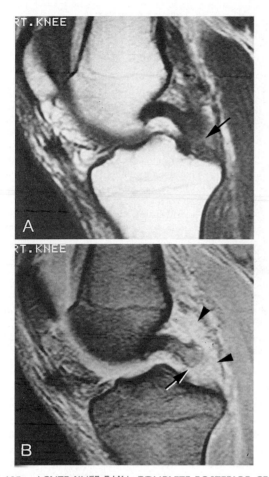

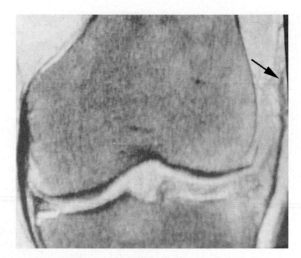

Figure 6.106.   LATERAL COLLATERAL LIGAMENT TEAR: KNEE. MRI, T2*-Weighted Coronal Knee. The thin, low signal intensity of the lateral collateral ligament is displaced laterally and does not attach at its femoral insertion (arrow). These findings are consistent with a grade III sprain.

Figure 6.105.   ACUTE KNEE PAIN: COMPLETE POSTERIOR CRUCIATE LIGAMENT (PCL) TEAR. A. MRI, T1-Weighted Sagittal Knee. Note the diffuse, intermediate signal intensity at the distal aspect of the posterior cruciate ligament (arrow). Its insertion on the proximal tibia is not definitely visualized. **B. MRI, T2*-Weighted Sagittal Knee.** The distal portion of the PCL is retracted in a proximal fashion away from its insertion on the tibia (arrow). Note the hyperintense signal within and surrounding the ligament (arrowheads), representing hemorrhage and edema. COMMENT: Complete tears of the posterior cruciate ligament usually do not occur as isolated injuries and require a significant force to create a complete tear. (Courtesy of Frank E. Seidelmann, DO; Kingsley A. Orraca-Tetteh, MD; and Matthew M. Brown, RT(R), Advanced MRImaging, Richmond Heights, Ohio)

MRI Findings

Partial tears are seen as focal or diffuse swelling of the ligament with intermediate signal intensity on T1-weighted images, becoming hyperintense with T2-weighting. In cases of complete rupture, there is obvious discontinuity or a gap of the ligament on both T1- and T2-weighted images. These findings can be seen in the sagittal plane, and are confirmed on coronal slices. (Fig. 6.104) Avulsions of the ligament occur at either the femoral or tibial attachment and are better visualized on the sagittal slices. (Fig. 6.105) Focal bone detachments or avulsion (*flake*) fractures are frequent additional findings at either attachment site. (8,19)

LATERAL COLLATERAL LIGAMENT

The lateral aspect of the knee is divided into three structural layers. The outermost layer consists of the iliotibial band, while the quadriceps retinaculum and patellofemoral ligaments comprise the middle layer. The deepest layer consists of the lateral joint capsule. The lateral collateral ligament, or fibular collateral ligament, is 5 to 7 cm long. It is extracapsular and free from meniscal attachments in its course from the lateral femoral epicondyle to its conjoined insertion into the biceps femoris tendon and fibular head. (6)

The lateral collateral ligament is a major contributor to the lateral stability of the knee joint. Injuries to the lateral collateral ligament (LCL) are far less common than injuries to the medial side. However, they are more difficult to diagnose clinically and are more disabling. Sprains of the LCL are accompanied by hemorrhagic edema surrounding the ligament, which is hyperintense on T2- and T2*-weighted images (Fig. 6.106). A partial tear is seen as a focal enlargement or deformity of the ligament on both T1- and T2-weighted images. When the ligament is completely ruptured, there is a typical wavy irregularity of the ligament contour, surrounded by fluid. Other lesions such as ACL and meniscal tears, as well as bone bruises, may also accompany these injuries. (20–22)

MEDIAL COLLATERAL LIGAMENT

The medial collateral ligament (MCL), or tibial collateral ligament, is 8 to 10 cm long and extends from its medial epicondylar origin to attach 4 to 5 cm inferior to the tibial plateau and posterior to the pes anserinus insertion. (6) The MCL is composed of two layers; one superficial and one deep. These layers are separated by a small bursa and a thin layer of peribursal fat that helps reduce friction during knee flexion.

Valgus stress to the flexed knee represents the major mechanism of MCL injury. Coronal and axial MR images reliably display MCL sprains and the associated hemorrhage or edema. Partial tears result in varying degrees of incomplete ligament disruption. Complete tears are often displaced and are better visualized on T2- and T2*-weighted images. (Fig. 6.107) Frequent additional findings include meniscocapsular separation and medial meniscal and ACL tears. (23)

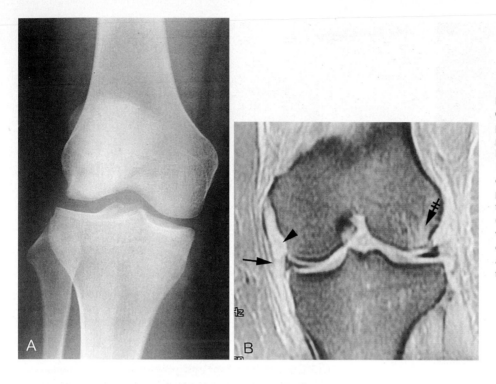

Figure 6.107.   COMPLETE TEAR OF THE MEDIAL COLLATERAL LIGAMENT: KNEE. This football player complained of knee pain following a "clipping" injury. **A. AP Knee.** This exam is normal. **B. MRI, T2*-Weighted Coronal Knee.** Observe the interruption of the thin, low signal intensity medial collateral ligament (arrow). The ligament is displaced from the medial tibial condyle by a collection of high signal intensity hemorrhage and edema (arrowhead). Also note the hyperintense signal within the subchondral bone of the lateral femoral condyle, consistent with a bone contusion (crossed arrow). (Courtesy of Kenneth B. Reynard, MD, Center for MRI, Ltd., Denver, Colorado)

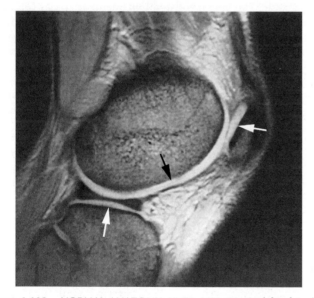

Figure 6.108.   NORMAL ANATOMY: KNEE. MRI, T2*-Weighted Sagittal Knee. This pulse sequence allows superb visualization of the hyperintense hyaline articular cartilage (arrows). Note the low signal intensity of the fatty marrow. On this far lateral sagittal image, slices are taken through the body of the meniscus creating an unseparated *bow-tie* appearance of the lateral meniscus.

THE ARTICULAR CARTILAGE

Because of its multiplanar capabilities and its ability to produce soft tissue contrast better than plain film or CT, MRI is ideal for imaging the articular cartilage. (17,18,24–28) The assessment of traumatic or degenerative cartilage lesions is important, especially for preoperative planning. MRI is an accurate means for detecting and staging moderate and advanced patellar cartilage lesions. (17) The detection of damage to the cartilage in degen-

erative and inflammatory arthritides may be helpful in the application of effective therapy.

MR imaging of the cartilage with thin slices is recommended to avoid volume averaging artifacts. High spatial resolution and tissue contrast between fluid and cartilage is necessary for accurate assessment of generalized cartilage thinning, focal lesions at the cartilaginous surface, and secondary changes in the subchondral bone. The optimum plane of imaging is perpendicular to the cartilaginous surface of interest. Several MR sequences can been used to image the cartilage. Spin-echo T1-weighted images adequately display morphologic changes in the cartilage. T2- and T2*-weighted images provide an arthrographic effect, allowing the detection of cartilaginous surface defects, sclerosis, and subchondral edema. Proton density-weighted images are also helpful in that they provide some T2-weighted properties coupled with good anatomic detail.

With T2*-weighted sequences both cartilage and fluid appear hyperintense and are difficult to differentiate. (29–33) (Fig. 6.108) More recently, fat-suppressed spin-echo techniques have been used to assess both surface and internal cartilaginous lesions with satisfactory results. (34–36)

CHONDROMALACIA PATELLAE

Chondromalacia patellae is defined as pathologic softening of the patellar cartilage and is probably associated with patella alta and patellar tracking disorders. There are two different processes that can affect the patellar cartilage: *surface degeneration*, which is an age-related process, and *basal degeneration*, which is a breakdown of the cartilage that begins with fibrillation of the cartilaginous fibers. Chondromalacia patellae is usually progressive in nature and in most cases advances to a severe irreversible stage. (37)

Four stages of chondromalacia patellae have been described. Three of these stages are well demonstrated on T1-, T2-, and T2*-weighted axial images. (17,18) MRI is not sensitive to stage I le-

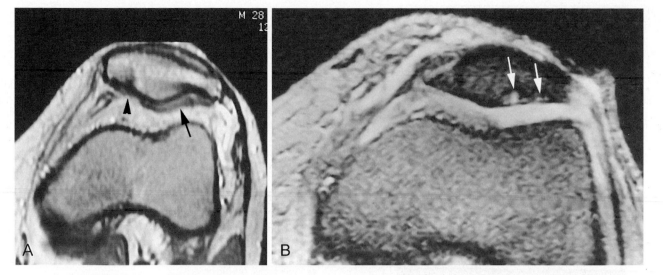

Figure 6.109.   CHONDROMALACIA PATELLA: GRADES III AND IV. A. MRI, Proton Density-Weighted Axial Knee. The normal retropatellar cartilage is intermediate in signal intensity and abuts the patellar cortex (arrow). Observe the marked loss of cartilage on the medial facet (arrowhead). The high signal intensity joint fluid now approximates the posterior patellar cortex. These findings are consistent with grade III chondromalacia patella.

B. MRI, T2*-Weighted Axial Knee. There is thinning, irregularity, and erosion of the retropatellar cartilage. The high signal intensity joint fluid is seen extending into several subchondral cysts (arrows). This finding represents grade IV chondromalacia patella. (Courtesy of Kenneth B. Reynard, MD, Center for MRI, Ltd., Denver, Colorado)

sions. Stage II changes are seen as *blisterlike* foci of hypointense signal involving the basal layer of cartilage. At this stage the cartilage surface remains intact. In stage III lesions focal, hypointense areas are observed, which represent cartilage irregularity (ulceration) or loss of the normal, sharply defined free margin of the cartilage. Stage IV changes include cartilaginous erosions extending to the bone surface, reactive subchondral sclerosis, and cyst formation. These findings appear as foci of hypointensity with the exception of the cysts, which are hyperintense on T2- and T2*-weighted images. (6,17,26) (Fig. 6.109)

OSGOOD-SCHLATTER'S DISEASE

This disorder consists of partial avulsion of the tibial tuberosity at the insertion of the patellar tendon. It occurs during adolescent growth (usually in young athletes) and manifests with anterior knee pain and local tenderness just below the patella. Conventional x-rays are often equivocal, but may show the bony fragmentation at the proximal tibial apophysis and blurring of the patellar tendon. There is a great deal of normal variance to the appearance of the tibial apophysis, which may appear fragmented but have nothing to do with the patient's symptoms. (See Chapter 3) Sagittal MR images using standard spin-echo sequences better display both the soft tissue and bone abnormalities at an early stage. (38,39)

It is important to remember that Osgood-Schlatter's disease is a form of tendinitis that is associated with incomplete fusion of the tibial apophysis. (38,39) A great deal of fluid (edema) must be present to cause patellar tendon blurring on plain film radiographs. Conversely, minute fluid accumulation at the distal attachment of the patellar tendon is well depicted with MRI, appearing as a focal area of high signal intensity on T2- and T2*-weighted images. (Fig. 6.110) The demonstration of apophyseal fragmentation with secondary tendinitis may be helpful in determining whether a patient has *active* Osgood-Schlatter's disease. (38,39)

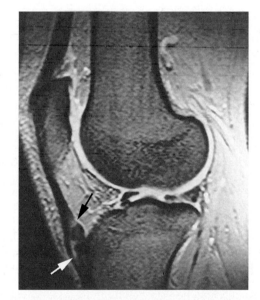

Figure 6.110.   CHRONIC KNEE PAIN: OSGOOD-SCHLATTER'S DISEASE. MRI, T2*-Weighted Sagittal Knee. There is fragmentation of the tibial tubercle with adjacent high signal intensity edema at the patellar tendon insertion (arrows). In addition, cephalad migration of the patella is noted (patella alta). These findings are consistent with chronic but active Osgood-Schlatter's disease. (Courtesy of Frank E. Seidelmann, DO; Kingsley A. Orraca-Tetteh, MD; and Matthew M. Brown, RT(R), Advanced MRImaging, Richmond Heights, Ohio)

JUMPER'S KNEE

This condition consists of focal inflammation of the patellar tendon origin (patellar tendinitis). It is an overuse injury, that results from repetitive stress like jumping. Professional athletes are frequently affected. The MR images display focal or segmental deformity and enlargement of the tendon at its proximal at-

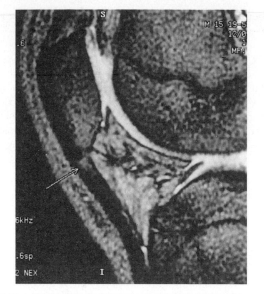

Figure 6.111.   CHRONIC KNEE PAIN: JUMPER'S KNEE. This young male soccer player began experiencing infrapatellar pain several weeks ago. **MRI, T2*-Weighted Sagittal Knee.** There is a focal hyperintense signal within the proximal insertion of the patellar tendon (arrow), consistent with patellar tendinitis (jumper's knee). (Courtesy of Frank E. Seidelmann, DO; Kingsley A. Orraca-Tetteh, MD; and Matthew M. Brown, RT(R), Advanced MRImaging, Richmond Heights, Ohio)

tachment. The affected area appears hyperintense on sagittal T2- and T2*-weighted images, contrasting the normally hypointense tendon. (38,39) (Fig. 6.111)

BUMPER OR FENDER FRACTURE (OCCULT TIBIAL PLATEAU FRACTURE)

This type of fracture occurs secondary to a forceful thrust of the lateral femoral condyle (which is stronger than the tibial plateau) downward onto the tibial plateau. This is called the *bumper* or *fender* fracture because the tibial plateau is at the approximate height of an automobile bumper. This eponym is retained although only 25% of the lateral tibial plateau fractures are caused by accidents where the knee is struck by an automobile. Eighty percent of the tibial plateau fractures are located in the lateral tibia. The fracture line in undisplaced fractures may be obliquely oriented and is often difficult to visualize on the routine anteroposterior or lateral radiographs of the knee.

MR imaging may be very helpful in the assessment of occult tibial plateau fracture in patients that present with knee pain following direct trauma to the lateral knee. These injuries are characterized by a hypointense spiderlike area of marrow edema in the lateral tibial plateau on coronal and sagittal T1-weighted images. On the T2- and T2*-weighted images, this area becomes hyperintense in contrast to the adjacent hypointense fracture line(s). (Fig. 6.112) This characteristic spiderlike pattern of marrow edema is also seen with bone contusions of the tibial plateau (usually the lateral tibial metaphysis). While their edema patterns are identical, the absence of the fracture line confirms a contusion rather than a fracture.

MYOSITIS OSSIFICANS

Myositis ossificans (MO) frequently occurs secondary to a solitary traumatic muscle injury, but can also be seen in young athletes with a history of recurrent muscle tears. Other causes include long-term immobilization resulting from paralysis or coma, connective tissue metaplasia, ossification of a hematoma and burns. (40) It presents as a soft tissue mass that undergoes progressive ossification. The lesion may cause muscular contraction and reduced range of motion of the hip. (38,40) Peripheral new bone formation appears 6 to 8 weeks after trauma in the areas of hemorrhage. After 6 months, peripheral compact bone with a central core of lamellar bone may be observed. (40) This creates the classic appearance of a dense peripheral calcified shell with a more radiolucent central matrix that is best depicted with CT. The main radiologic and pathologic differential diagnosis to MO is sarcoma. In comparison, soft tissue sarcomas are typically more dense centrally and have a more radiolucent peripheral edge. If the lesion is biopsied, the histologic similarities of MO and osteosarcoma may be misleading and result in an erroneous diagnosis because the pathologist is often unaware of the lesion's radiographic features. Therefore, MO is a *leave-me-alone* lesion and should *never* be biopsied.

The value of MRI in the assessment of myositis is to provide information regarding the extent of the lesion. The degree to which the lesion has matured determines its MR appearance. In the early phase, before ossification takes place, the T1-weighted images show an ill-defined lesion that is isointense with muscle. With T2-weighting the lesion becomes brighter than fat. Other signs include fluid-fluid levels on T1-weighted images and bone marrow edema adjacent to the area of myositis, detected on both T1- and T2- weighted images. (41–43)

In subacute myositis with early peripheral ossification, the central portion of the lesion has an intermediate signal intensity (isointense with muscle) on T1-weighted sequences and appears hyperintense with T2-weighting. A well defined, hypointense rim can be seen around the lesion on T1-weighted images. Chronic lesions often have low signal intensity on both T1- and T2-

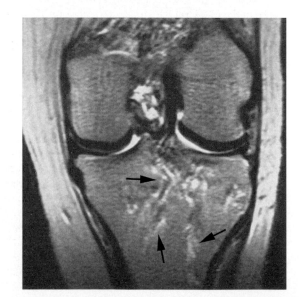

Figure 6.112.   OCCULT FRACTURE WITH SURROUNDING BONE MARROW EDEMA: TIBIA. This skier injured his knee and was unable to bear weight. Radiographs were performed immediately and were normal. His knee pain persisted. **MRI, T2-Weighted Coronal Knee.** Note the numerous, linear, high signal intensity areas (arrows) radiating from the proximal tibial cortex into the metaphysis. These findings are consistent with an occult tibial plateau fracture and surrounding marrow edema. (Courtesy of The Children's Hospital, Department of Radiology, Denver, Colorado)

weighted images, consistent with dense ossification and fibrosis. (42,43) In some cases the T1-weighted images may show hyperintense areas, representing fatty marrow, and hypointense ill-defined regions, consistent with cortical bone within and surrounding the lesion. (43)

A similar traumatic circumstance may produce the *cortical irregularity syndrome*. This lesion represents a fibroosseous response to a ligamentous or tendinous periosteal avulsion injury and occurs most frequently at the distal femur. (44) The MR appearance is typical of a fluid-filled cystic lesion—hypointense to the adja-

cent musculature on T1-weighted images and becoming very hyperintense with T2-weighting. (Fig. 6.113)

OSTEONECROSIS AND RELATED DISORDERS

Osteonecrosis of the knee can occur in individuals with the appropriate risk factors listed in Table 6.3 (p. 430). (Fig. 6.114) The MR appearance of osteonecrosis in the knee is similar to changes seen in the femoral and humeral heads and consists of a serpiginous low signal intensity border surrounding central

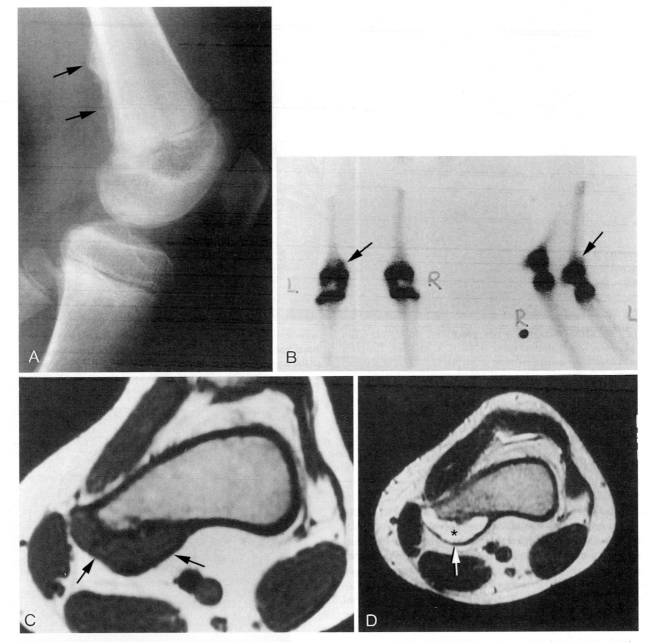

Figure 6.113. MYOSITIS OSSIFICANS: A LEAVE-ME-ALONE LESION. This 12-year-old male injured his knee playing football and continued playing while injured. The following radiograph is 3 months postinjury. **A. Lateral Knee**. Observe the solid, wavy periosteal new bone formation along the posterior surface of the distal femoral metaphysis (arrows). **B. Bone Scan, Bilateral Knee**. There is a small area of abnormal radiopharmaceutical uptake within the left distal femur (arrows). A presumptive diagnosis of osteosarcoma was made, and the patient was scheduled for biopsy. **C. MRI, T1-Weighted Axial Knee**. Note the eccentric, homogeneous, low signal in-

tensity mass on the posterior surface of the femur (arrows). This region is well encapsulated and is suggestive of a benign process. **D. MRI, T2-Weighted Axial Knee**. The cortical outline (arrow) is clearly defined and encloses the high signal intensity hemorrhagic edema (*). These findings are consistent with the *cortical irregularity syndrome*, a condition resulting from traumatic periostitis. COMMENT: The amount of uptake on the bone scan was far less than would be expected with osteosarcoma. (Courtesy of Frank Sivo, DC, North Miami, Florida)

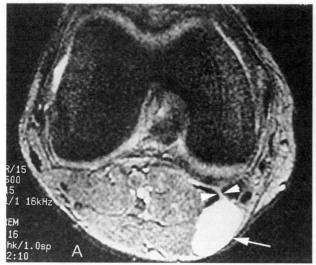
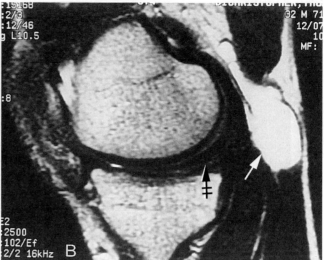

Figure 6.118.   BAKER'S CYST. A. MRI, T2*-Weighted Axial Knee. B. MRI, T2-Weighted Fast Spin-Echo Sagittal Knee. There is a large Baker's cyst posterior to the femoral condyle (arrow). Characteristically, uncomplicated cysts exhibit very hyperintense signal. The axial images show a tract connecting the cyst to the joint capsule (arrowheads). Also, there is a faint, horizontal, high signal intensity area coursing through the substance of the posterior horn of the medial meniscus (crossed arrow). It communicates with the articular surface, consistent with a grade III tear. COMMENT: Baker's cysts are often associated with tears of the posterior horn of the medial meniscus. Prior to the availability of MRI, arthrography was the standard imaging modality for the evaluation of meniscal tears. The accuracy and noninvasive character of MRI has led to the replacement of arthrography for most knee pathology. (Courtesy of Alan M. Lesselroth, MD, Mountain Diagnostics, Las Vegas, Nevada)

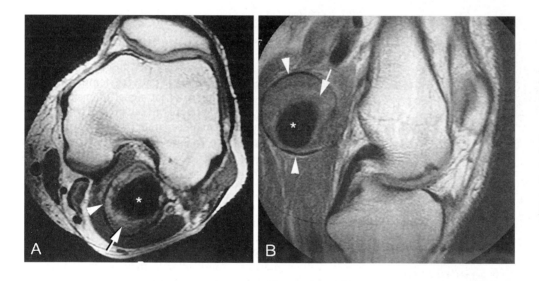

Figure 6.119.   POPLITEAL ARTERY ANEURYSM. A. MRI, T1-Weighted Axial Knee. B. MRI, T1-Weighted Sagittal Knee. The vessel is divided into a true lumen (*) and mural thrombus (arrow). The thin signal void surrounding the aneurysm (arrowheads) represents the atherosclerotic calcified wall that was identified on the plain films (not shown). COMMENT: The contrast between fast-flowing blood in the vessels and surrounding soft tissues permits MRI to be utilized in the evaluation of blood vessels. Changes in the size of the lumen are easily detected with MRI.

Popliteal Artery Aneurysm

Popliteal artery aneurysm may be demonstrated on MR images as hyperintense signal produced by slow blood flow within the dilated popliteal artery. Lamellated areas of variable signal intensity are seen surrounding the flow void or hyperintense slow flow. (Fig. 6.119) Hypointensity may occur within the aneurysm due to fibrin, hemosiderin, fast flow, flow void, and associated hypointense vessel walls. (1) Hyperintensity may be present within the lesion and is often the result of chronic pooled blood, slow flow, and associated edema. (1)

A good clinical examination should render a high suspicion of a popliteal artery aneurysm and the expense of MRI is not justified in establishing the diagnosis. Diagnostic ultrasound (where applicable) is far more cost effective in the detection of aneurysms.

Pigmented Villonodular Synovitis

Pigmented villonodular synovitis (PVNS) is an uncommon inflammatory disorder of synovial tissue. Its etiology is unknown, but it is considered by most to be a benign synovial neoplasm. The majority of the patients are young or middle-aged adults.

Synovitis occurs as a result of recurrent bleeding into the lesion. Connective tissue hyperplasia and hemosiderin deposition characterize the microscopic appearance. Gross examination reveals large, folded masses that are red and brown in color. PVNS occurs in any location where synovial tissue is found; however, the most common sites involve the lower extremities, particularly the knee (Fig. 6.120) and hip (Fig. 6.121). Notably, these masses, when closely approximated to a bony surface, produce an *outside-in* or *apple core* extrinsic pressure erosion (gouge defect). These bony defects are far more prevalent in the tightly compartmen-

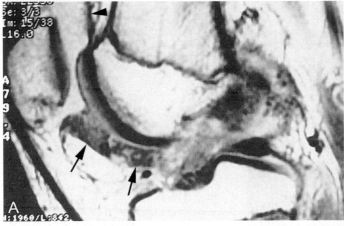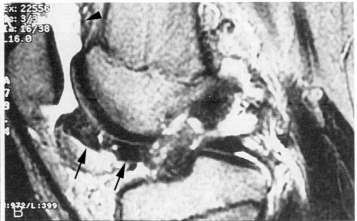

Figure 6.120. PIGMENTED VILLONODULAR SYNOVITIS (PVNS): PEDIATRIC KNEE. This 13-year-old male patient complained of chronic intermittent knee pain with swelling. **A. MRI, Proton Density-Weighted Sagittal Knee. B. MRI, T2-Weighted Sagittal Knee. Observe** the heterogeneous low signal intensity masses on the proton density-weighted image that remain unchanged on the T2-weighted image (arrows). Also note the distension of the suprapatellar bursa (arrowheads) secondary to a joint effusion. COMMENT: PVNS most commonly occurs in the knee joint. In the diffuse form, MR findings include soft tissue masses of mixed signal intensity with focal hypointense areas. The hypointense areas are seen on all pulse sequences and are the result of the paramagnetic effect of hemosiderin. (Courtesy of Joel B. Levine MD, and Keith R. Burnett, MD, Long Beach, California)

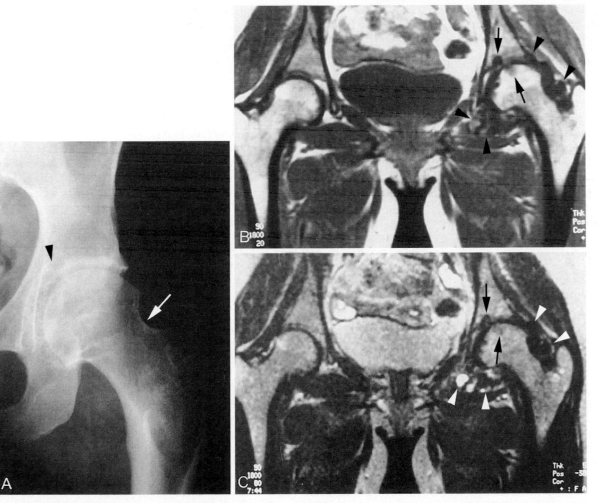

Figure 6.121. PIGMENTED VILLONODULAR SYNOVITIS (PVNS): HIP. This 26-year-old female patient presented with hip pain and stiffness. **A. AP Spot Hip.** Note the subtle erosion of the lateral femoral neck (arrow) and acetabular cortex (arrowhead). **B. MRI, Proton Density-Weighted Coronal Pelvis. C. MRI, T2-Weighted Coronal Pelvis.** There are discrete articular erosions on both sides of the affected hip joint (arrows). Note the nodular synovial masses adjacent to the femoral neck and inferior aspect of the femoral head (arrowheads). These masses are heterogeneous with intermediate and low signal intensity areas on the proton density-weighted image. The intermediate signal intensity areas become hyperintense with T2-weighting and are consistent with recent hemorrhage. The portions of the masses that maintain their hypointense signal on both images represent hemosiderin deposition. COMMENT: The etiology of PVNS is controversial. Early diagnosis, however, permits conservative surgical treatment with total synovectomy and curettage of the osteolytic foyers. Bone grafts are employed for filling the sites of osteolysis. A delay in diagnosis will result in arthrodesis and total joint arthroplasty. The sensitivity of MR imaging may obviate the need for radical management options in PVNS. (Courtesy of Joseph N. Fiore, DC, Pasadena, Maryland)

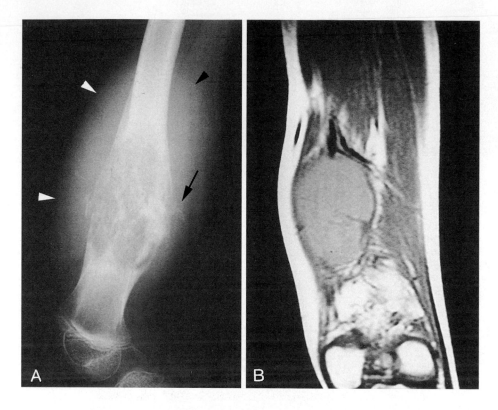

Figure 6.122. OSTEOSARCOMA: GROWING PAINS? This teenager complained of a mass in the thigh with persistent pain. **A. Lateral Femur.** Note the predominantly lytic expansile lesion of the distal femur. A spiculated periosteal reaction (arrow) and a large soft tissue mass were identified (arrowheads). **B. MRI, Proton Density-Weighted Coronal Femur.** Notice the well-defined, intermediate signal intensity neoplastic mass. (Courtesy of Vicky L. Youngman, DO, Denver, Colorado)

talized joints such as the hip, ankle, wrist, and hand. The knee is a loosely compartmentalized joint and is least likely to show extrinsic bony erosions. The treatment of choice in patients with PVNS is synovectomy. Eventually, a total joint replacement may be necessary if this process recurs or if there is significant damage to the articular cartilage. (45–47)

MRI Findings. The presence of hemosiderin in a hemorrhagic effusion can be detected with high sensitivity using T1- and T2-weighted MR images. (48) Low signal intensity masses are seen on all pulse sequences because of the paramagnetic effect of the hemosiderin within the hyperplastic synovium. Hemorrhage, reparative granulation tissue, and synovial fluid are displayed as intermediate or high signal areas on T2- and T2*-weighted images, depending on the relative amounts of these tissues present within the lesion.

OSTEOSARCOMA

Osteosarcoma is the second most common primary malignant bone neoplasm in the general population and is the most common primary malignant bone tumor in childhood. The reader is referred to Chapter 11 for a complete description of the various clinical and histologic classifications of this malignant tumor. Osteosarcomas most frequently affect the metaphyseal portion of the large tubular bones. The radiographic features vary with the histologic type and include areas of sclerosis (bone proliferation) and lucency (bone destruction).

MR imaging is ideally suited to assess the extent of marrow infiltration and soft tissue invasion using both spin-echo and gradient-echo pulse sequences. (Fig. 6.122) Osteosarcomas are typically heterogeneous, and the various cellular constituents of the tumor (e.g., fibrous, chondroid, blastic, or telangiectatic components) can modify the lesions' signal characteristics. (49) Generally, these lesions are low in signal intensity on T1-weighted im-

ages and become hyperintense when T2-weighted techniques are used. CT is better at determining whether cortical disruption has occurred, specifically when the lesion contains large amounts of bone proliferation (sclerosis), which is seen on MRI as a signal void (appearing identical to the cortex of normal bone). (Fig. 6.123) MRI, however, is better at determining the longitudinal extent of marrow infiltration. This information is necessary in surgical planning and in monitoring tumor response to chemotherapy.

THE ANKLE

INJURY TO TENDONS AND LIGAMENTS

Ligament sprains of the ankle joint are among the most commonly reported sports-related injuries. MRI provides valuable information in the evaluation of these injuries. The normal intact tendons and ligaments demonstrate low signal intensity on all pulse sequences. (1) Evaluation of these structures frequently presents a diagnostic challenge because of their variable orientation. The discussion in this text is limited to injury of the lateral collateral ligaments, Achilles tendon, and tibialis posterior tendon. Discussion of additional tendon and ligament injuries is beyond the scope of this text.

LATERAL COLLATERAL LIGAMENT INJURY

Eighty-five percent of ligamentous injuries to the ankle affect the lateral collateral ligaments. (2) This group of ligaments is comprised of the anterior talofibular, calcaneofibular, and posterior talofibular ligaments. Of these the anterior talofibular ligament (ATFL) is the most frequently injured. Involvement of the calcaneofibular and posterior talofibular ligaments is much less common and is almost always associated with an ATFL tear. (3,4)

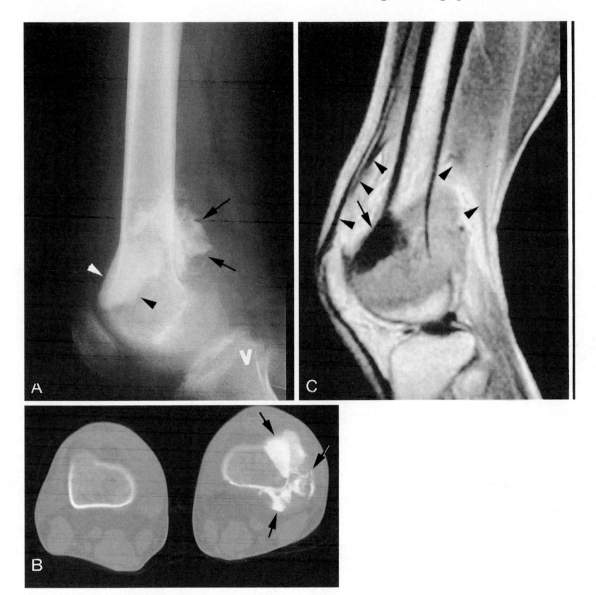

Figure 6.123. OSTEOSARCOMA: KNEE PAIN AND AN ENLARGING MASS. This 25-year-old male complained of pain and an enlarging mass around the left knee. **A. Lateral Knee.** There is a poorly defined calcified, soft tissue mass (arrows) and osteoblastic response (arrowheads) involving the distal femoral metaphysis. **B. CT, Bone Window Bilateral Axial Thigh.** Observe the dense mass arising from the left femoral marrow and cortex with extension into the soft tissues of the thigh (arrows). **C. MRI, T1-Weighted Sagittal Knee.** Note the low signal intensity in the marrow corresponding to the dense intramedullary osteoblastic tumor (arrow). The soft tissue extent of the tumor mass is clearly evident (arrowheads). COMMENT: MRI is the most accurate imaging modality for the evaluation and staging of musculoskeletal tumors.

Coronal, sagittal, and axial images using a dedicated extremity coil with T1- and T2-weighted spin-echo sequences are often adequate for evaluation. Axial sections with the foot in full dorsiflexion and full plantar flexion have been described as the most useful images for the assessment of the commonly injured ankle ligaments. (2) Three-dimensional (3-D) volume acquisition images may be obtained and can be reconstructed in any orthogonal plane to provide additional information regarding ligamentous integrity.

Generally, the MR appearance of any ankle ligament injury is similar, but varies slightly with the particular ligament involved. For example, tears of the ATFL may appear as partial or complete disruption or absence of the ligament, while tears of the deltoid ligament usually reveal evidence of edema and hemorrhage without complete disruption. (1) Acute tears demonstrate a high signal intensity area on T2- and T2*-weighted images and slightly hyperintense or isointense tendon thickening with T1-weighting. Conversely, chronic and healed tears are observed as thickened, hypointense areas within the ligament on all pulse sequences.

ACHILLES TENDINITIS AND RUPTURE

The Achilles tendon is the largest tendon in the body and is formed by the confluence of the gastrocnemius and soleus muscle complex. (1) Inflammation and/or rupture of this tendon is most often experienced as a result of overuse or direct trauma. Acute rupture occurs as a sequela to forced dorsiflexion of the foot against a contracting force generated by the calf muscles. This is most frequently seen in middle-aged male athletes with very large calf muscles. A predisposition to disruption of the Achilles tendon can occur as a result of weakened connective tissue in patients with underlying systemic disease processes such as diabetes, gout, rheumatoid arthritis, among others. (5) Clinical examination alone may not provide the definitive means for diagnosing Achilles tendon tears. Up to 25% of Achilles tendon tears, either partial or complete, are missed on physical examination. (1)

The normal Achilles tendon is uniformly low in signal intensity on all MR pulse sequences. The MRI findings of Achilles tendinitis include focal or fusiform thickening of the Achilles tendon

and diffuse increased signal intensity on T2-weighted images. Tears most frequently occur 2 to 6 cm proximal to the tendon's calcaneal insertion and are best demonstrated on sagittal and axial images. Complete rupture of the Achilles tendon results in discontinuity and a disrelationship of the low signal intensity tendon margins. (Fig. 6.124) An irregular appearance of the torn tendinous segments with redundancy and retraction is common. (Fig. 6.125) Subacute hemorrhage and edema are observed in the adjacent soft tissues as areas of high signal intensity on T2- and T2*-weighted images. High signal intensity within the substance of the tendon with T2-weighting suggests tendinitis or partial tear. (3,4)

The anatomic information gained from MRI helps to guide the clinician in determining whether conservative management

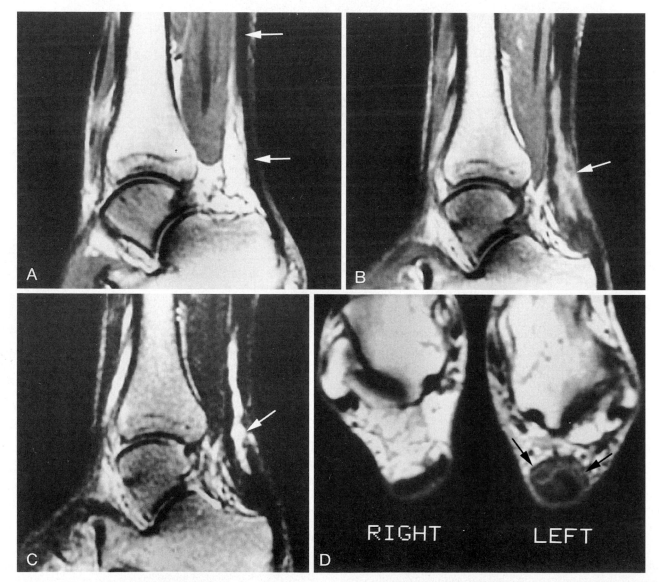

Figure 6.124.   ACHILLES TENDON TEAR: COMPLETE. This patient experienced a "pop" and severe ankle pain while playing tennis. **A. MRI, T1-Weighted Sagittal Ankle, Normal.** The smooth and well-defined low signal intensity of the Achilles tendon is noted (arrows) extending to its insertion on the calcaneus. **B. MRI, T1-Weighted Sagittal Ankle. C. MRI, T2-Weighted Sagittal Ankle**. There is an irregular, hyperintense signal interrupting the normally low signal intensity Achilles tendon. This high signal area becomes very hyperintense with T2-weighting and is consistent with a complete tear. **D. MRI, T1-Weighted Bilateral Axial Ankle.** There is a large circumferential collection of intermediate signal intensity edema surrounding the thickened left Achilles tendon (arrows). The normal contralateral side is observed as a crescentric, homogeneous, hypointense structure. COMMENT: Twenty-five percent of all Achilles tendon tears are missed on physical examination. MR represents the definitive imaging modality to provide this diagnosis.

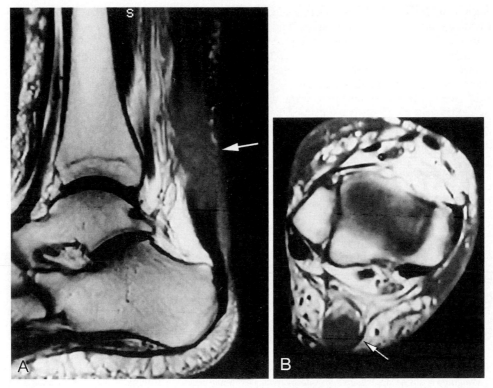

Figure 6.125. ACHILLES TENDON TEAR: COMPLETE. A. MRI, T1-Weighted Sagittal Ankle. B. MRI, T1-Weighted Axial Ankle. There is thickening and replacement of the normally low signal intensity Achilles tendon with an intermediate circumferential collection of edema (arrows). Note the distortion of the tendon's contour. (Courtesy of David L. Berens, MD, Buffalo MRI, Buffalo, New York)

with serial casting will be effective. Complete tears with significant separation of the tendon often require surgical intervention. (Fig. 6.126) MRI has become the *gold standard* in assessing Achilles tendon injuries and differentiating those tears that may respond to conservative management from those that require surgery.

TIBIALIS POSTERIOR TENDON INJURIES

Rupture of the tibialis posterior tendon may occur spontaneously or can be associated with prior synovitis, trauma, or steroid injection. (1) These injuries are most frequently seen in females in their fifth to sixth decade. (1)

Normally, the tendon appears uniformly low in signal on all pulse sequences and is best demonstrated in the coronal plane and on axial images that extend inferior to the medial malleolus. The tendon is located anterolateral to the flexor digitorum longus tendon. (1) Fluid in the tendon sheath, demonstrating increased signal intensity on T2-weighted images, may be observed in patients who have had chronic tenosynovitis of the tibialis posterior tendon. Type I posterior tibialis tendon tears are seen as a thickened tendon of heterogeneous signal intensity. Thinning of the tendon is consistent with a type II (partial) tear. (6) (Fig. 6.127) Type III tears exhibit complete disruption of the tendon and may be seen with or without abnormal morphology of the torn margins. (1) The site of the rupture is usually 6 cm proximal to its navicular insertion at the musculotendinous junction. MRI, using both axial and coronal slices, assists the clinician in determining whether a suspected tear is partial or complete.

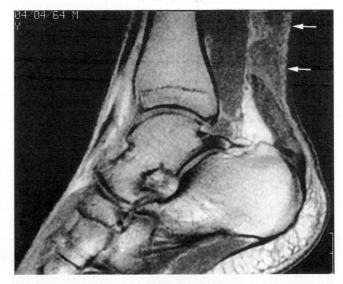

Figure 6.126. ACHILLES TENDON TEAR: COMPLETE. MRI, Proton Density-Weighted Sagittal Ankle. Note the intermediate signal intensity collection of hemorrhage and reparative tissue replacing the homogeneously low signal of the Achilles tendon (arrows). Observe the retraction and enlargement of the distal portion of the tendon. COMMENT: MRI is helpful in evaluating the torn tendon margins for surgical planning.

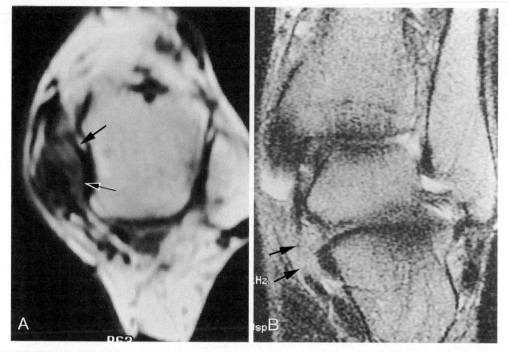

Figure 6.127. POSTERIOR TIBIALIS TENDON TEAR: TYPE II. This 57-year-old female complained of swelling and ankle pain following trauma 2 months earlier. **A. MRI, T1-Weighted Axial Ankle.** Observe the intermediate signal intensity surrounding the posterior tibialis tendon (arrows) suggestive of a tear. **B. MRI, T2-Weighted Coronal Ankle.** Note the hyperintense signal within the partially disrupted posterior tibialis tendon (arrows). COMMENT: Thickening and inflammatory changes are characteristic of a type I posterior tibialis tendon injury. In type II (partial) tears the tendon is attenuated, predisposing it to further rupture. Complete discontinuity and gapping with retraction of the fibers are the hallmark features of type III tendon tears.

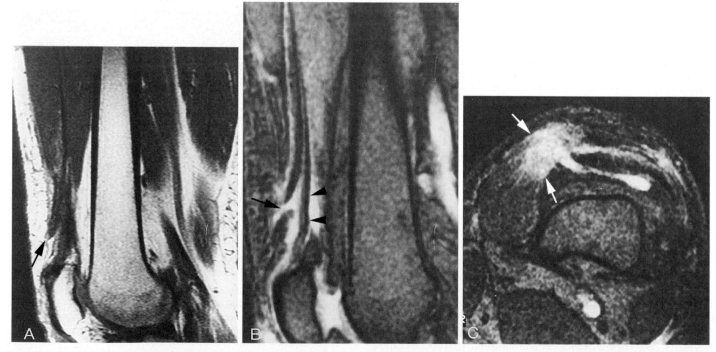

Figure 6.128. ACUTE GRADE III MUSCLE TEAR OF THE ANTEROME-DIAL THIGH. A. MRI, T1-Weighted Sagittal Thigh. B. MRI, T2*-Weighted Sagittal Thigh. Note the complete tear of the rectus femoris tendon (arrows). In addition, the vastus intermedius muscle (arrowheads) is attenuated. The hyperintense signal seen adjacent to this area represents acute hemorrhage. **C. MRI, T2*-Weighted Axial Thigh.** Note the large hyperintense signal intensity within the anterior thigh musculature (arrows), consistent with acute hemorrhage. (Courtesy of Frank E. Seidelmann, DO; Kingsley A. Orraca-Tetteh, MD; and Matthew M. Brown, RT(R), Advanced MRImaging, Richmond Heights, Ohio)

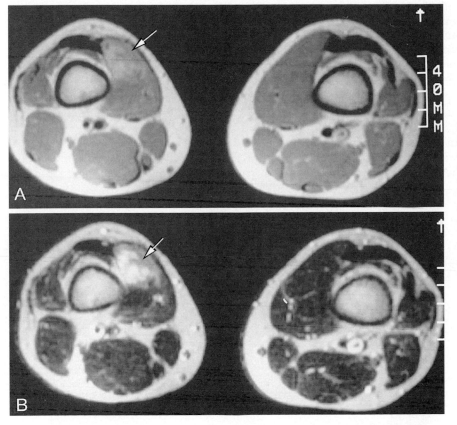

Figure 6.129. ACUTE MUSCLE HEMATOMA: ATH-LETIC INJURY. A. MRI, T1-Weighted Bilateral Axial Femur. Normal skeletal muscle displays intermediate to low signal intensity on these images. Note the minimally increased signal intensity in the right medial thigh (arrow). **B. MRI, T2-Weighted Bilateral Axial Femur.** Observe the markedly hyperintense area within the right medial thigh (arrow), consistent with an acute hematoma. COMMENT: The signal intensity of chronic hematomas demonstrates reduced signal with T2-weighting because of the hemosiderin content of the mass. Repeat MR imaging may be helpful in determining the time frame in which an athlete may return to training without threat of reinjury.

Figure 6.130. MUSCLE CONTUSION: CALF. This injury was sustained following a direct blow. **MRI, T2-Weighted Axial Leg.** There is intramuscular hemorrhage and edema within the gastrocnemius and soleus muscles of the left calf (arrows). Compare this high signal intensity area with the normal contralateral side. COMMENT: MRI is capable of evaluating a wide range of muscular injuries and their complications. Examples include contusion, hematoma, delayed-onset muscle soreness, tendinitis, and tendon tears.

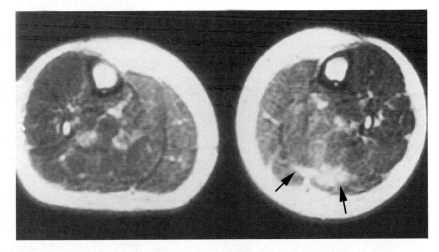

POSTTRAUMATIC MUSCLE DISORDERS

The orthopedic grading system used to grade most ligament injuries (grades I to III) also applies to most muscle injuries. MRI is capable of differentiating muscle strains (grade I), partial or complete musculotendinous tears (grades II and III, respectively), (Fig. 6.128) and intramuscular hematomas. (1) (Fig. 6.129) Most muscle injuries are never imaged and respond well to conservative therapy. In the elite or highly motivated professional athlete, however, MRI provides valuable information concerning the grade of injury, effect of treatment, and ultimately, when that athlete may return to full activity. This recent advance in MR technology provides prognostic information that has reduced the risk of recurrent sports-related muscle injuries resulting from premature high-level participation.

Muscle injuries are characterized by edema and/or underlying hemorrhage, which demonstrates high signal intensity on T2-weighted images. (2–4) (Fig. 6.130) STIR techniques improve lesion detection by suppressing adjacent intramuscular fat and amplifying the hemorrhagic signal intensity generated from the injury site.

GANGLION

A ganglion is a benign cystic lesion that usually occurs on or around a tendon or tendon sheath. Ganglia are most frequently seen in the wrist and hand. Although the exact pathogenesis is unknown in most instances, ganglia may occur in an intramuscular or intraarticular location as a result of significant injury. MRI reveals signal characteristics that are typical of encapsulated fluid collections seen elsewhere—low to intermediate signal intensity on the T1-weighted images that becomes very hyperintense with T2-weighting. (Fig. 6.131)

STRESS FRACTURE

Stress fractures are caused by abnormal repetitive loading of a normal bone. (7) The distal tibia and calcaneus are the most common ankle bones involved. MRI is capable of detecting these

injuries prior to their detection with conventional radiographs. The fracture line appears low in signal on both T1- and T2-weighted images. (3) On T1-weighted images the associated marrow edema is very apparent and is seen as a diffuse hypointense area, contrasting with the hyperintense fatty marrow. The lesion becomes hyperintense with T2-weighting. The fracture line is usually perpendicular to the articulating surface and can be long and serpiginous or short and straight.

OSTEOCHONDRITIS DISSECANS

Osteochondral lesions of the talus most frequently involve the talar dome and are more common in women in their second to

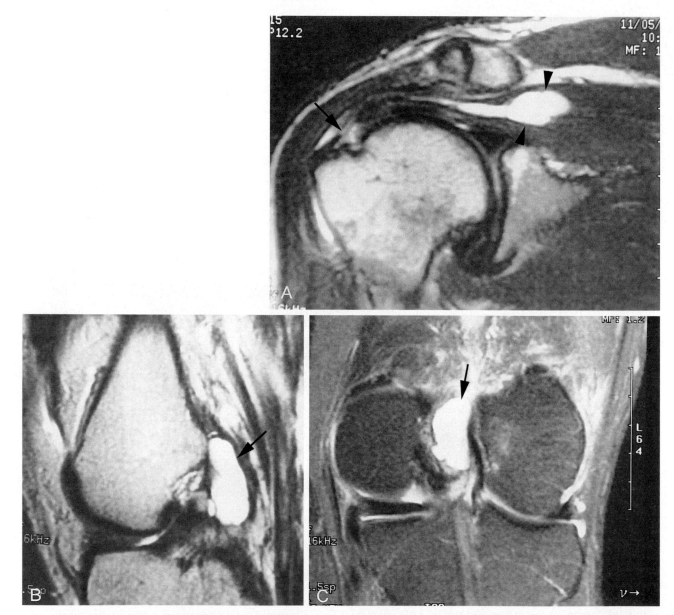

Figure 6.131. GANGLION CYST: A POSTTRAUMATIC ETIOLOGY. A. MRI, T2-Weighted Fast Spin-Echo Coronal Oblique Shoulder. There is a complete tear of the rotator cuff tendon (arrow) with minimal tendon retraction. Also note the high signal intensity fluid collection representing an intramuscular ganglion (arrowheads) within the supraspinatus muscle. **B. MRI, T2-Weighted Fast Spin-Echo Sagittal Knee. C. MRI, Fat-Suppressed T2-Weighted Fast Spin-Echo Coronal Knee.** The high signal intensity posterior to the distal femur represents an intraarticular ganglion (arrow). The inter-

condylar location of the ganglion is clearly demonstrated on the coronal image. COMMENT: Ganglions are benign, well-encapsulated synovial herniations. The etiology of these lesions is usually unknown; however, they may occur secondary to trauma. Ganglions are most frequently identified in the wrist, hand, and foot. (**A** Courtesy of Michael D. Smith, MD, Radiology Imaging Associates, P.C., Englewood, Colorado; **B** and **C** Courtesy of James L. Quale, MD, Radiology Imaging Associates, P.C., Englewood, Colorado)

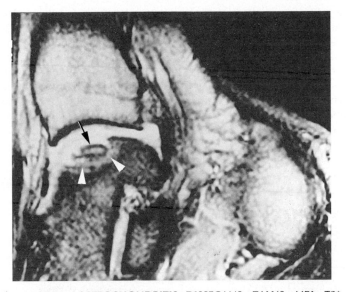

Figure 6.132. OSTEOCHONDRITIS DISSECANS: TALUS. MRI, T2*-Weighted Sagittal Ankle. Observe the large osteochondral fragment (arrow) within the defect of the talar dome. The hyperintense joint fluid completely surrounds the fragment, indicating this lesion is active and potentially unstable (arrowhead). COMMENT: MRI directs the management and treatment of osteochondritis dissecans. Bone and cartilage fragments displaying increased signal intensity at their interface with the subchondral bone frequently become unstable.

fourth decade of life. (5,8) In athletes, the middle one third of the lateral border of the talar dome and the posterior one third of the medial talar border are the most common sites of injury. (5) An associated tear of the lateral collateral ligament may also be seen.

MR imaging of the ankle joint in the sagittal and coronal planes adequately displays the lesion and provides information concerning the integrity of the overlying cartilage and fragment stability. (9) (Fig. 6.132) These lesions are accurately assessed with standard spin-echo (T1- and T2-weighted) and gradient-echo (T2*-weighted) techniques. The osteochondral fragment is low in signal on T1-, T2-, and T2*-weighted pulse sequences, while the osteochondral defect in the talus usually becomes hyperintense with T2-weighting. (Fig. 6.133) As in the knee, when the lesion is surrounded by high signal intensity articular fluid, the lesion is considered active and potentially unstable.

THE SHOULDER

Magnetic resonance imaging of the shoulder is indicated for evaluation of numerous disorders, including sports- and work-related injuries, inflammatory processes, and nontraumatic shoulder pain with negative plain radiographs. The following conditions are some of the most common disorders of the shoulder in which MRI greatly aids in establishing the definitive diagnosis.

SHOULDER IMPINGEMENT SYNDROME

Impingement syndrome is a condition caused by repetitive compression of the supraspinatus tendon and subacromial bursa under the coracoacromial arc. This is a common cause of shoulder

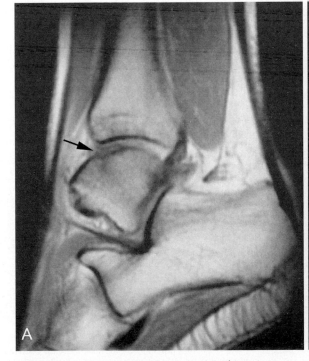

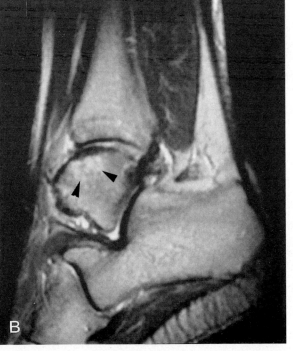

Figure 6.133. OSTEOCHONDRITIS DISSECANS: TALUS. This patient was clinically diagnosed with an ankle sprain, but her pain persisted. **A. MRI, T1-Weighted Sagittal Ankle. B. MRI, T2-Weighted Sagittal Ankle**. There is irregularity and minimal flattening of the talar dome (arrow). In addition, an area of low signal intensity is noted within the subchondral bone on the T1-weighted image. This area becomes hyperintense with T2-weighting (arrow-heads). COMMENT: Magnetic resonance imaging is more sensitive than radiography in the diagnosis of subtle osteochondral lesions. Its greatest attribute lies in evaluating the stability of the osteochondral fragment. The presence of edema surrounding the fragment suggests instability (likely to become free within the joint). The patient's physical activity and management must be altered accordingly.

dysfunction, particularly in athletes. This clinical entity begins as the space for the bursa and tendon becomes reduced. Repetitive injuries to the rotator cuff tendon occur causing tendinitis or tears and/or subacromial-subdeltoid bursitis. Rotator cuff tendinitis may induce fibrosis and secondary rupture. (1–3) Bigliani (4) has defined three different types and shapes of the acromion as seen on the plain film radiographic outlet projection and sagittal oblique MR images. These three types are:

Type I: The acromion is flat.
Type II: The acromion is curved.
Type III: The acromion is hooked.

A type III (hooked) acromion is associated with a much greater risk of developing rotator cuff tendinopathy. Acromioclavicular joint arthrosis with inferiorly oriented osteophytes further decreases the coracoacromial space, increasing the potential for impingement syndrome. This can often be determined by plain film radiography prior to the MRI examination.

Clinical information is crucial in establishing the correct diagnosis of this condition. MR imaging with T1- and T2-weighted pulse sequences in the coronal plane may augment the clinical findings; however, the definitive diagnosis is established on clinical grounds. Seeger (2,5) classifies the features of shoulder impingement syndrome into three categories based on their MRI appearance using coronal oblique slices:

Type I: Subacromial bursitis with normal signal intensity of the supraspinatus muscle and tendon on the T1-weighted images. On T2*-weighted images diffuse hyperintense signal may be seen within the tendon.
Type II: Partial tear of the rotator cuff tendon with a relatively high signal intensity area on the T1-weighted images that becomes hyperintense with T2-weighted pulse sequencing. No muscle retraction is observed. (Fig. 6.134)
Type III: Complete rotator cuff tear with retraction of the supraspinatus muscle. A very hyperintense signal intensity area within the supraspinatus tendon is seen on the conventional

T2-weighted images. This is considered pathognomonic for a rotator cuff tear. (Fig. 6.135)

ROTATOR CUFF TENDINITIS

Rotator cuff tendinitis is frequently a sports-related injury. It occurs in athletes who actively participate in volleyball, tennis, racquetball, handball, baseball, or any sport that requires repeated abduction and external rotation of the shoulder joint. MRI findings include intermediate signal within the substance of the tendon on the T1- and proton density-weighted images. This area may become hyperintense, hypointense or remain intermediate in its signal intensity on T2- or T2*-weighted images, depending on the chronicity of the lesion. (Fig. 6.136) In addition, thickening of the tendon may also be observed. (6)

ROTATOR CUFF TEARS

The rotator cuff is composed of four muscles: supraspinatus, infraspinatus, teres minor, and the subscapularis (**SITS** is a frequently used mnemonic that is helpful in remembering the muscles that contribute to the rotator cuff). They originate from the scapula and their tendons insert on the tuberosities of the humeral head. These muscles cross the glenohumeral joint, and together they form a musculotendinous hood that provides dynamic stability to the shoulder joint. (1,7) There is a *critical zone* of hypovascularity within the distal supraspinatus tendon. This hypovascular region is due to a poor anastomosis of the vessels that supply the surrounding musculoskeletal structures. Accordingly, this portion of the rotator cuff tendon is predisposed to tears and is a common site for hydroxyapatite crystal deposition (calcific tendinitis). (8) (Fig. 6.137)

MR imaging of the shoulder using T1-and T2-weighted pulse sequences in the sagittal and coronal oblique planes offers superb visualization of the rotator cuff tendons, in particular the distal supraspinatus tendon. The images obtained from a patient with a history of repetitive trauma to the shoulder should be carefully

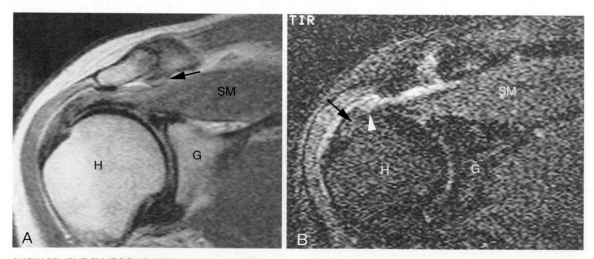

Figure 6.134. IMPINGEMENT SYNDROME WITH CHRONIC ROTATOR CUFF TENDINITIS AND A PARTIAL TEAR. A. MRI, T1-Weighted Coronal Shoulder. Arthrosis is noted at the acromioclavicular articulation with an inferiorly projecting osteophyte that impinges on the supraspinatus tendon (arrow). Diffuse hyperintense signal is noted within the substance of the tendon. **B. MRI, Short T1 Inversion Recovery (STIR) Coronal Shoulder.** Note the hyperintense signal within the substance of the supraspinatus tendon (arrow). A small bursal surface tear of the rotator cuff tendon is also noted (arrowhead). (*H*, Humeral head, *G*, Glenoid, *SM*, Supraspinatus Muscle). (Courtesy of Frank E. Seidelmann, DO; Kingsley A. Orraca-Tetteh, MD; and Matthew M. Brown, RT(R), Advanced MRImaging, Richmond Heights, Ohio)

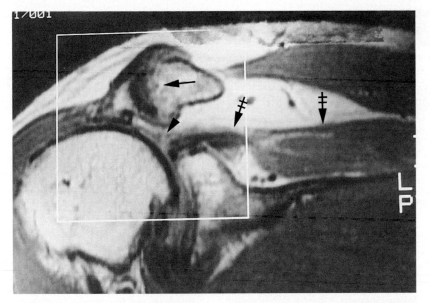

Figure 6.135.   IMPINGEMENT SYNDROME: PAIN WITH ABDUCTION OF THE SHOULDER. MRI, T1-Weighted Coronal Oblique Shoulder. There is hypertrophic deformity of the acromioclavicular joint (arrow). Note the intermediate signal intensity (arrowhead) within the atrophied and retracted rotator cuff (crossed arrows). There is also superior subluxation of the humeral head. These findings are consistent with complete rotator cuff tear. COMMENT: Entrapment of the subacromial bursa and supraspinatus ten-

dons may result in shoulder impingement syndrome. One cause of entrapment is acromioclavicular joint arthrosis. During abduction the supraspinatus tendon becomes trapped between osteophytes along the inferior acromioclavicular joint and the greater tuberosity of the humeral head. With attrition and eventual rupture of the supraspinatus tendon the action of the unopposed deltoid allows superior subluxation of the humerus.

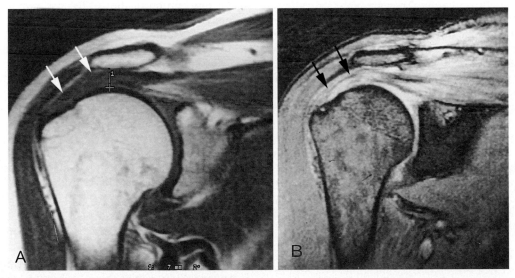

Figure 6.136.   CHRONIC SHOULDER PAIN: ROTATOR CUFF TENDINITIS. A. MRI, T1-Weighted Coronal Shoulder. Note the slightly hyperintense signal of the supraspinatus tendon (arrows) without evidence of focal signal alteration or morphologic change. The acromiohumeral distance is narrowed. **B. MRI, T2-Weighted Coronal Shoulder**. Diffuse hyperintense signal

is noted within the rotator cuff tendon (arrows) without evidence of frank tearing. (Courtesy of Frank E. Seidelmann, DO; Kingsley A. Orraca-Tetteh, MD; and Matthew M. Brown, RT(R), Advanced MRImaging, Richmond Heights, Ohio)

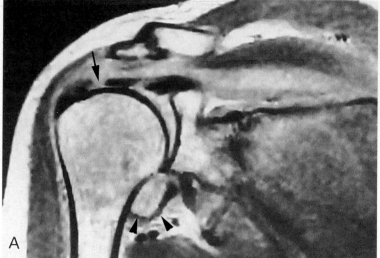

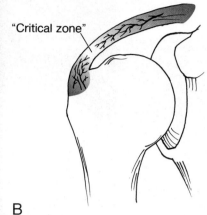

Figure 6.137. ROTATOR CUFF TENDON TEAR: COMPLETE. A. MRI, Proton Density-Weighted Coronal Oblique Shoulder. Observe the increased signal intensity within the rotator cuff tendon, representing a full-thickness tear (arrow). A hyperintense joint effusion is also present within the axillary recess (arrowheads). **B. Schematic Diagram: "Critical Zone."** The diagram illustrates the critical hypovascular zone of the supraspinatus tendon. This zone occurs just proximal to the rotator cuff insertion on the greater tuberosity of the humerus and predisposes the tendon to inflammation, secondary to overuse. (Courtesy of David L. Berens, MD, Buffalo MRI, Buffalo, New York)

evaluated to exclude associated lesions of the humeral head and glenoid labrum. (1,9,10)

Rotator cuff tears are most frequently associated with acute trauma or chronic repetitive injuries. They are common and are usually caused by repetitious lifting and/or activities that demand external rotation and abduction of the shoulder girdle (e.g., in baseball pitchers and weight lifters). Partial or complete tears of the rotator cuff (supraspinatus) tendon may produce sudden shoulder pain, reduced muscular strength, and articular dysfunction. Most tears are secondary to overuse and are part of a spectrum of rotator cuff disease that begins with tendinitis and progresses to a partial or complete tear. Cases of complete tear may be associated with anterior dislocation of the glenohumeral joint. These injuries are mainly seen in athletes who repeatedly throw and serve, such as baseball pitchers and tennis, and volleyball players. Other sport activities such as swimming and skiing also predispose to this type of injury. It is important to keep in mind that in athletes (either professional or amateur) over the age of 35 rotator cuff tears may occur secondary to degeneration. (1,11,12)

MRI Findings. MRI is the modality of choice for the diagnosis of rotator cuff lesions. High-resolution MR imaging in the sagittal and coronal oblique planes with spin-echo T1- and T2-weighted pulse sequences are commonly employed. MR arthrography (intraarticular injection of saline with or without a small amount of gadolinium) increases the overall sensitivity of the examination and is particularly useful in demonstrating small partial rotator cuff tears and capsular injury (discussed later in the text). Tears are visualized as moderately hyperintense defects in the tendon on T1-weighted images. The presence of hyperintense fluid at the site of the tear on T2-weighted images supports the diagnosis. Additional signs of complete tear include muscle retraction (often with the musculotendinous junction being pulled back past the normal 12 o'clock position on the humeral head), fluid in the subacromial-subdeltoid bursa, and disappearance of the peribursal

fat plane. (1,9) (Fig. 6.138) These findings are best depicted on the coronal oblique images. An additional secondary sign of complete tear of the rotator cuff is seen on plain films, with the humeral head gliding cephalically and resting closely under the acromion process. (Fig. 6.139) This narrows the subacromial arch and subsequently reduces the space available for the supraspinatus tendon. This occurs as a result of the unopposed action of the deltoid muscle, the major abductor of the shoulder.

A significant added benefit to the use of MR imaging of the shoulder is in the evaluation of partial tears of the rotator cuff. Partial tears exhibit signal changes identical to complete tears, but the abnormal signal focus does not span the entire width of the tendon. It is clear that partial tears on the bursal (superior) surface of the rotator cuff are best demonstrated with MRI and not with arthrography. (11) (Fig. 6.136) Prior to the use of MRI, these lesions could only be visualized arthroscopically or at surgery.

BURSITIS

Numerous different inflammatory conditions may result in subacromial and/or subdeltoid bursitis. For example, complete tears of the rotator cuff tendon establish communication of the subacromial bursa with the glenohumeral joint cavity, often resulting in hemorrhage or fluid accumulation within the bursa. Bursitis may also occur in patients with inflammatory disorders such as rheumatoid arthritis. On MR images, fluid or hemorrhage in the bursa appears hyperintense with T2-weighting and emits a low to intermediate signal on T1-weighted images. (1,10,11)

BICIPITAL TENDINITIS

Tenosynovitis of the biceps tendon is considered a degenerative disorder and is frequently associated with chronic rotator cuff disease. (13) MRI assists in accurately assessing the bicipital tendon and its surrounding synovial sheath. The presence of increased fluid within the synovial sheath is suggestive of tenosyn-

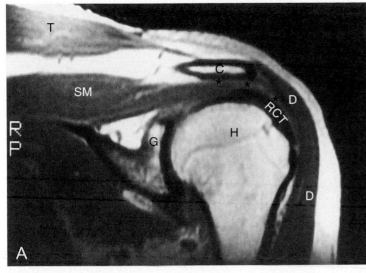
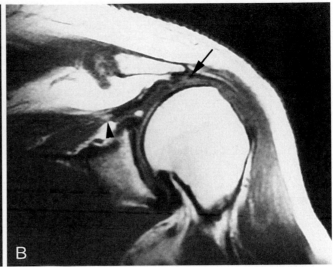

Figure 6.138.   ROTATOR CUFF TENDON TEAR. A. MRI, T1-Weighted Coronal Oblique Shoulder. Note the normal appearance of the supraspinatus muscle (*SM*), trapezius (*T*), rotator cuff tendon (*RCT*), deltoid (*D*), distal clavicle (*C*), subacromial subdeltoid bursa (asterisks), glenoid of the scapula (*G*), and humeral head (*H*). **B. MRI, T1-Weighted Coronal Oblique Shoulder.**

Observe the abnormal intermediate signal intensity disrupting the rotator cuff tendon (arrow). Retraction of the musculotendinous junction of the supraspinatus muscle (arrowhead) and superior subluxation of the humeral head are also present. (Courtesy of Mr. Richard J. Stevens, Medical Advances, Inc., Milwaukee, Wisconsin)

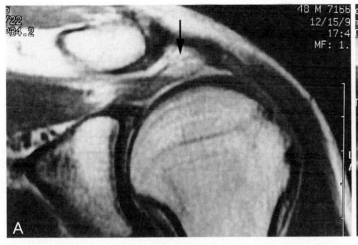
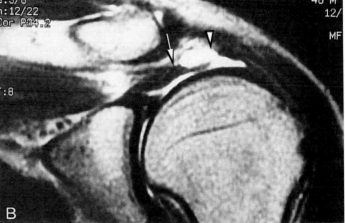

Figure 6.139.   ROTATOR CUFF: COMPLETE TEAR WITH RETRACTION. A. MRI, T1-Weighted Coronal Oblique Shoulder. There is increased signal intensity disrupting the rotator cuff tendon (arrow) indicating a full-thickness tear. **B. MRI, T2-Weighted Fast Spin-Echo Coronal Oblique Shoulder.** Observe the retraction of the musculotendinous junction of the supraspinatus

muscle, confirming a complete tear (arrow). Also note the high signal intensity at the distal end of the rotator cuff tendon (arrowhead) and superior subluxation of the humeral head. (Courtesy of Alan M. Lesselroth, MD, Mountain Diagnostics, Las Vegas, Nevada)

ovitis, but is generally considered a nonspecific finding and is often unreliable. A hyperintense signal intensity area within the biceps tendon itself on T2-weighted images is a more accurate sign indicating bicipital tendinitis. (14) (Fig. 6.140)

Progressive bicipital tendinitis is often a precursor to complete rupture of the biceps tendon. When complete rupture of the long head of the biceps tendon occurs, a classic *Popeye* muscle bulge in the upper arm is frequently observed. Complete tears without retraction may occur and should be evaluated with MRI. This provides a noninvasive method for assessing the margins of the tear. These nondisplaced tears are best treated conservatively, but occasionally require surgical intervention. (14)

SHOULDER INSTABILITY

Instability of the glenohumeral joint is most frequently associated with previous anterior dislocation. The anterior instability pattern is most common, while posterior and multidirectional instability are infrequently encountered. The unstable shoulder may manifest itself clinically as recurrent dislocation, pain, and weakness of the arm. Disability may result if proper treatment is not applied in a timely fashion. The vast majority of glenohumeral dislocations occur anteroinferiorly. A frequent finding in patients with recurrent dislocation is the *Hill-Sach's defect*, located at the posterolateral aspect of the humeral head (see Chapter 9

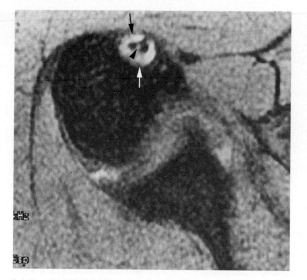

Figure 6.140.   BICIPTAL TENDINITIS. MRI, T2*-Weighted Axial Shoulder. Note the hyperintense edema within the synovial sheath of the biceps tendon (arrows). In addition, an area of high signal (arrowhead) is noted within the substance of the homogeneously low signal intensity biceps tendon. (Courtesy of Frank E. Seidelmann, DO; Kingsley A. Orraca-Tetteh, MD; and Matthew M. Brown, RT(R), Advanced MRImaging, Richmond Heights, Ohio)

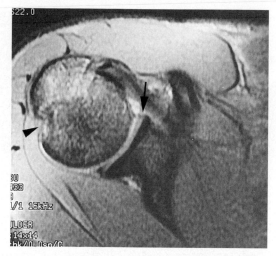

Figure 6.141.   SHOULDER PAIN: PREVIOUS ANTERIOR DISLOCATION. MRI, T2*-Weighted Axial Shoulder. The anterior labrum is not seen on this image, suggesting a displaced labral tear. Its normal location is indicated by the arrow. Note the Hill-Sach's compression fracture involving the postero-lateral aspect of the humeral head (arrowhead). The absence of marrow edema adjacent to the defect is consistent with an old injury. (Courtesy of Anthony S. Piana, DC, Hamden, Connecticut)

for a complete discussion of *Hill-Sach's defect*). These lesions are sometimes difficult to visualize with standard shoulder radiographs, but are seen well on axial MR images as focal depressions in the contour of the humeral head at the level of the coracoid process. (1–3,5,10,15–17) (Fig. 6.141)

THE BANKART LESION

Avulsion of the glenohumeral ligament labral complex from the glenoid rim is known as a *Bankart lesion*. This lesion may involve only the inferior glenohumeral ligament or may be associated with injury to the labrum or osseous glenoid. (Fig. 6.142) The osseous Bankart lesion is seen on plain film radiography. Advanced imaging is necessary to visualize the soft tissue component of this lesion. The Bankart lesion is classically associated with recurrent anterior shoulder dislocations and instability.

MRI Findings. The normal labrum is predominantly low in signal intensity on all pulse sequences. Areas of high signal within the labrum are suggestive of injury; however, other clinical and imaging findings (i.e., abnormal labral morphology, dislocation of the labrum, adjacent edema) must also support this appearance because an identical appearance has been seen in some asymptomatic individuals. The normal interposition of hyaline cartilage at the anterior labrum should not be confused with labral detachment or avulsion. This cartilage interposition is linear and not accompanied by edema, deformity, erosion, or other signs of instability. When labral lesions are present, a careful evaluation of the adjacent glenohumeral (capsular) ligaments is necessary to exclude associated capsular injury. (Fig. 6.143)

SUPERIOR LABRUM, ANTERIOR AND POSTERIOR LESION

Superior Labrum, Anterior and Posterior (SLAP) lesions are injuries that affect the superior portion of the glenoid labrum in the region of the biceps tendon insertion. (15) These lesions gen-

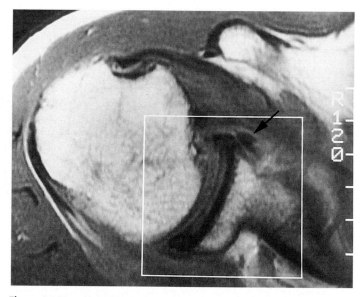

Figure 6.142.   ANTERIOR GLENOID LABRAL TEAR: UNSTABLE SHOULDER. MRI, T1-Weighted Axial Shoulder. There is interruption and rotational displacement of the anterior glenoid labrum (arrow). COMMENT: Tears of the glenoid labrum often present with functional instability. CT arthrography has been the primary imaging modality for the evaluation of shoulder instability (and labral tears). MR imaging has now replaced CT arthrography in the evaluation of labral pathology.

erally occur in young patients and are often associated with repetitive throwing or falling on an outstretched arm. These injuries are best depicted on the coronal oblique MR images and consist of superior labral fraying and/or detachment with variable biceps tendon involvement. Snyder (16) has described simple fraying and fragmentation of the biceps labral complex along with bucket-handle tears. SLAP lesions are less common than the Bankart avulsions and are most frequently associated with recurrent posterior shoulder subluxation and instability. (16)

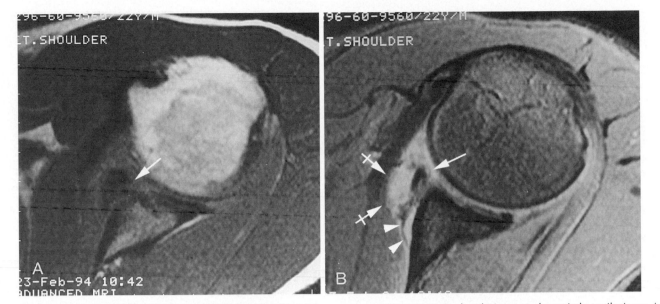

Figure 6.143. ACUTE ANTERIOR HUMERAL DISLOCATION. This adult male patient sustained an acute anteroinferior shoulder dislocation during a rugby tournament. **A. MRI, T1-Weighted Axial Shoulder. B. MRI, T2*-Weighted Axial Shoulder.** There is an osteocartilaginous fracture (arrow) involving the anterior portion of the glenoid (Bankart fracture). The low signal intensity anterior capsule is stripped from its osseous insertion (arrowheads) and is surrounded by hyperintense hemorrhage and edema (crossed arrows). COMMENT: Bankart lesions may be entirely cartilaginous, involving only the labral cartilage or may involve both the cartilage and the osseous glenoid. Capsular injuries to the glenoid labrum and anterior capsule are best visualized on axial MR images when a large amount of edema is present. The excess joint fluid provides the necessary contrast to adequately evaluate the capsular ligaments.

Previously, CT arthrography was considered the examination of choice for evaluating the unstable shoulder. MRI has replaced all other imaging modalities for most shoulder pathologies by virtue of its noninvasive nature and multiplanar capabilities. Dedicated shoulder coils must be employed to optimize spatial resolution and soft tissue contrast. MR arthrography is more sensitive than plain MRI in the detection of most soft tissue disorders involving the capsular-labral complex. Its invasive nature, however, precludes it from routine use.

OSTEONECROSIS

Osteonecrosis of bone is defined as death of the osseous cellular components in marrow caused by vascular compromise. Causes of osteonecrosis include trauma, hemoglobinopathies (such as sickle cell anemia), alcoholism, and excessive use of corticosteroids, among others. (10) Occasionally, osteonecrosis occurs with no apparent etiology and has been termed *spontaneous* or *idiopathic* osteonecrosis. A predilection for the ends of the long bones has been identified, with the femoral head, humeral head, and distal femur being the most common sites. (10)

Often plain films show no significant signs until there is advanced disease. The MR findings of bone infarction on spin-echo images include areas of low signal intensity with very irregular, serpiginous margins. These areas of low signal intensity are observed in the subchondral bone and may extend into the metaphysis.

THE ELBOW

Magnetic resonance imaging of the elbow is indicated in cases of trauma, infection, inflammatory processes, and other pathologies with subtle or absent radiographic findings. MR has the ability to display the cartilage, bone marrow, and periarticular soft tissues (ligaments, muscles, and tendons), including the neurovascular structures. This section discusses a few of the more common pathologies of the elbow and their MRI manifestations.

TENDINITIS

Extensor tendinitis (*tennis elbow*) is the most common traumatic injury of the elbow in athletes. (1) This entity, also called lateral epicondylitis, results from repetitive pronation and supination of the forearm with the wrist in extension. This injury is frequently seen in discus throwers, golfers, and tennis players. The pathologic process involves inflammation, mucinoid degeneration, and reactive granulation of the extensor carpi radialis brevis tendon. (2) The diagnosis of tennis elbow is mainly clinical. (3) Findings include local tenderness over the lateral epicondyle, which is reproduced with active dorsiflexion of the wrist against resistance and forearm supination. Medial epicondylitis is not as common as lateral and is associated with the common flexor pronator muscle group. Forceful flexion of the joint (as required of baseball pitchers) is a common cause.

Standard radiographs are usually negative, except for soft tissue swelling around the elbow. MR imaging should only be employed following a delayed or failed response to conservative management. Coronal and axial images using a dedicated extremity coil provide adequate visualization of the extensor carpi radialis brevis tendon and its insertion. Thickening of the tendon sheath is frequently seen and appears hyperintense on T2-weighted images. Intraarticular and periarticular fluid collections may also be observed with MRI. (4)

MEDIAL COLLATERAL LIGAMENT

The medial collateral ligament of the elbow has been referred to as the triangular ulnar collateral ligament and consists of three strong bands. (5) The anterior band, which is the strongest; the posterior band; and the transverse or oblique band, which is the weakest. The medial collateral ligament is seen on T1-weighted images as low signal intensity striations with interposed fat (high signal intensity areas) at its humeral origin. (6) Medial collateral ligament injuries are frequently found in baseball pitchers, as was seen in the recent career-ending injury for Nolan Ryan. MRI findings include a thickened, irregular ligament with hyperintense areas within the fibers on T2-weighted coronal images. (6) (Fig. 6.144) Acute tears are frequently surrounded by edema and hemorrhage, which appear hyperintense on both T2- and T2*-weighted images.

LATERAL COLLATERAL LIGAMENT

The radial collateral ligament is often referred to as the lateral collateral ligament. Tears of this ligament are not as common as the medial collateral ligament. (5) The MR findings of these injuries are similar in appearance to those involving the medial collateral ligament.

OSTEOCHONDRITIS DISSECANS

The most frequent cause of osteochondritis dissecans of the elbow is trauma. Clinical manifestations include pain and limited range of motion in extension. Some cases are diagnosed by means of standard radiographs. However, MRI is recommended when x-ray findings are inconclusive or if additional information regarding the integrity of the cartilage or the size and location of the dissected fragment is needed. (4,7) Sclerotic changes at the

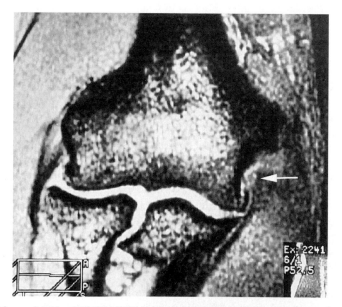

Figure 6.144. ULNAR COLLATERAL LIGAMENT TEAR: ELBOW. After pitching a 91-mph fast-ball, this major league baseball pitcher heard and felt a "snap" with a sudden onset of elbow pain. **MRI, Gradient-Echo 3-D Volume Acquisition Coronal Elbow**. There is a sharply defined complete interruption of the ulnar collateral ligament (arrow) with adjacent increased signal intensity (edema). COMMENT: MRI is an ideal modality for the localization and characterization of elbow ligament injuries. Ligament discontinuity and surrounding inflammatory edema are well visualized using a combination of T1- and T2-weighted MR images. The reformation capabilities of 3-D volume acquisitions allow accurate evaluation of ligaments that course through one or more anatomic planes. (Courtesy of The University Hospital, Department of Radiology, Denver, Colorado)

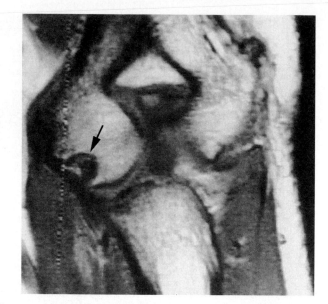

Figure 6.145. OSTEOCHONDRITIS DISSECANS: REPETITIVE VALGUS STRESS OF THE ELBOW. Observe the well-defined focal low signal intensity defect of the capitellum (arrow), consistent with osteochondritis dissecans. COMMENT: Activities that result in repetitive valgus stress may lead to compression of the capitellum and radial head. Ischemic injury may result and produce an osteochondral defect.

margin of the parent bone are frequently observed on plain film x-rays and correlate with the low signal intensity rim surrounding the osteochondral defect on the MR images. MRI helps in determining the stability of the osteochondral fragment. In unstable cases (i.e., loose fragment) there is disruption of the overlying cartilage and fluid between the defect and the host bone. Conversely, stable fragments do not exhibit intraarticular hyperintense fluid completely surrounding the fragment. (Fig. 6.145) These findings are well visualized using both spin-echo and T2*-weighted pulse sequences in orthogonal (coronal and sagittal) planes. (4,7,8)

THE WRIST

INTRODUCTION

The wrist is one of the most frequently injured joints in the human body. Its complex anatomy presents a diagnostic challenge to both the clinician and radiologist. Computed tomography provides excellent detail of cortical and medullary abnormalities, but soft tissue and bone marrow abnormalities are often not adequately delineated. The spatial resolution and superb soft tissue contrast of MRI permits visualization of the small ligaments of the wrist, including the scapholunate ligament and the triangular fibrocartilage complex. Intrinsic bone marrow lesions such as occult fracture and early osteonecrosis are also well demonstrated with MRI. This section reviews the pathologies of the wrist that are most likely to require magnetic resonance examination to establish the definitive diagnosis. Magnetic resonance of the wrist should be performed with a dedicated wrist coil using 3 mm or less slice thickness.

TRAUMATIC BONE LESION (OCCULT FRACTURE)

By definition an occult fracture is a cortical or bone marrow infraction that is not evident on plain films. These lesions, how-

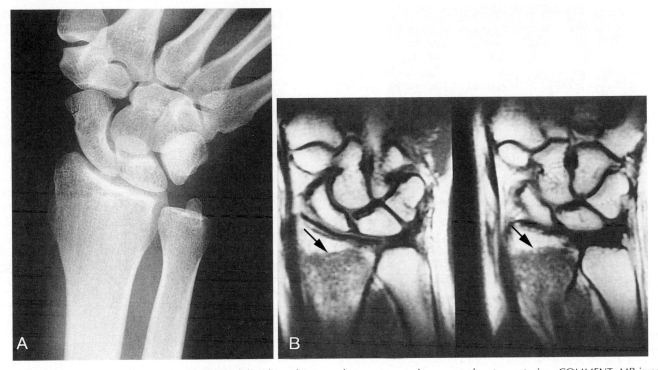

Figure 6.146. BONE CONTUSION OF THE WRIST. While riding a bicycle, this patient fell onto an outstretched wrist. **A. PA Ulnar Deviation Wrist.** No evidence of fracture is visualized. MRI was subsequently performed the same day. **B. MRI, T1-Weighted Coronal Wrist.** There is decreased signal intensity confined to, and completely filling, the medullary cavity of the distal radius to the physeal scar (arrows). These findings are indicative of bone marrow edema secondary to contusion. COMMENT: MR imaging is the only imaging modality that readily demonstrates bone contusion and trabecular microfractures. This information is helpful in demonstrating the magnitude of injury to a patient, particularly in medicolegal circumstances. (Courtesy of John D. Bailey, RT, MRI Center of Austin, Austin, Texas)

ever, are often visible with MRI and scintigraphy. (1,2) With MRI, the edema is seen in and around the fracture as an ill-defined and hypointense area on T1-weighted and proton density images that becomes hyperintense with T2-weighting. Medullary bone contusions or edema have a similar appearance, but lack the distinct fracture line. (Fig. 6.146) The edema in these injuries often reabsorbs, and the clinical symptoms resolve within a period of 6 weeks. (1,2)

SCAPHOID FRACTURE

Scaphoid (carpal navicular) fractures account for 50% of all carpal fractures. (3) Clinically, patients with scaphoid fractures will complain of pain over the anatomic snuffbox. Conventional radiographs of the wrist, which should include an ulnar deviation view, often assist in demonstration of the fracture line. These fractures occur through the waist of the scaphoid in over 70% of cases. The proximal pole is fractured in 20% of cases, and 10% of these injuries involve the distal pole. (3)

Both nuclear scintigraphy and MRI will be abnormal in patients with occult scaphoid fractures prior to visible, plain film findings. MRI, however, has greater spatial resolution and is therefore more accurate in defining the specific location and extent of the injury. Fractures are observed as low signal intensity areas on T1-weighted images that become hyperintense with T2-weighting. (3) (Fig. 6.147)

OSTEONECROSIS

Osteonecrosis may occur at any carpal bone as a result of traumatic disruption of the blood supply. The scaphoid and the lunate

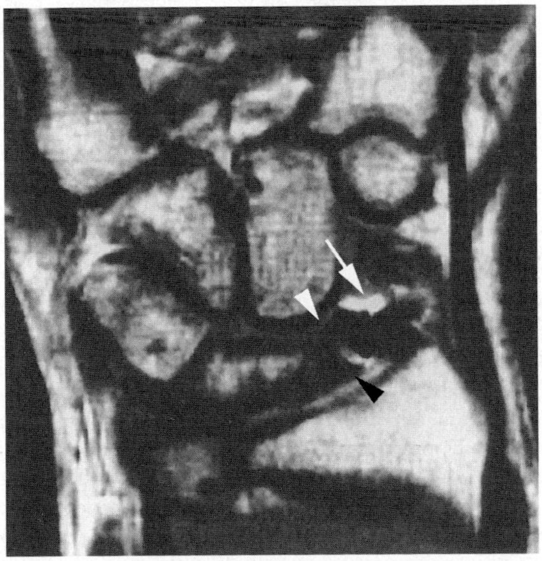

Figure 6.147. SCAPHOID FRACTURE WITH ISCHEMIC NECROSIS. MRI, Proton Density-Weighted Coronal Wrist. Observe the fracture through the waist of the scaphoid, represented as an area of hyperintense fluid (arrow). The low signal intensity of the proximal pole of the scaphoid is consistent with osteonecrosis (arrowheads). COMMENT: MRI is the most sensitive imaging modality to detect occult fracture and early osteonecrosis of the scaphoid.

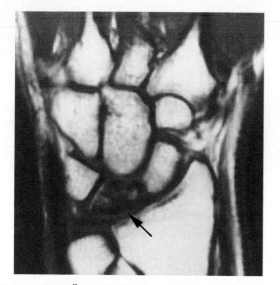

Figure 6.148. KIENBÖCK'S DISEASE: LUNATE. MRI, T1-Weighted Coronal Wrist. Note the homogeneous low signal intensity of the carpal lunate suggesting osteonecrosis. COMMENT: Osteonecrosis of the lunate (Kienböck's disease) is often the sequelae of trauma to the wrist. Collapse, fragmentation, and sclerosis (the snow-capped appearance) are the classic plain film findings.

(Kienböck's disease) are the most frequently affected carpal bones. Osteonecrosis of the scaphoid is usually the sequela of a traumatic injury to the waist or proximal pole and occurs in 10 to 15% of all scaphoid fractures. (3) (Fig. 6.147) MRI demonstrates the extent of the necrotic process more accurately than conventional radiography (4–6) and is equally as sensitive as nuclear scintigraphy. (7,8) When only T1-weighted sequences are used, the MR sensitivity in diagnosing necrosis is about 87.5%; with the addition of the T2-weighted sequences, the specificity is 100% (7). Therefore T1- and T2-weighted coronal and axial images should be used to best display the characteristics of the lesion. In the early stages T2-weighted sequences demonstrate regions of increased signal intensity. This area can be surrounded by hypointense signal, which is believed to represent the interface between nonviable (dead) bone and reparative granulation tissue. (9) In advanced cases the necrotic zone has a homogeneous, hypointense signal on both T1- and T2-weighted images. (Fig. 6.148)

CARPAL LIGAMENT RUPTURE

Magnetic resonance imaging has become a reliable modality for displaying the carpal ligaments. There are two groups of ligaments in the wrist: the *intrinsic* ligaments, which connect one carpal bone to another (e.g., scapholunate ligament); and the *extrinsic* ligaments, which arise from the pericarpal area to insert at the carpus (e.g., radioscaphoid ligament). When ligament injury is suspected clinically, MRI may be useful in substantiating the physical examination findings. The use of a dedicated wrist coil must be employed to limit the field of view and obtain the high signal-to-noise ratio necessary to optimally visualize the complex anatomy of this joint. Coronal images using spin-echo T1-weighted and T2- or T2*-weighted pulse sequences with 3 mm slice thickness can be used to visualize the ligaments. Three-dimensional (3-D) volume imaging sequences are capable of obtaining thinner slices (1 mm or less) and provide greater spatial resolution.

Intercarpal ligament disruptions are seen as areas of discontinuity and are frequently associated with an adjacent high signal intensity area (edema) on T2-weighted images. (10) (Fig. 6.149) The presence of increased fluid in the midcarpal joint can be a sensitive but nonspecific sign of either scapholunate and/or lunatotriquetral ligament tear. (7,11,12) These structures may be very difficult to visualize because of their small size. In addition, the lunatotriquetral ligament courses in an oblique fashion, often making it difficult to image. Consequently, *arthrography* of the wrist remains the *gold standard* in evaluating the integrity of the small intercarpal ligaments.

TRIANGULAR FIBROCARTILAGE

The triangular fibrocartilage complex (TFCC) is a major contributor to the stability of the wrist. It is located between the distal ulna and the proximal carpal row (lunate and triquetrum) and is comprised of the fibrocartilaginous disc, meniscal homologue, dorsal and volar radioulnar ligaments, ulnar collateral ligament, and the sheath of the extensor carpi ulnaris tendon. (13) The articular disc is seen as a triangular signal void arising from the medial aspect of the distal radius and approximating the ulnar styloid process. The TFCC appears as an elongated triangle with the apex directed toward the radius.

MRI is unique in that it is capable of displaying both degenerative and posttraumatic lesions of the TFCC. Clinical findings of an acute TFCC tear include pain and "popping" along the ulnar aspect of the wrist joint. The central portion of the triangular fibrocartilage (TFC) ligament is thin and is the most common site for degenerative tears. An irregular or linear area of increased signal that communicates with the articular surface on T2*- or T2-weighted pulse sequences is the classic MR finding of a traumatic TFCC tear. (Fig. 6.150) These usually occur within 2 to 3 mm of the radial insertion (7,14) or close to the ulnar attachment. (14)

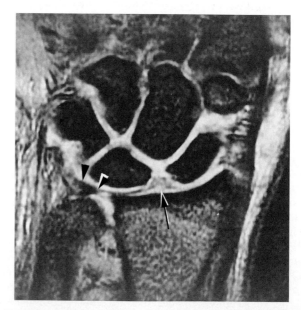

Figure 6.149. SCAPHOLUNATE LIGAMENT TEAR: WRIST. MRI, T2*-Weighted Coronal Wrist. Note the widened scapholunate joint space with a poorly defined scapholunate ligament (arrow). Observe the intact triangular fibrocartilage complex (arrowheads). (Courtesy of Frank E. Seidelmann, DO; Kingsley A. Orraca-Tetteh, MD; and Matthew M. Brown, RT(R), Advanced MRImaging, Richmond Heights, Ohio)

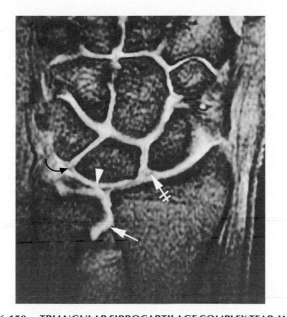

Figure 6.150. TRIANGULAR FIBROCARTILAGE COMPLEX TEAR: WRIST. MRI, T2*-Weighted Coronal Wrist. Note the normal hyperintense articular fluid extending into the distal radioulnar joint (arrow). This fluid escapes proximally through the vertical tear in the lateral portion of the triangular fibrocartilage (arrowhead). Observe the normal scapholunate (crossed arrow) and lunatotriquetral (curved arrow) ligaments. (Courtesy of Frank E. Seidelmann, DO; Kingsley A. Orraca-Tetteh, MD; and Matthew M. Brown, RT(R), Advanced MRImaging, Richmond Heights, Ohio)

Occasionally, there is an associated avulsion fracture of the styloid process. Fluid collection in the radiocarpal and the distal radioulnar joints has been described as an important secondary sign of acute TFCC tear. (7,14,15) Degenerative tears of the TFCC are often seen in asymptomatic individuals and appear on T2- and T2*-weighted coronal images as a hyperintense area of intrameniscal signal that does not communicate with the articular surface.

CARPAL TUNNEL SYNDROME

Carpal tunnel syndrome (CTS) involves motor and sensory dysfunction of the median nerve. This occurs as a result of compression of the median nerve as it passes through the carpal tunnel. Causes include fracture, infection, various infiltrative disease processes, and localized soft tissue pathology. Carpal tunnel syndrome is usually found in patients between the ages of 30 and 60 with a high female-to-male ratio (as high as 5:1). (16) Bilateral symptoms are present in over 50% of cases. (16)

Clinical symptoms include pain and paresthesias that are worse at night and often wake the patient. These symptoms follow the classic distribution of the median nerve and thus affect the palmar aspect of the thumb, index finger, and middle finger and the radial half of the ring finger. Muscle atrophy and loss of function are late findings. Positive Tinel's and Phalen's signs are strong neurologic indicators of CTS.

Anatomy of the Carpal Tunnel

The carpal tunnel can be broken down into its proximal and distal components. The proximal portion of the tunnel is at the level of the pisiform while the distal aspect of the tunnel occurs at approximately the level of the hamate.

The carpus has a concave bony contour along its volar surface

and is covered by the flexor retinaculum. The bony carpus forms the floor and walls of the carpal tunnel, with the rigid flexor retinaculum representing its roof. The flexor tendons of the hand and forearm as well as numerous neurovascular structures traverse through the tunnel, deep to the retinaculum.

The median nerve is round or oval at the level of the distal radius and becomes elliptical in shape at the pisiform and hamate. The morphologic appearance and position of the median nerve are altered during flexion and extension of the wrist.

Etiology

There are numerous causes of carpal tunnel syndrome. Fracture (e.g., Colles', hook of the hamate, proximal metacarpal) and tenosynovitis (repetitive strain injury) of the flexor tendons are some of the traumatic causes. Synovial hyperplasia is frequently seen in inflammatory arthritides (such as gout, pseudogout, rheumatoid arthritis, and amyloidosis) and results in an increased volume of tissue within the carpal tunnel, producing subsequent median nerve compression. Tumors of the median nerve (fibromas, neural sheath tumors) and other space occupying lesions such as lipomas and ganglions may encroach on the carpal canal producing carpal tunnel syndrome. Other known causes of CTS involve bilateral soft tissue thickening that may occur with pregnancy, acromegaly, hypothyroidism, and diabetes mellitus. (17)

Electrodiagnostic Testing for Carpal Tunnel Syndrome

The definitive means for establishing the diagnosis of CTS is nerve conduction testing. Plain film radiographs seldom offer any information that contributes to the diagnosis. The use of MRI in the diagnosis of carpal tunnel syndrome should be guided by clinical history and physical findings. MRI is indicated when conservative management has failed, electrodiagnostic testing is equivocal, or physical examination demonstrates a mass or fullness in the carpal region near the carpal tunnel.

MRI Findings

Both coronal and axial MR images of the wrist provide valuable information in determining the presence of median nerve damage or deficit. (18)

The following changes in the median nerve are present in CTS, regardless of the etiology. (7) (Fig. 6.151)

1. Diffuse swelling or segmental enlargement of the median nerve, best evaluated at the level of the pisiform.
2. Flattening of the median nerve, best demonstrated at the level of the hamate.
3. Palmar bowing of the flexor retinaculum, assessed at the level of the hamate.
4. Increased signal intensity within the median nerve at any level. This finding is well demonstrated on axial T2- and T2*-weighted and inversion recovery (STIR) images. (19)

THE TEMPOROMANDIBULAR JOINT
INTRODUCTION

Imaging of the temporomandibular joint (TMJ) continues to be a technologically challenging task. Plain film x-rays, in both the open- and closed-mouth positions, render basic information con-

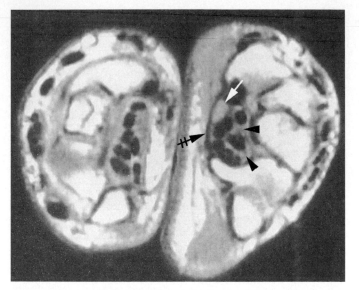

Figure 6.151. CARPAL TUNNEL SYNDROME. This 42-year-old female experienced weakness and tingling of the right wrist. **MRI, T2-Weighted Bilateral Axial Wrist**. There is increased signal intensity and swelling of the right median nerve (arrow). In addition, there is increased fluid between the flexor tendons within the tunnel (arrowheads) and slight bowing of the flexor retinaculum (crossed arrows). COMMENT: The nerve conduction velocity test has approximately an 80% sensitivity for carpal tunnel syndrome. If negative, an MRI examination should be utilized for further evaluation.

cerning the integrity of the joint. However, high-quality images are difficult to obtain because of the complex anatomy of this area. Bilateral open- and closed-mouth tomographic projections were used in the early years in evaluating the TMJ. Later, fluoroscopy, with and without intraarticular contrast, was employed to indirectly visualize joint pathology and to assess function. Arthrography allows indirect characterization of disc morphology, but is an invasive procedure with associated morbidity and limitations in accuracy. (1) More recently, sagittally reformatted computed tomography (CT) images following arthrography have been used to evaluate the TMJ. This technique, however, does not provide the spatial resolution necessary to accurately delineate the disc and surrounding ligaments. MR imaging has rapidly replaced these modalities. (2–5) Its noninvasive nature, lack of ionizing radiation, and multiplanar capability make MRI the ideal imaging technique for evaluating the structure and function of the TMJ. (6–8)

TECHNICAL CONSIDERATIONS

Sagittal images using T1- and T2*-weighted pulse sequences are utilized in the evaluation of the articular disc and surrounding ligaments of the TMJ. Surface coil technology allows the field of view to be limited, providing the necessary signal-to-noise ratio. Thin slices through the articulation may be obtained using 3-D volume acquisitions. The reformation capabilities of 3-D techniques reduce the need for coronal images; however, when the joint capsule or supporting ligaments are in question, coronal slices should be acquired. The examination should be performed in the full open- and closed-mouth positions to document meniscus position and degree of reduction. (1)

INTERNAL DERANGEMENT OF THE TEMPOROMANDIBULAR JOINT

Clinical symptoms of internal derangement include craniofacial and cervicocranial pain syndromes, myofascial pain, joint dysfunction and crepitus, and dental malocclusion. (1) The scope of this discussion concerning the temporomandibular joint is limited to meniscal displacement and perforation.

Meniscal Displacement

Internal derangement (displacement of the articular meniscus or disc) is the most common imaging finding in the TMJ. The discs often display surface irregularity, fissuring, fibrillation, and fraying, all of which may be identified with MRI. Injury to the bilaminar zone of the meniscus may allow anterior displacement of the disc in the open- or closed-mouth position. A rotational component to the meniscal displacement may also exist. (1)

A grading system characterizing disc morphology and displacement has been described. (9) A grade I disc demonstrates anterior displacement without visible morphologic change. (Fig. 6.152) Anterior displacement of an abnormally shaped disc characterizes a grade II disc lesion. (Fig. 6.153) Helms et al. (10) found that 95% of joints with grade II discs exhibited evidence of osteoarthritis, while only 17% of joints with grade I disc lesions showed similar changes.

Disc Perforation

Arthrography remains the best imaging modality to evaluate perforations of the TMJ meniscus. Most patients with a perforated meniscus also have a dislocation. MRI demonstrates the dislocation and adequately outlines the damage to the meniscus. (1)

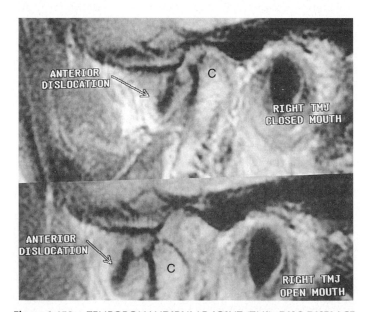

Figure 6.152. TEMPOROMANDIBULAR JOINT (TMJ): DISC DISPLACEMENT. MRI, Proton Density-Weighted Sagittal TMJ. The upper image (closed mouth) reveals complete anterior displacement of the low signal intensity intraarticular disc (arrow). The lower image (open mouth) displays anterior translation of the mandibular condyle (C) and no change in the position of the intraarticular disc. COMMENT: MRI is considered the *gold standard* for evaluating internal derangement of the TMJ.

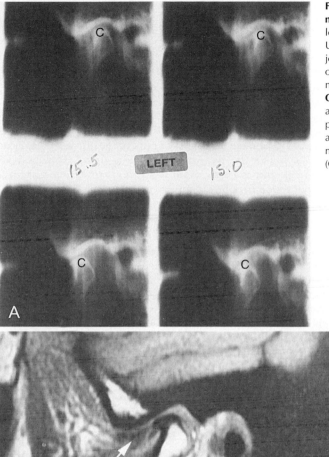

Figure 6.153.   TEMPOROMANDIBULAR JOINT (TMJ): A DISC THAT SLIPS. A. To-mography Closed Mouth (Uppers); Opened Mouth (Lowers) Lateral TMJs. Note the location of the mandibular condyle *(C)* in the glenoid during the closed position. Upon opening, the condyle translates and rotates anteriorly. Observe the asymmetric joint space narrowing and osteophyte formation on the mandibular condyle anteriorly. **B. MRI, T1-Weighted Sagittal Closed Mouth TMJ.** Note the anterior displacement of the disc in the closed mouth position (arrow). **C. MRI, T1-Weighted Sagittal Open Mouth TMJ.** There is anterior displacement of the disc (arrow), which remains anteriorly displaced regardless of the position of the mandible. COMMENT: MRI may provide assessment of TMJ dynamics, serving as a functional complement to anatomic assessment. A cine loop format displays the simulation of continuous motion during mouth opening and closing. The current modality of choice to assess the TMJ is MRI. (Courtesy of Kennon E. Rude, DC, Boulder, Colorado)

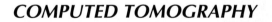

COMPUTED TOMOGRAPHY

HISTORICAL PERSPECTIVES

In 1972 Godfried Hounsfield of EMI Limited in London introduced the first generation of computed tomography equipment that consisted of an x-ray source, radiation detectors, and electronic devices mounted on a frame or gantry that surrounded the patient being imaged. (1) The computed tomography (CT) image depicts a thin slice of anatomy obtained from multiple x-ray absorption measurements made around the periphery of the body. Contrary to conventional tomography, where the image of a thin section of anatomy is made by blurring out information from unwanted areas above and below the plane of interest, the CT image is constructed by using data taken only from the region of interest. The x-ray tube and detectors were designed to move continuously across the patient.

Hounsfield won the Nobel prize for medicine in 1979 for the discovery of computed tomography. The first clinical prototype EMI head scan (Mark I) was installed in early 1972 at Atkinson Morley's Hospital in London. (1) It proved to be an immediate success, and an improved version was introduced at that year's meeting of the Radiological Society of North America. (2) The scanner consisted of a stationary anode x-ray tube cooled by circulating oil. (2) The first EMI head scanner in America was placed at the Mayo Clinic in July of 1973. (2)

The EMI scanner was designed for brain scanning, and its applications were limited to the head. (2) In the United States a dentist named Ledley became intrigued with the possibility of applying the technique to other regions of the body. (2) He parlayed this interest into funding for construction of the first whole-body scanner. (2) The first clinical unit was named the ACTA scanner, and it was installed at the University of Minnesota in 1973. (2) Anatomic motion remained a significant problem in applications of this scanner to regions other than the head and extremities. (2)

Since the development of the first-generation CT scanners, there have been major technical advancements that have dramatically increased the speed of scanning and quality of image reconstruction. (2) Fourth-generation CT scanners have since been developed, and, most recently, an *ultra fast* (helical/spiral) CT scanner has been introduced. Douglas Boyd and collaborators designed this unit to image the heart. By successfully steering a

small, focal-spot-size electron beam at four fixed tungsten target rings, an artifact-free image of the heart can be obtained in as little as 17 ms, with a single breathhold.

Glossary of Terms

Attenuation: the absorbed energy of an x-ray beam after it passes through a given substance. Each tissue examined has a specific attenuation or x-ray photon absorption value.

Gantry: a round or square housing for the x-ray tubes and scintillation detectors. The patient is placed in the open center of the gantry. Most CT scanners allow angulation of the gantry up to 30°. (Fig. 6.154)

Hounsfield unit (HU): the unit of radiographic density in computed tomography. Hounsfield units reflect the attenuation properties of a given tissue, relative to those of water and air. By assigning constant HU values to air (-1000 HU) and water (0 HU), a relative scale of radiographic densities (gray scale) is generated. The computer then assigns an HU value for each tissue voxel based on its attenuation coefficient. This is expressed as a specific shade of gray on the resultant CT image.

Photon detector cells (scintillation detectors): high-efficiency photodiodes that absorb and register the attenuated photon beam following its passage through the patient. The photon energy registered by the scintillation detector is processed by the computer to produce the CT image.

Pixel: tiny two-dimensional squares that represent attenuation characteristics from a three-dimensional volume of tissue (voxel). Each pixel is comprised of multiple attenuation coefficients that are averaged to create a mean measurement of tissue density (expressed in Hounsfield units).

Voxel: a volume of tissue projected into the pixel from which the Hounsfield unit is derived.

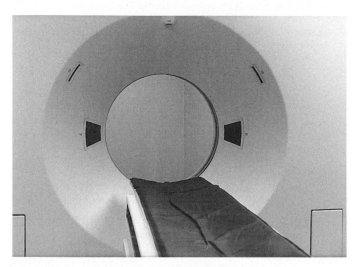

Figure 6.154.   GANTRY OF A COMPUTERIZED TOMOGRAPHIC SCANNER. The CT gantry houses the x-ray tube and photon detectors. The couch is padded for patient comfort and can be vertically adjusted. Its movement in and out of the gantry is precisely controlled allowing the exact location of each tomographic slice to be determined. Laser-assisted patient placement aids in the overall accuracy of the examination. Most gantries angle up to 30° to provide angled slices through the intervertebral discs.

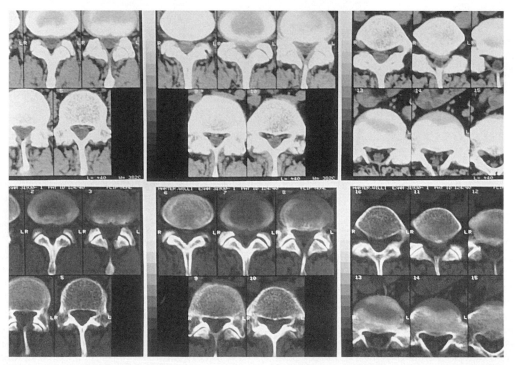

Figure 6.155.   NORMAL CT SCAN: BONE AND SOFT TISSUE WINDOWS. CT Axial Lumbar. These images display the distinction between bone and soft tissue window settings. Soft tissue windows (top row) are iden- tified by a gray appearance to the soft tissues and poor distinction between cortical and medullary bone, whereas bone windows (bottom row) are iden- tified by dark soft tissues and optimum cortical and medullary differentiation.

Window level: an arbitrary number chosen by the operator to limit the shades of gray to optimally display a specific attenuation value (tissue density).

Window width: a preselected range of attenuation values chosen by the operator to visualize a range of tissue densities. The window level represents the median density. For example, if the window level is set at 200 HU and the window width is 800, the resultant image would display Hounsfield units that measure +600 to −200. Any density greater than +600 or −200 would appear as white or black on the image, respectively. (Fig. 6.155)

Soft tissue window: window level and width that optimize the attenuation values of soft tissues. Differentiation of cortical and medullary bone is often not possible on these images.

Bone window: window level and width that optimize the attenuation values of bone, allowing cortical and medullary differentiation. The subtle attenuation coefficients of the soft tissues are not appreciated and have a dark gray appearance.

TECHNICAL CONSIDERATIONS

Fourth-generation computed tomography equipment places the photon detector cells in fixed positions around the patient, while the x-ray source rotates within the surrounding gantry. (Fig. 6.156) These CT units efficiently capture the continuous flow of x-ray energy through the use of 1000 or more photon detectors composed of scintillation crystals and photodiodes. (3)

The anatomic information received from the photon detectors is processed through a series of complex mathematical equations. This information is then manipulated into numerous tiny pixels. Each pixel is assigned an attenuation value (Hounsfield unit) and arranged in a matrix to form the final axial CT image. (Fig. 6.157) This image is then viewed on a monitor (cathode ray tube or CRT). The window level and width can be adjusted to change the image characteristics and highlight specific tissue attributes before the hard copy is produced.

On most systems, collimation as fine as 1 mm is now available. This feature, coupled with the use of a sharp reconstruction kernel, permits acquisition of detailed images of high-contrast ob-

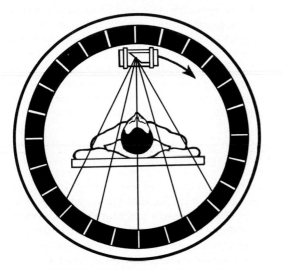

Figure 6.156.   ROTATE CT SCANNER. This diagram displays a fourth generation rotating scanner with stationary detector elements in the ring surrounding the patient. The tube and fan beam rotate around the patient as radiation is directed into the region of interest. The detectors measure the residual photon energy, and the computers then encode the attenuation characteristics necessary for image formation.

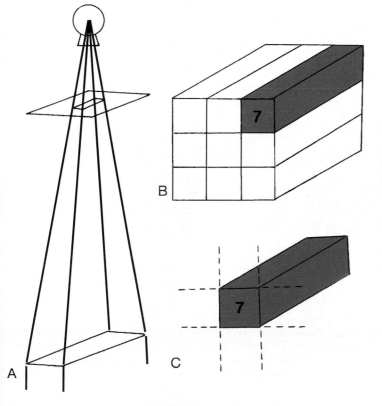

Figure 6.157.   IMAGE FORMATION. A. Collimation of The Fan X-Ray Beam. Precise collimation is employed so that a very thin fan beam of x-rays is used to scan thin sections of the body. **B. Voxels and Pixels.** Each photon detector deciphers a volume of tissue (voxel). The shaded box represents a voxel. The number "7" represents the attenuation coefficient of that volume of tissue and is known as a pixel. **C. Image Matrix.** The CT image is formed from a volume of data received from the detectors and processed by the computer for display on the CRT or hard copy. The shaded rectangular box represents a voxel and the shaded square at the end of the voxel is the picture element or pixel. Each image represents a matrix or composite of pixels. Each pixel represents the attenuation coefficient of a given volume of tissue.

jects like trabecular bone and the parenchyma of the lungs. (4–7) All CT information is acquired in the axial plane except for smaller body parts such as facial bones, wrist, and feet where sagittal or coronal images can be obtained. Sagittal or coronal images of the spine are created by manipulating the stored computer data from the axial images. This *reconstruction* or *reformatting* process is analogous to first viewing a loaf of bread slice by slice, in a transverse or axial orientation, then stacking each slice on top of one another and slicing vertically through the loaf to obtain a *coronal* or *sagittal* perspective. (Fig. 6.158) These reconstructed images are significantly less detailed than the axial images from which they were derived. True multiplanar imaging is best obtained using MRI, when applicable.

Helical/spiral CT scanners provide rapid data acquisition, resulting in fewer breathholds per scan compared with conventional CT. Accordingly, the greatly reduced scan time decreases motion artifact while increasing resolution. At present, a 1-second scan speed is possible, and faster speeds are limited only by photon flux from the x-ray tube and the conversion efficiency of the detector elements. A quicker examination time also improves overall patient comfort and provides a faster, more thorough assessment of acute patients. With helical CT a continuous volume of data over a specific anatomic region is obtained. Coupled with better image registration from the reduced scan time, this feature greatly enhances the quality of reconstructed images.

Currently, the major applications for three-dimensional helical CT are related to imaging of bone structures for surgical planning (e.g., for posttraumatic lesions in areas of complex osseous anatomy, such as the pelvis and facial skeleton) and the vascular system. (8)

Intrathecal, intradiscal, or intravenous injection of radiopaque contrast prior to examining a patient with CT may help in the assessment of certain conditions. Intravenous contrast may assist in delineating soft tissue lesions that may be difficult or impossible to see with noncontrast scans. In addition, the pattern of vascular enhancement may provide insight into the histology of a given lesion and allows differentiation of recurrent disc herniation from reparative scar in the post-surgical patient.

The radiation dose for a 30 to 36-slice standard CT scan of the lumbar spine is approximately 3 to 5 rads. By comparison, five plain film radiographs of the lumbar spine in an average-sized patient using a 100 kilohertz (kHz) true high-frequency generator, a 12:1 grid ratio, and 600-speed rare-earth film-screen combination results in a total patient dose of approximately 1 rad. However, a single phase generator, a 12:1 ratio, and a 400-speed rare earth film-screen combination on the same sized patient in the lumbar spine renders a total patient dose of approximately 2½ rads.

CONTRAINDICATIONS

Few contraindications to the use of computed tomography exist. As with other modalities that utilize ionizing radiation, patient dose should be kept to a minimum and children should not be scanned without strong clinical indication. Hypersensitivity to iodine products, delayed renal clearance, and congestive heart failure contraindicate the use of contrast infusion. Blood urea nitrogen and creatinine laboratory values should be assessed prior to intravenous contrast use. The presence of metallic objects near the area of interest may result in significant image artifact from

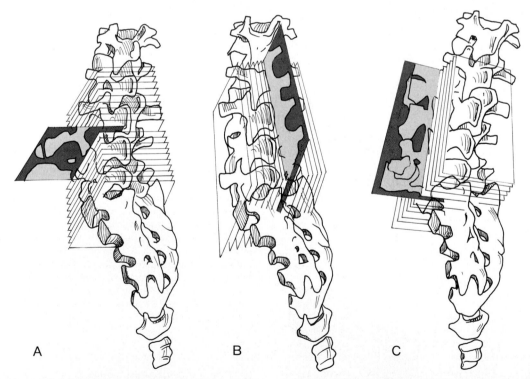

A   B   C

Figure 6.158. IMAGE RECONSTRUCTION (REFORMATION). A. Axial Images. The data used to produce a CT image are obtained in an axial format. **B. Sagittal Images. C. Coronal Images.** The numerical data used to produce the axial images can be used to create sagittal and coronal reformation images. COMMENT: The reformation process is analogous to a loaf of sliced bread. The slices of bread represent the axial images that are initially obtained by the CT scanner. If those slices are stacked one on top of another, that entire loaf of bread may be sliced vertically, producing a different (sagittal or coronal) perspective.

beam scattering. Better detail may be obtained from MR in some instances. Claustrophobia may occur in a very small percentage of the patients scanned.

NORMAL ANATOMY

Computed tomography utilizes x-ray technology to provide images oriented in the axial plane. By altering the window width and window level, one can *"target"* a specific tissue to be optimally visualized. Normally, both soft tissue and bone windows are performed for complete evaluation of a body region. (Fig. 6.159) CT is best utilized to evaluate the cortex and surrounding periosteum. MRI provides superior spatial and contrast resolution and is therefore best at evaluating the bone marrow and contents of the neural canal. (Fig. 6.160)

INDICATIONS FOR MUSCULOSKELETAL IMAGING

Computed tomography may be employed in the assessment of numerous pathologic conditions. Several broad categories of disease are discussed in this section, including traumatic, infectious, vascular, neoplastic, congenital, arthritic, and metabolic disorders.

TRAUMA

Traumatic lesions of the musculoskeletal system are frequently well demonstrated on conventional radiographs. In areas of complex anatomy such as the facial bones, spine, and pelvis, (Fig. 6.161) however, significant bony infractions may be occult or inadequately demonstrated on plain films. (Fig. 6.162) The use of CT is warranted when radiographs are equivocal or when suspicious clinical findings are not substantiated by the present plain film study. (Fig. 6.163) In cases of comminuted fractures, reconstructed computed tomography provides valuable information concerning the location of bone fragments and their re-

lationship to articulating surfaces. This information is crucial in the preoperative evaluation of intraarticular fractures of any joint. Occult fractures of the bone marrow, however, are better displayed on magnetic resonance (MR) images.

Axial and reconstructed sagittal CT slices offer a clear assessment of the vertebral column. In spinal trauma CT helps to exclude or confirm the presence of small bone fragments near the spinal cord by eliminating overlapping structures that may obscure the fractures on plain x-rays. (Fig. 6.164) In addition to fractures of the vertebral column, atlantoaxial rotatory subluxations and facet malalignments are well demonstrated by CT. (9) (Figs. 6.165, 6.166) When cord compression and/or intramedullary lesions are suspected clinically, the CT examination must be complemented by magnetic resonance imaging. MRI clearly displays posttraumatic cord injury, including edema and hemorrhage. CT does not have the necessary contrast resolution to adequately evaluate suspected spinal cord injury.

Computed tomography is also useful in the diagnosis of traumatic lesions of the orbits (e.g., blowout fractures), paranasal sinuses, and facial bones (e.g., tripod and Lefort fractures). (9–12) Three-dimensional reconstruction of the axial images is beneficial in unraveling the overlapping anatomy of the facial skeleton and in preoperative planning. Injury to other complex osseous structures, including the wrist, ankle (Fig. 6.167), shoulder (Fig. 6.168), and sternoclavicular joints, as well as the pelvic articulations, may be effectively evaluated with CT. The anatomic features of spondylolysis are also well demonstrated with CT. (Fig. 6.169)

Posttraumatic, calcified, soft tissue lesions (e.g., myositis ossificans, calcified hematomas) should also be assessed with CT. (Fig. 6.170) The differential diagnosis is especially important, and includes malignancy, infection, and aneurysm. Calcifications are seen with MRI as signal voids and are difficult to evaluate accurately. Computed tomography better demonstrates the extent and location of the calcifications (periosteal, parosteal, or intramuscular) and is the imaging modality of choice for these calcified lesions. Magnetic resonance can be useful in showing the uncal-

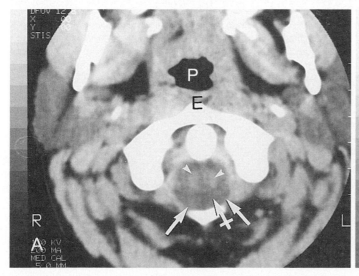

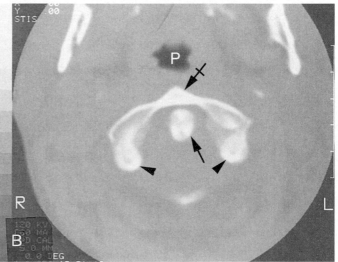

Figure 6.159. NORMAL ANATOMY: COMPUTED TOMOGRAPHY. A. CT, Soft Tissue Window, Axial C1. Soft tissue windows provide good contrast resolution between the various soft tissues, but suboptimally define the bony structures. Note the borders of the dural sac (arrows), which contain the spinal cord (arrowheads) and the lower attenuation cerebrospinal fluid (crossed arrow). Air is observed in the pharynx and esophagus.

B. CT, Bone Window, Axial C1. By adjusting the window level and expanding the window width, the same numerical data can be displayed with different image characteristics. The bones demonstrate better spatial and contrast resolution, whereas the soft tissues are now poorly differentiated. Note the dens (arrow), lateral masses (arrowheads), and anterior tubercle (crossed arrow) of C1. (*P*, Pharynx; *E*, Esophagus)

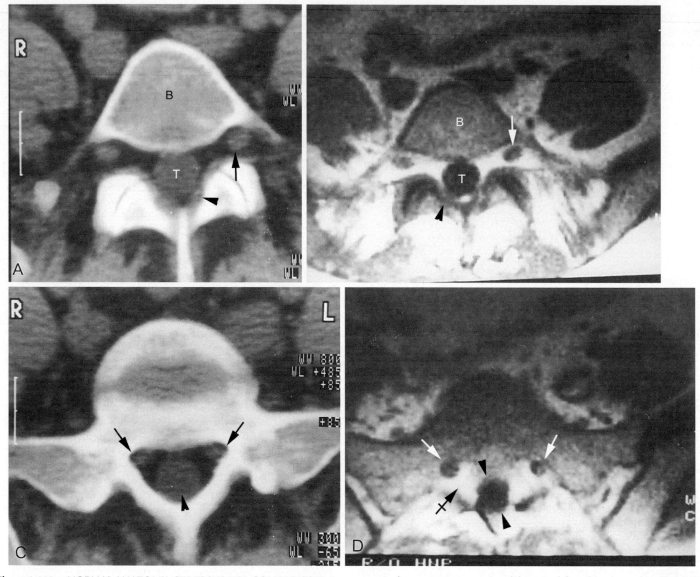

Figure 6.160.   NORMAL ANATOMY: CT VERSUS MRI; COMPARISON. A. CT, Bone Window Axial L5. Note the vertebral body (*B*), thecal sac (*T*), nerve root exiting the lateral recess (arrow), and ligamentum flavum (arrowhead). **B. MRI, T1-Weighted Axial L5.** The same structures are again identified as in **A**. The epidural fat has bright signal on MRI compared with its low attenuation on CT. **C. CT, Bone Window Axial L5-S1**. Note the normal and sym-metrical nerve roots (arrows) and the round thecal sac (arrowhead). **D. MRI, T1-Weighted Axial Sacrum.** The descending nerve roots (arrows) and the thecal sac (arrowheads) are of low signal intensity and are easily contrasted by the high signal intensity of the surrounding epidural fat (crossed arrow). (Courtesy of James J. Holland, DC, FACO, Sacramento, California)

Figure 6.161.   ATYPICAL JEFFERSON'S FRACTURE. CT, Bone Window Axial Atlantoaxial Joint. There is a fracture of the anterior and posterior ring of C1 (arrows) with minimal displacement of the lateral masses. In addition, there is a small cortical avulsion from the posterior aspect of the odontoid (arrowhead). COMMENT: The typical Jefferson fracture represents discontinuity of the anterior and posterior arches, thus resulting in displacement of the lateral masses. (Courtesy of The Wood River Memorial Township Hospital, Department of Radiology, Wood River, Illinois)

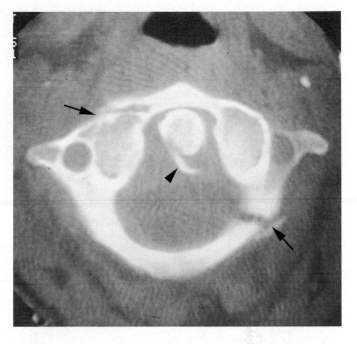

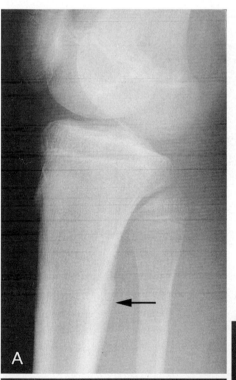

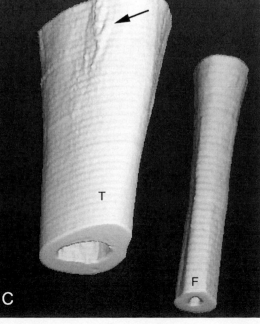

Figure 6.162. STRESS FRACTURE: TIBIA. A. Lateral Knee. There is a localized increase in cortical density on the posterior tibia (arrow), suspicious for a stress fracture. **B. CT, Bone Window Sagittal Reformation Tibia**. Axial CT slices were reformatted into a sagittal image and display focal eccentric cortical thickening along the posterior tibial cortex (arrows). **C. CT, Bone Window 3-D Reformation Tibia**. This reconstruction shows the cortical thickening on the tibial cortex (arrow). These findings are consistent with a stress fracture. COMMENT: The posterior border of the proximal tibial metaphysis is a common site for stress fracture of the lower extremity (*T*, Tibia, *F*, Fibula).

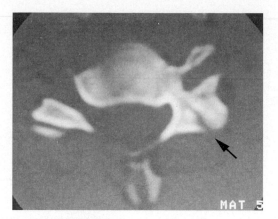

Figure 6.163.   PILLAR FRACTURE: A FREQUENTLY MISSED INJURY OF THE CERVICAL SPINE. This patient developed severe neck pain after his vehicle was struck from behind. Radiographs (not shown) were normal. **CT, Bone Window Axial Cervical.** Note a fracture line extending into the left articular pillar (arrow). COMMENT: Since axially oriented fractures can be missed on CT, coronal reformation is often necessary to detect these lesions. (Courtesy of The Wood River Memorial Township Hospital, Department of Radiology, Wood River, Illinois)

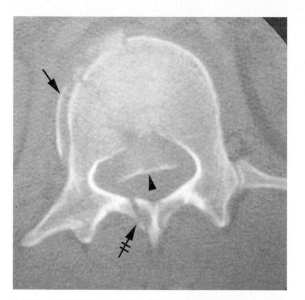

Figure 6.164.   BURST FRACTURE WITH RETROPULSION. This patient was injured as a result of a fall from a height of several stories. **CT, Bone Window Axial Lumbar.** There is impaction of the L1 vertebral endplate resulting in a double cortical contour (arrow) anteriorly. Another fracture of the posterior vertebral body is noted with retropulsion of a large fragment into the spinal canal (arrowhead). In addition, there is a fracture of the posterior neural arch (crossed arrow). The patient developed paraplegia as a result of the spinal cord injury. COMMENT: CT has revolutionized the evaluation of acute spinal trauma to the degree that many who have entered hospitals paralyzed have been discharged with no neurologic deficit. A major advantage of spinal CT is guidance for the surgeon to the specific anatomic location and the eventual treatment of complicated burst fractures of the spine.

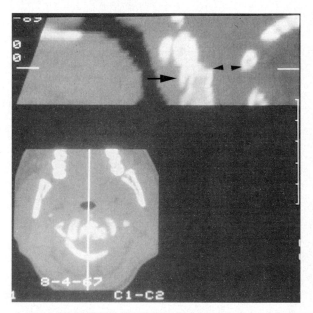

Figure 6.165.   ODONTOID FRACTURE: TYPE III. CT, Bone Window Sagittal Reformation Atlantoaxial Joint. The reformatted sagittal image demonstrates anterior displacement of a type III odontoid fracture (arrow). As a result of the anterior displacement, there is narrowing of the anteroposterior diameter of the spinal canal at C1-C2 (arrowheads). The reformatted image is obtained from the axial image shown below. (Courtesy of The Wood River Memorial Township Hospital, Department of Radiology, Wood River, Illinois)

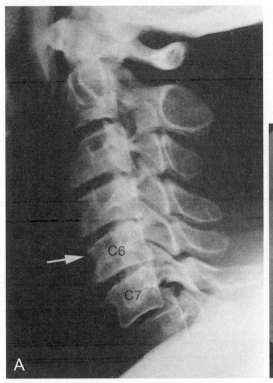

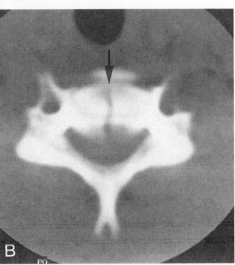

**Figure 6.166.   VERTICAL VERTEBRAL BODY FRACTURE AND FACET DIS-
LOCATION: CERVICAL SPINE. A. Lateral Cervical.** There is a bilateral interfacetal dislocation with resulting anterolisthesis of C6 on C7. In addition,
a small defect in the cortex of the superior C5 endplate is noted (arrow)
suggesting a minor compression deformity. **B, CT, Bone Window Axial Cer-**
vical. Note the vertical fracture line coursing through the vertebral body
(arrow), which was not apparent on the radiograph. COMMENT: CT is an
ideal modality for the evaluation and detection of fractures in the vertebral
column. (Courtesy of Steven P. Brownstein, MD, Springfield, New Jersey)

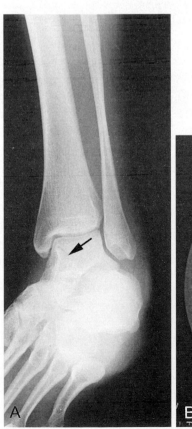

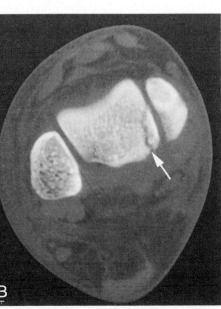

**Figure 6.167.   TALAR DOME FRACTURE: A CHALLENGING
DIAGNOSIS.** This 20-year-old female presented with pain and
swelling of her right ankle following a fall. The initial plain films
(not shown) were read normal by an outside facility. **A. Medial
Oblique Ankle.** Subsequent examination revealed a subtle curvilinear lucency (arrow) traversing the medial talar dome of the
right ankle, suggesting a fracture. **B. CT, Bone Window Axial
Right Ankle.** There is clear evidence of a minimally displaced
fracture involving the medial aspect of the talar dome (arrow).
COMMENT: CT of the ankle provides superior contrast resolution over plain films radiographs and is particularly helpful in
the evaluation of subtle fractures of the ankle. (Courtesy of The
Western States Chiropractic College, Department of Radiology,
Portland, Oregon)

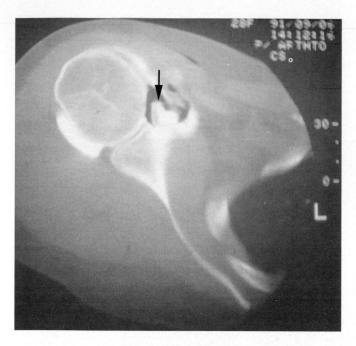

Figure 6.168. BANKART FRACTURE: SHOULDER INSTABILITY. This 25-year-old male sustained an injury in a rugby match and experienced pain and recurrent clicking in his shoulder. **CT, Bone Window Axial Double Contrast Arthrogram Shoulder.** Note the fracture and displacement of the anterior rim of the osseous glenoid and the cartilaginous labrum (arrow). COMMENT: The Bankart lesion may also present without osseous insult. These injuries involve only the cartilaginous labrum and/or anterior capsule and require CT arthrography or MRI for visualization.

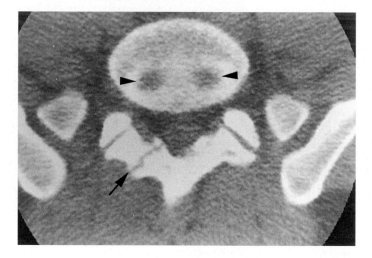

Figure 6.169.   UNILATERAL PARS DEFECT: SPONDYLOLYSIS. CT, Bone Window Axial Lumbar L5-S1. Note the unilateral pars defect (arrow). Incidentally, the *owl's eyes appearance* is noted on the undersurface of the L5 vertebral endplate. This represents the paired parasagittal indentations from nuclear impression, a normal variant. This appearance should not be confused with pathology. (Courtesy of W. Michael Spurlock, DC, Morehead, Kentucky)

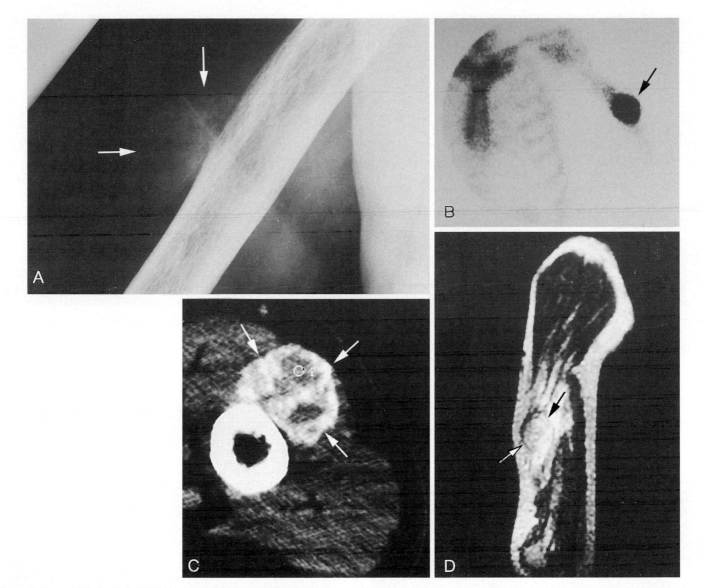

Figure 6.170.   MYOSITIS OSSIFICANS: A MISDIAGNOSIS. This 67-year-old male patient presented with an enlarging mass in his left arm without a history of trauma. **A. AP Humerus.** The plain film radiograph demonstrates a poorly defined calcific mass (arrows) immediately adjacent to the humeral cortex. **B. Bone Scan, Anterior Humerus.** Markedly increased radionuclide activity is present in the soft tissues of the arm (arrow). A biopsy was performed and suggested the presence of a sarcoma. An amputation was scheduled, but the patient fortunately sought a second opinion. **C. CT, Soft Tissue Window Axial Humerus.** Note the increased density in the perimeter of the lesion (arrows) and relatively lucent center. This is the classic appearance of myositis ossificans posttraumatica and *not* a diagnosis requiring biopsy or amputation. **D. MRI, T1-Weighted Coronal Humerus.** Note the well-defined margins of the lesion (arrows) and lack of soft tissue invasion, indicating its benign nature. COMMENT: An appropriate diagnostic imaging protocol, with CT preceding scintigraphy, would have likely obviated biopsy and eliminated the reckless diagnosis of sarcoma and the threatened amputation. (Courtesy of James L. Quale, MD, Radiology Imaging Associates, P.C., Englewood, Colorado)

cified intramuscular hematomas, which are often not evident on CT scans. Biopsy of questionable calcific lesions in the soft tissues should be avoided until a CT is performed. Careful inspection of the CT appearance of myositis ossificans will show a central lucency with a dense periphery versus the dense epicenter and lucent periphery of sarcoma.

INFECTION

Infectious processes such as discitis, osteomyelitis, and Brodie's abscess can be evaluated with computed tomography, showing cortical and juxtacortical involvement, as well as cloaca and sequestrum formation. Associated soft tissue involvement is common and may be seen as blurring of the fascial planes. This finding is frequently missed or not apparent on radiographs and is better appreciated with CT. In cases of spinal infections, endplate destruction and paravertebral masses are easily detected on axial CT images. (13–16) (Fig. 6.171) Disc space infections are more commonly seen in children and in adults who have previously undergone laminectomy or discectomy procedures. (9,17) Sclerosis, irregularities of the destroyed vertebral endplates, and narrowing of the disc space represent the typical signs of discitis on CT images, along with displacement of the epidural fat in the spinal canal from abscess. In addition, the subtle osseous erosions

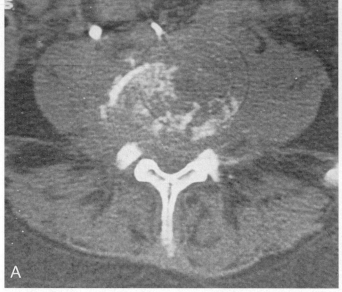

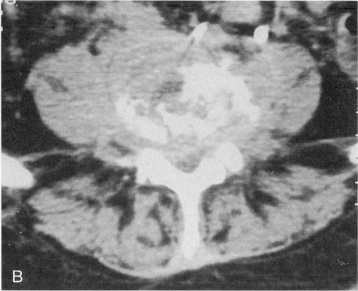

Figure 6.171.   SPONDYLODISCITIS: A DIABETIC WITH SEVERE BACK PAIN. A. CT, Bone Window Axial Lumbar. B. CT, Soft Tissue Window Axial Lumbar. There is widespread destruction of the vertebral body with para- spinal soft tissue extension. COMMENT: Spondylodiscitis usually occurs in the immunocompromised population, including diabetics, the elderly, and HIV patients.

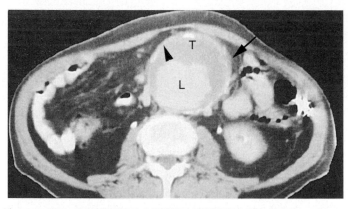

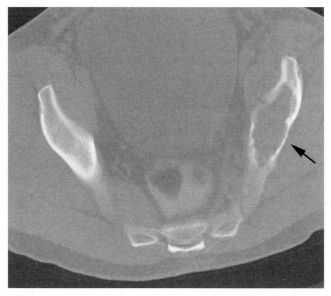

Figure 6.172.   ABDOMINAL AORTIC ANEURYSM. This elderly male pre- sented with visible abdominal pulsations and focal prominence of the um- bilicus. **CT, Soft Tissue Window Axial Abdomen.** Note the pronounced an- eurysmal dilatation of the abdominal aorta (arrow). Atherosclerotic plaquing was noted in the wall of the aneurysm (arrowhead). The variation in atten- uation within the aneurysm is due to peripheral thrombus formation and contrast-enhanced flowing blood. Incidentally, note the opacification of the bowel structures and ureters due to oral and intravenous contrast adminis- tration. (*T*, Thrombus, *L*, Lumen of the abdominal aorta). (Courtesy of The Wood River Memorial Township Hospital, Department of Radiology, Wood River, Illinois)

Figure 6.173.   PLASMACYTOMA: ILIUM. CT, Bone Window Axial Pelvis. There is an expansile osteolytic lesion in the marrow of the left ilium with no reactive sclerosis (arrow). This infiltrative lesion has produced endosteal erosion, but has not violated the outer cortex. COMMENT: Plasmacytoma, the solitary form of multiple myeloma, usually presents in the pelvis, ribs, and proximal femur.

and soft tissue abnormalities associated with infections of the sacroiliac and hip joints are readily apparent with CT. Nuclear scintigraphy and MRI are often helpful in the complete assessment of suspected osteomyelitis.

VASCULAR

Aneurysms of the intracranial or intrathoracic vessels should be evaluated with CT (pre- and postcontrast images are indicated if dissection or rupture is suspected). Abdominal aortic aneurysms are nicely displayed with CT; however, ultrasound is a more cost-effective and non-invasive method to obtain virtually the same information. (Fig. 6.172)

NEOPLASMS

A complete description of the CT characteristics of musculoskeletal tumors is beyond the scope of this text. Our purpose is to emphasize the importance of computed tomography in the diagnosis of some common benign and malignant neoplasms. CT is useful in further evaluating lesions seen on conventional radiographs or MRI scans, as well as in the detection of neoplastic processes previously unseen in areas of overlapping anatomy such as the vertebral column, pelvis (Fig. 6.173) and facial skeleton. (Fig. 6.174) Although MRI has replaced most indications for CT in the evaluation of soft tissue neoplasms, the osseous characteristics and calcified regions of a neoplastic process are still best demonstrated by CT. (Fig. 6.175) For example, CT is valuable in determining whether matrix calcification and endosteal scalloping are present in a suspected chondroid or fibrous lesion. In addition, Hounsfield measurements provide helpful information concerning a lesion's composition. Lipomas, for instance, have an attenuation value similar to subcutaneous fat, while aneurysmal bone cysts may exhibit a fluid-fluid level with differing Hounsfield values. The reactive sclerosis surrounding an osteoid osteoma often obscures the lucent tumorous nidus, making the plain film diagnosis of this benign neoplasm difficult. (Fig. 6.176) CT is

better suited than any other imaging modality to provide a detailed assessment of the bony cortex, especially when overt findings of cortical neoplasm (including osteoid osteoma), bony expansion, periosteal reaction, or subtle fracture are present. Malignant bone tumors are typically characterized by bone destruction and an ill-defined soft tissue mass (more common in primary malignant bone tumors). (9) (Fig. 6.177) The use of intravenous contrast may help in determining the extension of the tumor. In cases of meningeal carcinomatosis or metastasis to the spine, MRI is the procedure of choice.

CONGENITAL

Computed tomography can be utilized for the evaluation of congenital malformations such as closure defects of the neural arch (e.g., spina bifida occulta and manifesta), cervical spondylolysis, and facet asymmetry. In addition, congenital spinal stenosis is well visualized with CT by accurately measuring the transverse and sagittal dimensions of the spinal canal. In achondroplasia the short, thickened pedicles and laminae are responsible for this stenosis, which is most apparent in the lower lumbar spine. Four normal spinal canal configurations have been described. (Fig. 6.178) In the lumbar spine 10 to 20% of the normal population have the trefoil-shaped canal, which has a propensity to develop central or lateral recess stenosis.

ARTHRITIDES

The typical manifestations of degenerative joint disease in the peripheral articulations include asymmetric joint space narrowing, osteophytes, subchondral sclerosis, and cysts (geodes). These features are usually detectable on conventional plain films. CT provides a more accurate assessment of the degenerative changes in the spine and their relationship to the neural structures. Moreover, computed tomography is particularly useful in assessing spinal canal and lateral recess stenosis.

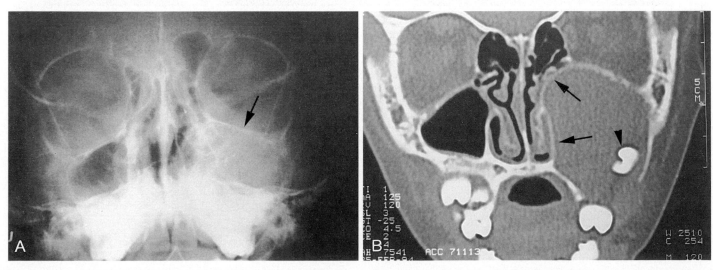

Figure 6.174.   DENTIGEROUS CYST: MAXILLARY SINUS. A. Water's Sinus View. There is a large soft tissue density occupying the left maxillary sinus and elevating the orbital floor (arrow). **B. CT, Bone Window Sinus**. Notice the replacement of the normally air-filled left maxillary sinus by the soft tissue mass. There is obliteration of the maxillary sinus floor and medial expansion into the nasal cavity (arrows). Also observe the elevation of the orbital floor by the mass that contains a tooth (arrowhead). These findings are highly suggestive of a dentigerous cyst. COMMENT: Dentigerous cyst is the most common cyst to arise in the mandible and frequently includes a tooth. (Courtesy of The University Hospital, Department of Radiology, Denver, Colorado)

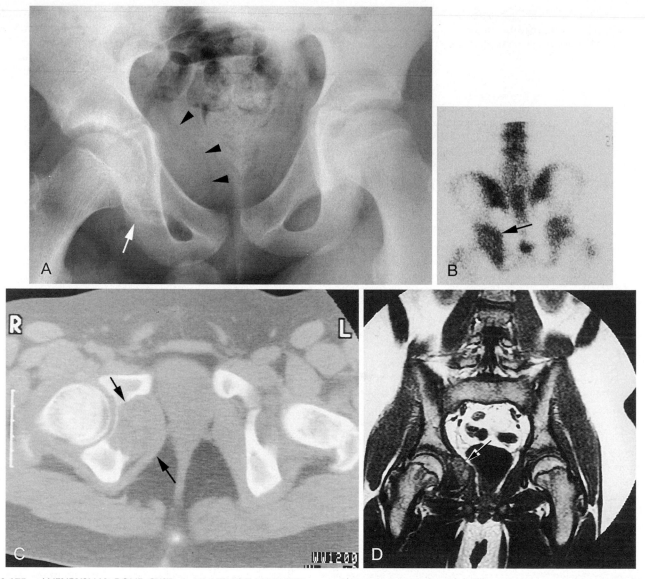

**Figure 6.175.   ANEURYSMAL BONE CYST: A MULTIMODALITY PER-
SPECTIVE.** This 11-year-old male presented with acute onset of right hip
pain and was suddenly unable to bear weight. **A. AP Pelvis**. There is an
expansile mass associated with a thin shell of cortical bone (arrow) arising
from the right ischium. A component of the mass is seen displacing the pelvic
soft tissues (arrowheads). **B. Bone Scan, Posterior Pelvis**. Note the increased
radiotracer activity corresponding to the expansile mass in the region of the
right ischium (arrow). **C. CT, Bone Window Axial Pelvis**. There is an eccentrically positioned, destructive mass (arrows) arising from the right ischium

with expansion into the pelvis. The articular cortex of the acetabulum is not
violated by the tumor. **D. MRI, T1-Weighted Coronal Pelvis**. Observe the
low signal intensity mass arising from the right ischium (arrow). This mass
compresses the lateral wall of the bladder. COMMENT: Computed tomography greatly enhances one's ability to perceive the extent of significant
pathology in flat bones. Often, plain film radiographs may fool the observer
regarding the actual size of the lesion. (Courtesy of The Children's Hospital,
Department of Radiology, Denver, Colorado)

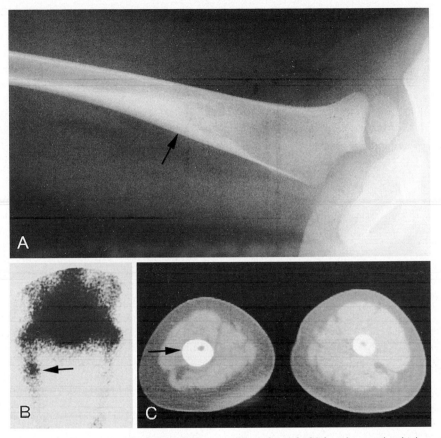

Figure 6.176.   OSTEOID OSTEOMA: "ELUSIVE" NIDUS. A. Lateral Hip. Notice the thickened medial cortex (arrow) in this 2-year-old male with hip pain. The nidus is not always visible on plain film, as in this case. **B. Bone Scan, Anterior Pelvis.** Note the focal increased uptake in the proximal right femur (arrow) representing the osteoid osteoma. **C. CT, Soft Tissue Window Bilateral Axial Thigh.** Observe the thickened cortex in the posterior right femur (arrow). COMMENT: Contiguous, thin CT slices are required to locate the tiny lucent nidus of an osteoid osteoma (usually 1 cm or less). (Courtesy of The Children's Hospital, Department of Radiology, Denver, Colorado)

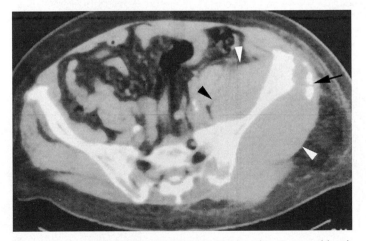

Figure 6.177.   HISTIOCYTIC LYMPHOMA: ILIUM. This 41-year-old male presented with pain and swelling of the left posterior pelvis. **CT, Soft Tissue Window Axial Pelvis.** Note the cortical destruction and debris of the left posterolateral ilium (arrow). In addition, a soft tissue mass surrounds the left ilium (arrowheads).

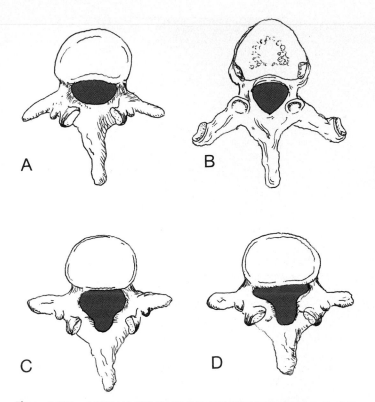

Figure 6.178.   NORMAL SPINAL CANAL CONFIGURATIONS. A. Oval. B. Triangular. C. Deltoid. D. Trefoil (3-Leaf Clover). These configurations are normal, but the possibility of lateral recess stenosis from parasagittal or far lateral disc herniation or degenerative stenosis is more frequently seen with the trefoil shaped spinal canal. The oval-shaped canal is most frequently seen in the cervical region. The triangular shape is most frequently observed in the thoracic spine, and the deltoid and trefoil shapes are commonly seen in the lumbar region.

Degenerative disease affects both the osseous and soft tissue components of the vertebral column. Frequently, degenerative stenosis results from a combination of hypertrophic changes that involve the intervertebral disc, discovertebral margin, apophyseal joints, and supporting ligaments. (Fig. 6.179) The bony changes (osteophytes) may be identified on radiographs, but their exact orientation and degree of encroachment into the canal is often not appreciated on plain films. Significant disc trauma often results in injury to the annular fibers and subsequent osteophyte formation. This process generally requires at least 1 year, but more often, 2 or more years are necessary before these changes are visible on plain films. Occasionally, earlier changes may be seen with CT. In addition, disc lesions (bulges, herniations) and ligament hypertrophy (PLL and ligamentum flavum) often play a major role in canal stenosis and remain undetectable on radiographs. (Fig. 6.180) For these reasons CT is more accurate than plain films in evaluating suspected spinal stenosis.

In the lumbar region spinal stenosis is suggested if the interpediculate distance is less than 12 mm or if the area of the spinal canal, at the level of the pedicles, is less than 1.5 square cm. (18) In the cervical spine, stenosis is present when the sagittal canal distance is 10 mm or less. (9) If clinical symptoms are not present, however, small canal diameter measurements alone are of little clinical significance.

CT images can also demonstrate changes that take place at the facet joints and at the lateral recess, resulting in spinal nerve root compression and radicular symptoms. (Fig. 6.181) The lateral recess is medial to the pedicle and posterior to the vertebral body. Its posterior border is the articular process. As the nerve root sleeve leaves the thecal sac, it passes through the lateral recess before it enters the intervertebral foramen (IVF). Frequently, facet imbrication from decreased disc height and hypertrophic facet disease act concurrently to create lateral recess and/or IVF en-

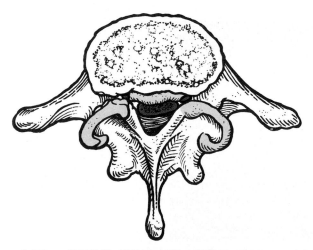

Figure 6.179.   CENTRAL CANAL AND LATERAL RECESS STENOSIS: SCHEMATIC DIAGRAM. This diagram illustrates an axial projection of a lumbar vertebra at the level of the lateral recess. There is reduction of the AP diameter of the central canal by a bulging disc anteriorly and hypertrophic ligamentum flavum posteriorly. The nerve roots in the lateral recess are mechanically compressed by the degenerative changes arising from the posterior body and apophyseal joints.

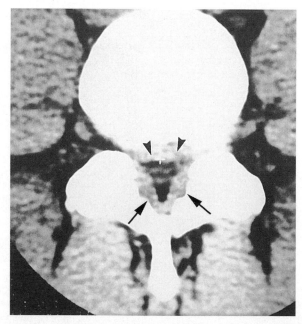

Figure 6.180.   STENOSIS FROM LIGAMENTUM FLAVUM HYPERTROPHY. CT, Soft Tissue Window Axial L3-L4. The thickened ligamentum flavum (arrows) and posterior disc bulge (arrowheads) narrow the central spinal canal. The thecal sac is compressed by the combined effects of these abnormalities.

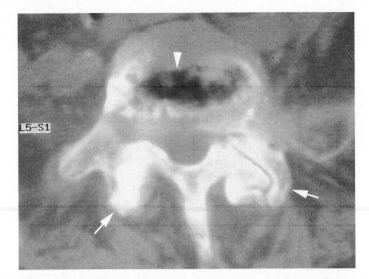

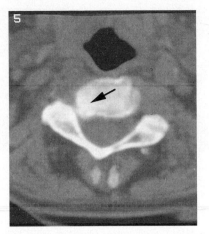

Figure 6.183.   NEUROFORAMINAL STENOSIS: A BONY CAUSE. A. CT, Bone Window Axial Cervical. Note the hypertrophic degenerative changes involving the right von Luschka joint (arrow) of this midcervical vertebral segment with resultant encroachment into the neural foramen. (Courtesy of The Wood River Memorial Township Hospital, Department of Radiology, Wood River, Illinois)

Figure 6.181.   DEGENERATIVE SPINAL STENOSIS. CT, Bone Window Axial L5-S1. There is marked arthrosis of the apophyseal joints (arrows) leading to degenerative spondylolisthesis and central canal stenosis. Intradiscal gas (vacuum phenomenon) is also identified within the L5-S1 disc (arrowhead). COMMENT: Degenerative spondylolisthesis occurs in a small percentage of patients with degenerative disease of the vertebral column. Most patients with degenerative spondylolisthesis fall in the Three F category; **F**emale, Above **F**orty Years, **F**our (L4).

croachment. This has been referred to as *up-down* stenosis. (19) (Fig. 6.182) In the cervical spine, uncinate process osteophytes also contribute to narrow the IVF. (Fig. 6.183) Compression of the corresponding nerve is frequently seen on the axial and sagittally reformatted images as displacement or obliteration of the epidural fat surrounding the nerve root. Stenosis of the lateral recess is often associated with central spinal stenosis.

Patients with lateral recess stenosis of the lumbar spine (*lateral nerve root entrapment syndrome*) frequently present with symptoms of *intermittent neurogenic claudication*. The typical patient complains of back and leg pain that is initiated by walking or other weight-bearing activity. The leg pain is usually greater than the back pain and is classically alleviated by sitting. This must be distinguished clinically from intermittent vascular claudication. Since the symptoms associated with both neurogenic and vascular claudication can begin with activity and abate with rest, their differentiation may be difficult. Lower extremity pain secondary to vascular claudication almost always begins and remains below the knee. Concurrent low back pain may also be present but separate from the cause of the leg pain. Neurogenic claudication generally does not occur when the patient rides a stationary bike (since the spine is in slight flexion, increasing the spinal canal size), while vascular claudication manifests with any physical activity, independent of the position of the spine.

Inflammatory arthritides are often adequately evaluated with plain film radiographs. A thorough clinical assessment, including a complete history and physical examination, as well as appropriate laboratory tests, is necessary and will usually provide adequate information for the diagnosis. When the findings are inconclusive or equivocal, CT may be employed to assist in the diagnostic workup. Computed tomography is primarily utilized in this capacity to image the early erosive changes of sacroiliitis that occur most frequently in the seronegative spondyloarthropathies (ankylosing spondylitis, enteropathic spondylitis, psoriatic arthritis, Reiter's syndrome). (Fig. 6.184) Later, these changes are accompanied by subchondral reactive sclerosis, gross marginal irregularity, and subsequent ankylosis.

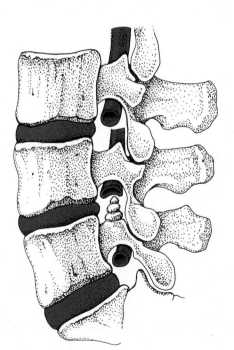

Figure 6.182.   UP-DOWN STENOSIS: SCHEMATIC DIAGRAM. The loss of disc height and hypertrophic degenerative changes of the superior articulating facet have reduced the osseous dimensions of the intervertebral foramen. The combination of these factors results in an increased likelihood of mechanical nerve root compression and lateral nerve entrapment syndrome.

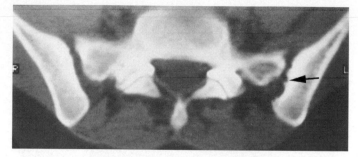

Figure 6.184. ANKYLOSING SPONDYLITIS: SACROILIAC JOINTS. CT, Bone Window Axial Sacrum. Note the widening of the left sacroiliac joint resulting from erosions along the articular surfaces of the ilium and sacrum (arrow). COMMENT: The early changes associated with the inflammatory arthropathies affecting the sacroiliac joints are better evaluated using CT because of its superior sensitivity over plain film radiography. CT is the imaging modality of choice to evaluate all pathologic abnormalities relating to the integrity of the sacroiliac joint. (Courtesy of Gary L. Boog, DC, Lancaster, New Hampshire)

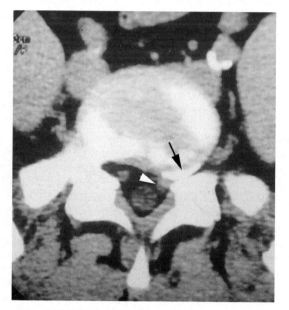

Figure 6.185. CALCIFIED HERNIATED NUCLEUS PULPOSUS. This patient suffered from chronic low back pain and sciatica. **CT, Soft Tissue Window Axial L5-S1.** Note the calcified disc fragment projecting from the left posterolateral margin of the L5 disc (arrow), which posteriorly displaces the adjacent S1 nerve root (arrowhead).

DISC HERNIATION

Disc herniation is one of the frequent indications for a CT evaluation of the spine in communities where MRI is not available. Herniations generally occur at the posterior or posterolateral aspect of the annulus fibrosus, where the posterior longitudinal ligament is smallest and the annulus is thinnest. The attenuation of the herniated fragment is generally between 90 and 120 HU, but may be as low as 60 HU. (20) The lack of epidural fat in the cervical and thoracic neural canal prohibits adequate CT visualization of disc herniations in those regions, unless intrathecal con-

trast is administered (CT myelography). Conversely, the abundance of fat in the lumbar spinal canal at L4-L5 and L5-S1 usually allows adequate soft tissue contrast for the diagnosis of disc herniation without prior intrathecal contrast injection. (Fig. 6.185) Evaluation of the relationship of the protruding disc material to the nerve roots (including the dorsal root ganglion) in the lower lumbar spine is frequently possible with CT. MRI has replaced CT and CT myelography as the imaging modality of choice for disc herniations at any spinal region. The multiplanar capability, contrast resolution, and lack of harmful biologic effects, along with superior physiologic information regarding the bone marrow and disc hydration, have made MRI an indispensable modality in the diagnostic workup of most spinal pathologies.

BONE DENSITOMETRY

Bone mineral density (BMD) values are necessary for predicting which patients with osteoporosis are at risk for spontaneous fracture of the weight-bearing skeleton. Quantitative computed tomography (QCT) can selectively measure the trabecular compartment of the vertebrae and is widely used for the assessment of BMD in patients with osteoporosis. It is also used to monitor changes in BMD during and after treatment. (21–23) Some reports have emphasized the superiority of QCT over posteroanterior dual x-ray absorptiometry (PA-DXA) in helping to discriminate between healthy women and those with osteoporosis. (21,24)

MEDICOLEGAL IMPLICATIONS
Computed Tomography

- Caution should be exercised when using this modality, as with any modality that uses ionizing radiation.
- Overutilization and inappropriate use should be avoided.
- Patients with diabetes, renal compromise, and congestive heart failure should be cautiously evaluated prior to the administration of intravenous contrast.
- Blood urea nitrogen and creatinine laboratory tests should be performed on every patient prior to the use of intravenous contrast. If these tests are abnormal, contrast infusion is contraindicated.

CT MYELOGRAPHY

HISTORICAL PERSPECTIVES

In 1976 Ditcher and Steeling reported the value of water-soluble contrast in association with computed tomographic examination of the spine. (25) Computed tomographic myelography (CTM) delineates the borders of the thecal sac from adjacent soft tissue and bone. (Fig. 6.186) Evaluation of intradural pathology utilizing CTM was a significant advancement in spinal

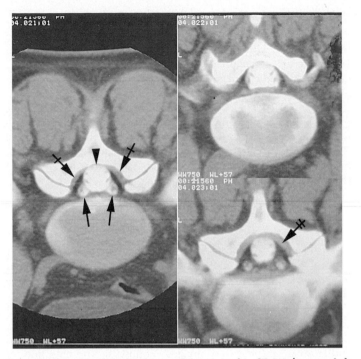

Figure 6.186. CT MYELOGRAM: NORMAL L5-S1. CT Myelogram, Soft Tissue Window Axial L5-S1. The normal appearance of the L5-S1 level shows the contrast-filled nerve roots (arrows) and thecal sac (arrowhead). Note the normal rootlets, which are of relatively low attenuation when compared with the contrast within the adjacent thecal sac. The spinal canal, neural foramina, and ligamentum flavum (crossed arrows) are normal. (Courtesy of The Wood River Memorial Township Hospital, Department of Radiology, Wood River, Illinois)

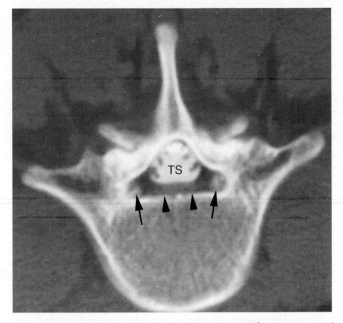

Figure 6.187. CT MYELOGRAM: NORMAL L5. CT Myelogram, Bone Window Axial L5 Level. Note the normal contrast-filled thecal sac. The relatively low attenuation nerve roots are noted in their normal lateral position. The S1 nerve roots (arrows) are seen within the lateral recess of the neural canal. The epidural venous plexus is seen along the posterior margin of the vertebral body (arrowheads). (*TS*, Thecal Sac.)

imaging. Reconstruction images allow sagittal and/or coronal evaluation, producing a three-dimensional perspective. CTM provides valuable information in the evaluation of degenerative disc disease, spinal stenosis, spinal cord or nerve root compression, and postoperative pain. However, the emergence of MRI as the diagnostic imaging modality of choice for spinal disorders will continue to reduce the clinical utility of CTM and myelography.

TECHNICAL CONSIDERATIONS

The CTM examination is performed 4 to 6 hours following a lumbar myelogram and immediately after a cervical myelogram. (26) This time delay serves to dilute the concentration of the contrast within the subarachnoid space and varies considerably between radiology departments. A fixed number is not universally accepted, and may be as short as 2 to 3 hours in other radiology departments. The patient is usually imaged in the prone position so that gravity layers the contrast within the subarachnoid space against the posterior vertebral body margin.

In the lumbar spine CTM is useful in evaluating the nerve root sheaths, cauda equina, pathology of surrounding bone and joints (including spinal canal stenosis), and postoperative changes. (27,28) (Fig. 6.187) CTM of the cervical spine demonstrates the size and shape of the central canal and provides direct visualization of the thecal sac, spinal cord and nerve root sleeves, as well as the surrounding osseous and soft tissue anatomy. (Fig. 6.188)

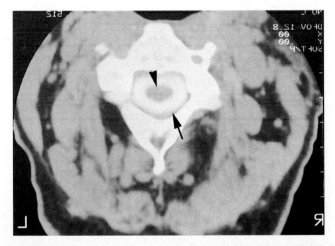

Figure 6.188. CT MYELOGRAM: NORMAL UPPER CERVICAL SPINE. CT Myelogram, Soft Tissue Window Axial Cervical. Observe the normally rounded appearance of the contrast-filled thecal sac (arrow). The contrast agent completely fills the subarachnoid space and surrounds the spinal cord (arrowhead).

CLINICAL INDICATIONS

Degenerative Joint Disease

Degenerative spinal stenosis is the primary clinical indication for CTM. The contrast resolution achieved with CT provides an accurate assessment of both the bony and soft tissue changes seen with degenerative spinal stenosis. With the addition of contrast medium the spinal cord and nerve roots and their relationship to the surrounding osteoligamentous structures are well delineated. (Fig. 6.189) Reformatted CTM images provide information regarding the size and shape of the neural foramina and filling of the nerve root sleeves.

Herniated Nucleus Pulposus (HNP)

Disc herniations may result in distortion and displacement of the epidural fat, thecal sac, spinal cord, and nerve roots. Axial CT without contrast does not provide optimal contrast resolution between these structures, particularly in the cervical and thoracic regions. The introduction of intrathecal contrast allows improved or complete filling of a nerve root sleeve and enhancement of the internal margin of the thecal sac. (Fig. 6.190) While improved resolution by means of intrathecal contrast greatly increases the diagnostic accuracy over plain CT, the evaluation of radiculopathy secondary to disc herniation in both the lumbar and cervical spine is best imaged by MRI. The use of CT myelography for the evaluation of disc herniation will likely evolve into a supplementary role, employed only when MRI or plain CT is equivocal or contraindicated. (Figs. 6.191, 6.192)

Inflammatory and Neoplastic Disorders

Inflammatory and neoplastic disorders may also be assessed with CTM. Intradural inflammation is known as *arachnoiditis* and is often associated with postsurgical intradural scar tissue. The characteristic adhesion or clumping of nerve roots is well visualized with CTM.

Just as CTM replaced myelography as the initial diagnostic examination for intraspinal tumors, MRI is now the imaging modality of choice in diagnosing and monitoring these neoplasms. The capacity of MRI to accurately define extradural and intradural pathology is widely recognized. The reader is referred to the preceding MRI section of this chapter for additional discussion regarding this topic.

Nerve Root Avulsion

Nerve root avulsions most frequently involve the lower cervical nerve roots and result from a severe force directed to the neck and shoulder region. Two paralysis patterns have classically been described with nerve root avulsions: Erb-Duchenne paralysis involving the C5-C6 nerve roots and Klumpke's paralysis involving the C7-C8 nerve roots. These conditions are best evaluated with CT myelography using sagittal and coronal reformatted images. Following the injection of intrathecal contrast, extravasation from the torn nerve root sleeve is observed. Often, the nerve root is avulsed from the spinal cord and is no longer present within its dural sleeve. (29)

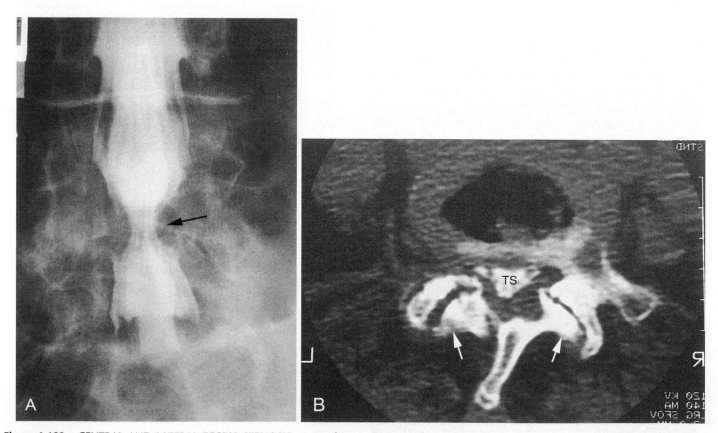

Figure 6.189.   CENTRAL AND LATERAL RECESS STENOSIS. A. Myelogram, AP Lumbar. Note the symmetric extradural compression of the thecal sac producing an hourglass deformity at L4-L5 (arrow). **B. CT Myelogram,** **Bone Window Axial Lumbar**. Marked hypertrophic degenerative changes are present in the apophyseal joints (arrows) resulting in encroachment and deformity of the thecal sac. (*TS*, Thecal Sac).

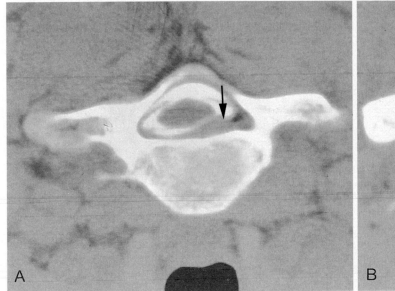
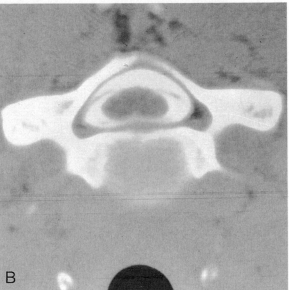

Figure 6.190. HERNIATED NUCLEUS PULPOSUS: CERVICAL SPINE. A. CT Myelogram, Soft Tissue Window Axial Cervical. Observe the ventral deflection of the dura by a paramidline disc herniation (arrow). **B. CT Myelogram, Soft Tissue Window Axial Cervical Normal.** Note the normal volume of subarachnoid space surrounding the spinal cord and the apposition of the dura and posterior vertebral body. COMMENT: The CT myelogram is often performed with the patient prone to approximate the thecal sac to the vertebral body. This posture enhances the detection of subtle disc lesions.

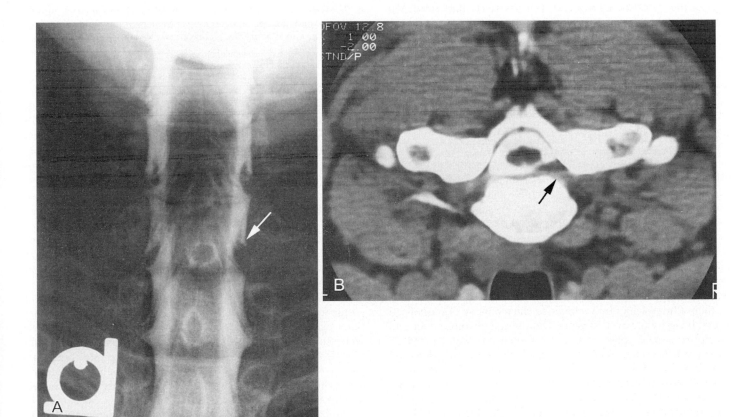

Figure 6.191. HERNIATED NUCLEUS PULPOSUS (HNP): CERVICAL SPINE. A. Myelogram, PA Cervical. There is a unilateral nerve root filling defect on the right at C7-T1 (arrow). **B. CT Myelogram, Bone Window Axial C7-T1.** Notice the extradural effacement of the thecal sac on the right produced by the disc herniation (arrow).

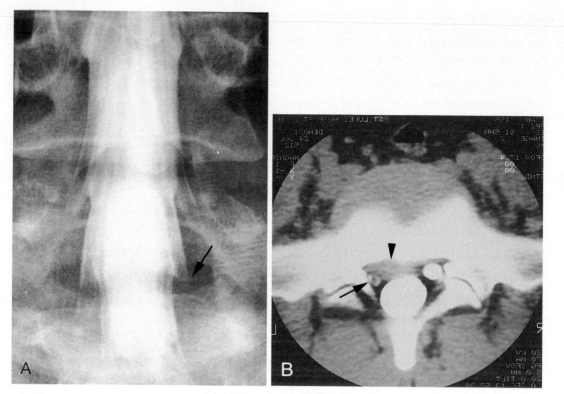

Figure 6.192.   HERNIATED NUCLEUS PULPOSUS: LUMBAR SPINE. This patient experienced low back pain with radiation into the left lower extremity. The Achilles deep tendon reflex was absent on the left. **A. Myelogram, PA Lumbosacral.** Note the poor filling of the left S1 nerve sheath (arrow).

B. CT Myelogram, Soft Tissue Window Axial L5–S1. There is posterior displacement and reduced filling of the left S1 nerve root sheath (arrow) as a result of the posterolateral disc herniation (arrowhead). (Courtesy of Leonard A. Suiter, DC, St. Louis, Missouri)

MYELOGRAPHY

HISTORICAL PERSPECTIVES

The workhorse of specialized spinal imaging prior to the evolution of CT and MRI was plain film myelography. Myelography provided indirect visualization of spinal canal contents by introducing a radiographic contrast agent into the subarachnoid space. Utilization of a positive or negative (gas) contrast agent allowed indirect assessment of the thecal sac, nerve roots, and spinal cord contours. Effacement or compression of these contrast-filled tracts may be caused by any of numerous space-occupying lesions, including disc herniation, tumor, hematoma, osteophyte, inflammation, and developmental anomaly.

Plain film myelography remained the mainstay of specialized spinal imaging for over 50 years. Dandy first introduced air into the subarachnoid space as a contrast agent in 1919. (1) In 1922 Sicard and Forestier, while treating sciatica with an iodized oil (Lipiodol), accidentally injected the agent into the subarachnoid space. This is thought to be the first reported myelogram, albeit inadvertent. (2) Mixter and Barr used Lipiodol myelography for the preoperative localization of lesions and assessment of spinal pain. (3) They were the first to report on the clinical significance of the intervertebral disc herniation using this imaging technique. The untoward effects of intrathecal Lipiodol (which included meningeal irritation and arachnoiditis) prompted the search for a safer contrast agent.

In the early 1940s iophendylate (Pantopaque) was developed.

It was less viscous and toxic than Lipiodol and soon became the contrast agent of choice for myelographic examinations for the next 30 years. Although this new contrast material was less viscous than its predecessors, it was still of a high enough density to obscure dural defects, preventing their recognition on the posteroanterior projection. (4)

While severe acute reactions were unusual with Pantopaque, arachnoiditis and, more frequently, headache, nausea, and vomiting were associated with its use. (5) Following the completion of the exam, it was necessary to mechanically remove this agent from the subarachnoid space. Invariably, not all of the contrast agent was extracted, creating the potential for continued toxic reactions to this foreign material.

The first nonionic water-soluble contrast agent (metrizamide [Amipaque]) was introduced in the late 1970s. Meningeal irritation was far less common with this new agent. Second-generation, water-soluble agents, including iohexol (Omnipaque) and iopamidol (Isovue), replaced metrizamide in the late 1980s and have proven to be less toxic to the central nervous system. Use of room air or carbon dioxide as a myelographic contrast agent has been largely abandoned. (6)

Nonionic, water-soluble agents are currently employed for intrathecal contrast imaging. Overall, a significant reduction in morbidity has been realized through the use of these newer contrast agents. (7) This contrast medium is introduced through small needles and is completely eliminated by transarachnoid diffusion into the blood stream and renal excretion. Partial removal of the contrast agent has been recommended, but is not felt by most to be necessary. (8) Severe adverse reactions such as seizures, hallucinations, and confusion are rare, occurring far less frequently than with metrizamide. Mild transient side effects, including headaches, nausea, vomiting, and dizziness, are common in patients undergoing cervical myelography using iohexol (Omnipaque). Bed rest with the head raised is recommended when adverse postmyelographic reactions are reported. Another important advantage of modern water-soluble agents is the better radiographic definition of the nerve root sleeves and intraarachnoid structures.

The disadvantages of myelography have been its invasiveness and lack of diagnostic specificity, caused by the nature of myelographic pattern detection. Myelography displays neural compression indirectly via changes in the contour of the contrast-filled subarachnoid space. The specific nature of a compressive or adhesive process requires additional diagnostic differentiation. CT or MRI is necessary to characterize the specific nature of the pathology.

Patients who undergo myelography should be encouraged to increase their fluid intake prior to the examination. Depending on when the examination is scheduled, meals may be restricted. Premedication is generally not required unless a large dose of contrast material is required or there is a seizure history. Evaluation of the bleeding time, prothrombin time, and partial thromboplastin time is necessary within 2 weeks of the myelogram. Abnormal bleeding is a contraindication to lumbar puncture. (6)

Following the examination, the patient is placed on bed rest with the head elevated for 3 to 4 hours. This allows the contrast medium to be absorbed. If CT scanning is scheduled after myelography, it will typically be delayed between 3 to 5 hours. In addition to patient safety and comfort, the delay reduces the concentration of intrathecal contrast medium, thereby improving visualization of intraarachnoid structures. All patients undergoing myelography are placed in observation for at least 6 hours following the examination to monitor untoward effects. (9) There has recently been a trend in imaging centers and hospitals to perform outpatient myelograms. While the risks and adverse reactions have been dramatically reduced, some risks remain and patients should be kept under observation for a 24-hour period.

The frequency of myelographic examinations has markedly diminished. For nerve root, spinal cord, and cauda equina examinations, myelography has been largely supplanted by CT and MRI.

Glossary of Terms

Arachnoiditis: inflammation of the meningeal covering of the spinal cord. A potential complication of the myelographic examination, the incidence of arachnoiditis has decreased with the introduction of modern nonionic water-soluble agents.

Contrast agent: a substance that provides radiographic contrast. In myelography, contrast is injected into the subarachnoid space of the spinal cord. Modern contrast agents are nonionic and water-soluble. Unlike their fat-soluble predecessors, water-soluble contrasts diffuse into the vascular system and are excreted through the kidneys, reducing CNS toxicity.

Extradural pattern: a myelographic pattern produced by pathologies that impress or indent the dural membrane. A variety of etiologies, including disc herniation, osteophyte, ligamentum flavum hypertrophy, hematoma, abscess, and neoplasm, may produce this appearance. A high-grade extradural block may completely obstruct the flow of contrast through the subarachnoid space.

Intradural extramedullary pattern: a myelographic pattern produced by a lesion that arises in the subarachnoid space. The mass is displayed as a round, well-defined defect in the contrast column. The spinal cord is typically displaced.

Intradural intramedullary pattern: a myelographic pattern produced by a lesion that arises within the substance of the spinal cord. For this pattern to be visualized, the spinal cord must be enlarged. Often, gradual tapering and narrowing of the contrast column is observed. Ependymoma and astrocytoma are the most common lesions that produce this pattern.

Intrathecal: this term is synonymous with the subarachnoid space. This potential space lies between the arachnoid and the pia mater. Contrast injected into this space mixes with cerebrospinal fluid and allows the contours of the spinal cord and nerve root sleeves to be visualized.

Lumbar puncture: this is the preliminary procedure that is performed prior to the introduction of the myelographic agent. Approximately 15 mL of CSF is withdrawn, and contrast is then injected. A needle enters the subarachnoid space between the L2-L3 or L3-L4 levels.

Myelography: a radiographic examination that introduces positive contrast into the subarachnoid space via a lumbar or cervical puncture. This procedure allows visualization of the inner margin of the thecal sac and nerve root sheaths. Fluoroscopy is used to assess the characteristics of the contrast column. Appropriate radiographic projections are then obtained in the region of interest. Following myelography, computed tomography may be performed to obtain additional detail and contrast.

Water-soluble contrast: a contrast agent that is nonionic and displays lower osmolality since it does not undergo ionic dissociation (Omnipaque and Isovue). These agents are considerably less neurotoxic than their fat-soluble predecessors (e.g., Pantopaque).

MYELOGRAPHIC PROCEDURES

Myelographic techniques require the injection of a contrast agent into the subarachnoid space by either a lumbar puncture (usually at L2-L3 or L3-L4) or a lateral cervical puncture with the spinal needle inserted at the C1-C2 level. (4) The needle is inserted under fluoroscopic guidance to confirm its position. The stylet is then removed to check for return of CSF. A small amount of CSF is obtained and sent for analysis. Fluoroscopy is used to visualize the myelographic contrast agent as it is slowly injected into the subarachnoid space. In the lumbar puncture the table may be tilted in a head-down direction, causing the contrast to flow to the thoracic and cervical regions. Radiographs of the lumbar region are obtained in the prone, lateral decubitus, and oblique positions (steep and shallow angulation). Anteroposterior, lateral, oblique, and swimmer's lateral views of the cervical and upper thoracic spine are performed when the contrast column is directed into this area. The accidental introduction of contrast into the brain, as could occur when the table is tilted head-down, should be avoided because it increases the incidence of adverse reactions. (6)

CLINICAL INDICATIONS

Clinical indications for myelography include the unavailability of CT or MRI, multilevel stenosis, and multilevel spinal disease. Currently, suspicion of disc herniation *is not* a clinical indication for myelography.

THE ABNORMAL MYELOGRAM

Myelography delineates the inner margin of the thecal sac throughout the cervical, thoracic, and lumbar spine. The spinal cord size, shape, and position are outlined by the contrast column. The size, course, and configuration of dural root sleeves are also delineated.

Variations in normal anatomy such as asymmetry and deformity of the thecal sac permit localization of space-occupying lesions to one of three anatomic areas: *extradural, intradural extramedullary,* and *intradural intramedullary.* Lesion classification by location within the spinal canal is necessary to arrive at a reasonable differential diagnosis.

EXTRADURAL

Extradural lesions reside outside the thecal sac but within the bony confines of the neural canal. (Fig. 6.193) They produce a

pattern of dural compression and, with extensive deformity, complete obstruction. (Fig. 6.194) The most common etiology of the extradural defect is intervertebral disc herniation. (Figs. 6.195, 6.196) Other extradural pathologies include posteriorly oriented degenerative osteophytes, ligamentum flavum hypertrophy, hematoma, metastasis, and abscess. (Fig. 6.197)

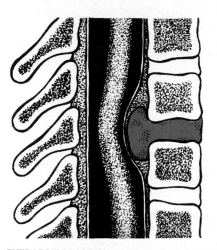

Figure 6.193.   EXTRADURAL LESION: SCHEMATIC DIAGRAM. This pattern refers to deformation and indentation of the dural membrane from an extradural source. The spinal cord may be displaced. Etiologies producing this pattern include disc herniation, degenerative stenosis, spinal tumor, hematoma, and abscess.

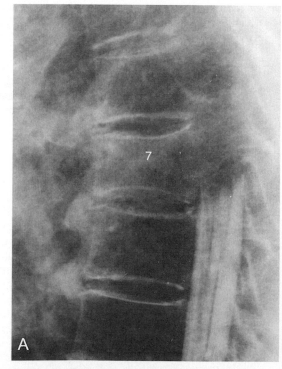

Figure 6.194.   MULTIPLE MYELOMA: A PATHOLOGIC FRACTURE. This elderly male complained of midthoracic pain that was worse at night. **A. Myelogram, Lateral Thoracic.** Notice the mild compression deformity of the superior endplate of T7 and the adjacent complete extradural obstruction of the myelographic column. **B. MRI, T1-Weighted Sagittal Thoracic.** This image reveals decreased signal intensity (arrow) in association with a mild compression deformity of the vertebral body. Additionally, there is mild ventral and dorsal expansion of the vertebral body, which has produced the extradural compression noted in **A**. A paraspinal soft tissue mass, which was proven to be myeloma, is noted anterior to the fracture (arrowhead).

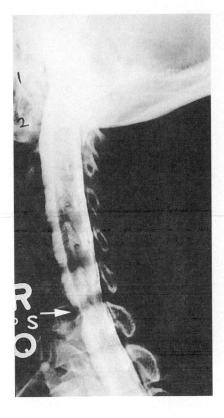

Figure 6.195.   HERNIATION OF THE C6-C7 NUCLEUS PULPOSUS. Myelogram, Oblique Cervical. Observe the ventral defect in the myelographic contrast column, the result of a herniated disc at C6-C7 (arrow). COMMENT: Extradural defects most commonly arise as a result of osteophyte or disc herniation.

Figure 6.196.   HERNIATED NUCLEUS PULPOSUS: LUMBAR SPINE. A. Myelogram, Left Posterior Oblique Lumbar. Observe the abrupt termination of the contrast-filled left S1 nerve root at the level of the L5-S1 disc (arrow) indicating a herniation. **B. Myelogram, Right Posterior Oblique Lumbar.** The normal, contrast-filled right S1 nerve root (arrow) is shown for comparison. COMMENT: In patients with a large spinal canal, the sensitivity of myelography is diminished. The dura in these individuals does not closely approximate the herniation; therefore the contrast column is not compressed.

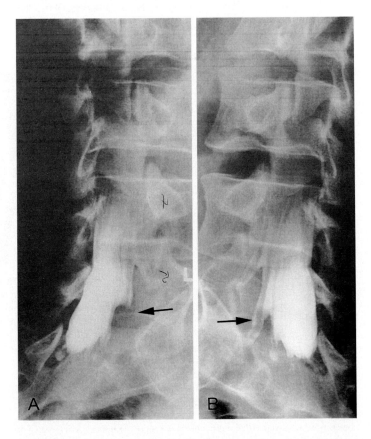

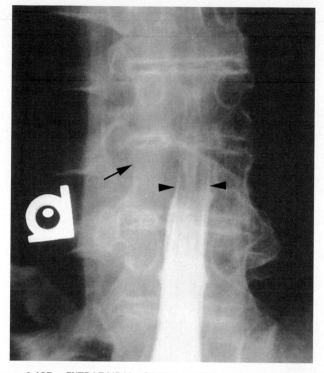

**Figure 6.197. EXTRADURAL OBSTRUCTION: METASTATIC CARCI-
NOMA.** This elderly male presented with a Brown-Sequard syndrome. **Myelogram, AP Thoracic.** There is absence of the left T10 pedicle (arrow) and
high-grade obstruction of the myelographic column (arrowheads). At surgery, the extradural space was filled with metastatic tumor resulting in complete obstruction of the subarachnoid space.

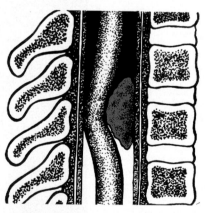

**Figure 6.198. INTRADURAL EXTRAMEDULLARY LESION: SCHEMATIC
DIAGRAM.** There is a well-defined lesion in the subarachnoid space. Observe the displacement of the spinal cord from the intradural lesion. This
pattern is observed with neural tumors such as meningioma and
neurofibroma.

INTRADURAL EXTRAMEDULLARY

Intradural extramedullary lesions exist within the dura but outside the spinal cord. (Fig. 6.198) Most of these lesions are benign tumors of neurogenic origin, most commonly neurofibroma (Fig. 6.199) and meningioma. (Fig. 6.200) Intradural extramedullary tumors are seen as intraspinal masses within the thecal sac, compressing and contralaterally displacing the spinal cord.

INTRADURAL INTRAMEDULLARY

Intradural intramedullary lesions represent the third classic myelographic pattern. (Fig. 6.201) The most common malignant neoplasms, astrocytoma and ependymoma, are frequently seen in the thoracic region. Ependymomas of the filum terminale, lipomas, and syrinx may also present with this abnormal myelographic pattern and demonstrate localized fusiform expansion of the spinal cord with thinning and spreading of the contrast column along the lateral margins of the cord. (Fig. 6.202) If the lesion produces complete obstruction, cervical instillation of contrast may be necessary to outline the upper level of the lesion. (4) Difficulty may be encountered in distinguishing intramedullary from extramedullary lesions, particularly when the latter results in bulging of the cord or obstruction within the canal. Currently, complete obstructions are unusual because the water-based contrast agents tend to diffuse past an obstructive lesion.

Today, myelography plays a minor role in spinal imaging. It is relegated to patient evaluation when MRI is equivocal or cannot be performed. It enhances the accuracy of CT, and when they are combined, the resulting examination is termed CT myelography (CTM). (10) CTM is still employed for the evaluation of suspected arachnoiditis. Patients presenting with a clinical picture suggestive of a cervical, thoracic, or lumbar disc herniation should no longer initially undergo myelography, but instead should be evaluated with MRI. Although the past decade has seen a marked reduction in the amount of myelographic procedures ordered, far too many needless myelograms are still being performed. The advances in noninvasive imaging procedures will continue to influence the future of spinal imaging.

MEDICOLEGAL IMPLICATIONS
Myelography

- This procedure is contraindicated in individuals who are being treated medically with tricyclic antidepressants, monoamine oxidase inhibitors, and phenothiazine compounds. These patients should be referred for MRI.

- Patients with a history of seizures require prophylactic medication prior to the examination.

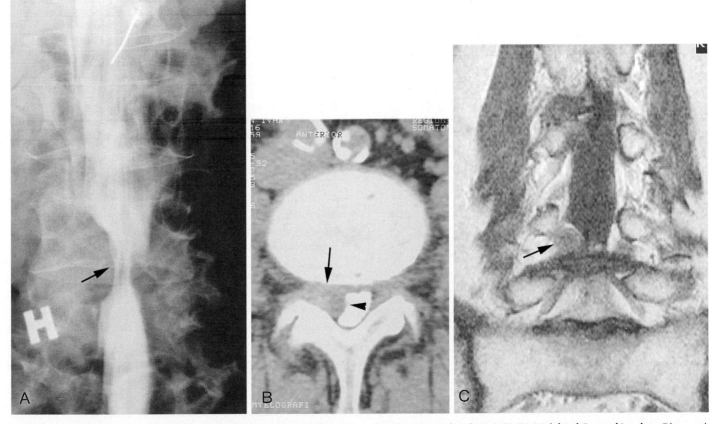

Figure 6.199. SCHWANNOMA: DISC HERNIATION LOOK-ALIKE. A. Myelogram, AP Lumbosacral. There is a large extradural defect on the myelogram at L4-L5 (arrow). **B. CT Myelogram, Soft Tissue Window Axial Lumbar.** Note the large, smoothly marginated, extradural mass that slightly expands the L4-L5 neural foramen (arrow) and deforms the contrast-filled thecal sac (arrowhead). **C. MRI, T1-Weighted Coronal Lumbar.** Observe the homogenous intermediate signal intensity mass (arrow) deflecting the thecal sac toward the midline. These findings are consistent with an extradural schwannoma. COMMENT: Schwannomas, as well as the other tumors of the nerve sheath, may erode bone and enlarge the intervertebral foramen.

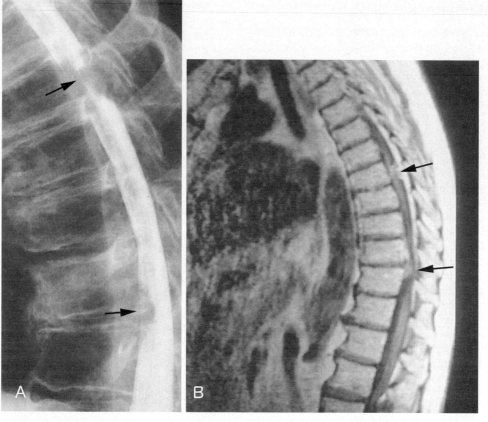

Figure 6.200.   MULTIPLE MENINGIOMAS. A. Myelogram, Lateral Thoracic. Notice the well-defined intradural filling defects at two levels in the thoracic spine (arrows). **B. MRI, T1-Weighted Contrast-Enhanced Sagittal Thoracic**. Observe the mild hyperintense signal of the intradural masses within the thoracic spinal cord (arrows). COMMENT: Meningioma and neurofibroma are the most common intradural extramedullary neoplasms. Meningiomas seldom erode pedicles or vertebral bodies. The absence of these findings may help to differentiate meningioma from neurofibroma.

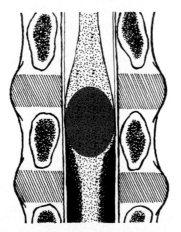

Figure 6.201.   INTRADURAL INTRAMEDULLARY LESION: SCHEMATIC DIAGRAM. Notice the diffuse enlargement of the spinal cord with bilateral tapering and narrowing of the contrast column surrounding the lesion. Etiologies producing this pattern include astrocytoma, ependymoma, arteriovenous malformation, and syrinx. These lesions are best demonstrated on anteroposterior or posteroanterior views.

- This procedure is contraindicated in patients who exhibit clinical signs of dehydration. All patients should be encouraged to increase fluid consumption 12 hours prior to the examination to ensure that they are well hydrated. This helps diminish the neurotoxic effects of the contrast.

- Improper injection techniques may produce nerve root injury, arachnoiditis, pulmonary oil emboli, epidermoid formation, or perforation of the annulus fibrosus (and subsequent disc herniation).

- Headaches, dizziness, nausea, and vomiting are common adverse reactions that subside with time.

- Meningitis-like symptoms, radiculitis, hyperreflexia, and cerebral or spinocerebellar symptoms (seizures, CNS ischemia, and visual and auditory changes) may occur because of the neurotoxic effects of the contrast.

- All patients should be screened for iodine sensitivity prior to the examination.

DISCOGRAPHY

HISTORICAL PERSPECTIVES

The application of discography in the diagnosis of low back pain syndromes was first described in 1948 by Hirsch and Lind-

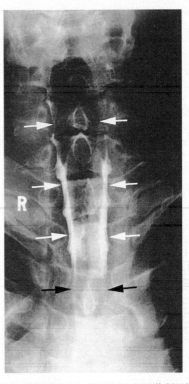

Figure 6.202.   SYRINGOMYELIA: "SHAWL-LIKE" SENSORY LOSS. This 34-year-old female had a 5-year history of recurrent right glenohumeral joint dislocation. **Myelogram, AP Cervicodorsal.** The myelogram demonstrates symmetric tapering (arrows) of the contrast column from the lower cervical spine extending to the upper thoracic region. This was the result of an enlarged spinal cord secondary to a congenital syrinx. COMMENT: Syrinx of the cervical cord may result in a neurotrophic arthropathy of the glenohumeral joints with subsequent instability. (Courtesy of Paul H. Young, MD, St. Louis, Missouri)

blom. (1,2) Injecting contrast into the nucleus of cadaveric discs demonstrated annular changes in the form of radial tears. Falconer and Erlacher described pain provocation with stimulation of the intervertebral disc. (3,4) Fernstrum stressed both neurogenic (compressive) and discogenic (inflammatory) causes of back and leg pain. (5)

Discography is an imaging technique that evaluates the integrity of the intervertebral disc. This examination assesses the morphology and physiology of the disc by injecting water-soluble contrast material into the nucleus pulposus. It is particularly useful in evaluating patients when surgery is contemplated for lumbar spine pain and/or radiculopathy and coupled with negative or equivocal CT or MRI examinations. Discography in the cervical spine is limited because of its unreliable results. (6) Fernstrum concluded that discography was valuable in evaluating patients who had spinal pain without evidence of disc herniation. (5)

Glossary of Terms

Annular fissure: interruption or tear of the annulus fibrosus that occurs as a result of trauma or disc degeneration.

CT discography: the combination of discography with computed tomography. This provides a more accurate assessment of intradiscal contrast distribution.

Discogram: a contrast examination that is performed by injecting a small volume of contrast agent into the nucleus pulposus. The morphology of the nucleus pulposus is indirectly evaluated and correlated with the patient's clinical response to the injection. When the patient's clinical symptoms are reproduced during injection of either the contrast or saline the examination is provocation positive, hence the term *Provocational Discogram.*

Extravasation: the escape of a material from a site or compartment. In discography this refers to the escape of radiopaque contrast from the confines of the disc.

STRUCTURE AND PATHOPHYSIOLOGY OF THE INTERVERTEBRAL DISC

The intervertebral disc provides the dual function of structural support and articular mobility. To accommodate these tasks, a variety of histologic tissues must be integrated. The dense collagen fibers and fibrocartilage of the annulus fibrosus surrounds the centrally positioned nucleus pulposus and inserts into the hyaline cartilage of the vertebral endplate. Along the periphery these fibers (Sharpey's fibers) attach directly into the cortical bone of the endplate.

The biomechanical behavior of the intervertebral disc is related to its hydration status. (7) The factors responsible for age-related changes within the disc are related to its biochemical constituents. Aging results in a decline in the proteoglycan concentration and an increase in the ratio of keratin sulfate to chondroitin sulfate. As the collagen and the collagen-proteoglycan binding of the nucleus pulposus increases, a decline in the water-binding capacity occurs, resulting in a dehydrated, fibrous, and rigid intervertebral disc. (8) These biochemical imbalances lead to a functionally impaired disc that exhibits altered load distribution through its individual components (nucleus pulposus and annulus fibrosus). Even the normal repetitive forces initiated by the activities of daily living produce cartilage fibrillation and annular fissuring. Through these tears the nucleus pulposus may progressively migrate toward the perimeter of the annulus and provoke pain. When fissures extend to the outer margin of the annulus fibrosus, herniation of the nucleus pulposus may follow. A variety of factors, including the speed of degeneration, the extent of annular fissuring and healing, and the magnitude of weight-bearing loads affect the extent of the herniation. (9)

Bogduk has proposed that disc-space narrowing is a consequence of nuclear degradation following endplate fracture. (8) Microfractures deform the endplate of the vertebral body and interrupt the vascular channels that deliver nutrients to the endplate and disc. Endplate fractures may also initiate an autoimmune response, further degrading the nuclear matrix.

PATHOGENESIS OF DISC PAIN

The etiology of low back pain is not explained simply on the basis of disc herniation and nerve root compression. Disc herniation may be the causative factor in only 5% of low back pain complaints. (10) There is a growing recognition that herniations and other disruptive disc lesions, as well as spinal cord and nerve root compression, may remain asymptomatic. (11,12) A direct cause-and-effect relationship between annular tears and pain provocation is yet to be established, since radial tears are common in asymptomatic individuals and may be age-related. (13)

Pain fibers have been identified in the outer one third of the posterior annular fibers of lumbar discs. Wiberg (14) demonstrated that pressure on the posterior annular fibers could provoke back pain. Coppes et al. (15) have shown nerve fibers in the nucleus pulposus of degenerated discs. New models of back pain emphasize chemical mediators. Proinflammatory by-products from the intervertebral disc such as phospholipase A_2 may initiate an inflammatory reaction in the annulus, sensitizing the surrounding tissues, including the disc and dorsal root ganglion. These inflammatory mediators may trigger a chemical neuritis, even in the absence of visible neurologic compression. (16,17) Nociceptive activity, however, cannot be elicited by mechanical stimulation without previous damage to the nerve root. (18) Pain arising in association with the nerve roots occurs in a narrow band and is characteristically sharp, lancinating, and frequently associated with paresthesia. In contrast, somatic pain arising from joints, muscles, ligaments, and the intervertebral disc produces dull and poorly localized pain in the back, pelvis, and thigh. (8)

Jinkins (19) describes a vertebrogenic syndrome consisting of local and referred pain, radicular pain and paresthesia, autonomic reflex alterations, muscular dysfunction, and altered viscerosomatic reflexes. He has suggested that the efferent autonomic fibers are driving afferent pain fibers, resulting in referred pain and dysfunction.

A comprehensive understanding of the role that the intervertebral disc plays in spinal and radicular pain remains elusive. Because of this, the invasive nature of discography and its true usefulness in back pain patients is still disputed, despite a recent resurgence of interest.

DISCOGRAPHY PROCEDURES

Patients selected for discographic examination are evaluated using fluoroscopy. The region of interest is prepped and draped.

The asymptomatic or less symptomatic side is selected for injection. Following local anesthesia, the initial spinal needle is advanced using fluoroscopic guidance until it penetrates the annulus and enters the disc substance. A smaller needle is then inserted through the larger needle. Once the smaller needle is in position, normal saline is injected and the volume is recorded. Following the saline injection, water-soluble contrast is injected into the disc. The radiographic appearance of the discogram and the presence or absence of a pain response is noted. (20)

Computed tomography performed after discography provides a high-resolution assessment of intradiscal herniation routes, sites of maximal protrusion, and herniation size. (21)

CLINICAL INDICATIONS

Clinical indications for discography include the need for definitively establishing the presence of discogenic pain and isolating a specific symptomatic level. An additional application is the end-stage evaluation of a complex spinal complaint that is being considered for surgical intervention.

THE ABNORMAL DISCOGRAM

The normal contrast-filled nucleus pulposus appears with an amorphous unilocular, bilocular, or double-wafer configuration. (Fig. 6.203) These patterns are usually confined to a central or slightly posterior location within the disc space, but may be altered slightly depending on the patient's position. (22) (Fig. 6.204) Discograms are considered abnormal when morphologic changes within the disc are observed or when the injection of either saline or contrast provokes a pain response (Provocational Discogram). (Fig. 6.205) The diagnostic significance of this response is confirmed when symptoms are relieved following injection of local

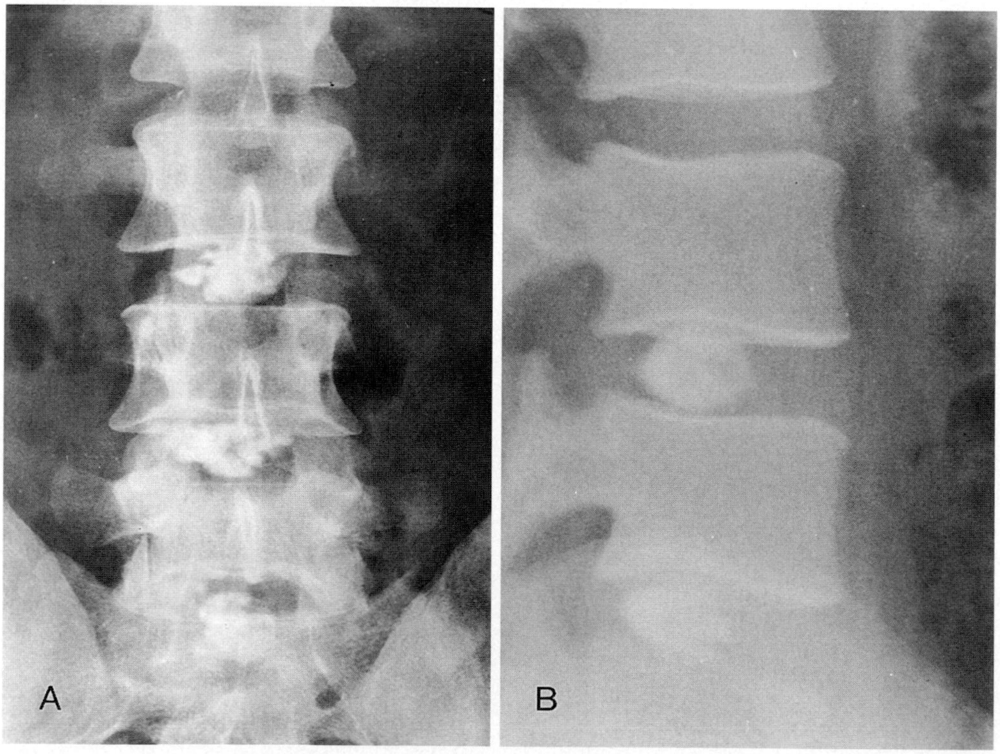

Figure 6.203.   NORMAL DISCOGRAM. A. AP Lumbar Spine Discogram. B. Lateral Lumbar Spine Discogram.
Observe the opacification of the nucleus pulposus of the 3rd, 4th, and 5th lumbar discs.

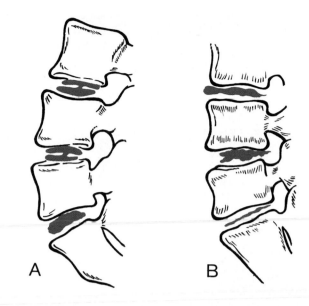

A   B

Figure 6.204. NORMAL AND ABNORMAL DISCOGRAMS. A. Normal Lateral Discogram: Schematic Diagram. The illustration demonstrates the normal appearance of the contrast-filled nucleus pulposus. The upper two discs demonstrate the bilocular pattern, characterized by two horizontal bars connected vertically. The lower disc reveals a nuclear pattern that is homogenous and amorphous. **B. Abnormal Lateral Discogram: Schematic Diagram**. This diagram demonstrates a series of contrast-filled abnormal discs. The upper disc displays flattening of the nucleus with anterior dissection and herniation. The middle disc also displays flattening of the nucleus with posterior extension of contrast, consistent with a minimal herniation. The lower nucleus pulposus is flattened and depicts complete bidirectional dissection through annular fissures, a finding characteristic of disc degeneration.

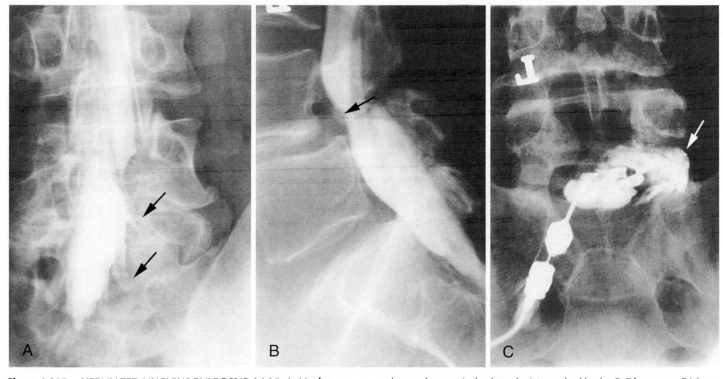

A   B   C

Figure 6.205.   HERNIATED NUCLEUS PULPOSUS: L4-L5. A. Myelogram, PA Lumbar. Note the extradural defects on the lateral margins of the contrast column that have amputated the exiting nerve root sleeves (arrows). **B. Myelogram, Lateral Lumbar** . Extradural compression of the ventral margin of the contrast column is noted immediately posterior to the L4-L5 disc space and ascends posteriorly along the L4 vertebral body. **C. Discogram, PA Lumbar L5-S1**. The contrast material injected through the centrally positioned needle tip has extravasated posterolaterally. (Courtesy of Robert L. Mattin, DC, Perth, Western Australia)

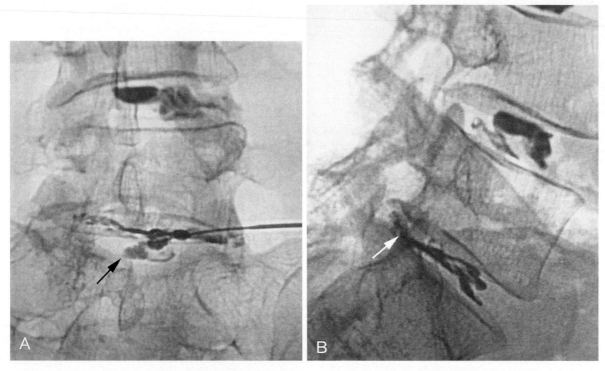

Figure 6.206.   SUBTRACTION DISCOGRAM: DEGENERATIVE DISC DISEASE. A. Discogram AP Lumbar. B. Discogram Lateral Lumbar. There is marked posterior migration of the discographic agent into the posterior annular fibers of the L5-S1 disc (arrow). This finding is representative of discal degeneration. COMMENT: The injection of saline during discography may provoke pain similar, or identical to, the patient's chief complaint (*provo-* *cational discogram*). Further confirmatory evidence of a specific level of discogenic pain is obtained if symptoms diminish with injection of an anesthetic agent. Often, multiple discograms are necessary to determine the level(s) and extent of surgical intervention necessary. This modality is unique in that it provides both morphologic information and clinical correlation. (Courtesy of James M. Cox, DC, DACBR, Fort Wayne, Indiana)

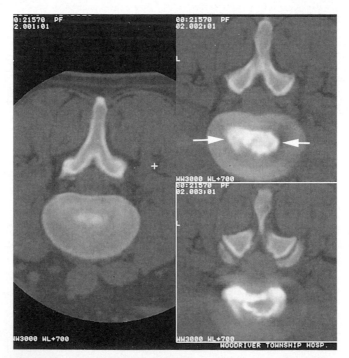

Figure 6.207.   CT DISCOGRAM: NORMAL. CT Discogram, Bone Window Axial Lumbar. The nucleus pulposus is normal in both its position and appearance (arrows) . This image demonstrates no evidence of annular tear or dissection of the nucleus pulposus. (Courtesy of The Wood River Memorial Township Hospital, Department of Radiology, Wood River, Illinois)

anesthetic into the disc. Dissection and annular disruption are observed when the contrast escapes the confines of the nuclear area extending anteriorly, posteriorly (Fig. 6.206) or through intraosseous routes into the vertebral body (Schmorl's nodes). Reproduction of the patient's pain pattern on pressurization of the disc is a key finding that, when elicited, provides physiologic information concerning a specific level of spinal anatomy, often correlating with the patient's clinical findings. This pain response is positive and significant even in structurally intact discs.

In the past, discography was occasionally performed prior to spinal arthrodesis to evaluate the integrity of the discs adjacent to the fusion level. (23) Magnetic resonance imaging has replaced discography in this capacity because MRI is capable of providing this information noninvasively.

Vanharanta classified CT discograms into four grades of nuclear penetration. (23) (Fig. 6.207) Radial fissures that penetrate the outer one third of the posterior annulus are more likely to stimulate nociceptive nerve endings and become symptomatic on injection of discographic contrast. (24) (Fig. 6.208)

The enormous diagnostic challenge of assessing spinal pain syndromes is assisted by discography, especially when coupled with computed tomography. (Fig. 6.209) In a reasonably safe and reliable manner, discography provides a unique anatomic and physiologic description of the disc.

MEDICOLEGAL IMPLICATIONS
Discography

- Septic spondylitis may occur if a sterile field is not maintained during this procedure.

- All patients should be screened for iodine sensitivity prior to the examination.

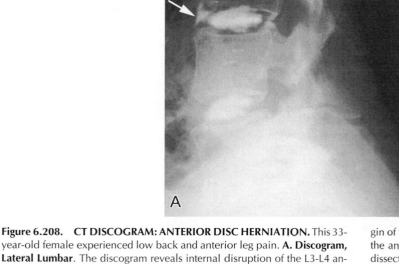
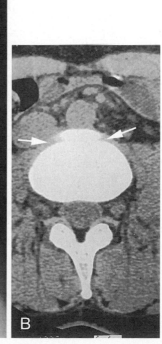

Figure 6.208.   CT DISCOGRAM: ANTERIOR DISC HERNIATION. This 33-year-old female experienced low back and anterior leg pain. **A. Discogram, Lateral Lumbar**. The discogram reveals internal disruption of the L3-L4 annular fibers with dissection of the contrast agent (arrow) to the anterior margin of the disc. **B. CT Discogram, Soft Tissue Window Axial L3-L4**. Observe the anterior herniation of nuclear material at the L3-L4 level with contrast dissecting underneath the anterior longitudinal ligament (arrow). (Courtesy of James M. Cox, DC, DACBR, Fort Wayne, Indiana)

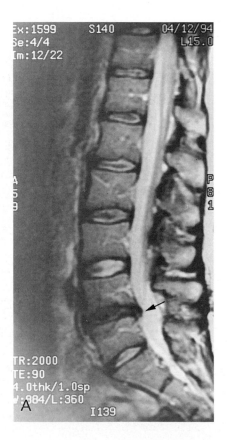

Figure 6.209.   RECURRENT LOW BACK PAIN: DISC VERSUS POSTSURGICAL SCAR. This patient is status postdiscectomy at L4-L5 four years prior. **A. MRI, T2-Weighted Sagittal Lumbar**. There is loss of the normal disc signal intensity at L4-L5 with a small posterior disc herniation (arrow). **B. MRI, T1-Weighted Noncontrast Axial Lumbar. C. MRI, T1-Weighted Contrast-Enhanced Axial Lumbar**. Note the small, central, contained disc herniation at L4-L5 which demonstrates minimal enhancement on the postcontrast images (arrows). **D. AP Discogram. E. Lateral Discogram**. Upon injection of the contrast into the L4-L5 disc space, the patient experienced localized back pain identical to her chief complaint. Note the extravasation of the contrast posterior to the vertebral margins (arrow). The intradiscal contrast also extends laterally and anteriorly to the peripheral annular fibers. **F. CT Discogram, Bone Window. G. CT Discogram, Soft Tissue Window**. The contrast is observed extending anteriorly to the outer annular fibers (arrow) and posteriorly beyond the posterior vertebral margins (arrowhead), abutting the ventral aspect of the thecal sac. Observe the low-attenuation area within the right lamina, consistent with a postsurgical fat graft (crossed arrow). COMMENT: This case nicely demonstrates the use of discography. When MRI is equivocal or does not display information that correlates with the patient's symptoms, a discogram is often employed to determine whether a given disc abnormality is the exact cause of the patient's symptoms. (Courtesy of Donald E. Freuden, DC, FACO, Denver, Colorado)

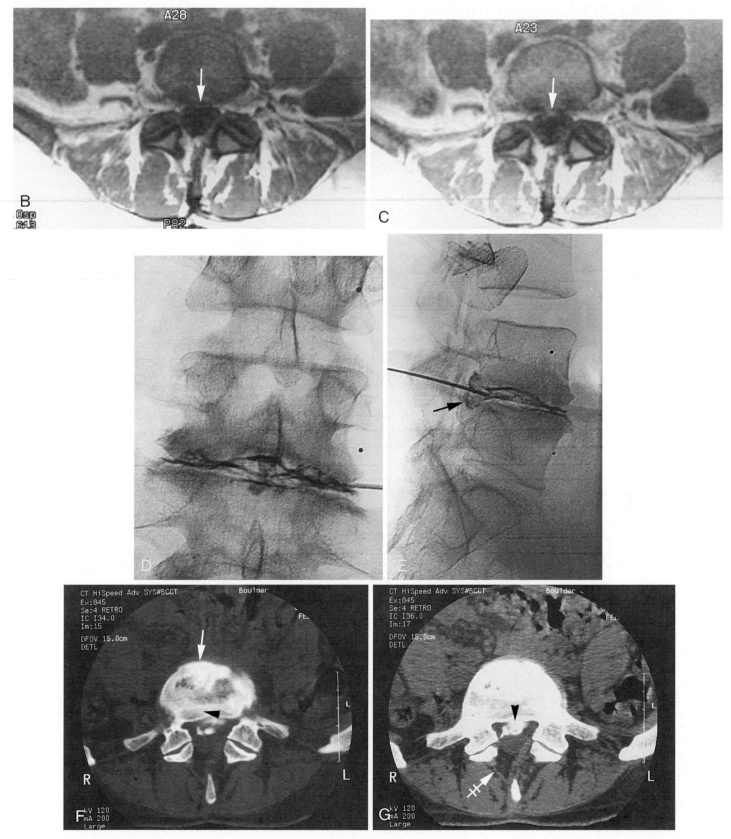

Figure 6.209B–G.

NUCLEAR MEDICINE

HISTORICAL PERSPECTIVES

A major landmark in the development of nuclear science was the classic experiment of Ernest Rutherford in 1919 at the Cavendish Laboratory in Cambridge, England. (1) Rutherford placed a small amount of radium in a container filled with oxygen and mounted a zinc sulfide screen nearby. Alpha particles emitted by the radium struck the zinc sulfide screen and produced on its surface pinpoints of light called *scintillations*, which could be observed and even counted by viewing the screen through a microscope. Rutherford and an associate, James Chadwick, deduced that the underlying process, which must have been occurring inside the container, was not the production of x-rays but rather positively charged nuclear particles, or protons. When an alpha particle emitted by the radium struck a nitrogen nucleus containing seven protons, one proton was ejected. The remainder of the nitrogen atom and the alpha particle joined together to form a new atom with eight protons, an oxygen atom. Rutherford had thus achieved the goal of the medieval alchemists: the transmutation of elements.

For the next decade laboratories in many countries engaged in a scientific race to be the first to develop *particle accelerators* or *atom smashers* capable of speeding up subatomic particles to the energies required for effective nuclear bombardment.

In the United States Ernest O. Lawrence in 1931 at the University of California Radiation Laboratory developed the cyclotron, the first of the circular accelerators. (2) The evolution of this new technology led to the application of radioisotope material to the study of human tissue. The first tracer study in clinical medicine that used radioactivity was the work of Blumgard, Weiss, and Yens in Boston in 1926. (3) The first biologic experiments using a new artificial radioisotope were reported in 1935 by Hevesy and Chiewitz (4), 12 years after Hevesy invented the tracer technique using a naturally radioactive isotope.

For the past 25 years the major radionuclide used in clinical work has been technetium. Technetium-99m was discovered by Perrier and Segre in 1937. (5) Radionuclide scanning of the liver, thyroid, lung, spleen, and other organs has revolutionized the evaluation of many body systems.

Glossary of Terms

ALARA principle: this principle states that procedures should not only maintain radiation doses within legal limits, but extend beyond to **As Low As Reasonably Achievable.**

Annihilation radiation: the radiation that arises from a collision between two particles with opposite charges. These particles are typically the positron and the electron. Their collision will result in annihilation and release of radiation into two oppositely directed 510 keV gamma rays. This radiation mechanism is employed in positron emission tomography (PET) scans.

Collimator: this device limits the radiation field entering the gamma camera crystal similar to a radiographic grid. There are a variety of collimator configurations such as converging, diverging, and pinhole. Collimator slits confine the gamma radiation in a uniform direction. This important device improves image quality.

Critical organ: the organ first subjected to the legally defined maximum permissible radiation exposure. The bladder is the critical organ in the technetium methylene diphosphonate (^{99m}Tc-MDP) bone scan examination.

Decay: the logarithmic disintegration of a radioactive substance into its daughter products.

Disintegration: the process of radioactive decay that results in spontaneous emission of particles from the nucleus.

Dose: the quantity of radiation that is delivered to a specific tissue site. In nuclear imaging the units of measurement are typically microcuries.

Flare phenomenon: increased tracer activity in a malignant lesion following chemotherapy. This phenomena represents healing at the lesion site and is accompanied by clinical improvement.

Gamma camera: this device is synonymous with a scintillation camera. It consists of a collimator, crystal, and photomultiplier (PM) array. Gamma radiation is directed into the collimator where it activates photons in the NaITL crystal. The photon scintillations are detected by the PM tubes and are electronically encoded for position (X, Y pulses). A photon (Z pulse) that is in a selected energy range is accepted after sampling by the pulse height analyzer.

Gamma rays: photons of gamma radiation.

Isotope: chemical elements that have the same atomic number but different atomic mass. Iodine for example, has several isotopes, including iodine-125 and iodine-131.

Pertechnetate (TcO$_4$): the standard compound formed as technetium is extracted from a generator by passing saline through it.

Photon: a quantum of electromagnetic energy.

Photopenia: the reduction of normal photon activity that is identified on a bone scan. This finding often accompanies ischemic or rapidly destructive lesions in the skeleton.

Positron: a particle that is equal to the mass of an electron, but maintains a positive electronic charge. When it contacts a negatively charged electron, annihilation radiation of 510 keV is emitted and detected by coincidence counters. This is the principle of positron emission tomography (PET).

Positron emission tomography (PET): an imaging modality that uses positron emitting radionuclides to produce annihilation radiation. The gamma rays emitted by the annihilation event are localized by detector systems called coincident circuits. Photon localization is displayed in the same manner as scintigraphy.

RAD: a unit of radiation absorption; 1 rad = 100 erg per gram.

Radioactive half-life: the time interval at which the radioactivity of a given sample will decrease to one half its initial value. The half-life of ^{99m}Tc-MDP is 6 hours.

Radiopharmaceutical: a radioactively labeled compound that is injected into the blood stream. The compound circulates and is deposited into the target tissue. Additional synonyms are radionuclide isotope and radionuclide agent. The most commonly employed radiopharmaceuticals in skeletal imaging are (listed in decreasing order):

Technetium-99m methylene diphosphonate (^{99m}Tc-MDP)

Gallium-67 (Ga-67)

Indium-111 oxine–tagged white blood cells (In-111)

Scintigraphy: this term is synonymous for a nuclear medicine procedure such as the bone scan. The term is derived from the decay of the radionuclide and its resultant gamma radiation or scintillations. The scintillations are detected by the gamma camera, processed by a computer, and displayed as an image. The number of scintillations corresponds to the concentration of the isotope.

Single Photon Emission Computed Tomography (SPECT): this technology employs one or more gamma cameras to tomographically record radiation in a defined plane. An image may be displayed in a multiplanar format (e.g., coronal, axial, sagittal). The SPECT exam provides increased localization of the radiopharmaceutical uptake. Its utility is maximized in difficult regions such as the spine, TMJ, and hip joint.

Super scan: a bone scan that displays diffuse axial metastatic disease so extensive and uniform that it mimics a normal exam. The pronounced skeletal uptake creates high contrast between bone and soft tissue. Uptake in the urinary system (kidneys and bladder) is faint because less radiotracer is available for excretion.

Three-phase bone scan: the three phases of a bone scan are the angiogram or flow phase, blood pool, and delayed or bone phase. The phases represent the temporal course of the radiopharmaceutical tracer.

Uptake: an accumulation of the radiopharmaceutical within the target tissue such as bone. A *hot spot* represents an increase in radiopharmaceutical deposition. A *cold spot* results from abnormally diminished radiopharmaceutical uptake, or photopenia.

INTRODUCTION

Diagnostic nuclear medicine is a vital tool in the diagnostic imaging armamentarium. Images are generated as the uptake and distribution of administered radiopharmaceuticals are detected. Although other imaging modalities may give a better analysis of structural integrity, nuclear medicine can often provide vital information regarding tissue perfusion, physiology, and biochemistry. Physiologic and metabolic changes often precede gross structural alteration of diseased tissue by hours, days, or even weeks. Nuclear medicine evaluation can therefore be a key factor in determining early diagnosis and proper treatment protocols and in establishing an accurate prognosis.

Nuclear medicine is a field of diagnostic imaging that encompasses various techniques and numerous applications. Radionuclide bone imaging and nuclear cardiology account for the majority of nuclear imaging studies. New procedures and applications, however, are constantly being developed. Radionuclide functional brain imaging, cholescintigraphy for the assessment of acute cholecystitis, and radiolabeled monoclonal antibodies for tumor detection are examples of the evolving diagnostic applications of nuclear imaging. Planar scintigraphy, single photon emission computed tomography (SPECT), and positron emission tomography (PET) are nuclear imaging techniques that are briefly discussed in this chapter.

Radionuclide bone scanning is presently the most frequently performed nuclear medicine technique, accounting for over half the studies performed in nuclear medicine departments. (6) Bone scanning techniques are employed in the evaluation of soft tissue, bone, and joint disorders. Fractures, infections, arthritides, tumors, and osteonecrosis are among the many disorders imaged by skeletal scintigraphy. Although the physiologic sensitivity of radionuclide bone scanning is a major advantage, this modality offers limited anatomic information and diagnostic specificity. To increase anatomic specificity, radiographs, computed tomography (CT), or magnetic resonance imaging (MRI) is often performed in conjunction with the bone scan to obtain the necessary anatomic information. (Fig. 6.210)

Skeletal scintigraphy radiopharmaceuticals were first introduced in the early 1960s with strontium-85, strontium-87, and fluorine-18. (7,8) Strontium-85 is an avid bone-seeking radiotracer with a long half-life and high radiation dose. These high-risk factors limited its use only to malignant conditions. Fluorine-18 sodium chloride displayed rapid blood clearance and high skeletal affinity, but its half-life was too short, limiting its application for scintigraphy. ^{99m}Tc-MDP polyphosphate compounds were successfully prepared and introduced in 1971 by Subramanian and McAfee. (9) Those early pharmacologic agents were tripolyphosphates. They were followed by pyrophosphates and today by diphosphonates. Diphosphonates have faster blood clearance and higher skeletal uptake than previous generations of pharmacologic agents. (10)

THREE-PHASE BONE SCAN: EXAMINATION PROCEDURE

Most radionuclide bone scans are performed in three phases (*three-phase bone scan*). These phases represent the distribution of the tracer over the course of time. The intravenous injection of the radiopharmaceutical agent initiates the three-phase bone scan. Phase one is known as the *flow phase* or *radionuclide angiogram* because of the intravascular location of the agent. Rapid sequential images are obtained over the region of interest every 2 to 3 seconds for 30 seconds. Approximately half of the radiotracer diffuses from the vascular to the extravascular space in 2 to 4 minutes. (6) The second phase is known as the *blood-pool phase* and occurs when the tracer is located in the extravascular space. A diffusion pattern is obtained by imaging the whole body or region of interest 5 minutes after injection. *Delayed* static images are obtained in the third phase or *bone scan phase* between 2 and 4 hours following the injection. (Fig. 6.211) These delayed images represent clearance of the tracer from the vessels and soft tissues and concentration into the skeleton. (Fig. 6.212) Twenty-four-hour scans are sometimes employed to evaluate osteomyelitis. (11)

ABSORBED PATIENT DOSE

The exact radiation dose absorbed by the patient in a three-phase bone scan is difficult to determine. A number of complex factors, including tracer biodistribution, organ pathology, and renal function, influence the dose. Approximately 50% of the injected dose is taken up by the skeleton within 2 to 6 hours. With normal renal excretion, 50 to 60% of the tracer is eliminated within 24 hours of injection. Urine concentration of the radionuclide in the bladder exposes it to a higher dose than other organs. The bladder therefore is the *critical* or *target organ*, receiving the highest dose. This dose may be reduced by preexam hydration of the patient and frequent voiding following the completion of the exam. (12) The whole body dose of a bone scan is approximately 0.13 rads. (13) In contrast, the average dose for a standard CT scan of the lumbar spine is 3 to 5 rads. There is often metabolic uptake of pertechnetate (which resembles iodine) in the following human tissue: choroid plexus, thyroid gland, salivary glands, stomach, and breast.

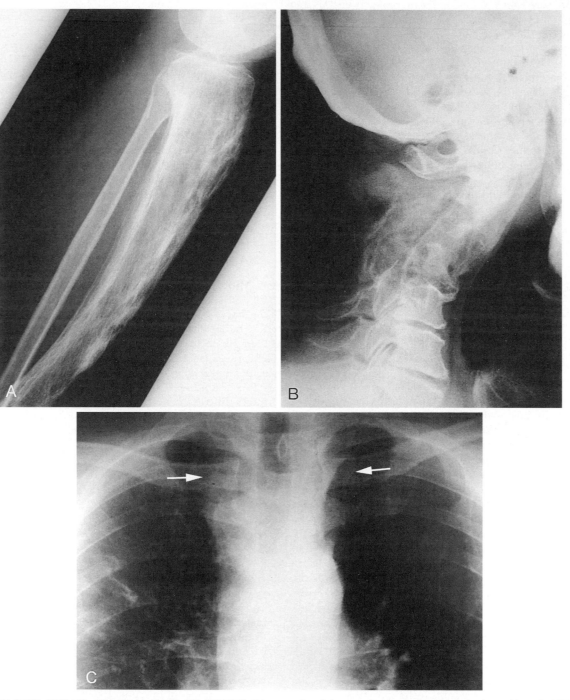

Figure 6.210. PAGET'S DISEASE: UNUSUAL CASE OF "LYTIC" IN-VOLVEMENT IN THE SPINE. This 57-year-old male presented with bilateral paresthesia and numbness in the lower extremities. **A. Lateral Leg.** Note the characteristic appearance of Paget's disease affecting the tibia. **B. Neutral Lateral Cervical.** The lytic phase of Paget's disease is seen involving C2 through C4. **C. PA Chest.** The manubrium is also affected by the disease (arrows). **D. AP Lumbar.** The T12 vertebral body demonstrates the characteristic "ivory" appearance of pagetic bone (arrow). A compression defor-mity of the pagetic L3 vertebral body is also evident. **E. MRI, T1-Weighted Sagittal Cervical.** Note the diffuse low signal intensity marrow replacement involving the neural arch and vertebral bodies of C2 through C4. **F. 99mTc-MDP Bone Scan, Anterior Whole Body (Left) and Posterior Whole Body (Right).** Increased tracer activity is present in T12 and L3, as noted on the plain film (see **D**). Abnormal activity is also identified in the tibia, pelvis, manubrium, scapula, and upper cervical spine. (Courtesy of Gary L. Smith, DC, DACBR, Portland, Oregon)

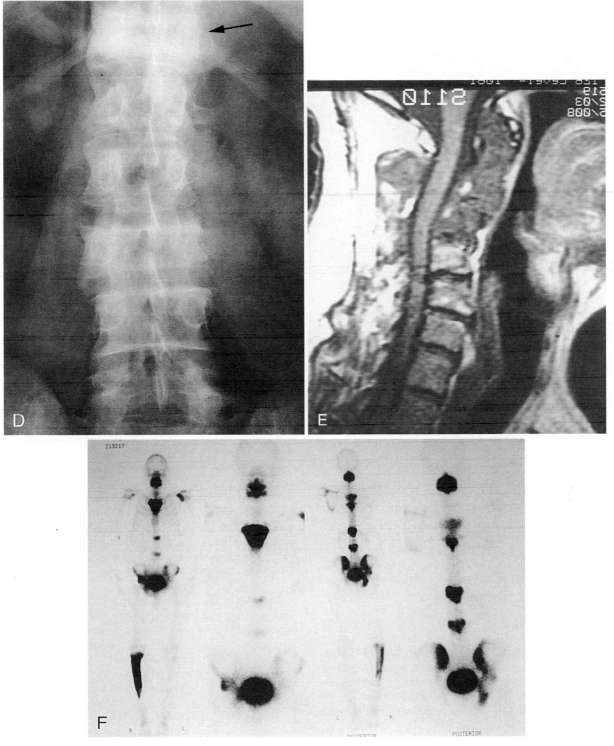

Figure 6.210D–F.

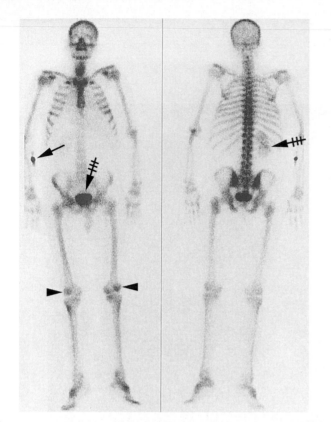

Figure 6.211. WHOLE BODY BONE SCAN: NORMAL ADULT. ^{99m}Tc-MDP **Bone Scan, Anterior Whole Body (Left) and Posterior Whole Body (Right).** This is the third phase of the three phase bone scan procedure. It displays symmetric skeletal uptake across the midline. An injection site is noted in the right midforearm (arrow), a normal finding. Note the normally increased activity in the sacroiliac joints and vertebral column, a reflection of higher rates of bone turnover. Clinically insignificant increased uptake is often observed in the knee joints of older individuals (arrowheads), secondary to degenerative arthritis. Accumulation of the radiopharmaceutical agent in the urinary tract (kidney and bladder) is normal (crossed arrows). COMMENT: Bone scanning is a highly sensitive means of detecting a wide range of musculoskeletal disorders. This procedure, however, frequently requires an anatomic imaging modality like CT or MRI for correlative purposes. (Courtesy of Timothy Schneider, DC, St. Louis, Missouri)

CONTRAINDICATIONS

The safety of scintigraphy is reflected in the limited circumstances that contraindicate its use. Pregnancy is a relative contraindication since transplacental transmission of radiopharmaceuticals is possible. The risk:benefit ratio should clearly warrant the use of a scintigraphic exam during pregnancy, as in a workup for skeletal metastases. (14) If a scintigraphic exam is performed, breast milk will carry isotope activity for several days following the exam. Formula feeding is recommended under these circumstances. (13)

IMAGE PRODUCTION

Nuclear medicine techniques employ radioactive tracer agents (radiopharmaceuticals) that are placed into the body by injection, ingestion, or inhalation. The radiopharmaceutical emits gamma rays that are detected by an instrument and transformed into electrical signals that ultimately generate a computer image of the tracer agent activity and concentration. Because the gamma rays

have high energy, very little is attenuated by the body and the exact distribution and intensity of the tracer in the body is reflected in the images. The intensity, pattern symmetry, and other anatomic characteristics of the organ or tissue are then evaluated. The distribution of radiopharmaceutical uptake, whether increased, delayed, or decreased, provides for a highly sensitive image of normal variation and pathophysiology.

The essential technical elements that are employed in the production of a nuclear medicine image are:

1. A pharmacologic agent that distributes into the organ tissue or compartment of interest.
2. A radionuclide that emits gamma radiation of sufficient energy to escape the target tissue or compartment (e.g., vascular, ventricular, intestinal compartments) and reach a detector. The radiopharmaceuticals are used in tiny trace amounts.
3. A gamma ray detector with computer processing, image production, and recording systems.

RADIOPHARMACEUTICAL AGENTS

A *radiopharmaceutical* chemically combines a radionuclide and a pharmacologic agent. A *radionuclide* is an element that emits gamma radiation while undergoing radioactive decay. The optimal radiopharmaceutical must be an efficient diagnostic agent, easy to produce, safe, and available at a reasonable cost. The ideal agent for bone scanning should emit principally gamma radiation, exhibit a convenient half-life, possess the appropriate chemical properties (e.g., stability and low toxicity) and be taken up by metabolically active bone tissue.

Gamma radiation, unlike beta or alpha particles, yields relatively high energy photons in a range between 70 to 500 kiloelectron volts (keV). Most nuclear imaging detector systems operate in this energy range. This energy is sufficient to pass through body tissues relatively unattenuated for detection by a gamma camera. The half-life of a radiopharmaceutical (the period necessary for half the radionuclei to decay) must be long enough to provide ample time for its preparation and administration. The half-life must be short enough, however, to limit patient radiation levels to values that are as low as reasonably achievable (*ALARA principle*). (15)

Following their administration, radiopharmaceutical agents are designed to be preferentially localized to particular targets; these might be organs, tissues, anatomic spaces, or metabolic pathways. Physiologic differences between normal and pathologic tissue produce different patterns of radiopharmaceutical uptake and distribution. The resultant image may show areas of increased gamma emission called *hot spots*. Areas of decreased gamma emission are known as *cold spots*.

Dozens of radiopharmaceuticals are now employed in nuclear imaging. The most widely used radionuclide is ^{99m}Tc-MDP. Its half-life of 6 hours and principal photon energy of 140/keV are convenient and have resulted in widespread use. The diphosphonate class of compounds labeled with ^{99m}Tc-MDP are utilized almost exclusively for bone imaging.

Since the early 1970s and into the 1980s, Indium-111 (^{111}In) and Gallium-67 (^{67}Ga) were employed to detect infection, inflammation and certain tumors such as lymphoma and hepatocellular carcinoma. (16,17) (Fig. 6.213) Today these agents are most commonly used for tumor localization, the evaluation of fever of unknown origin, AIDS, and inflammatory disorders of the lungs, abdomen (peritonitis), and pelvis. They are also used to differ-

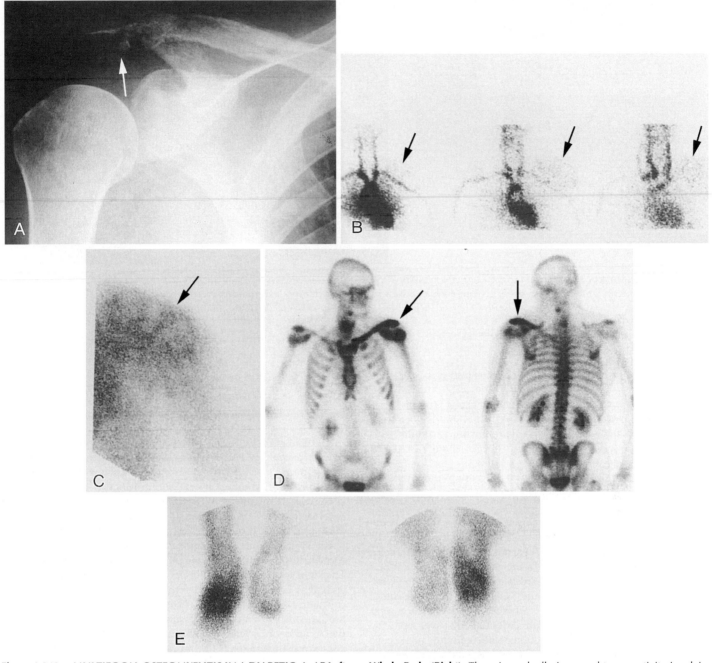

Figure 6.212.   MULTIFOCAL OSTEOMYELITIS IN A DIABETIC. A. AP Left Shoulder. Notice the destruction and debris involving the acromioclavicular joint (arrow). **B. Bone Scan (Angiogram Phase), Upper Torso and Neck.** Increased vascular perfusion is present involving the soft tissues of the left shoulder (arrows). **C. Bone Scan (Blood Pool Phase), Left Shoulder.** Note the diffusely increased tracer activity, consistent with hyperemia (arrow). **D. Bone Scan (Delayed Images), Anterior Whole Body (Left) and Posterior Whole Body (Right).** There is markedly increased tracer activity involving the clavicle and acromioclavicular and glenohumeral joints (arrows), suggestive of osteomyelitis. **E. Bone Scan, Dorsal Bilateral Foot (Left) and Plantar Bilateral Foot (Right).** There is diffuse increased tracer activity in the right, mid and forefoot, consistent with osteomyelitis. (Courtesy of Michael A. Fox, MD, Memphis, Tennessee)

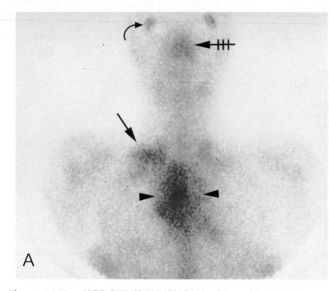

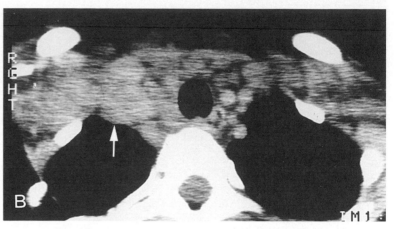

Figure 6.213. HODGKIN'S LYMPHOMA: GA-67 SCAN POSITIVE FOR TUMOR. A. Bone Scan, Anterior Chest. Areas of abnormally increased radiotracer activity, consistent with tumor, are observed in the right supraclavicular (arrow) and mediastinal (arrowheads) regions. Sites of activity involving the nasopharynx (crossed arrow) and lacrimal glands (curved arrow) on Ga-67 scans are normal. **B. CT, Soft Tissue Window Axial Chest.** Observe the soft tissue mass (arrow) present in the right mediastinum. COMMENT: Lymphoma demonstrates a pronounced affinity for Ga-67. (Courtesy of Timothy Schneider, DC, St. Louis, Missouri)

entiate osteomyelitis and postoperative complications suggestive of infection. (18)

Gallium-67 citrate uptake is maximized at sites of tumor, infection, or inflammation. The administered Ga-67 binds with iron-binding proteins to form a complex that attaches to a tumor surface or enters the focus of an infection. Approximately 10 to 20% of the injected gallium is excreted through the gastrointestinal tract (the critical organ) within 24 hours. Scans are then typically obtained 48 hours after injection. The half-life of Ga-67 is 78 hours. (19)

Indium-111 oxine leukocyte imaging is performed 18 to 24 hours after administration of autologous labeled white blood cells (WBCs). The In-111 labels leukocytes, monocytes, red blood cells, platelets, and plasma proteins. Tissue uptake of labeled WBCs indicates an inflammatory or infectious response. Indium-111 leukocyte scintigraphy is sensitive and specific for the detection of pulmonary, abdominal, and pelvic infections. (19) Concerns over the high dose (13 to 20 rads) and potential infection from the withdrawal, handling, and reinjection of labeled white blood cells have prompted the development of new agents, which include immunoglobulins and labeled antigranulocyte antibody agents. (20,21)

TRACER MECHANISMS

The precise mechanism of skeletal uptake of the radiopharmaceutical with ^{99m}Tc-MDP is not fully understood. The radiopharmaceutical is thought to localize preferentially because of a combination of increased blood flow and increased surface area on the hydroxyapatite (bone) crystal. (22,23) The agent is adsorbed or bound onto the mineral portion of the bone crystal and collagen, concentrating at sites of new-bone formation. Increased functional demand on the skeleton results in new bone formation, increasing the volume of crystal formed. This functional histologic response precedes the gross structural (radiographic) changes by several weeks or months. The ability of bone scanning to detect these early physiologic or pathologic altera-

tions accounts for its utility in the imaging of subtle skeletal disorders.

PLANAR SCINTIGRAPHY

In planar scintigraphy the gamma radiation emitted by a radiopharmaceutical that is administered intravenously is detected by a gamma or scintillation camera. The gamma camera consists of a collimator, coupled with a sodium iodide–thallium (NaITl) crystal detector and photomultiplier technology. The scintillation detector radiates visible light when struck by gamma photons. Photomultiplier tubes transform these light photons into electronic signals. Following amplification, the density and spatial coordinates of the photons are plotted by a computer. (Fig. 6.214) The detector/computer interface generates high-resolution images that correspond to the radiopharmaceutical location and concentration. Modern planar scintigraphic imaging systems simultaneously image the anterior and posterior aspects of the whole body or provide overlapping static views of a region. Images are then stored on film by means of a multiformat camera. (24)

High concentrations (increased activity) of the radiopharmaceutical photons are displayed as a dark area. The absence of photons (photopenia) produces a corresponding area of decreased activity, resulting in lighter areas on the image. Contrast in the image is influenced by technologic factors, tissue uptake, and attenuation by overlying tissue.

SINGLE PHOTON EMISSION COMPUTED TOMOGRAPHY (SPECT)

The image contrast and resolution of planar scintigraphy may be enhanced by introducing the tomographic characteristics of single photon emission computed tomography (SPECT) imaging. Planar imaging summates all planes of isotopic (point source) tracer activity to form an image. The modern multihead rotating SPECT camera systems display tracer activity in only

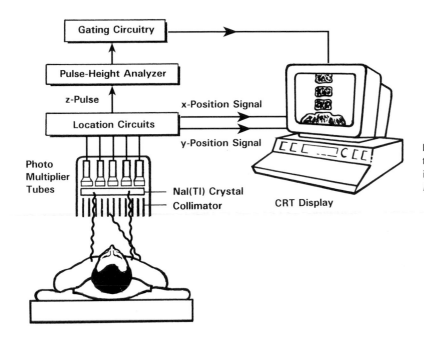

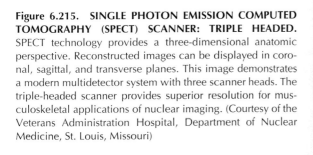

Figure 6.214.   GAMMA CAMERA SYSTEM. This diagram illustrates the principles of gamma-ray emission, collimation, detection, localization, and image display. (Modified from Wolbarst AB: *Physics of Radiology*, Norwalk, Appleton and Lange, 1993)

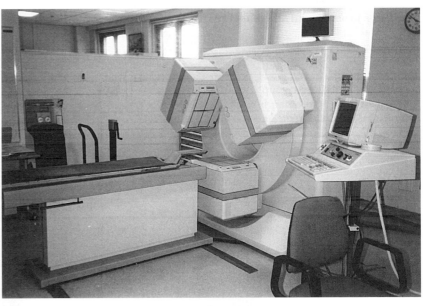

Figure 6.215.   SINGLE PHOTON EMISSION COMPUTED TOMOGRAPHY (SPECT) SCANNER: TRIPLE HEADED. SPECT technology provides a three-dimensional anatomic perspective. Reconstructed images can be displayed in coronal, sagittal, and transverse planes. This image demonstrates a modern multidetector system with three scanner heads. The triple-headed scanner provides superior resolution for musculoskeletal applications of nuclear imaging. (Courtesy of the Veterans Administration Hospital, Department of Nuclear Medicine, St. Louis, Missouri)

the selected image plane. Like CT scanning, a multiplanar format provides the potential for axial, coronal, or sagittal views. This results in increased image contrast, as well as variable spatial orientation and improved resolution. (25) Applications include evaluation of the musculoskeletal system, heart, brain, and abdomen. (26)

In SPECT technology, between one and four gamma or scintillation cameras on a rotating gantry are used to provide images in a selected tissue plane. The cameras travel in a circular or elliptical motion, allowing more accurate imaging of the patient with improved spatial resolution and sensitivity. (Fig. 6.215) SPECT images may be displayed in a three-dimensional format like CT and MRI. (Fig. 6.216) This multiplanar capability greatly enhances diagnostic accuracy, particularly in the evaluation of spinal pain. In the musculoskeletal system, clinical challenges such as tumor surveillance, symptomatic spondylolysis, (Fig. 6.217) apophyseal joint pain, and pseudoarthrosis following spi-

nal fusion are a few examples of conditions addressed by SPECT imaging. The technical advantages of SPECT, provided by its tomographic capability, significantly enhance the diagnostician's ability to accurately localize and identify a wide range of musculoskeletal lesions. (27–30)

NORMAL BONE SCAN

In the normal adult three-phase bone scan, activity is highest in the most metabolically active parts of the skeleton. During pediatric osseous development, all zones of epiphyseal and apophyseal activity avidly take up the tracer agent. Generally, the distal femur, proximal tibia, and proximal humerus are the most metabolically active bones and therefore exhibit the greatest amount of normal tracer uptake.

Regions of the skeleton subject to maximal mechanical stress contain a high ratio of trabecular to cortical bone. These areas

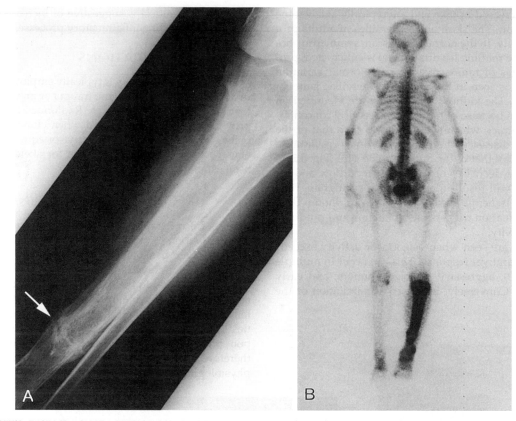

Figure 6.219. PAGET'S DISEASE: CHARACTERISTICALLY HOT BONE SCAN. A. AP Leg. Note the Pagetic involvement of the proximal tibia and the pseudofracture in the midshaft of the tibia (arrow). **B. ⁹⁹ᵐTc-MDP Bone Scan, Posterior Whole Body.** There is marked diffuse radionuclide uptake involving the entire right tibia. COMMENT: Paget's disease frequently extends to the subarticular margin of one end of a long or short tubular bone. (Courtesy of Dawn E. Bedrosian, MD, Denver, Colorado)

osteonecrosis, and tumors. (Fig. 6.222) Skeletal scintigraphic techniques may also be employed to evaluate prostheses, bone grafts, complications of trauma or surgery, and tumor recurrence and post-therapeutic response. (34,35) (Fig. 6.223) In addition, overuse or acute musculoskeletal injury may provoke an increase in the radiopharmaceutical uptake of muscles (rhabdomyolysis), tendons, bursae, and ligaments. Three-phase bone scanning techniques may also be used to assess vascular perfusion and the viability of soft tissues and to differentiate cellulitis from septic arthritis and osteomyelitis. (36) (Fig. 6.224)

The limited diagnostic specificity of radionuclide scintigraphy frequently requires a multimodality approach to imaging. In this regard scintigraphy parallels the application of the erythrocyte sedimentation rate (ESR). The elevated ESR, like an abnormal scintigram, is a sensitive indicator of disease, but requires correlative testing (additional lab work, radiographs, CT scan) to provide specificity. (Fig. 6.225) The accuracy of MR imaging is competitive with scintigraphy across a wide range of diagnoses. (37,38) Unlike MRI, nuclear scintigraphy provides a whole-body evaluation, whereas MRI is a regional modality. It is likely that complementary roles for MRI and scintigraphy will continue to exist for many diagnostic questions.

TRAUMA

Acute or chronic trauma may result in the complete or incomplete disruption of bone and cartilage. Plain film radiography remains the initial diagnostic imaging modality in the trauma workup. If clinical concerns remain after equivocal or negative findings on the initial radiographs, radionuclide scintigraphy should be considered to assess the musculoskeletal system and exclude radiographically occult osseous and/or soft tissue injury. The increased blood flow associated with bone repair results in marked radiopharmaceutical accumulation. Nuclear scintigraphy plays an important role in the child-abuse workup, in the follow-up of traumatic complications such as fracture nonunion, and in the assessment of tumor response to therapy. (39,40)

Occult fractures are not immediately apparent with plain film radiography, but demonstrate an increased perfusion on the angiogram phase of the scintigraphic examination. Additionally, there is increased radiotracer accumulation on the blood pool images and intense, poorly defined accumulation on the delayed images. (22) (Fig. 6.226)

Matin has outlined the scintigraphic presentation of fractures in their various phases following injury. (41) The acute phase, lasting 3 to 4 weeks, produces increased flow activity, blood pool accumulation, and on a bone scan a broad, intense zone of radiopharmaceutical uptake concentrating in the fracture line. Fractures, including those seen in the elderly, can be scintigraphically detected at initial presentation. Abnormal tracer uptake is observed within 24 hours of fracture in 95% of nonosteoporotic patients under the age of 65. In patients older than 65 the site of injury may initially be scintigraphically normal, but it will exhibit abnormal radiotracer uptake within 72 hours in 95% of patients. (41)

The subacute phase of fracture, lasting 8 to 12 weeks, reveals

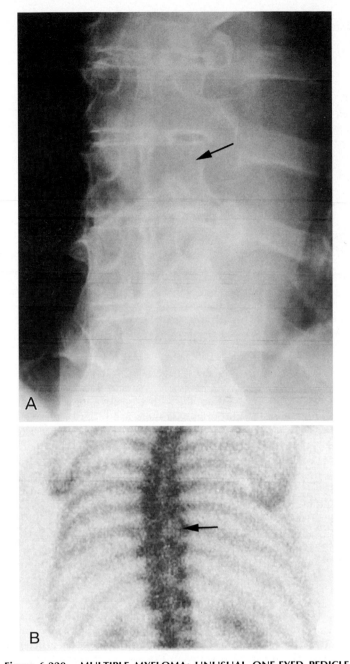

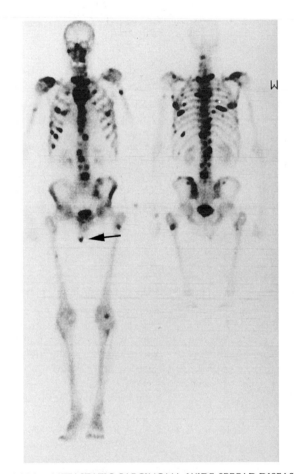

Figure 6.220.   MULTIPLE MYELOMA: UNUSUAL ONE-EYED PEDICLE SIGN. A. AP Thoracic. Observe the absence of the T7 pedicle (arrow). **B. ^{99m}Tc-MDP Bone Scan, Posterior Thoracic**. This scan demonstrates photopenia corresponding to the T7 segment (arrow). COMMENT: It is unusual for multiple myeloma to involve the pedicle. More commonly, osteolytic metastatic carcinoma will target the pedicle. (Courtesy of The Deaconess West Hospital, Department of Radiology, St. Louis, Missouri)

Figure 6.221.   METASTATIC CARCINOMA: WIDE-SPREAD DISEASE. This 72-year-old non-smoker presented with chest pain and a known diagnosis of bronchogenic carcinoma. **^{99m}Tc-MDP Bone Scan, Anterior Whole Body (Left) and Posterior Whole Body (Right).** Observe the numerous areas of markedly increased tracer activity in the spine, ribs, pelvis, and proximal long bones. Urine contamination in the patient's undergarments (arrow) is a frequent artifactual finding in elderly patients. (Courtesy of Timothy Schneider, DC, St. Louis, Missouri)

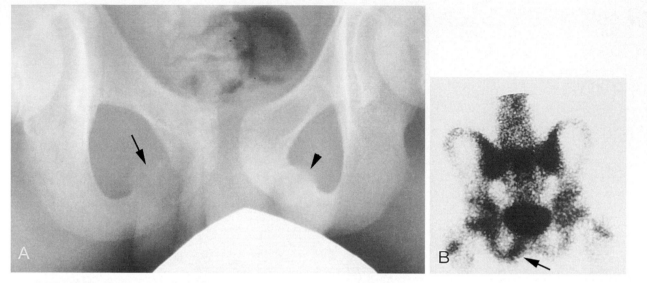

Figure 6.222.   OSTEOMYELITIS OF THE ISCHIOPUBIC SYNCHONDRO-SIS: DIFFERENTIATION FROM ITS NORMAL VARIANT. A. AP Pelvis. Note the focal lytic destruction involving the right ischiopubic synchondrosis (arrow). The contralateral side is normal (arrowhead). **B. ⁹⁹ᵐTc-MDP Bone Scan, Posterior Pelvis.** There is diffusely increased radiotracer activity in-volving the right ischium (arrow). COMMENT: The normal developing is-chiopubic synchondrosis was erroneously identified years ago by Van Neck as avascular necrosis. (Courtesy of The Children's Hospital, Department of Radiology , Denver, Colorado)

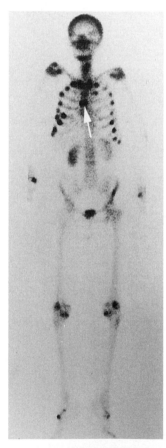

Figure 6.223.   ACUTE CHEST PAIN: IATROGENIC FRACTURES. ⁹⁹ᵐTc-**MDP Planar Bone Scan, Anterior Whole Body.** This elderly patient received an extended period of aggressive chest compression during CPR. Note the numerous areas of radiotracer uptake within the anterolateral portions of all of the ribs and the distal sternum (arrow). These findings are consistent with iatrogenically induced fractures. (Courtesy of Michael A. Fox, MD, Memphis, Tennessee)

a more diffuse persistent uptake with a focally intense area at the fracture line. In the chronic phase there is a progressive decline in the intensity of the abnormal radiotracer activity over 1 to 2 years, particularly in the weight-bearing bones (spine, femur, tibia). Following long-bone injury, scintigraphic activity returns to normal in 64% of patients at 1 year, 91% at 2 years, and 95% at 3 years. (42) Focal areas of abnormal radiopharmaceutical localization may persist as a result of chronic remodeling and degenerative repair.

Compression fractures of the spine reveal a horizontal band of increased tracer activity, typically affecting the superior endplate. (43) (Fig. 6.227) Scintigraphic activity in vertebral fractures normalized in 59% of patients within 1 year, 90% in 2 years, and 97% in 3 years. (44)

STRESS FRACTURE

Stress fractures are classified as either fatigue or insufficiency injuries. These fractures differ in their affected patient populations and presenting clinical histories. The basic pathophysiology involved in these chronic injuries is, however, very similar. Osteoclastic resorption, the initial event in the bone remodeling that occurs in response to repetitive loading, weakens the cortical bone. (45) Osteoblastic activity is subsequently initiated and bone remodeling follows. If the source of the stress is reduced, remodeling is successful and healing follows. If it is not, a complete fracture will evolve. Stimulation of the periosteum results in pain, but radiography in the early stages is frequently negative.

Stress remodeling or indeterminate stress lesions are indicated by abnormally increased activity on bone scans of patients who have been symptomatic between 4 and 8 weeks, but have negative radiographs. Stress fractures may be scintigraphically difficult to differentiate from occult fractures or bone bruises. A thorough history and careful physical examination must be correlated with the scintigraphic findings.

The bone scan, however, becomes positive at approximately

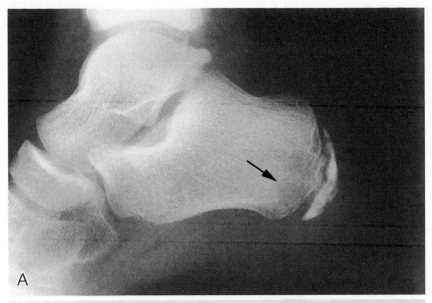

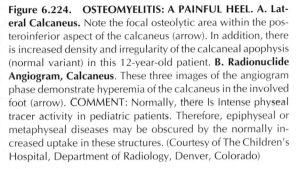

Figure 6.224. OSTEOMYELITIS: A PAINFUL HEEL. A. Lateral Calcaneus. Note the focal osteolytic area within the posteroinferior aspect of the calcaneus (arrow). In addition, there is increased density and irregularity of the calcaneal apophysis (normal variant) in this 12-year-old patient. **B. Radionuclide Angiogram, Calcaneus.** These three images of the angiogram phase demonstrate hyperemia of the calcaneus in the involved foot (arrow). COMMENT: Normally, there is intense physeal tracer activity in pediatric patients. Therefore, epiphyseal or metaphyseal diseases may be obscured by the normally increased uptake in these structures. (Courtesy of The Children's Hospital, Department of Radiology, Denver, Colorado)

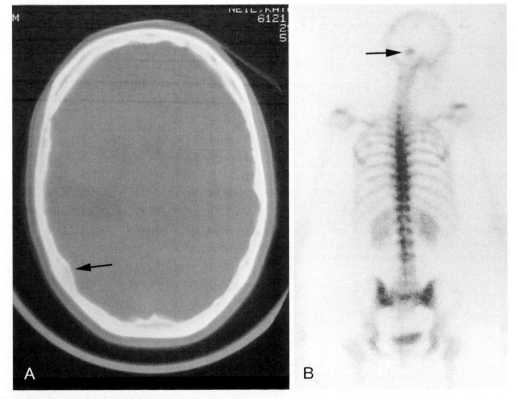

Figure 6.225. FIBROUS DYSPLASIA: A GREAT IMITATOR. This 37-year-old female complained of chronic headaches. **A. CT, Bone Window Axial Skull**. Observe the subtle expansion of the right diploic space (arrow). **B. 99mTc-MDP Bone Scan, Posterior Whole Body.** There is focal increased tracer activity on the calvarium (arrow) corresponding to the site of the lesion on the CT image. COMMENT: Fibrous dysplasia may show mild radiotracer uptake or no uptake or may be cold. This appearance, when correlated with the plain films and clinical findings, should exclude metastatic disease. (Courtesy of Kort W. Harshman, DC, Springfield, Missouri)

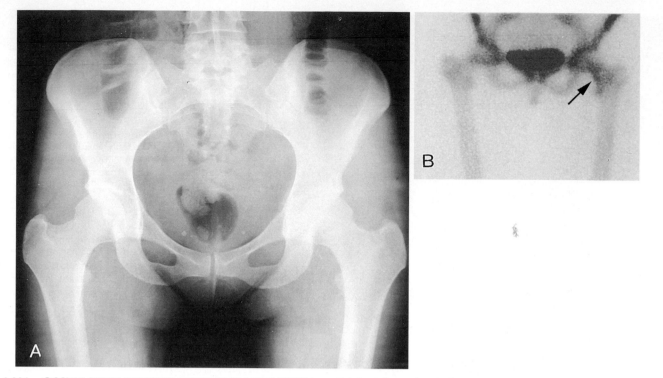

Figure 6.226. OCCULT STRESS FRACTURE: HIP PAIN IN A MARATHON RUNNER. This 31-year-old female runner presented with left hip pain. **A. AP Pelvis.** These radiographs are normal. **B. ⁹⁹ᵐTc-MDP Bone Scan, Anterior Pelvis**. A linear band of increased activity is noted involving the medial femoral neck, consistent with a stress fracture (arrow). (Courtesy of The Deaconess West Hospital, Department of Radiology, St. Louis, Missouri)

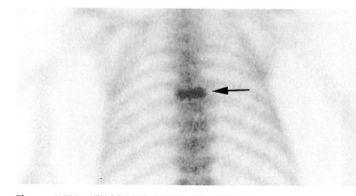

Figure 6.227. THORACIC SPINE COMPRESSION FRACTURE: HOT BONE SCAN. ⁹⁹ᵐTc-MDP Bone Scan, Posterior Thoracic. Increased radionuclide activity is seen at the T6 level (arrow) suggesting a recent injury. COMMENT: Compression fractures in the spine often result in increased tracer activity for as long as one year and occasionally up to 2 years. MRI, demonstrating bone marrow edema, is the most accurate and sensitive imaging modality in distinguishing the age of a compression fracture (old versus new). (Courtesy of The Deaconess West Hospital, Department of Radiology, St. Louis, Missouri)

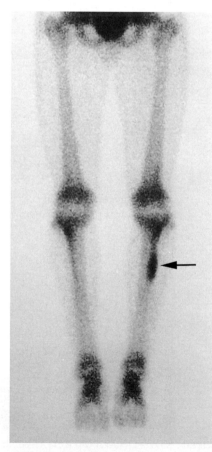

Figure 6.228. STRESS FRACTURE: LEG PAIN IN AN ADOLESCENT ATHLETE. ⁹⁹ᵐTc-MDP Bone Scan, Bilateral Lower Extremity. Note the increased fusiform tracer activity in the right lateral tibia (arrow), consistent with a stress fracture. (Courtesy of The Deaconess West Hospital, Department of Radiology, St. Louis, Missouri)

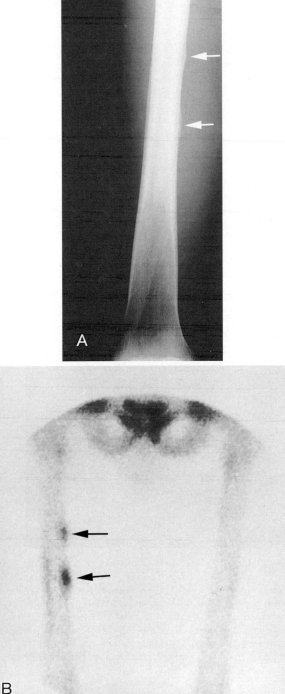

the same time symptoms of a stress fracture develop. Focal fusiform uptake within a long bone in the proper clinical setting is diagnostic of a stress fracture. (46) (Fig. 6.228) In addition, a diffuse increase in osseous activity is observed surrounding the stress fracture, which reflects the acceleration of osseous remodeling. Eventually, uptake becomes more focal and intense. Plain film radiographs usually reveal the stress fracture 2 to 12 weeks following its demonstration on the bone scan and 3 or 4 weeks after the onset of symptoms. (Fig. 6.229)

Insufficiency fractures have been described in the lower extremities, sacrum, ilium, and pubis. Insufficiency fracture of the osteoporotic sacrum reveals a butterfly appearance on bone scan (*Honda sign*) with the alae of the sacrum and the sacral body representing the wings and trunk of the butterfly, respectively. (22) (Fig. 6.230) When plain film radiographs are normal, unexplained, intractible pain in the lumbosacral or sacroiliac region should prompt the consideration of radionuclide scanning. Subtle areas of marrow abnormality, however, can be normal on planar bone scans and demonstrate abnormal hyperintense signal intensity on T2-weighted or STIR MR images. (Fig. 6.231)

Radionuclide scintigraphy permits differentiation between stress fractures and shin splints or tibial stress syndrome (soleus syndrome). Shin splints produce pain and tenderness along the medial border of the tibia as a result of disruption of Sharpey's fibers from the soleus muscle–tendon complex. (47) This periostitis produces an elongated linear pattern of activity in the posteromedial tibial cortex, in contrast to the more focal accumulation seen with stress fractures. (48) Scintigraphy is also of assistance in the diagnosis and management of active versus quiescent spondylolysis in athletes. (Fig. 6.232) MRI of the pars may show bone marrow edema in active lesions in the radiographic or preradiographic phase of spondylolysis. (See Chapter 5) (Fig. 6.233) Healing of this lesion is reflected by reduced tracer activity. (49) This information is beneficial for patient management and can guide the return to athletic training.

Figure 6.229. MULTIPLE STRESS FRACTURES: SYNCHRONOUS PRESENTATION. This athlete was evaluated for thigh pain. **A. AP Femur.** Observe the focal periostitis involving the medial diaphysis of the femur (arrows). **B. ^{99m}Tc-MDP Bone Scan, Anterior Femur.** Note two focal zones of increased activity, consistent with synchronous stress fractures of the femur (arrows). COMMENT: Stress fractures in the femoral diaphysis are rare. (Courtesy of Thomas E. Hyde, DC, DACBSP, North Miami, Florida)

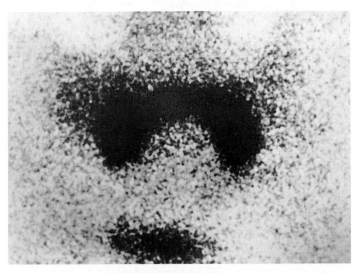

Figure 6.230. SACRAL INSUFFICIENCY FRACTURES: HONDA SIGN. This elderly patient had severe pain in the region of the sacral base with a normal radiographic examination. **^{99m}Tc-MDP Bone Scan, Posterior Pelvis.** Observe the "H"-like pattern of tracer uptake in the sacrum. COMMENT: Persistent lumbosacral pain in geriatric patients with osteoporosis and negative radiographs warrants consideration of radionuclide scintigraphy to exclude insufficiency fractures from a more sinister disease process such as neoplasm.

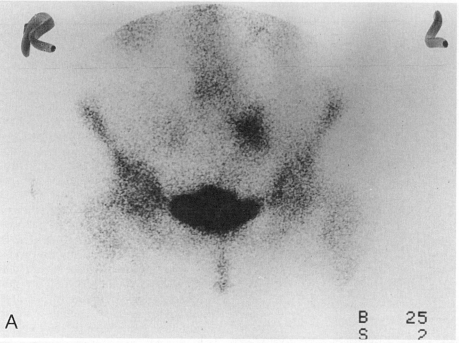

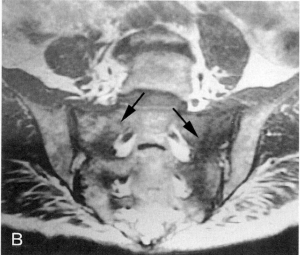

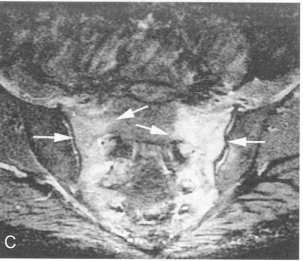

Figure 6.231.   HIDDEN TUMOR OR INSUFFICIENCY FRACTURE OF THE SACRUM? This 77-year-old female presented with a history of mastectomy and long-standing lumbosacral pain that was treated conservatively with continued progression of symptoms. Plain films (not shown) were normal. **A. ⁹⁹ᵐTc-MDP Planar Bone Scan, AP Pelvis.** Note the localized radiopharmaceutical uptake in the region of the left sacroiliac joint. **B. MRI, T1-Weighted Coronal Sacrum. C. MRI, Gradient-Echo Coronal Sacrum**. Note the diffuse low signal intensity within both the right and left portions of the sacrum. These areas become very hyperintense on the gradient-echo images and are consistent with marrow edema adjacent to insufficiency fractures

(arrows). COMMENT: The bilateral nature of this case on MRI shows the sensitivity of magnetic resonance versus bone scan, which only demonstrated unilateral abnormality. Elderly patients with chronic lumbosacral pain that is unresponsive to conservative management should be further evaluated to exclude insufficiency fractures of the sacrum. This patient was initially thought to have metastatic disease and biopsy of the sacrum proved to be representative of an insufficiency fracture. (Courtesy of Ian F. Murray, MD and Dan K. Westmoreland, MD, Park Avenue Diagnostic Center, Memphis, Tennessee)

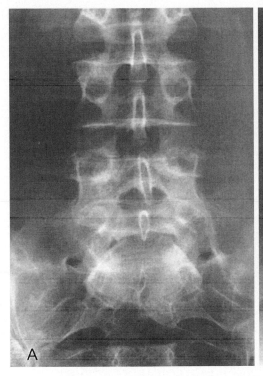

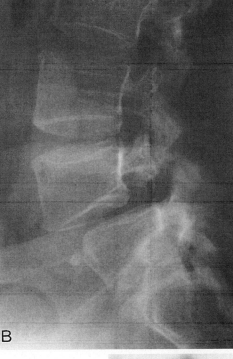

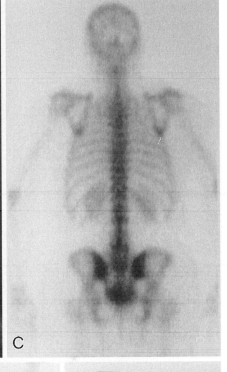

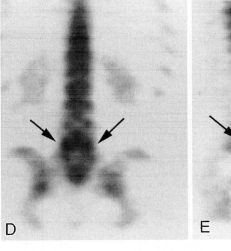

Figure 6.232.   SPONDYLOLYTIC SPONDYLOLISTHESIS: NEGATIVE PLANAR BONE SCAN WITH POSITIVE SPECT. This 37-year-old female dancer presented with localized persistent low back pain. **A. AP Lumbar. B. Lateral Lumbar.** Plain films reveal a 30% anterolisthesis of L4 on a transitional L5 segment. **C. ^{99m}Tc-MDP Planar Bone Scan, Posterior Whole Body. Normal. D. SPECT, Coronal Lumbar. E. SPECT, Sagittal Lumbar.** Note the bilaterally increased tracer activity involving the L4 pars (arrows). This radiopharmaceutical uptake demands a reduction in physical activity, especially in extension, to reduce or eliminate the patient's pain. (Courtesy of Vastoni Deuksar, MD and Alan M. Lesselroth, MD, Mountain Diagnostics, Las Vegas, Nevada)

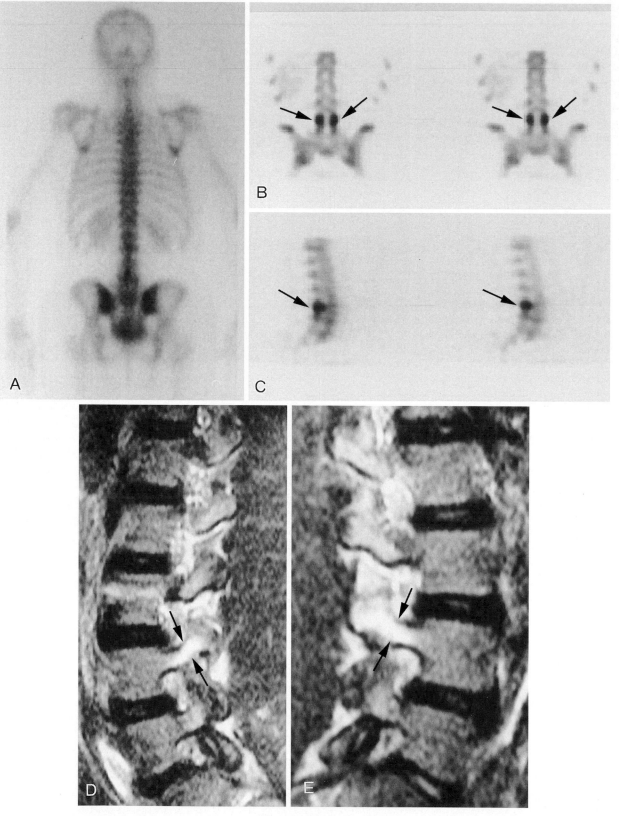

Figure 6.233A–E.

BONE BRUISE

The presence of localized extremity pain following trauma, normal radiographs, and a small area of increased tracer accumulation on bone scans is consistent with a bone bruise. The bone bruise does not display the fusiform appearance of stress fracture or linear pattern of shin splints, but rather a focal area of ill-defined radiotracer uptake. (22) This injury is felt to comprise minimal intraosseous bleeding with periosteal elevation and repair. Additional etiologies have been suggested, including transient osteoporosis, focal reflex sympathetic dystrophy, and trabecular microfractures. (50) The abnormal radiopharmaceutical accumulation may represent evidence of increased bone turnover or remodeling. The pathophysiology and clinical significance of bone bruises remains to be established. (51) MRI is the *most* sensitive imaging modality in the detection of bone bruises.

OSTEONECROSIS

Osteonecrosis is the result of skeletal ischemia. The ischemic event can be related to trauma such as fracture or dislocation, or to a wide range of pathologic states that disrupt the vascular supply of bone. These include collagen vascular diseases, corticosteroid use, radiation injury, alcoholism, diabetes, hyperlipidemia, hemoglobinopathies, Gaucher's disease, and Caisson disease. The hip is the most common site of involvement. (Fig. 6.234) Other common sites include the knee, (Fig. 6.235) shoulder, and carpal navicular bone. Osteonecrosis may be asymptomatic, but is typically associated with acute aching pain that is often worse at night. (36)

In early osteonecrosis the radiographic examination is often normal. Nuclear scintigraphy may show decreased or absent up-take. Later, after the bone has become revascularized and begins to remodel, bony demineralization and spotty sclerosis are demonstrated radiographically and increased radiotracer uptake is identified on the bone scan. If the necrotic process progresses, collapse, deformity, and flattening of the joint surface may become evident radiographically. This stage is characterized on the scintigram by a *rim* of increased radiopharmaceutical uptake surrounding a photopenic zone. This finding parallels the double line sign of osteonecrosis, a sign often observed with MRI. Finally, the typical plain film features of degenerative arthrosis become apparent. Bone scanning at this point reveals intense uptake on both sides of the articulation. The use of SPECT in the evaluation of osteonecrosis has greater sensitivity than conventional or planar imaging. (44)

CT may be helpful in evaluating the stages of osteonecrotic destruction. Magnetic resonance imaging, however, is the *most sensitive* means of early detection of osteonecrosis. (52)

REFLEX SYMPATHETIC DYSTROPHY SYNDROME (SUDECK'S ATROPHY)

This syndrome represents an exaggerated neurovascular response to traumatic or surgical injury and leads to severe pain, vasomotor instability, and trophic disturbances. The term *sympathetically maintained pain syndrome* has been recently used to describe these patients. (22,53,54) Reflex sympathetic dystrophy syndrome (RSDS) produces a characteristic scintigraphic pattern consisting of diffuse increased uptake that is usually most pronounced in a periarticular location. (Fig. 6.236) The sensitivity and specificity for RSDS using radionuclide imaging varies by location. The sensitivity of the delayed image pattern in the hand is

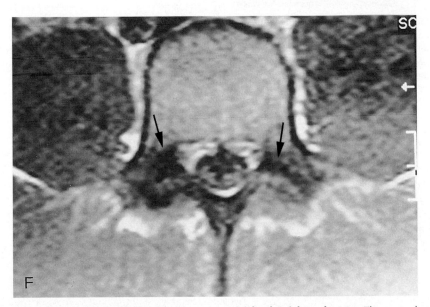

Figure 6.233. PRERADIOGRAPHIC PHASE OF SPONDYLOLYSIS: A CHALLENGING CASE STUDY. This 16-year-old football player had back pain for 3 months with no radiographic evidence of spondylolysis in the lumbar spine on plain films (not shown). **A. 99mTc-MDP Planar Bone Scan, Posterior Spine.** This examination was normal. **B. SPECT Scan, Coronal Lumbar. C. SPECT Scan, Sagittal Lumbar.** There is markedly increased activity in the L4 pars/pedicle junction bilaterally (arrows). **D. MRI, T2-Weighted Far Lateral Sagittal Lumbar (Right). E. MRI, T2-Weighted Far Lateral Sagittal Lumbar (Left).** A hyperintense signal in the pars/pedicle area is revealed and is consistent with bone marrow edema (arrows). **F. MRI, T1-Weighted Axial Lumbar, L4.** There are decreased signal intensity areas in the posterior elements of the L4 vertebrae (arrows) consistent with bone marrow edema. COMMENT: This patient is in the preradiographic phase of spondylolysis. His planar bone scan was normal, but SPECT was positive in the area of the L4 pars. The MRI reveals bone marrow edema indicating the active nature of the pars lesion. The patient was placed in a custom-made Boston overlap brace in near zero lordosis. His deep-seated low back pain resolved after being braced for only 2 weeks. The reader is referred to Chapter 5 for a more detailed discussion of this topic. (Courtesy of Richard L. Green, DC, Winthrop, Massachusetts)

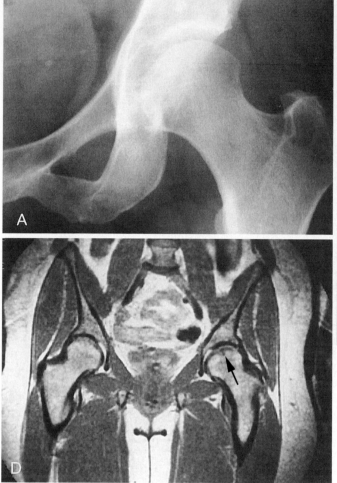

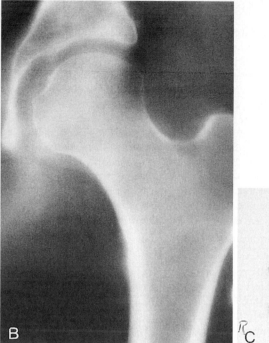

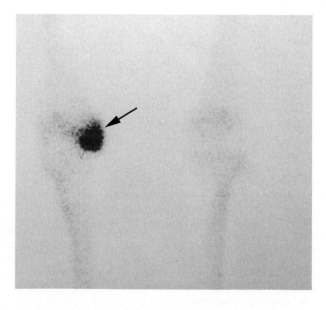

Figure 6.234.   OSTEONECROSIS: A HIDDEN CAUSE OF HIP PAIN. This 50-year-old female had a motor vehicle accident 2 years prior in which she sustained hip trauma. **A. AP Spot Hip. B. AP Tomogram Hip.** These examinations were normal. **C. ^{99m}Tc-MDP Bone Scan, Anterior Pelvis**. Note the mildly increased radiotracer uptake within the left femoral head. This exam was erroneously read as normal. **D. MRI, T1-Weighted Coronal Pelvis**. There is a well-circumscribed zone of low signal intensity in the left femoral head (arrow) confirming the diagnosis of osteonecrosis. COMMENT: The most sensitive imaging modality in the assessment of osteonecrosis is MRI, which is the *gold standard* for detection of osteonecrosis. (Courtesy of Donald E. Freuden, DC, FACO, Denver, Colorado)

Figure 6.235.   OSTEONECROSIS: SONK LESION. A. ^{99m}Tc-MDP Bone Scan, Bilateral AP Knee. Note the focal area of increased radiotracer uptake in the medial aspect of the right distal femur (arrow). COMMENT: SONK (**S**pontaneous **O**steo**N**ecrosis of the **K**nee) refers to idiopathic osteonecrosis which affects the medial femoral condyle in the adult. (Courtesy of The Deaconess West Hospital, Department of Radiology, St. Louis, Missouri)

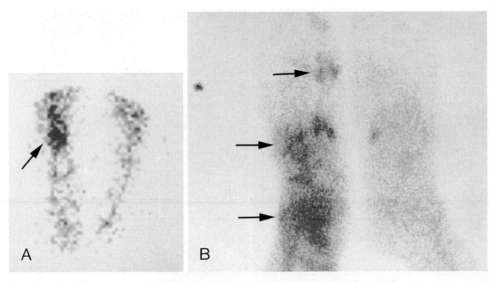

Figure 6.236.   REFLEX SYMPATHETIC DYSTROPHY SYNDROME (RSDS): SEVERE POSTTRAUMATIC FOOT PAIN. This patient sustained an ankle fracture and presented months later with residual progressive right foot pain. **A. ^{99m}Tc-MDP Bone Scan (Angiogram Phase), Bilateral Dorsal Foot.** Note the areas of increased radiotracer activity in the right foot (arrow). **B. ^{99m}Tc-** **MDP Bone Scan, Bilateral Plantar Foot.** Tracer activity is increased in the right hindfoot, midfoot, and proximal interphalangeal joint (arrows). These findings are consistent with the vasomotor instability seen with RSDS. (Courtesy of The Deaconess West Hospital, Department of Radiology, St. Louis, Missouri)

96% and in the foot is 100%. Specificity in the foot has been reported at 80% and in the hand at 97%. (53)

OSTEOMYELITIS

Although plain film radiography may be diagnostic for the evaluation of a suspected musculoskeletal infection, its sensitivity for early disease is low. (55) The characteristic radiographic findings of early osteomyelitis require 1 to 3 weeks to develop. This radiographic latent (occult) period is dependent on location and is approximately 10 days in the extremities and 21 days in the spine. (Fig. 6.237) Frequently, coexisting disorders may mimic or duplicate both the clinical and radiographic features of osteomyelitis. Such disorders are particularly frequent in diabetic patients, and consist of peripheral vascular disease, cellulitis, and neurotrophic arthropathy. (56) The failure to provide a prompt and accurate diagnosis of osteomyelitis will likely result in significant morbidity.

Three-phase radionuclide scintigraphy allows evaluation of the vascular flow and uptake in soft tissues and is a sensitive means of identifying skeletal infections. (57) Accordingly, its sensitivity in the evaluation of osteomyelitis has been reported between 90 and 100%, with a specificity of 73 to 79%. (19) The addition of a fourth phase, provided by a static 24-hour image obtained with identical counts and settings, significantly increases the specificity. (11)

The positive scintigraphic findings in soft tissue infection consist of increased uptake on the radionuclide angiogram and blood pool phases and diffuse uptake on delayed images. Septic arthritis also produces findings of increased activity on the radionuclide angiogram and blood pool images, but with marked periarticular uptake on the delayed images. (Fig. 6.238) If radionuclide scintigraphy is performed within 24 to 48 hours of the onset of symptoms, a *cold spot* or *photopenic zone* may result. This finding is seen only in the course of hematogenous osteomyelitis, particularly in children. It is caused by the localized occlusion of the capillary vasculature, which causes impedance of

radiopharmaceutical access. Osteomyelitis in children may be multifocal and may mimic neoplasm, thus requiring a biopsy. (58) The differential diagnosis of osteomyelitis and septic arthritis may require additional radionuclide imaging with *Ga-67-citrate* or *In-111–labeled white blood cells.* (Fig. 6.239) Diabetic patients, complex trauma victims, and postsurgical patients pose the greatest difficulty in the differentiation between osteomyelitis and septic arthritis. (57,59–61) Needle aspiration of the joint or open surgical biopsy may be the most expedient means of confirming the diagnosis.

The presence of increased activity on bone or joint images may also result from traumatic or inflammatory joint disorders such as seropositive arthritis (e.g., rheumatoid) and seronegative spondyloarthropathies (e.g., Reiter's syndrome, psoriatic arthritis, and ankylosing spondylitis). (See Chapter 10) (36,62–64) (Fig. 6.240) The presence of these conditions is generally suspected on clinical grounds and confirmed by laboratory testing and radiographs. Radionuclide scintigraphy is employed only in special clinical circumstances.

Gallium-67-citrate has been employed in the localization of both infectious and inflammatory (aseptic) lesions. (Fig. 6.241) Like ^{99m}Tc-MDP, it is taken up by bone, but it also localizes in regions of infection. Ga-67 displays high specificity for *acute* osteomyelitis because of its affinity for bacterial and cellular debris in addition to leukocytes. (13,65)

Gallium-67 has proven valuable in the evaluation of young children with suspected osteomyelitis because of the high incidence of false ^{99m}Tc-MDP negative bone scans. (19) It may be employed when the bone scan is inconclusive or demonstrates a photopenic area. The accuracy of combined bone-gallium imaging in evaluating osteomyelitis is not likely to be compromised by prior skeletal injury or other skeletal lesions. (66)

Chronic osteomyelitis may occasionally be exacerbated by a superimposed acute infection. When this occurs, it is necessary to distinguish the chronic process from the acute exacerbation. Plain film radiography lacks the necessary sensitivity required to accurately evaluate this complication. (57) Since bone turnover is

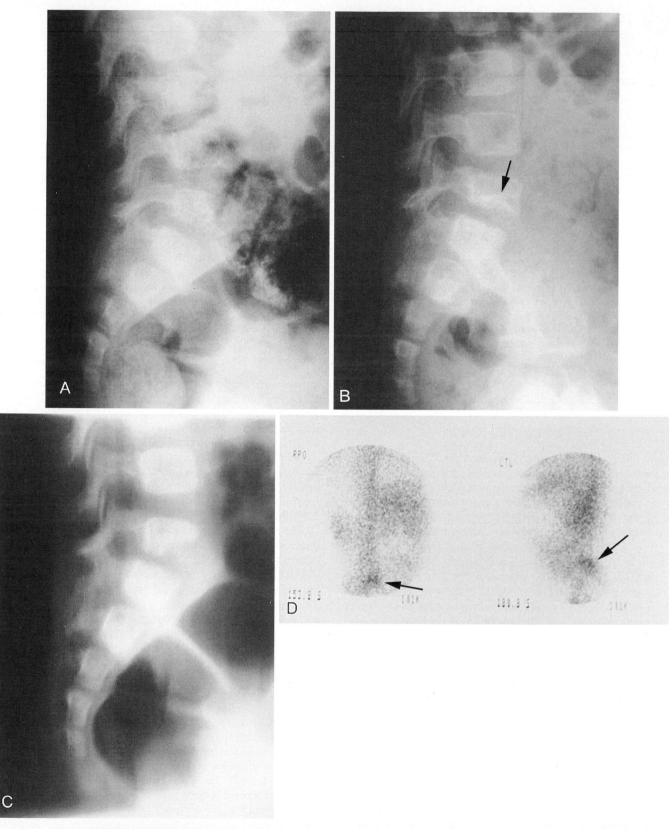

Figure 6.237. SEPTIC DISCITIS: LUMBAR SPINE. This pediatric patient had a 3-week history of fever and refused to bear weight. **A. Lateral Lumbar.** This exam was normal. **B. Lateral Lumbar.** A 2-week follow-up radiograph revealed destructive changes involving the inferior endplate of L5. **C. Tomography, Lateral Lumbar.** Note the enhanced visualization of the destructive changes and the narrowed disc space. **D. ⁹⁹ᵐTc-MDP Bone Scan, AP (Left) and Lateral (Right) Lumbar.** Diffusely increased tracer activity is noted corresponding to the lumbosacral junction (arrows). (Courtesy of The Children's Hospital, Department of Radiology, Denver, Colorado)

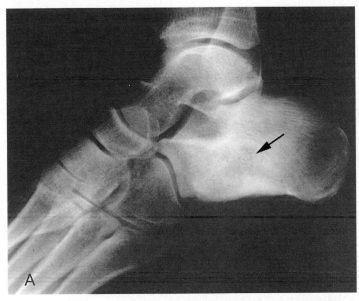

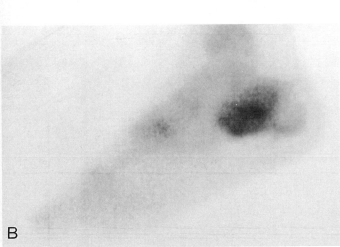

Figure 6.238.   OSTEOMYELITIS: CHRONIC HEEL PAIN. A. Lateral Calcaneus. Observe the ill-defined osteolysis in the calcaneus, surrounded by reactive sclerosis (arrow). These findings suggest chronic osteomyelitis.

B. ^{99m}Tc-MDP Bone Scan, Medial Right Foot. There is marked tracer uptake involving the calcaneus. (Courtesy of The Deaconess West Hospital, Department of Radiology, St. Louis, Missouri)

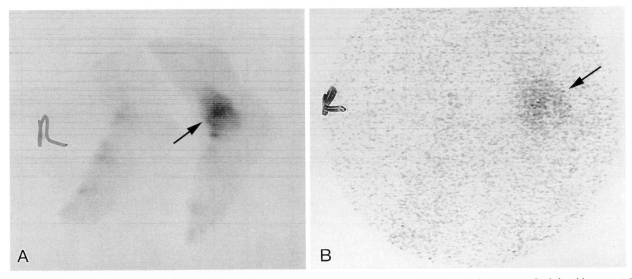

Figure 6.239.   ACUTE OSTEOMYELITIS: PERSISTENT ANKLE PAIN. A. ^{99m}Tc-MDP Bone Scan, Bilateral Ankle. There is focal increased tracer activity in the left ankle (arrow). **B. In-111 WBC Scan, Bilateral Ankle.** There is increased radiopharmaceutical activity in the left ankle (arrow). The combined findings of these exams are consistent with osteomyelitis. (Courtesy of Timothy Schneider, DC, St. Louis, Missouri)

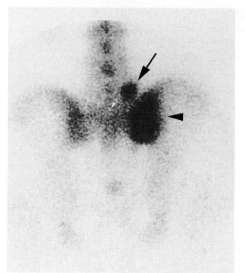

Figure 6.240.   INFECTIOUS SACROILITIS: IV DRUG USER. Bone Scan, Posterior Pelvis. Note the focal area of increased uptake at the L5-S1 apophyseal joint (arrow). There is also markedly increased radiopharmaceutical activity involving the right sacroiliac joint (arrowhead). COMMENT: IV drug use predisposes these individuals to infections in the "S" joints. These are the **S**acroiliac, **S**ymphysis pubis, **S**ternoclavicular, and **S**pinal articulations. (Courtesy of Dawn E. Bedrosian, MD, Denver, Colorado)

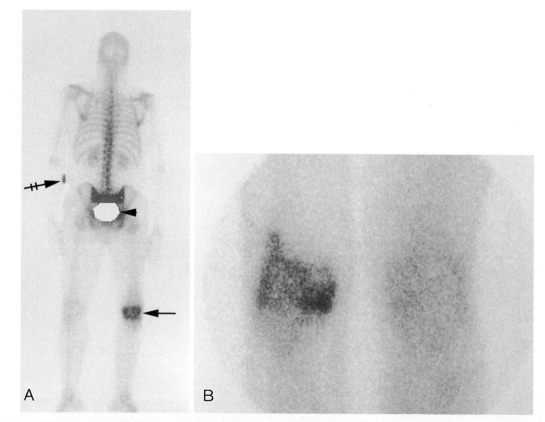

Figure 6.241.   OSTEOMYELITIS: MONOARTHRITIS. A. ^{99m}Tc-MDP Bone Scan, Posterior Whole Body. Marked radiopharmaceutical uptake is present at the right knee (arrow). The photopenic zone over the pelvis is due to shielding (arrowhead) used to improve skeletal resolution by eliminating bladder counts. Note the increased activity in the left forearm, consistent with the injection site (crossed arrow). **B. Ga-67 Scan, Bilateral Anterior Knee.** The 72-hour scan yields diffusely increased tracer activity involving the right knee, indicating an infectious disease process. (Courtesy of The Deaconess West Hospital, Department of Radiology, St. Louis, Missouri)

present in both *acute* and *chronic* osteomyelitis, bone scintigraphy by itself is also ineffective in assessing chronic osteomyelitis. The resolution of this diagnostic dilemma rests in the combined use of ^{99m}Tc-MDP and Ga-67-citrate. (57) The acute infectious process reveals avid gallium uptake, exceeding the usual technetium uptake seen with chronic osteomyelitis. Therefore a Ga-67 pattern of skeletal distribution that does not coincide with the pattern of ^{99m}Tc-MDP is suggestive of recurrent osteomyelitis. (67)

The In-111 leukocyte scan circumvents the osteogenic mechanism and traces the migration of white blood cells into an inflammatory process. (Fig. 6.242) Epstein recommended In-111 leukocyte imaging as the initial nuclear scan in the workup of active head and neck infections. (68) Indium-111 leukocyte imaging has a reported sensitivity of 90 to 95% in acute osteomyelitis, but this varies by location. In central skeletal locations such as the spine 53% sensitivity was reported. Chronic osteomyelitis results in a lower concentration of the labeled leukocytes in active bone marrow. This factor reduces the sensitivity for detection of chronic osteomyelitis in the axial skeleton. (69) The high radiation dose associated with In-111 leukocyte imaging precludes its widespread use in pediatric evaluation for osteomyelitis.

Photopenia occurs in over half of the patients undergoing In-111–labeled leukocyte scans performed to rule out osteomyelitis in the spine. (70) This decreased uptake must be differentiated from other causes such as metastasis, Paget's disease, surgical defects, radiation, fractures, and antibiotic therapy. The role of MR imaging in the evaluation of osteomyelitis is increasing be-cause of its superb contrast resolution and sensitivity to bone marrow and soft tissue changes. (37)

PROSTHESIS EVALUATION

A differential diagnosis that includes septic loosening, aseptic loosening, heterotopic ossification, trochanteric bursitis, or fracture should be considered in patients with prior total hip arthroplasty and hip pain. (Fig. 6.243) Aseptic prosthetic loosening is the most frequent diagnosis in this clinical setting. Plain film radiographs are helpful in excluding fracture, heterotopic bone formation, and loosening of the bone-cement interface (71); however, plain films are unable to distinguish between aseptic and septic loosening. Distinction between these two causes of loosening is imperative because surgical intervention is necessary when infection is present, but is not usually required with aseptic loosening. Radionuclide imaging techniques are widely used and have played an important role in the investigation of septic loosening (71), but needle aspiration of the joint or open surgical biopsy may be required.

SKELETAL NEOPLASMS

Plain film radiography is the initial modality employed for the imaging of suspected skeletal neoplasms. Early detection of lytic skeletal tumors, however, is difficult because 30 to 50% demineralization must occur before the lesion is radiographically demonstrable. (72) Radionuclide scintigraphy is considerably more

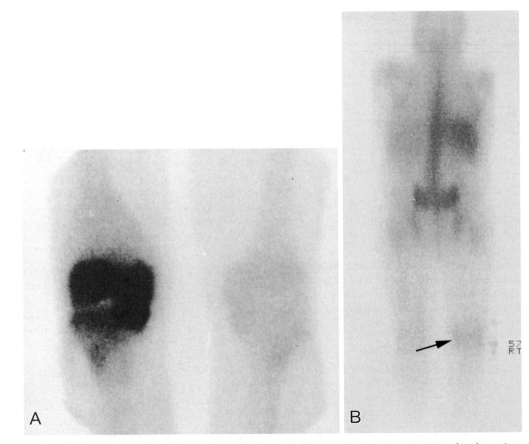

Figure 6.242.   SEPTIC ARTHRITIS: KNEE. A. Bone Scan, Bilateral Anterior Knee. There is a marked increase of tracer uptake on both sides of the knee joint, highly suggestive of septic arthritis. **B. In-111 WBC, Posterior Whole Body.** Radiotracer activity is increased in the region of the right knee (arrow) supporting the diagnosis of infection. (Courtesy of The Deaconess West Hospital, Department of Radiology, St. Louis, Missouri)

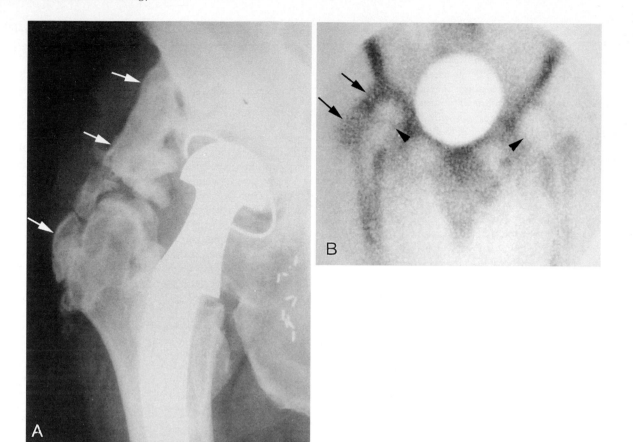

Figure 6.243.   HETEROTOPIC BONE: POSTOPERATIVE HIP PAIN. A. AP Right Hip. A total hip prosthesis is implanted with prominent heterotopic ossification bridging the ilium and femur (arrows). **B. ⁹⁹ᵐTc-MDP Bone Scan, Anterior Pelvis**. Increased activity associated with the heterotopic bone is demonstrated (arrows). Also, note the bilateral photopenia of the femoral prostheses (arrowheads). (Courtesy of The Deaconess West Hospital, Department of Radiology, St. Louis, Missouri)

sensitive than plain film radiography in the detection and determination of the extent of a skeletal lesion. (59) Bone-seeking radiopharmaceuticals localize in skeletal lesions very early in the pathologic process. Scintigraphic techniques are helpful for early benign and malignant tumor detection, and they have played a major role in the differential diagnosis, posttreatment assessment, and surveillance for tumor recurrence, but many of these applications have more recently been eclipsed by MRI.

Radionuclide skeletal scintigraphy is the most commonly performed nuclear imaging procedure in the United States for the diagnosis and follow-up of patients with malignant disease. Although imaging modalities such as CT and MRI are also used to assess soft tissue and bone tumors, the total-body survey capacity of radionuclide scintigraphy remains a significant advantage and is important in clinical staging.

Benign Skeletal Neoplasms

Benign skeletal neoplasms are often incidentally detected on plain film radiographs or are noted with whole-body scintigraphy. No definitive scintigraphic criteria exist to distinguish benign from malignant neoplasms. Matin has suggested three parameters to help distinguish benign lesions of bone from those that are malignant. (40) These nonspecific parameters include lesion uptake, location, and the multiplicity of lesions. Many benign neoplasms may reveal mild to moderate radiotracer uptake. (44)

These include nonossifying fibromas, fibrous cortical defects, bone cysts, enchondromas, and stable osteochondromas. Benign lesions displaying marked uptake include osteoid osteoma, giant cell tumor, growing osteochondroma, bone cysts with pathologic fracture (e.g., simple bone cyst, aneurysmal bone cyst), fibrous dysplasia, Paget's disease (Fig. 6.244), and bone infarction. (73) Osteoid osteomas usually display a characteristic round focus of intense uptake. (74)

Primary Malignant Neoplasms

Radionuclide scintigraphy has played a significant role in the diagnosis, staging, and follow-up of osseous and soft tissue neoplasms. Despite its limited specificity, a bone scan is a standard diagnostic test for the early diagnosis of malignant osseous involvement. Soft tissue sarcomas may involve the skeleton secondarily, resulting in abnormal scintigraphic activity locally or at distant osseous sites. (75,76)

Radionuclide scintigraphy may reveal evidence of soft tissue extension, paraneoplastic syndrome, or pulmonary or distant osseous metastases. (77,78) Primary malignant tumors of bone reveal their presence by the intense radiotracer uptake and increased activity on blood pool images. This is related to the neovascularity and hyperemia associated with the tumor. Radionuclide scintigraphy does not, however, sufficiently define the extent of the primary tumor for surgical planning. The neovas-

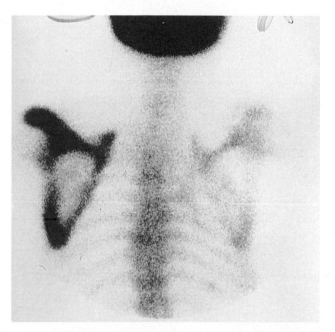

Figure 6.244. PAGET'S DISEASE: SCAPULA AND OCCIPUT. ^{99m}Tc-MDP **Bone Scan, Posterior Cervicothoracic Spot.** The entire left scapula is outlined by increased tracer activity. Incidentally, diffuse uptake is noted in the posterior occiput. COMMENT: Paget's is one cause of generalized increased calvarial thickness. (Courtesy of The Deaconess West Hospital, Department of Radiology, St. Louis, Missouri)

cularity and reactive bone changes typically obscure and overstate the lesion's borders. MRI and CT play significant roles in further characterizing the extent of the lesion within bone and adjacent soft tissues. (13) Scintigraphy is helpful when metastasis from a primary osseous neoplasm is suspected in a distal skeletal location.

Multiple Myeloma

Nuclear scintigraphy should not be performed in an attempt to initially diagnose or to determine the extent to which a patient is affected by multiple myeloma. A radiographic skeletal survey is more useful and accurate. Scintigraphy is recommended only as a baseline examination in the assessment of fracture activity (age of lesion). Multiple myeloma stimulates the production of an osteoclast activating factor (OAF). This enhances osteoclastic activity, causing bone destruction to occur at a much greater rate than the reactive osteoblastic activity. This results in a normal scintigram until the lesion is large enough to be identified as an area of photon deficiency. (Fig. 6.245) Photopenic areas (cold spots) may also be seen in aggressively lytic neoplasms such as the bubbly metastases of renal cell and thyroid carcinoma, as well as neuroblastoma. (72) These highly aggressive lesions lack significant reparative osteoblastic response to counteract the lysis, resulting in a reduced radiopharmaceutical concentration.

Skeletal Metastasis

The extremely high sensitivity (95 to 97%) of skeletal scintigraphy and the ability to image the entire skeleton in a single examination have made it the imaging procedure of choice for the detection of osseous metastatic carcinoma. (13) It often provides the initial evidence of bone metastasis from a carcinoma, since lesions may otherwise remain undetected radiographically for

months or years. Bone scans are also frequently utilized for baseline evaluation in initial staging, for monitoring the response to treatment for both chemotherapy and radiotherapy, and in the detection of complications such as pathologic fracture and osteonecrosis. (38) However, MRI is equally as sensitive and more specific than bone scan in detecting metastases. Unfortunately, whole-body MRI as a staging survey is not practical.

The typical scintigraphic pattern of metastatic carcinoma displays *diffuse multifocal lesions* randomly scattered throughout the axial skeleton. (Fig. 6.246) The differential diagnosis includes fracture, Paget's disease, osteomyelitis, metabolic bone disease, and occasionally osteoarthritis. (73) Osteoarthritis is a frequent cause of multiple focal lesions on a radionuclide scintigram. These lesions usually demonstrate a less-intense area of tracer uptake than metastasis, but occasionally they may be large enough to obscure an adjacent area of malignancy. This is particularly problematic in the vertebral column where apophyseal arthrosis and spondylosis provoke significant tracer uptake. This circumstance warrants the use of tomographic scintigraphy (SPECT) for more accurate localization of the abnormal uptake. (28) The presence of acute or even antecedent trauma involving the ribs is also a clinical challenge. Rib fractures arising from a traumatic event typically demonstrate a linear scintigraphic pattern. This nonrandom or linear pattern virtually excludes metastatic disease, which displays a random distribution of tracer activity. (79) (Fig. 6.247)

Paget's disease is often an incidental finding and can usually be differentiated from metastasis by correlation with plain film radiographs and/or the distribution of the involved bones. (See Chapter 11) (Fig. 6.248, 6.249) When there is a solitary site of tracer uptake on a radionuclide scintigram in a patient with a known primary malignancy, it is generally considered to be metastatic disease until proven otherwise. In a patient with a known primary neoplasm, the probability of a focal hot spot in the axial skeleton or proximal extremities being indicative of metastatic disease is quite high. When the identical circumstance arises in the skull or distal extremities (elbow to hand, knee to foot), this percentage is reduced to below 50%. (73) Solitary rib lesions are far less likely to be metastatic disease than multiple lesions. Tumeh found only 10% of solitary rib lesions to be metastatic, myeloma was more common. (80) Plain film radiographic correlation is mandatory when scintigraphy reveals a solitary lesion in a patient with a known malignancy. Negative or equivocal plain film radiography, in this circumstance, requires confirmation by CT, MRI, or biopsy.

Diffuse, widespread metastatic disease may present with an intense scintigraphic pattern known as the *super scan*. (44) This diffuse and relatively uniform activity throughout the axial skeleton may simulate a normal bone scan; however, because of the increased skeletal accumulation of tracer, there is minimal or absent *renal* activity. In addition, there is an unusually high bone to soft tissue background ratio with an increased ratio of uptake in the axial versus appendicular skeleton. Radiographic correlation is another means of avoiding this catastrophic pitfall. Diffuse osseous metastases producing the *super scan* most often arise from malignant primary neoplasms in the breast and prostate.

Healing metastatic lesions in bone increase the radiotracer accumulation in response to reactive new bone formation. This is known as the *flare phenomenon*. (81) With the administration of chemotherapy, the bone scan may appear to worsen or flare, suggesting increased metabolic activity. The flare phenomenon occurs in patients undergoing cyclic chemotherapy and actually

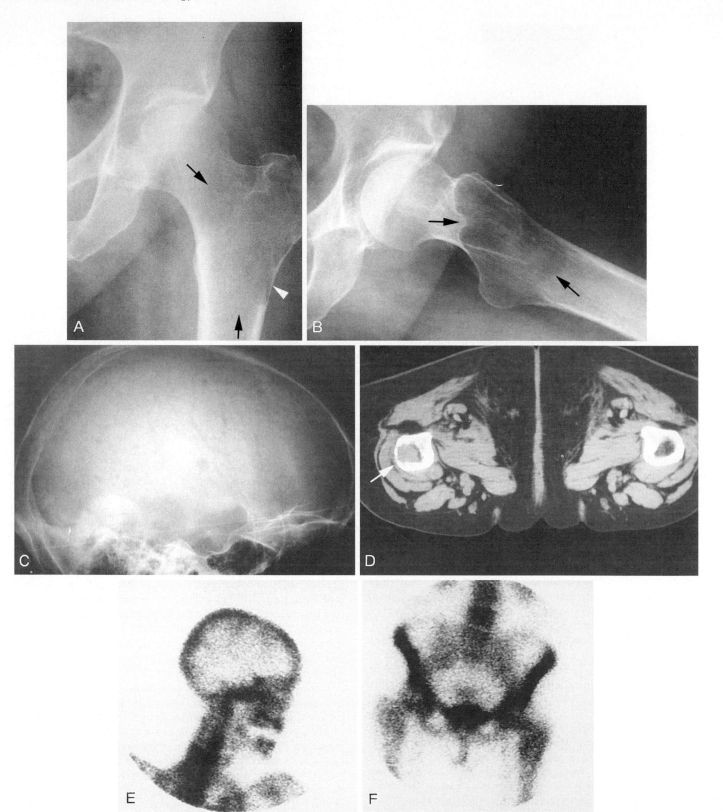

Figure 6.245.   MULTIPLE MYELOMA: NEGATIVE BONE SCAN. This 76-year-old female complained of left hip pain. **A. AP Hip. B. Lateral Frogleg Hip.** Observe the radiolucent appearance (arrows) and subtle endosteal scalloping (arrowhead) of the proximal femoral metaphysis. **C. Lateral Skull**. The skull demonstrates multiple punched-out lesions. **D. CT, Soft Tissue Window Axial Hip.** Note the thinning of the femoral cortex (arrow) and the tumor-filled marrow. **E. ⁹⁹ᵐTc-MDP Bone Scan, Skull. F. ⁹⁹ᵐTc-MDP Bone Scan, Anterior Pelvis**. Both the skull and pelvis are unremarkable. COMMENT: Bone scans are classically false-negative in multiple myeloma since lesions do not typically provoke an osteoblastic reparative response. (Courtesy of William E. Litterer, DC, DACBR, Fellow, ACCR, Elizabeth, New Jersey)

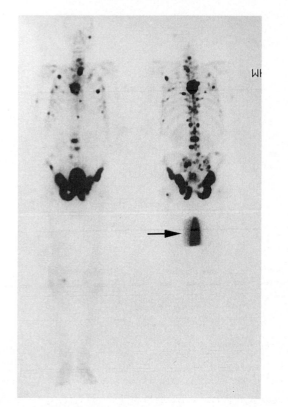

Figure 6.246. METASTATIC CARCINOMA: HISTORY OF BREAST CANCER. This 34-year-old female presented with severe back pain. She underwent a previous mastectomy for breast carcinoma, but denied radiation and chemotherapy. Two serial 6-month bone scans were negative. **^{99m}Tc-MDP Bone Scan, Anterior Whole Body (Left) and Posterior Whole Body (Right).** Observe the numerous foci of increased tracer activity in the axial skeleton, which are the result of metastatic malignancy. The patient was catheterized and the bladder was emptied to increase image quality. Note the urine-filled bag (arrow) and empty bladder on the posterior scan. (Courtesy of Timothy Schneider, DC, St. Louis, Missouri)

represents a favorable response to treatment. Radiographic correlation with evidence of increased sclerosis may be present within 2 to 6 months. With progressive healing, the flare phenomenon will decrease over time. Serial examinations may be necessary to confirm the flare phenomenon and differentiate this appearance from progressive disease, which demonstrates increased, rather than decreased, tracer activity with time.

Metastatic deposits may be so aggressive that they completely replace areas of the skeleton, producing photon-deficient lesions or cold spots similar to those seen with myeloma. An area with little or no tracer uptake, often surrounded by a rim of increased uptake, may indicate a *cold* metastatic lesion. In addition, early metastatic invasion may not stimulate reactive bone formation, resulting in a false-negative radionuclide scan. (59)

Osseous metastasis from breast carcinoma often presents as a solitary lesion. When such a scintigraphic lesion is observed in the sternum, there is a very high probability that metastatic disease exists. (82) The recurrence of breast cancer is usually first identified in the skeleton, frequently in the thoracic spine.

Prostatic carcinoma is the most common malignancy among men in the United States. The advent of prostate-specific antigen (PSA) testing has provided a sensitive means of detection in pa-

tients who are at high risk for prostate cancer. Radionuclide scintigraphy should be employed in patients in whom the PSA is elevated, those who display the appropriate symptomatology, and in patients who have been hormonally treated. In patients with proven prostate carcinoma, bone scanning also plays a role in prognosis. It determines whether bone metastasis has occurred and to what extent the skeleton is involved. (73)

In bronchogenic carcinoma, osseous metastases may develop from direct extension or via hematogenous routes. A positive radionuclide bone scan is a poor prognostic sign in patients with bronchogenic carcinoma. (72) Metastatic carcinoma beyond the elbow or knee (acral metastasis) is unusual, with the exception of aggressive bronchogenic carcinoma. On occasion, it may be isolated to the hands or feet, presenting radiographically as a *blowout* lesion. (83)

POSITRON EMISSION TOMOGRAPHY (PET)

Positron emission tomography (PET) is an emerging technique in nuclear medicine that also provides a tomographic format for biochemical and physiologic imaging. PET has been utilized in the assessment of brain neurophysiology and cardiac perfusion and has also shown promise in oncologic applications. (84,85) PET has also been shown to be superior to some standard imaging techniques in nuclear medicine. Its major disadvantages include its higher cost (two or three times the cost of a planar bone scan) and significant technical challenges. Advances in these areas could lead to the development of less expensive systems and expand the role of PET imaging in nuclear medicine.

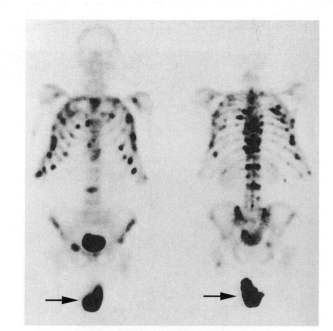

Figure 6.247. METASTATIC CARCINOMA: PROGRESSIVE LOW BACK PAIN. This elderly male had a history of treated small cell carcinoma of the lung and presented with low back pain. **^{99m}Tc-MDP Bone Scan, Anterior Whole Body (Left) and Posterior Whole Body (Right).** There are widespread sites of markedly increased tracer activity, consistent with skeletal metastasis. A urine filled bag from a draining catheter is noted inferior to the pelvis (arrows). (Courtesy of Timothy Schneider, DC, St. Louis, Missouri)

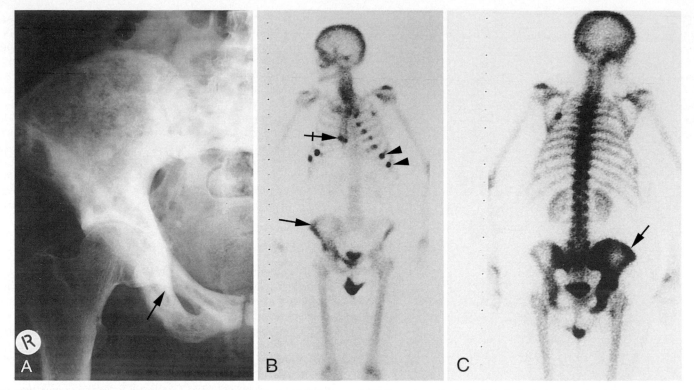

Figure 6.248.   PAGET'S DISEASE: THE GREAT IMITATOR. A. AP Pelvis. Notice the characteristic *cotton wool* appearance of pagetic bone and obliteration of Kohler's teardrop (arrow), one of the first signs of Paget's disease affecting the pelvic brim. **B. ⁹⁹ᵐTc-MDP Bone Scan, Anterior Whole Body.** There is increased activity in the right ilium (arrow). The linear pattern of increased activity on the anterior ribs (arrowheads) and at the tip of the sternum (crossed arrow) is consistent with recent fracture repair. **C. ⁹⁹ᵐTc-**

MDP Bone Scan, Posterior Whole Body. Increased activity occupying nearly the entire right hemipelvis represents Paget's disease (arrow). Abnormal increased activity over the calvarium is also noted. COMMENT: The linear pattern of rib fractures present in this case helps differentiate it from metastatic disease which usually displays a nonlinear (random) pattern of increased radiotracer activity. (Courtesy of Dawn E. Bedrosian, MD, Denver, Colorado)

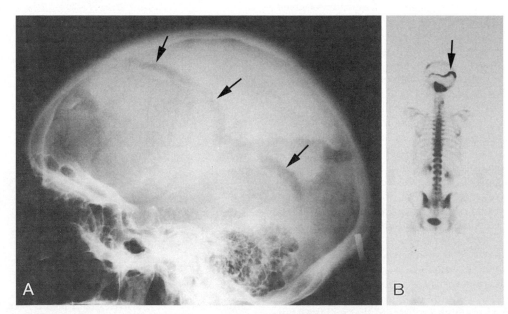

Figure 6.249.   PAGET'S DISEASE: UNUSUAL BONE SCAN. A. Lateral Skull. These plain films demonstrate a linear zone of radiolucency traversing the calvarium (osteoporosis circumscripta) (arrows). **B. ⁹⁹ᵐTc-MDP Bone Scan, Posterior Whole Body.** A band of increased tracer activity is noted

traversing the calvarium, consistent with the advancing edge of the lytic phase of Paget's disease (arrow). An additional area of abnormal uptake is seen at the skull base (arrowhead). (Courtesy of The University Hospital, Department of Radiology, Denver, Colorado)

PET scanners require radiopharmaceuticals that emit positrons. A positron is a positively charged electron (antimatter) that instantly collides with an electron, annihilating both particles. This high-energy collision emits two oppositely directed gamma rays. The radiation is measured by rings of detectors encircling the patient. The geometrically placed detectors record coincident radiation counts and, like SPECT, display them in a tomographic plane. (Fig. 6.250) The resolution of modern PET scanners is about 3 mm, which is superior to both planar and SPECT imaging. (13) PET imaging involves technical issues of immense complexity. The half-life of these agents (seconds to minutes) is so short that a cyclotron must be maintained on site for their production. This is one factor that accounts for the high cost of PET imaging. A significant barrier is also imposed by the limited reimbursement of PET examinations, since the majority are classified as investigational.

The clinical applications of PET imaging in the musculoskeletal system have focused on the evaluation of bone and soft tissue tumors and are currently investigational. (84) The most common radiopharmaceutical in this application is fluorine-18 (^{18}F) fluorodeoxyglucose (FDG). Imaging with FDG provides information concerning the distribution and magnitude of glucose metabolism. It is this metabolic basis of PET imaging that distinguishes it from other imaging techniques. In preliminary trials signifi-

cantly increased tracer uptake was seen in high-grade malignant soft tissue lesions, thus allowing differentiation from low-grade and benign neoplasms. It is likely that PET imaging will increase its impact on nuclear imaging in spite of its cost and technical challenges. (85)

MEDICOLEGAL IMPLICATIONS
Nuclear Medicine

- Caution should be exercised when using this modality, as with any modality that uses ionizing radiation.
- Overuse and inappropriate use should be avoided.
- Use in children, during pregnancy, and during breast-feeding should only occur when absolutely necessary.
- Dehydration is a direct contraindication.
- Radiopharmaceutical injection should be performed prior to dialysis.

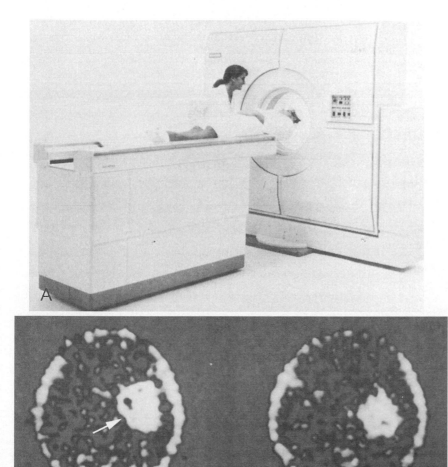

Figure 6.250. PET SCANNER. A. Typical PET Scanner. The patient couch and gantry are shown. Superficially, this appears much like the typical hardware of a CT scanner. **B. PET Brain Scan.** This PET image shows abnormal uptake within the brain resulting from a high-grade brain neoplasm (arrow). This examination was performed using F-18 fluorodeoxyuridine. (Courtesy of Siemens Medical Systems, Inc. and Eisenberg RL: Radiology: An Illustrated History. St. Louis, Mosby-Year Book, 1992.)

REFERENCES

MAGNETIC RESONANCE IMAGING

Introduction

1. **Bloch F, Hansen WW, Packard ME:** *Nuclear induction.* Phys Rev 69:127, 1946.
2. **Purcell EM, Torrey HC, Pound RV:** *Resonance absorption by nuclear magnetic moments in a solid.* Phys Rev 69:37, 1946.
3. **Eisenberg RL:** *Radiology. An Illustrated History.* St. Louis, Mosby-Year Book, 1992.
4. **Damadian RV:** *Tumor detection by nuclear magnetic resonance.* Science 117:1151, 1971.
5. **Moon RB, Richards JH:** *Determination of intracellular pH by ^{31}P magnetic resonance.* J Biol Chem 48:7276, 1973.
6. **Lauterbur PC:** *Image formation by induced local interactions: Examples employing nuclear magnetic resonance.* Nature 242:190, 1973.
7. **Damadian R, Minkhoff L, Goldsmith M, et al:** *Field focusing nuclear magnetic resonance (FONAR): Visualization of a tumor in a live animal.* Science 194:1430, 1976.
8. **Damadian R, Goldsmith M, Minkhoff L:** *NMR in cancer. XVI. FONAR image of the live human body.* Physiol Chem Phys 9:97, 1977.
9. **Rinck PA:** *Magnetic Resonance in Medicine: The Basic Textbook of the European Magnetic Resonance Forum.* Oxford, Blackwell Scientific Publications, 1993.
10. **Norfray JF, Rosen B, Taveras JM:** *Newer Pulse Sequences in Magnetic Resonance Imaging: Their Uses and Acronyms.* In: Taveras JM, Ferrucci JT, eds.: *Radiology: Diagnosis, Imaging, Intervention.* Vol. 3, Ch. 26A, Philadelphia, JB Lippincott, 1994.
11. **Lufkin RB:** *The MRI Manual.* Chicago, Year Book Medical Publishers, 1990.
12. **Partain CL, Patton JA:** *Magnetic Resonance Imaging Systems.* In: Taveras JM, Ferrucci JT, eds.: *Radiology: Diagnosis, Imaging, Intervention.* Vol. 1, Ch. 33, Philadelphia, JB Lippincott, 1988.
13. **Guebert GM, Pirtle OL, Yochum TR:** *Essentials of Diagnostic Imaging.* St. Louis, Mosby-Year Book, 1995.
14. **Stoller DW:** *Magnetic Resonance Imaging in Orthopaedics and Sports Medicine.* Philadelphia, JB Lippincott, 1993.

The Spine

1. **Roemer PB, Edelstein WA, Hayes CE, et al:** *The NMR phased array.* Magn Reson Med 16:192, 1990.
2. **Yousem DM, Schnall MD:** *MR examination for spinal cord compression: Impact of a multicoil system on length of study.* J Comput Tomgr 15:598, 1991.
3. **VanderMeulen P, Groen JP, Tinus AM, et al:** *Fast field echo imaging: An overview and contrast calculations.* Magn Reson Imaging 6:355, 1988.
4. **Gomori JM, Holland GA, Grossman RI, et al:** *Fat suppression by section-select gradient reversal on spin echo MR imaging.* Work in progress. Radiology 168:493, 1988.
5. **Felmlee JP, Ehman RL:** *Spatial presaturation: A method for suppressing flow artifacts and improving depiction of vascular anatomy in MR imaging.* Radiology 164:559, 1987.
6. **Haacke EM, Lenz GW:** *Improving MR image quality in the presence of motion by using rephasing gradients.* AJR 148:1251, 1987.
7. **Fitz CR, Harwood-Nash PC:** *The tethered conus.* Am J Roentgenol Radium Ther Nucl Med 125:515, 1975.
8. **Nakamura T:** *Diagnosis and treatment of tethered spinal cord syndrome based on experience of 77 cases.* Nippon Seikeigek Gakkai Zasshi 58:1237, 1984.
9. **Maehara T, Tanohata K, Noda M, et al:** *Medically treated steroid-induced epidural lipomatosis.* Neuroradiology 30:281, 1988.
10. **Yamada S, Zinke DE, Sanders D:** *Pathophysiology of "tethered cord syndrome."* J Neurosurg 54:494, 1981.
11. **Kaplan JO, Quencer RM:** *The occult tethered conus syndrome in the adult.* Radiology 137:387, 1980.
12. **DeLaPaz RL, Floris R, Norman D, et al:** *MRI of tethered spinal cord and caudal lipoma.* AJNR 7:550, 1986.
13. **Kuharik MA, Edwards MK, Grossman CB:** *Magnetic resonance evaluation of pediatric spinal dysraphism.* Pediatr Neurosci 12:213, 1986.
14. **Gillespie R, Faithfull DK, Roth A, et al:** *Intraspinal anomalies in congenital scoliosis.* Clin Orthop 93:103, 1973.
15. **McMaster ML:** *Occult intraspinal anomalies and congenital scoliosis.* J Bone Joint Surg (Am) 66:588, 1984.
16. **Nokes SR, Murtheh FR, Jones JD, et al:** *Childhood scoliosis.* MR Imaging Radiol 164:791, 1987.
17. **Coonrad RW, Richardson WJ, Oakes WJ:** *Left thoracic curves can be different.* Orthop Trans 9:126, 1985.
18. **Barnes PD, Brody JD, Jaramillo D, et al:** *Atypical idiopathic scoliosis: MR imaging evaluation.* Radiology 186:247, 1993.
19. **Yochum TR, Barry MS, Gould SJ, et al:** *Wrong sided scoliosis: When left isn't right.* JNMS 2:195, 1994.
20. **Pomeranz SJ:** *Craniospinal Magnetic Resonance Imaging.* Philadelphia, WB Saunders, 1989.
21. **Pillay PK, Awad IA, Little JR, et al:** *Surgical management of syringomyelia: A five-year experience in the area of magnetic resonance imaging.* Neurol Res 13:3, 1991.
22. **Elster AD, Chen MY:** *Chiari I malformations: Clinical and radiological reappraisal.* Radiology 183:347, 1992.
23. **Charry O, Koop S, Winter R, et al:** *Syringomyelia and scoliosis: A review of 25 pediatric patients.* J Pediatr Orthop 14:309, 1994.
24. **Nabors MW, Pait TG, Byrd EB, et al:** *Updated assessment and current classification of spinal meningeal cysts.* J Neurosurg 68:366, 1988.
25. **McArdle CB, Crofford MJ, Mirfakhraee M, et al:** *Surface coil MR of spinal trauma: Preliminary experience.* AJNR 7:885, 1986.
26. **Tarr RW, Drolshagen LF, Kerner TC, et al:** *MR imaging of recent spinal trauma.* JCAT 11:412, 1987.
27. **Stoller DW:** *Magnetic Resonance Imaging in Orthopaedics and Sports Medicine.* Philadelphia, JB Lippincott, 1993.
28. **Yuh WTC, Zachar CK, Barloon TJ, et al:** *Vertebral compression fractures: Distinction between benign and malignant causes with MR imaging.* Radiology 172:215, 1989.
29. **Melville GE, Taveras JM:** *Traumatic injuries of the spinal cord and nerve roots.* In: Taveras JM, Ferrucci JT, eds.: *Radiology: Diagnosis, Imaging, Intervention.* Vol. 3, Ch. 104, Philadelphia, JB Lippincott, 1993.
30. **Shoukimas GM:** *Magnetic resonance imaging of the spine and spinal cord.* In: Taveras JM, Ferrucci JT, eds.: *Radiology: Diagnosis, Imaging, Intervention.* Vol. 3, Ch. 112, Philadelphia, JB Lippincott, 1993.
31. **Gundry CR, Heithoff KB:** *Epidural hematoma of the lumbar spine: 18 surgically confirmed cases.* Radiology 187:427, 1993.
32. **Enzmann DR, DeLaPaz RL, Rubin JB:** *Magnetic Resonance Imaging of the Spine.* St. Louis, CV Mosby, 1990.
33. **Kulkarni MV, McArdle CB, Kopanicky D, et al:** *Acute spinal cord injury: MR imaging at 1.5 T.* Radiology 164:837, 1987.
34. **Fletcher BD, Scoles PV, Nelson AD:** *Osteomyelitis in children: Detection by magnetic resonance.* Work in progress. Radiology 150:57, 1984.
35. **Kahn DS, Pritzker KPH:** *The pathophysiology of bone infection.* Clin Orthop 96:12, 1973.
36. **deRoos A, vanMeerten EL, Bloem JL, et al:** *MRI of tuberculous spondylitis.* AJR 147:79, 1986.
37. **Kricun R, Shoemaker EI, Chovanes GI, et al:** *Epidural abscess of the cervical spine. MR findings in five cases.* AJR 158:1145, 1992.
38. **Danner RL, Hartman BJ:** *Update of spinal epidural abscess: 35 cases and review of the literature.* Rev Infect Dis 9:265, 1987.
39. **Algra PR, Heimans JJ, Valk J, et al:** *Do metastases in vertebrae begin in the body or the pedicles? Imaging study in 45 patients.* AJR 158:1275, 1992.
40. **Parizel PM, Baleriaux D, Rodesch G, et al:** *Gd-DTPA-enhanced MR imaging of spinal tumors.* AJR 152:1087, 1989.
41. **Laredo JD, Reizine D, Bard M, et al:** *Vertebral hemangiomas: Radiological evaluation.* Radiology 161:183, 1986.
42. **Shapiro R:** *Myelography,* ed 4. Chicago, Year Book Medical Publisher, 1984.
43. **Rasmussen TB, Kernohan JW, Adson AW:** *Pathological classification, with surgical considerations of intraspinal tumors.* Ann Surg 111:513, 1940.
44. **Ruben JM, Aisen AM, DiPietro MA:** *Ambiguities in MR imaging of tumoral cysts in the spinal cord.* JCAT 10:395, 1986.
45. **Dillon WP, Norman D, Newton TH, et al:** *Intradural spinal cord lesions: GD-DTPA-enhanced MR imaging.* Radiology 170:229, 1989.
46. **Valk J:** *Gadolinium-DTPA in MR of spinal lesions.* AJNR 9:345, 1988.
47. **Sze G, Krol G, Zimmerman RD, et al:** *Intramedullary disease of the spine: Diagnosis using gadolinium-DTPA enhanced MR imaging.* AJNR 9:847, 1988.
48. **Sloof JL, Kernohan JW, MacCarty CS:** *Primary Intramedullary Tumors of the Spinal Cord and Filum Terminale.* Philadelphia, WB Saunders, 1964.
49. **Rubinstein LJ:** *Tumors of the central nervous system. Atlas of Tumor Pathology,* Series 2, Fascicle 6, Washington D.C.: Armed Forces Institute of Pathology, 1972.
50. **Stechison MT, Tasker RR, Wortzman G:** *Spinal meningioma en plaque: Report of two cases.* J Neurosurg 67:452, 1987.
51. **Bull JWD:** *Spinal meningiomas and neurofibromas.* Acta Radiol 40:283, 1953.
52. **Vesalius A:** *De humani corporis fabrica libri septem.* Basileae: Ex officina J Oporini, 1543.
53. **Virchow RL:** *Untersuchungen uber die entwickelung des schadelgrundes im gesunden und krankhaften zustande, und den einfluss derselben auf schadelform, gesichtsbildung und gehirnbau.* Berlin, G. Reimer, 1857.
54. **vonLuschka H:** *Die halbgelenke des menschlichen korpers.* Berlin, G. Reimer, 1858.
55. **Kocher T:** *Die verletzungen der wirbelsaule zugleich als beitrag zur physiologie des menschlichen ruckenmarks.* Mitt Grenzgeb Med Chir 1:420, 1896.
56. **Middleton GS, Teacher JH:** *Injury of the spinal cord due to rupture of an intervertebral disc during muscular effort.* Glasgow Med J 76:1, 1911.
57. **Goldthwait JE:** *The lumbosacral articulation. An explanation of many causes of "lumbago," "sciatica" and "paraplegia."* Boston Med and Surg J 164:365, 1911.
58. **Elsberg CA:** *Experiences in spinal surgery, observations upon sixty laminectomies for spinal disease.* Surg Gynecol Obstet 16:117, 1913.
59. **Sicard JA:** *Les sciatiques; sciatiques par blesures de guerre; sciatiques medicale.* Marseille-Med 53:2, 1918.
60. **Cotunio D:** *De ischiade nervosa connentorius, 1764.* In: Armstrong JR, ed.: *Lumbar Disc Lesions: Pathogenesis and Treatment of Low Back Pain and Sciatica.* Baltimore, Williams & Wilkins, 1958.
61. **Schmorl G:** *Uber knorpelknoten an der hinterflache der wirbelbandscheiben.* Fortschr Geb Rontgenstrahlen 40:629, 1929.
62. **Dandy WE:** *Loose cartilage from intervertebral disc simulating tumor of the spinal cord.* Arch Surg 19:660, 1929.
63. **Mixter WJ, Barr JS:** *Rupture of the intervertebral disc with involvement of the spinal cord.* N Engl J Med 211:210, 1934.
64. **Franson RC, Saal JS, Saal JA, et al:** *Human disc phospholipase A_2 is inflammatory.* Spine 17S:129, 1992.
65. **Bobest M, Furo I, Tompa K, et al:** *Nuclear magnetic resonance study of intervertebral discs. A preliminary report.* Spine 11:709, 1986.
66. **Aguet J, Lane B:** *Imaging of degenerative disk disease of the lumbar spine.* Postgrad Radiol 7:241, 1987.

67. **Giles LGF:** *Anatomical Basis of Low Back Pain.* Baltimore, Williams & Wilkins, 1989.
68. **Post MJD:** *Computed Tomography of the Spine.* Baltimore, Williams & Wilkins, 1984.
69. **Jensen MC, Brant-Zawadski MN, Obuchowski N, et al:** *Magnetic resonance imaging of the lumbar spine in people without back pain.* N Engl J Med 331:69, 1994.
70. **Czervionke LF:** *Lumbar intervertebral disc disease.* Neuroimaging Clin North Am 3:465, 1993.
71. **Cacayorin ED, Kieffer SA:** *The Herniated Intervertebral Disc.* In: Taveras JM, Ferrucci JT, eds.: *Radiology: Diagnosis, Imaging, Intervention.* Vol. 3, Ch. 105, Philadelphia, JB Lippincott, 1991.
72. **Modic MT, Masaryk T, Boumphrey F, et al:** *Lumbar herniated disc and canal stenosis: Prospective evaluation by surface coil MR, CT and myelography.* AJNR 7:709, 1986.
73. **Ross JS, Modic MT, Masaryk JT:** *Tears of the annulus fibrosus: Assessment with Gd-DTPA-enhanced MR imaging.* AJNR 10:1251, 1989.
74. **Beltran J, Chandnani V, McGhee RA Jr:** *Gadopentetate dimeglumine—enhanced MR imaging of the musculoskeletal system.* AJR 156:457, 1991.
75. **Schelinger D, Manz HJ, Vidica B, et al:** *Disc fragment migration.* Radiology 175:831, 1990.
76. **Williams AL, Haughton VM, Daniels DL, et al:** *Differential diagnosis of extruded nucleus pulposus.* Radiology 148:141, 1983.
77. **Wiesel SW, Tsourmas N, Feff HL, et al:** *A study of computer assisted tomography: The incidence of positive CAT scans in an asymptomatic group of patients.* Spine 9:549, 1984.
78. **Holt EP Jr:** *The question of lumbar discography.* J Bone Joint Surg (Am) 50:720, 1968.
79. **Aprill C, Bodguk N:** *High-intensity zone: A diagnostic sign of painful lumbar disc on magnetic resonance imaging.* Br J Radiol 65:361, 1992.
80. **Macnab I:** *The Mechanism of Spondylogenic Pain.* In: Hirsch C, Zotterman Y, eds.: *Cervical Pain; Proceedings of the International Symposium Held Wenner-Gren Center, Stockholm, January 25–27, 1971.* New York, Pergamon Press, 1972.
81. **Smyth MJ, Wright V:** *Sciatica and the intervertebral disc: An experimental study.* J Bone Joint Surg (Am) 40:1401, 1958.
82. **Hasue M:** *Pain and the nerve root: An interdisciplinary approach.* Spine 18:2053, 1993.
83. **Raff J:** *Some observations regarding 905 patients operated upon for protruded lumbar intervertebral discs.* Am J Surg 97:388, 1959.
84. **Haldeman S, Rubinstein SM:** *Cauda equina syndrome in patients undergoing manipulation of the lumbar spine.* Spine 17:1469, 1992.
85. **Modic MT, Masaryk TJ, Ross JS:** *Imaging of degenerative disc disease.* Radiology 168:177, 1988.
86. **Kirkaldy-Willis WH, Burton CV, Heithoff KB, et al:** *Lateral spinal nerve entrapment.* Pain Management, 3:93, 1990.
87. **Kjerulf TD, Terry DW, Boubelik RJ:** *Lumbar synovial or ganglion cysts.* Neurosurg 19:415, 1986.
88. **Mercader J, Munoz Gomez J, Cardenal C:** *Intraspinal synovial cysts: Diagnosis by CT. Follow-up and spontaneous remission.* Neuroradiol 27:346, 1985.
89. **Harsch GR, Sypert GW, Weinsten PR, et al:** *Cervical spine stenosis secondary to ossification of the posterior longitudinal ligament.* J Neurosurg 67:349, 1987.
90. **Murakami N, Murgora T, Sobue I:** *Cervical myelopathy due to ossification of the posterior longitudinal ligament.* Arch Neurol 35:33, 1978.
91. **Gado MB:** *The Spine.* In: Lee JK, et al, eds.: *Computed Body Tomography with MRI Correlation,* ed 2. New York, Raven Press, 1989.
92. **Quencer RM, Tenner M, Rothman L:** *The postoperative myelogram: Radiographic evaluation of arachnoiditis and dural/arachnoidal tears.* Radiology 123:667, 1977.
93. **Ross JS, Modic MT, Masaryk TJ, et al:** *Postoperative lumbar spine.* Semin Roentgenol 23:125, 1988.
94. **Ross JS, Masaryk TJ, Modic MT:** *Gadolinium-DTPA-enhanced MR imaging of the postoperative lumbar spine: Time, course and mechanism of enhancement.* AJNR 10:37, 1989.
95. **Hueftle MG, Modic MT, Ross JS, et al:** *Lumbar spine: Postoperative MR imaging with GD-DTPA.* Radiology, 167:817, 1988.
96. **Ross JS, Masaryk TJ, Modic MT, et al:** *MR imaging of lumbar arachnoiditis.* AJNR 8:885, 1987.

Multiple Sclerosis

1. **Nesbit GM, Forbes GS, Cheithauer BW, et al:** *Multiple sclerosis: Histopathologic and MR and/or CT correlation in thirty-seven cases at biopsy and three cases at autopsy.* Radiology 180:467, 1991.
2. **Wallace CJ, Seland TP, Fong TC:** *Multiple sclerosis: The impact of MR imaging.* AJR 158:849, 1992.
3. **McFarlin DE, McFarland HF:** *Multiple sclerosis.* N Engl J Med 20:307, 1246, 1982.
4. **Swanson JW:** *Multiple sclerosis: Update in diagnosis and review of prognostic factors.* Mayo Clin Proc 64:577, 1989.
5. **Bartel DR, Markand ON, Kolar OJ:** *The diagnosis and classification of multiple sclerosis: Evoked responses and spinal fluid electrophoresis.* Neurology 33:611, 1983.
6. **Poser CM, Paty DW, Scheinberg L, et al:** *New diagnostic criteria for multiple sclerosis: Guidelines for research protocols.* Ann Neurol 13:227, 1983.
7. **Herndon RM, Brooks B:** *Misdiagnosis of multiple sclerosis.* Semin Neurol 5:94, 1985.
8. **Rudnick RA, Schiffer RB, Schwertz KM, et al:** *Multiple sclerosis: The problem of incorrect diagnosis.* Arch Neurol 43:578, 1986.
9. **Rudnick RA:** *Helping patients live with multiple sclerosis. What primary care physicians can do.* Postgrad Med 88:197, 1990.

10. **Schumacher GA, Beebe GW, Kibler RF, et al:** *Problems of experimental trials of therapy in multiple sclerosis.* Ann NY Acad Sci 122:552, 1965.
11. **Marie MP, Chatelin C:** *Sur certains symptomes vraisemblablement d'origine radiculaire chez les blesses du crane.* Rev Neurol (Paris) 2:336, 1917.
12. **Lhermitte J, Bollack, Nicolas M:** *Les douleurs a type d decharge electrique consecutives a la flexion cephalique dans la sclerose en plaques. Un cas de forme sensitive de la sclerose multiple.* Rev Neurol (Paris) 2:56, 1924.
13. **Kanchandani R, Howe JG:** *Lhermitte's sign in multiple sclerosis: A clinical survey and review of the literature.* J Neurol Neurosurg Psychiatry 45:308, 1982.
14. **Coleman RJ, Russon L, Blanshard K, et al:** *Useless hand of Oppenheim—magnetic resonance imaging findings.* Postgrad Med J 69:149, 1993.
15. **Gutrecht JA, Zamani AA, Slagado ED:** *Anatomic-radiologic basis of Lhermitte's sign in multiple sclerosis.* Arch of Neurol 50:849, 1993.
16. **Traynelis VC, Hitchon PW, Yuh WT, et al:** *Magnetic resonance imaging and post-traumatic Lhermitte's sign.* J Spinal Disorders 3:376, 1990.
17. **Grossman RI, Braffman BH, Brorson JR:** *Multiple sclerosis: A serial study of gadolinium-enhanced MR imaging.* Radiology 169:117, 1988.
18. **Colosimo M, Amatruda A, Cioffi RP:** *Magnetic resonance imaging in multiple sclerosis: An overview (review).* Italian J of Neurol Sciences 13:113, 1992.
19. **Koopmans RA, Li DK, Oger JJ, et al:** *Chronic progressive multiple sclerosis: Serial magnetic resonance brain imaging over six months.* Ann Neurol 26:248, 1989.
20. **Ormerod IE, Miller DH, McDonald WI, et al:** *The role of NMR imaging in the assessment of multiple sclerosis and isolated neurological lesions. A qualitative study.* Brain 110:1579, 1987.
21. **Runge VM, Price AC, Kirschner HS, et al:** *The evaluation of multiple sclerosis by magnetic resonance imaging.* RadioGraphics 6:203, 1986.
22. **Horowitz AL, Kaplan RD, Grewe G, et al:** *The ovoid lesion: A new MR observation in patients with multiple sclerosis.* AJNR 10:303, 1989.
23. **Wallace CJ, Seland TP, Fong TC:** *Multiple sclerosis: The impact of MR imaging.* AJR 158:849, 1992.
24. **Oppenheimer DR:** *The cervical cord multiple sclerosis.* Neuropathol Appl Neurobiol 4:151, 1978.
25. **Miller DH, Barkhof F, Nauta JJ:** *Gadolinium enhancement increases the sensitivity of MRI in detecting disease activity in multiple sclerosis.* Brain 116:1077, 1993.
26. **Kidd D, Thorpe JW, Thompson AJ, et al:** *Spinal cord MRI using multi-array coils and fast spin echo. II. Findings in multiple sclerosis.* Neurol 43:2632, 1993.
27. **Stude DE, Mick T:** *Clinical presentation of a patient with multiple sclerosis and response to manual chiropractic adjustive therapies.* J Manipulative Physiol Ther 16:595, 1993.
28. **Filippini G, Comi GC, Cosi V, et al:** *Sensitivities and predictive values of paraclinical tests for diagnosing multiple sclerosis.* J Neurol 241:132, 1994.
29. **Meurice A, Flandroy P, Dondelinger RF, et al:** *A single focus of probable multiple sclerosis in the cervical spinal cord mimicking a tumour.* Neuroradiol 36:234, 1994.
30. **Dean G, Bhigjee AI, Bill PL, et al:** *Multiple sclerosis in black South Africans and Zimbabweans.* J of Neurol, Neurosurg & Psychiatry 57:1064, 1994.
31. **Barkhof F, Tas MW, Frequin ST, et al:** *Limited duration of the effect of methylprednisolone on changes on MRI in multiple sclerosis.* Neuroradiol 36:382, 1994.
32. **Uncini A, DiMuzio A, Thomas A, et al:** *Hand dystonia secondary to cervical demyelinating lesion.* Acta Neurol Scand 90:51, 1994.

The Hip

1. **Shellock FG, Morris E, Deutsch AL, et al:** *Hematopoietic bone marrow hyperplasia: High prevalence on MR images of the knee in asymptomatic marathon runners.* AJR 158:335, 1992.
2. **Catto M:** *Pathology of Aseptic Bone Necrosis.* In: Davidson JK, ed.: *Aseptic Necrosis of Bone.* Amsterdam, Excerpta Medica, 1976.
3. **Milgram JW:** *Osteonecrosis.* In: Milgram JW, Gruhn JS, eds.: *Radiologic and Histologic Pathology of Nontumorous Diseases of Bones and Joints.* Northbrook, Northbrook Publishing, 1990.
4. **Osteaux M, DeMeirleir K, Shahabpour M:** *Magnetic Resonance Imaging and Spectroscopy in Sports Medicine.* Berlin, Springer-Verlag, 1991.
5. **Turner DA, Templeton AC, Selzer PM, et al:** *Femoral capital osteonecrosis: MR finding of diffuse marrow abnormalities without focal lesions.* Radiology 171:135, 1989.
6. **Mitchell DG, Rao VM, Dalinka M, et al:** *Hematopoietic and fatty bone marrow distribution in the normal and ischemic hip: New observations with 1.5-T MR imaging.* Radiology 161:199, 1986.
7. **Lang P, Jergesen HE, Moseley ME, et al:** *Avascular necrosis of the femoral head: High-field strength MR imaging with histologic correlation.* Radiology 169:517, 1988.
8. **Seiler JG III, Christie MJ, Homra L:** *Correlation of the findings of magnetic resonance imaging with those of bone biopsy in patients who have stage I or stage II ischemic necrosis of the femoral head.* J Bone Joint Surg (Am) 71:28, 1989.
9. **Steinberg MA:** *Management of avascular necrosis of the femoral head—An overview.* In Vassett FH, ed. Instr Course Lect, 37:41, 1988.
10. **Beltran J, Knight CT, Zuelzer WA, et al:** *Core decompression for avascular necrosis of the femoral head: Correlation between long-term results and preoperative MR staging.* Radiology 175:533, 1990.
11. **Kramer J, Hoffman S Jr, Engel A, et al:** *Bone marrow edema in transient osteoporosis: Initial stage of avascular necrosis of the hip.* Radiology 181(suppl):136, 1991 (abstract).
12. **Berquist TH, Ehman RL, Richardson ML, et al:** *Miscellaneous Conditions and Future Potential.* In: Berquist TH, ed.: *Magnetic Resonance of the Musculoskeletal System.* New York, Raven Press, 1987.
13. **Bloem JL:** *Transient osteoporosis of the hip: MR imaging.* Radiology 167:753, 1988.

14. **Higer HP, Grimm J, Pedrosa P, et al:** *Transitorische osteoporose oder femurkopf-necrose fruhdiagnose mit der MRT.* Rofo Fortschr Geb Rontgenstr Nuklearmed 50:407, 1989.
15. **Takatori Y, Kokubo T, Ninomiya S, et al:** *Transient osteoporosis of the hip: Magnetic resonance imaging.* Clin Orthop 271:190, 1991.
16. **Hauzeur JP, Hanquinet S, Genevois PA, et al:** *Study of magnetic resonance imaging in transient osteoporosis of the hip.* J Rheumatol 18:1211, 1991.
17. **Potter H, Moran M, Schneider R, et al:** *Magnetic resonance imaging in diagnosis of transient osteoporosis of the hip.* Clin Orthop 280:223, 1992.
18. **Daniel WW, Sanders PC, Alarcon GS:** *The early diagnosis of transient osteoporosis by magnetic resonance imaging. A case report.* J Bone Joint Surg (Am) 74:1262, 1992.
19. **Modic MT, Pflanze W, Feiglin DH, et al:** *Magnetic resonance imaging of musculoskeletal infections.* Radiol Clin North Am 24:247, 1986.
20. **Richardson ML, Kilcoyne RF, Gillespy T III, et al:** *Magnetic resonance imaging of musculoskeletal neoplasms.* Radiol Clin North Am 24:259, 1986.
21. **Mink JH, Deutsch AL:** *Occult cartilage and bone injuries of the knee: Detection, classification and assessment with MR imaging.* Radiology 170: 823, 1989.
22. **Hauzeur JP, Pasteels JL, Schoutens A, et al:** *The diagnostic value of magnetic resonance imaging in non-traumatic osteonecrosis of the femoral head.* J Bone Joint Surg (Am) 71:641, 1989.
23. **Chan TW, Dalinka MK, Steinberg ME, et al:** *MRI appearance of femoral head osteonecrosis following core decompression and bone grafting.* Skeletal Radiol 20:103, 1991.
24. **Wilson AJ, Murphy WA, Hardy DC, et al:** *Transient osteoporosis: Transient bone marrow edema?* Radiology 167:757, 1988.
25. **VandeBerg BE, Malghem JJ, Labaisse MA, et al:** *MR imaging of avascular necrosis and transient marrow edema of the femoral head.* RadioGraphics 13:501, 1993.
26. **Curtis PH, Kincaid WE:** *Transitory demineralization of the hip in pregnancy.* J Bone Joint Surg (Am) 41:1327, 1959.
27. **Lequesne M:** *Transient osteoporosis of the hip: A nontraumatic variety of Sudeck's atrophy.* Ann Rheum Dis 27:463, 1968.
28. **Rosen RA:** *Transitory demineralization of the femoral head.* Radiology 94:509, 1970.
29. **Dunstan CR, Evans RA, Somers NM:** *Bone death in transient regional osteoporosis.* Bone 13:161, 1992.
30. **Stoller DW:** *Magnetic Resonance Imaging in Orthopaedics and Sports Medicine.* Philadelphia, JB Lippincott, 1993.
31. **Madewell JE, Moser RP Jr, Sweet DE:** *Soft Tissue and Joint Tumors (Benign and Malignant).* In: Taveras JM, Ferrucci JT, eds.: *Radiology: Diagnosis, Imaging, Intervention.* Vol. 5, Ch. 102, Philadelphia, JB Lippincott, 1987.
32. **Pomeranz SJ:** *Gamuts and Pearls in MRI.* Cincinnati, Images Unlimited, 1990.
33. **Sundaram M:** *Aneurysmal Bone Cyst.* In: Taveras JM, Ferrucci JT, eds.: *Radiology: Diagnosis, Imaging, Intervention.* Vol. 5, Ch. 81, Philadelphia, JB Lippincott, 1992.
34. **Beltran J, Simon DC, Levy M, et al:** *Aneurysmal bone cyst: MR imaging at 1.5T.* Radiology 158:689, 1986.
35. **Cohen EK, Kressel HY, Frank TS, et al:** *Hyaline cartilage–origin bone and soft tissue neoplasms: MR appearance and histologic correlation.* Radiology 167:477, 1988.

The Knee

1. **Pomeranz SJ:** *Orthopedic and Sports Medicine MRI review lecture notes.* Cincinnati: MRI Education Foundation, 1993.
2. **Crues JV, Stoller DW:** *The Menisci.* In: Mink J, ed.: *MR Imaging of the Knee,* ed 2. New York, Raven Press, 1993.
3. **Smillie IS:** *Surgical Pathology of the Menisci.* In: *Injuries of the Knee Joint.* London, England, Livingstone, 1970.
4. **Crues JV, Ryu R:** *MRI of the knee. II.* Surg Rounds Orthop, May 1989.
5. **Crues JV, Ryu R:** *Knee.* In: Stark DD, Bradley WG, eds. *Magnetic Resonance Imaging.* St. Louis, Mosby-Year Book, 1992.
6. **Stoller DW:** *Magnetic Resonance Imaging in Orthopaedics and Sports Medicine.* Philadelphia, JB Lippincott, 1993.
7. **Newman AP, Daniels AU, Burks RT:** *Principles and decision making in meniscal surgery.* Arthroscopy 9:33, 1993.
8. **O'Donoghue DH:** *Surgical treatment of injuries to the ligaments of the knee.* JAMA 169:1423, 1959.
9. **Mink JH, Reicher MA, Crues JV:** *MRI of the Knee.* New York, Raven Press, 1987.
10. **Vellet AD, Marks PH, Fowler PJ, et al:** *Occult post-traumatic osteochondral lesions of the knee: Prevalence, classification, and short-term sequelae evaluated with MR imaging.* Radiology 170:271, 1991.
11. **Gentili A, Seeger LL, Yao L, et al:** *Anterior cruciate ligament tear: Indirect signs at MR imaging.* Radiology 193:835, 1994.
12. **Robertson PL, Schweitzer ME, Bartolozzi AR, et al:** *Anterior cruciate ligament tears: Evaluation of multiple signs with MR imaging.* Radiology 193:829, 1994.
13. **Lee JK, Yao L, Phelps CT, et al:** *Anterior cruciate ligament tears: MR imaging compared with arthroscopy and clinical tests.* Radiology 166:861, 1988.
14. **Remer EM, Fizgerald SW, Friedman H, et al:** *Anterior cruciate ligament injury: MR imaging diagnosis and pattern injury.* RadioGraphics 12:901, 1992.
15. **Tung GA, Davis LM, Wiggins ME, et al:** *Tears of the anterior cruciate ligament: Primary and secondary signs at MR imaging.* Radiology 188:661, 1993.
16. **McCauley TR, Moses M, Kier R, et al:** *MR diagnosis of tears of anterior cruciate ligament of the knee: Importance of ancillary findings.* AJR 162:115, 1994.
17. **Hayes CW, Sawyer RW, Conway WF:** *Patellar cartilage lesions: In vitro detection and staging with MR imaging and pathologic correlation.* Radiology 176:479, 1990.
18. **Yulish BS, Montanez J, Goodfellow DB, et al:** *Chondromalacia patellae: Assessment with MR imaging.* Radiology 164:763, 1987.
19. **Clendenin MB, DeLee JC, Heckman JD:** *Interstitial tears of the posterior cruciate ligament of the knee.* Orthopedics 3:764, 1980.

20. **Munk PL, Helms CA, Genant HK, et al:** *MRI of the knee: Current status, new directions.* Skeletal Radiol 18:569, 1989.
21. **Stoller DW:** *MRI of the knee.* Perspect Radiol 1:21, 1988.
22. **Munk PL:** *MR imaging of the knee: An overview.* Canad Assoc Radiol J 40:296, 1989.
23. **Turner DA, Prodromos CC, Petasnick JP, et al:** *Acute injury of the ligaments of the knee: MRI evaluation.* Radiology 154:717, 1985.
24. **Karnoven RL, Negendank WG, Fraser SM, et al:** *Articular cartilage defects of the knee: Correlation between magnetic resonance and gross pathology.* Ann Rheum Dis 49:672, 1990.
25. **Gylys-Morin VM, Hajek PC, Sartoris DJ, et al:** *Articular cartilage defects: Detectability in cadavers knees with MR.* AJR 148:1153, 1987.
26. **Hayes CW, Conway WF:** *Evaluation of articular cartilage: Radiographic and cross-sectional imaging techniques.* RadioGraphics 12:409, 1992.
27. **McCauley TR, Kier R, Lynch KJ, et al:** *Chondromalacia patellae: Diagnosis with MR imaging.* AJR 158:106, 1992.
28. **Handelberg F, Shahabpour M, Casteleyn PP:** *Chondral lesions of the patella evaluated with computed tomography, magnetic resonance imaging and arthroscopy.* Arthroscopy 6:24, 1990.
29. **Konig H, Sauter R, Deimling M, et al:** *Cartilage disorders: Comparison of spin echo, CHESS, and FLASH sequence MR images.* Radiology 164:753, 1987.
30. **Spritzer CE, Vogler JB, Martinez S, et al:** *MR imaging of the knee: Preliminary results with a 3-DFT GRASS pulse sequence.* AJR 150:597, 1988.
31. **Reiser MF, Bongartz G, Erleman R, et al:** *Magnetic resonance in cartilaginous lesions of the knee joint with three-dimensional gradient echo imaging.* Skeletal Radiol 17:465, 1988.
32. **Mah ET, Langlois SLP, Lott CW, et al:** *Detection of articular cartilage defects using magnetic resonance imaging: An experimental study.* Aust NZ J Surg 60:977, 1990.
33. **Yao L, Sinha S, Seeger LL:** *MR imaging of joints: Analytic optimization of GRE techniques at 1.5T.* AJR 158:339, 1992.
34. **Recht MP, Kramer J, Marcelis S, et al:** *Abnormalities of articular cartilage in the knee: Analysis of available MR techniques.* Radiology 187:473, 1993.
35. **Chandnani VP, Ho C, Chu P, et al:** *Knee hyaline cartilage evaluated with MR imaging: A cadaveric study involving multiple imaging sequences and intra-articular injection of gadolinium and saline solution.* Radiology 178:557, 1991.
36. **Ho C, Cervilla V, Kjellin I, et al:** *Magnetic resonance imaging in assessing cartilage changes in experimental osteoarthrosis of the knee.* Invest Radiol 27:84, 1992.
37. **Goodfellow J, Hungerford DS, Woods C:** *Patello-femoral joint mechanics and pathology.* J Bone Joint Surg (Br) 58:291, 1976.
38. **Osteaux M, DeMeirleir K, Shahabpour M:** *Magnetic Resonance Imaging and Spectroscopy in Sports Medicine.* Berlin Heidelberg, Springer-Verlag, 1991.
39. **Bodne D, Quinn SF, Murray L, et al:** *Magnetic resonance images of chronic patellar tendinitis.* Skeletal Radiol 17:24, 1988.
40. **Resnick D:** *Bone and Joint Imaging.* Philadelphia, WB Saunders, 1989.
41. **Laurin NR, Powe JE, Pavlovsky WF, et al:** *Multimodality imaging of early heterotopic bone formation.* Canad Assoc Radiol J 41:93, 1990.
42. **Kransdorf MJ, Meis JM, Jelinek JS:** *Myositis ossificans: MR appearance with radiologic pathologic correlation.* AJR 157:1243, 1991.
43. **DeSmet AA, Norris MA, Fisher DR:** *Magnetic resonance imaging of myositis ossificans: Analysis of seven cases.* Skeletal Radiol 21:503, 1992.
44. **Mirra JM:** *Bone Tumors. Diagnosis and Treatment.* Philadelphia, JB Lippincott, 1980.
45. **McMaster PE:** *Pigmented villonodular synovitis with invasion of the bone.* J Bone Joint Surg (Am) 42:1170, 1960.
46. **Jelinek JS, Kransdorf MJ, Utz JA, et al:** *Imaging of pigmented villonodular synovitis with emphasis on MR imaging.* AJR 152:337, 1989.
47. **Chung SMK, Janes JM:** *Diffuse pigmented villonodular synovitis of the hip.* J Bone Joint Surg (Am) 47:293, 1965.
48. **Stoller DW, Genant HK:** *Magnetic resonance imaging of the knee and hip.* Arthritis Rheum 33:441, 1990.
49. **Seeger LL, Eckardt JJ, Bassett LW:** *Cross-sectional imaging in the evaluation of osteogenic sarcoma: MRI and CT.* Semin Roentgenol 24:174, 1989.

The Ankle

1. **Stoller DW:** *Magnetic Resonance Imaging in Orthopaedics and Sports Medicine.* Philadelphia, JB Lippincott, 1993.
2. **Schneck CD:** *MR imaging of the most commonly injured ankle ligaments.* Radiology 184:499, 1992.
3. **Deutsch AL, Mink JH, Kerr R:** *MR of the Foot and Ankle.* New York, Raven Press, 1992.
4. **Pavlov H:** *Imaging of the foot and ankle.* Radiol Clin North Am 28:991, 1990.
5. **Bernt AL, Harty M:** *Transchondral fractures (osteochondritis dissecans) of the talus.* J Bone Joint Surg (Am) 41:988, 1959.
6. **Rosenberg ZS, Cheung Y, Jahss MH, et al:** *Rupture of the posterior tibial tendon: CT and MR imaging with surgical correlation.* Radiology 169:229, 1988.
7. **Daffner RH:** *Stress fractures: Current concepts.* Skeletal Radiol 2:221, 1977.
8. **Pappas AM:** *Osteochondrosis dissecans.* Clin Orthop 158:59, 1981.
9. **Greco A, McNamara MT, Escher RM, et al:** *Spin echo and STIR MR imaging of sports-related muscle injuries at 1.5T.* JCAT 15:994, 1991.

The Shoulder

1. **Osteaux M, DeMeirlier K, Shahabpour M:** *Magnetic Resonance Imaging and Spectroscopy in Sports Medicine.* Berlin, Springer-Verlag, 1991.

2. **Seeger LL, Gold RH, Bassett LW:** *Shoulder instability: Evaluation with MR imaging.* Radiology 168:695, 1988.
3. **Kieft GJ, Bloem JL, Rozing PM, et al:** *Rotator cuff impingement syndrome: MR imaging.* Radiology 166:211, 1988.
4. **Bigliani LU, Morrison DS, April EW:** *Morphology of the acromion and its relationship to rotator cuff tears.* Orthop Trans 10:459, 1986.
5. **Seeger LL, Gold RH, Bassett LW, et al:** *Shoulder impingement syndrome: MR findings in 53 shoulders.* AJR 150: 343, 1988.
6. **Rafii M, Firooznia H, Sherman O, et al:** *Rotator cuff lesions: Signal patterns at MR imaging.* Radiology 177: 817, 1990.
7. **Middleton WD, Kneeland JB, Carrera GF, et al:** *High-resolution MR imaging of the normal rotator cuff.* AJR 148:559, 1987.
8. **Yochum TR, Rowe LJ:** *Essentials of Skeletal Radiology,* ed 1. Baltimore, Williams & Wilkins, 1987.
9. **Mitchell MJ, Causey G, Berthoty DP, et al:** *Peribursal fat plane of the shoulder: Anatomic study and clinical experience.* Radiology 168:699, 1988.
10. **Seeger LL:** *Magnetic resonance imaging of the shoulder.* Clin Orthop 244:48, 1989.
11. **Neer CS, Craig EV, Fukuda H:** *Cuff-tear arthropathy.* J Bone Joint Surg (Am) 65:1232, 1983.
12. **Anderson TE:** *Rehabilitation of common shoulder injuries in athletes.* J Musculoskel Med 5:15, 1988.
13. **Erickson SJ, Fitzgerald SW, Quinn SF, et al:** *Long bicipital tendon of the shoulder: Normal anatomy and pathologic findings on MR imaging.* AJR 158:1091, 1992.
14. **Kieft GJ, Dijkmans BA, Bloem JL, et al:** *Magnetic resonance imaging of the shoulder in patients with rheumatoid arthritis.* Ann Rheum Dis 49:7, 1990.
15. **Cartland JP, Crues JV, Stauffer A, et al:** *MR imaging in the evaluation of SLAP injuries of the shoulder: Findings in 10 patients.* AJR 159: 787, 1992.
16. **Snyder SJ, Karzel RP, DelPizzo W, et al:** *SLAP lesions of the shoulder.* Arthroscopy 6:274, 1990.
17. **Kieft GJ, Bloem JL, Rozing PM, et al:** *MR imaging of recurrent anterior dislocation of the shoulder: Comparison with CT arthrography.* AJR 150:1083, 1988.

The Elbow

1. **Collins HR:** *Sports Injuries: Mechanisms, Prevention and Treatment.* Baltimore, Williams & Wilkins, 1985.
2. **Coel M, Yamada CY, Ko J:** *MR imaging of patients with lateral epicondylitis of the elbow (tennis elbow): Importance of increased signal of the anconeus muscle.* AJR 161:1019, 1993.
3. **Nirsch RP:** *Tennis elbow.* Orthop Clin North Am 43:787, 1973.
4. **Osteaux M, DeMeirleir K, Shahabpour M:** *Magnetic Resonance Imaging and Spectroscopy in Sports Medicine.* Berlin, Springer-Verlag, 1991.
5. **Williams PL:** *Gray's Anatomy,* ed 37. Edinburgh, Churchill Livingstone, 1989.
6. **Murphy BJ:** *MR imaging of the elbow.* Radiology 184: 525, 1992.
7. **Mesgarzadeh M, Sapega AA, Bonakdarpour A, et al:** *Osteochondritis dissecans: Analysis of mechanical stability with radiography, scintigraphy and MR imaging.* Radiology 163:775, 1987.
8. **Ehman RL, Berquist TH, McCleod RA:** *Imaging of the musculoskeletal system: A 5-year appraisal.* Radiology 166:313, 1988.

The Wrist

1. **Yao L, Lee JK:** *Occult intraosseous fracture: Detection with MR imaging.* Radiology 167:749, 1988.
2. **Mink JH, Deutsch AL:** *Occult cartilage and bone injuries of the knee: Detection, classification and assessment with MR imaging.* Radiology 170:823, 1989.
3. **Mazet R Jr, Hohl M:** *Fractures of the carpal scaphoid.* J Bone Joint Surg (Am) 48:82, 1963.
4. **Beltran J, Herman LJ, Burk JM, et al:** *Femoral head avascular necrosis. MR imaging with clinical-pathologic and radionuclide correlation.* Radiology 166:215, 1988.
5. **Coleman BG, Kressel HY, Dalinka MK, et al:** *Radiographically negative avascular necrosis: Detection with MR imaging.* Radiology 168:525, 1988.
6. **Desser TS, McCarthy S, Trumble T:** *Scaphoid fractures and Kienbock's disease of the lunate: MR imaging with histopathologic correlation.* Magn Res Imag 8:357, 1990.
7. **Stoller DW:** *Magnetic Resonance Imaging in Orthopaedics and Sports Medicine.* Philadelphia, JB Lippincott, 1993.
8. **Curtis DJ:** *Injuries of the wrist: An approach to diagnosis.* Radiol Clin North Am 19:625, 1981.
9. **Beltran J:** *MRI: Musculoskeletal System.* Philadelphia, JB Lippincott, 1990.
10. **Barry MS, Kettner NW, Pierre-Jerome C:** *Carpal instability: Pathomechanics and contemporary imaging.* Chiropractic Sports Medicine 5:38, 1991.
11. **Schweitzer ME, Brahme SK, Hodler J, et al:** *Chronic wrist pain: Spin echo and short term inversion recovery MR imaging and conventional and MR arthrography.* Radiology 182:205, 1992.
12. **Zlatkin MB, Greenan T:** *Magnetic resonance imaging of the wrist.* Magn Reson Q, 8:65, 1992.
13. **Resnick D, Niwayama G:** *Diagnosis of Bone and Joint Disorders,* ed 2. Philadelphia, WB Saunders, 1988.
14. **Golimbu CN, Firooznia H, Melone CP Jr, et al:** *Tears of the triangular fibrocartilage of the wrist: MR imaging.* Radiology 173:731, 1989.
15. **Cerofolini E, Luchetti R, Pederzini L, et al:** *MR evaluation of triangular fibrocartilage complex tears in the wrist: Comparison with arthrography and arthroscopy.* JCAT 14:963, 1990.
16. **Coyle MP:** *Nerve Entrapment Syndromes in the Upper Extremity.* In: Dee R, ed.: *Principles of Orthopedic Practice,* Vol. 1, New York, McGraw-Hill, 1989.
17. **Middelton WD, Kneeland JB, Kellman GM, et al:** *MR imaging of the carpal tunnel: Normal anatomy and preliminary findings in the carpal tunnel syndrome.* AJR 148:307, 1987.
18. **Zeiss J, Skie M, Ebraheim N, et al:** *Anatomic relations between the median nerve and flexor tendons in the carpal tunnel: MR evaluation in normal volunteers.* AJR 153:533, 1989.
19. **Healy C, Watson JD, Longstaff A, et al:** *Magnetic resonance imaging of the carpal tunnel.* J Hand Surg (Br) 15:243, 1990.

The Temporomandibular Joint

1. **Stoller DW:** *Magnetic Resonance Imaging in Orthopaedics and Sports Medicine.* Philadelphia, JB Lippincott, 1993.
2. **Jacobs JM, Manaster BJ:** *Digital subtraction arthrography of the temporomandibular joint.* AJR 148:344, 1987.
3. **Ross JB:** *Arthrography compared with MRI for TMJ intracapsular soft tissue diagnosis.* TMJ Update 7:31, 1989.
4. **Helms CA, Kaplan P:** *Diagnostic imaging of the temporomandibular joint: Recommendations for the use of various techniques.* AJR 154:319, 1990.
5. **Rao VM, Farole A, Karasick D:** *Temporomandibular joint dysfunction: Correlation of MR imaging, arthrography and arthroscopy.* Radiology 174:663, 1990.
6. **Chossegros C, Cheynet F, Moulin G, et al:** *Indications for imagery in dysfunctional temporomandibular pathology.* Rev Stomatol Chir Maxillofac 95:173, 1994.
7. **Watt-Smith S, Sadler A, Baddeley H, et al:** *Comparison of arthrotomographic and magnetic resonance images of 50 temporomandibular joints with operative findings.* Br J Oral Maxillofac Surg 31:139, 1993.
8. **Paesani D, Westesson PL, Hatala M, et al:** *Prevelance of temporomandibular joint internal derangement in patients with craniomandibular disorders.* Am J of Orthodontics and Dentofacial Orthop 101:41, 1992.
9. **Helms CA, Doyle GW, Orwig D, et al:** *Staging of internal derangements of the TMJ with magnetic resonance imaging: Preliminary observations.* Journal of Craniomandibular Disorders 3:93, 1989.
10. **Helms CA, Kaban LB, McNeill C, et al:** *Temporomandibular joint: Morphology and signal intensity characteristics of the disk at MR imaging.* Radiology 172:817, 1989.

COMPUTED TOMOGRAPHY

1. **Hounsfield GN:** *Computerized transverse axial scanning (tomography) I. Description of a system.* Br J Radiol 46:1016, 1973.
2. **Eisenberg RL:** *Radiology: An Illustrated History.* St. Louis, Mosby-Year Book, 1992.
3. **Colsher JG, Pelc NJ:** *Computerized Tomography Systems and Performance.* In: Taveras JM, Ferrucci JT, eds.: *Radiology: Diagnosis, Imaging, Intervention.* Vol. 1, Ch. 31, Philadelphia, JB Lippincott, 1987.
4. **Heiken JP, Brink JA, Vannier MW:** *Spiral (helical) CT.* Radiology 189:647, 1993.
5. **Zeman RK, Fox SH, Silverman PM, et al:** *Helical (spiral) CT of the abdomen.* AJR 160:719, 1993.
6. **Polacin A, Kalender WA, Marchal G:** *Evaluation of section sensitivity profiles and image noise in spiral CT.* Radiology 185:29, 1992.
7. **Crawford CR, King KF:** *Computed tomography scanning with simultaneous patient translation.* Med Phys 17:967, 1990.
8. **Rubin GD, Dake MD, Napel SA, et al:** *Three-dimensional spiral CT angiography of the abdomen: Initial clinical experience.* Radiology 186:147, 1993.
9. **Haaga JR, Alfidi RJ:** *Computed Tomography of the Whole Body.* Vol. 1, ed 2. St. Louis, CV Mosby, 1988.
10. **Smith B, Regan WF:** *Blow-out fracture of the orbit: Mechanism and correction of internal orbital fracture.* Am J Opthalmol 44:733, 1957.
11. **Gentry LR, Manor WF, Turski PA, et al:** *High-resolution CT analysis of facial struts in trauma. 1. Normal anatomy.* AJR 140:523, 1983.
12. **Gentry LR, Manor WF, Turski PA, et al:** *High-resolution CT analysis of facial struts in trauma. 2. Osseous and soft-tissue complications.* AJR 140:533, 1983.
13. **Madsen JR, Rosenberg AE:** *Case Records of the Massachusetts General Hospital: A 27-Year-Old Woman with Pain in the Neck and Shoulder and Clumsiness of the Hand. Case Study 16-1992.* N Engl J Med 326:1070, 1991.
14. **Devereaux MD, Hazelton RA:** *Pyogenic spinal osteomyelitis—its clinical and radiological presentation.* J Rheumatol 10:491, 1983.
15. **Lifeso RM:** *Pyogenic spinal sepsis in adults.* Spine 15:1265, 1990.
16. **Osenbach RK, Hitchon PW, Menezes AH:** *Diagnosis and management of pyogenic vertebral osteomyelitis in adults.* Surg Neurol 33:266, 1990.
17. **Burke DR, Brant-Zawadski M:** *CT of pyogenic spine infection.* Neuroradiology 27:131, 1985.
18. **Ullrich CG, Binet EF, Sanecki MG, et al:** *Quantitative assessment of the lumbar spinal canal by computed tomography.* Radiology 134:137, 1980.
19. **Williams AL:** *CT diagnosis of degenerative disc disease: The bulging annulus.* Radiol Clin North Am 21:289, 1983.
20. **Teplick JG, Haskin ME:** *Computed tomography of the postoperative lumbar spine.* AJR 141:865, 1983.
21. **Guglielmi G, Grimston SK, Fisher KC, et al:** *Osteoporosis: Diagnosis with lateral and posteroanterior dual x-ray absorptiometry compared with quantitative CT.* Radiology 192:845, 1994.
22. **Genant HK, Block JE, Steiger P, et al:** *Appropriate use of bone densitometry.* Radiology 170:817, 1989.
23. **Cann CE:** *Quantitative CT for determination of bone mineral density: A review.* Radiology 166:509, 1988.
24. **Pacifici R, Rupich R, Griffin M, et al:** *Dual energy radiography versus quantitative computer tomography for the diagnosis of osteoporosis.* J Clin Endocrinol Metab 70:705, 1990.

25. **DiChiro G, Schellinger D:** *Computed tomography of spinal cord after lumbar intrathecal introduction of metrizamide (computer-assisted myelography).* Radiology 120:101, 1976.
26. **Resnick D, Niwayama G:** *Diagnosis of Bone and Joint Disorders,* ed 2. Philadelphia, WB Saunders, 1988.
27. **Heithoff KB, Herzog RJ:** *Computed Tomography (CT) and Enhanced CT of the Spine.* In: Frymoyer JW: *The Adult Spine: Principles and Practice.* New York, Raven Press, 1991.
28. **Heilbronner R, Fankhauser H, Schnyder P, et al:** *Computed tomography of the postoperative intervertebral disc and lumbar spinal canal: Serial long-term investigation in 19 patients after successful operation for lumbar disc herniation.* Neurosurgery 29:1, 1991.
29. **Melville GE, Taveras JM:** *Traumatic Injuries of the Spinal Cord and Nerve Roots.* In: Taveras JM, Ferrucci JT, eds.: *Radiology: Diagnosis, Imaging, Intervention.* Vol. 3. Ch. 104, 1993.

MYELOGRAPHY

1. **Dandy WE:** *Roentgenography of the brain after the injection of air into the spinal canal.* Ann Surg 70:397, 1919.
2. **Sicard JA, Forestier J:** *Methode generale d'exploration radiologique par l'huile iodee (Lipiodol).* Bull et Mem Soc d Hop de Paris 46:463, 1922.
3. **Mixter WJ, Barr JS:** *Rupture of the intervertebral disc with involvement of the spinal canal.* N Engl J Med 211:210, 1934.
4. **Burton CV:** *Lumbosacral arachnoiditis.* Spine 3:24, 1978.
5. **Shapiro R:** *Myelography,* ed 4. Chicago, Year Book Medical Publishers, 1984.
6. **Schick RM:** *Myelographic techniques.* Postgrad Radiol 9:40, 1989.
7. **Lipman JC, Wang AM, Brooks ML, et al:** *Seizure after intrathecal administration of iopamidol.* AJNR 9:787, 1988.
8. **Aprill CN:** *Myelography.* In: Frymoyer JW: *The Adult Spine,* New York, Raven Press, 1991.
9. **Kuuliala IK, Goransson HJ:** *Adverse reactions after iohexol lumbar myelography: Influence of postprocedural positioning.* AJR 149:389, 1987.
10. **Jackson RP, Becker GJ, Jacobs RR, et al:** *The neuroradiographic diagnosis of lumbar herniated nucleus pulposus: I. A comparison of computed tomography (CT), myelography, CT-myelography, discography and CT-discography.* Spine 14:1356, 1989.

DISCOGRAPHY

1. **Hirsch C:** *An attempt to diagnose the level of a disc lesion clinically by disc puncture.* Acta Orthop Scand 18:132, 1948.
2. **Lindblom K:** *Diagnostic puncture of the intervertebral discs in sciatica.* Acta Orthop Scand 17:231, 1948.
3. **Falconer MA, McGreorge M, Begg AC:** *Observations on the cause and mechanism of symptom-production in sciatica and low-back pain.* J Neurol Neurosurg Psychiatry 11:13, 1948.
4. **Erlacher PR:** *Nucleography.* J Bone Joint Surg (Br) 34:204, 1952.
5. **Fernstrom U:** *A discographical study of ruptured lumbar intervertebral discs.* Acta Chirurgica Scand 258:1, 1960.
6. **Ghelman B:** *Discography.* In: Kricun ME: *Imaging Modalities in Spinal Disorders.* Philadelphia, WB Saunders, 1988.
7. **Bobest M, Furo I, Tompa K, et al:** *1 H nuclear magnetic resonance study of intervertebral discs. A preliminary report.* Spine 11:709, 1986.
8. **Bogduk N, Twomey LT:** *Clinical Anatomy of the Lumbar Spine,* ed 2. Melbourne, Churchill Livingstone, 1991.
9. **Aguet J, Lane B:** *Imaging of degenerative disk disease of the lumbar spine.* Postgrad Radiol 7:241, 1987.
10. **Stevens RL, Ryvar R, Robertson WR, et al:** *Biological changes in the annulus fibrosus in patients with low-back pain.* Spine 7:223, 1982.
11. **Teresi LM, Lufkin RB, Reicher MA, et al:** *Asymptomatic degenerative disk disease and spondylosis of the cervical spine: MR imaging.* Radiology 164:83, 1987.
12. **Jensen MC, Brant-Zawadzki MN, Obuchowski N, et al:** *Magnetic resonance imaging of the lumbar spine in people without back pain.* N Engl J Med 331:69, 1994.
13. **Kieffer SA, Stadlan EM, Mohandas A, et al:** *Discographic-anatomical correlation of developmental changes with age in the intervertebral disc.* Acta Radiol Diagn (Stockh) 9:733, 1969.
14. **Wiberg G:** *Back pain in relation to the nerve supply of the intervertebral disc.* Acta Orthop Scand 19:211, 1947.
15. **Coppes MH, Marani E, Thomeer RT, et al:** *Innervation of annulus fibrosus in low back pain (letter).* Lancet 336:189, 1990.
16. **McCarron RF, Wimpee MW, Hudkins PG, et al:** *The inflammatory effect of nucleus pulposus. A possible element in the pathogenesis of low-back pain.* Spine 12:760, 1987.
17. **Saal JS, Franson RC, Dobrow R, et al:** *High levels of inflammatory phospholipase A_2 activity in lumbar disc herniations.* Spine 15:674, 1990.
18. **Howe JF, Loeser JD, Calvin WH:** *Mechanosensitivity of dorsal root ganglia and chronically injured axons: A physiological basis for the radicular pain of nerve root compression.* Pain 3:25, 1977.
19. **Jinkins JR:** *The pathoanatomic basis of somatic and autonomic syndromes originating in the lumbosacral spine.* Neuroimaging Clin North Am 3:443, 1993.
20. **Aprill CN:** *Myelography.* In: Frymoyer JW ed.: *The Adult Spine.* New York, Raven Press, 1991.
21. **Ninomiya M, Muro T:** *Pathoanatomy of lumbar disc herniation as demonstrated by computed tomography/discography.* Spine 17:1316, 1992.

22. **Schnebel BE, Simmons JW, Chowning J, et al:** *A digitizing technique for the study of movement of intradiscal dye in response to flexion and extension of the lumbar spine.* Spine 13:309, 1988.
23. **Vanharanta H, Sachs BL, Spivey MA, et al:** *The relationship of pain provocation to lumbar disc deterioration as seen by CT/discography.* Spine 12:295, 1987.
24. **Hartman JT, Kendrick JI, Lorman P:** *Discography as an aid in evaluation for lumbar and lumbosacral fusion.* Clin Orthop 81:77, 1971.

NUCLEAR MEDICINE

1. **Eisenberg RL:** *Radiology: An Illustrated History.* Mosby-Year Book, 1992.
2. **Wagner H:** *Nuclear Medicine.* New York, HP Publishers, 1975.
3. **Blumgart HL, Yens OC:** *Studies on the velocity of blood flow.* J Clin Invest 4:1, 1927.
4. **Hevesy G, Chiewitz D:** *Radioactive indicators in the study of phosphorus metabolism in rats (letter).* Nature 136:754, 1935.
5. **Perrier C, Segre E:** *Radioactive isotopes of element 43 (letter).* Nature 140:193, 1937.
6. **Holder LE:** *Clinical radionuclide bone imaging.* Radiology 176:607, 1990.
7. **Charkes ND, Sklaroff DM:** *Early diagnosis of metastatic bone cancer by photoscanning with strontium-85.* J Nucl Med 5:168, 1964.
8. **Charkes ND:** *Some differences between bone scans made with ^{87m}Sr and ^{85}Sr.* J Nucl Med 10:491, 1969.
9. **Subramanian G, McAfee JG:** *A new complex of ^{99m}Tc for skeletal imaging.* Radiology 99:192, 1971.
10. **Davis MA, Jones AL:** *Comparison of ^{99m}Tc-labeled phosphate and phosphonate agents for skeletal imaging.* Semin Nucl Med 6:19, 1976.
11. **Alazraki N, Dries D, Datz F, et al:** *Value of a 24-hour image (four-phase bone scan) in assessing osteomyelitis in patients with peripheral vascular disease.* J Nucl Med 26:711, 1985.
12. **O'Connor MK, Brown ML, Hung JC, et al:** *The art of bone scintigraphy—technical aspects.* J Nucl Med 32:2332, 1991.
13. **Thrall JH, Ziessman HA:** *Nuclear Medicine: The Requisites.* St. Louis, CV Mosby, 1995.
14. **Maguire C, Florence S, Powe JE, et al:** *Hepatic uptake of technetium-99^m HM-PAO in a fetus.* J Nucl Med 31:237, 1990.
15. **Guebert GM, Pirtle OL, Yochum TR:** *Essentials of Diagnostic Imaging.* St. Louis, Mosby-Year Book, 1995.
16. **Lavender JP, Lowe J, Barker JR, et al:** *Gallium-67 citrate scanning in neoplastic and inflammatory lesions.* Br J Radiol 44:361, 1971.
17. **Segal AW, Arnot RN, Thakur ML, et al:** *Indium-111-labelled leukocytes for localization of abscesses.* Lancet 2:1056, 1976.
18. **Corstens FH, Oyen WJ, Becker WS:** *Radioimmunoconjugates in the detection of infection and inflammation.* Semin Nucl Med 23:148, 1993.
19. **Alazraki NP:** *Radionuclide imaging in the evaluation of infections and inflammatory disease.* Radiol Clin North Am 31:783, 1993.
20. **Buscombe JR, Oyen WJ, Grant A, et al:** *Indium-111-labeled polyclonal human immunoglobulin: Identifying focal infection in patients positive for human immunodeficiency virus.* J Nucl Med 34:1621, 1993.
21. **Buscombe JR, Lui D, Ensing G, et al:** *^{99m} Tc- human immunoglobulin (HIG)—first result of a new agent for the localization of infection and inflammation.* Eur J Nucl Med 16:649, 1990.
22. **Holder LE:** *Bone scintigraphy in skeletal trauma.* Radiol Clin North Am 31:739, 1993.
23. **McDougall IR, Rieser RP:** *Scintigraphic techniques in musculoskeletal trauma.* Radiol Clin North Am 27:1003, 1989.
24. **Wolbarst AB:** *Physics of Radiology.* Norwalk, Appleton & Lange, 1993.
25. **Collier BD Jr, Hellman RS, Krasnow AZ:** *Bone SPECT.* Semin Nucl Med 17:247, 1987.
26. **Hellman RS, Collier BD:** *Single photon emission computed tomography: A clinical experience.* In: Freeman LM, Weissmann HS, eds.: Nuclear Medicine Annual 1987. New York, Raven Press, 1987.
27. **Murray IP, Dixon J:** *The role of single photon emission computed tomography in bone scintigraphy.* Skeletal Radiol 18:493, 1989.
28. **Buscombe JR, Towsend CE, Kouris K, et al:** *Clinical high resolution skeletal single photon emission tomography using a triple-headed gamma camera.* Br J Radiol 66:817, 1993.
29. **Ryan PJ, Taylor M, Grevitt M, et al:** *Bone single-photon emission tomography in recent meniscal tears: An assessment of diagnostic criteria.* Eur J Nucl Med 20:703, 1993.
30. **Podoloff DA, Kim EE, Haynie TP:** *SPECT in the evaluation of cancer patients: Not quo vadis; rather, ibi fere summus.* Radiology 183:305, 1992.
31. **Collier BD Jr, Fogelman I, Brown ML:** *Bone scintigraphy: II. Orthopedic bone scanning.* J Nucl Med 34:2241, 1993.
32. **Collier BD, Kir KM, Mills BJ, et al:** *Bone scan: A useful test for evaluating patients with low back pain.* Skeletal Radiol 19:267, 1990.
33. **Fogelman I, Collier BD, Brown ML:** *Bone scintigraphy: III. Bone scanning in metabolic bone disease.* J Nucl Med 34:2247, 1993.
34. **Sweeney DC, Greenberg JS, McAfee JG, et al:** *Benign bone lesions simulating metastases on Tc-99^m diphosphonate imaging.* Clin Nucl Med 17:134, 1992.
35. **Brown ML:** *The role of radionuclides in the patient with osteogenic sarcoma.* Semin Roentgenol 24:185, 1989.
36. **Tumeh SS:** *Scintigraphy in benign bone disease.* Postgrad Radiol 7:183, 1987.
37. **Modic MT, Pflanze W, Feiglin DH, et al:** *Magnetic resonance imaging of musculoskeletal infections.* Radiol Clin North Am 24:247, 1986.
38. **Bates D, Ruggieri P:** *Imaging modalities for evaluation of the spine.* Radiol Clin North Am 29:675, 1991.

39. **Conway JJ, Collins M, Tanz RR, et al:** *The role of bone scintigraphy in detecting child abuse.* Semin Nucl Med 23:321, 1993.
40. **Matin P:** *Bone scanning of trauma and benign conditions.* In: Freeman LM, Weissmann HS, eds. Nuclear Medicine Annual 1982. New York, Raven Press, 1982.
41. **Matin P:** *Bone scintigraphy in the diagnosis and management of traumatic injury.* Semin Nucl Med 13:104, 1983.
42. **Matin P:** *Basic principles of nuclear medicine techniques for detection and evaluation of trauma and sports medicine injuries.* Semin Nucl Med 18:90, 1988.
43. **Bahk YW, Kim OH, Chung SK:** *Pinhole collimator scintigraphy in differential diagnosis of metastasis, fracture, and infections of the spine.* J Nucl Med 28:447, 1987.
44. **VandeStreek PR, Carretta RF, Weiland FL:** *Nuclear medicine approaches to musculoskeletal disease. Current status.* Radiol Clin North Am 32:227, 1994.
45. **Rockett JF, Magill HL, Moinuddin M, et al:** *Scintigraphic manifestation of iliotibial band injury in an endurance athlete.* Clin Nucl Med 16:836, 1991.
46. **Matheson GO, Clement DB, McKenzie DC, et al:** *Scintigraphic uptake of ^{99m}Tc at non-painful sites in athletes with stress fractures: The concept of bone strain.* Sports Med 4:65, 1987.
47. **Michael RH, Holder LE:** *The soleus syndrome. A cause of medial tibial stress (shin splints).* Am J Sports Med 13:87, 1985.
48. **Rupani HD, Holder LE, Espinola DA, et al:** *Three-phase radionuclide bone imaging in sports medicine.* Radiology 156:187, 1985.
49. **Papanicolaou N, Wilkinson RH, Emans JB, et al:** *Bone scintigraphy and radiography in young athletes with low back pain.* AJR 145:1039, 1985.
50. **Lagier R, Chamay A:** *Localized Sudeck's dystrophy and distal interphalangeal osteoarthritis of a finger: Anatomicoradiologic study.* J Hand Surg Am 9:328, 1984.
51. **Kettner NW, Pierre-Jerome C:** *Magnetic resonance imaging of the wrist: Occult osseous lesions.* J Manipulative Physiol Ther 15:599, 1992.
52. **Baker L, Blanco J, Young S:** *MRI of avascular necrosis of the hip.* Radiol Rep 2:222, 1990.
53. **Kozin F, Soin JS, Ryan LM, et al:** *Bone scintigraphy in the reflex sympathetic dystrophy syndrome.* Radiology 138:437, 1981.
54. **Derbekyan V, Novales-Diaz J, Lisbona R:** *Pancoast tumor as a cause of reflex sympathetic dystrophy.* J Nucl Med 34:1992, 1993.
55. **Schauwecker DS:** *The scintigraphic diagnosis of osteomyelitis.* AJR 158:9, 1992.
56. **Larcos G, Brown ML, Sutton RT:** *Diagnosis of osteomyelitis of the foot in diabetic patients: Value of 111-In-leukocyte scintigraphy.* AJR 157:527, 1991.
57. **Tumeh SS, Tohmeh AG:** *Nuclear medicine techniques in septic arthritis and osteomyelitis.* Rheum Dis Clin North Am 17:559, 1991.
58. **Howman-Giles R, Uren R:** *Multifocal osteomyelitis in childhood. Review by radionuclide bone scan.* Clin Nucl Med 17:274, 1992.
59. **Brown ML, Collier BD Jr, Fogelman I:** *Bone scintigraphy: 1. Oncology and infection.* J Nucl Med 34:2236, 1993.
60. **Jacobson AF, Harley JD, Lipsky BA, et al:** *Diagnosis of osteomyelitis in the presence of soft-tissue infection and radiologic evidence of osseous abnormalities: Value of leukocyte scintigraphy.* AJR 157:807, 1991.
61. **Boyd SJ, Nour R, Quinn RJ, et al:** *Evaluation of white cell scintigraphy using indium-111 and technetium-99^m labeled leukocytes.* Eur J Nucl Med 20:201, 1993.
62. **Briggs RC, Kolbjornsen PH, Southall RC:** *Osteitis pubis, Tc-99^m MDP, and professional hockey players.* Clin Nucl Med 17:861, 1992.

63. **Battafarano DF, West SG, Rak KM, et al:** *Comparison of bone scan, computed tomography, and magnetic resonance imaging in the diagnosis of active sacroiliitis.* Semin Arthritis Rheum 23:161, 1993.
64. **Rosenthall L:** *Nuclear medicine techniques in arthritis.* Rheum Dis Clin North Am 17:585, 1991.
65. **Lisbona R, Derbekyan V, Novales-Diaz J, et al:** *Gallium-67 scintigraphy in tuberculous and nontuberculous infectious spondylitis.* J Nucl Med 34:853, 1993.
66. **Sorsdahl OA, Goodhart GL, Williams HT, et al:** *Quantitative bone gallium scintigraphy in osteomyelitis.* Skeletal Radiol 22:239, 1993.
67. **Tumeh SS, Aliabadi P, Weissman BN, et al:** *Chronic osteomyelitis: Bone and gallium scan patterns associated with active disease.* Radiology 158:685, 1986.
68. **Epstein JS, Ganz WI, Lizak M, et al:** *Indium 111-labeled leukocyte scintigraphy in evaluating head and neck infections.* Ann Otol Rhinol Laryngol 101:961, 1992.
69. **Schauwecker DS:** *Osteomyelitis: Diagnosis with In-111-labeled leukocytes.* Radiology 171:141, 1989.
70. **Palestro CJ, Kim CK, Swyer AJ, et al:** *Radionuclide diagnosis of vertebral osteomyelitis: Indium-111-leukocyte and technetium-99^m-methylene diphosphonate bone scintigraphy.* J Nucl Med 32:1861, 1991.
71. **Weissman BN:** *Current topics in the radiology of joint replacement surgery.* Radiol Clin North Am 28:1111, 1990.
72. **Jazmati B, Tumeh S:** *Scintigraphy of malignant bone disease.* Postgrad Radiol 8:140, 1988.
73. **Brown ML:** *Bone scintigraphy in benign and malignant tumors.* Radiol Clin North Am 31:731, 1993.
74. **Papanicolaou N:** *Osteoid osteoma: operative confirmation of complete removal by bone scintigraphy.* Radiology 154:821, 1985.
75. **Goshen E, Mozes M, Mercer R, et al:** *A discrepancy between bone scan and MRI concerning the involvement of adjacent bone in soft tissue sarcoma.* Clin Nucl Med 18:759, 1993.
76. **Anez LF, Gupta SM, Berger D, et al:** *Scintigraphic evaluation of multifocal hemangioendothelioma of bone.* Clin Nucl Med 18:840, 1993.
77. **Stokkel MP, Valdes Olmos RA, Hoefnagel CA, et al:** *Tumor and therapy associated abnormal changes on bone scintigraphy: Old and new phenomena.* Clin Nucl Med 18:821, 1993.
78. **Palestro CJ, Swyer AJ, Kim CK, et al:** *Infected knee prosthesis: diagnosis with In-111 leukocyte, Tc-99^m sulphur colloid, and Tc-99^m MDP imaging.* Radiology 179:645, 1991.
79. **Harris AE, Toney MA:** *Bridging rib fractures. Scintigraphic and radiographic findings.* Clin Nucl Med 18:915, 1993.
80. **Tumeh SS, Beadle G, Kaplan WD:** *Clinical significance of solitary rib lesions in patients with extraskeletal malignancy.* J Nucl Med 26:1140, 1985.
81. **Coleman RE, Mashiter G, Whitaker KB, et al:** *Bone scan flare predicts successful systemic therapy for bone metastases.* J Nucl Med 29:1354, 1988.
82. **Kwai AH, Stomper PC, Kaplan WD:** *Clinical significance of isolated scintigraphic sternal lesions in patients with breast cancer.* J Nucl Med 29:324, 1988.
83. **Kosuda S, Gokan T, Tamura K, et al:** *Radionuclide imaging of two patients with metastasis to a distal phalanx of the hand.* Clin Nucl Med 11:659, 1986.
84. **Adler LP, Blair HF, Makley JT, et al:** *Noninvasive grading of musculoskeletal tumors using PET.* J Nucl Med 32:1508, 1991.
85. **Hoffman JM, Hanson MW, Coleman RE:** *Clinical positron emission tomography imaging.* Radiol Clin North Am 31:935, 1993.

7

Principles of Radiologic Interpretation

Lindsay J. Rowe and Terry R. Yochum

"In radiography, as in photography, microscopy, and many other observations, the appearance which seems the most obvious does not always correspond with the real condition."
Anonymous

GENERAL CONSIDERATIONS

Conventional radiographic procedures (plain film) are the most frequently utilized imaging modality in the evaluation of the skeletal system. (1) Contemporary technologic advancements have resulted in additional modalities being utilized with each method providing its own specific area of pre-eminence. (2) Skeletal radiology is frequently the cornerstone to the diagnosis and appropriate management of a broad spectrum of conditions treated by numerous members of the health professions including medicine, chiropractic, osteopathy, physiotherapy and podiatry. (3-6) This chapter will outline the essentials of skeletal imaging, anatomy, and physiology and provide a working framework to enhance interpretive skills.

TECHNICAL CONSIDERATIONS

Numerous methods of investigating the skeletal system are available. (Table 7.1) Each modality has its own area of specific use and specialized information. Usually, a number of these are used in combination to provide the necessary information for arriving at an accurate diagnosis.

PLAIN FILM RADIOGRAPHY

Applications. This is the most widely utilized skeletal imaging method. No contrast media is used to enhance various body structures. The visualization of these components is dependent on the natural contrast between the five radiographic densities—

Table 7.1.   Skeletal Imaging Modalities

	Biomechanics	Pathology
CONVENTIONAL IMAGING		
Plain film radiography	+	+++
Stress radiography	+++	+++
Tomography	+	+++
Xeroradiography	−	+++
CONTRAST IMAGING		
Arthrography	+	+++
Angiography	−	+++
Lymphangiography	−	+++
Myelography	+	+++
Discography	+	+++
Sinography	−	+++
RADIOISOTOPIC IMAGING		
Bone scan	−	+++
ADVANCED IMAGING		
Ultrasound	+	++
Cineroentgenology	+++	+
Computed tomography	+	+++
Magnetic resonance	+	+++

+++ High sensitivity
++ Sensitive
+ Low sensitivity
− No application

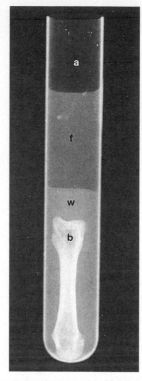

Figure 7.1.   NORMAL RADIOGRAPHIC DENSITIES. There are four naturally occurring radiodensities as shown in this x-ray of a test tube: air (*a*), fat (*f*), water (*w*), and bone (*b*). Note the distinctive difference in density of each component.

air, fat, water, bone, and metal. (Figs. 7.1, 7.2) A basic premise in plain film evaluation is the absolute necessity of having a minimum of two views, preferably perpendicular to each other. (Fig. 7.3) These should be supplemented with additional projections, such as oblique, angulated, or stress studies, as clinically indicated. (7) (Figs. 7.4, 7.5)

Considerable conflict has arisen in more recent times as to the indications for when skeletal radiography should be obtained—particularly in the spine—as concerns for radiation safety, public health, and rising health care costs have gained momentum. Guidelines have been developed to assist in the imaging decision-making process. (8–12) (Table 7.2)

Applications of skeletal radiographs are many. They are often the initial investigations of skeletal abnormalities and provide pivotal information as to what additional imaging modality may be indicated or contraindicated. Recognition of a definite diagnosis is frequently possible or at least a short list of differential diagnoses can be determined. In addition, plain films are important for comparison of changes in the disease process over time or with therapy, and provide chance detection of unsuspected bony and soft tissue abnormalities. Biomechanical information can be gleaned from functional stress radiographs obtained at extremes of motion, on weight bearing or with compression-distraction forces applied. (13)

Advantages. Conventional radiographic studies are readily available, relatively inexpensive, and noninvasive. They depict anatomic details in a format that is readily understandable and requires relatively few anatomic computations for the understanding of three-dimensional relationships. A key benefit is the demonstration of bony landmarks and the ability to assess contiguous structures over considerable length.

Disadvantages. The major drawbacks consist of lack of soft tissue discrimination, diminished sensitivity in detecting bone den-

sity changes, resolution of small lesions, radiographic latent period, variability and effect of exposure differences, technical artifacts, and exposure to ionizing radiation.

Soft tissue depiction is limited to definition of anatomic planes determined largely by surrounding fat. Diagnostic sensitivity can be limited with up to 30 to 50% loss of bone density and a lesion size of at least 1 to 5 cm often necessary before being visible on a radiograph. (14–16) In this context the patient may have extensive histologic disease and have a normal appearing radiograph. (Fig. 7.6) Similarly, the time interval from when the disease process manifests clinically, until it becomes visible radiographically, can be quite long. This is referred to as the *radiographic latent period*. Osteomyelitis in a peripheral bone takes a minimum of 10 to 14 days before it can be seen on the plain film, whereas in the spine this can take 21 days. Tumors may be expected to be slower than infections to manifest, though aggressive lesions can manifest within 4 to 6 weeks.

TOMOGRAPHY

The word *tomography* is derived from the Greek *tomos*, which means "a cutting." Tomography involves visualizing a selected anatomic layer and has been called *laminography* and *zonography*. Essentially, it permits the detailed examination of anatomy and abnormalities that are inaccessible by conventional radiography, allowing selective imaging at any selected level in the body. The level to be imaged is set at the fulcrum between the x-ray tube and film cassette, which move in opposite directions during the exposure. (Fig. 7.7) The movement may be linear or hypocycloidal. The effect is to produce a sharp, in-focus image at the level

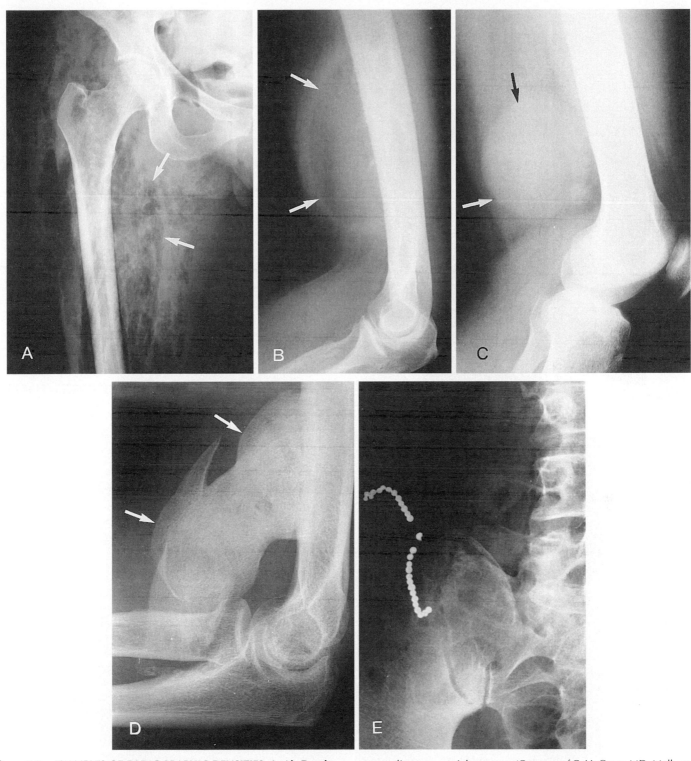

Figure 7.2.   EXAMPLES OF RADIOGRAPHIC DENSITIES. A. Air Density. Observe the radiolucent densities within the soft tissues of the thigh in this patient with gas gangrene (arrows). **B. Fat Density.** A well-demarcated radiolucent mass is present within the soft tissues of the anterior arm (arrows). This appearance is characteristic of the benign fatty tumor lipoma. **C. Water Density.** Posterior to the distal femoral shaft is a round, well-circumscribed mass of the same density as the surrounding muscle (arrows). The diagnosis was malignant synovial sarcoma. (Courtesy of C. H. Quay, MD, Melbourne, Australia) **D. Bone Density.** A smooth bony growth extends from the anterior arm (arrows). Observe the smooth cortical margin and internal trabecular pattern characteristic of posttraumatic myositis ossificans. **E. Metal Density.** Numerous round metallic densities appear aligned in an ''S'' shaped configuration in the right lower quadrant of the abdomen. These represent ingested shot pellets lodged in the appendix.

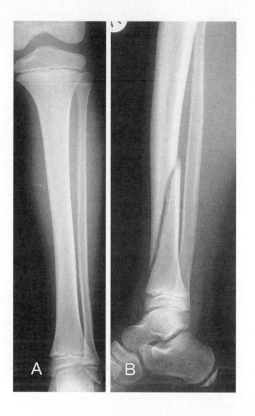

Figure 7.3.   **DEMONSTRATION OF MINIMUM RADIOGRAPHIC PRO-
CEDURE. A. Anteroposterior View: Tibia and Fibula.** No abnormality is
evident. **B. Lateral View: Tibia and Fibula.** An oblique fracture line is seen
in the tibia which was not visible on the AP view. COMMENT: No radiographic study is complete without a minimum of two views perpendicular
to each other.

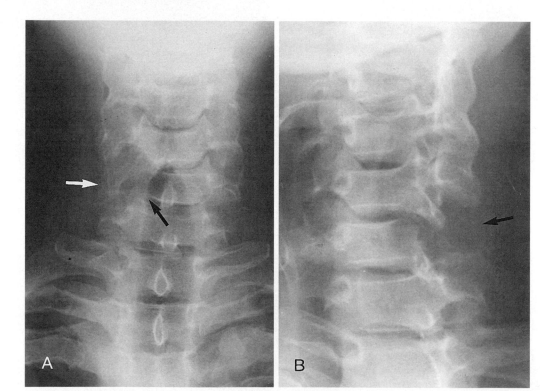

Figure 7.4.   **USE OF SUPPLEMENTARY SPINAL RADIOGRAPHS. A. Anteroposterior View: Lower Cervical Spine.** A subtle destructive lesion is
present in the sixth cervical pedicle and articular pillar (arrows). **B. Oblique
View: Lower Cervical Spine.** The destruction is now clearly depicted (arrow).
This is a characteristic lesion of osteolytic metastatic carcinoma.

COMMENT: Cervical pedicles, foramina, and articular pillars require
oblique films for proper visualization and evaluation. Lumbar obliques serve
the purpose of demonstrating abnormalities of the pedicle, facets, and pars
region.

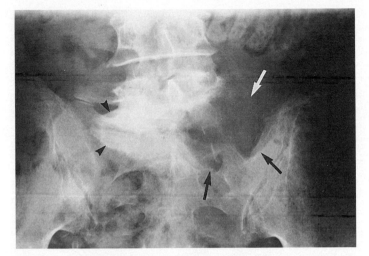

Figure 7.5. ANGULATED LUMBOSACRAL VIEW. Matching the sacral base angle has greatly improved the depiction of the sacrum, sacroiliac joint, and the fifth lumbar body and disc space. Observe the osteolytic destruction of the sacral ala (arrows) from metastatic carcinoma and the large degenerative osteophytes on the contralateral side (arrowheads). COMMENT: This is an excellent projection to evaluate for pathology in any patient with low back pain.

Table 7.2   Guidelines for Obtaining Skeletal Radiographs*
PROBABLE INDICATORS
Trauma—recent, old
Unexplained weight loss
Night pain
Neuromotor deficit
Inflammatory arthritis
History of malignancy
Fever of unknown origin (>100° F)
Abnormal blood finding
Deformity (scoliosis, etc.)
Failure to respond to therapy
Medicolegal implications
POSSIBLE INDICATORS
>50 years of age
Drug or alcohol abuse
Corticosteroid use
Unavailability of alternate imaging
Unavailable/lost/technically inadequate previous studies
Outdated previous studies
Research
Constitutional/systemic disease
Recent immigration
Therapeutic risk assessment (contraindications)
Therapeutic response
NON INDICATORS
Patient education
Routine screening
Habit
Discharge status assessment
Routine biomechanical analysis
Pre-employment status
Physical limitations of patient
Inadequate equipment
Non trained personnel
Financial gain
Recent high level radiation exposure
Pregnancy

*Most of these proposed guidelines have been based on the literature relating to assessment of spinal disorders.

of the fulcrum while blurring out those structures above and below. Sequential films are taken at varying fulcrum levels to totally evaluate the structure in question.

Applications. This procedure is especially useful in evaluations of such complex structures as the skull and spine, as well as in delineating the site, characteristics, and extent of a bony abnormality. (Fig. 7.8)

Advantages. Tomography is beneficial when overlying structures obscure a lesion by removing them from view. Subtle fractures and early bone destruction can be identified when plain films are normal. Complex anatomic deformities of the spine and pelvis can be readily analyzed with tomography.

Disadvantages. High radiation dose is the single greatest handicap because multiple exposures are required. In addition, long exposure times are required to allow for tube-cassette motion, which allows for patient motion artifacts. Enough slices must be obtained at thin intervals; otherwise lesions will be overlooked. Soft tissue planes are more readily identifiable, but internal structure is not visible as a rule.

XERORADIOGRAPHY

The system is different from conventional radiography in that it uses an electrically charged selenium plate as the "cassette." When x-rays strike the plate, the charge is lost. A fine blue powder is blown onto the plate and adheres to the charged regions. The powder is then fused by heat onto paper to produce the image. The selenium plate is then washed and recharged, ready for the next use.

Applications. Xeroradiography has been mainly utilized for examination of the breast (mammography), though some applications in skeletal imaging have been found. (Fig. 7.9) It is especially useful in the detection of foreign bodies and soft tissue problems.

Advantages. The major advantage of the procedure is the exquisite edge enhancement between different densities of bone and soft tissue allowing far more detail than conventional films. (17) In bone lesions it is useful in differentiating cartilaginous and osteogenic bone tumors as well as clearly demonstrating changes such as calcification in soft tissues. (17)

Disadvantages. Specific x-ray apparatus, cassettes, film, and processor are required. Of greatest concern are the high levels of radiation exposure required. Its use in contemporary skeletal imaging and mammography has been largely overtaken by other modalities.

CONTRAST EXAMINATIONS

The major contrast examinations that may be used in the evaluation of skeletal disease include arthrography, angiography, lymphangiography, myelography, discography, and sinography.

Arthrography

Contrast opacification of joint cavities is a useful procedure in the evaluation of joint disease. Air is often combined with the injected water-soluble media to provide a double contrast arthrogram that provides better evaluation of the articular surfaces, me-

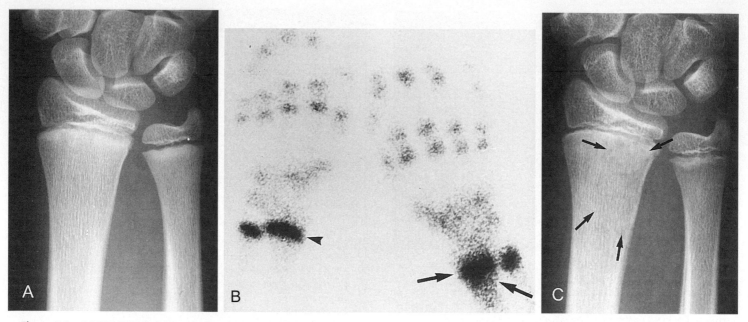

Figure 7.6. LIMITATIONS OF PLAIN FILM EXAMINATIONS. A. Initial Anteroposterior View: Wrist. Despite swelling, pain, and a slight fever, the radius shows no radiographic abnormality. **B. Radioisotope Bone Scan at Initial Presentation.** Note the increased area of blackness ("hot spot") in the corresponding symptomatic radius (arrows) as compared to the normal side (arrowhead). **C. Ten Days Later: Anteroposterior View, Wrist.** Observe the motheaten-type radiolucencies within the radial metaphysis (arrows). These are early plain film findings in osteomyelitis. COMMENT: This study demonstrates the sensitivity of the bone scan to increased bone activity, even when the plain film is normal. Plain films require at least 30 to 50% destruction of bone before one can demonstrate the lesion, while bone scans will be positive with 3 to 5% destruction. Additionally, the need to re-x-ray when signs and symptoms persist is demonstrated. (Courtesy of David P. Thomas, MD, Melbourne, Australia)

Figure 7.7. PRINCIPLES OF TOMOGRAPHY. The film and x-ray tube move synchronously in opposite directions. Note that during the motion the fulcrum (open circle) remains in clear focus, while areas above and below will be blurred and rendered almost invisible.

nisci, and synovium. (Fig. 7.10) The most common joint examined by this procedure is the knee. Other joints less frequently injected include the shoulder, hip, and wrist. In addition, tendon sheaths (tenography) and bursae (bursography) are examined by the same method. Injection into the spinal facet joints is often done prior to the injection of antiinflammatory or analgesic agents. (18)

Applications. Clearly the major area is in identifying intraarticular derangements of menisci, or cartilage, ligamentous, and synovial abnormalities. Loose bodies, tears in cartilages, ligament tears, arthritic processes, and extension into adjacent tissues can all be clarified.

Advantages. It is a readily available technique that allows assessment of joint integrity and intraarticular components. Radiolucent structures such as cartilage are identifiable.

Disadvantages. Drawbacks include the invasive nature of the procedure, operator and interpreter dependency, demonstration of only surfaces of structures, and possible oversight of small lesions.

Angiography

The introduction of a water-soluble contrast agent into an artery (arteriogram) or vein (venogram) can add vital information to the understanding of the disease process and its subsequent management.

Applications. The procedure is used mainly in the evaluation of bone tumors, vascular disease, traumatic skeletal injuries, and avascular necrosis. In bone tumors the size and aggressiveness of the lesion can be assessed by the degree of neovascularity, speed of media removal, and local structure invasion. Traumatic injuries may tear, distort, obstruct, dilate, or produce anomalous connections in vessels, which will be demonstrated only by angiography.

Advantages. The isolation of arterial supply, the extent of the lesion, and its relationship to adjacent structures aid greatly in the surgical management.

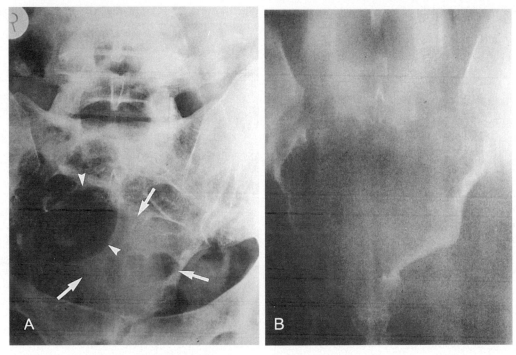

Figure 7.8.   DEMONSTRATION OF TOMOGRAPHY. A. Anteroposterior View: Sacrum. Close scrutiny of the lower sacrum reveals destruction of the sacral foramina, cortices, and trabecular patterns (arrows). Note the obscuring gas shadow (arrowheads). **B. Tomography, Anteroposterior View: Sacrum.** The degree of sacral destruction is now more clearly depicted. The overlying confusing gas shadows are eliminated by this form of study. Diagnosis: Chordoma. (Courtesy of David P. Thomas, MD, Melbourne, Australia)

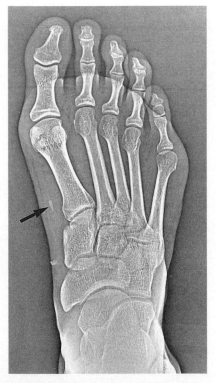

Figure 7.9.   XERORADIOGRAPHY. Although seen here in a black and white reproduction, the image is a light blue and is mounted on paper. Observe the exquisite bone and soft tissue detail, as well as the foreign body glass artifact (arrow).

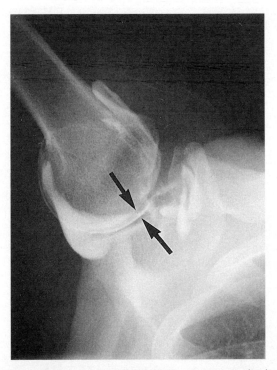

Figure 7.10.   ARTHROGRAM: SHOULDER. Contrast media has been placed into the glenohumeral joint and adjacent bursa. Note the lucent zone paralleling the surface of the humeral head (arrows), representing the articular cartilage.

Disadvantages. Drawbacks include the requirement of specialized equipment in a specialized facility, the invasiveness of the procedure, potential complications (hematoma, infection, embolization), along with relatively high radiation doses incurred.

Lymphangiography

Evaluation of the lymphatic system can be achieved by the injection of an oil-based medium. The procedure requires the injection of a blue-green dye between one or more webs of the toes, followed one hour later by an incision on the dorsum of the foot to identify a large lymphatic channel. Once identified, the channel is cannulated and an oil-based medium is injected slowly over 1 to 3 hours. Approximately 24 hours later the contrast medium will be identifiable within the lower extremity, inguinal, iliac, and paraaortic nodes. The media may remain visible for many months.

Applications. The major disorders evaluated with lymphangiography include lymphoma, metastasis, and lymphatic obstruction.

Advantages. The lymph nodes and lymphatic channels are assessed according to location, size, shape, and configuration for evidence of abnormality. In addition, flow characteristics can be identified.

Disadvantages. The main deterrents to the use of lymphangiography is the incision on the dorsum of the foot, length of time for the procedure, and the frequent difficulties in interpreting findings.

Myelography

Contrast examination of the spine and spinal cord is achieved by injection into the subarachnoid space, usually in the lumbar spine at the second or third lumbar level. The contrast media is a nonionic water-soluble compound.

Applications. This procedure aids in the diagnosis of disc, vertebral canal, spinal cord, and nerve root disease. (Fig. 7.11)

Advantages. It is especially useful in determining multilevel spinal stenosis and injury at the junction of the nerve root and spinal cord.

Disadvantages. This invasive procedure carries the risk of infection and iatrogenic complications, such as damage to nerve roots and dural tears. If bleeding occurs upon injection, the risk for arachnoiditis increases. Postmyelogram headache is encountered in about 40% of cases; those who experience headaches prior to myelography will develop a postmyelographic headache 60% of the time, while non premyelographic headache patients only develop postmyelographic headache 30% of the time. (19) Anaphylaxis, while uncommon, can be a life-threatening complication. In view of these problems and limitations, MRI is considered the technique of choice in the investigation of the spinal cord and its surrounding intraspinal structures. (20) A more complete discussion of myelography is offered in Chapter 6.

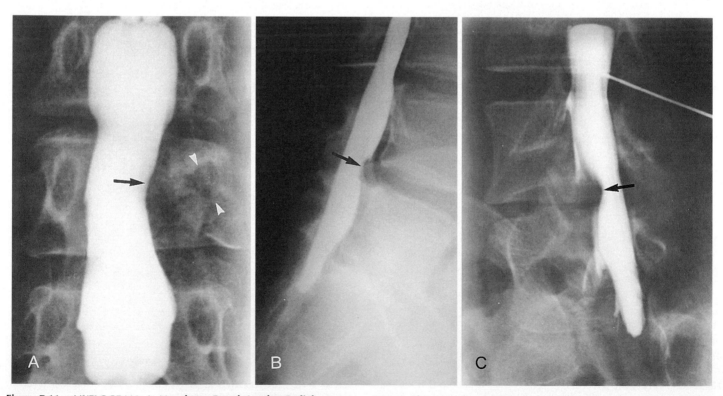

Figure 7.11. MYELOGRAM. A. Neoplasm: Fourth Lumbar Pedicle. Note the destruction of the pedicle and adjacent vertebral body (arrowheads), with adjacent displacement of the contrast column by the soft tissue mass (arrow). These are characteristic findings of osteolytic metastatic carcinoma. **B and C. Disc Protrusion: Fourth Lumbar Disc.** Observe the smooth indentation in the myelographic column (arrow).

Discography

Placement of water-soluble contrast media into the intervertebral disc under fluoroscopic control allows assessment of each disc injected.

Applications. Injection of an opaque medium into the intervertebral nucleus pulposus (discography) has been used to evaluate discal pathology. Four aspects of the injected disc are assessed: the volume of contrast that can be injected (degenerative discs accept more than 2ml of contrast), the pain response of the patient on injection (*provocational study*), the pattern of contrast distribution (fissuring, extravasation, pooling), and the amount of resistance to injection. (20)

Advantages. The procedure allows not only a morphologic analysis but also the functional aspect of *pain provocation*. The reproduction of symptoms upon injection is interpreted as a positive isolating factor for identifying discogenic pain. (21) When combined with CT (CT discography), the extent and orientation of internal annular tears (internal disc disruption) can be determined, such lesions are not routinely definable by any other means, including MRI. (22)

Disadvantages. Specialized equipment and a specialized facility are required to carry out the procedure. Use of fluoroscopy increases the radiation dose for the procedure. As an invasive procedure the usual risks for infection (0.1 to 0.2%), nerve root damage, dural trauma and tears, chemical meningitis, exacerbation or worsening pain, and allergic reactions do exist. The issue of whether discography can precipitate or accelerate disc degeneration is unclear at this stage, though most reports do not support the hypothesis that the procedure is a deleterious factor. (23) A detailed discussion of this procedure is offered in Chapter 6.

Sinography

This is a selective technique applied in the evaluation of bone infections that are associated with a draining external sinus. The sinus is catheterized and the contrast media injected to show the origin and extent of the infection.

RADIONUCLIDE IMAGING

The principle of nuclear imaging hinges on the selective uptake of certain compounds by different organs of the body. Tissues that can be imaged include the brain, heart, lung, kidneys, and skeleton. In bone imaging (bone scan) the most common isotope used is technetium-99m methylene diphosphate (^{99m}Tc-MDP).

The procedure is performed by injecting 15 to 20 millicuries of technetium-99m intravenously and waiting various time periods from 30 minutes to 2 hours for concentration in bony areas of increased blood flow and osteoblastic activity. This is the typical "triphasic" (three phase) study; an initial "flow study," a slightly delayed "blood pool study," and some hours later a "delayed study." An imaging device—the gamma camera—is placed over the patient and records the bone-emitted gamma rays as the isotope undergoes degeneration to a lower energy level. These rays are filtered by a pinhole collimator, transformed into light, and an image is transposed onto a polaroid or radiographic film. Projections of the entire body in the posteroanterior and anteroposterior planes are performed. In addition, selected spot projections over questionable locations are also obtained. Regions of increased uptake will show as dark spots ("hot spots"). Nor-

mally, the isotope will collect more in the long bone metaphyses, thyroid, bladder, kidneys, sternum, costochondral junctions, spine, sacroiliac joints and at the injection site. (24) (Fig. 7.12) The isotope half-life is six hours and is readily excreted by the kidneys. The combination of tomography and isotopic bone scans (Single Photon Emission Computed Tomography, SPECT) allows accurate assessment of regions within bone or where bones overlap, such as the pars interarticularis in the lumbar spine.

Applications. The indications for a bone scan include the detection of skeletal metastasis and other tumors, infection, arthritis, fracture, and avascular necrosis. This is especially useful in diagnosing occult, stress, and recent fractures, in addition to those whose plain films are normal but have pain of undetermined origin. (Fig. 7.13) Bone scanning of the spine can be helpful in both the diagnosis and therapeutic decision making process, helping to identify degeneration, pseudoarthrosis in spinal fusions, spondylolisthesis, fracture, infection, tumor, and metabolic disorders. It is not useful for evaluating spinal stenosis, disc herniation, or postlaminectomy. (25)

Advantages. Only 3 to 5% bone destruction is necessary for pathologic bone destruction to be visible on a bone scan, representing up to ten times an increased sensitivity factor over plain film radiography. Early, clinically unsuspected bone disease, such as metastasis, can be readily identified.

Disadvantages. Diagnostically, the image obtained is quantitative only—it is a measure of activity. Therefore, the scan of a

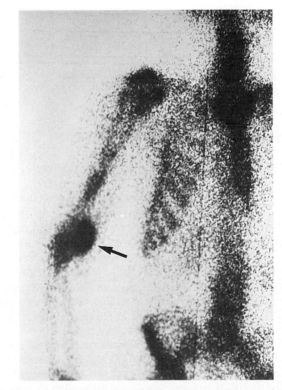

Figure 7.12.   NORMAL RADIOISOTOPIC BONE SCAN. Note the normal increased uptake in the metaphysis of the humerus, sternum, costochondral junctions, lumbar spine, ilium, and sacroiliac joints. The dense region in the elbow is the site of the intravenous injection of the isotope (arrow). COMMENT: Bone scans are evaluated for asymmetry in uptake since, normally, metabolically active regions will concentrate the isotope. (Courtesy of Thomas E. Hyde, DC, DACBSP, North Miami, Florida)

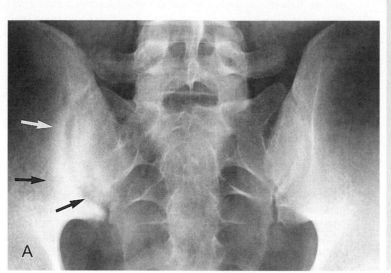

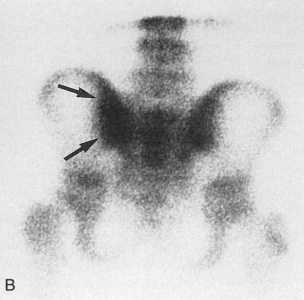

Figure 7.13.   ABNORMAL RADIOISOTOPIC BONE SCAN. A. Anteroposterior View: Sacroiliac Joints. Unilateral sacroiliitis (arrows) is evidenced by loss of the sacral and iliac articular margins, with prominent reactive sclerosis. **B.** Observe the increased isotopic uptake ("hot spot") over the corresponding sacroiliac joint (arrows). COMMENT: Although the diagnosis is not definitive on these findings, the scan confirms the presence of increased bone activity. The diagnosis following aspiration of the joint was infection due to *Staphylococcus aureus.* (Courtesy of Gerald A. Fitzgerald, MD, Sydney, Australia)

neoplasm may appear identical to infection, with further correlation providing the definitive diagnosis. Some skeletal lesions remain inactive or show areas of no uptake on bone scans. This may occur in rapidly destructive processes and in multiple myeloma. A more complete discussion of radionuclide imaging is offered in Chapter 6.

ULTRASOUND

Ultrasonography is frequently utilized in diagnosing abdominal, pelvic and vascular disease. In problems of the skeletal system ultrasound has a limited scope but can be selectively used in certain situations.

Applications. Soft tissue masses—defining whether the mass is cystic or solid—cellulitis, abscess and hematoma are amenable lesions for ultrasonographic investigation. Integrity of peripherally located tendons, especially the rotator cuff and achilles tendon can also be assessed. Neonatal and pediatric hip evaluation can be extremely rewarding in the early detection of congenital hip dysplasia, congenital hip dislocation, and intraarticular effusion. In the spine, ultrasound has limited use in the evaluation of spinal stenosis, disc herniation, and paraspinal soft tissue abnormalities. (26,27) Ultrasound provides a method of evaluating spondylolisthesis without the use of ionizing radiation. (28)

Advantages. Visualization of soft tissues adjacent to the peripheral articulations (e.g., shoulder, knee) is where it becomes increasingly useful. It can be rapidly performed, is noninvasive, does not involve ionizing radiation and can provide a dynamic evaluation of the soft tissue. Ultrasound can be very useful in guiding biopsy or joint aspiration techniques. A useful application is the display of vascular integrity and flow.

Disadvantages. The internal characteristics of bone are not able to be imaged. Similarly, tissues close to bone may be obscured. Metal implants greatly inhibit detailed visualization of the adjacent soft tissues. The accuracy of the examination is extremely operator dependent.

VIDEOFLUOROSCOPY

Visualization of dynamic motion of body structures through fluoroscopy and recording the images has been a source of fascination for decades. Until the 1980s the method of recording has been with 16 or 35 mm film and was referred to as "cineradiography." With the advent of videorecording the transcription process has become greatly simplified. In the spine, motion patterns have been evaluated in normal and abnormal conditions, though its clinical efficacy has not been fully elucidated. (11,29) No consensus on normal standards of motion patterns exists, with a wide range of normal variations described.

Applications. Motion of internal organs, passage of introduced contrast agents, and joint function have been the major applications. Assessment of joint instability, such as at the atlantoaxial joint in the presence of odontoid anomalies, has been shown to be useful in preoperative evaluations. Effects of fusion (arthrodesis) on joint motion can be appreciated as can failure of the fusion procedure. Accurate assessment of joint function requires digitization. (11,29)

Advantages. Dynamic characteristics of joint mechanics are visualized throughout the entire range of motion. Recording of the images allows the movement sequence to be slowed for frame-by-frame analysis and digitization for accurate appraisal.

Disadvantages. Radiation dose can be high if multiple planes are imaged. (30,31) The procedure itself is not lengthy, but the subsequent analysis requires considerable time. There is a paucity of literature upon which to base meaningful estimations of motion magnitude and patterns. (32) The expense and training necessary to do good fluoroscopic studies renders this modality most suited to the laboratory and not to routine clinical use. (11,29)

COMPUTED TOMOGRAPHY

The essential components of a CT system include a circular scanning gantry housing the x-ray tube and image sensors, a table for the patient, an x-ray generator, and a computerized data processing unit. The patient lies on the table and is placed inside the gantry. The x-ray tube is rotated 360° around the patient while the computer collects the data and formulates a transverse image or "slice." Each cross-sectional slice represents a thickness of between 0.5 to 1.3 cm of body tissue. In order to produce an optimal examination multiple sequential slices are obtained. In the lumbar spine 20 to 25 sequential slices produce an average total study dose of 1 to 3 rads. (33) Contemporary computers are capable of producing multiplanar reconstructions (sagittal, coronal, oblique and three-dimensional). (34)

Applications. Although computed tomography (CT) has had its greatest impact in the evaluation of the central nervous system, various uses have been found in skeletal imaging. (35) Following its introduction in 1973 by Hounsfield, many technical advances have occurred to improve resolution and diagnostic capability. (36,37) Skeletal applications include assessment of neoplasms, trauma, infections, metabolic disease, and spinal syndromes. (35) (Fig. 7.14) Bone mass determinations for osteoporosis can be readily achieved (quantitative bone mineral analysis). Combination with other modalities such as myelography (CT myelography), discography (CT discography), and angiography (CT enhanced scan) adds greatly to the analysis of spinal syndromes.

Advantages. Exquisite depiction of bony and soft tissue anatomy is possible. Manipulation of the acquired data allows alter-ations in relative density (windows), measurements of density or distances (cursor), and display in multiple planes (multiplanar imaging).

Disadvantages. Large patients and motion produce technically degraded images. Metal implants produce "star"-shaped artifacts (blooming) while penetration of thick bones adjacent to low attenuation soft tissues produces beam hardening. The averaging of densities throughout the thickness of the slice may result in inaccurate representation of tissue densities (volume averaging). The radiation dose can be relatively high and scanning times lengthy. (See Chapter 6.)

MAGNETIC RESONANCE IMAGING

Magnetic resonance imaging (MRI) is alternatively known as MR or nuclear magnetic resonance (NMR). The patient is placed in a magnetic field that displaces mobile hydrogen atoms that can be measured and formed into an image. Those structures that have a high water content—such as the liver, spleen, muscles, and heart—produce the highest image details. The nucleus pulposus of the disc is readily identified in normal and degenerative conditions. When bone is examined it is actually the marrow that forms the image, due to the low levels of osseous water and high levels of fat.

Applications. The utilization of MR is widening rapidly. (38) (Fig. 7.15) Soft tissues are exquisitely captured and easily identifiable. Shoulder rotator cuff tendon integrity is a key area of investigation. Because the bone marrow is imaged directly, MRI is extremely sensitive in detecting marrow disease. (39) The internal architecture of the joints is seen with dramatic detail. In the spine,

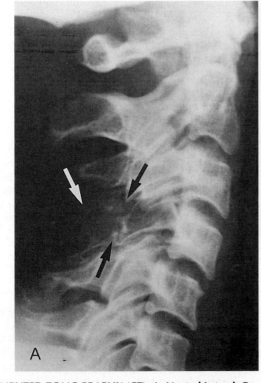
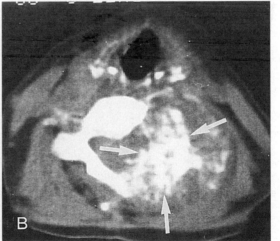

Figure 7.14.   COMPUTED TOMOGRAPHY (CT). A. Neutral Lateral: Cervical Spine. Lytic destruction of the fourth cervical spinous, lamina, and articular pillar is observed (arrows). The diagnosis was aneurysmal bone cyst (ABC). **B. Computed Tomogram.** A selected image of the lesion confirms the anatomical location of the tumor in the posterior arch (arrows). Additional information is gained about its size, internal matrix, and soft tissue extension.

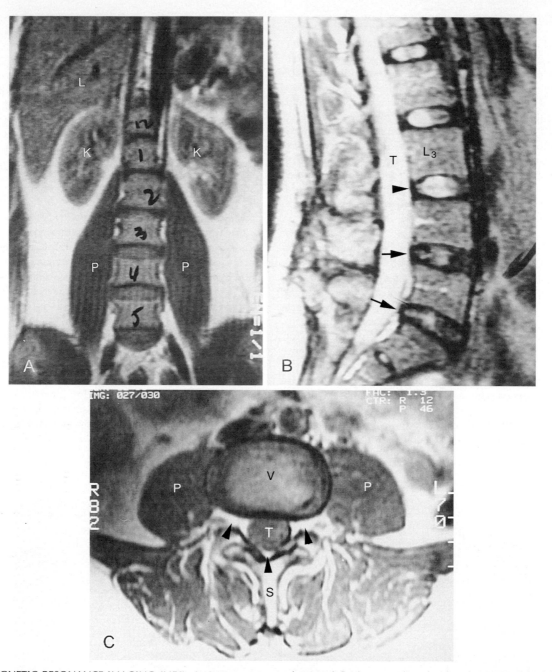

Figure 7.15.   MAGNETIC RESONANCE IMAGING (MRI). A. Anteroposterior View. Exquisite detail of the liver (*L*), kidneys (*K*), and psoas muscle (*P*) is obtained. The surrounding white ("high signal") tissue is fat. **B. Lateral View.** Note the intense white appearance of the normally hydrated nucleus pulposus and straight contour of the posterior annulus fibers (arrowhead). In comparison the dehydrated degenerated discs show a blackened internal structure ("low signal intensity") and a bulging convex posterior annulus margin (arrows). The vertical white structure posteriorly represents the ce- rebrospinal fluid surrounding the thecal sac (*T*). **C. Axial View.** A cross-sectional view through the mid L5 vertebral body and intervertebral foramen demonstrates the L5 vertebral body (*V*), psoas muscle (*P*), thecal sac (*T*) and spinous process (*S*). The high signal intense epidural fat is seen symmetrically surrounding the thecal sac and exiting nerve roots (arrowheads). COMMENT: MRI is dependent on the presence of the hydrogen proton to produce an image. The bone marrow is visible due to its high water content.

the structure and hydration of the disc are represented clearly as are the cord, nerve roots, and intrinsic canal contents such as the epidural fat, ligamentum flavum, and facet joints. (40) (Fig. 7.15 B and C) The use of intravenous contrast (gadolinium) shows areas of increased vascularity including regions of neoplasm and inflammation.

Advantages. Complications are few and can be avoided. Soft tissue contrast resolution is excellent; direct multiplanar imaging without reconstruction, use of non-ionizing radiation, and direct accurate characterization of pathologic tissue are its strengths.

Disadvantages. Claustrophobia is a common problem due to being inside the noisy small tunnel for protracted times. The presence of some metallic clips, especially intracranially, may prevent use of MR. Joint replacements are not a contraindication to MR, however pacemaker patients should not go into the proximity of the scanner. The expense of the study, availability, and extensive equipment and housing requirements do inhibit its use. (See Chapter 6)

SKELETAL ANATOMY AND PHYSIOLOGY

SKELETAL DEVELOPMENT

Bone is derived from mesodermal tissue. The first bone to ossify in the body is the clavicle. Two processes of bone formation occur—*intramembranous and enchondral.*

Intramembranous Ossification

Initially, a model is formed from condensed mesenchymal cells. These cells then differentiate into two forms: (1) fibroblasts, producing collagen fiber membranes; and (2) osteoblasts, producing osteoid. Subsequently, bone is formed in this fibrous membrane. There is no preformed stage of cartilage. Bones formed by this process include the parietal and temporal bones, squama, and tympanic parts of the temporal bone, upper occipital squamosa, vomer, medial pterygoid, and upper face. The clavicles and mandible are also membranous bones but later develop secondary cartilaginous centers. In normal bones the width of bone is largely controlled by this method, due to the activity of the periosteum (appositional bone growth).

Enchondral Ossification

From the condensed mesenchymal model cartilage cells (chondroblasts and chondrocytes) form and produce a cartilage cast of the definitive bone. Subsequently, this cartilage template is transformed to bone as peripheral capillaries penetrate and induce the formation of osteoblasts. This peripheral collar of new bone then extends bidirectionally along the long axis of the bone. A similar but separate process occurs within epiphyseal centers. This process is responsible for the formation of all tubular bones, vertebrae, ethmoids, and inferior conchae. This method of ossification is primarily used to lengthen long bones after birth, until skeletal maturity.

BONE STRUCTURE

The anatomic structure of bone includes various divisions—epiphysis, physis, zone of provisional calcification, metaphysis, and diaphysis. (Fig. 7.16) In addition, two types of bone are identifiable—*cortical* and *medullary.* These are encased by an outer covering of invisible periosteum.

Epiphysis

The end of a growing bone is called an *epiphysis.* Initially composed of cartilage, there is gradual ossification that eventually

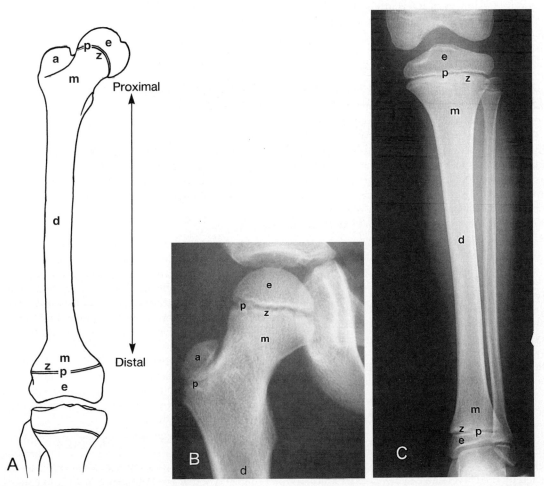

Figure 7.16. GROWING BONE, ANATOMICAL DIVISIONS. A. Diagrammatic Representation. B and C. Radiograph. Observe the epiphysis (*e*), phy- sis (*p*), zone of provisional calcification (*z*), metaphysis (*m*), diaphysis (*d*), and apophysis (*a*).

fuses with the shaft at the end of the growth period. Its primary function is to produce and support the articular cartilage. Pathologically, an epiphysis is prone to dysplasia, ischemia, arthritic deformation, and specific neoplasms such as chondroblastoma and giant cell tumor. Apophyses of bone should also be thought of as epiphyses despite their function as muscle attachments.

Physis

The cartilage growth plate between the epiphysis and metaphysis is known as the *physis*. Alternate terms include *epiphyseal plate*, *epiphyseal growth plate*, and *bone growth center*. There are layers of progressively maturing cartilage and developing bone. Adjacent to the physis a stable zone of resting cells is found, followed by sequential zones of proliferation and hypertrophy. These layers are responsible for providing longitudinal growth of a long bone and remain radiolucent during skeletal development. Altered hormonal or vascular dynamics may decrease or increase growth, producing abnormalities of length such as dwarfism and giantism.

Zone of Provisional Calcification (ZPC)

At the junction of the physis and metaphysis a thin line of increased density is identifiable. This represents the region of calcification of the physis cartilage which is the precursor to bone formation. Calcium disorders, such as rickets, will disturb the appearance of this line. Residuals of intermittent growth arrest from systemic disease may be seen later in life as transverse, opaque metaphyseal lines (growth arrest lines).

Metaphysis

Between the zone of provisional calcification and diaphysis lies the metaphysis. The metaphysis is the most metabolically active region of a bone and, as a result, is the most common site for tumors and infections of bone. In this location calcified cartilage is transformed into definitive weight-bearing stress trabeculae (primary trabeculae) and supporting transverse or oblique trabeculae (secondary trabeculae). Additionally, as part of this process the constricting tubulation of the bone occurs by periosteal resorption. Abnormalities of tubulation result in underconstriction or undertubulation of the metaphysis (Erlenmeyer flask deformity). (Fig. 7.17)

Diaphysis

This lies between both metaphyses and is the longest part of the bone. It is also known as the shaft of the bone. The most notable feature of the diaphysis is the thickened cortex and decreased medullary space. Its main function is to provide mechanical strength and contain the bone marrow. Abnormalities of the diaphysis include marrow diseases such as multiple myeloma, Ewing's sarcoma, non-Hodgkin's lymphoma, adamantinoma, and infection.

Cortex

The densest and strongest of all bone is the cortex. It is constructed of densely packed compact lamellar bone and osteons and is interconnected by the Haversian canal systems. Externally, it is enveloped by the periosteum and lined internally with endosteum. Its thickness and integrity are a strong radiological in-

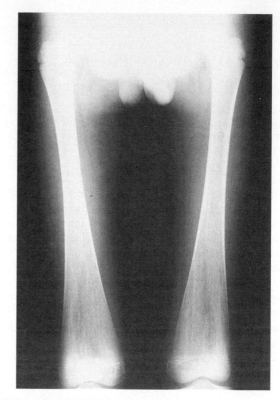

Figure 7.17. ERLENMEYER FLASK DEFORMITY. A lack of the normal metaphyseal/diaphyseal constriction is characteristic of this deformity, due to a undertubulation of the metaphysis. Although present in a number of disorders, this is most notable in Gaucher's disease.

dicator in the diagnosis of bone tumors, infections, and other disorders.

Medulla

The internal cavity of bone is traversed by thin, interconnecting trabeculae (spongiosa) and contains the bone marrow. In children red marrow predominates in all bones. Adults exhibit red marrow only in the axial skeleton, epiphyses, and metaphyses.

Periosteum

A thin membrane of tissue envelops the diaphysis and metaphysis of bone and is called the *periosteum*. Epiphyseal periosteum does not exist. In children periosteum is attached only at the metaphysis, while in adults a firm attachment is made at the metaphysis and diaphysis. Histologically, two layers are evident—an outer fibrous and an inner cambium layer. The fibrous layer functions to provide the mechanical means of attachment of itself, tendons, and ligaments by way of Sharpey's fibers. The inner cambium layer is metabolically labile, containing osteoblastic and osteoclastic potential. This inner zone may therefore produce or resorb bone, in response to a pulling away from the underlying bone by pus, blood, or tumors, and is an important indicator of bone disease.

Endosteum

All trabeculae and inner cortical margins are covered with a single layer that has both osteoclastic and osteoblastic properties. At the cortex a balance between the outer periosteum and inner endosteum maintains cortical thickness.

BONE METABOLISM

Bone metabolism is a complex and dynamic process. Many factors are responsible in promoting or reducing bone activity. The discussion to follow focuses on the effects of minerals and hormones active in normal and abnormal conditions.

Bone Minerals

The major bone minerals are calcium and phosphorus, which usually exist in bone at a ratio of 2:1.

Calcium. Calcium plays numerous roles in body metabolism, including muscle and nerve function. Within bone, calcium forms many different complexes, especially with phosphorus. The main calcium–phosphorus complex is that of crystalline hydroxyapatite—$Ca_{10}(PO_4)_6(OH)_2$. Less than 1% of bone calcium is readily available for turnover at any particular time. The most active sites are at the Haversian canal linings and resorption cavities. The major factors controlling calcium deposition include mechanical stress, vitamin D, parathormone, trace minerals, and alkaline phosphatase.

Phosphorus. Serum levels of phosphorus are inversely related to calcium. The role of phosphorus is to allow precipitation of calcium at the bone crystal surface.

Hormones

Parathormone (PTH). Produced by the parathyroid gland, PTH functions to increase serum calcium by promoting bone, kidney, and gut resorption of calcium. In bone this is accomplished by increasing osteoclastic activity. In addition, phosphorus levels are decreased.

Calcitonin. Its origin is uncertain, though the thyroid and parathyroid glands are likely sites. It is directly antagonistic to PTH by acting to decrease serum calcium levels by reversed effects on the skeleton, kidney, and gut.

Estrogen. Produced by the ovarian follicle, its presence stimulates bone production by inducing protein anabolic activity. It closely controls longitudinal growth and maturity.

Androgen. This is the male counterpart of estrogen. It is produced in the testes and adrenal cortex and controls longitudinal growth and maturity.

Growth Hormone (GH). Arising from the acidophilic cells of the anterior pituitary, GH controls the chondrocyte proliferation and hypertrophy at the growth plate. An absence of GH in the growing period produces dwarfism; an excess of GH produces giantism. If an excess is present in an adult, acromegaly results, with increased membranous ossification in the skull and mandible and subperiostally in long bones. Additionally, joint cartilage proliferates and degenerates prematurely.

Glucocorticoids. The most important glucocorticoid with effects on bone is hydrocortisone. It induces protein catabolism and phosphorus excretion and therefore encourages osteoclasis. Strong gluconeogenic influences also have the potential to produce diabetes.

THE CATEGORICAL APPROACH TO BONE DISEASE

To assist the correlation of film findings with probable diagnoses the mnemonic "CATBITES" proposed by Howe is useful. (41) Each letter corresponds to a specific category of skeletal disease: **C**:Congenital; **A**:Arthritis; **T**:Trauma; **B**:Blood; **I**:Infection; **T**:Tumor; **E**:Endocrine; **S**:Soft tissue. (Table 7.3) An attempt

Table 7.3. The Categories of Bone Disease ("CATBITES")
Congenital
Arthritis
Trauma
Blood (Hematologic)
Infection
Tumor
Endocrine, Nutritional, Metabolic
Soft Tissue

to approach a given abnormality by using this framework will greatly simplify the process of including and excluding different entities.

CONGENITAL

This includes localized and generalized skeletal anomalies. Localized anomalies include segmentation defects in the spine (block vertebrae, hemivertebrae), pelvic faults such as congenital hip dysplasia and limb variations such as polydactyly. Generalized congenital dysplasias include achondroplasia, osteopetrosis, and cleidocranial dysplasia.

ARTHRITIS

Joint afflictions manifest by alterations in various articular components, including the bony ends, articular surfaces and cartilage, joint cavities, and periarticular soft tissues. By identifying these changes in the joint a diagnosis can often be reached. The "**ABCs**" method (**A**lignment, **B**one, **C**artilage, **S**oft tissues) is directly applicable to the analysis of joint disease. Alignment disturbances such as ulnar deviation of the digits in the hand suggests rheumatoid arthritis, whereas anterolisthesis of a vertebral body suggests a defect in the posterior arch such as spondylolysis, facet joint arthrosis, or fracture-dislocation. Bone changes are key markers of joint disease; juxtaarticular osteopenia suggests inflammatory arthropathy such as rheumatoid arthritis, whereas sclerosis indicates a mechanical arthropathy, most commonly degenerative joint disease. Cartilage effects are reflected in joint space integrity, with uniform loss of joint space being found in inflammatory joint disease, whereas nonuniform loss is a sign of degenerative causes. Soft tissue clues may include swelling (inflammatory arthritis, rheumatoid arthritis), masses (deposition arthropathies, gout, amyloid) or calcification (calcinosis, scleroderma).

TRAUMA

Traumatic injuries include fractures, subluxations, dislocations, and soft tissue abnormalities such as myositis ossificans.

BLOOD

This category encompasses those abnormalities that are characterized by their origins within the bone marrow, such as the various hemolytic anemias or an absence of blood supply typified by epiphyseal avascular necrosis (osteonecrosis).

INFECTION

Disorders of infective processes in bone (osteomyelitis) and joints (septic arthritis) may be difficult to differentiate from tumors but usually can be suggested, given pertinent clinical features, and recognized by key radiologic signs.

TUMOR

Neoplastic conditions, whether benign or malignant, can be recognized by their destructive and productive features. The recognition that a lesion has neoplastic characteristics excludes other categories as being possible considerations except in isolated instances.

ENDOCRINE, NUTRITIONAL, METABOLIC

This is a broad category that contains a number of entities such as nutritional osteopenias (scurvy, rickets, etc.) and parathyroid and hormonal diseases.

SOFT TISSUES

Systematic analysis of the soft tissues can reveal abnormalities of clinical significance. Masses can be clues to tumors such as lipoma, myomas, and neuromas; arthropathies such as rheumatoid, gout, or amyloid; traumatic lesions such as hematoma; and infections such as an abscess or cellulitis. Calcifications may be linked to dermatomyositis, lupus, or scleroderma, parasitic infestation, tumor, or myositis ossificans.

RADIOLOGIC PREDICTOR VARIABLES

A number of methodologies in the assessment of skeletal abnormalities have been suggested. (42,43) A computer-assisted approach based on standard criteria has also been developed. (44,45) A systematic step-by-step analysis is the optimum method to arrive at an appropriate diagnosis. (Table 7.4) One of the most important decisions based on the accumulated data is to differentiate between slow and aggressive lesions. (Table 7.5)

Table 7.4.   Radiologic Predictor Variables

PRELIMINARY ANALYSIS
Clinical data: age, sex, race, history
Number of lesions
Symmetry of lesions
Systems involved
ANALYSIS OF THE LESION
Skeletal location
Position within bone
Site of origin
Shape
Size
Margination
Cortical integrity
Behavior of the lesion
Matrix
Periosteal response
Soft tissue changes
Joint changes
SUPPLEMENTARY ANALYSIS
Other radiologic procedures
Laboratory examination
Biopsy

Table 7.5.   Radiologic Criteria of Benign and Aggressive Lesions

	Benign	Aggressive Primary	Aggressive Secondary
Age (Decades)	123	1234567	4567
Size:			
0–6 cm	+++	+	+
6+ cm	+	+++	+++
Monostotic	+++	+++	++
Polyostotic	+	+	+++
Cortical destruction	−	+++	+++
Periosteal reaction			
Solid	+++	+	−
Laminated	++	++	−
Spiculated	−	+++	+
Codman's	++	++	+
Destruction			
Geographic	+++	+	−
Motheaten	−	+++	+++
Permeative	−	+++	+++
Margins			
Sharp	+++	+	+
Imperceptible	−	+++	+++
Matrix	+++	++	−
Soft tissue mass	−	+++	+
Joint space	−	−	−

− Absent
+ Occasionally
++ Common
+++ Very common

PRELIMINARY ANALYSIS
Clinical Data

Age.   Many disorders exhibit peak ages and age ranges of occurrence. For example, bone tumors such as osteosarcoma, Ewing's sarcoma, and aneurysmal bone cyst are most common under the age of 20 years. Over 50 years of age, disorders such as Paget's disease, metastasis, and multiple myeloma become more common. Knowledge of these age predilections greatly assists in forming diagnostic possibilities.

Sex.   Similarly, some disorders exhibit a sex predominance. Examples of male prevalences include Paget's disease, gout, ankylosing spondylitis, Reiter's syndrome (46), and hemophilia. Female-dominated disorders include osteoporosis, systemic lupus erythematosus, osteitis condensans ilii, and rheumatoid arthritis.

Race.   Certain racial populations are predisposed to some skeletal diseases. Sickle cell anemia in blacks and thalassemia in Italian and other Mediterranean populations are classic examples.

History.   An accurate current history is vital to radiologic interpretation. Specific information such as the history of trauma, previous diagnosis and associated conditions, and pain and swelling often dictates the follow-up procedures necessary to confirm or disprove the suspected diagnosis.

Number of Lesions

Numerous disorders may be polyostotic (multiple bones) or monostotic (single bone). (Table 7.6) Polyostotic bone disease includes congenital dysplasias, fibrous dysplasia, Paget's disease, metastatic disease, multiple myeloma, and histiocytoses. (Fig. 7.18) Solitary sites of involvement are usually indicative of a bone tumor or infection. This is an important feature to demonstrate, since the differential possibilities change greatly according to the number of sites affected.

Symmetry of Lesions

Symmetrical and equally distributed skeletal lesions are usually due to disseminated diseases that interfere with bone function and metabolism, such as hyperparathyroidism, osteomalacia, osteoporosis, and leukemia. Asymmetric, haphazardly arranged lesions suggest chance seeding of lesions, such as in metastasis and Paget's disease.

Determination of Systems Involved

If only bone involvement is present, then numerous disorders can be excluded, such as hyperparathyroidism and metastasis. Singular involvement of bone is distinctive of benign bone tumors, occasionally Paget's disease, and selected congenital disorders.

ANALYSIS OF THE LESION

Careful scrutiny of a lesion according to the following criteria will aid in arriving at a diagnosis and will provide clinical insight into its present and possible future behavior.

Skeletal Location

Statistical evaluations of bone lesions, especially tumors, reveal a frequent site predilection. (Table 7.7) For example, most cases of chordoma selectively involve the sacrum and skull base, while osteosarcoma is predominantly encountered around the knee. Knowledge of these common sites of occurrence aid greatly in making a diagnosis.

Table 7.6. Monostotic Versus Polyostotic Bone Disease		
	Monostotic	Polyostotic
CONGENITAL	Block vertebra	Bone dysplasia
	Polydactyly	Achondroplasia
TRAUMATIC	Localized injury	Battered child
		Severe injury
ARTHRITIS	Degenerative joint disease	Rheumatoid arthritis
TUMOR	Osteoid osteoma	Multiple myeloma
	Osteosarcoma	Metastasis
INFECTION	Staphylococcal	Salmonella
HEMATOLOGIC	Perthes disease	Sickle cell anemia
NUTRITIONAL	None	Hyperparathyroidism
METABOLIC		Rickets, scurvy
ENDOCRINE		

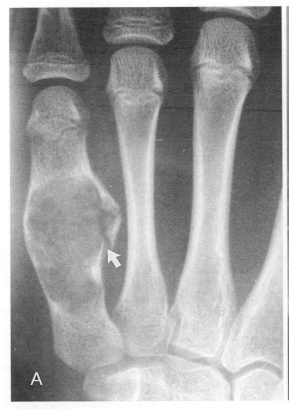
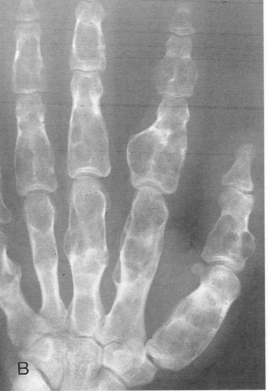

Figure 7.18. MONOSTOTIC AND POLYOSTOTIC BONE DISEASE. A. Monostotic Lesion. A solitary osteolytic lesion is present in the fifth metacarpal. Observe the pathologic fracture in this enchondroma (arrow). **B. Polyostotic Lesions.** Multiple expansile osteolytic lesions are seen through-out all metacarpals and phalanges. Similar changes were present in the opposite hand, feet, and long bones in this patient with multiple enchondromatosis (Ollier's disease).

Table 7.7.   Most Common Locations of Bone Tumors

	Tumor	Skeletal Sites
MALIGNANT	Adamantinoma	Mandible, tibia
	Chondrosarcoma	Pelvis, scapula, sternum, femur, humerus
	Chordoma	Sacrococcygeal, skull base, C2 body
	Ewing's sarcoma	Pelvis, femur, humerus
	Fibrosarcoma	Femur, tibia
	Multiple myeloma	Pelvis, spine, sternum, femur, humerus
	Osteosarcoma	Femur, tibia, humerus
	Parosteal sarcoma	Femur
	Non-Hodgkin's lymphoma	Femur, humerus, pelvis, spine
QUASIMALIGNANT	Giant cell tumor	Femur, tibia, radius
BENIGN	Aneurysmal bone cyst	Femur, tibia, humerus, neural arch
	Bone island	Pelvis, femur
	Chondroblastoma	Humerus, femur
	Chondromyxoid fibroma	Tibia, rib, ulna
	Enchondroma	Metacarpal, phalanges, metatarsals, femur
	Fibrous cortical defect	Femur, tibia
	Hemangioma	Spine, skull
	Nonossifying fibroma	Femur, tibia
	Osteoblastoma	Femur, humerus, neural arch
	Osteochondroma	Femur, tibia, humerus
	Osteoid osteoma	Femur, tibia, neural arch
	Osteoma	Sinuses, skull
	Simple bone cyst	Humerus, femur, calcaneus

Table 7.8.   Tumor Positions in Bone

	Benign	Malignant
EPIPHYSEAL	Chondroblastoma Giant cell tumor	Giant cell tumor
EPIPHYSEAL—METAPHYSEAL	Aneurysmal bone cyst Giant cell tumor	Giant cell tumor Metastasis
METAPHYSEAL	Bone island Enchondroma Fibrous cortical defect Nonossifying fibroma Osteoid osteoma Osteochondroma Simple bone cyst	Chondrosarcoma Fibrosarcoma Metastasis Osteosarcoma
METAPHYSEAL—DIAPHYSEAL	Chondromyxoid fibroma Nonossifying fibroma Osteoid osteoma	Chondrosarcoma Metastasis Osteosarcoma Multiple myeloma
DIAPHYSEAL	Osteoid osteoma Latent bone cyst	Adamantinoma Ewing's sarcoma Metastasis Multiple myeloma Non-Hodgkin's lymphoma

Position Within Bone

Specific lesions are found in the various anatomic divisions of bone. (Table 7.8) (Fig. 7.19) In the epiphysis congenital dysplasia, ischemic necrosis, and neoplasms such as chondroblastoma and giant cell tumor occur. Metaphyseal lesions are the most common due to the high metabolic rate and high vascularity of the region. Diaphyseal disorders usually are related to marrow disease such as multiple myeloma, Ewing's sarcoma, and non-Hodgkin's lymphoma ("round cell" tumors).

Site of Origin

Important clues to the diagnosis can be obtained by attempting to designate the tissue site of origin within the bone. (Fig. 7.20)

Medullary.   These lesions are mostly centric in location. There may be evidence of scalloping and thinning of the cortex from the endosteal surface, a sign that is often found associated with fibrous and cartilaginous lesions. (Fig. 7.20A)

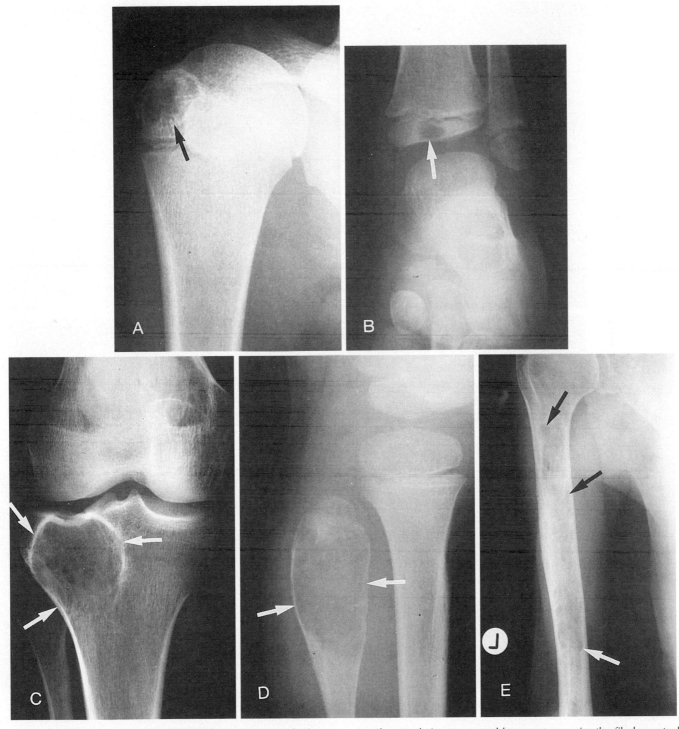

Figure 7.19.   LOCATIONS OF LESIONS WITHIN BONE. A. Apophysis. An apophysis is analogous to an epiphysis and is therefore prone to developing similar lesions. Observe the osteolytic lesion in the greater tuberosity of this 10-year-old patient, a chondroblastoma (arrow). **B. Epiphysis.** A well-defined osteolytic lesion is evident within the distal tibial epiphysis of this 7-year-old patient, also a chondroblastoma (arrow). **C. Epiphyseal-Metaphyseal.** Within the lateral tibial epiphysis and metaphysis a sharply circumscribed abnormality is present—a giant cell tumor (arrows). **D. Metaphysis.** An ex- pansile, osteolytic, aneurysmal bone cyst occupies the fibular metaphysis (arrows). Note that the epiphysis is unaffected. **E. Diaphysis.** Multiple, sharply demarcated, osteolytic lesions are present throughout the humeral diaphysis. Note the inner cortical destruction (endosteal scalloping), indi- cating the medullary origins of the tumor (arrows); in this case, multiple myeloma. COMMENT: Knowledge of locational predispositions greatly en- hances the observer's diagnostic accuracy.

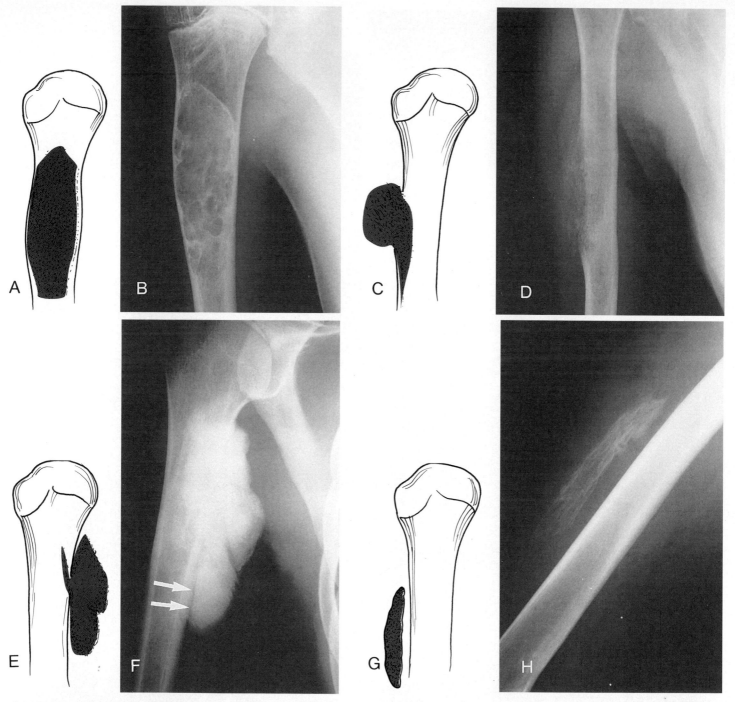

Figure 7.20.   SITES OF ORIGIN. A and B. Medullary. Note the central location, slight expansion, thin but intact cortex, and scalloped endosteal margin. Diagnosis: *Simple bone cyst* (unicameral bone cyst). **C and D. Cortical.** Note the eccentric location, cortical destruction, and periosteal new bone formation. Diagnosis: *Ewing's sarcoma.* **E and F. Periosteal.** A dense soft tissue mass is the dominant feature, with no evidence of bone destruc-

tion. Observe the thin, separating, radiolucent cleft between the mass and cortex (arrows) indicating its extracortical origin. Diagnosis: *Periosteal osteosarcoma.* (Courtesy of Friedrich H. W. Heuck, MD, Stuttgart, West Germany) **G and H. Extraosseous.** A well-demarcated soft tissue lesion is visible which demonstrates cortical and trabecular bone. Diagnosis: *Traumatic myositis ossificans* of the anterior thigh.

Cortical. The most distinctive feature is the frequent eccentric position in at least one projection of the lesion. (Fig. 7.20B) Notably, there is usually destruction, distortion, or expansion of the cortical bone. These lesions commonly provoke an overlying periosteal response. Cortical lesions are more readily identifiable than medullary lesions. (Fig. 7.21)

Periosteal. These are typified by their close apposition but definite separation from the majority of the underlying bone.

There is usually a notable lesion in the soft tissues but very little actual bony abnormality. (Fig. 7.20C)

Extraosseous. The abnormality is conspicuous by its distant location from the bone or adjacent cleft that separates the mass from the cortical surface. (Fig. 7.20D) Sites of origin include muscle, nerves, arteries, and synovium. A large extraosseous mass may produce an extrinsic pressure atrophy of bone conspicuous by the presence of a sclerotic rim.

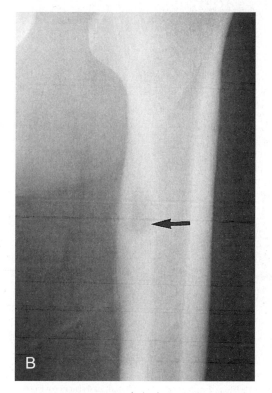

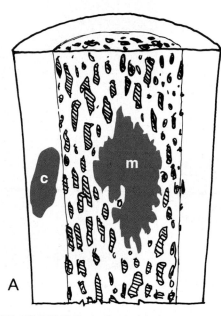

Figure 7.21.   VISIBILITY OF LESIONS. A. Cortical lesions (*c*) are more readily identified than medullary lesions (*m*) because of the surrounding compact bone. **B.** A localized cortical lesion in the femur is easily recognized (arrow). Diagnosis: Brodie's abscess. (Courtesy of Steven P. Brownstein, MD, Springfield, New Jersey)

Shape

Benign, slow-growing lesions are usually elongated along the axis of the bone ("long lesion in a long bone"). (Fig. 7.22) Typical examples include fibrous dysplasia, nonossifying fibroma, and unicameral bone cyst. Rapidly growing lesions can be pleomorphic and do not exhibit definitive morphologic shapes. Shapes of lesions must not be considered as a reliable differential sign between slow- and fast-developing abnormalities.

Size

Size of a lesion can be useful. Most benign tumors are under 6 cm in size at the time of discovery, while aggressive lesions tend to be larger. Exceptions to this rule include benign conditions such as aneurysmal bone cyst, simple bone cyst, giant cell tumor, and fibrous dysplasia, all of which may be very large at the initial examination.

Margination

The peripheral margins of a lesion closely reflect its growth rate. Two terms are used to describe this zone of transition into normal bone—*imperceptible* and *sharp*. (Fig. 7.23)

Imperceptible Margination.   Other terms that are commonly used include *poor, hazy,* and *ill-defined margins,* or *a wide zone of transition.* The gradation between the lesion and normal bone occurs gradually, with no distinct demarcating line or change in density. (Fig. 7.23A and B) This type of boundary is indicative of aggressive bone destruction such as that seen in infections and malignant tumors.

Sharp Margins.   Synonyms include *definite* and *sclerotic margins* or *a narrow zone of transition.* The interface between the lesion and normal bone is clearly identified and may be outlined by a

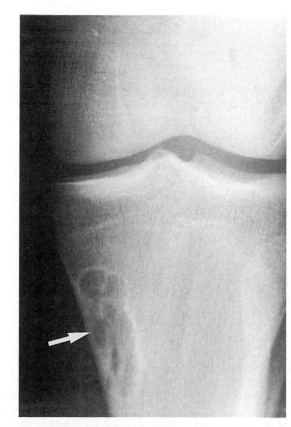

Figure 7.22.   LONG LESION IN A LONG BONE. This eccentrically placed, well-defined radiolucent lesion displays typical features of a slowly developing neoplasm which is distorted with long bone growth (arrow). Note that the length far exceeds its width. Diagnosis: Nonossifying fibroma.

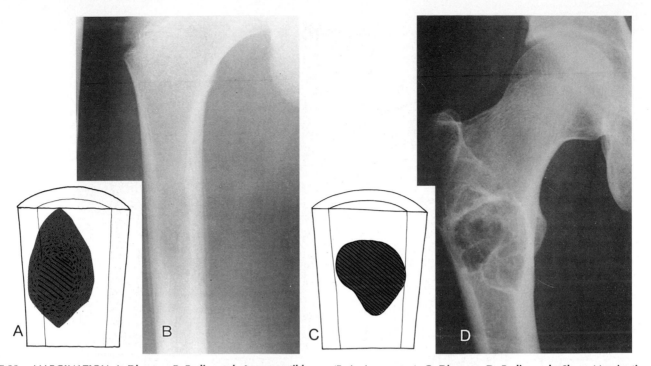

Figure 7.23.   MARGINATION. A. Diagram. B. Radiograph: Imperceptible Margination. A motheaten osteolytic lesion is present in the medullary cavity, with some adjacent endosteal destruction. It is difficult to perceive where the lesion begins and ends, which is typical of an aggressive abnormality (Ewing's sarcoma). **C. Diagram. D. Radiograph: Sharp Margination.** Conversely, this geographic lesion exhibits a conspicuous zone of transition accentuated by the sclerotic margin. This appearance usually denotes a contained, slowly growing lesion which, in this case, was fibrous dysplasia.

sclerotic line. (Fig. 7.23C and D) This type of bone abnormality is usually slow growing, such as in fibrous dysplasia and simple bone cyst.

Cortical Integrity

A key factor in assessing the growth rate of a bone lesion is the integrity of the cortex. A number of appearances may occur—thinning, thickening, expansion, destruction, and fracture. (Fig. 7.24)

Cortical Thinning.   Normally, the cortex gradually thins toward the metaphysis and remains uniform into the epiphysis. (Fig. 7.24A) Osteoporosis generally thins all cortices (pencil thin). Localized thinning is seen in lesions such as tumors. When the inside surface of the cortex is eroded and undulated, it is referred to as *endosteal scalloping* and is frequently seen in medullary tumors such as enchondroma and multiple myeloma. Thinning without loss of integrity usually denotes slow growth of the abnormality.

Cortical Thickening.   This may occur either locally or generally within a bone. (Fig. 7.24B) Localized causes include osteoid osteoma and stress fracture due to periosteal and endosteal appositional new bone. The classic disorder to thicken cortices is Paget's disease, due to disordered bone remodeling.

Cortical Expansion.   Bulging of an intact cortex outward is a sign of slow but continued growth. (Fig. 7.24C) The outer cortex represents a balance between continuous erosion from within and periosteal new bone on the outside. Generally, this is a sign of a benign lesion but can be seen in slow-growing malignant tumors.

Cortical Destruction.   Disruption of the cortical bone is a strong indicator of aggressive bone disease. (Fig. 7.24D) This is usually easier to identify than destruction within the medullary cavity. Manifestations of cortical destruction include loss of definition and identifiable permeative or motheaten lesions.

Fracture.   A sharp, irregular radiolucent line is visible, creating discontinuity of the cortical surface. (Fig. 7.24E)

BEHAVIOR OF LESION

Bone lesions are of three types—osteolytic, osteoblastic, or mixed. (Table 7.9)

Osteolytic Lesions

These are typified by their loss of localized bone structure and density. It is the subtle loss of bone density that is the most difficult to perceive of all patterns of bone disease. Neoplastic bone destruction is due to pressure or hyperemia-generated osteoclastic resorption, not direct tumor lysis. (47) As a result, these lesions are radiolucent on radiologic examination. Three patterns of bone destruction are identified—geographic, motheaten, and permeative—which may occur separately but usually in varying degrees of combination. (44,47) (Fig. 7.25)

Geographic Lesions.   Other terms used are circumscribed or uniformly lytic lesion. (Fig. 7.25A and B) The morphologic criteria of geographic lesions are that they are usually solitary, are greater than 1 cm, and have a sharp margin. Occasionally, multiple geographic lesions may occur. Internal septations (trabeculation) may isolate separate chambers, giving a "soap bubble" appearance. (Fig. 7.26) In general, geographic lesions are slower-growing abnormalities.

Motheaten Lesions.   Multiple, poorly marginated, small, or moderately sized (2 to 5 mm) lucencies are characteristic of this pattern. (Fig. 7.25C and D) Frequently, the margins of each lesion are ragged and irregular. Confluence with adjacent lesions is

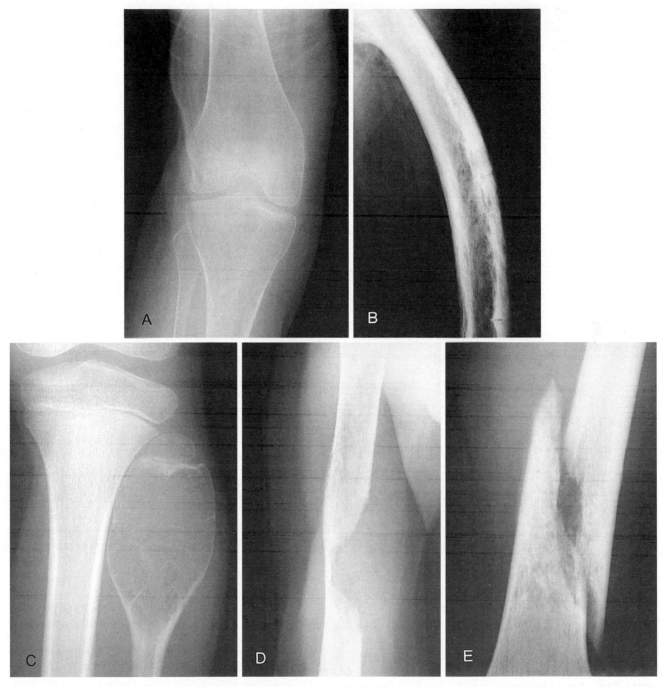

Figure 7.24.   CORTICAL INTEGRITY. A. Thinning. There is extreme thinning of all visible cortices (''pencil thin'') and generalized demineralization of all bones in this patient with *osteoporosis*. **B. Thickening.** The two cortices are grossly thickened, with compromise of the adjacent medullary space. Additionally, the bone is deformed and has transverse lucencies on its convex surface (pseudofractures), all consistent with the diagnosis of *Paget's disease.* **C. Expansion.** Note the thin bulging but intact cortex of the proximal fibula. This represents continued endosteal erosion and periosteal deposition, with continued growth of the lesion. Diagnosis: *Aneurysmal bone cyst.* **D. Destruction.** Disruption of the cortex is indicative of an aggressive bone lesion; in this case, from *metastatic carcinoma.* **E. Fracture.** An oblique fracture line and disruption of the cortex is readily identified through a *malignant* lesion.

Table 7.9. Radiologic Features of Lesion Behavior
OSTEOLYTIC BEHAVIOR
Geographic Lesion
Solitary
Greater than 1 cm
Sharp margin
Motheaten lesion
Multiple
2–5 mm
Ragged margins and coalescence
Imperceptible transition
Permeative Lesion
Multiple
Less than 1 mm
Imperceptible transition
OSTEOBLASTIC BEHAVIOR
Diffuse Lesion
Homogenously sclerotic ("ivory")
Obliterated corticomedullary junction
Localized Lesion
Single or multiple
Irregular, hazy border
Asymmetrical
MIXED BEHAVIOR
Both osteolytic and osteoblastic features

common. This type of destruction reflects an aggressive abnormality such as lytic metastatic bone disease or osteomyelitis.

Permeative Lesions. Numerous tiny, pinhole-sized lucencies (less than 1 mm) constitute the permeative pattern. (Fig. 7.25E and F) A wide zone of transition is evident. These lesions are frequently overlooked because of their size, and with progression may enlarge enough to become motheaten in character. They are usually seen in the most rapidly aggressive malignant bone tumors.

Osteoblastic Lesions

These show increased density due to an overproduction of bone or calcium laden tissue. (Fig. 7.27) These may be diffuse ivory-like or localized ("snowball"). Examples include blastic metastasis, osteosarcoma, and Paget's disease.

Mixed Lesions

Both lytic and blastic patterns are evident. (Fig. 7.28) The most common cause is mixed metastasis.

MATRIX

The dominant internal extracellular substance of a lesion is termed the matrix. Radiologically, the matrix can be determined based on its appearance. (48,49) (Table 7.10)

Fat. Intraosseous fat matrix (lipoma) cannot as a rule be suggested on plain films but occasionally may have central calcification. (Fig. 7.29) Soft tissue lipomas, however, can be identified due to the relatively low contrast with surrounding muscle. CT scanning will be definitive in both instances in identifying the low-density fat.

Cartilage. Cartilaginous matrix frequently calcifies in distinct patterns that are readily identifiable. (49) (Fig. 7.30)

Stippled Calcification. Small, discrete, spotty densities typify this variety. (Fig. 7.30A) It represents localized dense mineralization of hyaline cartilage. This type is best identified in enchondroma.

Flocculent Calcification. Larger but still spotty densities represent confluence of stippled regions. (Fig. 7.30B) As a result, floccules and stipples may be seen together.

Arc and Ring Calcification. Thin, eggshell-like curvilinear calcifications occur at the periphery of mature cartilage lobules. (Fig. 7.30C) This is usually seen in chondrosarcoma.

Osseous. Bone production by tumors shows varying degrees of density from diffuse to hazy or very dense (ivory-like). (Fig. 7.31) The most characteristic bone-producing tumor is osteosarcoma.

Fibrous. Fibrous matrix lesions are difficult to identify, since the internal density changes may be subtle. (Fig. 7.32) The most definitive feature is the "smoky" or hazy internal density. Some have referred to it as the *ground glass* appearance. (50) This type of matrix is usually identified in fibrous dysplasia.

PERIOSTEAL RESPONSE

Periosteal new bone is an important radiologic feature seen in many abnormalities, especially infection and tumor. Generally, a *radiographic latent period* of between 10 to 21 days following the initial stimulus is necessary before it can be identified on the radiograph. (51) The stimulus to produce periosteal new bone may be due to subperiosteal extensions of blood, pus, or tumor. These migrate beneath the periosteum by way of the Haversian canals, which freely intercommunicate throughout the cortex and into the medullary cavity. Additional bone-forming irritants include hyperemia, inflammation, and edema. The mechanisms active in these factors inducing periosteal new bone formation by the inner cambium layer are complex. Proposed mechanisms include the physical elevation of the periosteum away from the cortical bone, compensation to underlying destruction, tumor containment, hyperemia, and tumor-secreted osteogenic substances. (51) Whatever the stimulus, three basic periosteal patterns of new bone formation are encountered—*solid, laminated, and spiculated.* (Table 7.11) (Fig. 7.33)

Solid Response

A *solid* periosteal response is defined as a continuous layer of new bone that attaches to the outer cortical surface. (Fig. 7.33A and B) Variations of this pattern focus on its shape and external contour. For example, a localized reaction may render the external contour elliptical in shape. In some instances the surface may be undulating. Despite these deviations a solid pattern is readily identified and typically is related to a very slow form of irritation. Disorders associated include osteoid osteoma, stress fracture, venous stasis, and hypertrophic osteoarthropathy.

Laminated Response

Alternative terms include *lamellated, layered,* and *onion-skin.* The most conspicuous feature is the alternating layers of lucent and opaque densities on the external bone surface. (Fig. 7.33C and D) At times only a single lamination will be visible. This pattern can be interpreted as a cyclical variation in growth of the underlying lesion. Histopathologic studies show the radiolucent zones to be filled with prominent dilated blood vessels in loose connective tissue that has not ossified. (51,52) With time, a laminated response may transform to a solid form as the opaque bony

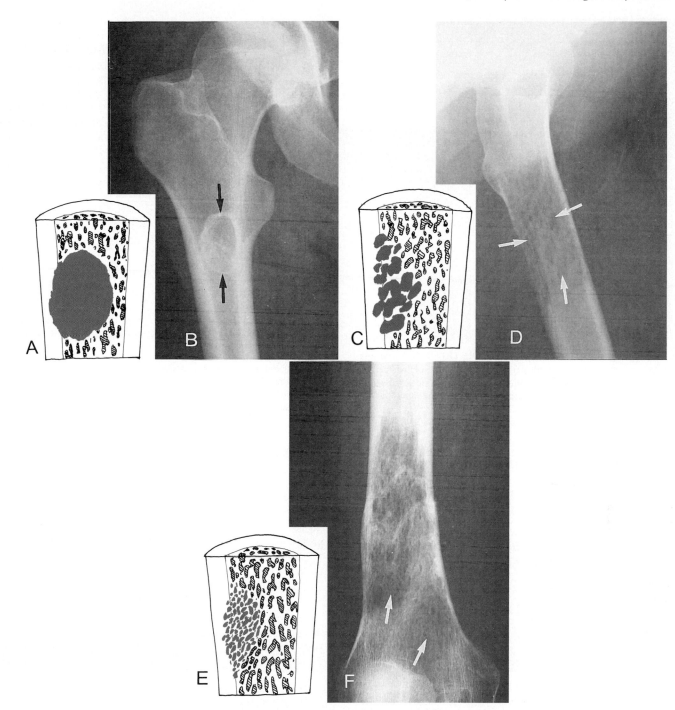

Figure 7.25.   PATTERNS OF OSTEOLYTIC DESTRUCTION. A. Diagram. B. Radiograph: Geographic. A solitary, well-demarcated lesion is seen in the proximal femur (arrows). Diagnosis: *Fibrous dysplasia.* **C. Diagram. D. Radiograph: Motheaten.** Multiple, poorly outlined radiolucencies are visible (arrows). Note the wide zone of transition. Diagnosis: *Metastatic carcinoma.* (Courtesy of Lawrence A. Cooperstein, MD, Pittsburgh, Pennsylvania). **E. Diagram. F. Radiograph: Permeative.** Numerous, tiny, pinhole-sized lesions can be seen (arrows). Diagnosis: *Non-Hodgkin's lymphoma.*

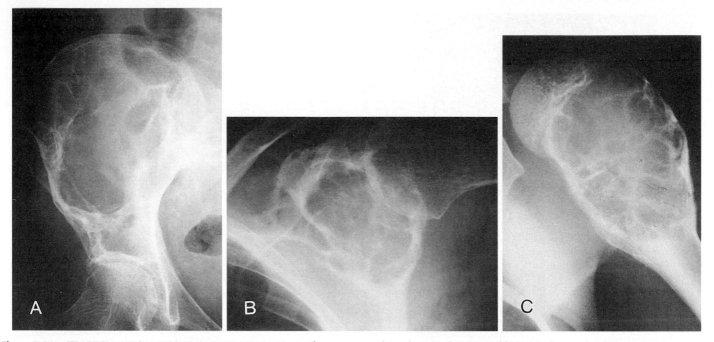

Figure 7.26.   TRABECULATION ("SOAP BUBBLE LESION"). A. Plasmacytoma. Observe the expansile, lightly septated appearance of this lesion in the ilium. **B. Chondrosarcoma.** A similarly appearing lesion involves the subglenoid region of the scapula. **C. Aneurysmal Bone Cyst.** Note the me- taphyseal expansile, septated lesion in the proximal humerus. COMMENT: A trabeculated lesion may be benign or malignant and is found in various bone neoplasms.

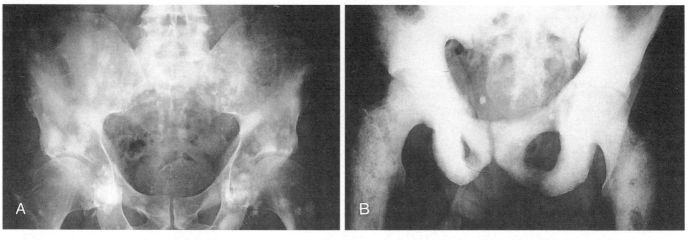

Figure 7.27.   OSTEOBLASTIC METASTATIC PATTERNS. A. Localized. Multiple osteoblastic lesions are seen throughout the pelvis ("snowball"). **B. Diffuse.** All bones demonstrate a generalized increase in bone density ("ivory-like"). COMMENT: The most common primary source for blastic lesions in males is carcinoma of the prostate and in females carcinoma of the breast.

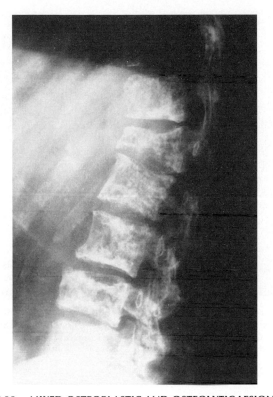

Figure 7.28.   MIXED OSTEOBLASTIC AND OSTEOLYTIC LESIONS. Multiple lytic and blastic changes are seen disseminated throughout the lumbar spine. Diagnosis: Mixed metastatic carcinoma. (Reprinted with permission: Yochum TR, et al: *A radiographic anthology of vertebral names.* J Manipulative Physiol Ther 8:87, June 1985)

Table 7.10.   Radiologic Features of Lesion Matrix

Matrix	Lesion
Fat	Lipoma
Lucent	
Calcification	
Cartilage	Enchondroma, chondrosarcoma
Lucent	
Calcification	
(stipples, floccules, arcs and	
rings)	
Osseous	Osteosarcoma, osteoma
Dense	
Fibrous	Fibrous dysplasia
Hazy (ground glass)	

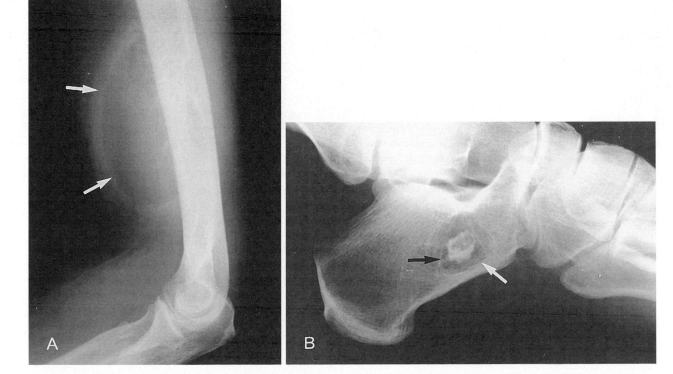

Figure 7.29.   FAT MATRIX. A. Soft Tissue Lipoma. Observe the radiolucent soft tissue lesion on the anterior arm (arrows). **B. Intraosseous Lipoma.** Note the radiolucent lesion (arrows) with central target calcification in the calcaneus. (Courtesy of Steven P. Brownstein, MD, Springfield, New Jersey)

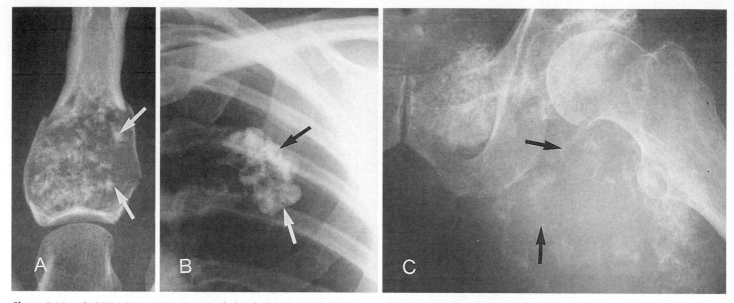

Figure 7.30.   CARTILAGE MATRIX. A. Stippled Calcification. The small, discrete opacities can be identified (arrows). Diagnosis: *Enchondroma* with pathologic fracture. **B. Flocculent Calcification.** Larger, more confluent densities are present at the anterior second rib (arrows). Diagnosis: *Osteochondroma.* **C. Arc and Ring Calcification.** Thin, curvilinear densities typify this type of calcification (arrows). Diagnosis: *Chondrosarcoma.*

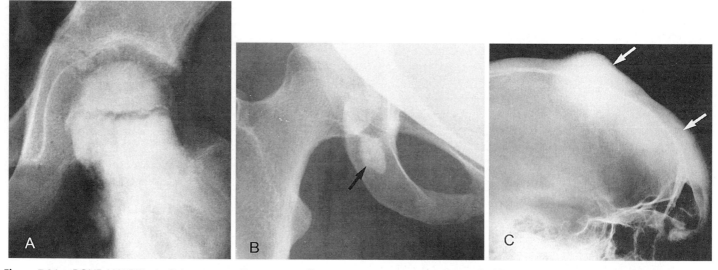

Figure 7.31.   BONE MATRIX. A. Osteosarcoma. Dense, wave-like new bone formation is evident in the proximal femoral metaphysis and epiphysis. **B. Bone Island.** A well-circumscribed, homogenous, opaque lesion is present in the ischium (arrow). The radiopaque density overlying the pelvic basin represents an ovarian shield. (Courtesy of Gary M. Guebert, DC, DACBR, St. Louis, Missouri). **C. Osteoma.** A smooth, dense, and wave-like calvarial overgrowth typifies this lesion of intramembranous bone (arrows).

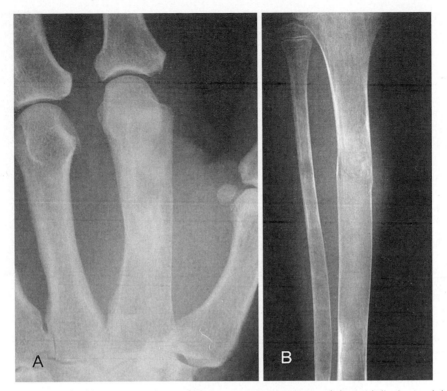

Figure 7.32. FIBROUS MATRIX. A. Note the blurred trabecular markings and the overall "smoky" appearance of the medullary portion of the diaphysis of the second metacarpal. **B.** Observe the cortical thinning and hazy trabecular pattern of the mid-diaphysis of the tibia and fibula. Note the pathologic fracture of the tibia (arrow). The diagnosis in **A** and **B** was fibrous dysplasia.

Table 7.11. Radiologic Features of Periosteal Response	
Pattern	**Lesion**
Solid	Osteoid osteoma
Homogenous, single attached layer	
Laminated	Ewing's sarcoma
Alternating layers of lucency and opacity	
Spiculated	Osteosarcoma
Radiating spicules	
Codman's Triangle	Any
Solid or laminated	

layers thicken and infringe on the adjacent connective tissue. The significance of the laminated response is varied, since it can be seen in slow and aggressive tumors as well as with infections. The classic associated disorder is Ewing's sarcoma.

Spiculated Response

Additional terms include *perpendicular, brushed whiskers,* and *hair-on-end.* (Fig. 7.33E and F) The term *sunburst* has been used to describe radiating spicules of bone from a point source. (Fig. 7.34) The most conspicuous finding is the fine, linear spiculations of new bone oriented perpendicularly away from the cortex. Each spicule is separated from the other by an interposed radiolucent region. (51,53) Frequently, the length of the spicules decreases peripherally away from the midpoint of the lesion. This pattern

of new bone formation is indicative of a very aggressive bone tumor, usually osteosarcoma.

Codman's Triangle

Other synonyms include *Codman's angle, periosteal cuff,* and *periosteal buttress.* First described by Ribbert in 1914, Codman associated the triangle of periosteal new bone at the peripheral lesion-cortex junction as due to subperiosteal extension of the lesion. (54) (Fig. 7.35) This had long been interpreted as a pathognomonic sign of a primary malignant bone tumor but is now known also to be seen accompanying benign tumors, infections, and many other disorders.

SOFT TISSUE CHANGES

Many diagnostic clues can be found in soft tissue changes. Signs of soft tissue abnormality include displaced overlying skin lines, displaced or obliterated myofascial planes, increased density, calcification, and air. (Fig. 7.36) When an adjacent cortex is disrupted in the presence of a soft tissue mass, the diagnosis of an aggressive primary bone tumor is almost certain. Notably, infectious lesions that extend into the soft tissue usually obliterate fascial fat lines due to edema, while tumors displace them.

JOINT CHANGES

Careful scrutiny of adjacent articulations when a bone lesion is found frequently renders helpful information. Generally speaking, tumors do not break the articular cortex, spread into the joint,

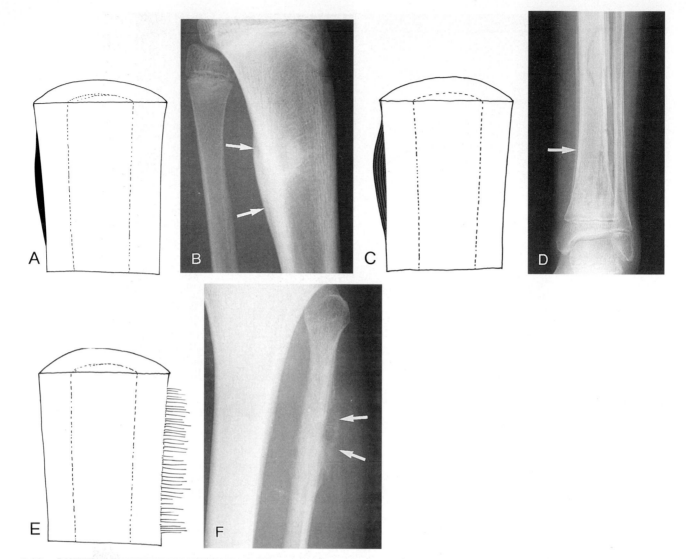

Figure 7.33.   PATTERNS OF PERIOSTEAL RESPONSE. A. Diagram. B. Radiograph: Solid Response. An elliptical, homogenous layer of bone is evident (arrows) adjacent to this stress fracture. **C. Diagram. D. Radiograph: Laminated Response.** Alternating lucent and opaque laminations are seen adjacent to a focus of osteomyelitis (arrow). **E. Diagram. F. Radiograph: Spiculated Response.** Radiating spicules of bone (arrows) characterize this aggressive osteosarcoma.

or involve the opposing articular cortex. This is in direct contrast to infections, which, when in close proximity to a joint, destroy the opposing articular cortices and intervening joint cartilage. (Figs. 7.37, 7.38) This rule applies to all articulations, including the sacroiliac and intervertebral discs.

Essentially, two forms of joint space loss occur—*non-uniform* and *uniform*. (Fig. 7.39) A nonuniform decrease in joint space is defined as only part of a single joint cavity demonstrating a loss in width. This type of localized joint compromise is distinctive for degenerative joint disease. A uniform loss of joint space conversely shows diminution throughout the entire articulation and is suggestive of an inflammatory arthropathy such as rheumatoid arthritis.

Also, certain arthritic disorders have associated bone lesions that may be misinterpreted as tumors. A good example is the subarticular degenerative cyst (geode) that simulates an epiphyseal neoplasm. (Fig. 7.40) The recognition of coexistent articular changes characteristic of degenerative joint disease, however,

makes this misdiagnosis less likely. Other arthritic conditions that may have confusing, coexistent bone lesions include rheumatoid arthritis, gout, and pigmented villonodular synovitis.

SUPPLEMENTARY ANALYSIS

Other Imaging Procedures

The combination of additional modalities with the plain film information will frequently allow a diagnosis to be established. The decision making process as to which modality to employ depends on the clinical scenario and plain film findings. Malignant bone disease, osteomyelitis, stress fractures, and other bone lesions that may be subtle are best investigated initially with bone scan followed by CT of any detected areas of abnormal uptake. Soft tissue, spinal cord-nerve root lesions, and intraarticular derangements are best imaged by MRI. In trauma CT or MRI are best suited.

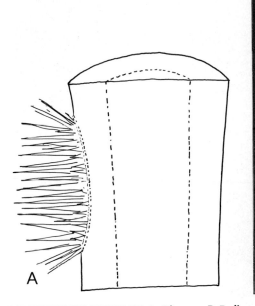

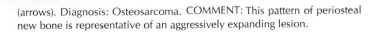

Figure 7.34.   SUNBURST PERIOSTEAL RESPONSE. A. Diagram. B. Radiograph. The periosteal spicules appear to radiate away from a point source (arrows). Diagnosis: Osteosarcoma. COMMENT: This pattern of periosteal new bone is representative of an aggressively expanding lesion.

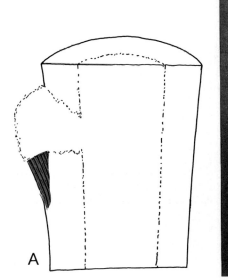

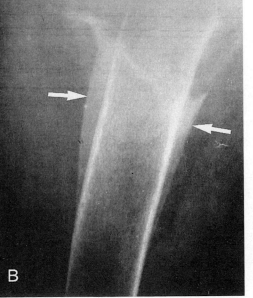

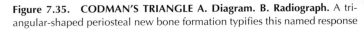

Figure 7.35.   CODMAN'S TRIANGLE A. Diagram. B. Radiograph. A triangular-shaped periosteal new bone formation typifies this named response (arrows) and is a significant but nonspecific finding in many disorders, including infection, neoplasm, and trauma.

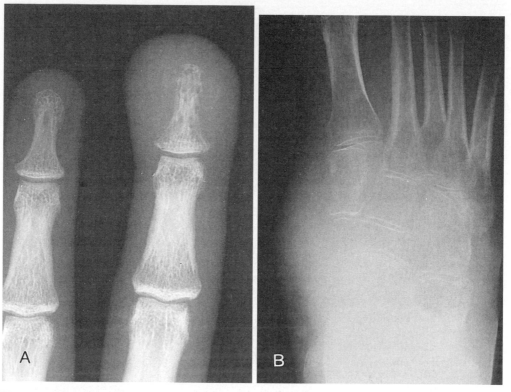

Figure 7.36.   SOFT TISSUE CHANGES. A. Ewing's Sarcoma. Observe the combination of motheaten bone destruction and soft tissue mass in this digit. **B. Malignant Synovioma.** Note the severe bone destruction and large soft tissue mass in the foot. COMMENT: The combination of bone destruction and soft tissue mass makes the diagnosis of primary malignant tumor or infection likely.

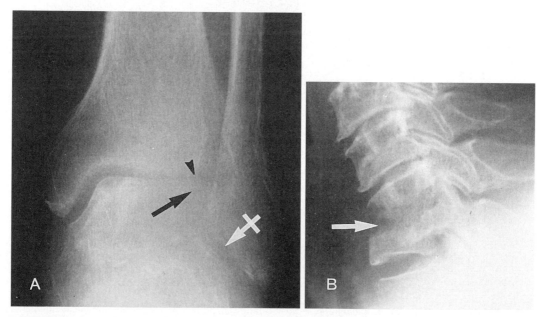

Figure 7.37.   JOINT INFECTION. A. Ankle. Note the destruction of the cortical outlines of the lateral talus (arrow), plafond of the tibia (arrowhead), and distal medial fibula (crossed arrow). **B. Cervical Spine.** Loss of the intervertebral disc height and contiguous vertebral endplates are evident at C6-C7 (arrow). COMMENT: Joint infections distinctively tend to involve both opposing articular cortices ("crossing the joint").

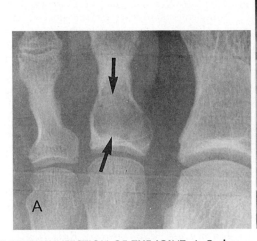
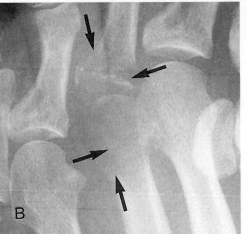

Figure 7.38.   TUMOR VERSUS INFECTION OF THE JOINT. A. Enchondroma. Note the loss of bone density extending to but not beyond the articular cortex (arrows). (Courtesy of David M. Walker, DPM, Melbourne, Australia) **B. Infection.** Observe the lytic destruction of the opposing metatarsal head and proximal phalanx (arrows). COMMENT: This demonstrates the tendency for neoplasms to respect the joint surfaces, while infections readily infiltrate and involve all joint components.

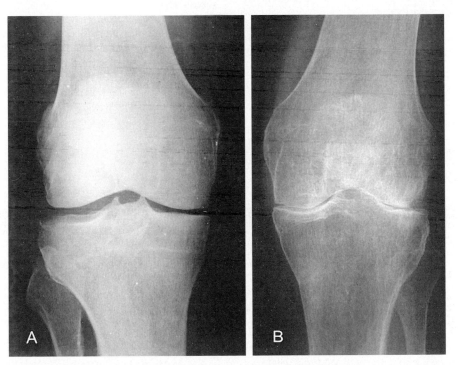

Figure 7.39.   PATTERNS OF JOINT SPACE LOSS. A. Nonuniform. A decreased joint space within the medial compartment of the knee characterizes degenerative joint disease. **B. Uniform.** A decreased joint space of both the medial and lateral compartments of the knee, in contrast, demonstrates typical inflammatory changes such as seen in rheumatoid arthritis. Also, observe the diffuse osteoporosis. COMMENT: No matter where the site of involvement is, the pattern of joint space loss frequently provides the clue to arriving at a definitive diagnosis.

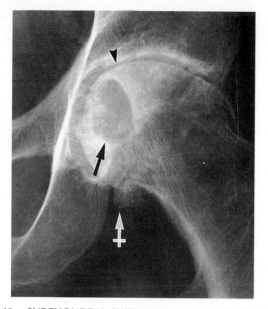

Figure 7.40. SUBCHONDRAL CYST MIMICKING NEOPLASM. The large geographic radiolucency within the femoral head has the appearance of a destructive neoplasm (arrow); however, close scrutiny of the adjacent narrowed joint space (arrowhead) and associated osteophytes (crossed arrow) makes the diagnosis of a degenerative subchondral cyst (geode) most likely. (Courtesy of Mahinder Lall, BSc (Hon) MSc, DC, Melbourne, Australia) COMMENT: This case demonstrates the importance of evaluating the joint in bone disease.

Laboratory Examination

Numerous laboratory parameters can be assessed in the evaluation of various skeletal disorders. This may include peripheral blood, plasma proteins, biochemistry, antibodies, chromosomes, bone marrow, urine, joint aspirates, microbiology, and histopathology.

An absolute minimum skeletal profile should include a complete blood count, erythrocyte sedimentation rate, serum calcium and phosphorus, serum alkaline and acid phosphatase, and total serum proteins. More specialized procedures are applied when a particular diagnostic entity is suspected or to be excluded. Standard values, while not universally uniform, provide the baseline for comparisons. (55) (Table 7.12)

Complete Blood Count (CBC).   A white cell count and differential, hematocrit, hemoglobin, red cell count, and other cellular features are evaluated.

Erythrocyte Sedimentation Rate (ESR).   An increased tendency of red blood cells to precipitate out due to increased concentrations of fibrinogen is noted in many disease states. As such, it represents a nonspecific index of disease, particularly those of an inflammatory nature such as infection. Even after resolution of the infection ESR levels do not return to normal for at least 3 weeks. (56)

C-Reactive Protein (CRP).   In normal individuals no C-reactive protein will be present. Any inflammatory change or tissue necrosis will increase the hepatic release of this protein. Like the ESR, it is not a specific sign for any particular disorder but remains as a general index of pathologic activity. It usually precedes changes in the ESR. A twofold increase in CRP levels, moderate leukocytosis with signs and symptoms of osteomyelitis suggests coexisting septic arthritis. (56)

Table 7.12. Normal Laboratory Values*

	Adult Values		Indication
	Male	**Female**	**Indication**
Acid phosphatase	0.5–2 (Bodansky)		Prostate metastasis
Alkaline phosphatase	2–4.5 (Bodansky)		Liver, bone disease
Calcium	8.5–10.5 mg/100 ml		Tumor, destruction
Complete blood count (CBC)			Anemia, tumor, infection
Hematocrit	42–52 ml/100 ml	37–47 ml/100 ml	
Hemoglobin	14–18 gm/100 ml	12–16 gm/100 ml	
Red blood cell (total)	4.6–6.2 mill/mm³	4.2–5.4 mill/mm³	
White blood cell (total)	4500–11000 mm³		
C-reactive protein (CRP)	Absent		Inflammation, tumor
Erythrocyte sedimentation rate (ESR)	0–15 mm/hr	0–20 mm/hr	Inflammation, tumor
Phosphorus	2–4.5 mg/100 ml		Tumor, destruction
Protein	6–8 gm/100 ml		Tumor
Total			
Fractions			
Albumin	3.5–5.5 gm/100 ml		
Globulin	1.5–3.0 gm/100 ml		Multiple myeloma
Special antigens			
HLA B27	6–8% of population		Seronegative arthritis
RA factor	3% of population		Rheumatoid arthritis
Uric acid	3–6 mg/100 ml		Gout

*Adapted from: Wallach J.: *Interpretation of Diagnostic Tests. A Handbook Synopsis of Laboratory Medicine*, 2 ed. Boston, Little, Brown & Co., 1974.

Serum Calcium. Serum calcium is normally kept within very strict limits. In disorders of bone destruction or increased para-thormone activity serum calcium will be elevated.

Serum Phosphorus. This is also an indicator of bone destruction and an important index of bone activity. It usually will show an inverse relationship to calcium levels.

Alkaline Phosphatase. This is a group of isoenzymes that are found in strong concentrations in bone, liver, spleen, kidney, intestine, and placenta. They are designated as "alkaline" because they exhibit optimal activity at a pH of 9. Their main clinical application is in the detection of liver or bone disease. In bone abnormalities such as Paget's or metastatic disease an increased alkaline phosphatase level is a direct reflection of increased osteoblastic activity.

Acid Phosphatase. Within the prostate, red blood cells and platelet isoenzymes of acid phosphatase are found. They are grouped together as "acid" since their optimal activity is at a pH of 5. The major disorders that demonstrate abnormal levels of the enzyme are in metastasis from prostatic carcinoma and Gaucher's disease. In prostate cancer it is usual for the prostate capsule to be disrupted before the serum acid phosphatase will be found in abnormal concentrations. It appears that the abnormal amounts of the enzyme are liberated by the bone and soft tissue metastatic lesions. As such, a patient may have carcinoma of the prostate yet still show normal acid phosphatase levels as long as the capsule remains intact.

Prostate specific antigen (PSA) is a tumor marker useful in the diagnosis, response to therapy, and relapse of carcinoma of the prostate. In the presence of a normal size gland a marked elevation of the PSA should be treated with a high suspicion for carcinoma. Benign prostate hypertrophy can produce less marked elevations. The course of the disease activity can be followed with serial PSA levels.

Total Protein. Protein levels are frequently altered in certain bone disorders, especially malignancy. A raised total serum protein often indicates metastatic disease or multiple myeloma. More specific examination of the various protein fractions will reveal a more definitive diagnosis. In multiple myeloma, for example, there is an overproduction of a specific immunoglobulin (mono-clonal gammopathy), which reverses the normal albumin-globulin ratio (A:G ratio) and on electrophoresis shows as an IgG or IgA spike. In the urine the presence of Bence-Jones proteins may be found in almost 40% of those with multiple myeloma.

Additional Studies. When indicated, certain laboratory examinations will provide additional data in the evaluation of a skeletal or rheumatologic disorder. Uric acid levels are of assistance in the evaluation of gout, chromosomal studies for dysplasias, and the special antigens such as HLA-B27 in seronegative arthritis and rheumatoid factor in inflammatory arthritis. More sophisticated studies include electrophoresis, calcium balance studies, renal function, synovial fluid and blood studies, and bioassay.

Biopsy

The definitive diagnosis frequently rests on the histologic evaluation of biopsy material. This can be obtained by numerous methods, including incisional and needle aspiration. (57) Frequently, the radiograph determines the site for biopsy and further follow-up procedures. (Fig. 7.41) In bone marrow evaluations the most common sites for obtaining specimens include the sternum and iliac crest.

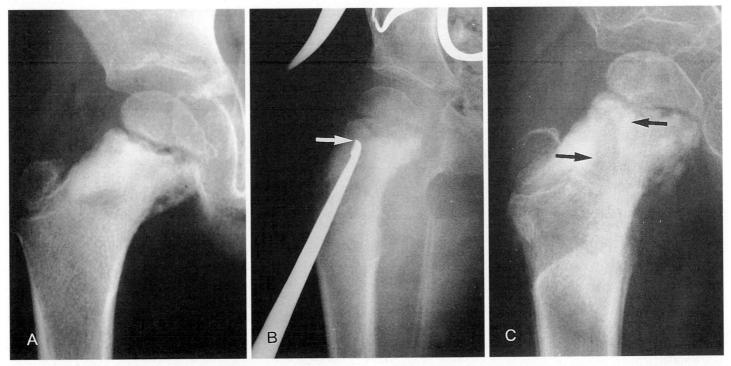

Figure 7.41. BIOPSY PROCEDURE. A. Initial Film. Based on the osteoblastic nature of the lesion, its location, and the age of the patient, a presumptive diagnosis of osteosarcoma was made. **B. Biopsy Film.** Note the position of the biopsy tool within the matrix of the tumor (arrow).

C. Postbiopsy Film. With the procedure completed, a residual linear lucency remains at the biopsy site (arrows). Final biopsy confirmed the diagnosis of *osteosarcoma*.

MEDICOLEGAL IMPLICATIONS
Radiologic Interpretation

- Expertise in radiologic interpretation is related to developing a knowledge base in anatomy, pathology and differential diagnosis; being exposed to a wide range of exemplary case materials; being able to correlate with clinical data; continuing education; and experience.

- The most common reasons for errors of interpretation include analysis on poor studies, lack of knowledge, perceptual errors, reading reports and not the film, and a failure to access second opinion reviews when required.

- Analysis on poor or inadequate studies has direct bearing on the ability to render diagnostic opinions. (58–60) Similarly inadequate or inappropriate projections detract greatly in diagnostic interpretations. An appropriate strategy to deal with these shortcomings should be addressed, which may include re-x-ray, additional views, or utilizing an alternative imaging modality. Inclusion of structures within the field of view that will be obscured due to exposure difficulties such as the lung field, abdomen, and spinal transitional zones requires use of the "hot light" or obtaining a well exposed projection.

- Lack of knowledge when interpreting images will result in missed diagnoses. Educational background, ongoing postgraduate training, literature access, ongoing utilization and interaction with peers are vital to maintaining acceptable standards of interpretive skills in radiology. (58) Diagnostic discordance rates between practitioners and those with specialty backgrounds vary. (61,62) Care should be taken to not attempt to interpret unfamiliar imaging modalities.

- Perceptual errors can result in missing or incorrectly identifying an abnormality. Inaccurate diagnoses and missed diagnoses in hospitals may be as high as 5 to 10%. (63,64) The interobserver reliability in the interpretation of images is known to often be wide. (65–67) The most common reason for a lawsuit is due to diagnostic error. (61,68–70) Mistakes can also be due to failure to recognize a normal variant, failure to continue the search after the first abnormality was found, and a lesion at the periphery of the study. (71) Taking the time to systematically review an imaging study is paramount to recognition of an abnormality, as is developing a search pattern in analyzing a study. Even a poorly illuminating view box can lead to errors.

- Previous reports should be obtained but not assumed to be correct. Awareness of the errors inherent in the interpretation of all imaging studies, no matter who performs the interpretation, is vitally important. These potential errors in interpretation place back onto all treating practitioners the responsibility to interpret every set of studies personally, not assume any available report is accurate, and to analyze the study on their own.

- Second opinions should be sought if abnormalities are deemed clinically relevant or if their significance is unclear, when the diagnosis is equivocal, and in medicolegal circumstances.

CAPSULE SUMMARY   Principles of Radiologic Interpretation

TECHNICAL CONSIDERATIONS

- *Plain Film:* Most commonly employed method. Based on differential absorption of x-rays by body tissues. Five densities—air, fat, water, bone, and metal. Minimum of two views, perpendicular to each other. Need 30 to 50% destruction to be visible on film.
- *Tomography:* Increased detail at fulcrum between moving tube and cassette.
- *Xeroradiography:* Enhanced sharpness but high dose. Used mainly in mammography.
- *Contrast Studies:* Arthrogram—joints; angiogram—vessels; lymphangiogram—lymph channels; myelogram—spinal subarachnoid space; discogram—intervertebral disc.
- *Radionuclide Imaging:* Technetium-99m methylene diphosphate (99m Tc-MDP) taken up selectively by osteoblasts. Only 3 to 5% destruction needed to be visible. Abnormal uptake regions referred to as "hot spots." Quantitative imaging only.
- *Computed Tomography:* Computer formulated cross-sectional images, bone and soft tissue details, reconstructions in any plane and three dimensional possible.
- *Magnetic Resonance Imaging:* Uses magnetic fields to create sectional images with exquisite details of soft tissue resolution.

SKELETAL ANATOMY AND PHYSIOLOGY

- *Intramembranous Ossification:* Bone formation from a fibroblastic membrane.
- *Enchondral Ossification:* Bone formation from a cartilaginous model.
- *Parts of a Bone:* Epiphysis, physis, metaphysis, diaphysis, apophysis, cortex, medulla, and periosteum. Epiphysis vulnerable to dysplasia and ischemia.
- *Metaphysis:* Most active part of a bone and is prone to tumors and infections.
- *Periosteum:* Has an inner, metabolically active layer that can lay down or take away cortical bone.
- Calcium and phosphorus are the most important bone minerals; usually in the form of hydroxyapatite (Ca10 (PO4)6 (OH)2).
- Hormones most active in bone metabolism are parathormone, calcitonin, estrogen, androgen, growth hormone, and glucocorticoids.

CATEGORICAL APPROACH TO BONE DISEASE

- Seven categories (CATBITES)—congenital, arthritis, trauma, blood (hematologic), infection, tumor, nutritional/metabolic/endocrine, soft tissue.

RADIOLOGIC PREDICTOR VARIABLES

- The evaluation of certain features of a lesion leads to the correct diagnosis or differential diagnosis:
  - Clinical data—age, sex, race, history
  - Number of lesions—polyostotic, monostotic
  - Symmetry of lesions
  - Systems involved
  - Skeletal location

- Position within bone—predilection to a bone site an important diagnostic clue. *Epiphysis:* giant cell tumor, chondroblastoma. *Diaphysis:* round cell tumors.
- Site of origin
- Shape—elongated lesions frequently due to slow growth and development during bone growth.
- Size
- Margination—imperceptible (aggressive), sharp (benign).
- Cortical integrity—thin, thick, expansion, destruction, and fracture.
- Behavior of lesion—lytic, blastic, or mixed. *Lytic* lesions will be either geographic (slow), motheaten, or permeative (rapid). *Geographic:* single, greater than 1 cm, sharp margins, and may be septated ("soap bubble"). *Motheaten:* multiple, 2 to 5 mm, imperceptible margins, and confluent. *Permea-*

tive: multiple, less than 1 mm, and imperceptible margins. Blastic lesions: diffuse (ivory) or localized (snowball).
- Matrix—fat, cartilage, bone, fibrous.
- Periosteal response—solid, laminated, spiculated.
- Codman's triangle—takes 10 to 21 days to appear.
- Soft tissue changes—displaced skin and muscle planes, increased density, calcification or air. When combined with broken cortex, primary malignant bone tumor is the most likely cause.
- Joint changes—arthritis, infection—rarely tumors.
- Supplementary procedures—other imaging modalities, laboratory, and biopsy. Most standard lab tests for bone include CBC (with differential), CRP, ESR, calcium, phosphorus, alkaline and acid phosphatase, prostate specific antigen (PSA), and serum proteins.

REFERENCES

1. **Kaye JJ:** Arthritis. *Role of radiography and other imaging techniques in evaluation.* Radiology 177:601, 1990.
2. **Modic MT, Herzog RJ:** *Spinal imaging modalities. What's available and who should order them.* Spine 19:1764, 1994.
3. **Rowe LJ:** Skeletal Radiology and Its Applications to the Practice of Chiropractic. *Master of Applied Science (Chiropractic) Thesis.* Royal Melbourne Institute of Technology University, Melbourne, Australia 1995.
4. **Rowe LJ:** *Imaging of Degenerative and Mechanical Disorders of the Lumbar Spine.* In: Giles LGF and Singer KJ, eds. *Clinical Anatomy and Management of the Lumbar Spine.* Melbourne: Butterworth Heineman, 1996.
5. **Rowe LJ, Howard B:** *The Role of Imaging in Clinical Practice.* In: Haldeman S, ed. *Modern Developments in Chiropractic.* New York: Appleton Lange, 1992.
6. **Schuerger SR:** *Introduction to critical review of roentgenograms.* Phys Ther 68:1114, 1988.
7. **Dupuis PR, Yong-Hing K, Cassidy JD, et al:** *Radiologic diagnosis of degenerative lumbar spinal instability.* Spine 10(3):287, 1985.
8. **Deyo R, Diehl A:** *Lumbar spine films in primary care: Current use and effects of selective ordering criteria.* J Gen Intern Med 1:20, 1986.
9. **Phillips RB:** *Plain film radiography in chiropractic.* J Manipulative Physiol Ther 15:47, 1992.
10. **Sherman R:** *Chiropractic x-ray rationale.* J Can Chiro Assoc 30:33, 1986.
11. **Schultz G, Phillips RB, Cooley J, et al:** *Diagnostic Imaging of the spine in chiropractic practice: Recommendations for utilization.* Chiro J Austr 22:141, 1992.
12. **Bigos SJ, Hansson T, Castillo RN, et al:** *The value of preemployment roentgenographs for predicting acute back injury claims and chronic back pain disability.* Clin Orthop 283:124, 1992.
13. **Friberg O:** *Functional radiography of the lumbar spine.* Ann Med 21:341, 1989.
14. **Ardran GM:** *Bone destruction not demonstrable by radiography.* Br J Radiol 24:107, 1951.
15. **Borak J:** *Relationship between the clinical and roentgenological findings in bone metastases.* Surg Gynecol Obstet 75:599, 1942.
16. **Lachman E:** *Osteoporosis: The potentialities and limitations of its roentgenologic diagnosis.* AJR 74:712, 1955.
17. **Paulus DD:** *Xeroradiography. An in-depth review.* CRC Crit Rev (Diagn Imag) March:309, 1980.
18. **Tress, Lau L:** *Depo—Medrol and facet joint injections.* Australas Radiol 35:291, 1991.
19. **Hallam DM, Sonne NM, Jensen GS, et al:** *Headache after lumbar iohexol myelography: The influence of a history of headaches and early ambulation.* Neuroradiology 35:319, 1993.
20. **Aprill CN:** *Diagnostic Disc Injection.* In: Frymoyer JW, ed. *The Adult Spine: Principles and Practice.* New York, Raven Press; 1991.
21. **Maezawa S, Muro T:** *Pain provocation at lumbar discography as analyzed by computed tomography/discography.* Spine 17:1313, 1992.
22. **Guyer RD, Ohnmeiss DD:** *The role of diskography and interdiskal therapy.* Current Opinion Orthop 5:49, 1994.
23. **Johnson RG:** *Does discography injure normal discs? An analysis of repeat discograms.* Spine 14:424, 1989.
24. **Bassett LW, Gold RH, Webber MM:** *Radionuclide bone imaging.* Radiol Clin North Am 19:(4) 645, 1981.
25. **Valdez DC, Johnson RG:** *Role of technetium-99m planar bone scanning in the evaluation of low back pain.* Skeletal Radiol 23:91, 1994.
26. **Porter RW, Ottowell E, Wicks M:** *Use of diagnostic ultrasound for spinal canal measurements.* J Bone Joint Surg (Br) (64)(2):249, 1977.
27. **Porter RW, Hibbert C, Wellman P:** *Backache and the lumbar spinal canal.* Spine 5:99, 1985.
28. **Hammond BR:** The Detection of Spondylolysis Using Lumbar Sonography. *PhD Thesis* University of Surrey, 1984.
29. **Breen AC, Allen R, Morris A:** *Spine kinematics: A digital videofluoroscopic technique.* J Biomed Eng 11:224, 1989.
30. **Howe JW:** *Observations from cineroentgenographic studies of the spinal column.* J Am Chiropractic Assn 7(10):65, 1970.
31. **Pennal GF, Garson SC, McDonald G, et al:** *Motion studies of the lumbar spine. A preliminary report.* J Bone Joint Surg (Br) 54:442, 1972.
32. **Bell GD:** *Skeletal applications of videofluoroscopy.* J Manipulative Physiol Ther 13:396, 1990.
33. **McCullough EC, Payne JT:** *Patient dosage in computed tomography.* Radiology 129:457, 1978.
34. **Rabassa AE, Guinto FC, Crow WN, et al:** *CT of the spine: Value of reformatted images.* AJR 161:1223, 1993.
35. **Murphey MD, Quale JL, Martin NL, et al:** *Computed radiography in musculoskeletal imaging: State of the art.* AJR 158:19, 1992.
36. **Hounsfield GN:** *Computerized transverse axial scanning (tomography) Part I: Description of system.* Br J Radiol 46:1016, 1973.
37. **Genant HK, Cann CE, Chapetz NI, et al:** *Advances in computed tomography of the musculoskeletal system.* Radiol Clin North Am 19(4):645, 1981.
38. **Han JS, Benson JE, Yoon YS:** *Magnetic resonance imaging in the spinal column and craniovertebral junction.* Radiol Clin North Am 22(4):805, 1984.
39. **Gerard EL, Ferry JA, Amrein PC, et al:** *Compositional changes in vertebral bone marrow during treatment for acute leukemia: Assessment with quantitative chemical shift imaging.* Radiology 183:39, 1992.
40. **Cotler HB:** *Clinical applications for magnetic resonance imaging of the spine.* Am Acad Orthop Surg (Instructional Course Lectures), XLI:257, 1992.
41. **Howe JW:** *A suggested approach to radiographic interpretation and reporting.* ACA Council Roentgenol, Roentgen Brief, 1982.
42. **Sherman RS:** *General principles of the radiologic diagnosis of bone disorders.* Radiol Clin North Am 8:173, 1970.
43. **Sherman RS:** *The nature of radiologic diagnosis in diseases of bone.* Radiol Clin North Am 8:227, 1970.
44. **Lodwick GS:** *Solitary malignant tumors of bone: The application of predictor variables in diagnosis.* Semin Roentgenol 1:293, 1966.
45. **Lodwick GS:** *Atlas of Tumor Radiology. The Bones and Joints,* Chicago, Year Book Medical Publishers, 1971.
46. **Kramer DM:** *Basic principles of magnetic resonance imaging.* Radiol Clin North Am 22 (4):765, 1984.
47. **Madewell JE, Ragsdale BD, Sweet DE:** *Radiologic and pathologic analysis of solitary bone lesions. Part I: Internal margins.* Radiol Clin North Am 19(4):715, 1981.
48. **Edeiken J, Hodes PJ, Caplan LH:** *New bone production and periosteal reaction* AJR 97:708, 1966.
49. **Sweet DE, Madewell JE, Ragsdale BD:** *Radiologic and pathologic analysis of solitary bone lesions. Part III: Matrix patterns.* Radiol Clin North Am 19(4):785, 1981.
50. **Greenfield GB:** Radiology of Bone Diseases, ed 3. Philadelphia, JB Lippincott, 1980.
51. **Ragsdale BD, Madewell JE, Sweet DE:** *Radiologic and pathologic analysis of solitary bone lesions. Part II: Periosteal reactions.* Radiol Clin North Am 19(4):749, 1981.
52. **Volberg FM Jr, Whalen JP, Krook L, et al:** *Lamellated periosteal reactions: A radiologic and histologic investigation.* AJR, 128:85, 1977.
53. **Brunschwig A, Harman PH:** *Studies in bone sarcoma. Part III: An experimental and pathological study of the role of the periosteum in formation of bone in various primary bone tumors.* Surg Gynecol Obstet 60:30, 1935.
54. **Codman EA:** *Registry of bone sarcoma.* Surg Gynecol Obstet 42:105, 1925.
55. **Wallach J:** *Interpretation of Diagnostic Tests. A Handbook Synopsis of Laboratory Medicine,* ed 2. Boston, Little, Brown & Co., 1974.
56. **Unkila-Kallio L, Kallio MJT, Peltola H:** *The usefulness of C-reactive protein levels in the identification of concurrent septic arthritis in children who have acute hematogenous osteomyelitis.* J Bone Joint Surg (Am) 76:848, 1994.
57. **Hajdu SI, Melamed MR:** *Needle biopsy of primary malignant bone tumors.* Surg Gynecol Obstet 133:829, 1971.
58. **Renfrew DL, Franken EA, Berbaum KS, et al:** *Error in radiology: classification and lessons in 182 cases presented at a problem case conference.* Radiology 183:145, 1992.

59. **Hopper KD, Rosetti GF, Edmiston RB, et al:** *Diagnostic radiology peer review: A method inclusive of all interpreters of radiographic examinations regardless of specialty.* Radiology 180:557, 1991.

60. **Levin DC:** *The practice of radiology by nonradiologists: cost, quality and utilization issues.* AJR 162:513, 1994.

61. **Vincent CA, Driscoll PA, Audley RJ, et al:** *Accuracy of detection of radiographic abnormalities by junior doctors.* Arch Emerg Med 5:101, 1988.

62. **Halvorsen JG, Kunian A:** *Radiology in family practice: a prospective study of 14 community practices.* Fam Med 22:112, 1990.

63. **Pringle RG:** *Missed fractures.* Injury 4:311, 1972.

64. **de Lacey G, Barker A, Harper J, et al:** *An assessment of the clinical effects of reporting accident and emergency radiographs.* Br J Radiol 53:304, 1980.

65. **Boden SD, Davis DO, Dina TS, et al:** *Abnormal magnetic-resonance scans of the lumbar spine in asymptomatic patients. A prospective investigation.* J Bone Joint Surg (Am) 72:403, 1990.

66. **Wiesel SW:** *The reliability of imaging (computed tomography, magnetic resonance imaging, myelography) in documenting the cause of spinal pain.* J Manipulative Physiol Ther 15:51, 1992.

67. **Weisel SW, Tsopurmas N, Feffer HL, et al:** *A study of computer-assisted tomography. The incidence of positive CT scans in an asymptomatic group of patients.* Spine 9:549, 1984.

68. **Tuddenham WJ:** *Visual search, image organization, and reader error in roentgen diagnosis.* Radiology 78:694, 1962.

69. **Morrish HF, Messenger OJ:** *Medicolegal encounters in Canadian radiology.* Can Assoc Radiol J 41:259, 1990.

70. **Hirtle RL:** *Chiropractic malpractice.* ACA J Chiro, October:35, 1987.

71. **Kline TJ, Kline TS:** *Radiologists, communication and Resolution 5: A medicolegal issue.* Radiology 184:131, 1992.

8

Skeletal Dysplasias

Margaret A. Seron, Terry R. Yochum, Michael S. Barry, and Lindsay J. Rowe

INTRODUCTION

The skeletal dysplasias are a vast and often confusing group of disorders that have been the subject of much curiosity and speculation over the years. Recently, with the advent of sophisticated genetic and laboratory studies, the various causes of skeletal dysplasias are becoming better understood. However, they still remain a heterogeneous group, with considerable variation noted even within specific entities.

By definition, skeletal dysplasias are the result of faulty development. Many are known to be the result of specific genetic mutations and are inherited. Many are congenital; fewer develop in adolescence or early adulthood.

This chapter addresses only the more commonly encountered skeletal dysplasias. It is important that these be accurately diagnosed, so that more serious conditions such as malignancy or toxicity can be ruled out, and so that serious sequelae of the dysplasia itself can be recognized and possibly prevented. Examples of such sequelae include the life-threatening dissecting aneurysm that often accompanies Marfan's syndrome and the paralysis that frequently develops due to congenital spinal stenosis in achondroplasia.

Related entities are grouped together for ease of understanding, and the groupings are arranged in alphabetical order.

ACHONDROPLASIA

GENERAL CONSIDERATIONS

Achondroplasia, the most common congenital dwarfism, is a hereditary, autosomal dominant disturbance in epiphyseal chondroblastic growth and maturation. The name *achondroplasia* was first used in 1878 by Parrot. (1) Other synonyms that have been used include *chondrodystrophia fetalis* (2), *chondrodystrophic dwarfism*, and *micromelia*.

The phenotypic appearance of this disorder is remarkably similar in all cases and is the result of a single mutant gene. The parents of achondroplastic dwarfs are normal in 90% of cases; it is thought that sporadic mutations account for 80% of achondroplastic births. (3) The offspring of the rare mating of two achondroplastics often manifest a severe form (homozygous) of this dysplasia, which is usually lethal within the first weeks of life.

CLINICAL FEATURES

Achondroplasia is one of the oldest growth disorders known to man. In ancient times these individuals were kept as advisors to emperors and entertainers to the wealthy. It is only since the nineteenth century that these people have been known to be normal except for their physical appearance. (4) Most obvious is their stature, which averages approximately 50 inches.

The characteristics of this dwarfing dysplasia are recognizable at birth. The long bones are markedly shortened, especially the more proximal ones (rhizomelia). The upper extremity is affected more than the lower. The cranium is large, with a prominent forehead and depressed nasal bridge. The base of the skull is constricted and the foramen magnum is small. Associated hydrocephalus may be obstructive or nonobstructive. (5) The length of the spinal column is relatively normal; thus the dwarfism is due primarily to limb shortening. The abdomen is protuberant and the buttocks are prominent. A thoracolumbar kyphosis often develops; the lumbar spine is hyperlordotic. A characteristic rolling gait is caused by the posterior tilt of the pelvis and posterior angulation of the hip joints. (6)

Additional clinical features include elbow deformities with limitation of supination and extension (7), flexion contractures of the hips, and genu varum. The characteristic *trident hand* is due to a widening of the space between the third and fourth digits (8) and the inability to approximate them in extension.

Achondroplastics may die at birth due to a difficult delivery, a small foramen magnum, or a constricted thorax. (6) However, the majority survive and enjoy normal life spans. During childhood sleep apnea and sudden death may result from compression of the brain stem at the craniocervical junction. (9–11) The most significant complication in adulthood is congenital spinal stenosis, often leading to paraplegia. Mental and sexual development are normal.

PATHOLOGIC FEATURES

In the past it was thought that achondroplasia was due to an endocrine abnormality, but exhaustive studies have found no disturbances of endocrine function. The major abnormality is failure of normal enchondral cartilage growth at the physis. Periosteal and membranous ossification are normal. Some enchondral ossification centers are affected more than others, particularly those at the base of the skull and at the ends of long bones.

RADIOLOGIC FEATURES

The most characteristic radiographic features are found in the skull spine, pelvis, and limbs. (12) Narrowing of the spinal canal is the pathologic hallmark of achondroplasia. (11) The base of the skull (which is formed by enchondral ossification) is small, often with a stenotic foramen magnum. Basilar impression is frequent. The cranium is large, though short in its anteroposterior dimension (brachycephaly). The frontal bones are prominent and the nasal bones are small. The mandible forms normally and, therefore, gives the impression of prognathism.

There is symmetric shortening of all long bones, with the proximal portions being most affected. (Fig. 8.1) The bone ends are often splayed, with metaphyseal cupping. (Fig. 8.2) Because peri-

osteal ossification proceeds normally, there is relative widening of the shafts. The ulna and tibia are often shorter than the radius and fibula. The tubular bones of the hands and feet are short and thick. (Fig. 8.3) The fingers are all the same length, with separation of the middle and ring fingers (*trident hand*). (Fig. 8.4) The

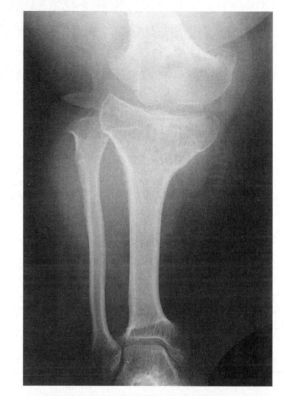

Figure 8.2.   ACHONDROPLASIA: LOWER LIMB. Observe the splayed and cupped metaphyses, as well as the shortening of the leg.

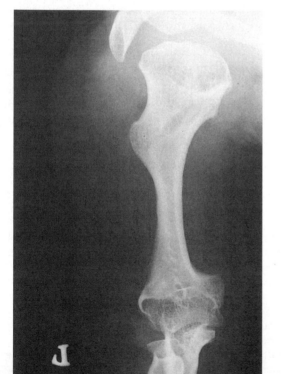

Figure 8.1.   ACHONDROPLASIA: HUMERUS. Note the shortening of the humerus. This shortening is most apparent in the proximal portions of the limbs. COMMENT: Achondroplasia is the most common form of dwarfism; the average height is 50 inches.

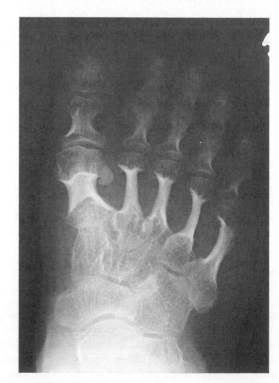

Figure 8.3.   ACHONDROPLASIA: FEET. Note the short, thick tubular bones. (Courtesy of David P. Thomas, MD, Melbourne, Australia)

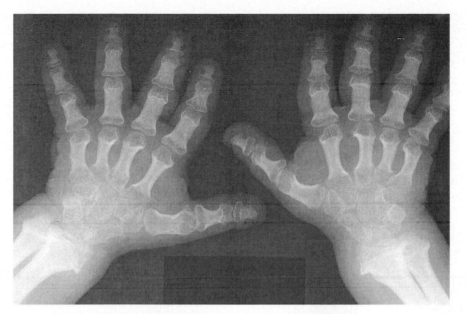

Figure 8.4. ACHONDROPLASIA: *TRIDENT* HANDS. Observe the characteristic *trident* hand, with separation of the third and fourth digits. Also note that the fingers are all the same length. (Courtesy of Bryan Hartley, MD, Melbourne, Australia)

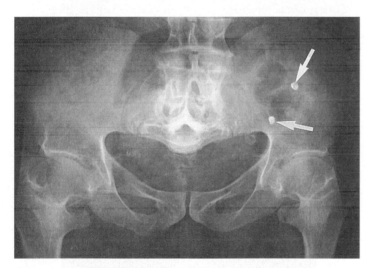

Figure 8.5. ACHONDROPLASIA: PELVIS. Observe the characteristic *champagne glass* pelvis. The ilii are short and flat. Also observe that the acetabular roofs are horizontally oriented. Of incidental notation is retention of barium in two colonic diverticuli (arrows).

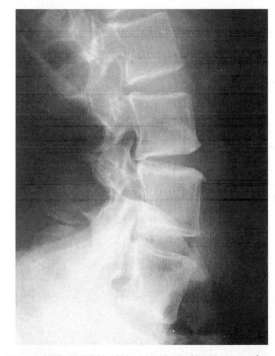

Figure 8.6. ACHONDROPLASIA: LUMBAR SPINE. Note the posterior scalloping of the vertebral bodies. The pedicles are short and thick and contribute to the development of lumbar spinal stenosis. COMMENT: These individuals are usually hyperlordotic.

ribs are quite short and often do not extend around the thorax. The scapulae may be squared inferiorly (13), with shallow glenoids. The entire pelvis is small. The ilia are shortened caudally and flattened, with small sciatic notches. The acetabulae are horizontally oriented and there is excessive thickening of the "Y" cartilage. (Fig. 8.5) The length of the spinal column is generally normal at birth, though mild platyspondyly may be seen. The amount of cartilage is increased, causing the height of the discs to equal that of the vertebral bodies. Posterior scalloping of the bodies is common. The interpedicular spaces decrease caudally in the lumbar region, whereas they increase from L1 to L5 in the normal individual. The pedicles are short and thick. (Fig. 8.6) The lumbar lordosis is often exaggerated, complicated by a horizontally oriented sacrum. An angular kyphosis often develops at the thoracolumbar junction, resulting from anteriorly wedged or *bullet-nosed* vertebrae. (14) (Fig. 8.7)

NEUROLOGIC COMPLICATIONS

Neurologic manifestations may be seen at any age. In the infant the small foramen magnum and hydrocephalus can lead to cord compression and sudden death. Sleep apnea is also well documented. (9,10) Spinal stenosis is a frequent neurologic complication. In fact, Holder et al. (4) consider achondroplasia to be the archetype of congenital spinal stenosis. Although the entire spine is involved, cord compression and resultant paraplegia de-

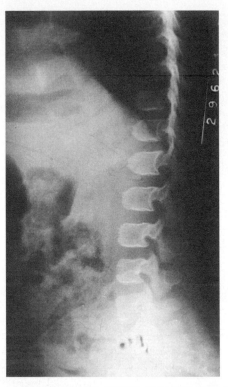

Figure 8.7.   ACHONDROPLASIA: SPINAL COLUMN. Note the increased disc height and *bullet-nosed* vertebrae. (Courtesy of Paul E. Siebert, MD, Denver, Colorado)

velop more commonly in the adult at the thoracolumbar and lumbar regions.

Several anatomic factors contribute to the development of spinal stenosis in achondroplastics. These include decreased interpedicular distance, along with thick and short pedicles and facets, which create a decrease in the transverse and AP canal dimensions of up to 50% at the L5 level. (6) There is often stenosis of the nerve root canal (lateral entrapment syndrome), which usually occurs at L5-S1. These conditions often require surgical decompressive laminectomies from T11 to L5. (4) (Figs. 8.8, 8.9) CT and MRI have proven to be useful in evaluating stenosis of the craniocervical junction (15), and lumbar spine. MRI is particularly useful for evaluating the brain stem, spinal cord, cauda equina, and exiting nerve roots. (11)

Four clinical syndromes have been described: (16)

1. Nerve root compression caused by disc herniation and osteophyte formation;
2. Transverse myelopathy gradually induced by severe kyphosis;
3. Acute traumatic transverse myelopathy with sudden paraplegia; and
4. Intermittent claudication of the cauda equina, possibly due to ischemia. These patients have symptoms suggesting vascular disease of the lower extremities associated with activity.

Achondroplasia has been confused with other dwarfing dysplasias. These include the mucopolysaccharidoses, trisomy, and spondyloepiphyseal dysplasia. However, careful biochemical

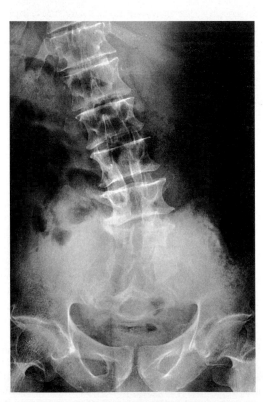

Figure 8.8.   ACHONDROPLASIA, LUMBAR SPINE: SURGICAL DECOMPRESSION. This patient has had laminectomies from L3 to L5 as treatment for the common complication of achondroplasia, spinal stenosis. (Courtesy of Douglas B. Hart, DC, Carina, Queensland, Australia)

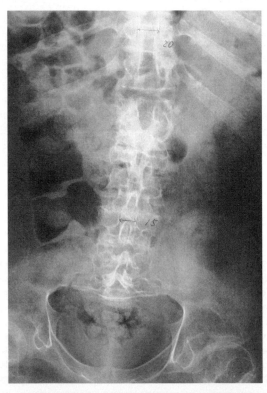

Figure 8.9.   ACHONDROPLASIA, LUMBAR SPINE: SURGICAL DECOMPRESSION. This patient has had decompression surgery from T11 through L1. Note the decreased interpedicular space throughout the lumbar spine. At L4, this distance measures 15 mm. The average normal measurement at L4 is 27 mm. (Courtesy of The Childrens Hospital, Dept. of Radiology, Denver, Colorado)

and radiographic evaluation of these individuals should readily reveal the proper diagnosis.

MEDICOLEGAL IMPLICATIONS
Achondroplasia

- Lumbar spine stenosis may produce nerve root compression and/or cauda equina syndrome. Therefore, spinal manipulative therapy must be preceded by a thorough clinical and radiographic evaluation for stenosis. If lower extremity neurologic signs or cauda equina–type symptoms are present, an MRI is indicated.

- Basilar impression and stenosis of the foramen magnum may produce spinal cord and lower brain stem compression resulting in apnea and sudden death. Other complications of foramen magnum stenosis include syringomyelia and communicating hydrocephalus secondary to obstruction of the basal cisterns and Sylvian aqueduct.

CLEIDOCRANIAL DYSPLASIA

GENERAL CONSIDERATIONS

Cleidocranial dysplasia is an uncommon autosomal dominant disorder that affects 0.5 per 100,000 live births. (1) It is characterized by faulty ossification of the intramembranous bones. Skull and clavicular anomalies, as well as midline defects, are classic features of this dysplasia. According to Soule (2), the first case was described by Cutter in 1870. (3) In 1898 the condition was recognized as an entity by Marie and Sainton and given the name *cleidocranial dysostosis*. (4) The condition is congenital and has an extremely varied presentation. Less frequently, cases are seen that do not have clavicular or cranial findings; in 1985 Silverman and Reiley supported the term *spondylo-megaepiphyseal-metaphyseal dysplasia* for the recessively inherited form of this disorder. (5)

CLINICAL FEATURES

The typical individual presents with a large head, small face, and drooping shoulders. Height is reduced in both males and females with cleidocranial dysplasia (6), but dwarfism is not a usual feature. The chest is frequently narrowed or cone-shaped. The patient's mental status is normal. Gait disturbances due to deformities of the hips and femora, and abnormal dentition with severe caries and periodontitis are the most common complaints. Hearing loss has been reported, apparently secondary to structural abnormalities of the ossicles. (7) Clavicular hypoplasia or agenesis produces extreme mobility of the shoulders. Often, the patient can touch the two acromial regions together under the chin. (Fig. 8.10) Laboratory findings are consistently normal.

RADIOLOGIC FEATURES

The radiographic signs are characteristic and leave little room for difficulty in diagnosis.

Skull

Early in infancy there is delayed or absent ossification of the calvarium. With time, multiple Wormian bones are formed in the sutures and often the metopic suture persists. Widening of the principal sutures (sagittal and coronal) gives a *hot cross bun* appearance. (8) (Fig. 8.11) There is marked brachycephaly with a widened interparietal diameter. The supraorbital region, temporal squama, and occipital bone are frequently thickened. The foramen magnum is deformed and enlarged, and there may be platybasia. (9)

The small face is the result of underdeveloped facial bones. Frequently, the nasal bones fail to ossify and the paranasal sinuses are hypoplastic. While the maxilla is small, the mandible is large and the mandibular suture closes late. A high arched or cleft palate is not uncommon. Delayed and defective dentition is a prominent and often symptomatic finding. (10)

Thorax

Anomalous clavicular development is a nearly constant finding. The clavicle is formed from three separate ossification centers (sternal, middle, and acromial). Since one or more of these centers can be affected, there is considerable variation in the clavicular involvement. (Fig. 8.12) In 10% of cases the clavicle is completely absent. A pseudarthrosis may develop when the middle portion is missing. The scapulae are often small, winged, or elevated. The shoulder girdle deformities allow great mobility of the shoulders. While the ribs are usually normal, the chest is narrow and cone-shaped.

Pelvis

The bones of the pelvis are small and underdeveloped, forming a small pelvic bowl. Commonly, there is a midline defect at the pubic symphysis, where the rami fail to approximate anteriorly. (Fig. 8.13) Early coxa valgus develops into coxa varus, possibly secondary to weight-bearing stresses on the poorly mineralized femoral neck. (5) Lateral notching of the capital femoral epiphysis has been reported. (11)

Spine

The vertebrae often show delayed mineralization, biconvex bodies, and spina bifida occulta (5), especially in the cervical and upper thoracic segments. (12) There is an increased incidence of spondylolysis in the lumbar spine. (1) Hyperlordosis, excessive kyphosis, and scoliosis are secondary to the neural arch defects and hemivertebrae.

Extremities

The most marked changes are found in the hands, where an accessory epiphysis for the base of the second metacarpal occurs, creating an elongated digit. The distal phalanges are hypoplastic and often pointed. (13) (Fig. 8.14) Similar changes may be found in the feet but are less common. The long tubular bones are less frequently involved but, occasionally, shortening of the radius with an abnormal wrist articulation is seen.

COMPLICATIONS

Hearing loss, severe dental problems, dislocations of the shoulders and hips, and scoliosis are troublesome but do not lead to a shortened life span.

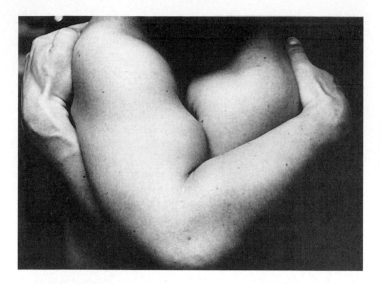

Figure 8.10.   CLEIDOCRANIAL DYSPLASIA: HYPERMOBILE SHOULDERS.
Extreme hypermobility of the shoulders is secondary to agenesis or hypoplasia
of the clavicles. This patient can approximate his shoulders under the chin.
(Courtesy of Kenneth E. Yochum, DC, St. Louis, Missouri)

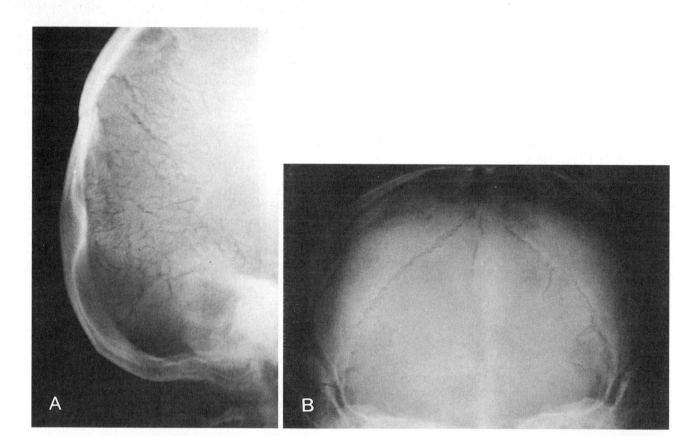

**Figure 8.11.   CLEIDOCRANIAL DYSPLASIA: SKULL INVOLVEMENT. A.
Lateral Occiput: Wormian Bones.** Note the numerous Wormian bones
throughout the occipital region. These sutural bones are fairly common in
cleidocranial dysplasia but are not pathognomonic, as they are found
in other disorders as well. (Courtesy of M. Bruce Farkas, DO, JD, Chicago,
Illinois) **B. Sutural Widening.** As in this patient, widening of the sutures and
persistence of the fetal sutures are common findings.

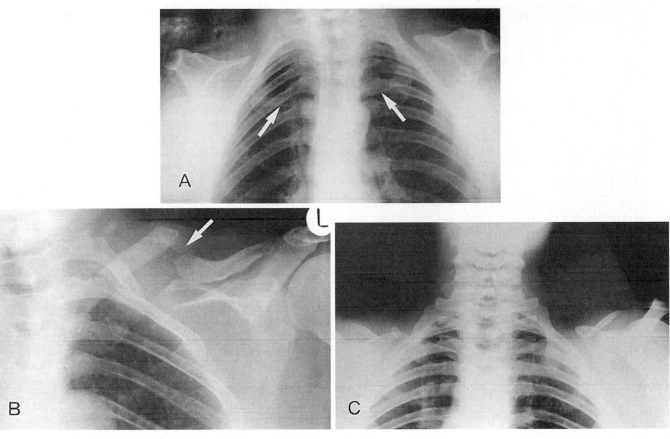

Figure 8.12. CLEIDOCRANIAL DYSPLASIA: CLAVICULAR INVOLVEMENT. A. There is agenesis of the middle and lateral portions of the clavicle, with only the medial portion present (arrows). **B.** Note the agenesis of the middle ossification center of the clavicle, with a pseudarthrosis (arrow).

C. All three ossification centers are present but are hypoplastic, with resultant pseudarthroses. COMMENT: In 10% of individuals with cleidocranial dysplasia the clavicles are completely absent.

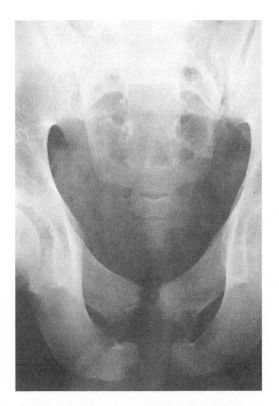

Figure 8.13. CLEIDOCRANIAL DYSPLASIA: PUBIC SYMPHYSIS. Note the midline diastasis of the pubic symphysis. (Courtesy of M. Bruce Farkas, DO, JD, Chicago, Illinois)

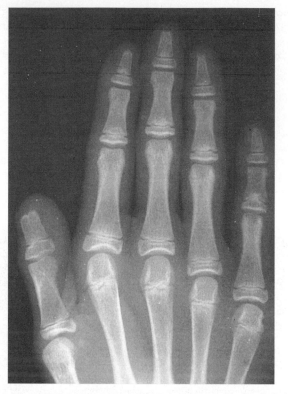

Figure 8.14. CLEIDOCRANIAL DYSPLASIA: HANDS. The distal phalanges are hypoplastic and flattened. (Courtesy of M. Bruce Farkas, DO, JD, Chicago, Illinois)

MEDICOLEGAL IMPLICATIONS
Cleidocranial Dysplasia

- Faulty dentition results in dental caries. If untreated, progression to osteomyelitis of the maxilla or mandible is possible.
- The narrow thorax in childhood may lead to respiratory distress.
- Although unusual, platybasia and basilar impression may crowd the brain stem and upper cervical spinal cord.

CRANIOSYNOSTOSIS
GENERAL CONSIDERATIONS

Craniosynostosis is the term used for premature closure or fusion of one or more of the sutures of the skull. It can be classified as primary or secondary. Primary craniosynostosis can occur as an isolated phenomenon or, more frequently, is seen in conjunction with other malformation syndromes, especially the acrocephalosyndactyly syndromes. Secondary craniosynostosis is found in rickets, hypophosphatasia, thyroid disorders, and hypercalcemia, and has also been seen following surgical decompression of intracranial contents. (1) Restraint of the fetal head may be one of the factors contributing to isolated closure of a suture. (2) Synostosis of the cranium may result from a primary resistance to stretching by the preosseous membranous sutures; thus, the sutures close prematurely owing to excessive toughness of the membranous suture. (3)

RADIOLOGIC FEATURES

The affected suture has a straight rather than a serrated radiolucent line. There may be osseous proliferation (sclerosis) at the suture line or frank osseous fusion. MRI and CT may be useful for evaluating associated abnormalities of the face and central nervous system. (4) The most commonly encountered pattern is isolated closure of the sagittal suture, seen in more than 50% of cases. (1) This pattern results in an increased anteroposterior diameter of the skull and a decreased biparietal diameter. Synostosis of both coronal sutures results in a skull that is short in its anteroposterior diameter. Unilateral closure of a coronal suture produces flattening of the orbit on the ipsilateral side. Isolated closure of the lambdoid suture leads to flattening of one side of the occiput. Isolated metopic closure results in a triangular forehead with hypotelorism. Accurate radiographic interpretation should identify the affected suture(s), rather than attempting to use the often confusing terminology that describes the abnormal shape of the skull.

THE EPIPHYSEAL DYSPLASIAS

The epiphyseal dysplasias are a diverse and overlapping group of entities. Often, differentiation between the various types is not easily made. For academic and teaching purposes, they will be described here in their more classic presentations, but it is important for the reader to realize that the clinical and radiographic features of any one case may not be clear-cut. The epiphyseal dysplasias covered in this text include chondrodysplasia punctata, dysplasia epiphysealis hemimelica (Trevor's disease), epiphyseal dysplasia multiplex, and spondyloepiphyseal dysplasia.

CHONDRODYSPLASIA PUNCTATA
GENERAL CONSIDERATIONS

Chondrodysplasia punctata is a type of epiphyseal dysplasia characterized by punctate or stippled calcification of multiple epiphyseal centers during the first year of life. This entity is rare and has been classified into two types: (a) an autosomal dominant form (Conradi-Hunermann syndrome) with a very heterogenous expression and a normal life expectancy and (b) a recessive form that is rhizomelic (proximal limb) and is frequently fatal in the first years of life. (1) Synonyms include stippled epiphyses, dysplasia epiphysealis punctata (2), chondrodystrophia fetalis calcificans, and chondrodystrophia calcificans congenita. (3)

CLINICAL FEATURES

Clinically, children with chondrodysplasia punctata appear similar to achondroplastic dwarfs. (4)

The lethal rhizomelic form features symmetric proximal limb shortening, joint contractures, mental retardation, cataracts, optic atrophy, and skin changes. The spine is normal on physical examination. (5) Most infants die in the first year of life, often as a result of respiratory failure (6) or recurrent infection. Less frequently, tracheal stenosis (7) or spinal cord compression is the cause of death. (8) Females are affected twice as often as males. (9,10)

The dominant form, Conradi-Hunermann syndrome, has asymmetric features, with less limb shortening and deformity. The intelligence is normal, but there are prominent spinal changes. There has been discussion that this form is actually composed of several different genetic disorders, ranging from a mild nondeforming type (Sheffield) (11) to dominant and recessive types carried on the X chromosome. (10,12) The dominant X-linked mode of transmission is lethal in males and females with this type have typical clinical features including extensive ichthyosiform skin lesions, cataracts at birth, nail abnormalities, and linear areas of alopecia. (10,13) The rare recessive X-linked mode of transmission predominates in male offspring and is characterized by asymmetric limb shortening, mental retardation, and small distal phalanges. (10) Sporadic cases of Conradi-Hunermann syndrome may result from women who received Coumadin and Warfarin (anticoagulant medication) during early pregnancy. (14–16) Anticonvulsant drugs have also been implicated as a cause of chondrodysplasia punctata. (17)

PATHOLOGIC FEATURES

The epiphyseal centers undergo mucoid degeneration, and hypervascularity is prominent. This leads to fragmentation of the epiphysis. Calcific and ossific punctate deposits are scattered through the fragments. These calcifications disappear in the first year of life and ossification will proceed, though often in an abnormal fashion, resulting in deformity.

RADIOLOGIC FEATURES

The appearance of stippled epiphyses is typical, but these often disappear within the first year of life. (4) Therefore, it is imperative that the diagnosis be made prior to the disappearance of these characteristic calcifications.

The roentgen findings in the two forms differ:

Lethal Recessive Type

The epiphyseal stippling is noted primarily in the hips, shoulders, knees, and wrists. There is symmetric shortening of the limbs, particularly proximally, and more frequently in the upper

extremities. The metaphyses are often flared, and the long bones are bowed. (Fig. 8.15) In most cases there are coronal clefts of the vertebrae, but stippling of the spine is usually absent and spinal deformity is not as severe as in the dominant Conradi-Hunermann syndrome. (18)

Conradi-Hunermann Syndrome

The stippling at the ends of long bones and in short tubular bones may be mild to severe, with occasional asymmetric limb shortening. The metaphyses and diaphyses are normal. (Fig. 8.16) The vertebral endplates and sometimes the centra are stippled, leading to abnormally shaped vertebrae and a resultant kyphoscoliosis. (Figs. 8.17, 8.18) Stippling may also affect the ends of the ribs, the hyoid bone, the thyroid cartilage,

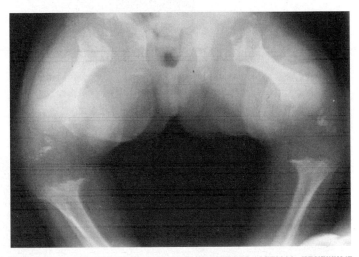

Figure 8.15. CHONDRODYSPLASIA PUNCTATA, LETHAL RECESSIVE FORM: EPIPHYSEAL STIPPLING. Along with epiphyseal stippling, there is symmetric limb shortening and the metaphyses are flared. COMMENT: These individuals usually die within the first year of life.

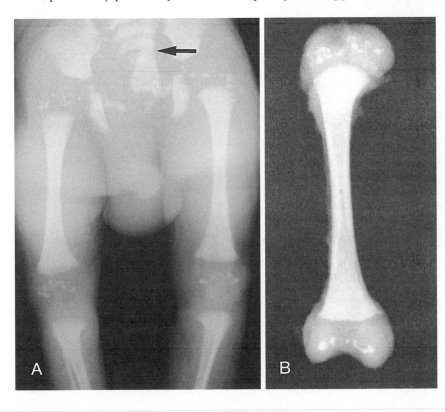

Figure 8.16. CHONDRODYSPLASIA PUNCTATA: CONRADI-HUNERMANN SYNDROME (DOMINANT FORM). A. Pelvis and Legs. Limb shortening is less commonly encountered, and stippling may be mild to severe. The artifact is a clamp for the newborn's umbilicus (arrow). **B. Autopsy Specimen.** Note that in this dominant form the metaphysis and diaphysis are normal. COMMENT: In this dominant form life expectancy is normal. This disorder may be associated with the use of Coumadin and Warfarin during pregnancy.

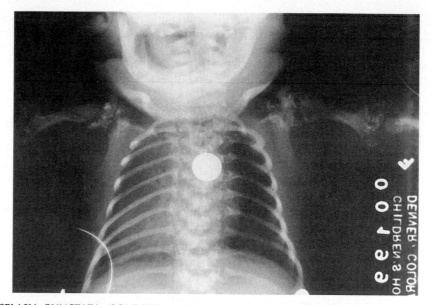

Figure 8.17.   CHONDRODYSPLASIA PUNCTATA, CONRADI-HUNER-MANN SYNDROME: SPINE AND UPPER EXTREMITIES. Observe the extensive vertebral stippling in this newborn. Irregular epiphyses are also noted in the shoulders and elbows. (Courtesy of The Childrens Hospital, Dept. of Radiology, Denver, Colorado)

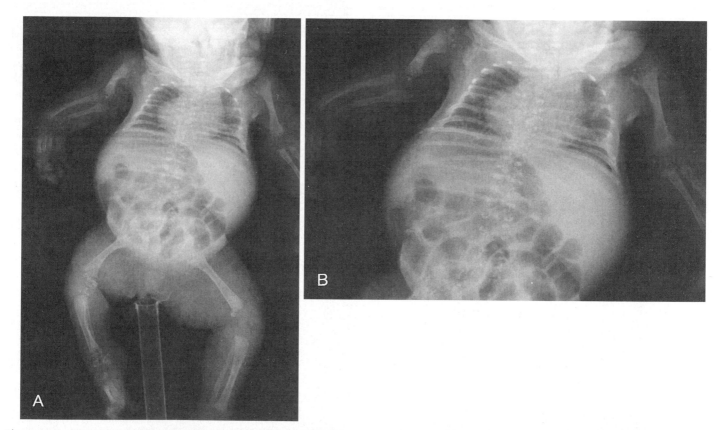

Figure 8.18.   CHONDRODYSPLASIA PUNCTATA, CONRADI-HUNER-MANN SYNDROME. A. Full Skeleton. B. Close Up of Spine and Shoulders. This newborn has the characteristic stippling throughout the spine and ex-tremities. COMMENT: This form of chondrodysplasia punctata has asymmetric limb shortening. (Courtesy of The Childrens Hospital, Dept. of Radiology, Denver, Colorado)

and the base of the skull. Laryngeal and tracheal calcifications may occur. The extent of calcification does not correlate with overall prognosis. (18)

MEDICOLEGAL IMPLICATIONS
Chondrodysplasia Punctata (Conradi-Hunermann)

- A thorough examination to exclude congenital cardiopulmonary complications is necessary.
- Hypoplasia of the dens and os odontoideum have been reported and may lead to atlantoaxial instability. Cervical spine flexion/ extension stress radiographs should be performed, particularly if neurologic signs are evident, or if spinal manipulation of the cervical region is being considered.

DYSPLASIA EPIPHYSEALIS HEMIMELICA
GENERAL CONSIDERATIONS

This uncommon bone dysplasia involving the epiphyses was originally reported by Mouchet and Belot in 1926, (1) and then again by Trevor in 1950, who gave it the name *tarsoepiphyseal aclasis*. (2) While still referred to as *Trevor's disease*, it was Fairbank

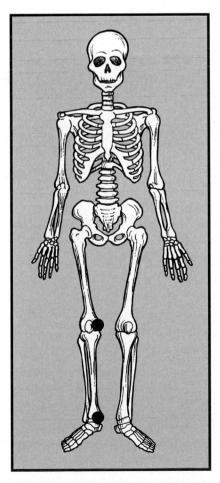

Figure 8.19. SKELETAL DISTRIBUTION DYSPLASIA EPIPHYSEALIS HEMIMELICA.

who suggested the name *dysplasia epiphysealis hemimelica*, as he felt that this entity was not a true aclasis, and there were cases where bones other than the tarsals were involved. (3) Aegerter and Kirkpatrick have suggested that it be called epiphyseal hyperplasia. (4)

Dysplasia epiphysealis hemimelica has no known etiology and is nongenetic. (5,6) This disorder may occur either as a solitary finding, or more commonly, affecting multiple bones. Azouz et al. have classified the dysplasia into three categories: localized form (monostotic involvement), classical form (more than one area in a single lower extremity), and a generalized or severe form (involvement of an entire lower extremity). (5) Dysplasia epiphysealis hemimelica has also been found in conjunction with other benign cartilaginous lesions of bone. Within one family some members displayed solitary dysplasia epiphysealis hemimelica, while others were found to have associated extraskeletal osteochondromas, typical osteochondromas, and intracapsular chondromas. (7) Dysplasia epiphysealis hemimelica has also been reported to coexist with the sclerosing bone dysplasias. (8)

CLINICAL FEATURES

Presenting during the first decade of life, dysplasia epiphysealis hemimelica is three times more common in males. (5) The disorder becomes symptomatic when the asymmetrical epiphyseal overgrowth interferes with normal joint range of motion. It is found predominantly in the lower extremity and is usually monomelic (one limb). (Fig. 8.19) The most commonly involved bones are the distal femur, distal tibia, and talus. (Fig. 8.20) The small bones of the hands and feet can also be affected, displaying premature ossification of the enlarged growth centers. (3,9,10,11) Involvement of the ulna has been reported. (12) (Fig. 8.21) Mendez et al. described a case with involvement of the entire capital femoral epiphysis and ipsilateral acetabular articular cartilage. (13) Functional impairment of the joint may be seen, along with varus and valgus deformities. Hard, bony swellings are noted clinically in the region of involvement, but pain is infrequent. Painful locking of the knee, regional muscular atrophy,

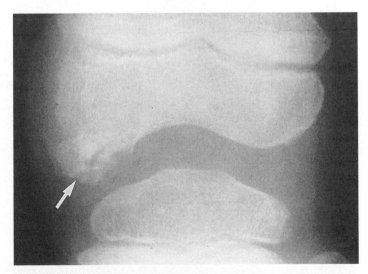

Figure 8.20. DYSPLASIA EPIPHYSEALIS HEMIMELICA: DISTAL FEMUR. Note the focal overgrowth of the medial femoral condyle (arrow). COMMENT: These overgrowths become symptomatic when there is interference with normal joint movement; varus and valgus deformities may develop in affected joints. (Courtesy of Gary M. Guebert, DC, DACBR, St. Louis, Missouri)

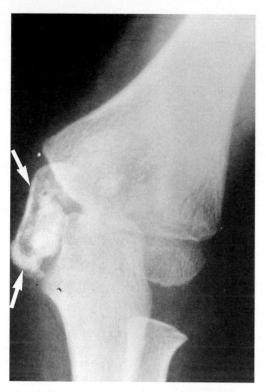

Figure 8.21. DYSPLASIA EPIPHYSEALIS HEMIMELICA: PROXIMAL ULNA. Note the less commonly encountered involvement of the proximal ulna (arrows). (Courtesy of Gary M. Guebert, DC, DACBR, St. Louis, Missouri)

and clumsy gait have been reported. (14) Shortening or lengthening of the limb may also be associated.

RADIOLOGIC FEATURES

Focal overgrowth of one half of an epiphysis in the lower extremity is the characteristic feature. (Fig. 8.22) The medial side of the epiphysis is affected twice as often as the lateral side. (6) (Fig. 8.23) The overgrowth is a bony mass covered with epiphyseal cartilage that is attached to the remainder of the epiphysis. The lesion is sometimes composed of multiple centers and may be separated from the epiphysis. Histologically, the lesions are identical to osteochondromas. With skeletal maturity, these osteocartilagenous masses fuse with the remainder of the epiphysis or, less frequently, remain as separate bodies. The distribution and roentgen appearance of this entity generally present no diagnostic dilemma.

EPIPHYSEAL DYSPLASIA MULTIPLEX
GENERAL CONSIDERATIONS

Epiphyseal dysplasia multiplex is a disorder with abnormalities of the epiphyses that are generally manifested in childhood and lead to severe degenerative changes. Most cases appear to be of autosomal dominant transmission, but varied severity is noted within families. Ribbing described the disorder in 1937, and Fairbank coined the term *dysplasia epiphysealis multiplex* in 1947. (1,2) Rubin believes epiphyseal dysplasia multiplex to be a tarda form of chondrodysplasia punctata. (3) Synonyms include *multiple*

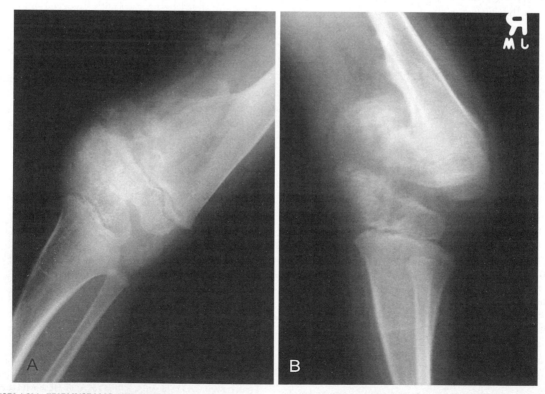

Figure 8.22. DYSPLASIA EPIPHYSEALIS HEMIMELICA. A. AP Knee. B. Lateral Knee. Note that the involvement of the distal femoral and proximal tibial epiphyses are confined to the medial half of these growth centers. Deformity of the distal femoral metaphysis is secondary to the changes in the epiphysis. COMMENT: This condition should not be confused with HME (hereditary multiple exostosis), which involves the metaphyses and spares the epiphyses. (Courtesy of The Childrens Hospital, Dept. of Radiology, Denver, Colorado)

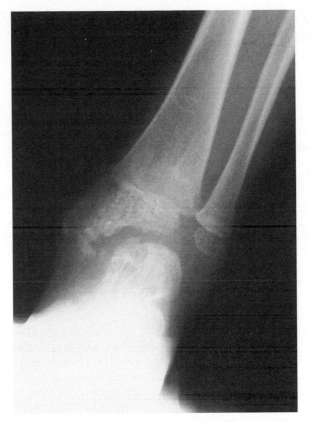

Figure 8.23. DYSPLASIA EPIPHYSEALIS HEMIMELICA: ANKLE. Observe the characteristic overgrowth of the distal tibial epiphysis. The changes are confined to the medial side of the growth center. COMMENT: The medial side of the epiphysis is affected twice as commonly as the lateral side in this condition. (Courtesy of The Childrens Hospital, Dept. of Radiology, Denver, Colorado)

epiphyseal dysplasia, *Fairbank-Ribbing disease*, and *dysplasia polyepiphysaire*.

CLINICAL FEATURES

Generally, the disorder is first noticed when the child begins to walk, with common complaints of a waddling gait and difficulty running. Milder cases may not become apparent until early adulthood, when premature joint degeneration occurs. Both sexes are equally affected. Mental status is normal. Most individuals are of short stature with a tendency toward dwarfism. (4,5) The hands and feet are short and stubby. Other findings include flexion deformities, genu valgum or varum, and, occasionally, coxa vara. Approximately 50% of cases reveal a tibiotalar slant produced by deformity of the lateral portion of the distal tibial epiphysis. (6) This sign is not pathognomonic, however, since it can also be seen in hemophilia and juvenile rheumatoid arthritis. The most frequent sites of epiphyseal involvement are the hips, knees, and ankles, with the shoulders and wrists being less commonly affected.

PATHOLOGIC FEATURES

Epiphyseal dysplasia multiplex appears to be caused by an abnormality of the epiphyseal chondrocytes. (7–9) The number of chondrocytes is decreased and their arrangement is abnormal, leading to delayed and disorderly ossification of the epiphyses.

RADIOLOGIC FEATURES

Development of the epiphyses is delayed (4,5) and their appearance is mottled with irregular mineralization during the second or third year of life. The involvement is bilateral and symmetric, with the hips, knees, and ankles most commonly involved. (Fig. 8.24) While growth is abnormal and delayed, maturation and fusion are usually normal. Frequently, the epiphyses will develop from multiple centers. Occasionally, the metaphyses are flared, most likely due to the abnormal epiphyses. The carpal and tarsal bones are hypoplastic, and the long tubular bones of the hands (and sometimes the feet) are short and thick. (Fig. 8.25)

Mature epiphyses have irregular articular surfaces. The affected femoral heads and condyles are flattened. (Fig. 8.26) Thus, coxa vara deformities are often complicated by slipped femoral capital epiphyses. (10) Approximately two thirds of patients exhibit spinal changes similar to Scheuermann's disease. (11,12) Anterior vertebral body wedging and scoliosis are often present. Less frequently there is platyspondyly. The irregular epiphyses lead to premature and often severe degeneration, especially in the hips and knees. Osteochondritis dissecans of the knee has been reported in two families with epiphyseal dysplasia multiplex. (4)

Several entities—including Legg-Calvé-Perthes' disease, Morquio's disease, and cretinism—may have similar roentgen findings. However, the symmetrical nature and characteristic joints of involvement should provide sufficient evidence for an accurate diagnosis of epiphyseal dysplasia multiplex.

MEDICOLEGAL IMPLICATIONS
Epiphyseal Dysplasia Multiplex

- Dens agenesis has been described. A complete cervical spine examination, including a standard radiographic series, should be performed prior to treatment of this area. If agenesis of the dens is present, flexion/extension stress radiographs should be performed.

- Hip and groin pain may occur secondary to slipped capital femoral epiphysis. When these symptoms are present, AP and frogleg radiographs should be performed. The delayed ossification center may prevent an early diagnosis. If there is a strong clinical suspicion of SFCE and the femoral head is not yet ossified, hip arthrography is recommended.

SPONDYLOEPIPHYSEAL DYSPLASIA
GENERAL CONSIDERATIONS

Spondyloepiphyseal dysplasia is a group of inheritable bone dysplasias with a wide range of expression. It is generally divided into *congenital* and *tarda* forms. Spondyloepiphyseal dysplasia congenita is recognized at birth and is usually transmitted by an autosomal dominant trait. (1) The tarda type is manifested only in males, usually in late childhood, and is transmitted in an

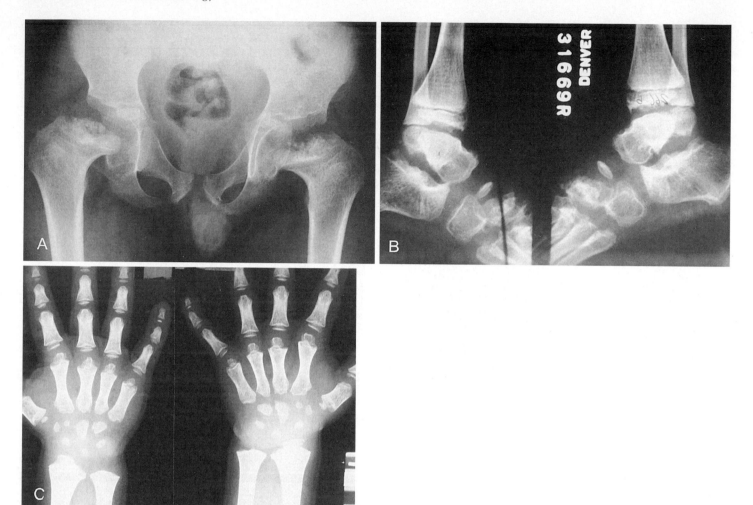

Figure 8.24.   EPIPHYSEAL DYSPLASIA MULTIPLEX. A. Pelvis. Observe the bilateral and symmetric involvement of the proximal femoral epiphyses. There is secondary flaring of the metaphyses. **B. Ankles.** The fragmentation and deformity of the distal tibiae and tarsals is symmetrical. **C. Hands.** The distal radial and ulnar epiphyses are deformed. Also note the deformity of the metacarpal growth centers. COMMENT: The irregular epiphyses lead to premature and severe degenerative arthritis, especially in the hips. (Courtesy of The Childrens Hospital, Dept. of Radiology, Denver, Colorado)

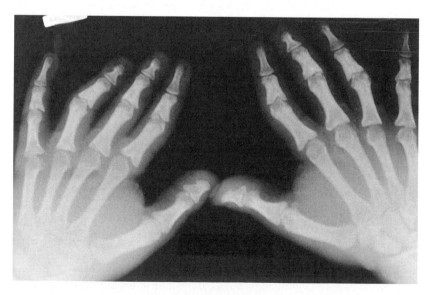

Figure 8.25.   EPIPHYSEAL DYSPLASIA MULTIPLEX: HANDS. Note the symmetrically short and thick tubular bones. There is irregularity of the phalangeal articular surfaces. The hands and feet are short and stubby.

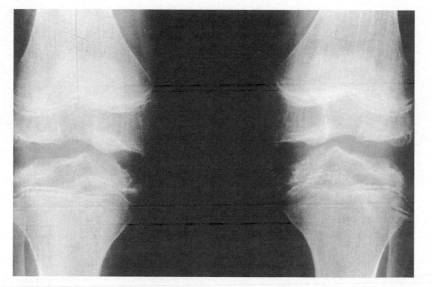

Figure 8.26. EPIPHYSEAL DYSPLASIS MULTIPLEX: KNEES. There is symmetric flattening of the femoral condyles and irregularity of the tibial plateaus. COMMENT: The irregular epiphyses often lead to premature and severe degenerative changes. (Courtesy of Jack Edeiken, MD, Houston, Texas)

X-linked recessive mode. (2) The tarda expression has also been reported in autosomal dominant and autosomal recessive transmissions. (3)

Spondyloepiphyseal Dysplasia Congenita

Clinical Features.   At birth, affected infants have short limbs, flat faces, and widely spaced eyes. (1) Other clinical features include a cleft palate, hearing loss, myopia, and retinal detachment. (4,5) The neck and spine are short, frequently with exaggerated kyphosis and lordosis. Scoliosis and pectus carinatum often are present. Poorly developed muscle tone contributes to genu valgum or varum and hip contractures. (6,7) The height attained ranges from 37 to 52 inches. (1) The hands and feet are normal.

Radiologic Features.   The most prominent features are found in the spine and pelvis. Ossification is delayed, and in the newborn there may be lack of ossification of the pubic bone, distal femur, proximal tibia, calcaneus, and talus. Ossification of the femoral head is greatly retarded throughout childhood, and marked coxa vara is common, complicated by premature osteoarthritis. The acetabular roofs are horizontal, and the iliac wings are short. In the spine the anterior vertebral bodies appear bulbous (*pear-shaped* vertebrae). (Fig. 8.27) With age, these flatten into platyspondyly and persist into adulthood. (8) The platyspondyly, along with thin discs, results in extreme shortening of the trunk. Often, several vertebral bodies at the thoracolumbar junction are hypoplastic. (9) Scoliosis and severe kyphosis and lordosis develop. Odontoid hypoplasia is common and occasional nonunion of the odontoid can be a cause of cervical instability. (10,11) The proximal long bones are often shortened (rhizomelia), with flared metaphyses. The articular surfaces are irregular, and carpal and tarsal maturation may be retarded.

The major entity which must be differentiated from spondyloepiphyseal dysplasia congenita is Morquio's syndrome. Morquio's syndrome is an autosomal recessive mucopolysaccharidosis, which is characterized by keratosulfaturia, corneal opacities, and spinal changes. Unlike spondyloepiphyseal dysplasia, the disc height is normal in Morquio patients and the vertebral bodies are flattened with central *beaking*.

Spondyloepiphyseal Dysplasia Tarda

Clinical Features.   Spondyloepiphyseal dysplasia tarda usually manifests between the ages of 5 and 10 and is found only in males. There is mild loss of stature, with the adult height varying from 52 to 62 inches. (12,13) Back pain is a frequent complaint, and premature osteoarthritis begins shortly after puberty.

Radiologic Features.   The short stature of affected individuals is due primarily to platyspondyly, which is most marked in the thoracic region. A characteristic configuration of the vertebral body is noted, in which there is hyperostotic bone deposited on the posterior two-thirds of the endplates. This is referred to as a *hump-shaped* or *heaping-up* vertebra. (14) (Fig. 8.28) The ring epiphyses do not ossify, and the disc spaces are thin. Mild kyphosis, scoliosis, and early degenerative changes are frequent. Early and marked osteoarthritis of the hips is the most prominent radiographic feature. Loss of joint space, spurring, and cyst formation result in deformity of the femoral head and neck. The pelvis is often small and there may be a broad thorax with sternal prominence. Degenerative changes are occasionally seen in the shoulders and less frequently in the knees and ankles.

MEDICOLEGAL IMPLICATIONS
Spondyloepiphyseal Dysplasia Congenita

• Hypoplasia of the dens with subsequent atlantoaxial dislocation has been reported in the congenita form. A standard three view radiographic series is recommended prior to manipulative treatment of the cervical spine in patients with this disorder. If dens hypoplasia is noted, flexion/extension stress radiographs should be obtained.

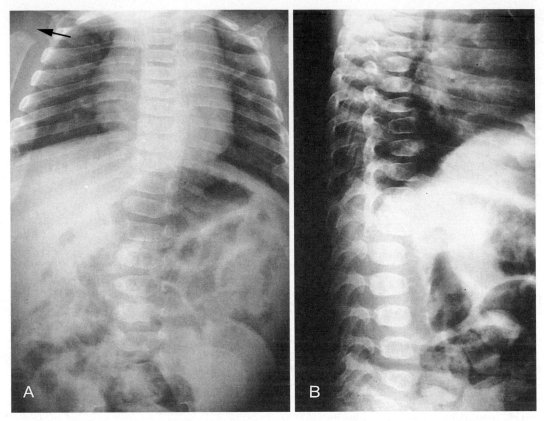

**Figure 8.27.   SPONDYLOEPIPHYSEAL DYSPLASIA: CONGENITA FORM.
A. AP Thoracolumbar Spine.** Note the delayed ossification of the proximal humeral epiphysis (arrow). **B. Lateral Thoracolumbar Spine.** Observe the mild bulbous appearance of the anterior vertebral bodies. This will flatten into platyspondyly and persist into adulthood. COMMENT: The platyspondyly, along with thin discs, results in extreme shortening of the trunk. (Courtesy of The Childrens Hospital, Dept. of Radiology, Denver, Colorado)

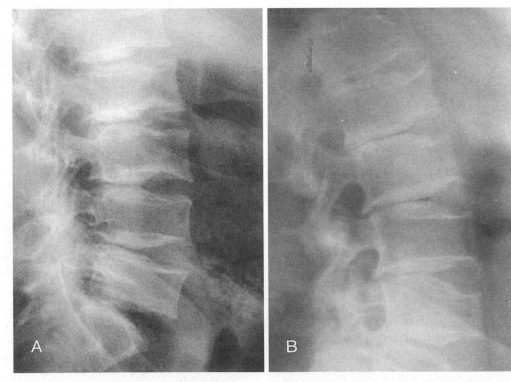

Figure 8.28.   SPONDYLOEPIPHYSEAL DYSPLASIA: TARDA FORM. A. Lumbar Spine. Hyperostotic bone is deposited on the posterior two-thirds of the vertebra, referred to as *hump-shaped* or *heaping-up* vertebra. (Courtesy of John R. Nolan, DC, Wanganui, New Zealand) **B. Lumbar Spine.** This patient also demonstrates a *heaping-up* configuration. COMMENT: Note the thinness of the disc. The changes in spondyloepiphyseal dysplasia lead to back pain and premature osteoarthritis.

FIBRODYSPLASIA OSSIFICANS PROGRESSIVA

GENERAL CONSIDERATIONS

Fibrodysplasia ossificans progressiva (1) is a rare, disabling disorder that leads to progressive ossification of striated muscles, tendons, ligaments, fascia, and aponeuroses. The occurrence is usually sporadic, but it may be inherited as autosomal dominant with a wide range of expression. (2) In 1692, Patin first described a case of a young woman who *turned to wood*. (3) Munchmeyer reported the first series of cases, and the disorder is sometimes referred to as *Munchmeyer's disease*. (4) Other synonyms include *fibrogenesis ossificans progressiva*, *myositis ossificans progressiva*, and *fibrositis ossificans progressiva*. The etiology of this disorder is unknown.

CLINICAL FEATURES

The initial findings of this disease are usually seen in the first years of life. There is no gender predominance. The most common presenting symptom is torticollis, with painful, hot, edematous masses in the sternocleidomastoid muscles. Involvement then progresses to the remaining soft tissues of the neck, shoulders, spine, and upper arms. Later in the course of the disease the lower extremities may be affected. Occasionally, these masses follow trivial trauma. Fever may accompany the acute phase. As the acute tenderness of the masses subsides, the lesions become smaller and harden, as ossification occurs. The extensive ossification leads to severely disabling restriction of joint movement. Involvement of the intercostal musculature interferes with respiration. Wasting follows ossification of the muscles of mastication. The smooth muscles of the tongue, larynx, diaphragm, heart, and sphincters are not involved. (1) An abnormal electrocardiogram has been reported. (5)

Seventy-five percent of patients with fibrodysplasia ossificans progressive have bilateral microdactyly of the first toe, with synostosis of the phalanges. A smaller percentage have similar anomalies of the thumbs. These congenital digital anomalies are present in 5% of the family members of fibrodysplasia ossificans progressiva patients, thus supporting the hereditary, but varied presentation theory of this disease. (6–8) Two sets of homozygous twins have been reported to have fibrodysplasia ossificans progressiva. (9,10)

LABORATORY FEATURES

Chemistry findings are generally noncontributory, with blood chemistry, serum alkaline phosphatase, renal function, and parathormone levels all within normal limits. (5)

PATHOLOGIC FEATURES

Early, the soft tissue masses are composed of edema and inflammatory exudate, forming a mass of collagen. Calcium salts then are deposited within the collagenous mass, eventually developing into an irregular mass of lamellar and woven bone. McKusick suggests that fibrodysplasia ossificans progressiva affects the interstitial tissues primarily, and that muscle involvement is secondary to pressure atrophy. (1) It has been suggested that the calcium salts are deposited due to lack of a circulating inhibitor (5), or due to a primary defect in the collagen. (1) Still other reports reveal abnormalities suggestive of a progressive myopathy. (11,12)

RADIOLOGIC FEATURES

The radiographic findings can be divided into two categories—digital anomalies and ectopic ossification.

Digital Anomalies

The digits are anomalous at birth, thus preceding the ectopic ossification. As previously stated, microdactyly of the first toe is present in 75% of individuals with fibrodysplasia ossificans progressiva and in 5% of unaffected family members. (Fig. 8.29) Another common finding is microdactyly of the thumbs. (Fig. 8.30) The microdactyly results from phalangeal shortening, synostosis, or rarely, absence. Short metacarpals, especially the first and fifth, may be found. Hallux valgus is nearly always present. (11) Other associated congenital anomalies include brachydactyly, clinodactyly, large epiphyses, and broad femoral necks. (Fig. 8.31)

Ectopic Ossification

During the acute inflammatory stage, the lesions appear radiographically as soft tissue masses. Swelling of the soft tissue planes is well demonstrated on CT scans and ossification can be detected on CT before it is apparent on plain radiographs. (13) As the collagen organizes, calcium salts are deposited. Linear and spheroid deposits of bone are seen as the process progresses to ossification. (Fig. 8.32) Eventually, columns of bone replace tendons, fascia, and ligaments and are seen in the muscles. (Fig. 8.33) Ossification of tendon and ligament insertions gives the appearance of exostoses. Sesamoid bones may fuse to the digits. In the

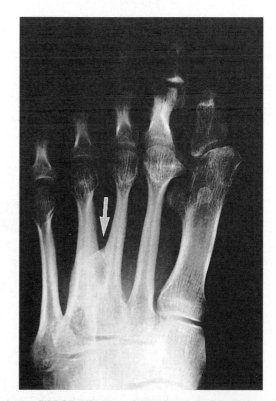

Figure 8.29. FIBRODYSPLASIA OSSIFICANS PROGRESSIVA: MICRODACTYLY OF THE GREAT TOE. Microdactyly of the great toe is present in 75% of individuals with fibrodysplasia ossificans progressiva and in 5% of unaffected family members. Also note the hallux valgus deformity and the synostosis of the third and fourth metatarsal bases (arrow).

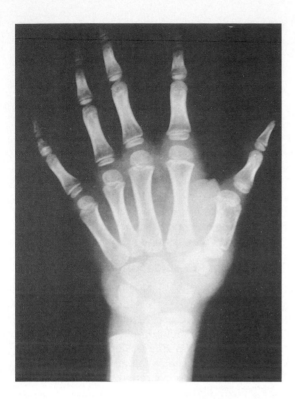

Figure 8.30. FIBRODYSPLASIA OSSIFICANS PROGRESSIVA: MICRODACTYLY OF THE THUMB. The microdactyly results either from phalangeal shortening or synostosis. In this case the first metacarpal is short as well.

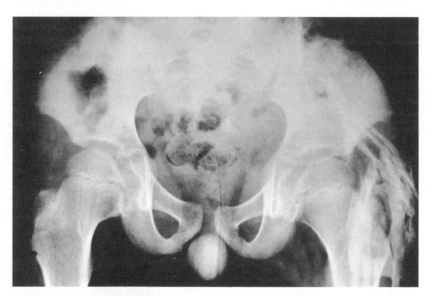

Figure 8.31. FIBRODYSPLASIA OSSIFICANS PROGRESSIVA, PELVIS: BROAD FEMORAL NECKS. Broad femoral necks are often associated with fibrodysplasia ossificans progressiva. Note the extensive ossification around the hip joint.

majority of cases, ossification of the soft tissues of the spine (i.e., interspinous ligament, supraspinous ligament, ligamentum nuchae, paraspinal muscles) (14) is followed by vertebral and apophyseal joint fusions. The intervertebral discs are hypoplastic and become calcified. The changes are similar to those seen in ankylosing spondylitis and contribute to the severe restriction

of mobility. Early ossification of the neck soft tissues results in premature fusion of the cervical spine growth centers with hypoplastic and ankylosed vertebral bodies. (Fig. 8.34) The diagnosis is readily made when congenital digital anomalies are present in association with widespread soft tissue ossification.

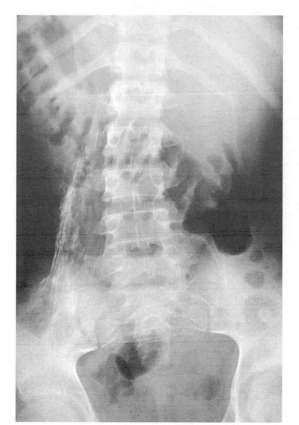

Figure 8.32. FIBRODYSPLASIA OSSIFICANS PROGRESSIVA: PSOAS MUSCLE OSSIFICATION. There is unilateral ossification of the psoas muscle. Eventually, columns of bone replace tendons, fascia, ligaments, and muscle, leading to severe disability.

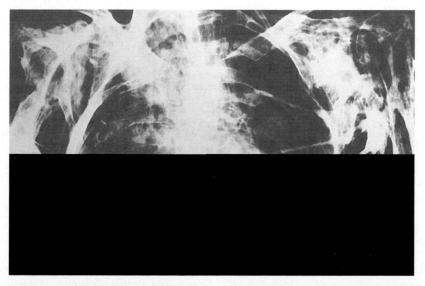

Figure 8.33. FIBRODYSPLASIA OSSIFICANS PROGRESSIVA: THORACIC AND AXILLARY INVOLVEMENT. Columns of bone traverse the axillary regions and extend around the chest. Involvement of the intercostal muscles interferes with respiration. Respiratory failure and cor pulmonale are severe complications.

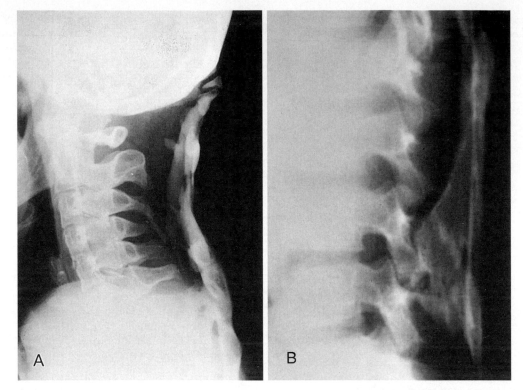

Figure 8.34. FIBRODYSPLASIA OSSIFICANS PROGRESSIVA: SPINE. A. Cervical Spine. Note the ossification extending caudally from the occiput along the spine. Also note the hypoplastic fused vertebral bodies. **B. Lumbar Spine.** The ossification extends into the lumbar region. COMMENT: The most common presenting symptom is torticollis. The muscles of the neck are inflamed and become progressively ossified. Premature fusion of the cervical spine growth centers leads to hypoplastic, ankylosed vertebral bodies. Involvement then progresses to the shoulders and upper arms.

MEDICOLEGAL IMPLICATIONS
Fibrodysplasia Ossificans Progressiva

- Manipulation is contraindicated. Even mild muscle trauma induces reparative ossification, accelerating the progressive nature of this disorder.

- Osteomalacia may develop in patients who have received drug therapy and may result in pathologic fractures.

- Progressive respiratory disease and subsequent cardiopulmonary failure are inevitable.

HOLT-ORAM SYNDROME
GENERAL CONSIDERATIONS

Holt and Oram first described the familial transmission of combined congenital cardiac deformities and anomalies of the arms and hands in 1960. (1) This uncommon autosomal dominant dysplasia has variable expressivity (2,3) but the skeletal anomalies do not involve the lower extremities. Synonyms include *heart-hand syndrome*, *cardio-limb syndrome*, and *cardiomelic syndrome*.

CLINICAL FEATURES

The cardiovascular changes most commonly manifest as a patent atrial septum, but ventricular septal defects (4) and anomalies of the great vessels are also encountered. Limited range of motion and/or dislocation of the elbow is associated with hypoplasia or absence of the radial head, radio-ulnar, and humero-ulnar synostosis. Hypoplasia or complete absence of the radius has been found (radial ray deficiency). (Fig 8.35) Holt-Oram is one of the more common causes of *radial ray deficiency* or *dysplasia*. Shoulder anomalies include hypoplastic humeri, clavicles and scapulae, and Sprengel's deformity. Chest wall anomalies include deficiency in the pectoral muscles, pectus excavatum, and pectus carinatum. Aplastic anemia has been reported. (5)

RADIOLOGIC FEATURES

Anomalies of the thumbs are the most common skeletal finding. (6) An extra phalanx in the first digit is frequent (*triphalangeal thumb*). Absence of the thumb has also been reported. Poznanski states that the carpal findings are most characteristic with some abnormality of the scaphoid being present in almost all cases. (7) Extra carpals are common and carpal fusions are occasionally seen. The middle phalanges of the fifth fingers are short and there is usually associated clinodactyly. (7)

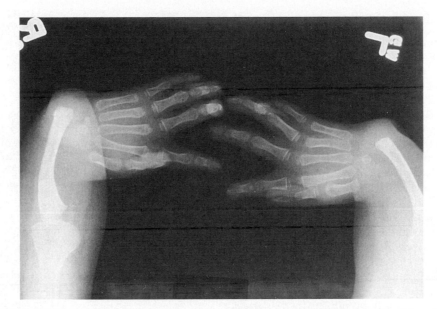

Figure 8.35. HOLT-ORAM SYNDROME: HANDS AND WRISTS. Note agenesis of the radius (radial ray deficiency). The case is unusual due to sparing of the thumbs. COMMENT: Anomalies of the thumbs are common in this syndrome, as well as cardiac deformities. (Courtesy of The Childrens Hospital, Dept. of Radiology, Denver, Colorado)

MEDICOLEGAL IMPLICATIONS
Holt-Oram Syndrome

- Cardiovascular complications are frequently seen and are typically congenital in nature. Careful clinical assessment of the cardiovascular system should be performed in all patients with this disorder.

INFANTILE CORTICAL HYPEROSTOSIS
GENERAL CONSIDERATIONS

Infantile cortical hyperostosis is an uncommon and puzzling disease of infants, nearly always presenting before the age of 5 months. It was first described by Caffey and Silverman in 1945 and is sometimes referred to as *Caffey's disease* or *Caffey's syndrome*. (1) Gender distribution is equal, and cases have been found throughout the world with no racial predilection. Familial involvement over several generations has been noted. (2) The incidence of the disease has been decreasing, especially sporadic cases, and the inherited mode of transmission may represent the major pattern of involvement seen today. (3)

CLINICAL FEATURES

Patients usually manifest a clinical triad of hyperirritability, swelling of the soft tissues, and palpable, hard masses over affected bones. Fever is nearly always present, along with an increased erythrocyte sedimentation rate and elevated serum alkaline phosphatase levels. More than half of Caffey's patients show reduced hemoglobin and red blood cell levels. (4) Anemia and a moderate leukocytosis may be present. Serologic and cul-ture tests for viral and bacterial agents have all been unrewarding. Pseudoparalysis, pleuritis, and pallor are additional clinical features. Remissions and exacerbations are common with some cases showing improvement with corticosteroid therapy. The soft tissue swelling and hard masses are extremely tender to palpation but lack warmth and discoloration. This swelling is most marked over the mandible. (5) The average age at onset is 9 weeks, but it has been present at birth and has even been recognized in utero. (6,7)

The severity and course of the disease are extremely variable. Most cases resolve within a few weeks to several months, but there have been cases persisting into adolescence. (8) Mild cases may go without clinical notice, while severe involvement can produce deformities that persist into adulthood. (9)

PATHOLOGIC FEATURES

Langer and Kaufman have described three stages of the disease: (a) an acute stage with lesions on the periosteum, (b) a subacute stage with reestablishment of the periosteum in a normal fashion, and (c) a late stage with bone remodeling where radiographs show cortical hyperostosis and residual bony bridges. (10)

Pathologic changes are initially seen in the periosteum, which swells, then loses its distinct margins and blends with the adjacent soft tissues. During this inflammatory stage the cortex undergoes resorption. As the disease progresses, connective tissue and trabeculae are laid down, sometimes enlarging the bone to profound proportions. Remodeling occurs with healing, but some bony deformities may persist.

The etiology of infantile cortical hyperostosis is still unknown. Most of the clinical and pathologic features suggest an infectious agent, most likely a virus. Similar findings in hamsters and cats have been reported. (4) The theory of a viral etiology is further supported by the lack of response to antibiotic and sulfonamide therapy. Familial incidence over several generations suggests the importance of genetic or inheritable factors. (5)

RADIOLOGIC FEATURES

Periosteal new bone formation takes place within the soft tissue swelling adjacent to the cortex. This new bone may be very dense and may increase to the extent that the bone doubles its original size. The hyperostosis usually persists for some time after evidence of soft tissue swelling has subsided. During the healing phase, the new bone formation may have a *laminated* appearance, but this is not noted during the acute stage.

The most commonly involved bones are the mandible, clavicle, and ribs, where involvement is frequently symmetric. (5) (Figs. 8.36, 8.37) The ulna is the most frequently involved of the long bones, often without concomitant involvement of the radius. (Fig. 8.38) With the exceptions of the vertebrae, phalanges, and round bones (carpals and tarsals), any bone of the skeleton may be involved. (4) In the past it was believed that infantile cortical hyperostosis never manifested without involvement in the mandible, but the familial cases are characterized by less mandibular involvement, more lower extremity involvement, and an earlier age of onset. (3)

The cortical hyperostosis is most prominent in the lateral arches of the ribs (11), and there may be associated ipsilateral pleural effusions and diaphragmatic eventration. The epiphyses

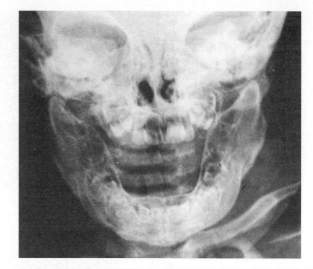

Figure 8.36. INFANTILE CORTICAL HYPEROSTOSIS: MANDIBULAR INVOLVEMENT. Note the bilateral mandibular hyperostosis, with soft tissue swelling. COMMENT: The most commonly involved bones are the mandible, clavicle, and ribs. (Reprinted with permission: Edeiken J: *Roentgen Diagnosis of Diseases of Bone*, ed 3. Baltimore, Williams & Wilkins, p 818, 1981)

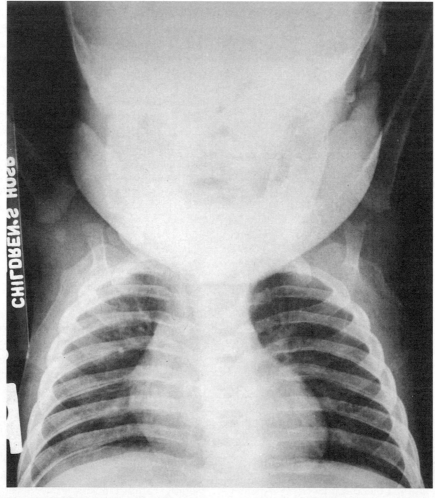

Figure 8.37. INFANTILE CORTICAL HYPEROSTOSIS: RIB AND MANDIBULAR INVOLVEMENT. There is symmetric hyperostosis of the ribs and mandible. (Reprinted with permission: Edeiken J: *Roentgen Diagnosis of Diseases of Bone*, ed 3. Baltimore, Williams & Wilkins, p 822, 1981)

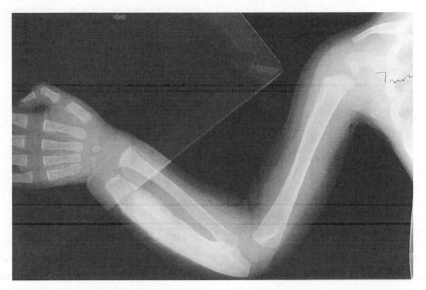

Figure 8.38.   INFANTILE CORTICAL HYPEROSTOSIS: ULNAR INVOLVE-MENT. Note involvement of the ulna, with sparing of the radius and hu-merus. The ulna is the most frequently involved long bone in infantile cortical hyperostosis.

are spared when long bone involvement occurs. (Fig. 8.39) In the skull, various presentations may occur. Thickening of the calvarium or destructive lesions may simulate histiocytosis or metastatic neuroblastoma. Involvement around the anterior fontanelle yields an appearance not unlike the bulging due to increased intracranial pressure. Scapular lesions have been mistaken for malignant tumors. Several cases with shoulder girdle involvement have presented with Erb's palsy. (12)

Residual changes—including facial asymmetry, disturbances in longitudinal growth, medullary expansion, and undertubulation of long bones—are often associated with severe and chronic cases. (13) Pressure from extreme hyperostosis may destroy the adjacent periosteum and lead to osseous bridging and local fusion of cortical walls. This is most frequently seen in the ribs and between the ulna and radius, or between the tibia and fibula. Radioulnar synostosis can lead to radial head dislocation. (14)

While the radiographic features of infantile cortical hyperostosis can raise the concern of child abuse, bone scans will usually show symmetric involvement of the mandible, clavicles, and ribs, leading to the correct diagnosis. (15)

MARFAN'S SYNDROME

GENERAL CONSIDERATIONS

Marfan's syndrome is an autosomal dominant entity consisting of long, slender tubular bones, ocular abnormalities, and aortic aneurysm. First described in 1896 by Marfan (1), it is now thought that his patient actually had congenital contractural arachnodactyly, a distinctly different, yet similar disorder. (2) Synonyms for Marfan's syndrome include *arachnodactyly* and *dolichostenomelia*. (3) Marfan's syndrome is not rare, occurring in 4 to 6 per 100,000 live births. (4,5) The majority of patients will have familial incidence, though some cases are sporadic.

CLINICAL FEATURES

No gender or racial predominance has been established. The severity of involvement varies greatly, but most individuals can be diagnosed clinically. The clinical manifestations defining Mar-

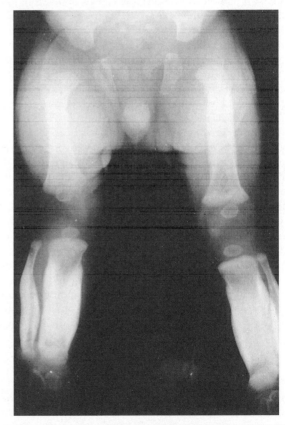

Figure 8.39.   INFANTILE CORTICAL HYPEROSTOSIS: LOWER EXTREMITIES. Note the symmetric involvement in the lower extremities, with sparing of the epiphyses.

fan's syndrome involve three systems: skeletal, ocular, and cardiovascular. (4) The extremities are markedly elongated, with very sparse soft tissue, owing to muscular hypoplasia and a scarcity of subcutaneous fat. The elongation of the tubular bones (the trunk is spared) is most marked in the distal portion of the extremities, especially the phalanges, metacarpals, and metatarsals. The lower extremity exhibits greater overgrowth than the upper. Underdevelopment and hypotonicity of the muscular system contributes to joint laxity and dislocation. Associated findings include hip dislocation, genu recurvatum, patellar dislocation, and pes planus. Persistent bilateral perilunate dislocations have been reported. (6) Generally, affected individuals are taller than 6 feet. Scoliosis is found in greater than 50% of patients with Marfan's syndrome. (4)

Classically, the skull reveals dolichocephaly. The face is elongated, with a high, arched palate and prominent jaw. Mental capacity is generally normal. Poor dentition is frequent, often with two rows of misplaced, long teeth. More than 50% of cases of Marfan's syndrome have dislocation of the ocular lens (ectopia lentis); this is the most common ocular abnormality. (7–9) Also frequently encountered are myopia and contracted pupils, which are secondary to the absence of the dilator muscle of the pupil. There may also be strabismus and retinal detachment. In adulthood cataracts may form secondary to lens detachment.

Some form of congenital heart disease is present in about one third of affected individuals. These complications are responsible for more than 95% of the discernible causes of death in patients with Marfan's syndrome and are the primary reason that these patients' life expectancy is halved. (10) Atrial septal defect is the most frequent congenital heart lesion. (9) Abnormal tunica media and cystic medial necrosis predispose to dissection and rupture of the aorta and pulmonary artery. Dilatation of the ascending aorta, along with abnormalities of the valves, leads to valvular incompetence and left-sided insufficiency referred to as the *floppy valve syndrome*. (2,11)

To allow proper diagnosis in less classical cases, clinical and radiographic tests have been described. Steinberg suggests the *thumb sign*, which refers to the protrusion of the flexed thumb beyond the confines of a clenched fist. (12) Radiographically, the metacarpal index (the ratio of the length to the width of the second through fifth metacarpal bones) is increased in Marfan patients. (13) Thoracic cage deformities (i.e., pectus excavatum, pectus carinatum, thoracic scoliosis) often develop early in life and can aid in the early diagnosis of Marfan's syndrome. (14)

Pathologically, Marfan's syndrome is a connective tissue disorder, with a failure to produce normal collagen. It appears to be the poor quality, rather than an insufficient quantity, of collagen which leads to the vast array of changes. The etiology is still unknown, and there are no consistently abnormal laboratory findings.

RADIOLOGIC FINDINGS

Elongation of the extremities without an increase in width is classic. There is no osteoporosis. The tubular bones of the hands and feet are particularly long, slender, and gracile; hence, the name *arachnodactyly* or *spider-like* fingers. (Fig. 8.40) The cortices are generally thinned, and the trabecular pattern is often delicate.

Acetabular protrusion, unilateral or bilateral, is found in nearly 50% of patients (5,15,16) and is thought to be secondary to weakened acetabular bone.

In the spine the findings include tall vertebrae (17) and often a severe scoliosis or kyphoscoliosis. The scoliosis is frequently a double major or right thoracic curve (4), which develops early in childhood. The spinal canal is widened in greater than 50%, especially in the lumbosacral region. There is posterior scalloping

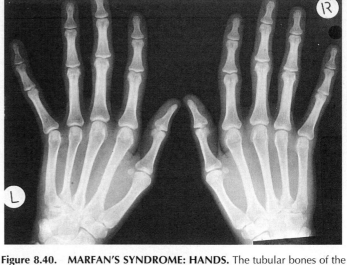

Figure 8.40. MARFAN'S SYNDROME: HANDS. The tubular bones of the hands and feet are long, slender, and gracile; hence, the name *arachnodactyly* or *spider-like* fingers. COMMENT: 50% of cases have ocular lens dislocations and cardiac abnormalities which contribute to shortened lifespans. Also encountered are dissecting aortic aneurysms. (Courtesy of Bryan Hartley, MD, Melbourne, Australia)

of the vertebral bodies, and thinning of the pedicles and lamina secondary to dural ectasia. (4,18) Occasionally, meningoceles and nerve root compression may be seen. (19)

A pectus excavatum deformity with elongated ribs is often encountered, and McKusick suggests that this finding is indicative of hereditary Marfan's syndrome. (9) Similar roentgen findings are seen in homocystinuria, an inheritable methionine metabolism disorder. However, the presence of osteoporosis, along with vertebral body flattening and mental retardation, aid in differentiating these two entities.

MEDICOLEGAL IMPLICATIONS
Marfan's Syndrome

- A complete cardiac examination should be performed to exclude congenital cardiac abnormalities.

- The spontaneous and abrupt onset of chest pain may indicate either aortic dissection (secondary to cystic medial necrosis) or pneumothorax. Computed tomography is indicated if aortic dissection is suspected.

- Faulty dentition is responsible for dental caries. If untreated, osteomyelitis of the maxilla or mandible may develop.

- Slipped capital femoral epiphysis has been described as a complication of this disorder. If suspected clinically, AP and frog-leg radiographs of the corresponding hip joint should be obtained.

- Laxity of the transverse ligament may be present, resulting in atlantoaxial hypermobility and possible dislocation. Manipulation of the upper cervical region should be performed with caution and only following a complete radiographic cervical spine series, including flexion/extension stress views.

METAPHYSEAL DYSPLASIA

GENERAL CONSIDERATIONS

First described by Pyle in 1931, metaphyseal dysplasia is a rare autosomal recessive disorder characterized by splaying or flaring of the ends of long bones. (1) Familial incidence has been reported. (2,3) Synonyms include *Pyle's disease* and *familial metaphyseal dysplasia*. In 1970, Gorlin described craniometaphyseal dysplasia as a distinct entity, separate from metaphyseal dysplasia. Craniometaphyseal dysplasia is a more severe disorder characterized by abnormal craniofacial features with cranial nerve involvement, infrequent hemi- or quadriplegia, and mental or motor retardation. (4)

CLINICAL FEATURES

Metaphyseal dysplasia is a benign condition, with general health unimpaired and a normal lifespan. (5) The disorder manifests at variable ages, most commonly in late childhood. Many patients are taller than normal, presenting with bulbous enlargements of the lower extremity joints and often with genu valgum. There are few clinical symptoms; occasionally, patients complain of joint pain or contractures (5) and muscular weakness. The process is apparently due to failure of subperiosteal remodeling in the metaphyses; the cause of this is thought to be chronic hyperemia of the perichondrial ring of osteoblasts. The hyperemia may be due to congenital hyperplasia of the perichondral ring arteries. (6)

RADIOLOGIC FEATURES

While clinical manifestations are not seen until late childhood, the skeleton of a newborn with Pyle's disease may be overly radiopaque, simulating osteopetrosis. (7) With growth, most bones assume a normal density, but there is failure of metaphyseal modeling, producing splaying or an *Erlenmeyer flask* deformity. (Fig. 8.41) The cortex in the involved area is thinner and is predisposed

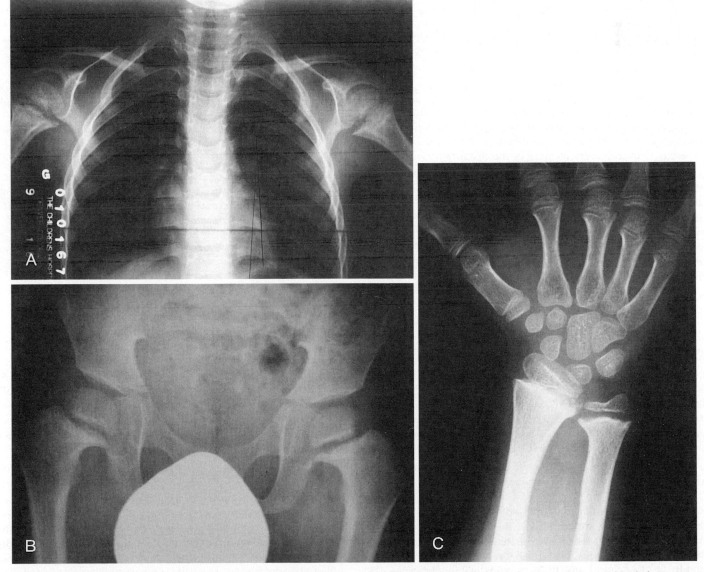

Figure 8.41.   METAPHYSEAL DYSPLASIA. A. Shoulders. Observe the flared metaphyses of the proximal humeri. **B. Pelvis.** The proximal metaphyses of the femora are splayed. **C. Wrist.** The distal radial and ulnar metaphyses are flared. (Courtesy of The Childrens Hospital, Dept. of Radiology, Denver, Colorado)

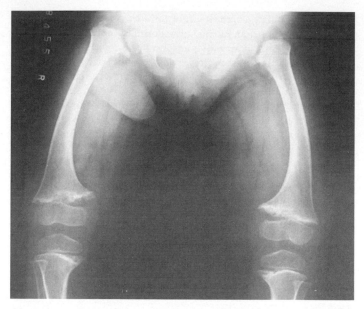

Figure 8.42.   METAPHYSEAL DYSPLASIA: LOWER EXTREMITIES. Note the flared metaphyses, resulting in an *Erlenmeyer flask* deformity. COMMENT: The lower extremity is more markedly affected than the upper in this dysplasia. (Courtesy of The Childrens Hospital, Dept. of Radiology, Denver, Colorado)

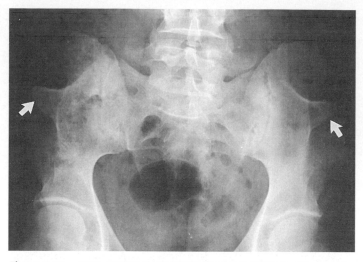

Figure 8.43.   NAIL-PATELLA SYNDROME: ILIAC HORNS. Observe the bilateral central posterior iliac horns, which are characteristic of this syndrome (arrows). COMMENT: An isolated finding of iliac horns, without nail and patellar findings, is referred to as Fong's disease.

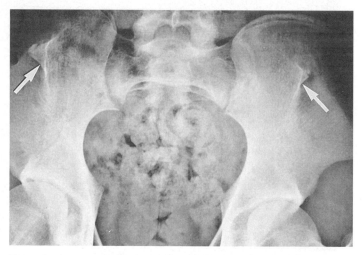

Figure 8.44.   NAIL-PATELLA SYNDROME: ILIAC HORNS. This patient demonstrates small posterior iliac horns (arrows).

to fracture. The lower extremity is more markedly affected than the upper. (Fig. 8.42) The most commonly involved bones are the distal femur, tibia (proximal and distal), and proximal fibula. In the upper extremity, involvement of the distal radius, ulna, and proximal humerus is most frequent. Occasionally, the hands and feet show metaphyseal flaring in the small tubular bones. There may be involvement of the sternal ends of the clavicles and ribs (3) or of the rami of the ischium and pubis. Craniofacial manifestations include hypoplasia of the sinuses (2) and hyperostosis of the calvarium and mandible, with ocular hypertelorism. (8) Vertebra plana or platyspondyly with increased density of the central bodies is also associated. (7)

NAIL-PATELLA SYNDROME

GENERAL CONSIDERATIONS

Nail-patella syndrome is an uncommon autosomal dominant disorder (1), and is also known as osteo-onychodysostosis, hereditary osteo-onychodysplasia (HOOD) syndrome, and Fong's syndrome. The presence of bilateral posterior iliac horns was first described by Kieser in 1939 (2) and Fong in 1946. (3) The association of iliac horns with other abnormalities of the nails, elbows, and knees was recognized by Mino et al. in 1948. (4) Kidney dysplasia with renal osteodystrophy (5) can lead to death in young adulthood.

CLINICAL FEATURES

This disorder manifests with dysplastic fingernails, small or absent patellae, bony deformities of the pelvis and elbows, iliac horns, numerous soft tissue abnormalities, and renal dysplasia. (6–8) Clinically, the manifestations become evident most frequently in the second and third decades of life. However, the radiographic findings of bilateral posterior iliac horns allows identification of this dysplasia at any age. (9)

Hypoplasia, or splitting of the nails, is most commonly seen on the thumb and index finger. Clinodactyly and short fifth metacarpals may also be found. There is often palpable absence of the patellae. The widespread soft tissue abnormalities include joint contractures, abnormal pigmentation of the iris, web formations of the hands and feet, and muscular hypoplasia.

Renal dysplasia can lead to life-threatening kidney disease. There may be proteinuria, hematuria, hypertension, and other forms of nephropathy. (5)

RADIOLOGIC FEATURES

A pair of central posterior iliac horns formed by separate ossification centers is the characteristic radiographic sign. (10) The iliac horns are pathognomonic and, if present signify the identification of this disorder, even in infancy. (11) (Figs. 8.43, 8.44) In a small percentage of cases, the paired horns may be absent. (12) Other abnormalities of the pelvis consist of dysplasia of the iliac wings with flaring or shortening. In the knees, the patellae may be absent or small and there may be asymmetric development of the femoral condyles leading to deformity, gait abnormalities, patellar instability and genu valgum. (9) The medial condyle of the distal humerus and the capitellum are occasionally hypoplastic, producing an increased carrying angle of the elbow and subluxation or dislocation of the radial head. (12)

The presence of a unilateral posterior iliac horn has been reported and is not associated with nail-patella syndrome. (13)

THE OSTEOPENIC DYSPLASIAS

When evaluating a patient from a radiographic perspective, it is often helpful to classify disorders into major categories according to their general radiographic appearance. This categorical approach can be helpful when assessing a patient with a skeletal dysplasia.

Those dysplasias that result in increased bone formation, or sclerosis, have been grouped together as the sclerotic dysplasias (e.g., osteopetrosis, osteopoikilosis). This group of disorders will be discussed later in this chapter, following this section, that describes those dysplasias that demonstrate a generalized decrease in bone density (osteopenia).

The osteopenic dysplasias are more numerous than the sclerotic variety. Only the more frequently encountered entities will be discussed in this section. These include Ehlers-Danlos syndrome, massive osteolysis of Gorham, the mucopolysaccharidoses (e.g., Hurler's syndrome, Morquio's syndrome) and osteogenesis imperfecta.

EHLERS-DANLOS SYNDROME
GENERAL CONSIDERATIONS

Ehlers-Danlos syndrome is a rare inherited connective tissue disorder characterized by skin fragility and hyperelasticity, articular hypermobility, and vascular fragility. (1–3) The eyes, and the

bronchopulmonary, genitourinary, cardiovascular, alimentary, and central nervous systems may also be affected by this disorder of mesenchymal tissue. (4)

Ehlers-Danlos syndrome is comprised of a group of interrelated disorders that share common clinical and biochemical abnormalities. Currently, ten types have been described in the literature (types I–X) and are differentiated by their mode of inheritance and clinical presentation. (5) The majority of cases are associated with an autosomal dominant pattern of inheritance with variable penetrance. (6) Autosomal recessive and X-linked recessive modes of inheritance have also been described.

The first description of this disorder was written by van Meekeren in 1682. (7) Numerous reports of individuals with *elastic* or *stretchable* skin surfaced in the dermatologic journals in the nineteenth century. In 1901, Ehlers described the vascular fragility and articular hypermobility that are characteristic features of this disorder. (8) The presence of subcutaneous fibrous tumors was first described in 1908 by Danlos. (9) The combined use of their names to describe this disorder is a tribute to their early efforts. Synonyms include *arthrochalasis multiplex congenita*, (5) *cutis hyperelastica* (10) and *dermatorrhexis* (11)

CLINICAL FEATURES

Ehlers-Danlos syndrome is comprised of ten interrelated disorders that share, to different degrees, the common clinical triad of joint hyperextensibility, fragile blood vessels, and cutaneous abnormalities. (5) Types I–III exhibit a variable pattern of complete multisystem involvement. Type III, for example, is characterized by the predominance of articular hypermobility. (3) Types IV–X are much less common than types I–III. (1) Type IV is the most serious form of Ehlers-Danlos syndrome and is characterized by extreme vascular fragility, minimal joint involvement, and thin skin that lacks the hyperextensible properties that are seen in the other forms of this disorder. (12)

Ehlers-Danlos syndrome most frequently affects Caucasian males, often of European descent. (13) These patients are often relatively tall and exhibit a characteristic gait. (2,3,6) Hyperextension of the hip joints compensates for genu recurvatum (Fig. 8.45)

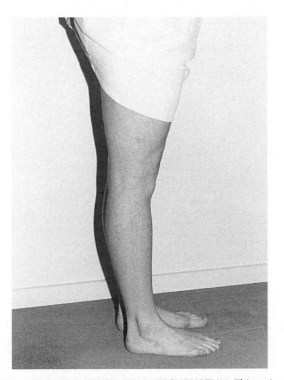

Figure 8.45. EHLERS-DANLOS: GENU RECURVATUM. This patient demonstrates knee extension beyond 180° (genu recurvatum). (Courtesy of John A.M. Taylor, DC, DACBR, Portland, Oregon)

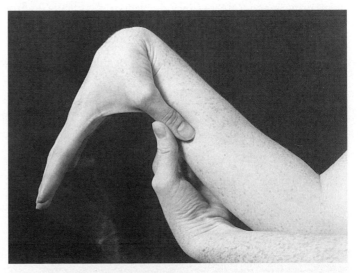

Figure 8.46. EHLERS-DANLOS: HYPERABDUCTION OF THE THUMB. Passive abduction hypermobility of the thumb is demonstrated by this patient. (Reprinted with permission: Taylor JAM, Greene-Deslauriers K, Tanaka DI: *Case report: Ehlers-Danlos syndrome.* J Manipulative Physiol Ther 13:273, 1990)

and is often accentuated by pes planus deformities. (6,7,13) Extreme wrist extension, hyperabduction of the thumb, (Fig. 8.46) and extension of the knees and elbows beyond 180° are often observed. Lop ears, redundant skin folds around the eyes, poor dentition, and a high, arched palate are the characteristic facial features of Ehlers-Danlos patients. (7,11,13,14) As in osteogenesis imperfecta, Ehlers-Danlos patients may have blue sclerae due to the thin corneal covering of the eye. The mental status of affected individuals is normal. (4)

Cutaneous manifestations include hyperelasticity, (Fig. 8.47) fragility, and subcutaneous nodules. The skin is thin and feels *velvety* or *chamois-like* to the touch. (6) Initially, it is hyperelastic and will retract to its normal position after being stretched. Later, as the skin ages and loses its elastic properties, permanent skin folds develop. (3) Bruises are often apparent on visual inspection of exposed areas. (3,6) Cutaneous lacerations often result from minor trauma and numerous large scars may be seen covered by thin skin. (3,6) This appearance has been described as the *cigarette paper* appearance. (4,7,15) The cutaneous nodules may be spherules, hematomas, or molluscoid fibrous tumors. The spherules are necrotic fat that is thought to represent the sequela of subclinical trauma. (14,15) Subcutaneous hematomas result from vascular fragility and subsequent bleeding diathesis. The molluscoid tumors are often noted at pressure points and are composed of proliferative connective tissue and fat. (14,15)

The ligamentous and capsular laxity result in recurrent joint dislocations, and eventually, premature degenerative arthritis. These extremely flexible individuals are sometimes employed as exhibitionists at local fairgrounds or with the circus. Their abilities have earned them descriptive titles such as the *Elastic Lady* and *Pretzel Man*. (7) The extensive flexibility these individuals exhibit has provided employment opportunities with the circus as a *rubber* man or woman.

Cardiovascular abnormalities include tetralogy of Fallot, aortic dissection, aneurysms, arteriovenous fistulas, varicose veins, and valvular abnormalities. (5) These complications are the most serious and may be life-threatening.

Bronchopulmonary abnormalities include spontaneous pneumothorax, bronchiectasis, and pulmonary hypertension. (5) Genitourinary abnormalities include bladder diverticula, hydronephrosis, and medullary sponge kidney. (5) Dilatation of the bowel, as well as spontaneous perforation and hemorrhage of the large bowel, may occur. (3,5)

PATHOLOGIC FEATURES

The primary causative abnormality involves faulty collagen synthesis and organization. (3) Previous studies have reported the elastic fiber content of the skin to be increased, (13,16) normal, (11) or decreased. (7,14) McKusick suggested that the alterations in the elastic fiber content are a reactive response to the abnormal size and appearance of the collagen fibrils. (7) Byers and Holbrook found numerous biochemical abnormalities in the type IV, VI–VIII, IX and X forms of Ehlers-Danlos syndrome. (17)

RADIOLOGIC FEATURES

The most characteristic radiographic findings of Ehlers-Danlos syndrome are seen in the soft tissues. Calcified subcutaneous spherules of necrotic fat tissue may be encountered. These spherules measure 2–15 mm in size and are most frequently observed in the pretibial soft tissues and along the forearms. (5–7,15) These non-laminated, ringlike calcifications do not resemble phleboliths and should not be confused with the characteristic *cigar shaped* intramuscular calcifications of cysticercosis. (5–7) The hematomas and molluscoid fibromas may also calcify. Heterotopic ossification may occur, particularly around the hip. Capsular and ligamentous laxity, which results in recurrent subluxations and/or dislocations, has been implicated as the cause for this ectopic bone formation. (3,18)

Spinal changes include platyspondyly and posterior vertebral body scalloping. (Fig. 8.48) The scalloping is a pressure-related

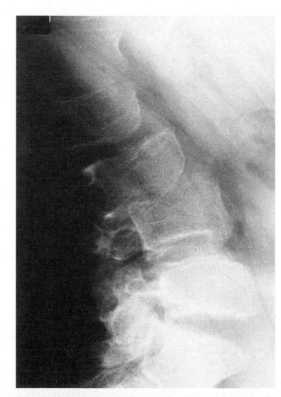

Figure 8.48.   EHLERS-DANLOS: SPINAL CHANGES. Observe the retrolistheses of L2 on L3 and L3 on L4. Platyspondyly is noted at L1, L2 and L3, and posterior vertebral body scalloping is seen at L3. The posterior vertebral body scalloping is secondary to CSF pulsations in an ectatic thecal sac. The presence of this finding must be differentiated from a mass within the neural canal. (Reprinted with permission: Taylor JAM, Greene-Deslauriers K, Tanaka DI: *Case report: Ehlers-Danlos syndrome.* J Manipulative Physiol Therapy 13:273, 1990)

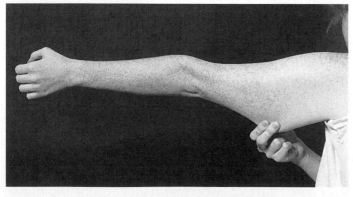

Figure 8.47.   EHLERS-DANLOS: SKIN HYPERELASTICITY. Skin hyperelasticity is seen in this patient. (Courtesy of John A.M. Taylor, DC, DACBR, Portland, Oregon)

phenomenon from cerebral spinal fluid (CSF) pulsations in an ectatic thecal sac. (3,5) Scoliosis and flattening of the thoracic sagittal curve may be seen. (5) Rarely, a thoracic lordosis may be present. (2,5) Spondylolysis and severe spondylolisthesis have been reported in association with the scoliosis. (19–21) Asymmetry of the thoracic cage and pectus excavatum or carinatum may also be present. (5) Acroosteolysis (resorption of the terminal tufts of the fingers) is seen in those patients who demonstrate the clinical findings of Raynaud's phenomenon. (19,20)

Numerous other congenital anomalies may be seen with Ehlers-Danlos syndrome. These include delayed ossification of the cranial vault, micrognathia, hypertelorism, clinodactyly of the fifth digit, elongation of the ulnar styloid process, radioulnar synostosis, arachnodactyly, club foot, and pes planus. (5)

MEDICOLEGAL IMPLICATIONS
Ehlers-Danos Syndrome

- Ligamentous laxity often results in recurrent joint dislocations.
- Cardiovascular complications include aneurysms and dissection of main arteries, including the aorta.
- Gastrointestinal complications include spontaneous rupture and hemorrhage of the bowel.
- The insidious onset of dyspnea and chest pain may occur secondary to spontaneous pneumothorax.
- Disc herniations are often seen in patients with this disorder and may produce radicular and/or cauda equina signs and symptoms.
- Osseous and soft tissue manipulations may produce vascular injury, resulting in vessel dissection and/or subcutaneous hematoma formation.

MASSIVE OSTEOLYSIS OF GORHAM
GENERAL CONSIDERATIONS

Gorham and colleagues first described a peculiar variety of massive osteolysis of bone in 1954. (1) Numerous cases have appeared in the literature since then and several names have been offered including *hemangiomatosis* (2), *massive osteolysis, disappearing bone disease,* and *vanishing bone disease.*

CLINICAL FEATURES

This disorder affects both sexes and can occur at any age, but usually becomes evident before the 5th decade. No family history has been found. Interestingly, some individuals relate a significant trauma prior to the onset of symptoms. Laboratory findings are generally unremarkable. The patient may present with acute onset of pain, or describe insidious progression of dull pain and soft tissue atrophy. Occasionally, patients present only after pathologic fracture and resultant deformity.

Any bone can be involved and the process often spreads to adjacent bones. The most commonly affected regions are the long bones, pelvis, (Fig. 8.49) thorax, and spine. The osseous destruction generally increases over a period of years, but the progression is unpredictable and prognosis is difficult. (3) Some cases eventually stabilize and a case of spontaneous recovery of bone

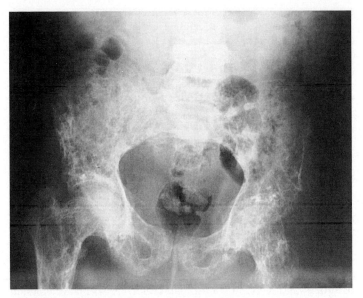

Figure 8.49.   MASSIVE OSTEOLYSIS OF GORHAM: PELVIS. Observe the dramatic *disappearing* bone appearance of the entire pelvis and proximal femora. (Courtesy of The Childrens Hospital, Dept. of Radiology, Denver, Colorado)

has been reported. (4) Clinical and radiographic improvement has occurred after radiation therapy. (5) Spinal cord transection with paraplegia (6) or even death have resulted from spinal involvement. Pulmonary complications may develop when the disease involves the thorax.

PATHOLOGIC FEATURES

The involved bone is soft and spongy with eroded cortices. Initially, bone is replaced by angiomatous tissue with unusually wide capillary-like vessels. (7) With progression of the disease, the angiomatous tissue is replaced with vascular fibrous tissue. The marrow spaces are hypervascular. The etiology of the disorder remains unknown. Gorham and Stout (2) suggested that the massive osteolysis represents a vascular derangement or a diffuse hemangiomatosis. The bone resorption appears to be the result of hypervascularity and is not related to increased osteoclastic activity.

RADIOLOGIC FEATURES

The radiographic findings of massive osteolysis are often dramatic. Initially, subcortical and intramedullary radiolucent foci are seen, often resembling patchy osteoporosis. Progressive destruction of bone occurs, resulting in numerous fractures and bony fragmentation. An entire portion of bone may disappear. The ends of the remaining bone typically become tapered. The process often extends to contiguous bones. Affected soft tissues become atrophied and frequently demonstrate calcification within thrombi (phleboliths). Advanced cases with the classic findings of disappearing bone are easily diagnosed. The differential diagnosis should include metastatic neuroblastoma, histiocytosis X, and lymphangiomatosis of bone. The pointed or tapered ends of bone, especially those developing after fracture, may mimic the pseudoarthrosis of neurofibromatosis or fibrous dysplasia.

MEDICOLEGAL IMPLICATIONS
Massive Osteolysis of Gorham

- The replacement of normal bone with the vascular lesions that characterize this disorder may sufficiently weaken the surrounding bone, resulting in pathologic fracture. Manipulation of joints adjacent to affected bone is contraindicated.

MUCOPOLYSACCHARIDOSES

The mucopolysaccharidoses are a group of inherited metabolic disorders that result in widespread skeletal, visceral, and mental abnormalities. A defect in metabolic degradation leads to the storage of mucopolysaccharide macromolecules in the nervous system and other body tissues. There is also excessive urinary excretion of mucopolysaccharides, which are components of connective tissue.

Brante was the first to use the term *mucopolysaccharidosis* in 1952 while describing a patient with gargoylism. (1) Further investigation has shown that the absence of certain enzymes causes the clinical and radiologic features that characterize the mucopolysaccharidoses (MPS). The MPS are classified into various types and there are additional diseases, such as the mucolipidoses and a gangliosidosis, that demonstrate similar clinical and radiologic findings. (2) McKusick (3) has classified these entities into six distinct syndromes:

MPS-I: Hurler (MPS-I-H)
  MPS-I-S: Scheie
  MPS-I-H-S: Hurler-Scheie
MPS-II: Hunter
MPS-III: Sanfilippo (subtypes A,B,C,D)
MPS-IV: Morquio (subtypes A,B)
MPS-VI: Maroteaux-Lamy
MPS-VII: Sly

This text will describe only two of these entities, MPS-I-H (Hurler's syndrome), and MPS-IV (Morquio's syndrome), which are more commonly encountered and are readily differentiated by their characteristic clinical and radiographic findings.

MPS-I: HURLER'S SYNDROME
GENERAL CONSIDERATIONS

Hurler's syndrome is a rare autosomal recessive (4) disorder of mucopolysaccharide metabolism that leads to excessive lipoid accumulation in the central nervous system (5) and other viscera. (6) It occurs in approximately 1 in 100,000 births. (7) The excessive mucopolysaccharides excreted in the urine are dermatan sulfate and heparin sulfate. Synonyms include *lipochondrodystrophy*, *gargoylism*, *osteochondrodystrophy*, and *dysostosis multiplex*.

CLINICAL FEATURES

Patients are usually normal at birth and remain so until after the first year of life. Facial features then begin to coarsen, with the development of a large head, widely set eyes (hypertelorism), a sunken nose, large lips, and a protruding tongue. Corneal opacities develop and the teeth are short and malformed. Mental deterioration ensues and deafness gradually develops. Hepatosplenomegaly produces a protuberant abdomen, and umbilical and inguinal hernias are common. As physical development ceases in the early years of life, affected individuals become dwarfed. A severe dorsolumbar kyphosis develops, along with multiple flexion contractures. The hands are *trident* and sometimes *clawed*. At about the same time, cardiomegaly and heart murmurs become evident. Death usually occurs in the second decade, often following pneumonia or cardiac failure.

RADIOLOGIC FEATURES

Changes seen in the skull include macrocephaly, frontal bossing, calvarial thickening, and premature closure of the sagittal and lambdoid sutures. Hydrocephalus is common. The sella turcica is enlarged and "J" shaped. (Fig. 8.50A) Often, the facial bones are small and the mandibular angle is widened. Spinal changes are fairly typical. A thoracolumbar kyphosis develops secondary to vertebral body hypoplasia. (Fig. 8.50B) The lower thoracic and upper lumbar bodies are small in their anterior-superior aspect and may be *beaked* inferiorly. The remaining vertebral centra may be oval due to convexity of the upper and lower surfaces. The pedicles are often long and slender. Atlantoaxial subluxation has been reported. (8) The ribs are overly wide, with tapered ends, producing a *paddle* or *spatulated* appearance. (Figs. 8.50C, 8.51) The ilia are flared, with obliquely directed acetabular roofs. Coxa valga or vara is common. Varus deformity of the humerus is characteristic. The tubular bones have widened diaphyses; this is more obvious in the upper extremities than in the lower. Often, the metacarpals and phalanges are short and wide, producing a *trident* hand. Osteoporosis is a frequent finding. (Fig. 8.50D)

Differential diagnosis from Morquio's syndrome is easily accomplished by observing the spinal differences, as well as the lack of hepatosplenomegaly in Morquio-type patients. While some resemblance to achondroplasia exists, the Hurler's patient is normal at birth and achondroplasia is easily discerned in the infant.

MEDICOLEGAL IMPLICATIONS
Hurler's Syndrome

- Dens hypoplasia resulting in atlantoaxial subluxation may occur. A standard (three view) radiographic series of the cervical spine should be performed prior to administering manipulative treatment to this area.

- Careful clinical evaluation of the cardiopulmonary system is recommended to uncover cardiomegaly and cardiac murmurs, which may affect individuals with this disorder and lead to cardiac failure.

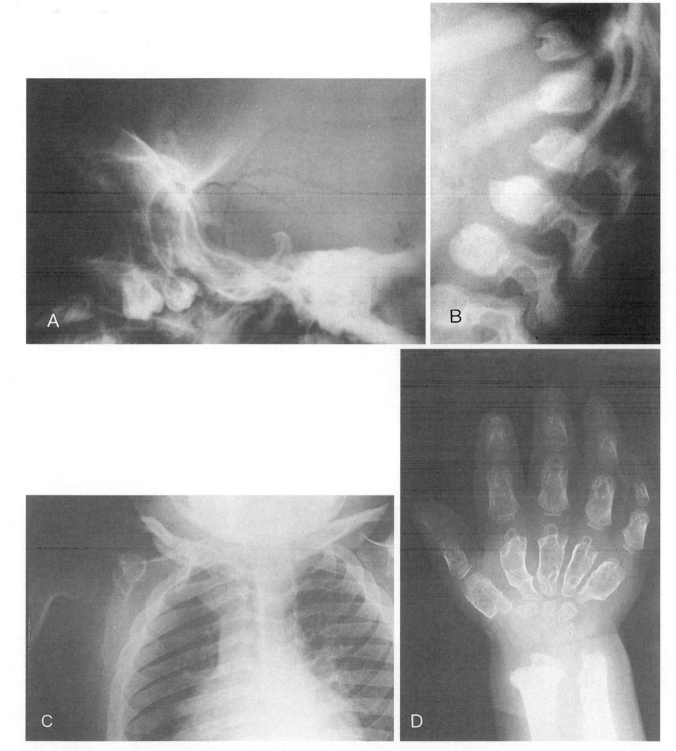

Figure 8.50.   HURLER'S SYNDROME. A. *J* Shaped Sella Turcica. A characteristic feature is an enlarged and *J* shaped sella. **B. Thoracolumbar Kyphosis.** The lower thoracic and upper lumbar vertebral bodies are small and are beaked inferiorly, resulting in a thoracolumbar kyphosis. **C. Paddle Ribs.** The ribs are overly wide, producing a *paddled* or *spatulated* appearance. Note the characteristic varus deformity of the humerus (arrows). **D. Hands.** The metacarpals and phalanges are short and wide. Note also the osteoporosis. (Courtesy of Bryan Hartley, MD, Melbourne, Australia)

MPS-IV: Morquio's Syndrome

GENERAL CONSIDERATIONS

Morquio's syndrome is an autosomal recessive disorder that occurs in approximately 1 in 100,000 births. (7) An error in mucopolysaccharide metabolism leads to keratosulfaturia, which is present at birth and establishes the diagnosis. Two forms of this dysplasia have been described (types A and B). Type B is the milder form and is differentiated from the more severe form by analysis of the enzyme deficiency. (9) Morquio (10) and Brailsford (11) independently described the syndrome in 1929. Synonyms include *chondrodystrophy*, *familial osteodystrophy*, *eccentro-osteochondrodysplasia*, *Morquio-Ullrich syndrome*, and *Morquio-Brailsford syndrome*. (12)

CLINICAL FEATURES

Patients often appear normal at birth, with the manifestation of skeletal changes becoming apparent only upon weight-bearing. During early childhood individuals develop marked dwarfism, dorsal kyphoscoliosis, weakness, and muscular hypotonia. Adult height rarely exceeds four feet. The sternum is usually horizontal and protuberant (pectus carinatum), the neck is short, and the head appears sunken into the chest. The nose is short, with a depressed bridge, and the eyes are wide-set. The maxillae are wide, with deformed, poorly spaced teeth. Fine corneal opacities develop around the age of 10. (13) Mental capacity is generally normal, but deafness often develops. Genu valgum and flexion contractures of the extremities are common. Enlarged wrists and deformed hands are noted. Atlantoaxial dislocations occur due to odontoid hypoplasia and may result in paraplegia and respiratory paralysis. Cardiomegaly results from aortic valvular involvement. (2) Most patients survive into the third and fourth decades.

RADIOLOGIC FEATURES

In early infancy, the vertebrae are slightly rounded with a small anterior beak. (14) By age 2 or 3, universal platyspondyly with central beaking is nearly pathognomonic. (Figs. 8.52, 8.53) Often, the first or second lumbar vertebra is posteriorly displaced and hypoplastic. The disc spaces are normal or increased. Atlantoaxial instability results from a hypoplastic or absent odontoid.

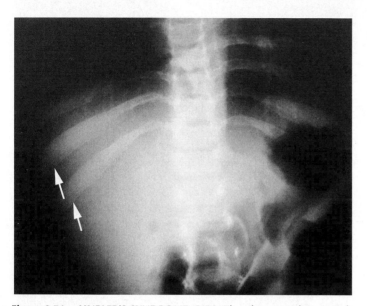

Figure 8.51.   HURLER'S SYNDROME: RIBS. The ribs are wide anteriorly (arrows) producing a *paddle* or *spatulated* appearance. (Courtesy of The Childrens Hospital, Dept. of Radiology, Denver, Colorado)

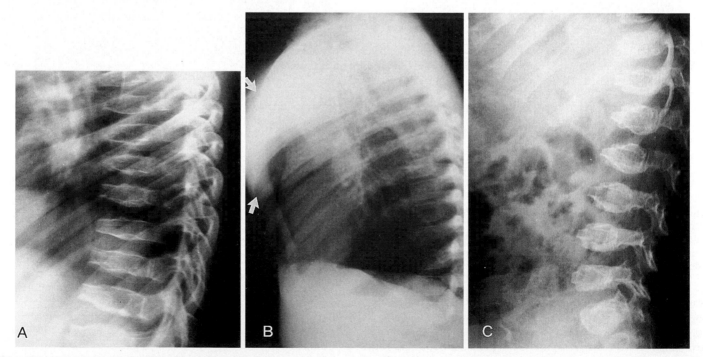

Figure 8.52.   MORQUIO'S SYNDROME: PLATYSPONDYLY WITH CENTRAL BEAKING AND PECTUS CARINATUM. A. Thoracic Spine. Note the flat vertebral bodies and central beaking. **B. Pectus Carinatum.** The sternum is horizontally oriented and protuberant (pectus carinatum) (arrows). **C. Lumbar Spine.** Note the characteristic central beaking in the lumbar spine. Also note that the disc heights are normal. (Courtesy of Leonard R. Levine, MD, Melbourne, Australia)

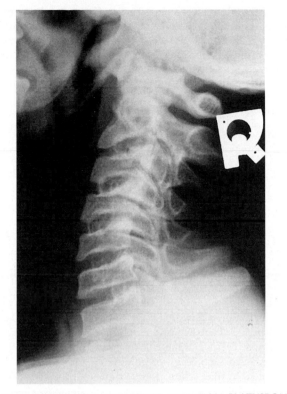

Figure 8.53.   MORQUIO'S SYNDROME: UNIVERSAL PLATYSPONDYLY OF THE CERVICAL SPINE. All cervical vertebrae are flat, but the discs are normal. (Courtesy of Andrew H. Jackson, Jr., DC, DACBR, Belleville, Illinois)

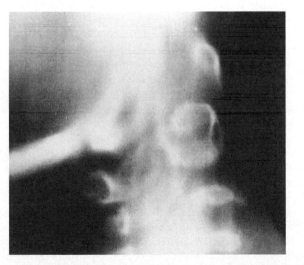

Figure 8.54.   MORQUIO'S SYNDROME: AGENESIS OF THE ODONTOID. This tomogram of the upper cervical spine demonstrates odontoid agenesis. COMMENT: Atlantoaxial instability results from hypoplasia or agenesis of the odontoid. (Courtesy of Andrew H. Jackson, Jr., DC, DACBR, Belleville, Illinois)

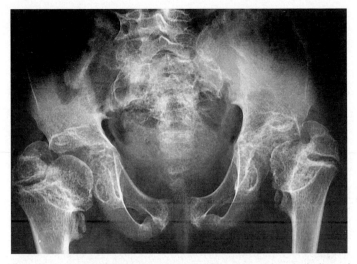

Figure 8.55.   MORQUIO'S SYNDROME: PELVIS. Note the poorly formed acetabulae and femoral heads. Hip dislocations are frequently encountered. (Courtesy of Leonard R. Levine, MD, Melbourne, Australia)

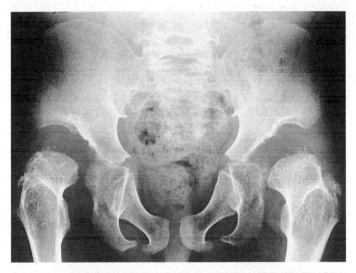

Figure 8.56.   MORQUIO'S SYNDROME, PELVIS: WIDENED FEMORAL NECKS. The femoral necks are widened. Also note the flared ilii. (Courtesy of Leonard R. Levine, MD, Melbourne, Australia)

(Fig. 8.54) The acetabuli and capital femoral epiphyses are hypoplastic and the hips are often unstable, leading to hip dislocation. (15) (Fig. 8.55) The femoral necks are wide (Fig. 8.56) and coxa valga or vara is common. The long tubular bones are short and thick, especially in the upper extremity. The hands and feet are deformed secondary to carpal, tarsal, and phalangeal growth disturbances.

The major entity that must be differentiated from Morquio's syndrome or MPS-IV is spondyloepiphyseal dysplasia. On close inspection the spinal changes are characteristic in each disorder, and the biochemical findings that are present in Morquio's syndrome are absent in spondyloepiphyseal dysplasia.

MEDICOLEGAL IMPLICATIONS
Morquio's Syndrome

• Dens hypoplasia or agenesis may occur, resulting in atlantoaxial subluxation or dislocation. Flexion/extension stress radiographs of the cervical region should be performed if hypoplasia or agenesis of the dens is seen on a standard (three view) cervical series. Respiratory paralysis secondary to atlantoaxial dislocation has been described.

- Congenital narrowing of the trachea may result in airway collapse during forward flexion of the head.

- A careful clinical evaluation of the cardiac system to exclude cardiac complications is recommended.

OSTEOGENESIS IMPERFECTA

GENERAL CONSIDERATIONS

Osteogenesis imperfecta is a generalized inheritable disorder of connective tissue with widespread abnormalities. The most serious involvement is in the skeleton, but changes in ligaments, skin, sclera, the inner ear, and dentition are also noted. The disease is thought to have an autosomal dominant transmission. Many synonyms have been used in the literature, including *osteopsathyrosis idiopathica*, (1) *mollities ossium*, (2) *fragilitas ossium*, (3) and *Lobstein's disease.*

There are four major clinical criteria for diagnosis: (a) osteoporosis with abnormal fragility of the skeleton (Fig. 8.57) (b) blue sclerae, (c) abnormal dentition (dentinogenesis imperfecta), (4) and (d) premature otosclerosi. (5,6) Only two of these need be present to confirm the diagnosis. Other findings include generalized ligamentous laxity, episodic diaphoresis (sweating) with abnormal temperature regulation, easy bruising, hyperplastic scars, and premature vascular calcification.

Osteogenesis imperfecta has been subdivided into two forms: the congenita form, with a high rate of stillborns and infant mortality; and the tarda form, often with a normal life expectancy.

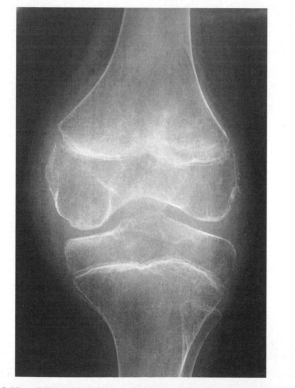

Figure 8.57.   OSTEOGENESIS IMPERFECTA: SEVERE OSTEOPOROSIS OF THE KNEE. Observe not only the severe osteoporosis but also the extreme thinness of the cortices, both of which contribute to the skeletal fragility of osteogenesis imperfecta. (Courtesy of David P. Thomas, MD, Melbourne, Australia)

Initially, this subdivision was based on the age at the time of first fracture, (5) but recently investigators have used the designations of congenita and tarda to refer to the presence or absence of osseous deformities at birth. (5,6) The presence or absence of bowing deformities of the long bones is useful as a guide to the severity of the disease. The tarda form is further subdivided into type I, with acquired bowing, and type II, with no bowing deformities. (4) These divisions of osteogenesis imperfecta are purely descriptive and are not based on the genetic patterns of inheritance.

In 1979 Sillence and colleagues offered a new classification based on clinical findings and genetic patterns of inheritance. (7) Type I, autosomal dominant with variable penetrance, is the most common form of osteogenesis imperfecta, and includes most patients with the tarda form. It is characterized by varying severity, blue sclera, dentinogenesis imperfecta, and premature otosclerosis. (8,9) Type II, autosomal recessive, is associated with severe neonatal fractures. This is a very heterogeneous category. (10) Most of these patients die in the perinatal period. Type III, mostly sporadic, but also autosomal dominant and recessive, is associated with severe progressive skeletal deformities, and most infants have fractures at birth. Dramatic dwarfism is also associated with this group. Type IV, autosomal dominant, has variable skeletal findings. Types I, II, and III all have blue sclera, while type IV has normal sclera. Beighton et al. have added a fifth category, characterized by blue sclera, dentinogenesis imperfecta, Wormian bones, and minimal skeletal fragility. (11) This new classification system offers enhanced typification of affected individuals; however, many patients have an atypical presentation and defy categorization.

CLINICAL FEATURES

The gender predominance of osteogenesis imperfecta is stated to be equal (12) or slightly increased in females. (6,13) It is found in all races. The severe congenita form is characterized by osseous fractures and deformities which often are observable in utero. (14) The skull is paper thin and soft. Death occurs in utero, during the birthing process, or shortly thereafter, usually following intracranial hemorrhage.

Osteogenesis imperfecta tarda is less severe and has a widely varied presentation. Fractures following trivial trauma occur during childhood, after puberty, and, more rarely, later in adulthood. (Fig. 8.58) Blue sclerae are found in the majority of individuals with osteogenesis imperfecta (over 90%) (5,6) and result from the appearance of the brown choroid when seen through the abnormal collagen in the thin sclera. (12) A white ring of normally colored sclera called *Saturn's ring* often surrounds the cornea. (4) Many patients have bluish-gray to yellowish-brown opalescent teeth, referred to as *dentinogenesis imperfecta*. While the enamel is normal, the dentin is malformed and defective, leading to easy chipping and severe caries. The otosclerosis, aside from early onset, is similar to idiopathic conduction deafness. The abnormal temperature regulation may be related to a disturbance in cellular ATPase. (15) A defect in platelet aggregation results in bleeding tendencies.

Many patients show some evidence of growth retardation. Severely affected individuals are dwarfed due to both the abnormal growth patterns and the severe fractures and deformities. (Fig. 8.59) The lower extremities are affected more than the upper. Kyphoscoliosis and bowing of the limbs contribute to the shortening. Bone fragility appears to decrease with increasing age. Females

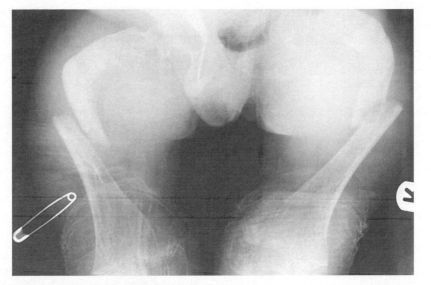

Figure 8.58. OSTEOGENESIS IMPERFECTA: MULTIPLE FRACTURES OF THE LOWER EXTREMITIES. Observe the bilateral midshaft fractures and the bowing deformity of the proximal femora. COMMENT: Fractures are more commonly encountered in the lower extremities in osteogenesis imperfecta. (Courtesy of Tyrone Wei, DC, DACBR, Portland, Oregon)

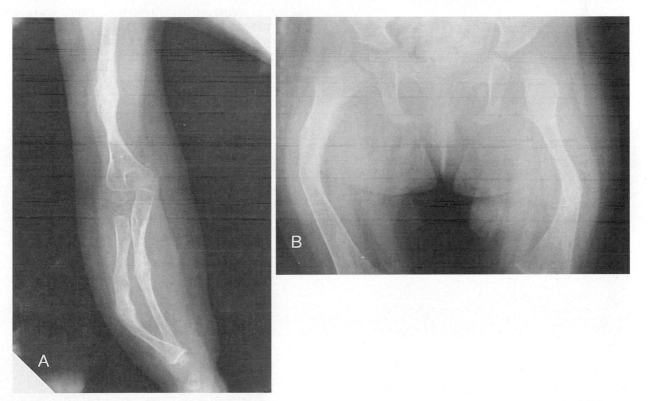

Figure 8.59. OSTEOGENESIS IMPERFECTA: BOWING DEFORMITIES. A. Upper Extremity. Multiple fractures have contributed to bowing deformities. **B. Femora.** Note the bilateral bowing deformities of the femora, occurring secondary to the fractures.

may especially show remission following puberty. Estrogen therapy has shown some benefit.

PATHOLOGIC FEATURES

Osteogenesis imperfecta is characterized by abnormal maturation of collagen affecting both intramembranous and enchondral bone formation. Primitive fetal collagen and bone are not replaced with mature lamellar and woven bone. An enzyme deficiency (ATPase) may be the cause of the abnormal connective tissue proteins. (5,12,15,16) The numerous fractures heal within a normal period of time but produce an exuberant callus which yields only a poor cellular matrix.

RADIOLOGIC FEATURES

The cardinal roentgen features of osteogenesis imperfecta are a diffuse decrease in bone density, pencil-thin cortices, and multiple fractures. Fairbank (17) has subdivided osteogenesis imperfecta into three groups based on radiographic findings: (a) thin and gracile bones, (Fig. 8.60) (b) short, thick bones, (Fig. 8.61) and (c) cystic bones. (Fig. 8.62) The thin and gracile type is most frequent and these are generally osteogenesis imperfecta tarda patients. Patients with the congenita form often have the *thick bone* radiographic appearance. This description, however, is a misnomer because, although the bone is wider than normal owing to fracture deformity, the cortices are paper thin and the overall density is diminished. The cystic type is rare and is characterized by osteopenic, flared metaphyses. This flared, cystic appearance may extend into the diaphyses. The radiographic subtypes are purely descriptive, and patients may be seen to change from one type to another.

Hanscom et al. have recently developed another classification, types A through F, based on six radiologic criteria: (a) vertebral contours, (b) bowing of long bones, (c) trefoil-shaped pelvis, (d) cystic changes in long bone metaphyses and epiphyses, (e) thickness of long bone cortices, and (f) thickness of rib cortices. (18–20) This new classification defines a narrower spectrum of disease than previous classifications and allows for determination of prognosis regarding spinal deformities, ambulation, and life span. This classification also aids in the treatment of scolioses in affected individuals.

Multiple fractures, often transverse and in the lower extremities, are the radiographic hallmarks of osteogenesis imperfecta. Subsequent healing with tumoral callus leads to shortening (the result of telescoping), bowing deformities, and pseudarthroses.

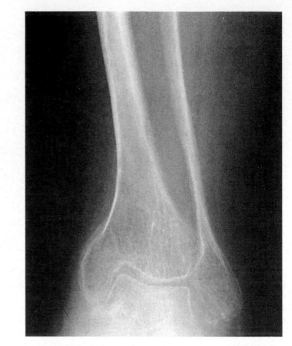

Figure 8.60.   OSTEOGENESIS IMPERFECTA, THIN AND GRACILE TYPE: TIBIA AND FIBULA. Observe the thin and gracile configuration of the bones of lower extremity. COMMENT: Thin and gracile bones are the most common type found in osteogenesis imperfecta.

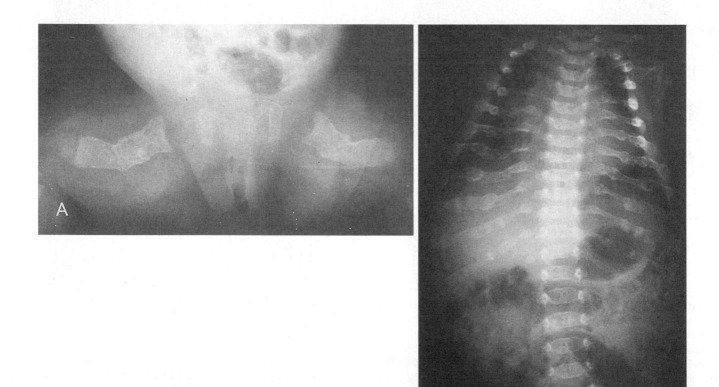

Figure 8.61.   OSTEOGENESIS IMPERFECTA: SHORT, THICK BONES. A. Femora. Note the short, thick appearance of the femora. **B. Ribs.** Multiple fractures also contribute to the thick appearance of the ribs. (Courtesy of Alf Turner, MIR, BAppSc (Chiro), DACBR, Bournemouth, England)

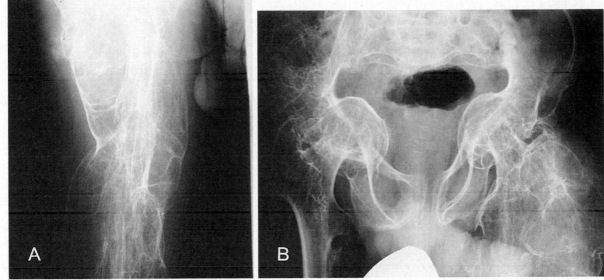

Figure 8.62.   OSTEOGENESIS IMPERFECTA: CYSTIC BONES. A. Femur. Note the expanded cystic nature of the femur. **B. Pelvis.** Observe, also, the bilateral protrusio acetabuli. COMMENT: Intraosseous hemorrhage is be-lieved to be the mechanism leading to the cystic appearance of bone in osteogenesis imperfecta.

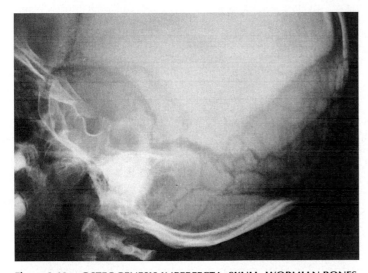

Figure 8.63.   OSTEOGENESIS IMPERFECTA, SKULL: WORMIAN BONES. Numerous small Wormian bones are found in the occipital region in this patient. COMMENT: Wormian bones are not pathognomonic of osteogenesis imperfecta and are found in several of the dysplasias. (Courtesy of C. H. Quay, MD, Melbourne, Australia)

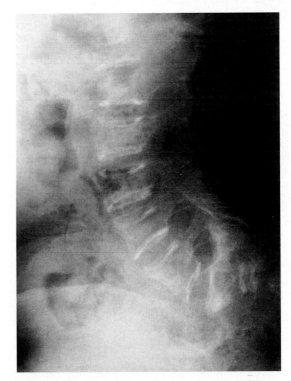

Figure 8.64.   OSTEOGENESIS IMPERFECTA, LUMBAR SPINE: BICONCAVE LENS VERTEBRA. Note the severe osteoporosis of the spine and the biconcave appearance of the vertebral bodies. (Courtesy of Tyrone Wei, DC, DACBR, Portland, Oregon)

The excessive callus formation (called *pseudotumors*) has been mistaken for osteosarcoma. (21)

Skull radiographs reveal persistent Wormian bones (Fig. 8.63) and enlarged sinuses. The calvarium is lucent and thin. Platybasia is a frequent finding and may be accompanied by basilar impression. Kyphoscoliosis is common, resulting from ligamentous laxity, osteoporosis, and fracture deformity. The vertebral bodies may be anteriorly wedged and often appear evenly flattened or biconcave (creating the *biconcave lens vertebra*). (22) (Fig. 8.64) Protrusio acetabuli may occur, and a shepherd's crook deformity of the proximal femur has been noted. (Fig. 8.65) Premature degenerative joint disease results from ligamentous laxity and multi-ple fractures of the articular surfaces. The differentiation of child abuse from osteogenesis imperfecta is generally readily accomplished based on other clinical findings. However, in those rare cases of type IV, who present with no blue sclera and mild skeletal changes, biopsy for collagen analysis may be helpful. (23)

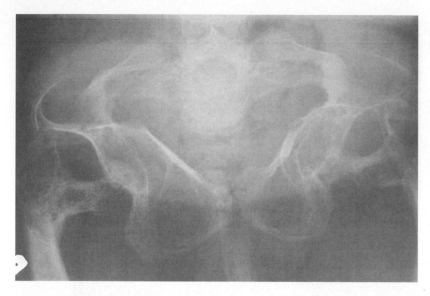

Figure 8.65. OSTEOGENESIS IMPERFECTA: PROTRUSIO ACETABULI. This patient has bilateral protrusio acetabuli and coxa vara. (Courtesy of Tyrone Wei, DC, DACBR, Portland, Oregon)

MEDICOLEGAL IMPLICATIONS
Osteogenesis Imperfecta

- Due to the overall bone fragility, osseous and deep soft tissue manipulations are contraindicated.

- Faulty dentition usually results in numerous dental caries. If untreated, maxillary or mandibular osteomyelitis may develop.

- Ligamentous laxity may produce joint hypermobility and instability. Recurrent dislocations and premature osteoarthritis are often seen.

- Basilar impression from bone softening may decrease the volume of the posterior fossa, leading to hydrocephalus and/or cerebellar compression.

- Patients with the congenita form of this dysplasia often exhibit severe spinal deformity (e.g., kyphoscoliosis), which may result in respiratory failure and/or paraplegia.

THE SCLEROSING DYSPLASIAS

This section is devoted to those skeletal dysplasias that cause an increase in bone density or sclerosis. The sclerosing bone dysplasias are due to disturbances in the formation and remodeling of bone. They are poorly understood and for most, the etiology is unknown. These conditions exhibit great variability in their clinical, radiologic, and histopathologic manifestations, as well as in their prognosis. Some demonstrate an overall increase in bone density, while others have a peculiar and often pathognomonic pattern of sclerosis. Only the more common sclerosing dysplasias are discussed in this section.

Several of the entities in this section are thought to be intimately related; these are osteopoikilosis, osteopathia striata, and melorheostosis. Patients have been reported who exhibit signs of all three of these disorders and when occurring together, they are termed *overlap syndromes*. (1) The remaining entities show no relationship to the others but are grouped here because of their sclerotic presentation.

MELORHEOSTOSIS

GENERAL CONSIDERATIONS

Melorheostosis is a rare, sclerosing bone dysplasia that was first described in 1922 by Leri and Joanny. (1) Synonyms include *Leri type of osteopetrosis, osteosi eberneizzante monomelica*, (2) and *flowing hyperostosis*. The name *melorheostosis* is of Greek derivation, meaning *limb, flow,* and *bone*, and aptly describes the hyperostotic appearance that has been likened to wax flowing down a lighted candle. (3)

CLINICAL FEATURES

The etiology is unknown, and there is no sex predilection. While most authors agree that melorheostosis is a congenital entity, most affected individuals do not manifest any symptoms until late childhood or early adolescence. The most common presenting symptom is pain, though some cases are found incidentally. (4) The onset is insidious with bone hyperostosis progressing through childhood into adult life. The disease has a slow, chronic course with periods of exacerbation and arrest. (5) Joint swelling and limitation of motion are seen and are usually more marked in adults than in children. (6) Joint contractures and deformities may ensue, with reported cases of genu varum and valgum, valgus deformities of the feet, and dislocation of the patella. Severe involvement in children may lead to premature epiphyseal closure, with resultant limb shortening.

Soft tissue changes are frequently present and include anomalous pigmentation, scleroderma-like atrophy of the skin, and muscular wasting. Pressure on adjacent vessels may contribute to lymphedema. The soft tissue changes may precede the osseous findings and have been demonstrated on thermography. (7) An association with arteriovenous malformations has been reported. (8) This disorder is most frequently monomelic and usually involves a lower limb. (9) (Fig. 8.66A–C) Often, the innominate or scapula corresponding to the involved limb is also affected. The process appears to begin proximally and progress distally. Other

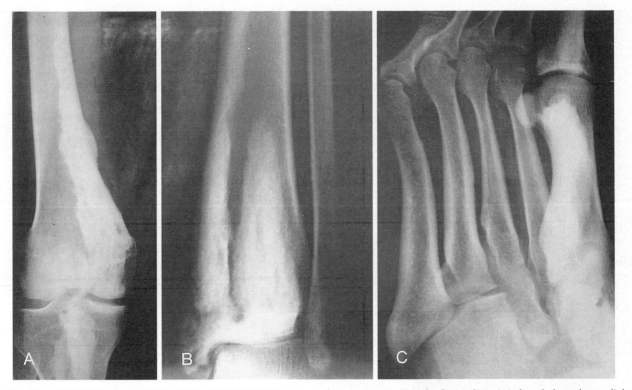

Figure 8.66. MELORHEOSTOSIS: LOWER LIMB INVOLVEMENT. A. Femur. Note the flowing, dense, cortical bone along the medial aspect of the femur. **B. Tibia.** Observe the dense bone formation that appears to flow distally down the tibia. **C. Foot.** The bone formation continues down the lower extremity into the foot, where it is found along the medial aspect of the tarsals and metatarsals. COMMENT:Melorheostosis is usually monomelic and is found in the lower limbs. (Courtesy of Steven P. Brownstein, MD, Springfield, New Jersey)

sites of involvement include the vertebrae, ribs, skull, and facial bones.

The histologic findings are nonspecific, with hyperostotic sclerotic bone and thickened trabeculae. The marrow space may contain fibrotic tissue. While many etiologic hypotheses have been offered, especially vascular insufficiency, the best explanation has been proposed by Murray and McCredie, who suggest that the lesions follow sclerotomes and myotomes that are supplied by an individual spinal sensory nerve. (10) Disease of a sensory nerve could result in the segmental distribution of this bone dysplasia and its associated soft tissue abnormalities. Laboratory findings are classically normal.

RADIOLOGIC FEATURES

Cortical thickening in a streaked or wavy pattern is the most marked roentgen feature. (Fig. 8.67) In children the hyperostosis is primarily endosteal; in adulthood, periosteal bone deposition is more dramatic. (11) The radiographic findings appear to reflect developmental errors at the sites of intramembranous and enchondral bone formation. (12) The hyperostotic bone protrudes under the periosteum and usually follows along one side of a long bone. (Figs. 8.68 and 8.69) Endosteal involvement may encroach upon the medullary space. Bony masses resembling osteochondromas extend into adjacent articulations. Involvement of the carpal and tarsal bones resembles the multiple bone islands that are seen in osteopoikilosis. In the pelvis and scapulae (flat bones) the sclerotic bone may be in the form of dense radiations from the joint. Heterotopic bone formation and soft tissue calcification are

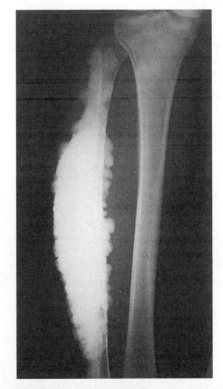

Figure 8.67. MELORHEOSTOSIS, FIBULA: WAVY NEW BONE FORMATION. Wavy, undulating, cortical bone formation appears to surround the fibula. This appearance has been referred to as *wax flowing down a lighted candle.* (Courtesy of Gilbert M. Meal, DC, Christchurch, Great Britain)

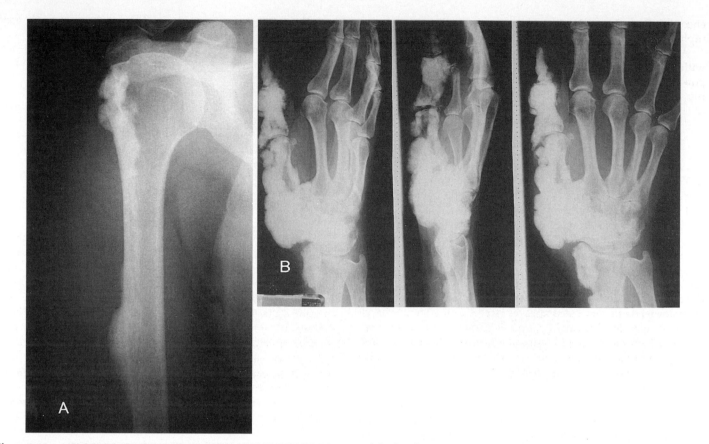

Figure 8.68.   MELORHEOSTOSIS: DISTRIBUTION ALONG ONE SIDE OF THE BONE. A. Humerus. The hyperostotic bone flows along one side of the humerus. **B. Hand.** Extensive involvement is seen along the lateral aspect of the hand. (Reprinted with permission: Yochum TR, et al: *Melorheostosis—A report of two patients.* ACA Council Roent, Roentgen Brief, April 1981)

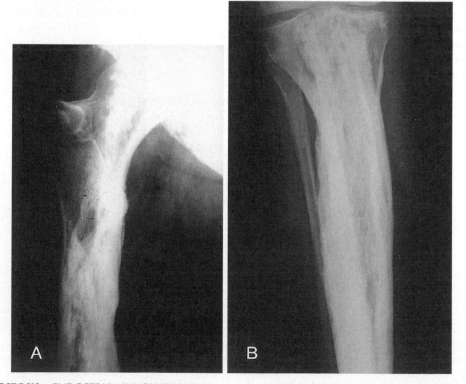

Figure 8.69.   MELORHEOSTOSIS: ENDOSTEAL INVOLVEMENT. A. Femur. Endosteal involvement of the femur encroaches on the medullary space. **B. Tibia.** Note that the medullary canal appears compromised due to endosteal bone formation. (Courtesy of Paul D. Sykes, DC, Adelaide, Australia)

encountered and may lead to joint ankylosis. (13) Bone scintigraphy shows increased tracer uptake in the involved area. (14)

A number of other disorders have been found in association with melorheostosis. These include linear scleroderma, osteopoikilosis, osteopathia striata, neurofibromatosis, tuberous sclerosis, and hemangiomas. (8,15–19,20)

OSTEOPATHIA STRIATA

GENERAL CONSIDERATIONS

Osteopathia striata is a rare and unusual entity first described in 1924 by Voorhoeve as a variant of osteopoikilosis. (1) In 1950 Fairbank applied the name *osteopathia striata*, (2) but the disease still bears the synonym *Voorhoeve's disease*. Characteristic findings are linear bands of dense bone in the metaphyses and diaphyses of long bones. While the etiology is unknown, a genetic mode of transmission may be involved, especially in light of its suspected variance from osteopoikilosis (an autosomal dominant disorder). (3) Curiously, patients with osteopathia striata often show evidence of other conditions that cause increased bone density, such as melorheostosis and osteopetrosis. (4,5) A limited study of individuals with focal dermal hypoplasia (Goltz syndrome) has revealed a high incidence of concomitant osteopathia striata. (6,7) Osteopathia striata has also been reported in association with several cases of cranial sclerosis. (8–10)

CLINICAL FEATURES

The majority of patients are asymptomatic, with osteopathia striata found incidentally on x-ray examination. Some individuals present with vague joint pain. (2) Laboratory findings are normal, and no age or sex predilection has been demonstrated.

RADIOLOGIC FEATURES

The primary areas of involvement are the major long bones of the body. Usually bilateral in distribution, (11,12) vertical radiopaque lines in the metaphysis extend for some distance into the diaphysis. More rarely, striations are seen crossing the epiphyseal line to involve the epiphysis. The length of these densities appears to be related to the growth rate of the bone; the long bone with the greatest growth potential (the femur) consistently demonstrates the longest striations. (13)

A fanlike pattern radiating from the acetabulum to the iliac crest is characteristic of involvement in the ilium and has been referred to as the *sunburst effect*. (14) (Fig. 8.70) Occasionally, densities are encountered in the small tubular bones of the hands and feet or the spine. Thickening and sclerosis of the base of the skull has been reported.

Osteopathia striata appears to reflect old bone remodeling and therefore, the lesions are not associated with increased scintigraphic activity. (15,16)

OSTEOPETROSIS

GENERAL CONSIDERATIONS

Osteopetrosis is a rare hereditary and familial bone abnormality characterized by the lack of resorption of normal primitive osteochondroid tissue. This persistence of osteochondroid inhibits the formation of normal mature adult bone with a medullary canal containing marrow tissue. (1) There appear to be at least four forms: (a) a benign, heterogenous form (2) that is autosomal dominant; (b) a severe malignant form that is autosomal recessive; (c) an intermediate recessive type; (3,4) and (d) a recessive type with tubular acidosis that is also known as *carbonic anhydrase II deficiency syndrome*. (5,6) Consanguinity apparently plays a role in the severe malignant form. (7) Synonyms include *Albers-Schönberg's disease*, *osteosclerosis*, *osteopetrosis generalisata*, *osteosclerosis generalisata*, *marble bones*, and *chalk bones*.

CLINICAL FEATURES

The severe forms of osteopetrosis are recognized in infancy; (8) often, the patient dies within the second year of life. Florid cases are inevitably stillborn. The clinical picture is one of severe anemia, hepatosplenomegaly, lymphadenopathy, thrombocytopenia, and failure to thrive. The dense, but extremely brittle, bones fracture easily. Involvement of the cranium may lead to optic nerve atrophy with blindness or other cranial nerve defects. The most frequent causes of death are massive hemorrhage and recurrent infection. Leukemia and sarcoma are known sequelae.

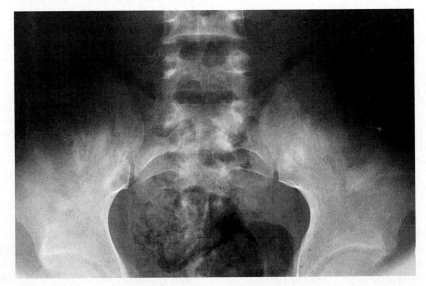

Figure 8.70.   OSTEOPATHIA STRIATA, PELVIS: *SUNBURST* EFFECT. The dense bone formation is seen in a fan-like pattern radiating from the acetab-ulum toward the iliac crest. This has been referred to as the *sunburst* effect of osteopathia striata. (Courtesy of Bryan Hartley, MD, Melbourne, Australia)

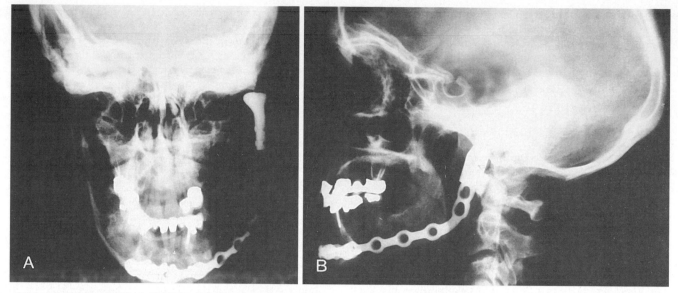

Figure 8.71. OSTEOPETROSIS: A UNIQUE COMPLICATION. A and B. Observe the sclerosis at the skull base. A hemimandibulectomy has been performed as a result of osteomyelitis of the mandible. COMMENT: Osteopetrosis prediposes a patient to the development of dental caries and abscess formation. Extensive involvement may lead to osteomyelitis of the mandible as a rare complication. (Courtesy of David F. Gendreau, DC, DACBR, Los Angeles, California)

Fifty percent of benign cases are asymptomatic. (5) They may be discovered incidentally when the patient is radiographed for some other reason, such as a fracture. Other cases present with anemia, facial palsies, deafness, and hepatosplenomegaly. Defective dentition with severe caries may lead to osteomyelitis of the maxilla or mandible. (10) (Fig. 8.71)

LABORATORY FINDINGS

Anemia is invariably present and does not correlate well with the degree of sclerosis. Some individuals with markedly increased density have mild anemia, while those with little change in bony density may have severe anemia. Myelophthisic, aplastic, and hypoplastic types of anemia are encountered. Often, thrombocytopenia is severe and leads to hemorrhage. The serum calcium levels may be elevated.

PATHOLOGIC FEATURES

Failure of the normal resorptive mechanism, which replaces calcified cartilage with mature bone, accounts for the bone changes. The osteoclasts may be unresponsive to parathyroid hormone and unable to resorb bone and cartilage. (11) The primitive calcified cartilage persists in abundance, and a medullary space is never allowed to form. This leads to anemia and extramedullary hematopoiesis, causing hepatosplenomegaly. MRI has been found to aid in the evaluation of marrow involvement. (12) Failure of remodeling also produces flared metaphyses (*Erlenmeyer flask deformity*). (Fig. 8.72)

While the bone is very radiopaque in appearance and hard to the touch, it is actually very brittle and subject to pathologic fracture. (Fig. 8.73) These are characteristically transverse, healing quickly but producing a callus of defective, osteopetrotic bone. Frequently, there are vertical or horizontal striations of normal bone interspersed with the more abundant primitive tissue, suggesting that the disease may have an intermittent nature.

RADIOLOGIC FEATURES

There is generalized sclerosis of the skeleton, and there may be a homogenous appearance of increased density, without trabeculation, and little or no differentiation between cortical and medullary regions. (Fig. 8.74) Frequently, however, there are striations producing a *bone within a bone* appearance, also referred to as *endobones*. (Fig. 8.75) The endobones represent fetal vestiges and contain embryonic strata that are normally removed. (13) One case has been reported that presented with alternating dense and radiolucent metaphyseal transverse lines as the only evidence of the disease. (14) The long bones have flared and elongated metaphyses; (Fig. 8.76) occasionally, the shafts may be widened. Involvement of the hands and feet parallel changes in the long bones, and tuftal erosion has been reported. (15) Characteristically, the ilium demonstrates multiple, dense curved lines paralleling the iliac crest. (Fig. 8.77) In the spine a number of presentations are seen. The vertebrae may be uniformly dense or, more commonly, there are dense bands adjacent to the endplates, with a more normal appearing midbody—the *sandwich vertebra*. (15) (Fig. 8.78) The *bone within a bone* appearance is also commonly seen in the vertebral bodies. (16) (Fig. 8.79) Spinal stenosis with myelopathy in the cervical spine has been reported. (17) Spondylolysis may be seen in the lumbar spine. (18,19) (Fig. 8.80) Skull changes include calvarial and basilar thickening and sclerosis, with poor sinus development. (Fig. 8.81) Endobones, or *bones within bones* are frequently seen in the occipital and sphenoid bones with CT scanning. (13) The skull changes may produce macrocephaly and hydrocephalus. Involvement of the mandible may result in prognathism. Complications include pathologic fractures (especially of the femur), hemorrhage, infection, blindness, and deafness. Leukemia and sarcoma are also known sequelae. Differential diagnosis includes idiopathic hypercalcemia and heavy metal poisoning.

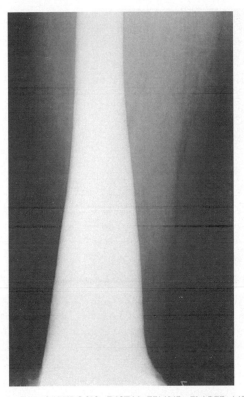

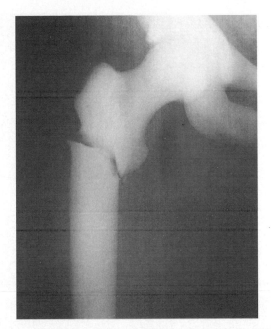

Figure 8.73. OSTEOPETROSIS, FEMUR: PATHOLOGIC FRACTURE. Observe the pathologic fracture through the subtrochanteric region of the femur. COMMENT: While the bone is very radiopaque in appearance, it is actually very brittle.

Figure 8.72. OSTEOPETROSIS, DISTAL FEMUR: FLARED METAPHYSIS (*ERLENMEYER FLASK DEFORMITY*). Note the uniformly dense appearance of the femur. Failure of remodeling produces flared metaphyses.

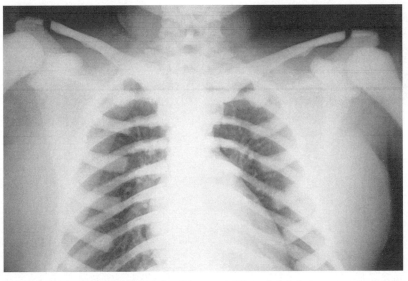

Figure 8.74. OSTEOPETROSIS, THORAX: HOMOGENEOUS INCREASED DENSITY. Note the homogeneous increased density without trabeculation or differentiation between cortical and medullary regions throughout the ribs.

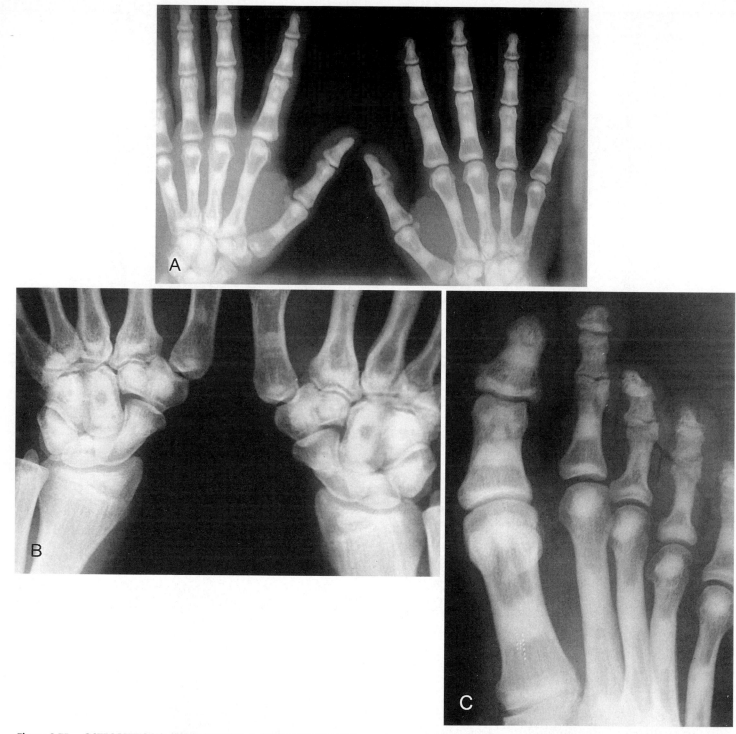

Figure 8.75.   OSTEOPETROSIS: *BONE WITHIN A BONE* **APPEARANCE. A. Hands.** Note the increased densities within the metacarpals and phalanges, producing a *bone within a bone* effect. **B. Wrists.** Note the areas of increased density within the carpal bones. **C. Foot.** The *bone within a bone* appearance here is similar to that seen in the small bones of the hand.

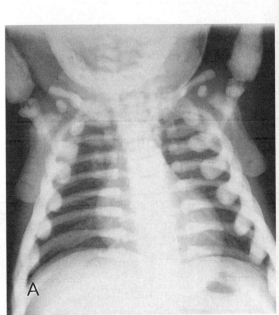

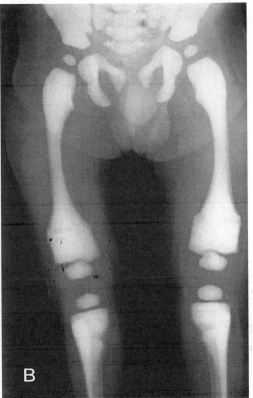

Figure 8.76.   OSTEOPETROSIS: FLARED METAPHYSES. A. Thorax. Note the flared metaphyses of the ribs and proximal humeri. **B. Lower Extremities.** There is a uniform increase in density and flared metaphyses in the distal femora. COMMENT: Anemia is invariably present in osteopetrosis but does not correlate well with the degree of sclerosis.

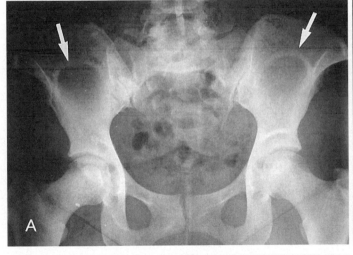

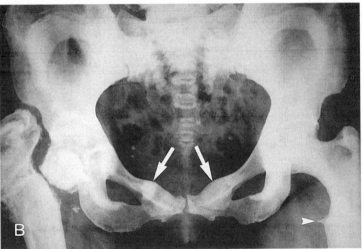

Figure 8.77.   OSTEOPETROSIS: CURVED LINE PARALLELING THE ILIAC CREST. A. Pelvis. Note the single curved line paralleling each iliac crest, with a *bone within a bone* appearance (arrows). A similar appearance is visualized in the femoral head and supra-acetabular region bilaterally. (Courtesy of Brian V. Lonsdale, DC, Geelong, Victoria, Australia) **B. Pelvis:** Pathologic Fracture of the Femur. Note the thick, dense bands paralleling the iliac crests and the pathologic subcapital fracture of the femur. Thickening of the pubic rami is secondary to previous fractures (arrows). Of incidental note is a musculotendinous exostosis at the lesser trochanter (arrowhead).

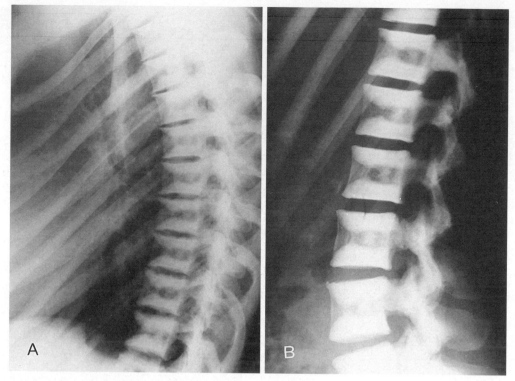

Figure 8.78. OSTEOPETROSIS: *SANDWICH* VERTEBRAE. A. Thoracic Spine. Note the dense bands along the superior and inferior endplates, referred to as the *sandwich* vertebra. **B. Lumbar Spine.** Another patient with *sandwich* vertebrae of the lumbar spine. (Courtesy of Bryan Hartley, MD, Melbourne, Australia)

MEDICOLEGAL IMPLICATIONS
Osteopetrosis

- Patients exhibiting persistent hip pain must be evaluated to exclude ischemic necrosis of the femoral head.

- Thickening of the osseous structures may narrow the foramina of the skull base, resulting in neurovascular compression. Most commonly, the optic and acoustic nerves are affected by long-standing compression. The resulting nerve atrophy produces irreversible blindness and deafness.

- Dental caries occur secondary to faulty dentition. If untreated, osteomyelitis of the maxilla or mandible may develop.

- Pathologic fractures may occur secondary to bone fragility. Osseous manipulation may be contraindicated in patients that exhibit generalized involvement throughout the skeleton.

- Anemia, recurrent infections, and leukemia are known complications that the treating physician must consider.

OSTEOPOIKILOSIS
GENERAL CONSIDERATIONS

This uncommon but interesting bone disorder was first described by Albers-Schönberg (1) and by Ledoux-Lebard and Chabaneux (2) in the early 1900s. Osteopoikilosis is characterized by small round or ovoid radiopacities appearing in the juxtaarticular regions of bone. It would appear to be autosomal dominant in transmission and has been found to become more prominent in succeeding generations in some cases. (3–6) Synonyms include *osteopathia condensans disseminata* and *spotted bones*.

CLINICAL FEATURES

The majority of cases are asymptomatic and found on radiographic studies taken for other reasons. Although it can be seen at any age, it is rarely detected before age 3. (7) Males are affected more frequently than females. (8) In approximately 25% of cases cutaneous abnormalities are present, including dermatofibrosis lenticularis disseminata (9,10), keloid formation (11,12), and scleroderma-like lesions. (13) In 15 to 20% of cases there may be mild joint pain, with or without joint effusion. (14) Laboratory findings are normal.

PATHOLOGIC FEATURES

While the etiology of this disorder is still unknown, the lesions appear to reflect spongy bone remodeling related to mechanical stress, but unrelated to healing secondary to microfractures. (15) The lesions may represent foci of bone that failed to become cancellous during the course of growth and differentiation. (8) It has been suggested that osteopoikilosis, because of its diffuse nature, hereditary mode of transmission, and association with cutaneous abnormalities, may be a manifestation of a metabolic connective tissue disorder. (15)

The lesions are foci of compact lamellar bone containing haversian systems. Histologically, osteopoikilotic bone closely re-

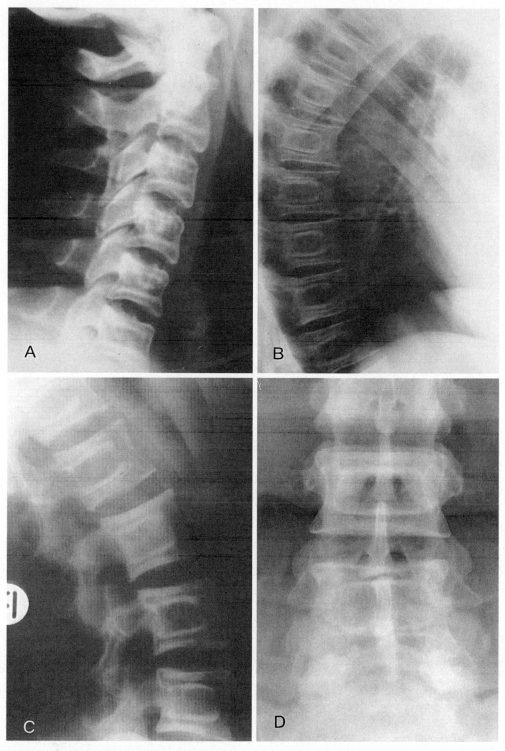

Figure 8.79.   OSTEOPETROSIS: *BONE WITHIN A BONE* APPEARANCE.
A. Cervical Spine. Note the sclerotic lines paralleling the cervical spine endplates. (Courtesy of Robin R. Canterbury, DC, DACBR, Davenport, Iowa) **B. Thoracic Spine.** Note the appearance of tiny vertebrae within larger vertebral bodies. **C. Lateral Lumbar Spine.** Note the *bone within a bone* effect, similar to the cervical and thoracic vertebral bodies. **D. AP Lumbar Spine.** Observe the *bone within a bone* appearance as viewed frontally. (**B-D,** Courtesy of Brian V. Lonsdale, DC, Geelong, Victoria, Australia)

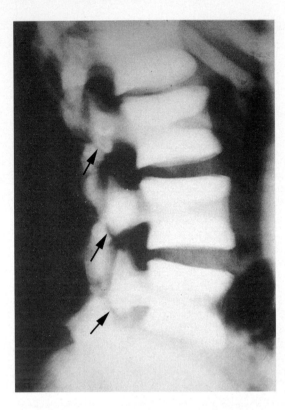

Figure 8.80.   OSTEOPETROSIS: LUMBAR SPINE. Observe the presence of spondylolysis (pars defects) at L2, L3 and L4 (arrows). (Reprinted with permission of European Journal of Chiropractic, *Khanchandani*, BA: 37, 1989)

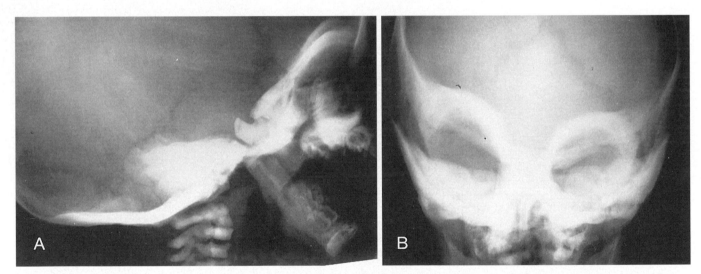

Figure 8.81.   OSTEOPETROSIS: SKULL INVOLVEMENT. A. Lateral Skull. Observe the basilar thickening and sclerosis. Also note involvement of the facial bones. **B. AP Skull.** Observe the involvement of the facial bones and basilar region, as viewed frontally.

sembles the solitary bone island. However, while bone islands are sometimes found to be metabolically active on bone scans, this is not a regular feature of osteopoikilosis, and is rarely seen. (16)

RADIOLOGIC FEATURES

Multiple small radiopacities found scattered in epiphyseal and metaphyseal regions are generally pathognomonic. (Fig. 8.82) The lesions are symmetric, with a predilection for the long tubular bones, carpals, and tarsals. (Fig. 8.83) In the pelvis and scapula the densities are found adjacent to the acetabulum and glenoid. (Fig. 8.84) Rarely, lesions are found in the skull, spine, ribs, and clavicles. (Fig. 8.85) Occasionally, their size may change, with reports of disappearance and reappearance in children and, more rarely, in adults. (17) Generally, the size ranges from 1 to 10 mm in diameter. Rarely, larger lesions are found. Most commonly, they are uniformly dense but occasionally exhibit lucent centers. Infrequently, the sclerotic areas in osteopoikilosis become more radiopaque with age. (18)

Osteopoikilosis has been found in association with both osteopathia striata and melorheostosis, and it has been suggested that these are related conditions. (19) It is of interest that a patient who had both osteopoikilosis and osteosarcoma has been described. Since osteosarcoma is related to active osteogenesis, it has been proposed that perhaps the chronic remodeling of osteopoikilosis resulted in degeneration into the malignant osteogenic tumor. (20–22)

The considerations for differential diagnosis include blastic metastasis, tuberous sclerosis, and mastocytosis. However, to aid in the definitive diagnosis, a radiographic skeletal survey will demonstrate the symmetric juxtaarticular distribution and uniform size so characteristic of osteopoikilosis.

PROGRESSIVE DIAPHYSEAL DYSPLASIA

GENERAL CONSIDERATIONS

Progressive diaphyseal dysplasia is a rare congenital, familial, and hereditary disorder characterized by cortical thickening and sclerosis of mainly the long tubular bones. Camurati, in 1922 (1), and Engelmann, in 1929 (2), were the first to describe this disorder, and it is frequently referred to as *Engelmann-Camurati* or *Engelmann's disease*. In 1948, Neuhauser coined the term *progressive diaphyseal dysplasia* (PDD), describing the predilection for the diaphyses and the progressive nature of the disease. (3) It is now considered an autosomal dominant entity, but the expression is extremely variable.

CLINICAL FEATURES

Progressive diaphyseal dysplasia usually manifests in the first decade. Males are affected more frequently than females. (4) Often, the patient presents clinically with a waddling gait and poor muscular development. Profound weakness is found primarily in the lower extremities, and there is malnutrition. Tenderness over the involved long bones may be noted. (5) Occasionally, the serum alkaline phosphatase level (6) and erythrocyte sedimentation rate are elevated. CPK has also been found to be elevated in some patients. (7) Anemia is not a regular feature. The disease progression is slow and unpredictable, but the involvement is always symmetric. (8) The clinical signs of weakness and malnutrition often resolve following adolescence. The radiographic features persist and are the most prominent findings of this disorder.

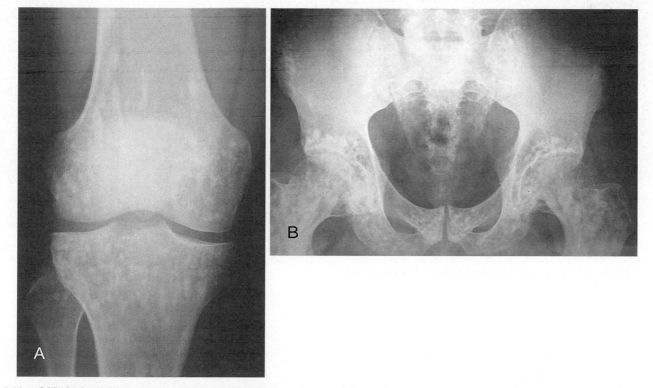

Figure 8.82.   OSTEOPOIKILOSIS: METAPHYSEAL AND EPIPHYSEAL RADIOPACITIES. A. Knee. Note the clustering of small opacities in the metaphyseal and epiphyseal regions. **B. Pelvis.** Also note the small roundish densities that are found surrounding the acetabulae and proximal femora. (Courtesy of Brian V. Lonsdale, DC, Geelong, Victoria, Australia)

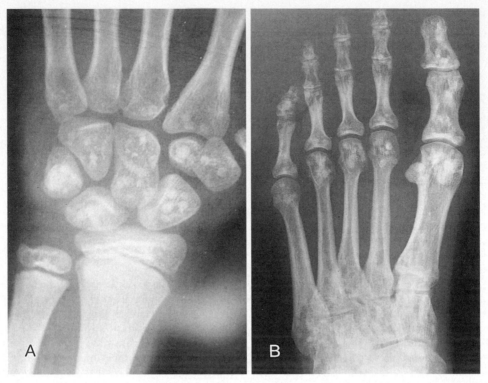

Figure 8.83. OSTEOPOIKILOSIS: INVOLVEMENT OF THE HANDS AND FEET. A. Wrist. Small roundish radiopacities resembling bone islands are seen in the carpal and proximal metacarpal bones in this patient. **B. Foot.** All of the visualized bones of the foot show roundish radiopacities. (Courtesy of Bryan Hartley, MD, Melbourne, Australia)

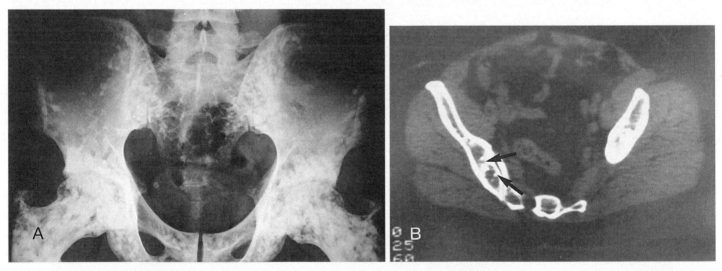

Figure 8.84. OSTEOPOIKILOSIS: PELVIC INVOLVEMENT. A. AP Pelvis: Plain Film. Note the diffuse involvement of osteopoikilosis, with radiopacities scattered throughout the pelvis and proximal femora. **B. CT Scan: Mid-pelvis.** The small densities are located in the medullary portion of the innominates (arrows). (Courtesy of Bryan Hartley, MD, Melbourne, Australia)

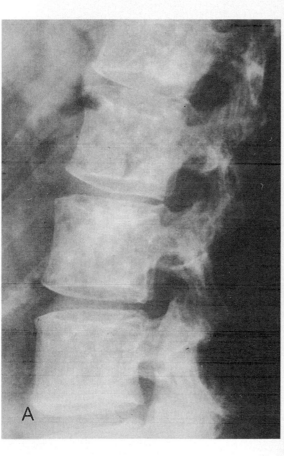

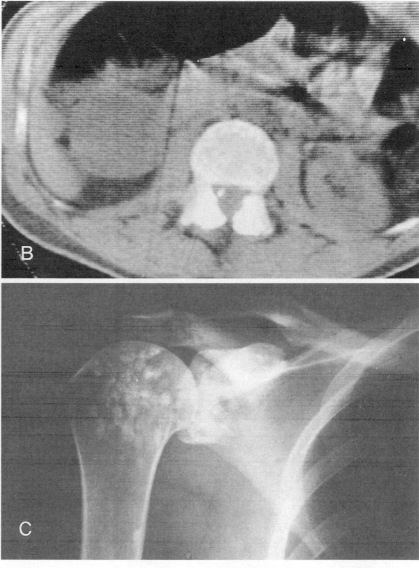

Figure 8.85. OSTEOPOIKILOSIS: SPINAL INVOLVEMENT. A. Lateral Lumbar Spine. Note the diffuse involvement of the lumbar vertebrae. **B. CT Scan: Lumbar Segment.** A CT scan of the same patient reveals the presence of these radiopacities in the spongy bone of the vertebral body. **C. Shoulder.** Also observe in this patient clustering of densities within the glenoid and proximal humerus. COMMENT: Osteopoikilosis rarely involves the skull, spine, ribs, and clavicles. (Courtesy of Bryan Hartley, MD, Melbourne, Australia)

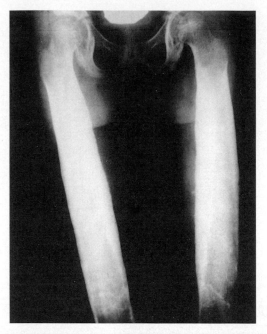

Figure 8.86. PROGRESSIVE DIAPHYSEAL DYSPLASIA, FEMORA: SYMMETRIC DIAPHYSEAL INVOLVEMENT. Note the symmetric fusiform widening of the femoral diaphyses.

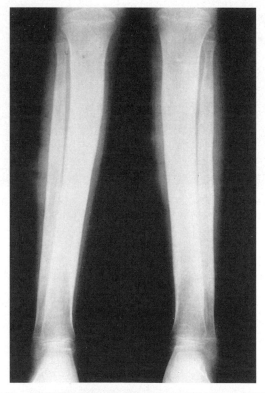

Figure 8.87. PROGRESSIVE DIAPHYSEAL DYSPLASIA, LOWER LEGS: SPARING OF THE METAPHYSES AND EPIPHYSES. There is symmetric widening and sclerosis of the tibial and fibular diaphyses, with sparing of the metaphyses and epiphyses.

Pathologically, the classic feature is greatly increased osteoblastic activity, with new bone formation. CT scans have shown that the endosteal involvement is more pronounced than the periosteal involvement. (8) A sparse vascular supply to the region of

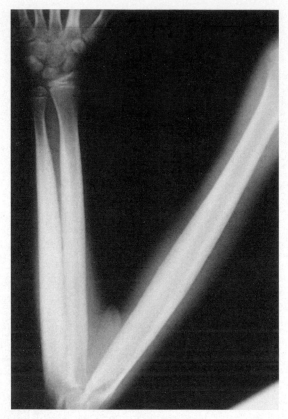

Figure 8.88. PROGRESSIVE DIAPHYSEAL DYSPLASIA, UPPER EXTREMITY: RELATIVE ELONGATION OF THE LONG BONES. Along with widening and increased density of the diaphyses, there is a relative elongation of the long bones. Also note the poor muscular development.

involvement has been suggested as the stimulus for the marked new bone formation. (9,10)

RADIOLOGIC FEATURES

Neuhauser and associates present an excellent description of the roentgen features. (3) The skeleton is involved in a symmetric distribution with fusiform widening of the diaphyseal portions of long bones. (Fig. 8.86) The metaphyses and epiphyses are generally spared. (Fig. 8.87) New bone is produced by the cortex, widening the diameter of the diaphysis, while encroaching on the medullary canal. There may be relative elongation of the bone as well. (Fig. 8.88) The new bone formation begins in the midshaft, progressing proximally and distally but ending abruptly, without involving the metaphysis.

The most commonly involved bones are the femur, tibia, radius, ulna, and humerus. (Fig. 8.89) While all long bones may be affected, the pelvic, carpal and tarsal bones are usually spared. (Fig. 8.90) The skull may show basilar sclerosis and, less commonly, calvarial hyperostosis. Exophthalmos is seen with severe involvement of the skull. (8) The ribs, clavicles, and spine occasionally display similar changes in bone density. When the spine is involved, the sclerosis affects the posterior aspect of the vertebral body and the posterior arches, but without stenosis. (8) Complications may occur and include increased intracranial pressure and encroachment on the cranial nerves. The distribution and radiographic features of progressive diaphyseal dysplasia do not generally offer a diagnostic dilemma.

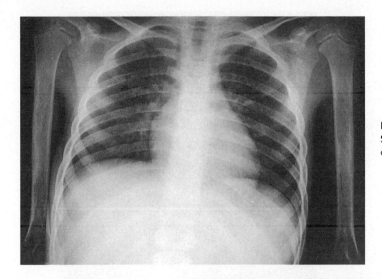

Figure 8.89. PROGRESSIVE DIAPHYSEAL DYSPLASIA: CHEST AND SHOULDERS. Note the symmetric widening of the humeral shafts. (Courtesy of The Childrens Hospital, Dept. of Radiology, Denver, Colorado)

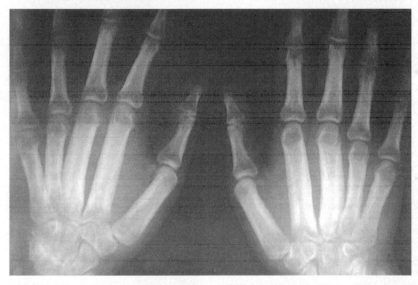

Figure 8.90. PROGRESSIVE DIAPHYSEAL DYSPLASIA: BILATERAL HAND INVOLVEMENT. Note the widening and increased density of the metacarpals bilaterally. COMMENT: The hands and feet are frequently spared in progressive diaphyseal dysplasia.

MEDICOLEGAL IMPLICATIONS
Progressive Diaphyseal Dysplasia

- Progressive bone thickening at the skull base may result in clinical signs of increased intracranial pressure and/or cranial nerve encroachment. If these signs are present, evaluation with CT and/or MRI is recommended.

PYKNODYSOSTOSIS

GENERAL CONSIDERATIONS

Defined in 1962 by Maroteaux and Lamy, (1) pyknodysostosis is thought to be the dysplasia that afflicted the French painter, Toulouse-Lautrec. (2) This condition is transmitted by an auto-somal recessive trait (3) and is characterized by increased bone density, dwarfism, and skeletal fragility. Though considered a distinct entity by most, similarities with osteopetrosis and cleidocranial dysplasia do exist.

CLINICAL FEATURES

Individuals manifest disproportionate short stature in early childhood and rarely exceed 5 feet in height as adults. Additional loss of stature may be due to multiple fractures occurring during the patient's lifetime. (4) The disorder is twice as common in males as in females. (5) The facial appearance is characteristic, with a beaked nose, prognathic jaw, small face, and a prominent forehead. Failure of closure of the cranial sutures produces an enlarged head. Dentition is anomalous, and the palate is high and arched. Lowered intelligence has been noted in approximately 10% of cases. (6) The hands and feet are stubby, with spoon-shaped nails (koilonychia) and finger clubbing. Laboratory find-

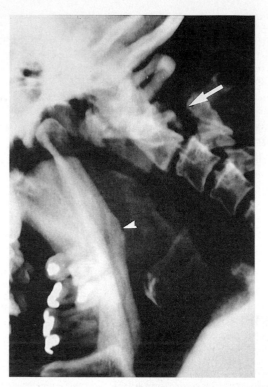

Figure 8.91. PYKNODYSOSTOSIS, LATERAL MANDIBLE: RECEDING JAW. Hypoplasia of the mandible with an obtuse angle (arrowhead) produces a receding jaw. Abnormal dentition and nonunion of a hangman's fracture (arrow) are also noted.

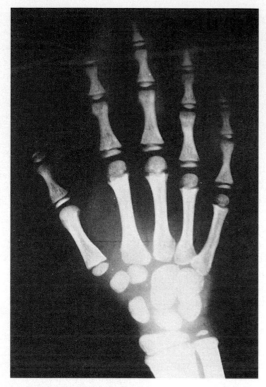

Figure 8.92. PYKNODYSOSTOSIS, HAND: TERMINAL TUFT HYPOPLASIA. Note the acroosteolysis, which is a consistent finding in pyknodysostosis. There is also a generalized increase in bone density.

ings are consistently normal. Unlike osteopetrosis, the medullary canal is maintained in patients with pyknodysostosis; (5) therefore, anemia and splenomegaly are not associated with this dysplasia. (7)

RADIOLOGIC FEATURES

A generalized increase in bone density is seen, with preservation of the medullary canal. This osteosclerosis is most prominent in the long bones, which are subject to transverse pathologic fractures. Stress fractures of weight-bearing bones, as well as fractures of the clavicle and mandible, are often seen. (6) Numerous abnormalities are found in the skull. The cranial sutures remain open, with a wide anterior fontanelle; also, numerous Wormian bones are seen. The facial bones and sinuses are hypoplastic. Mandibular hypoplasia with an obtuse angle results in a receding jaw. (8) (Fig. 8.91) Retention of the deciduous teeth is often present, with unerupted or malformed permanent teeth. Platybasia is frequent. Hypoplasia or absence of the lateral ends of the clavicles and terminal tufts of the fingers and toes (acroosteolysis) is a consistent finding. (Fig. 8.92) In the pelvis there may be shallow and obliquely roofed acetabulae and coxa valga. Bowing and overgrowth of the radius (Madelung's deformity) contribute to abnormal radioulnar articulations. Spinal abnormalities include hyperlordosis, scoliosis, kyphosis (9), and block vertebrae, especially at the craniovertebral and lumbosacral regions. (10) *Spool-shaped* vertebrae (6) and persistence of anterior infantile notching are frequently present. Primary spondylolysis of C2 has been reported. (11) Spondylolisthesis of the lower lumbar vertebrae is also seen. (9,12) The lack of anemia and the preservation

of the medullary canal help to distinguish pyknodysostosis from osteopetrosis. The short stature and dense bones of pyknodysostosis are absent in cleidocranial dysplasia.

MEDICOLEGAL IMPLICATIONS
Pyknodysostosis

- Osseous manipulation is contraindicated due to bone fragility.
- Platybasia, along with sclerosis and thickening of the skull base, may diminish the osseous dimensions of the posterior fossa resulting in encroachment on the cerebellum and/or brain stem.
- Dental caries may occur due to faulty dentition. If untreated, osteomyelitis of the maxilla or mandible may develop.
- The long uvula and diminutive facial bones may obstruct the nasal pharynx, resulting in hypoventilation (apnea) during sleep.

TUBEROUS SCLEROSIS
GENERAL CONSIDERATIONS

Tuberous sclerosis is a rare, autosomal dominant, multisystem disorder of neuroectodermal origin. It belongs to a unique group of diseases known as the *phakomatoses*. This group of neuroectodermal disorders is characterized by tumors of the skin and central nervous system. The most frequently seen phakomatosis is neurofibromatosis. Tuberous sclerosis was first described by von Recklinghausen in 1862. (1) Bourneville, in 1880 (2), coined the term *tuberous sclerosis* after providing a detailed description of the clinicopathologic features. A myriad of clinical and radiographic features have been reported in association with this disorder. The classic clinical triad consists of mental retardation, epileptic seizures, and skin lesions, but one or more of these characteristics may be lacking. Synonyms include *Bourneville's disease* and *epiloia* (meaning *mindless epileptic*). (2)

CLINICAL FEATURES

Diagnosis of tuberous sclerosis is most often made during adolescence or early adulthood, but may be delayed until autopsy because of the paucity of symptoms. The most common clinical presentation is mental deficiency with epilepsy. (3) The seizures usually manifest in the first decade of life but are nonspecific. Lesions of the central nervous system are responsible for the epilepsy and mental retardation. (4) The characteristic skin lesion is the hamartoma, and hamartomas may involve many noncutaneous sites as well, including eyes, lungs, kidneys, liver, spleen, brain, heart, and bones.

Cutaneous Manifestations

The most widely recognized skin change is adenoma sebaceum (a hamartoma), which is present in 80–90% of cases. This is frequently evident in childhood but may not manifest until puberty or pregnancy. (5,6) The earliest skin manifestations are thought to be hypopigmented macules that occur on the legs and trunk. (7–10) These are oval or leaf-shaped, with irregular margins, and may be evident at birth. The presence of hypopigmented macules in infants makes the diagnosis of tuberous sclerosis probable, while their occurrence with seizures makes it highly probable. (4,8) Other cutaneous lesions include cafe au lait spots, shagreen, or peau-chagrin patches (20 to 50% of cases), gingival and periungual fibromas, and skin tags. Ocular abnormalities such as retinal phakomas (white patches) are seen at birth in approximately 52% of cases. (4)

Cranial Abnormalities

Intracerebral calcifications are found on x-ray examination in 50 to 80% of cases. (11) (Fig. 8.93) The most common locations are in the basal ganglia and paraventricular regions. The incidence increases with the patient's age. Cortical tubers and subependymal nodules (hamartomas) are common near the ventricles and may calcify. The calcifications may be multiple or singular and appear as discrete nodules or, occasionally, as linear conglomerates. Cerebellar calcifications are found in 10–15% of patients. (12,13) MRI has enhanced the ability to detect otherwise unapparent brain lesions. (4) Cranial ultrasonography has allowed for early diagnosis of tuberous sclerosis. (14)

Visceral Abnormalities

Hamartomas are found in many organs and, depending on the predominant tissue, are classified as myolipomas, angiomyomas, angiofibromas, adenomas, or rhabdomyomas. These lesions are rarely present at birth, but their incidence increases with age and they may grow slowly.

Renal hamartomas (angiomyolipomas) occur in 40 to 80% of

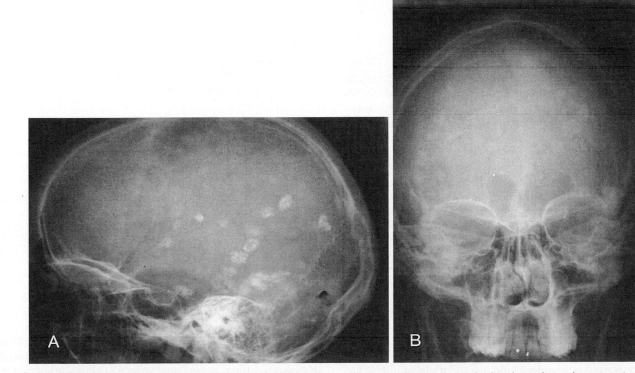

Figure 8.93. TUBEROUS SCLEROSIS: INTRACRANIAL CALCIFICATION. A. Lateral Skull. Note the numerous calcifications scattered throughout the skull. **B. PA Skull.** A frontal view of this patient's skull aids in localizing the calcifications primarily in the basal ganglia and paraventricular regions. (Courtesy of Bryan Hartley, MD, Melbourne, Australia)

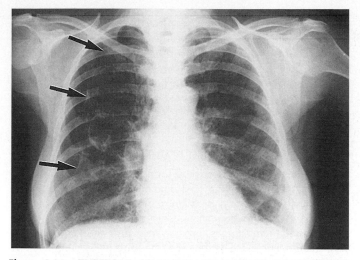

Figure 8.94.   TUBEROUS SCLEROSIS: PULMONARY INVOLVEMENT. Note the diffuse bilateral interstitial infiltrate. Tuberous sclerosis is one of the rare causes of *honeycomb* lung. Also note the right spontaneous pneumothorax (arrows). (Courtesy of Bryan Hartley, MD, Melbourne, Australia)

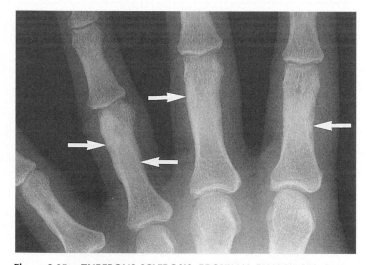

Figure 8.95.   TUBEROUS SCLEROSIS, PROXIMAL PHALANGES: SMALL TUBULAR BONE INVOLVEMENT. Note the irregular subperiosteal new bone and nodules along the proximal phalangeal shafts (arrows).

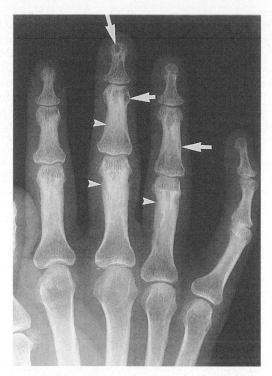

Figure 8.96.   TUBEROUS SCLEROSIS, HAND: PHALANGEAL CYSTS. Observe the small, well-defined cysts in the distal and middle phalanges (arrows). There is also subperiosteal new bone formation in the middle and proximal phalangeal shafts (arrowheads).

patients (15) and may cause them to present with flank pain and hematuria. The majority of renal hamartomas in tuberous sclerosis are bilateral, and 50% of individuals with renal angiomyolipomas may have no other manifestations of the disease. (11) Rarely, malignant degeneration of these benign neoplasms may occur. Renal artery tortuosity and aneurysms are not infrequent.

The rare cardiac involvement is usually with rhabdomyoma, and then it is commonly multiple. Colonic adenomas are infrequently seen. Fewer than 1% of patients with tuberous sclerosis have pulmonary manifestations; almost all are female. (16) The pulmonary system is typically involved late in the disease process and is characterized by a uniform and diffuse or basilar interstitial pattern, with or without progressive volume loss. (17,18) Tuberous sclerosis is a rare cause of *honeycomb* lung and it carries a poor prognosis. (Fig. 8.94) The insidious onset of acute dyspnea and chest pain may occur secondary to spontaneous pneumothorax.

Endocrine and metabolic dysfunctions are common in these patients, but poorly understood. Abnormal pituitary or adrenal function and thyroid disorders may be seen. Abnormal glucose tolerance tests and high levels of serum alkaline phosphatase have also been reported. (19)

RADIOLOGIC FEATURES

Skeletal lesions occur in approximately 50% of cases and have a varied presentation. (20) In addition to the intracranial calcifications, generalized thickening and hyperostosis of the cranial vault may be evident.

The tubular bones of the hands and feet frequently have cortical manifestations. (Fig. 8.95) Irregular subperiosteal new bone formation and nodules are common. Small, well-defined cysts are seen in the small tubular bones of the hand, particularly in the distal phalanges. (Fig. 8.96) The trabecular pattern may be coarsened.

The spine and innominate bones are often involved, with osteoblastic deposits of varied size and contour. (21) (Fig. 8.97) The reactive new bone may be in response to osseous hamartomas. (20) The areas of increased density may be diffuse or seen as discrete islands, and are most common in the vertebral bodies and pedicles and along the pelvic brim. (13) Cortical excrescences affecting the tibia in tuberous sclerosis patients have been referred to as *periosteal warts*. (22) Enlargement and sclerosis of a rib has been reported in association with tuberous sclerosis. (23)

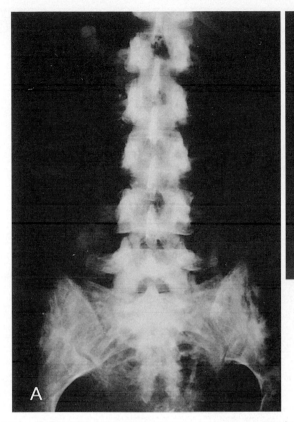

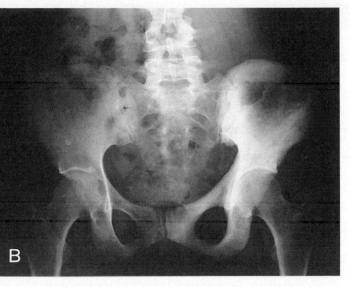

Figure 8.97.   TUBEROUS SCLEROSIS: SPINAL AND PELVIC INVOLVE-MENT. A. Lumbar Spine. Note the diffuse increased bone density and scle-rotic pedicles. **B. AP Pelvis.** Observe the unilateral innominate sclerosis. (Courtesy of Bryan Hartley, MD, Melbourne, Australia)

In a series of 12 patients with tuberous sclerosis, six had scoliotic curves ranging from 12° to 78°. (24)

The fatty component of most renal hamartomas may allow for their detection on plain radiographs, accompanied by kidney enlargement and contour irregularities. When present, the interstitial changes that occur in the lungs are apparent radiographically.

Complications of tuberous sclerosis include urinary tract infection, pulmonary disease (e.g., pneumothorax, hemoptysis, dyspnea, aspiration pneumonia), cor pulmonale, and neoplastic degeneration of the hamartomatous lesions.

MEDICOLEGAL IMPLICATIONS
Tuberous Sclerosis

- Renal and renal vascular complications are frequently seen in patients with this disorder. These include urinary tract infection, angiomyolipoma formation, renal artery aneurysm, and renal and perirenal hemorrhage. Back, flank, or abdominal pain may signify the occurrence of these complications. The replacement of normal renal parenchyma with numerous angiomyolipomas may result in chronic hypertension and renal insufficiency. This may eventually lead to renal failure.

- The insidious onset of acute dyspnea and chest pain may occur secondary to pneumothorax from chronic interstitial lung disease.

Table 8.1. The Skeletal Dysplasias: Major Clinical Features

Entity	Transmission	Major Clinical Features	Lifespan	Complications
Achondroplasia	Autosomal dominant	Rhizomelic dwarf Waddling gait Increased lumbar lordosis Large head, prominent forehead, depressed nasal bridge Spinal column normal length *Trident* hand	Normal	Back pain Spinal stenosis
Cleidocranial Dysplasia	Autosomal dominant	Large head, small face, drooping, hypermobile shoulders Abnormal gait Severe dental caries	Normal	Deafness Severe dental caries Hip and shoulder dislocations Scoliosis
Chondrodysplasia Punctata	Mild form: Autosomal dominant Lethal form: Autosomal recessive; increased in females	Mild dwarfing Normal mental status Rhizomelic dwarf Mental retardation Joint contractures	Normal Death in first years of life	Thoracic kyphoscoliosis Respiratory failure Recurrent infection
Dysplasia Epiphyseal Hemimelica	Thought to be hereditary	Monomelic limb deformity Functional impairment Valgus and varus deformity	Normal	Functional impairment of involved limb Rarely, limb shortening or elongation
Epiphyseal Dysplasia Multiplex	Autosomal dominant	Waddling gait Stubby hands and feet Flexion deformities Genuvalgum and varum deformities	Normal	Premature degenerative joint disease, especially of the hips and knees
Spondyloepiphyseal Dysplasia	Congenita form: Autosomal dominant	Short limbs, flat face, wideset eyes (hypertelorism) Increased thoracic kyphosis and lumbar lordosis, scoliosis, pectus carinatum, dwarfing	Normal	Scoliosis, increased lumbar lordosis, increased thoracic kyphosis
	Tarda form: Males only X-linked recessive	Mild loss of stature, back pain	Normal	Premature DJD
Fibrodysplasia Ossificans Progressiva	Autosomal dominant	Progressive ossification of striated muscles, with loss of motion and wasting	Death in 2nd-3rd decade	Respiratory failure Severe wasting Short thumbs and great toes
Holt-Oram Syndrome	Autosomal dominant	Cardiac deformities Dislocation of the elbow Limited range of motion Pectus excavatum & carinatum	Life is shortened when complications occur	Cardiac and major vessel abnormalities
Infantile Cortical Hyperostosis	Unknown May be viral	Hyperirritability; painful swellings Fever Exacerbations and remissions Increased ESR	Normal	Usually resolves without complications
Marfan's Syndrome	Autosomal dominant	Tall, slender individual with muscular hypoplasia; many have scoliosis Joint laxity and dislocations Lens dislocations, cataracts	Life is shortened when complications occur	Dissecting aneurysms Lens dislocations
Metaphyseal Dysplasia	Autosomal dominant	Tall individuals with bulbous enlargement of lower extremity joints	Normal	Rarely, fractures through thin cortices
Nail-Patella Syndrome	Autosomal dominant	Hypoplasia of nails on thumb and index fingers Joint contractures, muscular hypoplasia Renal dysplasia	Normal	Occasionally renal impairment Patellar and radial head dislocations

Table 8.1. *Continued*

Entity	Transmission	Major Clinical Features	Lifespan	Complications
Ehlers-Danlos Syndrome	Usually autosomal dominant	Joint hyperextensibility Fragile blood vessels Cutaneous abnormalities	Normal	Aortic dissection Aneurysms, valvular abnormalities Pulmonary hypertension
Massive Osteolysis of Gorham	Unknown	Pain and soft tissue atrophy in the involved area Progression is usual but prognosis is difficult	Life is shortened when complications occur	Spinal cord transection Paraplegia
Hurler's Syndrome	Autosomal recessive	Large head, hypertension, corneal opacities Mental deterioration, hepatosplenomegaly Severe dwarfing, dorsal kyphosis, flexion contractures Hydrocephalus	Death in 2nd decade	Cardiac failure, pneumonia
Morquio's Syndrome	Autosomal recessive	Marked dwarfism, dorsal kyphosis, muscular hypotonia Horizontal sternum, short neck Deafness, genu valgum, flexion contractures C1-C2 dislocations	Death in 3rd-4th decade	Paraplegia, respiratory failure Atlantoaxial subluxation
Osteogenesis Imperfecta	Autosomal dominant	Osteoporosis with skeletal fragility Blue sclera, abnormal dentition } Triad	Congenital form: stillborn or early death	Multiple fractures with severe deformity Hearing loss Pneumonia
Melorheostosis	Congenital	Pain over involved bone Joint contractures, restricted motion Skin abnormalities (scleroderma-like)	Normal	Rarely, premature epiphyseal closure with limb shortening
Osteopathia Striata	Congenital Probably genetic	Usually asymptomatic	Normal	None
Osteopetrosis	Benign form: Autosomal dominant	Often asymptomatic, defective dentition Rare, anemia, deafness	Usually normal	Pathologic fracture, hemorrhage, mandibular osteomyelitis
	Severe form: Autosomal recessive	Severe anemia, hepatosplenomegaly, failure to thrive Blindness	Death within 2 years of life	Massive hemorrhage, recurrent infections, anemia Rarely, leukemia and sarcoma
Osteopoikilosis	Autosomal dominant	Usually asymptomatic	Normal	None
Progressive Diaphyseal Dysplasia	Autosomal dominant in males	Waddling gait, poor muscular development Lower extremity weakness	Normal	Increased intracranial pressure Encroachment on neural canal
Pyknodysostosis	Autosomal recessive	Dwarfism Skeletal fragility Block vertebrae Characteristic facies: enlarged head, receding jaw Stubby hands and feet Anomalous dentition	Normal	Pathologic fracture
Tuberous Sclerosis	Autosomal dominant	Mental retardation, epileptic seizures Skin lesions	Normal or shortened from complications	Urinary tract infection, pulmonary disease Cor pulmonale Hamartomas, renal angiomyolipomas

Table 8.2. The Skeletal Dysplasias: Major Roentgen Features

Entity	Major Roentgen Features	Major Sites of Involvement	Bone Density
Achondroplasia	Symmetric limb shortening, especially proximal Relative widening of shafts, *champagne glass* pelvis, narrow thorax Posterior scalloping of vertebral bodies Narrowed interpedicular distance *Trident* hand	Skull, spine, pelvis, limbs Proximal long bones—rhizomelia Congenital spinal stenosis, especially lumbar	Normal
Cleidocranial Dysplasia	Persistent sutures, Wormian bones, agenetic or hypoplastic clavicles Hypoplastic facial bones Midline defects of pelvis, small pelvis Neural arch defects	Skull, clavicles, pelvis, spine	Normal
Craniosynostosis	Affected suture is a straight line often with sclerosis Deformity of skull secondary to premature suture closure	Skull	May be sclerotic along involved suture
Chondrodysplasia Punctata	Mild form: Fragmented epiphyses, normal metaphyses and diaphyses Vertebral stippling	Spine, limbs	Normal
	Lethal form: symmetric rhizomelic shortening due to fragmented epiphyses, flared metaphyses Rarely, spinal involvement	Hips, shoulders, knees, wrists	Normal
Dysplasia Epiphysealis Hemimelica	Focal overgrowth of one half of the epiphysis	Lower extremity predominates	Normal
Epiphyseal Dysplasia Multiplex	Bilateral symmetric epiphyseal irregularity Endplate irregularity Hypoplastic carpals and tarsals Flattened femoral heads and condyles	Hips, knees, and ankles	Normal

Spondyloepiphyseal Dysplasia	Congenita:
	  Delayed ossification
	  Rhizomelic dwarfing
	  Platyspondyly (short spine)
	  Irregular articular surfaces
		Spine, pelvis	Normal

	Tarda:
	  Heaping-up vertebrae
	  Narrowed discs
		Spine, pelvis	Normal

Fibrodysplasia Ossificans Progressiva	Ossification of striated muscle Short thumbs and great toes	Neck, trunk, pelvis, upper extremity	Normal or decreased
Holt-Oram Syndrome	Thumb anomalies: triphalangeal thumb or complete agenesis Carpal fusion, extra carpals Clinodactyly Radial ray deficiency	Thumbs, carpals, radius	Normal
Infantile Cortical Hyperostosis	Periosteal new bone formation	Mandible, clavicles, ribs	Normal or increased when acute
Marfan's Syndrome	Long, slender bones Thin cortices	Most marked in distal extremities but involves the entire skeleton	Normal

Table 8.2.   *Continued*

Entity	Major Roentgen Features	Major Sites of Involvement	Bone Density
Metaphyseal Dysplasia	Failure of metaphyseal remodeling with splaying or *Erlenmeyer flask* deformity	Distal femur, proximal and distal tibia, proximal fibula	Normal
Nail-Patella Syndrome	Bilateral, central posterior iliac horns Patella is small or absent	Ilium, patella, nails Kidney	Normal
Ehlers-Danlos Syndrome	Calcified subcutaneous spherules Heterotopic ossification Platyspondyly, posterior vertebral body scalloping	Soft tissues Spine	Decreased
Massive Osteolysis of Gorham	Dramatic bone destruction with pathologic fractures	Any bone	Decreased
Hurler's Syndrome	Frontal bossing, calvarial thickening, large, "J" shaped sella, dorsolumbar kyphosis Paddle ribs Flared ilia Coxa valga and vara	Entire skeleton	Decreased
Morquio's Syndrome	Universal platyspondyly, hypoplastic or agenetic odontoid Short, thick tubular bones	Entire skeleton	Normal
Osteogenesis Imperfecta	Severe osteoporosis with pencil-thin cortices Multiple fractures, especially lower extremities *Biconcave lens* vertebrae	Entire skeleton	Decreased
Melorheostosis	Streaked or wavy periosteal new bone *Wax flowing down a lighted candle* appearance	Lower extremity (usually monomelic) Often with innominate also involved	Increased
Osteopathia Striata	Vertical metaphyseal striations of increased density	Long bones	Increased
Osteopetrosis	Benign and Severe Form: Generalized sclerosis or *bone within a bone* *Sandwich* vertebrae	Entire skeleton	Increased
Osteopoikilosis	Multiple small radiopacities in metaphyseal and epiphyseal regions Usually symmetric	Long tubular bones, carpals, tarsals, pelvis, scapulae	Increased
Progressive Diaphyseal Dysplasia	Symmetric fusiform widening of the diaphyses	Femur, tibia, radius, ulna, humerus	Increased
Pyknodysostosis	Generalized increase in bone density with preservation of medullary canals	Most prominent in long bones	Increased
Tuberous Sclerosis	Intracranial calcifications Hyperostosis of cranium Periosteal new bone (warts) in tubular bones, coarsened trabeculae Osteoblastic deposits in spine and pelvis	Skin, viscera, skeleton	Increased

Table 8.3. Synonyms of Skeletal Dysplasias

Entity	Synonyms	Entity	Synonyms
Achondroplasia	Chondrodystrophia fetalis Chondrodystrophic dwarfism Micromelia	Ehlers-Danlos Syndrome	Arthrochalasis multiplex congenita Cutis hyperelastica Dermatorrhexis
Cleidocranial Dysplasia	Mutational dysostosis Cleidocranial dysostosis	Massive Osteolysis of Gorham	Gorham's disease Disappearing bone disease Vanishing bone disease Hemangiomatosis
Craniosynostosis	Craniostenosis		
Chondrodysplasia Punctata	Conradi-Hunermann syndrome Stippled epiphyses Dysplasia epiphysialis punctata Chondrodystrophia fetalis calcificans Chondrodystrophia calcificans congenita	Hurler's Syndrome	Lipochondrodystrophy Gargoylism Osteochondrodystrophy Dysostosis multiplex
		Morquio's Syndrome	Chondrodystrophy Familial osteodystrophy Eccentro osteochondrodysplasia Morquio-Ullrich syndrome Morquio-Brailsford's syndrome
Dysplasia Epiphysealis Hemimelica	Tarsoepiphyseal aclasis Trevor's disease Epiphyseal hyperplasia Articular chondromas		
Epiphyseal Dysplasia Multiplex	Multiple epiphyseal dysplasia Fairbank-Ribbing disease Dysplasia polyepiphysaire	Osteogenesis Imperfecta	Osteopsathyrosis idiopathica Mollities ossium Fragilitas ossium Lobstein's disease
Spondyloepiphyseal Dysplasia	None	Melorheostosis	Flowing hyperostosis Leri-type osteopetrosis Osteosi eberneizzante monomelica
Fibrodysplasia Ossificans Progressiva	Munchmeyer's disease Fibrogenesis ossificans progressiva Fibrositis ossificans progressiva	Osteopathia Striata	Voorhoeve's disease
Holt-Oram Syndrome	Heart-hand syndrome Cardio-limb syndrome Cardiomelic syndrome	Osteopetrosis	Albers-Schönberg's disease Osteosclerosis Osteopetrosis generalisata Osteosclerosis generalisata Marble bones Chalk bones
Infantile Cortical Hyperostosis	Caffey's disease Caffey's syndrome		
Marfan's Syndrome	Arachnodactyly Dolichostenomelia	Osteopoikilosis	Osteopathia condensans disseminata Spotted bones
Metaphyseal Dysplasia	Pyle's disease Familial metaphyseal dysplasia	Progressive Diaphyseal Dysplasia	Engelmann's disease Engelmann-Camurati disease
Nail-Patella Syndrome	Hereditary onycho osteodysplasia HOOD syndrome Fong's syndrome	Pyknodysostosis	None
		Tuberous Sclerosis	Bourneville's disease Epiloia

REFERENCES

ACHONDROPLASIA

1. **Parrot MJ:** *Sur la malformation achondroplasique et le dieu Ptah.* Bull Soc Anthropol Paris 1 (3rd ser):296, 1878.
2. **Kaufmann E:** *Untersuchungen Hber die sogenannte foetale Rachitis (Chondrodystrophy Foetalis).* Berlin, Georg Reimer, 1892.
3. **Caffey J:** *Pediatric X-Ray Diagnosis,* ed 7. Chicago, Year Book Medical Publishers, 1978.
4. **Holder JC, FitzRandolph RL, Flanigan S:** *The spectrum of spinal stenosis.* Curr Prob Diag Radiol 15:16, 1985.
5. **Wise BL, Sondheimer F, Kaufman S:** *Achondroplasia and hydrocephalus.* Neuropaediatrie 3:106, 1971.
6. **Edeiken J:** *Roentgen Diagnosis of Diseases of Bone,* ed 3. Baltimore, Williams & Wilkins, 1981.
7. **Bailey JA II:** *Elbow and other upper limb deformities in achondroplasia.* Clin Orthop 80:75, 1971.
8. **Marie P:** *L'achondroplasie dans l'adolescence et l'age adult.* Presse Med 8:17, 1900.
9. **Pauli RM, Scott CI, Wassman ER Jr, et al:** *Apnea and sudden unexpected death in infants with achondroplasia.* J Pediatr 104:342, 1984.
10. **Fremion AS, Garg BP, Kalsbeck J:** *Apnea as the sole manifestation of cord compression in achondroplasia.* J Pediatr 104:398, 1984.
11. **Wang H, Rosenbaum AE, Reid CS et al:** *Pediatric patients with achondroplasia: CT evaluation of the craniocervical junction.* Radiology 164:515, 1987.
12. **Saldino RM:** *Radiographic diagnosis of neonatal short-limbed dwarfism.* Med Radiogr Photogr 49:61, 1973.
13. **Fairbank T:** *An Atlas of General Affections of the Skeleton,* Baltimore, Williams & Wilkins, 1951.
14. **Murray RO, Jacobson HG:** *The Radiology of Skeletal Disorders,* ed 2. New York, Churchill Livingston, 1977.
15. **Hecht JT, Nelson FW, Butler IJ, et al:** *Computerized tomography of the foramen magnum: achondroplastic values compared to normal standards.* Am J Med Genet 20:355, 1985.
16. **Galanski M, Herrmann R, Knoche V:** *Neurological complications and myelographic features of achondroplasia.* Neuroradiology 17:59, 1978.

CLEIDOCRANIAL DYSPLASIA

1. **Taybi H, Lachman R:** *Radiology of Syndromes, Metabolic Disorders, and Skeletal Dysplasias,* ed 3. Chicago, Year Book Medical Publishers, 1983.
2. **Soule AB Jr:** *Mutational dysostosis (cleidocranial dysostosis).* J Bone Joint Surg (Am) 28:81, 1946.
3. **Cutter E:** *Descriptive Catalogue of the Warren Anatomical Museum,* (JBS Jackson) 21, No. 217, Boston, 1870.
4. **Marie P, Sainton P:** *Sur la dysostose cleidocranienne hereditaire.* Rev Neurol 6:835, 1898.
5. **Silverman F, Reiley M:** *Spondylo-megaepiphyseal-metaphyseal dysplasia: A new bone dysplasia resembling cleidocranial dysplasia.* Radiology 156:365, 1985.
6. **Jensen BL:** *Somatic development in cleidocranial dysplasia.* Am J Med Gen 35:69, 1990.
7. **Hawkins HB, Shapiro R, Petrillo CJ:** *The association of cleidocranial dysostosis with hearing loss.* AJR 125:944, 1975.
8. **Aegerter E, Kirkpatrick JA:** *Orthopedic Diseases,* ed 4. Philadelphia, WB Saunders, 1975.
9. **Keats TE:** *Cleidocranial dysostosis. Some atypical roentgen manifestations.* AJR 100:71, 1967.
10. **Anspach WE, Huepel RC:** *Familial cleidocranial dysostosis (cleidal dysostosis).* Am J Dis Child 58:786, 1936.
11. **Jarvis JL, Keats TE:** *Cleidocranial dysostosis. A review of 40 new cases.* AJR 121:5, 1974.
12. **Resnick D, Niwayama G:** *Diagnosis of Bone and Joint Disorders,* ed 2. Philadelphia, WB Saunders, 1988.
13. **Caffey J:** *Pediatric X-Ray Diagnosis,* ed 7. Chicago, Year Book Medical Publishers, 1978.

CRANIOSYNOSTOSIS

1. **Resnick D, Niwayama G:** *Diagnosis of Bone and Joint Disorders,* ed 2. Philadelphia, WB Saunders, 1988.
2. **Graham JM Jr:** *Craniostenosis: A new approach to management.* Pediatr Ann 10:258, 1981.
3. **Caffey J:** *Pediatric X-ray Diagnosis,* ed 7. Chicago, Year Book Medical Publishers, 1978.
4. **Carmel PW, Luken MG, Ascheri GF:** *Craniosynostosis: Computed tomographic evaluation of skull base and calvarial deformities and associated intracranial changes,* Neurosurgery 9:366, 1981.

CHONDRODYSPLASIA PUNCTATA

1. **Spranger J:** *The epiphyseal dysplasias.* Clin Orthop Rel Res 114:46, 1976.
2. **Bateman D:** *Two cases, and specimens from a third case, of punctate epiphyseal dysplasia.* Proc R Soc Med 29:745, 1936.
3. **Hunermann C:** *Chondrodystrophia calcificans congenital als abortive form der chondrodystrophie.* Z Kinderheilkd 51:1, 1931.
4. **Andersen PE Jr, Justesen P:** *Chondrodysplasia punctata. Report of two cases.* Skeletal Radiol 16:223, 1987.

5. **Sugarman GI:** *Chondrodysplasia punctata (rhizomelic type): Case report and pathologic findings.* Birth Defects 10:399, 1974.
6. **Cremin BJ, Beighton P:** *Dwarfism in the newborn: The nomenclature and genetic significance.* Br J Radiol 47:77, 1974.
7. **Kaufmann HJ, Mahoubi S, Sprackman TJ, et al:** *Tracheal stenosis as a complication of chondrodysplasia punctata.* Ann Radiol 1:203, 1976.
8. **Afshani E, Girdany BR:** *Atlanto-axial dislocation in chondrodysplasia punctata. Report of the findings in two brothers.* Radiology 102:399, 1972.
9. **Fairbank T:** *An Atlas of General Affections of the Skeleton,* Baltimore, Williams & Wilkins, 1951.
10. **Happle R, Matthias HH, Macher E:** *Sex linked chondrodysplasia punctata?* Clin Genet 11:73, 1977.
11. **Taybi H, Lachman RS:** *Radiology of Syndromes, Metabolic Disorders, and Skeletal Dysplasias,* Chicago, Year Book Medical Publishers, 1983.
12. **Sheffield LJ, Danks DM, Mayne V, et al:** *Chondrodysplasia punctata—23 cases of a mild and relatively common variety.* J Pediatr 86:916, 1976.
13. **Manzke H, Chrisophers E, Wiederman HR:** *Dominant sex-linked inherited chondrodysplasia punctata: A distinct type of chondrodysplasia punctata.* Clin Genet 17:97, 1979.
14. **Jacobson HG:** *Dense bone—too much bone: Radiological considerations and differential diagnosis.* Skeletal Radiol 13:1, 1985.
15. **Shaw WL, Emery J, Hall JG:** *Chondrodysplasia punctata and maternal warfarin use during pregnancy.* Am J Dis Child 129:360, 1975.
16. **Warkany J:** *A warfarin embryopathy?* Am J Dis Child 129:287, 1975.
17. **Silengo MC, Luzzatti L, Silverman FN:** *Clinical and genetic aspects of Conradi-Hunermann disease. A report of three familial cases and review of the literature.* J Pediatr 97:911, 1980.
18. **Resnick D, Niwayama G:** *Diagnosis of Bone and Joint Disorders,* ed 2. Philadelphia, WB Saunders, 1988.

DYSPLASIA EPIPHYSEALIS HEMIMELICA

1. **Mouchet A, Belot J:** *La tarsomegalie.* J Radiol Electrol 10:289, 1926.
2. **Trevor D:** *Tarso-epiphyseal aclasis: Congenital error of epiphyseal development.* J Bone Joint Surg (Br) 32:204, 1950.
3. **Fairbank TJ:** *Dysplasia epiphysealis hemimelica (tarso epiphyseal aclasis)* J Bone Joint Surg (Br) 38:237, 1956.
4. **Aegerter E, Kirkpatrick JA:** *Orthopedic Diseases,* ed 4. Philadelphia, WB Saunders, 1975.
5. **Azouz EM, Slomic AM, Marton D, et al:** *The variable manifestations of dysplasia epiphysealis hemimelica.* Pediatr Radiol 15:44, 1985.
6. **Keret D, Spatz DK, Caro PA, et al:** *Dysplasia Epiphysealis Hemimelica: Diagnosis and Treatment.* J Pediatr Orthop 12:365, 1992.
7. **Hensinger RN, Cowell HR, Ramsey PL, et al:** *Familial dysplasia epiphysealis hemimelica, associated with chondromas and osteochondromas. Report of a kindred with variable presentations.* J Bone Joint Surg (Am) 56:1513, 1974.
8. **Greenspan A, Steiner G, Sotelo D, et al:** *Mixed sclerosing bone dysplasia coexisting with dysplasia epiphysealis hemimelica (Trevor-Fairbank disease).* Skeletal Radiol 15:452, 1986.
9. **Keats TE:** *Dysplasia epiphysealis hemimelica (tarso epiphyseal aclasis).* Radiology 68:558, 1957.
10. **D'Angio GJ, Ritvo M, Ulin R:** *Clinical and roentgen manifestations of tarso-epiphyseal aclasis; review of the manifestations of tarso-epiphyseal aclasis; review of the literature and report of an additional case.* AJR 74:1068, 1955.
11. **Lamesch AJ, Jacquemart J:** *Dysplasia epiphysealis hemimelica of the carpal bones.* Bull Soc Sci Med Grand Duche Luxemb 125:84, 1988.
12. **Buckwalter JA, El-Khoury GY, Flatt AE:** *Dysplasia epiphysealis hemimelica of the ulna.* Clin Orthop Rel Res 135:36, 1978.
13. **Mendez AA, Keret D, MacEwen GD:** *Isolated dysplasia epiphysealis hemimelica of the hip joint.* J Bone Joint Surg (Am) 70:921, 1988.
14. **Caffey J:** *Pediatric X-Ray Diagnosis,* ed 7. Chicago, Year Book Medical Publishers, 1978.

EPIPHYSEAL DYSPLASIA MULTIPLEX

1. **Ribbing S:** *Studien über hereditare, multiple epiphysenstörungen.* Acta Radiol Suppl 34:1, 1937.
2. **Fairbank T:** *Dysplasia epiphysialis multiplex.* Br J Surg 34:225, 1947.
3. **Rubin P:** *Dynamic Classification of Bone Dysplasias,* Chicago, Year Book Publishers, 1964.
4. **Versteylen RJ, Zwemmer A, Lorie CA, et al:** *Multiple epiphyseal dysplasia complicated by severe osteochondritis dissecans of the knee.* Skeletal Radiol 17:407, 1988.
5. **Amir D, Mogle P, Weinberg H:** *Multiple epiphysial dysplasia in one family. A further review of seven generations.* J Bone Joint Surg (Am) 67:809, 1985.
6. **Leeds NE:** *Epiphyseal dysplasia multiplex.* AJR 84:506, 1960.
7. **Maroteaux P:** *Birth Defects Compendium,* New York, National Foundation, March of Dimes, Alan R Liss, 1979.
8. **Berg PK:** *Dysplasia epiphysialis multiplex.* AJR 97:31, 1966.
9. **Hoefnagel D, Sycamore LK, Russel SW, et al:** *Hereditary multiple epiphysial dysplasia.* Ann Hum Genet 30:201, 1967.
10. **Resnick D, Niwayama G:** *Diagnosis of Bone and Joint Disorders,* Philadelphia, WB Saunders, 1981.
11. **Hulvey JT, Keats T:** *Multiple epiphyseal dysplasia. A contribution to the problem of spinal involvement.* AJR 106:170, 1969.
12. **Hunt DD, Ponseti IV, Pedrine-Mille A, et al:** *Multiple epiphyseal dysplasia in two siblings.* J Bone Joint Surg (Am) 49:1611, 1967.

SPONDYLOEPIPHYSEAL DYSPLASIA

1. **Spranger JW, Langer LO Jr:** *Spondyloepiphyseal dysplasia congenita.* Radiology 94:313, 1970.
2. **Maroteaux P, Lamy M, Bernard J:** *La dysplasie spondyloepiphysaire tardive; description clinique et radiologigue.* Presse Med 65:1205, 1957.
3. **Genez BM, et al:** *Case report 487 Diagnosis: Spondyloepiphyseal dysplasia tarda (SDT) (presumptively proved).* Skeletal Radiol 17:306, 1988.
4. **Kozlowski K, Bittel D, Budzinska A:** *Spondylepiphyseal dysplasia congenita.* Ann Radiol 11:367, 1968.
5. **Roaf R, Longmore JB, Forrester RM:** *A childhood syndrome of bone dysplasia, retinal detachment and deafness.* Dev Med Child Neurol 9:464, 1967.
6. **Spranger JW, Langer LO Jr, Wiedemann HR:** *Bone Dysplasias. An Atlas of Constitutional Disorders of Skeletal Development,* Philadelphia, WB Saunders, 1974.
7. **Saldino RM:** *Radiographic diagnosis of neonatal short-limbed dwarfism.* Med Radiogr Photogr 49:61, 1973.
8. **Murray RO, Jacobson HG:** *The Radiology of Skeletal Disorders,* ed 2. New York, Churchill Livingston, 1977.
9. **Edeiken J:** *Roentgen Diagnosis of Diseases of Bone,* ed 3. Baltimore, Williams & Wilkins, 1981.
10. **LeDoux MS, Naftalis RC, Aronin PA:** *Stabilization of the cervical spine in spondyloepiphyseal dysplasia congenita.* Neurosurgery 28:580, 1991.
11. **Wynne-Davies CM, et al:** *Instability of the upper cervical spine.* Arch Dis Child 64:283, 1989.
12. **Langer LO Jr:** *Spondyloepiphyseal dysplasia tarda.* Radiology 82:833, 1964.
13. **Poker N, Finby N, Archibald R:** *Spondyloepiphyseal dysplasia tarda.* Radiology 85:474, 1965.
14. **Aegerter E, Kirkpatrick JA:** *Orthopedic Diseases,* Philadelphia, WB Saunders, 1975.

FIBRODYSPLASIA OSSIFICANS PROGRESSIVA

1. **Young JWR, Haney PJ:** *Case Report 314.* Skeletal Radiol 13:318, 1985.
2. **Rogers JG, Geho WB:** *Fibrodysplasia ossificans progressiva.* J Bone Joint Surg (Am) 61:909, 1979.
3. **McKusick VA:** *Heritable Disorders of Connective Tissue,* ed 4. St. Louis, CV Mosby, 1972.
4. **Resnick D, Niwayama G:** *Diagnosis of Bone and Joint Disorders,* Philadelphia, WB Saunders, 1981.
5. **Lutwak L:** *Myositis ossificans progressiva; mineral, metabolic and radioactive calcium studies of the effects of hormones.* Am J Med 37:269, 1964.
6. **Koontz AR:** *Myositis ossificans progressiva.* Am J Med Sci 174:406, 1927.
7. **VanCreveld S, Soeters JM:** *Myositis ossificans progressiva.* Am J Dis Child 62:1000, 1941.
8. **Riley HD Jr, Christie A:** *Myositis ossificans progressiva.* Pediatrics 8:753, 1951.
9. **Letts RM:** *Myositis ossificans progressiva. A report of two cases with chromosome studies.* Can Med Assoc J 99:856, 1976.
10. **Eaton WL, Conkling WS, Daeschner CW:** *Early myositis ossificans progressiva occurring in homozygotic twins; a clinical and pathological study.* J Pediatr 50:591, 1957.
11. **Fletcher E, Moss MS:** *Myositis ossificans progressiva.* Ann Rheum Dis 24:267, 1965.
12. **Smith DM, Zerman W, Johnston CC, et al:** *Myositis ossificans progressiva. Case report with metabolic and histochemical studies.* Metabolism 15:521, 1966.
13. **Reinig JW, Hill SC, Fang M, et al:** *Fibrodysplasia ossificans progressiva: CT appearance.* Radiology 159:153, 1986.
14. **Resnick D:** *Case report 240.* Skeletal Radiol 10:131, 1983.

HOLT-ORAM SYNDROME

1. **Holt M, Oram S:** *Familial heart disease with skeletal malformations.* Br Heart J 22:236, 1960.
2. **Kaufman RL, Rimoin DL, McAlister WH, et al:** *Variable expression of the Holt-Oram syndrome.* Am J Dis Child 127:21, 1974.
3. **Najjar H, Mardini M, Tabboa R, et al:** *Variability of the Holt-Oram syndrome in Saudi individulas.* Am J Med Genet 29:851, 1988.
4. **Harris LC, Osborne WP:** *Congenital absence or hypoplasia of the radius with ventricular septal defect: Ventriculo-radial dysplasia.* J Pediatr 68:265, 1966.
5. **Taybi H, Lachman RS:** *Radiology of Syndromes, Metabolic Disorders, and Skeletal Dysplasias,* ed 3. Chicago, Year Book Medical Publishers, 1990.
6. **Caffey J:** *Pediatric X-Ray Diagnosis,* ed 7. Chicago, Year Book Medical Publishers, 1978.
7. **Poznanski AK:** *The Hand In Radiologic Diagnosis,* Philadelphia, WB Saunders, 1974.

INFANTILE CORTICAL HYPEROSTOSIS

1. **Caffey J, Silverman WA:** *Infantile cortical hyperostoses; preliminary report on a new syndrome.* AJR 54:1, 1945.
2. **Clement AR, Williams JG:** *The familial occurrence of infantile cortical hyperostosis.* Radiology 80:409, 1963.
3. **Saul RA, Lee WH, Stevenson RE:** *Caffey's disease revisited. Further evidence for autosomal dominant inheritance with incomplete penetrance.* Am J Dis Child 136:56, 1982.
4. **Caffey J:** *Pediatric X-Ray Diagnosis,* ed 7. Chicago, Year Book Medical Publishers, 1978.
5. **Resnick D, Niwayama G:** *Diagnosis of Bone and Joint Disorders,* Philadelphia, WB Saunders, 1981.
6. **Bennet HS, Nelson TR:** *Prenatal cortical hyperostosis.* Br J Radiol 26:47, 1953.

7. **Barba WP II, Freriks DJ:** *The familial occurrence of infantile cortical hyperostosis in utero.* J Pediatr 42:141, 1953.
8. **Taj-Eldin S, Al-Jawak J:** *Cortical hyperostosis: Infantile and juvenile manifestations in a boy.* Arch Dis Child 46:564, 1971.
9. **Blank E:** *Recurrent Caffey's cortical hyperostosis and persistent deformity.* Pediatrics 55:856, 1975.
10. **Langer R, Kaufman HJ:** *Open quiz solution: Case report.* Skeletal Radiol 15:377, 1986.
11. **Gentry RR, Rust RS, Lohr JA, et al:** *Infantile cortical hyperostosis of the ribs (Caffey's disease) without mandibular involvement.* Pediatr Radiol 13:236, 1983.
12. **Holtzman D:** *Infantile cortical hyperostosis of the scapula presenting as an ipsilateral Erb's palsy.* J Pediatr 81:785, 1972.
13. **Milton LR, Elliott JH:** *Ocular manifestations of infantile cortical hyperostosis.* Am J Ophthalmol 64:902, 1967.
14. **Scott EP:** *Infantile cortical hyperostosis: Report of an unusual complication.* J Pediatr 62:782, 1963.
15. **Tien R, Barron BJ, Dhekne RD:** *Caffey's disease: Nuclear medicine and radiologic correlation: A case of mistaken identity.* Clin Nucl Med 13:583, 1988.

MARFAN'S SYNDROME

1. **Marfan AB:** *Un cas de deformation congenitale des quatre membres, tres prononcee par les extremities caracterisee par l'allongement des os avec un certain degre d'amincissement.* Bull Mem Soc Med Hop Paris, 3rd series, 13:220, 1896.
2. **Resnick D, Niwayama G:** *Diagnosis of Bone and Joint Disorders,* Philadelphia, WB Saunders, 1981.
3. **Achard C, Grenet H:** *Persistance de la lymphocytose arachnoidienne, et des douleurs dans un cas de zona.* Bull Mem Soc Med Hop Paris 19:1069, 1902.
4. **Magid D, Pyeritz RE, Fishman EK:** *Musculoskeletal manifestations of the Marfan syndrome: Radiologic features.* AJR 155:99, 1990.
5. **Kuhlman JE, Scott WW Jr, Fishman EK, et al:** *Acetabular protrusion in the marfan syndrome.* Radiology 164:415, 1987.
6. **Pennes DR, Braunstein EM, Shirazi KK:** *Carpal ligamentous laxity with bilateral perilunate dislocation in Marfan syndrome.* Skeletal Radiol 13:62, 1985.
7. **Burch FE:** *Association of ectopia lentis with arachnodactyly.* Arch Ophthalmol 15:645, 1936.
8. **Etter L, Glover LP:** *Arachnodactyly complicated by dislocation of lens and death from rupture of dissecting aneurysm of aorta.* JAMA 123:88, 1943.
9. **McKusick VA:** *Heritable Disorders of Connective Tissue,* St. Louis, CV Mosby, 1966.
10. **Murdoch JL, Walker BA, Halpren BL, et al:** *Life expectancy and causes of death in the Marfan syndrome.* N Engl J Med 286:804, 1972.
11. **Edeiken J:** *Roentgen Diagnosis of Diseases of Bone,* ed 3. Baltimore, Williams & Wilkins, 1981.
12. **Steinberg I:** *A simple screening test for the Marfan syndrome.* AJR 97:118, 1966.
13. **Parrish JG:** *Heritable disorders of connective tissue.* Proc R Soc Med 53:515, 1960.
14. **Obarski TP, Schiavone WA:** *Thoracic cage deformities in the early diagnosis of the Marfan syndrome and cardiovascular disease.* J Am Osteopathic Assoc 90:446, 1990.
15. **Wenger DR, Ditkoff TJ, Herring JA, et al:** *Protrusio acetabuli in Marfan's syndrome.* Clin Orthop Rel Res 147:134, 1980.
16. **Fast A, Otremsky Y, Pollack D, et al:** *Protrusio acetabuli in Marfan's syndrome: Report on two patients.* J Rheumatol 11:549, 1984.
17. **Greenfield GB:** *Radiology of Bone Diseases,* ed 3. Philadelphia, JB Lippincott, 1975.
18. **Nelson JD:** *The Marfan syndrome, with special reference to congenital enlargement of the spinal canal.* Br J Radiol 31:561, 1958.
19. **Pyeritz RE, Fishman EK, Bernhardt BA, et al:** *Dural ectasia is a common feature of the Marfan syndrome.* Am J Hum Genet 43:726, 1988.

METAPHYSEAL DYSPLASIA

1. **Pyle E:** *A case of unusual bone development.* J Bone Joint Surg (Am) 13:874, 1931.
2. **Hermel MB, Gershon-Cohen J, Jones DT:** *Familial metaphyseal dysplasia.* AJR 70:413, 1953.
3. **Bakwin H, Krida R:** *Familial metaphyseal dysplasia.* Am J Dis Child 53:1521, 1937.
4. **Gorlin RJ, Koszalka MF, Spranger J:** *Pyle's disease (familial metaphyseal dysplasia): A presentation of two cases and argument for its separation from craniometaphyseal dysplasia.* J Bone Joint Surg(Am) 52:347, 1970.
5. **Greenspan A:** *Sclerosing bone dysplasias-a target-site approach.* Skeletal Radiol 20:561, 1991.
6. **Caffey J:** *Pediatric X-ray Diagnosis,* ed 7. Chicago, Year Book Medical Publishers, 1978.
7. **Jacobson HG:** *Dense bone—Too much bone: Radiological considerations and differential diagnosis.* Skeletal Radiol 13:1, 1985.
8. **Mori PA, Holt JF:** *Cranial manifestations of familial metaphyseal dysplasia.* Radiology 66:335, 1956.

NAIL-PATELLA SYNDROME

1. **Looij B Jr, Slaa RL, Hogewind BL, et al.:** *Genetic counseling in hereditary osteo-onychodysplasia (HOOD, nail-patella syndrome) with nephropathy.* J Med Genet 25:682, 1988.
2. **Kieser W:** *Die sog. Flughaut beim Menschen. Ihre Beziehung zum Status dysraphicus und ihre Erblichkeit. (Dargestellt an der Sippe Fr.)* Z Menschl Vererb-u Konstitutionslehre 23:594, 1939.
3. **Fong EE:** *"Iliac horns" (symmetrical bilateral central posterior iliac processes); a case report.* Radiology 47:517, 1946.
4. **Mino RA, Mino VH, Livingstone RG:** *Osseous dysplasia and dystrophy of the nails. Review of the literature and report of a case.* AJR 60:682, 1988.

5. **Eisenberg KS, Potter DE, Bovill EG:** *Osteoonychodystrophy with nephropathy and renal osteodystrophy. A case report.* J Bone Joint Surg (Am) 54:1301, 1972.
6. **Hawkins CF, Smith DE:** *Renal dysplasia in a family with multiple hereditary abnormalities including iliac horns.* Lancet 1:803, 1950.
7. **Thompson EA, Walker ET, Weens HS:** *Iliac horns (an osseous manifestation of hereditary arthrodysplasia associated with dystrophy of the fingernails).* Radiology 53:88, 1949.
8. **Darlington D, Hawkins CF:** *Nail-patella syndrome with iliac horns and hereditary nephropathy.* J Bone Joint Surg (Br) 49:164, 1967.
9. **Resnick D, Niwayama G:** *Diagnosis of Bone and Joint Disorders,* ed 2. Philadelphia, W B Saunders, 1988.
10. **Edeiken J:** *Roentgen Diagnosis of Diseases of Bone,* ed 3. Baltimore, Williams & Wilkins, 1981.
11. **Williams HJ, Hoyer JR:** *Radiographic diagnosis of osteo- onychodysostosis in infancy.* Radiology 109:151, 1973.
12. **Garces MA, Muraskas JK, Muraskas EK, et al.:** *Hereditary onycho-osteo-dysplasia (HOOD syndrome): A report of two cases.* Skeletal Radiol 8:55, 1982.
13. **Wasserman D:** *Unilateral iliac horn (central posterior iliac process). Case report.* Radiology 120:562, 1976.

EHLERS-DANLOS SYNDROME

1. **Beighton P, Grahame R, Bird H:** *Ehlers-Danlos Syndrome.* In: *Hypermobility of the Joints.* Berlin, Springer-Verlag, 1983.
2. **Beighton P, Horan F:** *Orthopaedic aspects of Ehlers-Danlos syndrome.* J Bone Joint Surg (Br) 51:444, 1969.
3. **Resnick D, Niwayama G:** *Diagnosis of Bone and Joint Disorders,* ed 2. Philadelphia, WB Saunders, 1981.
4. **Rybka FJ, O'Hara ET:** *The surgical significance of Ehlers-Danlos syndrome.* Am J Surg 113:431, 1967.
5. **Taybi H, Lachman R:** *Radiology of Syndromes, Metabolic Disorders, and Skeletal Dysplasias,* ed 3. Chicago, Year Book Medical Publishers, 1983.
6. **Taylor JAM, Greene-Deslauriers K, Tanaka DI:** *Case report: Ehlers-Danlos syndrome.* J Manipulative Physiol Ther 13:273, 1990.
7. **Beighton P:** *McKusick's Heritable Disorders of Connective Tissue,* ed 5. St. Louis, CV Mosby Co, 1993.
8. **Ehlers E:** *Cutis laxa, neigung zu Haemorrhagien in der haut, lockerung mehrer artikuationen.* Derm Z: 8:173, 1901.
9. **Danlos H:** *Un cas de cutis laxa avec tumeurs par contusion chronique des coudes et des genoux.* Bull Soc Frac Derm Syph 19:70, 1908.
10. **Lapayowker MS:** *Cutis hyperelastica, the Ehlers-Danlos syndrome.* AJR 84:232, 1960.
11. **Brown A, Stock VF:** *Dermatorrhexis: Report of a case.* Am J Dis Child 54:956, 1967.
12. **Pope FM, Jones PM, Wells RS, et al:** *Ehlers-Danlos syndrome IV (acrogeria): New autosomal dominant and recessive types.* J R Soc Med 73:180, 1980.
13. **Coventry MB:** *Some skeletal changes in Ehlers-Danlos syndrome. A report of two cases.* J Bone Joint Surg (Am) 43:855, 1961.
14. **Svane S:** *Ehlers-Danlos syndrome. A case with some skeletal changes.* Acta Orthop Scand 37:49, 1966.
15. **Holt JF:** *The Ehlers-Danlos syndrome.* AJR 55:420, 1946.
16. **Freeman JT:** *Ehlers-Danlos syndrome.* Am J Dis Child 79:1049, 1950.
17. **Byers PH, Holbrook KA:** *Molecular basis of clinical heterogeneity in Ehlers-Danlos syndrome.* Ann NY Acad Sci 460:298, 1985.
18. **Katz I, Stuner K:** *Ehlers-Danlos syndrome with ectopic bone formation.* Radiology 65:352, 1955.
19. **Lewkonia RM, Pope FM:** *Joint contractures and acroosteolysis in Ehlers-Danlos syndrome type IV.* J Rheumatol 12:140, 1985.
20. **Newton TH, Carpenter ME:** *The Ehlers-Danlos syndrome with acro-osteolysis.* Br J Radiol 32:739, 1959.
21. **Beighton P, Thomas ML:** *The radiology of Ehlers-Danlos syndrome.* Clin Radiol 20:354, 1969.

MASSIVE OSTEOLYSIS OF GORHAM

1. **Gorham LW, et al:** *Disappearing bones: A rare form of massive osteolysis. Report of two cases, one with autopsy findings.* Am J Med 17:674, 1954.
2. **Gorham LW, Stout AP:** *Massive osteolysis (acute spontaneous absorption of bone, phantom bone, disappearing bone).* J Bone Joint Surg (Am) 37:985, 1955.
3. **Murray RO, Jacobson HG:** *The Radiology of Skeletal Disorders,* ed 2. New York, Churchill Livingston, 1977.
4. **Campbell J, Almond HGA, Johnson R:** *Massive osteolysis of the humerus with spontaneous recovery. Report of a case.* J Bone Joint Surg (Br) 57:238, 1975.
5. **Hanly JG, Walsh NM, Breshihan B:** *Massive osteolysis in the hand and response to radiotherapy.* J Rheumatol 12:580, 1985.
6. **Halliday DR, Dahlin DC, Pugh DG, et al:** *Massive osteolysis and angiomatosis.* Radiology 82:637, 1964.
7. **Resnick D, Niwayama G:** *Diagnosis of Bone and Joint Disorders,* ed 2. Philadelphia, WB Saunders, 1988.

MUCOPOLYSACCHARIDOSES

1. **Brante G:** *Gargoylism: A mucopolysaccharidosis.* Scan J Clin Lab Invest 4:43, 1952.
2. **Resnick D, Niwayama G:** *Diagnosis of Bone and Joint Disorders,* ed 2. Philadelphia, WB Saunders, 1988.
3. **McKusick VA:** *Heritable Disorders of Connective Tissue,* ed 4. St. Louis, CV Mosby, 1972.
4. **Lamy M, Maroteaux P, Bader JP:** *Etude genetique du gargoylisme.* J Genet Hum 6:156, 1957.

5. **Tuthill CR:** *Juvenile amaurotic idiocy; marked adventitial growth associated with skeletal malformations and tuberculomas.* Arch Neurol Psychiatr 32:198, 1934.
6. **Kressler RJ, Aegerter EE:** *Hurler's syndrome (gargoylism); summary of literature and report of case with autopsy findings.* J Pediatr 12:579, 1938.
7. **Eggli KD, Dorst JP:** *The mucopolysaccharidoses and related conditions.* Semin Roentgenol 21:275, 1986.
8. **Thomas SL, Childress MH, Quinton B:** *Hypoplasia of the odontoid with atlanto-axial subluxation in Hurler's syndrome.* Pediatr Radiol 15:353, 1985.
9. **Holzgrave W, Grobe H, von Figura K, et al:** *Morquio syndrome. Clinical findings of 11 patients with MPS IV-A and 2 patients with MPS IV-B.* Hum Genet 57:360, 1981.
10. **Morquio L:** *Sur une forme de dystrophie osseuse familiale.* Bull Soc Pediatr Paris 27:145, 1929.
11. **Brailsford JE:** *Chondro-osteo-dystrophy; roentgenographic and clinical features of a child with dislocation of vertebra.* Am J Surg 7:404, 1929.
12. **Zellweger H, Pnsetti IV, Pedrini V, et al:** *Morquio-Ullrich's disease.* J Pediatr 59:549, 1961.
13. **Fairbank T:** *An Atlas of General Affections of the Skeleton,* Baltimore, Williams & Wilkins, 1951.
14. **Grossman H, Dorst JP:** *Mucopolysaccharidosis and mucolipidosis.* In: H Kaufman Ed.: *Intrinsic Diseases of Bones (Progress in Pediatric Radiology,* Vol 4), Basel, S Karger, 1973.
15. **Dutton RV:** *A practical radiologic approach to skeletal dysplasias in infancy.* Radiol Clin North Am 25:1211, 1987.

OSTEOGENESIS IMPERFECTA

1. **Lobstein JGCFM:** *Lehrbuch der Pathologischen Anatomie Bd II,* Stuttgart, 1835.
2. **Ormerod EL:** *An account of a case of mollities ossium.* Br Med J 2:735, 1859.
3. **Gurlt E:** *Handbuch der Lehre von den KnochenbrHchen, Bd 1,* Berlin, 1862-1865.
4. **Resnick D, Niwayama G:** *Diagnosis of Bone and Joint Disorders,* Philadelphia, WB Saunders, 1981.
5. **Falvo KA, Root L, Bullough PG:** *Osteogenesis imperfecta: Clinical evaluation and management.* J Bone Joint Surg (Am) 56:783, 1974.
6. **Bauze RJ, Smith R, Francis MJO:** *A new look at osteogenesis imperfecta.* J Bone Joint Surg (Br) 57:2, 1975.
7. **Sillence DO, Senn A, Danks DM:** *Genetic heterogeneity in osteogenesis imperfecta.* J Med Genet 16:101, 1979.
8. **Sillence D:** *Osteogenesis imperfecta: An expanding panorama of variants.* Clin Orthop Rel Res 159:11, 1981.
9. **Resnick D, Niwayama G:** *Diagnosis of Bone and Joint Disorders,* ed 2. Philadelphia, W B Saunders, 1988.
10. **Byers PH, Bonadio JF, Steinmann B:** *Osteogenesis imperfecta: Update and perspective.* Am J Med Genet 17:429, 1984.
11. **Beighton P, Spranger J, Versveld G:** *Skeletal complications in osteogenesis imperfecta.* S Afr Med J 64:565, 1983.
12. **McKusick VA:** *Heritable Disorders of Connective Tissue,* ed 4. St. Louis, CV Mosby, 1972.
13. **Ibsen KH:** *Distinct varieties of osteogenesis imperfecta.* Clin Orthop Rel Res 50:279, 1967.
14. **Danelius G:** *Osteogenesis imperfecta intrauterin diagnostiziert.* Arch Gynaekol 154:160, 1933.
15. **Solomons CC, Miller EA:** *Osteogenesis imperfecta—New perspectives.* Clin Orthop Rel Res 96:229, 1973.
16. **Giordano A:** *Hereditary disease of the osteocartilagenous system; comparative morphological basis.* Acta Genet 7:155, 1957.
17. **Fairbank T:** *An Atlas of General Affections of the Skeleton,* Baltimore, Williams & Wilkins, 1951.
18. **Sillence DO:** *Osteogenesis imperfecta nosology and genetics.* Ann NY Acad Sci 543:1, 1988.
19. **Hanscom DA, Winter RB, Lutter L, et al:** *Osteogenesis imperfecta. Radiographic classification, natural history, and treatment of spinal deformities.* J Bone Joint Surg (Am) 74:598, 1992.
20. **Hanscom DA, Bloom BA:** *The Spine in Osteogenesis Imperfecta.* Orthop Clin of No Am 19:449, 1988.
21. **Jacobson HG:** *Dense bone—Too much bone: Radiological considerations and differential diagnosis.* Skeletal Radiol 13:1, 1985.
22. **Meschan I:** *Analysis of Roentgen Signs in General Radiology,* Vol 1, Philadelphia, WB Saunders, 1973.
23. **Ablin DS, Greenspan A, Reinhart M, et al:** *Differentiation of Child Abuse from Osteogenesis Imperfecta.* AJR 154:1035, 1990.

THE SCLEROSING DYSPLASIAS

1. **Greenspan A:** *Sclerosing bone dysplasias—a target-site approach.* Skeletal Radiol 20:561-583, 1991.

MELORHEOSTOSIS

1. **Leri A, Joanny J:** *Une affection non decrite des os. Hyperostose "en coulee" sur toute la longueur d'un membre ou "melorheostose."* Bull Mem Sco Hop Paris 46:1141, 1922.
2. **Putti V:** *L'osteosi eberneizzante monomelica (una nuova sindrome osteopatica).* Chir Organi Mov 11:335, 1927.
3. **Yochum TR, et al:** *Melorheostosis—A report of two patients.* ACA Council Roentgenol, Roentgen Brief, April 1981.
4. **Franklin EL, Matheson I:** *Melorheostosis; report on case with review of literature.* Br J Radiol 15:185, 1942.

5. **Campbell CJ, Papdemetriou T, Bonfiglio M:** *Melorheostosis. A report of the clinical roentgenographic and pathological findings in fourteen cases.* J Bone Joint Surg (Am) 50:1281, 1968.
6. **Younge D, Drummond D, Herring J, et al:** *Melorheostosis in children. Clinical features and natural history.* J Bone Joint Surg (Br) 61:415, 1979.
7. **Bied JC, Malsh C, Meunier P:** *La melorheostose chez l'adulte. A propos de deux cas dont l'un traite par un diphosphonate.* Rev Rhum Mal Osteoartic 43:193, 1976.
8. **Patrick JH:** *Melorheostosis associated with arteriovenous aneurysm of the left arm and trunk.* Skeletal Radiol 51:126, 1969.
9. **Jacobson HG:** *Dense bone—Too much bone: Radiological considerations and differential diagnosis.* Skeletal Radiol 13:1, 1985.
10. **Murray RO, McCredie J:** *Melorheostosis and the sclerotomes: A radiological correlation.* Skeletal Radiol 4:57, 1979.
11. **Dimar JR, Campion TS:** *Melorheostosis: Two case presentations and review of the literature.* Orthopaedic Review 16:615, 1987.
12. **Greenspan A:** *Sclerosing bone dysplasias-a target-site approach.* Skeletal Radiol 20:561, 1991.
13. **Dissing I, Zafirovski G:** *Para-articular ossifications associated with melorheostosis Leri.* Acta Orthop Scand 50:717, 1979.
14. **Whyte MP, Murphy WA, Siegel BA:** *99mTc-pyrophosphate bone imaging in osteopoikilosis, osteopathia striata and melorheostosis.* Radiology 127:439, 1978.
15. **Soffa DJ, Sire DJ, Dodson JH:** *Melorheostosis with linear sclerodermatous skin changes.* Radiology 114:577, 1975.
16. **Green A, Ellswood WH, Collins JR:** *Melorheostosis and osteopoikilosis—with a review of the literature.* AJR 87:1096, 1962.
17. **Abrahamson MN:** *Disseminated asymptomatic osteosclerosis with features resembling melorheostosis, osteopoikilosis, and osteopathia striata. Case report.* J Bone Joint Surg (Am) 59:991, 1968.
18. **McCarroll HR:** *Clinical manifestations of congenital neurofibromatosis.* J Bone Joint Surg (Am) 32:601, 1950.
19. **Hall GS:** *A contribution to the study of melorheostosis: Unusual bone changes associated with tuberous sclerosis.* Q J Med 12:77, 1943.
20. **Beauvais P, Faure C, Montagne JP, et al:** *Leri's melorheostosis: Three pediatric cases and a review of the literature.* Pediatr Radiol 6:153, 1977.

OSTEOPATHIA STRIATA

1. **Voorhoeve N:** *L'image radiologique non encore decrite de'une anomalie due squelette.* Acta Radiol 3:407, 1924.
2. **Fairbank HAT:** *Osteopathia striata.* J Bone Joint Surg (Br) 32:117, 1950.
3. **Jacobson HG:** *Dense bone—too much bone: Radiological considerations and differential diagnosis.* Skeletal Radiol 13:1, 1985.
4. **Abrahamson MN:** *Disseminated asymptomatic osteosclerosis with features resembling melorheostosis, osteopoikilosis, and osteopathia striata. Case report.* J Bone Joint Surg (Am) 50:991, 1968.
5. **Hurt RL:** *Osteopathia striata—Voorhoeve's disease. Report of a case presenting the features of osteopathia striata and osteopetrosis.* J Bone Joint Surg (Br) 35:89, 1953.
6. **Knockaert D, Dequecker J:** *Osteopathia striata and focal dermal hypoplasia.* Skeletal Radiol 4:223, 1979.
7. **Larreque M, Maroteaux P, Michey Y, et al:** *L'osteopathie striee, symptome radiologique de l'hypoplasia dermique en aives.* Ann Radiol 15:287, 1972.
8. **Resnick D, Niwayama G:** *Diagnosis of Bone and Joint Disorders,* ed 2. Philadelphia, W B Saunders, 1988.
9. **Hoeffel JC, Merle M:** *Osteopathia striata with cranial sclerosis.* Rontgen-Bl 43:465, 1990.
10. **Nakamura T, Yokomizo Y, Kanda S, et al.:** *Osteopathia striata with cranial sclerosis affecting three family members.* Skeletal Radiol 14:267, 1985.
11. **Carlson DH:** *Osteopathia striata revisited.* J Canad Assoc Radiol 28:190, 1977.
12. **Fairbank HAT:** *A case of unilateral affection of the skeleton of unknown origin.* Br J Surg 12:594, 1925.
13. **Gehweiler JA, Bland WR, Carden TS Jr, et al:** *Osteopathia striata—Voorhoeve's disease. Review of the roentgen manifestations.* AJR 118:450, 1973.
14. **Aegerter E, Kirkpatrick JA:** *Orthopedic Diseases,* ed 4. Philadelphia, WB Saunders, 1975.
15. **Greenspan A:** *Sclerosing bone dysplasias-a target-site approach.* Skeletal Radiol 20:561-583, 1991.
16. **Whyte MP, Murphy WA, Siegel BA:** *99mTc-pyrophosphate bone imaging in osteopoikilosis, osteopathia striata and melorheostosis.* Radiology 127:439, 1978.

OSTEOPETROSIS

1. **Zawisch C:** *Marble bone disease; a study of osteogenesis.* Arch Pathol 43:55, 1947.
2. **Andersen PE Jr, Bollerslev J:** *Heterogeneity of autosomal dominant osteopetrosis.* Radiology 164:223, 1987.
3. **Beighton P, Hamersma H, Cremin BJ:** *Osteopetrosis in South Africa. The benign, lethal and intermediate forms.* S Afr Med J 55: 659, 1979.
4. **Kahler SG, Burns JA, Aylsworth AS:** *A mild autosomal recessive form of osteopetrosis with recessive inheritance.* Am J Med Genet 17:451, 1984.
5. **Schwartz GJ, Brion LP, Corey HE, et al:** *Open quiz-solution:Case report 668.* Skeletal Radiol 20:447, 1991.
6. **Cumming WA, Ohlsson A:** *Intracranial calcification in children with osteopetrosis caused by carbonic anhydrase II deficiency.* Radiology 157:325, 1985.
7. **Nussey AM:** *Osteopetrosis.* Arch Dis Child 13:161, 1938.
8. **Beighton PH, Horan FT, Hamersma H:** *A review of the osteopetroses.* Postgrad Med J 53:507, 1977.
9. **Greenfield GB:** *Radiology of Bone Diseases,* ed 3. Philadelphia, JB Lippincott, 1980.
10. **Murray RO, Jacobson HG:** *The Radiology of Skeletal Disorders,* ed 2. New York, Churchill Livingstone, 1977.
11. **Shapiro F, Glimcher MJ, Holtrop ME, et al:** *Human osteopetrosis.* J Bone Joint Surg (Am) 62:384, 1980.
12. **Rao VM, Dalinka MK, Mitchell DG et al:** *Osteopetrosis: MR characteristics at 1.5 T.* Radiology 161:217, 1986.
13. **Elster AD, Theros EG, Key LL, et al:** *Cranial imaging in autosomal recessive osteopetrosis. I,II.* Radiology 183:129 and 137, 1992.
14. **Sear HR:** *A case of Albers-Schönberg's disease.* Br J Surg 14:657, 1927.
15. **Moss AA, Minzer F:** *Osteopetrosis: An unusual cause of terminal tuft erosion.* Radiology 97:631, 1970.
16. **Jacobson HG:** *Dense bone—too much bone: Radiological considerations and differential diagnosis.* Skeletal Radiol 13:1, 1985.
17. **McCleary L, Rovit RL, Murali R:** *Case report: Myelopathy secondary to congenital osteopetrosis of the cervical spine.* Neurosurgery 20:487, 1987.
18. **Khanchandani BA:** *Albers-Schönberg's disease with multiple-level lumbar spondylolysis: A case report.* Europ J of Chiropractic 37:5, 1989.
19. **Saha MM, Bhardwaj OP, Srivastava G, et al:** *Osteopetrosis with spondylolysis-four cases in one family.* Br J Radiol 43:738, 1970.

OSTEOPOIKILOSIS

1. **Albers-Schönberg H:** *Eine seltene, bisher nicht bekannte strukturanomalie des skelettes.* Fortschr Geb Roentgenstr Nuklear Med 23:174, 1915-1916.
2. **Ledoux-Lebard R, Chabaneix D:** *L'osteopoecilie forme nouvelle d'osteite condensante generalisee sans symptomes cliniques.* J Radiol Electrol Med Nucl 2:133, 1916-1917.
3. **Szabo AD:** *Osteopoikilosis in a twin.* Clin Orthop Rel Res 79:156, 1971.
4. **Wilcox LF:** *Osteopoikilosis.* AJR 30:615, 1933.
5. **Risseeuw J:** *Famili re osteopoikilie.* Ned Tijdschr Geneeskd 80:3827, 1936.
6. **Melnick JC:** *Osteopathia condensans disseminata (osteopoikilosis). Study of a family of four generations.* AJR 82:229, 1959.
7. **Busch KFB:** *Familial disseminated osteosclerosis.* Acta Radiol 18:693, 1937.
8. **Tong ECK, Samii M, Tchang F:** *Bone imaging as an aid for the diagnosis of osteopoikilosis.* Clin Nuclear Med 13:816, 1988.
9. **Sutherland CG:** *Osteopoikilosis.* Radiology 25:470, 1935.
10. **Windholz F:** *Gber famili re osteopoikilie und dermatofibrosis lenticularis disseminata.* Fortschr Geb Roentgenstru Nuklear Med 45:566, 1932.
11. **Buschke A, Ollendorff H:** *Ein fall von dermatofibrosis lenticularis disseminata und osteopathia condensans disseminata.* Dermatol Wochenschr 86:257, 1928.
12. **Raskin MM:** *Osteopoikilosis. Possible association with dystocia and keloid.* South Med J 68:270, 1975.
13. **Weissmann G:** *Scleroderma associated with osteopoikilosis.* Arch Intern Med 101:108, 1958.
14. **Bethge JFJ, Ridderbusch KE:** *Gber osteopoikilie und das neue krankheitsbild hyperostose bei osteopoikilie.* Ergeb Chir Orthop 49:138, 1967.
15. **Lagier R, Mbakop A, Bigler A:** *Osteopoikilosis: A radiological and pathological study.* Skeletal Radiol 11:161, 1984.
16. **Greenspan A:** *Sclerosing bone dysplasias-a target-site approach.* Skeletal Radiol 20:561, 1991.
17. **Holly LE:** *Osteopoikilosis: 5-year study.* AJR 36:512, 1936.
18. **Blank N, Lieber A:** *The significance of growing bone islands.* Radiology 85:508, 1965.
19. **Abrahamson MN:** *Disseminated asymptomatic osteosclerosis with features resembling melorheostosis, osteopoikilosis, and osteopathia striata. Case report.* J Bone Joint Surg (Am) 50:991, 1968.
20. **Mindell ER, Northup CS, Douglass HO Jr:** *Osteosarcoma associated with osteopoikilosis. Case report.* J Bone Joint Surg (Am) 60:406, 1978.
21. **Dahlin DC:** *Pathology of osteosarcoma.* Clin Orthop Rel Res 111:23, 1975.
22. **Resnick D, Niwayama G:** *Diagnosis of Bone and Joint Disorders,* Philadelphia, WB Saunders, 1981.

PROGRESSIVE DIAPHYSEAL DYSPLASIA

1. **Camurati M:** *Di un rara case di osteite simmetrica creditaria delgi arti inferiori.* Chir Organi Mov 6:662, 1922.
2. **Engelmann G:** *Ein fall von osteopathia hyperostotica (sclerotisans) multiplex infantilis.* Fortschr Geb Roentgenstru Nuklear Med 39:1101, 1929.
3. **Neuhauser EBD, Schwachmann H, Wittenborg M, et al:** *Progressive diaphyseal dysplasia.* Radiology 51:11, 1948.
4. **Jacobson HG:** *Dense bone—too much bone: Radiological considerations and differential diagnosis.* Skeletal Radiol 13:1, 1985.
5. **Sear HR:** *Engelmann's disease.* Br J Radiol 21:236, 1948.
6. **Bingold AC:** *Engelmann's disease: Osteopathia hyperostotica (sclerotisans) multiplex infantilis; progressive metaphyseal dysplasia.* Br J Surg 37:266, 1950.
7. **Naveh Y, Ludatschcer R, Alon U, et al:** *Muscle involvement in progressive diaphyseal dysplasia.* Pediatr 76:944, 1985.
8. **Kaftori JK, Kleinhaus U, Naveh Y:** *Progressive diaphyseal dysplasia (Camurati-Engelmann): Radiographic follow-up and CT findings.* Radiology 164:777, 1987.
9. **Singleton EB:** *Progressive diaphyseal dysplasia (Engelmann's disease).* Radiology 67:233, 1956.
10. **Aegerter E, Kirkpatrick JA:** *Orthopedic Diseases,* ed 4. Philadelphia, WB Saunders, 1975.

PYKNODYSOSTOSIS

1. **Maroteaux P, Lamy M:** *La pycnodysostosis.* Presse Med 70:999, 1962.
2. **Maroteaux P, Lamy M:** *The malady of Toulouse-Lautrec.* JAMA 191:715, 1965.
3. **Elmore S, Nance W, McGee B, et al:** *Pycknodysostosis with a familial chromosome anomaly.* Am J Med 40:273, 1966.

4. **Aegerter E, Kirkpatrick J:** *Orthopedic Diseases,* ed 4. Philadelphia, WB Saunders, 1975.
5. **Greenspan A:** *Sclerosing bone dysplasias-a target-site approach.* Skeletal Radiol 20:561, 1991.
6. **Murray RO, Jacobson HG:** *The Radiology of Skeletal Disorders,* ed 2. New York, Churchill Livingstone, 1977.
7. **Emami-Ahari Z, Zarabi M, Javid B:** *Pycknodysostosis.* J Bone Joint Surg (Br) 51:307, 1969.
8. **Dusenberry JF Jr, Kane JJ:** *Pycknodysostosis: Report of three new cases.* AJR 99:717, 1967.
9. **Floman Y, Gomori JM, Fast A:** *Isthmic spondylolisthesis in pycnodysostosis.* J Spinal Disorders 2:268, 1989.
10. **Elmore SM:** *Pycknodysostosis: A review.* J Bone Joint Surg (Am) 49:153, 1967.
11. **Currarino G:** *Primary spondylolysis of the axis vertebra (C2) in three children, including one with pyknodysostosis.* Pediatr Radiol 19:535, 1989.
12. **Resnick D, Niwayama G:** *Diagnosis of Bone and Joint Disorders,* ed 2. Philadelphia, WB Saunders, 1988.

TUBEROUS SCLEROSIS

1. **Gean AD, Taveras JM:** *The phakomatoses.* In: Taveras JM, Ferucci JT, eds,: *Radiology: Diagnosis-Imaging-Intervention.* Vol 3, Chap 35, Philadelphia, JB Lippincott, 1989.
2. **Bourneville DM:** *Contribution a l'etude de l'idiotie.* Arch Neurol 1:69, 1880.
3. **Edeiken J:** *Roentgen Diagnosis of Diseases of Bone,* ed 3. Baltimore, Williams & Wilkins, 1981.
4. **Resnick D, Niwayama G:** *Diagnosis of Bone and Joint Disorders,* ed 2. Philadelphia, W B Saunders, 1988.
5. **Lagos JC, Holman CB, Gomez MR:** *Tuberous sclerosis: Neuroroentgenologic observations.* AJR 104:171, 1968.
6. **Medley BE, McLeod RA, Houser OW:** *Tuberous sclerosis.* Semin Roentgenol 11:35, 1976.
7. **Bunde S:** *The significance of a white macule on the skin of a child.* Dev Med Child Neurol 12:805, 1970.
8. **Fitzpatrick TB, Sxabo G, Hori Y, et al:** *White leaf-shaped macules: Earliest visible signs of tuberous sclerosis.* Arch Dermatol 98:1, 1968.
9. **Gold AP, Freeman JM:** *Depigmented nevi: The earliest sign of tuberous sclerosis.* Pediatrics 35:1003, 1965.
10. **Hurwitz S, Braverman IM:** *White spots in tuberous sclerosis.* J Pediatr 77:587, 1970.
11. **Resnick D, Niwayama G:** *Diagnosis of Bone and Joint Disorders,* Philadelphia, WB Saunders, 1981.
12. **Ross AT, Dickerson WW:** *Tuberous sclerosis.* Arch Neurol Psychiatr 50:233, 1943.
13. **Green GJ:** *The radiology of tuberous sclerosis.* Clin Radiol 10:135, 1968.
14. **Frank LM, Chaves-Carballo E, Earley L:** *Early diagnosis of tuberous sclerosis by cranial ultrasonography.* Arch Neurol 41:1302, 1984.
15. **Crosett AD Jr:** *Roentgenographic findings in the renal lesion of tuberous sclerosis.* AJR 98:739, 1966.
16. **Babcock TL, Snyder BA:** *Spontaneous pneumothorax associated with tuberous sclerosis.* J Thorac Cardiovasc Surg 83:100, 1982.
17. **Dwyer JM, Hickie JB, Gravan J:** *Pulmonary tuberous sclerosis: Report of three patients and a review of the literature.* Q J Med 40:115, 1971.
18. **Malik SK, Pardee N, Martin CJ:** *Involvement of the lungs in tuberous sclerosis.* Chest 58:538, 1970.
19. **Sareen CK, Ruvalcaba RHA, Scotvold MJ, et al:** *Tuberous sclerosis. Clinical, endocrine, and metabolic studies.* Am J Dis Child 123:34, 1972.
20. **Jacobson HG:** *Dense bone—too much bone: Radiological considerations and differential diagnosis.* Skeletal Radiol 13:1, 1985.
21. **Komar NN, Gabrielsen TD, Holt JF:** *Roentgenographic appearance of lumbosacral spine and pelvis in tuberous sclerosis.* Radiology 89:701, 1967.
22. From *The Learning File,* Skeletal Section, SK-2617, with permission of the Center for Devices and Radiological Health, FDA, and the American College of Radiology, 1978.
23. **Nathanson N, Anvet NL:** *An unusual x-ray finding in tuberous sclerosis.* Br J Radiol 39:786, 1966.
24. **Madigan RR, Wallace SL:** *Scoliosis associated with tuberous sclerosis.* J Tenn Med Assoc 74:643, 1981.

Table 9.1.   Key Features to Identifying and Classifying a Fracture

Fracture Type
Skin penetration
Comminution
Mechanism (avulsion, impaction, etc.)
Complete/incomplete
Pathologic
Stress
Fracture Orientation
Oblique
Transverse
Spiral
Spatial Relationships
Alignment
Apposition
Rotation
Soft Tissue Involvement

Table 9.2.   Key Features to Identifying and Classifying Dislocations

Position
Relative to proximal bone
Type
Subluxation
Dislocation
Diastasis
Associated Fractures

Depressed Fracture.   This type of fracture represents an inward bulging of the outer bone surface. (1) Two characteristic sites for depressed fractures are the tibial plateau and frontal bone.

Compression Fracture.   There is decreased size of the involved bone due to trabecular telescoping, occurring primarily in the spine following a forceful hyperflexion injury. The vertebral endplates are driven toward each other, creating compression of the intervening spongy bone. (1)

The mechanism of injury in impaction and compression fractures is similar, with the term *compression fracture* used for fractures of the vertebrae and *impaction fracture* primarily for those bones of the appendicular skeleton, the most common of which is the femoral neck. (Fig. 9.5A and B)

Incomplete Fracture

Incomplete fractures are broken on only one side of the bone, leaving a buckling or bending of the bone as the only sign of fracture. (1) Angular deformity is common; however, no displacement is expected. The following represent various types of incomplete fracture.

Greenstick (Hickory Stick) Fracture.   This occurs primarily in infants and children under the age of 10 because of the relatively greater component of pliable woven bone. The bone bends applying tension to the convex side, producing a transverse fracture with the concave side remaining intact. (1) (Fig. 9.6A) Greenstick fractures heal without any complications in most instances.

Torus (Buckling) Fracture.   Due to compression forces the cortex bulges outward. (1) Most occur in the metaphysis, and are a very painful special variety of greenstick fracture. The term *torus* is derived from the Latin root meaning "to bulge." (Fig. 9.6B) This has been likened to the cap at the tip or base of a Greek column or pillar.

Infraction

This type of fracture is actually a form of impaction fracture that is only moderately severe in nature. (1) It is used to explain a minor localized break in the cortex, leaving minimal bone deformity.

Chip (Corner) Fracture

This represents a form of avulsion fracture that is usually limited, demonstrating the separation of a small chip of bone from the corner of a phalanx or other short or long tubular bone. (1) (Fig. 9.7)

Pathologic Fracture

A pathologic fracture is a fracture through a bone that is weakened by a localized or systemic disease process. Pathologic fractures are usually transverse and often appear quite smooth. (1) (Fig. 9.8A and B)

Stress (Fatigue) Fracture

A stress fracture is caused by repetitive stress, causing gradual formation of microfractures and, eventually, an interruption in the bone structure at a greater rate than can be offset by the re-

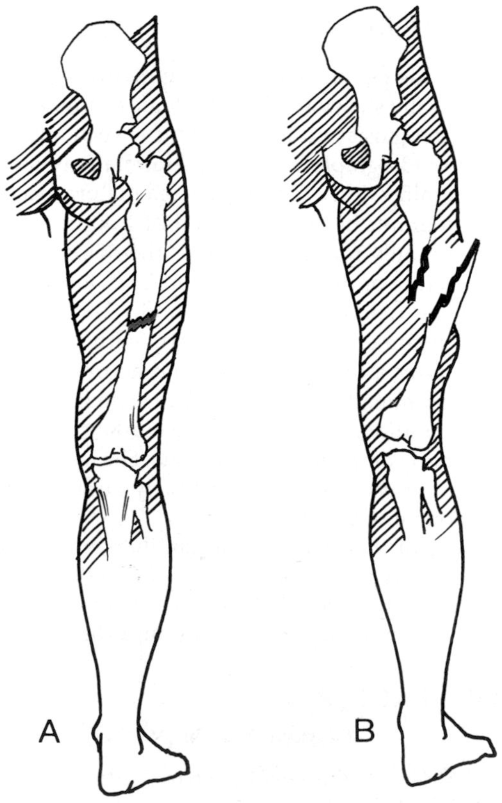

Figure 9.1.   FRACTURE AND SKIN RELATIONSHIPS. A. Closed Fracture B. Open Fracture.

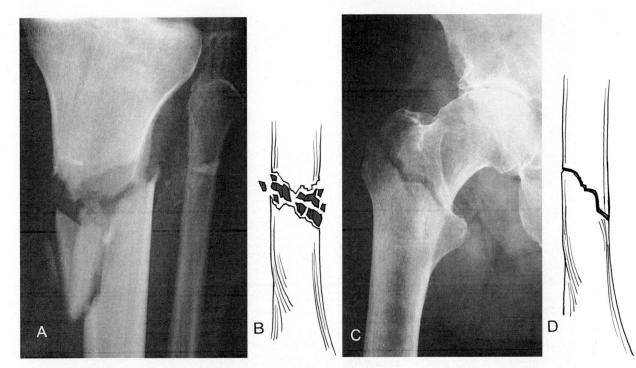

Figure 9.2.   COMMINUTED VERSUS NONCOMMINUTED FRACTURE. A. AP Tibia and Fibula. Observe the comminuted fracture of the proximal tibia. A "butterfly" fragment is visible on the medial surface. There is associated diastasis of the proximal tibiofibular articulation. **B. Diagram: Com-** **minuted Fracture. C. AP Femur.** Observe the singular radiolucency present within the intertrochanteric space of the proximal femur without fragmentation. **D. Diagram: Noncomminuted Fracture.**

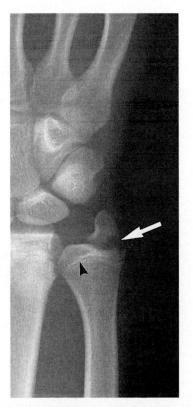

Figure 9.3.   AVULSION FRACTURE: WRIST. Observe the avulsion fracture of the distal ulnar styloid process (arrow). The growth plate of the distal ulna should not be confused with a fracture (arrowhead). An impacted fracture is visible at the distal radius.

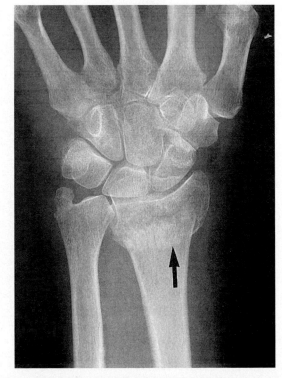

Figure 9.4.   IMPACTION FRACTURE: WRIST. There is an area of increased bone density (arrow) associated with this impaction fracture of the distal radius.

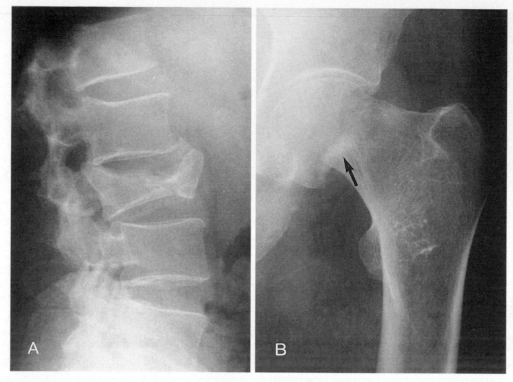

Figure 9.5.   COMPRESSION OR IMPACTION FRACTURE. A. Lateral Lumbar Spine. Observe the significant loss in height of the L3 vertebral body. This is an old compression fracture. **B. AP Hip**. Note the linear band of radiopacity, representing the area of impaction in this subcapital fracture (arrow).

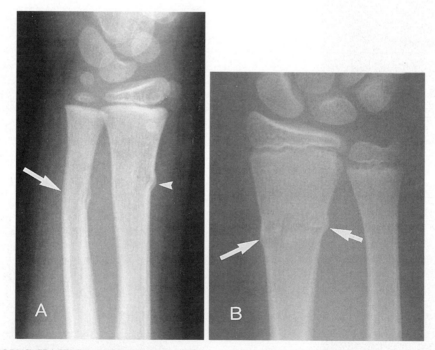

Figure 9.6.   GREENSTICK (TORUS) FRACTURE: FOREARM. A. PA Forearm. Observe the altered angulation of the distal ulna, representing a greenstick fracture (arrow). A torus fracture of the radius is also seen (arrowhead). **B. PA Wrist**. Note the bulging of the cortex of the distal radius consistent with a torus fracture (arrows).

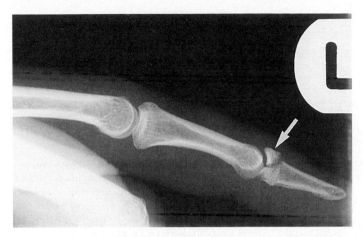

Figure 9.7.   CHIP FRACTURE: LATERAL FINGER. There is a chip fracture present at the base of the distal phalanx (arrow).

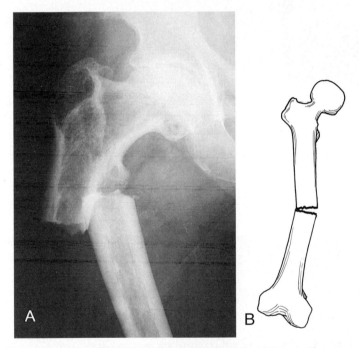

Figure 9.8.   PATHOLOGIC FRACTURE: FEMUR. A. AP Femur. There is a transverse fracture noted through the proximal diaphysis of the femur. Observe the cortical thickening and accentuated trabecular patterns consistent with Paget's disease. **B. Diagram: Pathologic Fracture.**

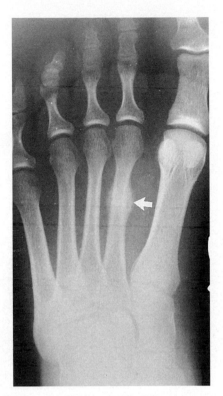

Figure 9.9.   STRESS FRACTURE: FOOT. Callus formation is noted surrounding the mid-diaphysis of the second metatarsal (arrow). A subtle transverse fracture line can be identified through the overlying callus formation. COMMENT: This is one of the most common sites for stress fractures and is most frequently found in increased physical activities related to walking, running, and jumping.

The phenomenon of "bone bruise" has only come to light with the application of MR imaging in traumatic injuries. It is presumed to represent hemorrhage and edema associated with trabecular microfractures, usually beneath an adjacent joint surface. (3) It appears as an area of high signal intensity on T2-weighted images and on T1-weighted images it appears as speckled areas of low signal intensity. (Fig. 9.10)

Pseudofracture

A pseudofracture is not a true fracture. It is thought that it actually represents an insufficiency fracture or is due to vascular pulsations. (3) Histologically, pseudofractures are discrete regions of uncalcified osteoid. Radiographically, they appear as linear lucencies on the convex surface of the bone that are oriented at 90° to the long axis of the bone. (Fig. 9.11) They are often multiple and found in association with bone-softening diseases such as Paget's disease, rickets, osteomalacia, and fibrous dysplasia. Various synonyms are applied to pseudofractures, including *Looser's lines*, *Milkman's syndrome*, *increment fractures*, and *umbau zonen*.

Stable and Unstable Fractures

Assessing stability of a fracture may require determination of a number of criteria, depending on location. In general, a stable fracture is one that does not move nor is likely to move during the healing phase. In the spine the major consideration is the threat to adjacent neurologic structures, especially the cord. A

parative process. (Fig. 9.9) It represents an actual fatigue failure of the bone. A stress fracture through a diseased bone is called an *insufficiency* fracture. (1,2)

Occult Fracture, Bone Bruise

An occult fracture is one in which the fracture gives clinical signs of its presence without any radiologic evidence. Often, follow-up radiologic examination, usually within seven to ten days, reveals resorption of bone at the fracture site or frank displacement. The most common occult fracture site involves the carpal navicular (scaphoid), with the ribs being the second most common site. Occult fractures in the spine are very rare.

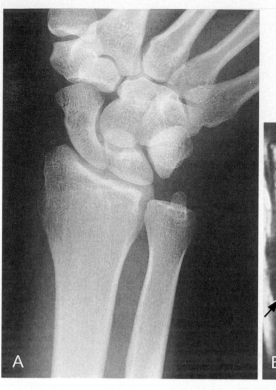

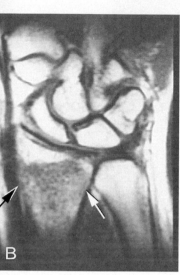

Figure 9.10.   BONE BRUISE. A. Plain Film PA View. No abnormality can be discerned in the radius. **B. MRI T1-Weighted Image**. A speckled region of low signal intensity is present in the metaphysis representing bone marrow edema (arrows). (Courtesy John Bailey, RT, Austin, Texas)

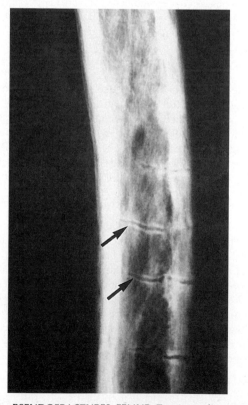

Figure 9.11.   PSEUDOFRACTURES: FEMUR. Transverse linear radiolucencies surrounded by a sclerotic margin are visible (arrows). These pseudofractures are present on the convex surface of the bowed femur as a complication to Paget's disease, recognizable by the thickened cortex, increased density, and accentuated trabecular lines.

stable spinal fracture has little probability of producing neurologic compromise.

FRACTURE ORIENTATION

Oblique Fracture

The oblique fracture commonly occurs in the shaft of a long tubular bone. (2) Its course is approximately 45° to the long axis of the bone.

Spiral Fracture

Torsion, coupled with axial compression and angulation, creates a spiral fracture. In contrast to the blunt-ended oblique fracture, the ends of a spiral fracture are pointed like a pen. (2)

Transverse Fracture

A transverse fracture runs at a right angle to the long axis of a bone. This type of fracture is uncommon through healthy bone, but is frequently seen in diseased bone (pathologic fracture). An example of this type of fracture is the "banana" transverse pathologic fracture associated with Paget's disease of bone. (2) (Fig. 9.8A and B)

SPATIAL RELATIONSHIPS OF FRACTURES

Alignment

The alignment of a fracture is described as the position of the distal fragment in relation to the proximal fragment. Fractures are in "good" alignment when there is no perceptible angulation in frontal and side views. The relationship of fracture fragments must be accurately described in the x-ray report, especially when reduction is anticipated. (1)

Apposition

The appositional state of the fracture site concerns the closeness of the bony contact at the fracture site. *Good apposition* means near complete surface contact of the fractured area. *Partial apposition* refers to partial bony contact. If the fractured ends are pulled apart by muscle force or therapeutic traction, it is referred to as *distraction*.

Rotation

Twisting forces on a fractured bone along its longitudinal axis produce rotational deformity. Inclusion of the proximal and distal joints on the film is necessary in determining rotation malposition. (1)

TRAUMATIC ARTICULAR LESIONS

Subluxation

Subluxation occurs when there is a partial loss of contact between the usual articular surface components of a joint. (Fig. 9.12A and B) The joint surfaces are incongruous, but a significant portion remains apposed. (2)

Dislocation (Luxation)

Dislocation refers to a complete loss of contact between the usual articular components of a joint. (Fig. 9.12C) When found associated with a fracture, it is referred to as a fracture dislocation. In the extremities a dislocated bone is always described in relation to the proximal bone. In the spine the dislocated segment is described relative to the segment below. (1)

Diastasis

Diastasis represents displacement or frank separation of a slightly movable joint (syndesmosis). (1) The most common locations for this to occur are the pubic symphysis, (Fig. 9.13) sutures of the skull, or the distal tibiofibular syndesmosis. A separated suture is a *diastatic* fracture. (2)

Chondral and Osteochondral Fractures

A fracture through a joint surface may result from shearing, rotary, or tangential impaction fractures. The fracture fragment may consist of cartilage only (chondral fractures) or cartilage and underlying bone (osteochondral fractures). (2) The condition of osteochondritis dissecans is an example of an osteochondral fracture seen to involve convex surfaces of the femoral condyles, talar dome, and capitulum.

EPIPHYSEAL FRACTURES

SALTER-HARRIS CLASSIFICATION

A classification system of growth plate injuries based on the radiologic findings was proposed by Salter and Harris in 1963. (4) This system has gained widespread acceptance, and is the standard for describing and predicting prognosis of epiphyseal injuries. Essentially, the components involved in the fracture determine its classification type. (Fig. 9.14) (Table 9.3)

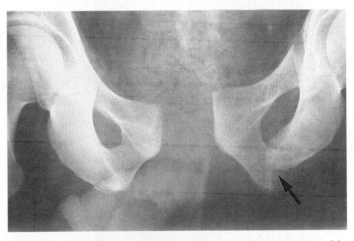

Figure 9.13. DIASTATIC FRACTURE: SYMPHYSIS PUBIS. Widening of the symphysis pubis is present. Additionally noted is a fracture through the ischiopubic junction (arrow).

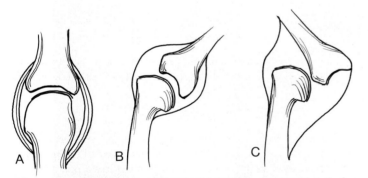

Figure 9.12. TRAUMATIC ARTICULAR LESIONS. A. Normal Articular Alignment. B. Subluxation. There is partial displacement of the articular components. **C. Dislocation.** There is total disrelationship of the articular components.

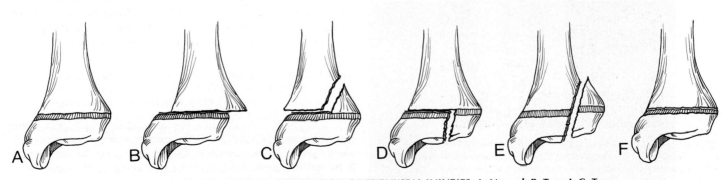

Figure 9.14. SALTER-HARRIS CLASSIFICATION OF EPIPHYSEAL INJURIES. A. Normal. B. Type I. C. Type II. D. Type III. E. Type IV. F. Type V.

Salter-Harris Type I

This represents isolated fracture through the growth plate. (Fig. 9.15A) Usually, the radiograph appears normal, with the diagnosis being made clinically because of tenderness over the epiphyseal plate and soft tissue swelling. This type of fracture can complicate scurvy, rickets, osteomyelitis, and hormone imbalance, presenting often as a slipped capital femoral epiphysis.

Salter-Harris Type II

This is a fracture through the displaced growth plate, which carries with it a corner of the metaphysis. (Fig. 9.15B) The me-

taphyseal fragment has been called the "Thurston-Holland sign." (5) This is the most common epiphyseal injury, comprising approximately 75% of cases. (6) The most common sites are the distal radius (50%), as well as the tibia, fibula, femur, and ulna. (6) The epiphyseal separation is usually easily reduced and the prognosis is generally favorable. (6)

Salter-Harris Type III

The fracture line is directed along the growth plate and then turns toward the epiphysis. (Fig. 9.15C) It results in intraarticular fracture that may require open reduction treatment. The most frequent site is the distal tibia. (6)

Salter-Harris Type IV

This is an obliquely oriented, vertical fracture that passes through the epiphysis, growth plate, and metaphysis. (Fig. 9.15D) The fracture fragment consists of a portion each of the metaphysis, growth plate, and epiphysis. The most common sites are the lateral condyle of the distal humerus in patients under 10 years of age, and the distal tibia in those over the age of 10. Prognosis is poor without expeditious open reduction and internal fixation and may result in permanent deformity. (4)

Table 9.3.   Salter-Harris Classification of Epiphyseal Injuries

Type	Fracture Site		
	Growth Plate	Metaphysis	Ephphysis
I	*		
II	*	*	
III	*		*
IV	*	*	*
V	Compression		

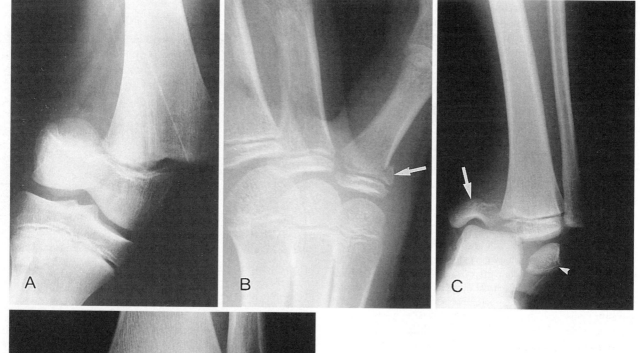

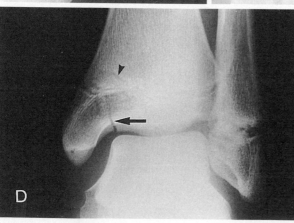

Figure 9.15.   SALTER-HARRIS CLASSIFICATION OF EPIPHYSEAL INJURIES: RADIOLOGIC FEATURES. A. AP Knee: Type I. Epiphyseal separation at the distal femur. **B. Fifth Digit of the Hand: Type II.** Epiphyseal separation with an additional metaphyseal fragment (Thurston-Holland fragment) (arrow). **C. AP Ankle: Type III.** Separation of the medial distal epiphysis (arrow) of the distal tibia, with an associated type I separation of the lateral malleolus (arrowhead). **D. AP Ankle: Type IV.** Fracture lines extend through the medial aspect of the tibial epiphysis (arrow), with extension into the adjacent metaphysis (arrowhead). A type I epiphyseal separation is present, affecting the distal fibula.

Salter-Harris Type V

This injury is the least common of all the Salter-Harris epiphyseal lesions, resulting in a compressive deformity of the growth plate. Initially, the radiographs are normal, until cessation of growth creates bone shortening or partial arrest, which leads to progressive angular deformity. (1) These children should be monitored for at least 2 years following injury to ensure that the normal growth of bone is occurring at the growth plate. The most common sites are the distal tibial and distal femoral epiphyseal centers. (6)

FRACTURE REPAIR

THREE PHASES OF HEALING

Circulatory or Inflammatory Phase

The initial circulatory or inflammatory phase is conveniently subdivided into three distinct phases—cellular (with hematoma), vascular, and primary callus—each phase lasting approximately 10 days. (7)

Cellular Phase. Trauma sufficient to cause fracture in bone also damages the overlying muscle, tendon, periosteum, numerous blood vessels, and marrow tissue, resulting in hematoma or clot formation. (8) The injured cells, as well as the hematoma, incite a cellular inflammatory response that is particularly prominent during the first 5 days of the fracture. Surviving cells in the area of injury, and new cells brought in by the granulation tissue, create a blastema of undifferentiated mesenchymal cells. This granulation tissue invades and replaces the hematoma. These cells are ultimately capable of modulating into the mature components of callus.

Vascular Phase. The cellular phase is promptly followed by the vascular phase. A specialized circulatory network develops around the fracture. This network consists of dilated tributaries of major vessels that form around the periphery of the injured area and a central swamplike area of wide-open capillaries, resulting in formation of a vascular spindle. Following injury, the blood flow of the entire limb is augmented, with active hyperemia at the edges of the injured area. The vigorous blood flow in the arteries and arterioles is slowed when it reaches the vascular "swamp," and passive hyperemia or congestion occurs. This passive hyperemia promotes active secretion of osteoid matrix by the mesenchymal cells that have migrated into the area.

The active hyperemia on the periphery of the vascular spindle, by reason of its high-speed and well-oxygenated blood flow, induces osteoclastic activity in the cortex surrounding the fracture, which is easily demonstrable on sequential radiographs. It also activates the vascular bed of the old growth plate and subchondral plate, producing radiographically identifiable subchondral and submetaphyseal resorption bands. Augmented circulation to the entire limb also produces hypertrichosis due to stimulation of hair follicles and tanning of the skin from stimulation of the melanocytes.

Trauma in the muscle and stripping of the periosteum add to the initial fracture hematoma. Periosteal cells adjacent to the fracture become activated, reproduce, and secrete a matrix about themselves that, in effect, "elevates" the periosteum. Simultaneously, changes take place in the injured muscle tissue outside the periosteum, with granulation tissue replacing muscle cells. These cells then give rise to mature callus. As the process continues, a new periosteum forms at the line of demarcation between the normal muscle and callus. This periosteal callus, when mineralized, may produce a Codman's triangle on radiographs.

Primary Callus Phase. Callus is the plastic exudate and tissue that develops around the ends of, and ultimately unites, the fracture fragments. (2) The term is derived from the Latin word *callum*, meaning "hard" or "thickened."

Once the vascular phase is well established, more and more "raw material" becomes available. Cellular elements arise from injured bone, connective tissue, marrow, and muscle to form undifferentiated mesenchymal cells. Whether these cells are modulated rhabdomyoblasts, fibroblasts, or osteoblasts or are new cells arising out of the necrotic tissue has not been resolved; nevertheless, muscle, connective tissue, and bone marrow are all essential in producing a blastema that accounts for approximately 70% of the callus in a femur shaft fracture. High-speed deposition of osteoid occurs in the form of coarsely woven bone, deposited in a more or less haphazard fashion in the area of the fracture. This osteoid becomes mineralized, and earliest radiographic visualization occurs after 14 days. Depending on the degree of motion and vascularization, cartilage is formed within the callus at the same time.

The development of this primitive material in the blastemal zone represents the formation of the primary callus. The first stage of fracture healing can be summarized as (a) necrosis, hematoma (approximately ten days), (b) vascular spindle formation (approximately ten days), and (c) primary callus.

Reparative or Metabolic Phase

This is the second phase of fracture healing and is characterized by a more orderly secretion of callus and the removal and replacement of coarsely woven osteoid by a more mature form of bone. The process is one of remodeling, mimicking the generalized remodeling processes that occur during normal growth and development. The callus can be divided into separate entities, separated more by nomenclature than by function, and are identifiable as sealing, buttressing, bridging, and uniting callus. Buttressing callus is adjacent to the outer surface of the cortex and is formed by the periosteum as well as surrounding skeletal musculature. Sealing callus fills the medullary cavity and arises from the marrow to "seal" it from the fracture site. Bridging callus unites the gap between the two buttress ends and uniting callus joins the cortical portions of the fractured bone. Clinical union is achieved when the callus is sufficiently developed to allow weight bearing or similar stress.

Remodeling or Mechanical Phase

The final phase in fracture repair is the remodeling or mechanical phase, which involves realignment and remodeling of bone and callus along lines of stress. Extra bone is deposited in stress lines and removed in areas in which stress is not applied (Wolff's law). The final stage of fracture healing is restoration of the medullary cavity and bone marrow.

The sequence of events in the healing of a fracture, as described previously, has definite practical consequences in the management of the patient.

Although a hematoma is not essential to the healing of a fracture, the hematoma plays a role in inducing granulation tissue response. The greater the response, the more cellular the granulation tissue and the better the ultimate callus. Therefore, the less disturbance of the hematoma, the better.

Large necrotic bone fragments will have to be removed by

phagocytic processes and may impede callus formation. Sequestered bone fragments may require removal to help the healing process. Injury induces increased vascularity, which promotes callus. Injured soft tissue should therefore be left alone. Muscle contributes extensively to formation of callus and is richly vascularized; it should be minimally disturbed, despite injury. Poor fracture healing usually occurs in bones with little or no adjacent musculature.

Clinical healing will precede anatomic reconstitution. Extensive remodeling will proceed for years after the fracture; therefore, realignment of fracture fragments should emphasize maintaining viable bone and all fragments within the field of the vascular spindle. Anatomic reconstitution will usually occur as a consequence of extensive remodeling and does not require exact replacement of fracture fragments.

RADIOLOGIC FEATURES OF FRACTURE HEALING

Within the first five days following fracture, resorption of the fracture line occurs, creating an increase in width of the actual fracture line. (Fig. 9.16A and B) In the following 10 to 30 days a "veil" of new bone formation occurs adjacent to the fracture site (callus). (Fig. 9.16C) Gradually, the callus formation is remodeled, filling in the previous area of cortical disruption. (Fig. 9.16D) This entire healing process takes 4 to 6 weeks in the young patient and 6 to 12 weeks in the geriatric patient.

COMPLICATIONS OF FRACTURE

Complications of fractures are multiple. (Table 9.4) These may arise at different times following injury and can be conveniently divided into immediate, intermediate, and delayed complications. (2)

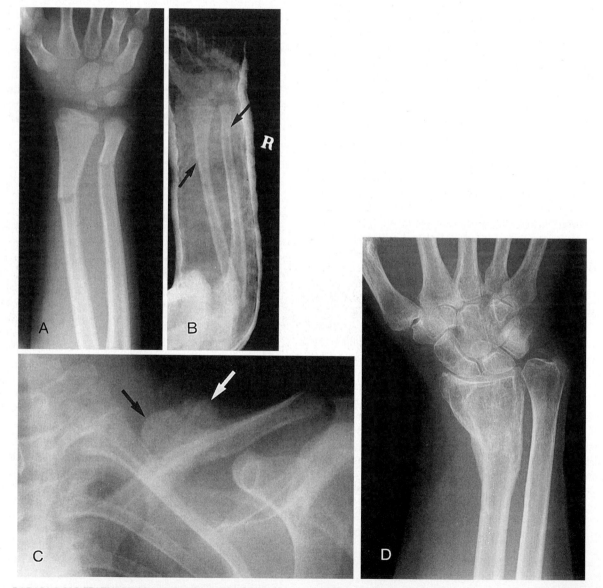

Figure 9.16.   RADIOLOGIC FEATURES OF FRACTURE HEALING. A. PA Forearm. There are complete fractures present in the distal diaphysis of the radius and ulna, with associated angular deformity. **B. Postreduction Film Through Case.** Observe the realignment at the fracture sites (arrows). There is no evidence of callus formation at the fracture site, distinctive of the early phase of fracture repair. **C. AP Clavicle: Healing Fracture.** Observe the ex-

uberant callus formation secondary to a healing fracture in the midclavicle (arrows). **D. PA Wrist: Healed Fracture.** There is complete absence of the fracture line in the distal metaphysis of the radius, with residual deformity noted. Of incidental notation is an old avulsion fracture of the distal ulnar styloid process.

Table 9.4.	Complications of Fractures

Immediate complications
Arterial injury
Compartment syndromes
Gas gangrene
Fat embolism syndrome
Thromboembolism
Intermediate complications
Osteomyelitis
Hardware failure
Reflex sympathetic dystrophy syndrome
Posttraumatic osteolysis
Refracture
Myositis ossificans
Synostosis
Delayed union
Delayed complications
Osteonecrosis
Degenerative joint disease
Lead arthropathy and toxicity
Osteoporosis
Aneurysmal bone cyst
Nonunion
Malunion

IMMEDIATE COMPLICATIONS

Arterial Injury

Vascular injury may accompany fractures, especially open and comminuted injuries. The popliteal artery is the most common artery to be injured following fractures of the distal femur or proximal tibia or knee dislocation. The second most common site is the superficial femoral artery at the adductor canal. Other less frequent sites include the brachial artery in supracondylar fractures of the humerus or elbow dislocation, aortic arch in sternal fractures, iliac arteries in pelvic fractures, and axillary artery in shoulder dislocations or upper rib fractures.

Compartment Syndromes

A continuing rise in pressure within a closed compartment due to edema and hemmorhage may compromise perfusion of contained muscles, resulting in permanent necrosis. The anterior tibial compartment of the leg and anterior forearm (Volkmann's contracture) are the most frequent regions of involvement.

Gas Gangrene

Any injury that penetrates the skin or intestine and compromises the blood supply can precipitate clostridium perfringens infection. This can occur within 1 to 3 days, with the buttocks and thighs the most frequent sites. The appearance of thin linear, parallel, streaks within muscle planes is characteristic.

Fat Embolism Syndrome

Fracture of a major bone may be associated with pulmonary fat embolism for one to five days after. Following fracture the cumulative effects of vasoactive substances and fat hydrolysis within the marrow act to mobilize emboli. (2,9) More than 50% of patients with fat embolism syndrome have multiple fractures including the femur; 30% involve the femur alone; 10% involve the tibia; 5% involve the pelvis and the remainder of smaller bones. (10)

Thromboembolism

Injuries that result in immobilization and bed rest can precipitate deep vein thrombosis, which can become a potentially lethal source of pulmonary emboli. Fractures of the hip, pelvis, and lower extremity are particularly prone to this complication.

INTERMEDIATE COMPLICATIONS

Osteomyelitis

Approximately 15% of open fractures, and those requiring internal fixation with plates and screws, go on to develop osteomyelitis. (11,12) It is a rare complication of closed fractures. The most common organism is *Staphylococcus aureus*, occurring in 60 to 70% of cases. (11) The most likely sites for secondary osteomyelitis are the femur and tibia. Most cases manifest within a month of occurrence of open fracture or open surgical reduction. (2) The dominant symptom is pain, and the radiologic features are destructive "moth-eaten" lesions, sequestra formation, and periosteal response near the fracture site. (Fig. 9.17C)

Hardware Failure

Failure of hardware applied to fractures can be due to loosening, breakage, bending, or migration. Loosening can be detected by widening of the metal-bone interface and movement. Migration of pins to distant sites by vascular transport can rarely occur to the heart, aorta, and great vessels. (13)

Reflex Sympathetic Dystrophy Syndrome

Severe and painful regional osteoporosis following rather trivial trauma is referred to as *reflex sympathetic dystrophy syndrome* (RSDS) or *Sudeck's atrophy*. This is a relatively rare complication of trauma to a limb. A more detailed discussion of this entity is found in Chapter 14.

Posttraumatic Osteolysis

Dissolution of bone following trauma is a poorly understood disorder peculiar to the distal clavicle and pubic bones. Posttraumatic osteolysis of the clavicle (PTOC) is the most common example and follows fracture of the clavicle, acromioclavicular joint trauma, or overuse syndromes of the shoulder—especially in athletes. (14,15) This is discussed in more detail later in the chapter.

Refracture

Disruption of the bone at the site of the original fracture is usually secondary to inappropriate immobilization, noncompliant patient, underlying tumor or infection, or through bone weakened by surgery such as a pin site.

Myositis Ossificans

Heterotopic bone formation at a site of trauma can occur alone or in combination with a fracture. It is recognizable as an increasingly confluent ossification in muscle tissue most commonly at the thigh or anterior arm. This is discussed in more detail later in this chapter.

Synostosis

Bony fusion between two adjacent bones is most frequent between bones closely apposed, such as the radius–ulna, tibia–fibula, and the small bones of the hands and feet. Such a complication may create significant functional loss of motion.

Delayed Union

Slow bony union across a fracture site may follow inappropriate immobilization, intrinsically poor vascularity, disease state (diabetes, malignancy, infection, malnutrition) and advancing age. A number of sites—such as the scaphoid, proximal femur and tibia—are known to often exhibit delayed union.

DELAYED COMPLICATIONS

Osteonecrosis

When bone is deprived of its blood supply, it will undergo necrosis. Synonyms for this condition include *avascular necrosis, ischemic necrosis, aseptic necrosis,* and *osteonecrosis.* The crucial factors in the development of posttraumatic osteonecrosis are the location of the fracture, the intrinsic vascularity of the bone, and appropriate early treatment. The most common sites in order of frequency for post-fracture avascular necrosis are the femoral head, humeral head, scaphoid, and talus. These and others are discussed in Chapter 13.

Degenerative Joint Disease

If a fracture is intraarticular, damage to the articular cartilage can occur. This is seen most commonly in weight-bearing joints such as the hip, knee, or ankle. Additionally, if the fracture changes the weight-bearing axis of the joint and alters the distribution of forces across the joint, degenerative changes may be initiated. The constellation of subsequent arthritic changes represent secondary degenerative joint disease (posttraumatic arthritis).

Lead Arthropathy and Toxicity

Gunshot wounds may not only produce comminuted fractures, but retention of lead can produce secondary toxic local and systemic effects. Lead within a joint precipitates a degenerative arthropathy. Systemic lead intoxication can follow lead pellet breakdown, especially when located near joints due to the acidity of the fluid and mechanical effects to fragment the metal. (16)

Osteoporosis

Following fracture healing there may be delayed return to full function due to pain, altered function, nerve palsy, or failure to mobilize. The return of bone density may subsequently be incomplete.

Aneurysmal Bone Cyst

Although uncommon, aneurysmal bone cyst has been documented to follow a traumatic event. (17,18) Conversion of a subperiosteal hematoma to the expansile tumor is the likely mechanism.

Nonunion

Nonunion is a failure to complete osseous fusion across the fracture site. Contributing factors of nonunion include distraction, inadequate immobilization, infection, or impaired circulation. The most common sites for nonunion are the midclavicle, ulna, and tibia. The radiographic signs of nonunion take a number of months to develop and include fracture rounding, lack of callus, sclerosis, and pseudoarthrosis. (Fig. 9.17A and B) (Table 9.5)

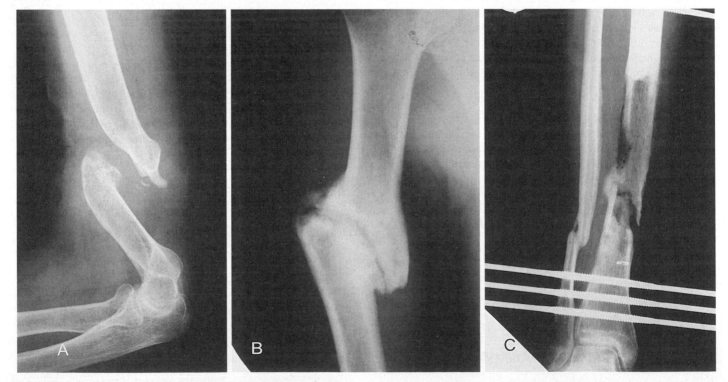

Figure 9.17. FRACTURE COMPLICATIONS. A. Nonunion: Lateral Humerus. A failure of union of the fracture sites is evidenced by rounding and sclerosis of the adjacent fracture margins. **B. Nonunion with Pseudarthrosis: Humerus.** A pseudarthrosis has formed as the result of failure of union of this fracture. Observe the exuberant sclerosis at the fracture margins. **C. Osteomyelitis: Tibia and Fibula.** Following removal of a tibial fixation plate, an extensive osteomyelitis has formed, as evidenced by a "moth-eaten" pattern of bone destruction and cortical disruption.

Pseudoarthrosis is precipitated by inadequate immobilization where motion between the fractured bony ends constantly shears the small vessels that grow into the fracture site in an attempt to heal. The callus produced is poorly vascularized and tends to produce cartilage instead of bone. Continued motion results in myxoid degeneration and liquefaction of the cartilage, with the formation of a pseudo-joint cavity. This pseudoarthrosis, once established, can be healed only by refracture, removal of the cartilaginous component, and the reestablishment of a vascular spindle with new callus formation.

Malunion

Union in poor anatomic position can produce severe loss of functional capacity, especially if joint mechanics are altered. Shortening of a limb can also result, which may create distant secondary compensations and stresses such as pelvic unleveling, spinal scoliosis, and altered gait mechanics.

FRACTURES OF THE SKULL AND FACIAL BONES

SKULL FRACTURES

General Comments

The anatomic complexity of the skull makes interpretation of skull radiographs difficult. Less than 10% of skull fractures are detected on plain film radiographs. (1,2) In many instances skull

Table 9.5.   Radiographic Signs of Fracture Nonunion

Rounding of the Fracture Margin
Lack of Callus Formation
Sclerosis of Fracture Margins
Pseudarthrosis

series are performed only for medicolegal reasons. Up to 15% of intracranial injuries, such as intracerebral or subdural hematomas, do not involve fractures. (3,4) (Fig. 9.18) The minimum routine radiographic study of the skull includes the PA Caldwell and AP Towne's, with right and left laterals. More specialized projections, such as the tangential or submentovertex views, may be helpful, along with computed tomography and magnetic resonance imaging as clinically indicated. In the presence of altered neurology (loss of consciousness, abnormal reflexes, sensory or motor changes), abnormal physical findings (palpable defect, ear discharge, discolored ear drum), and significant historical facts (loss of consciousness, vomiting, amnesia) the correlation with intracranial injury may be as high as 45%. In these circumstances plain films should be avoided in preference to CT scanning. (2,4) MR imaging in acutely injured patients is usually not indicated due to technical difficulties with life support systems attached, prolonged imaging times, insensitivity to early hematomas, and fractures. (4)

Linear Fracture

Up to 80% of all skull fractures are linear skull fractures. (4) These appear on the radiograph as sharp, irregular, radiolucent lines with no sclerotic rim. (Fig. 9.19A and B) Although their entire length cannot be determined, they are usually several centimeters long. Since their course may be straight, angular, or curvilinear, the linear fractures must be differentiated from vascular grooves or sutures. Fracture lines are more radiolucent than vascular grooves because they involve both the inner and outer table of the skull. Vascular grooves represent impressions of varying depth on either the inner or outer table and are therefore less sharp in appearance. Fractures will cross sutures, whereas vascular grooves will not. Radiolucent lines with serrated edges usually represent sutural lines rather than fractures. The skull bones most commonly fractured are the temporal or parietal bones.

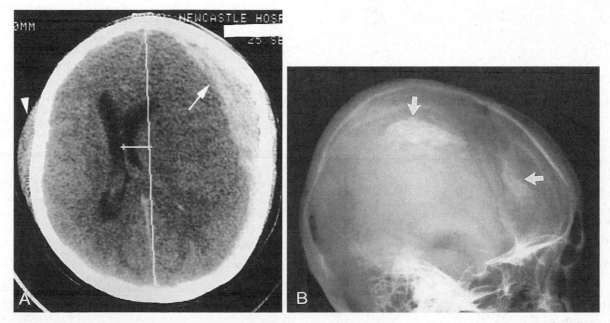

Figure 9.18.   SUBDURAL HEMATOMA: SKULL. A. CT Scan: Contrecoup Injury with Subdural Hematoma. Adjacent to the left lateral brain surface is a linear zone of high attenuation with a slightly concave medial border (arrow). Note the pronounced midline shift of the intracranial contents away from the hematoma. On the contralateral extracranial surface soft tissue swelling marks the point of injury (arrowhead). **B. Plain Film: Calcified Subdural Hematoma**. Thin plaque-like calcifications are seen adjacent to the parietal bones (arrows). This is a manifestation of a past subdural hematoma which has subsequently organized and calcified. (Courtesy of C. Ann Heller, MBBS, DACR, Newcastle, Australia)

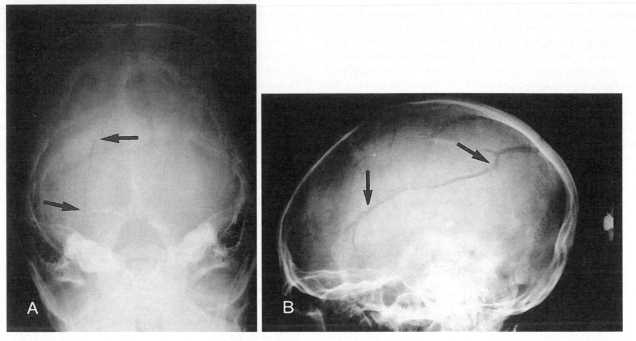

Figure 9.19.   LINEAR SKULL FRACTURES. A. Towne's View, Occipital Bone. A linear fracture line extends through the occipital bone (arrows).

B. Parietal Bone. A linear fracture extends from the posterior aspect of the cranial vault anteriorly (arrows).

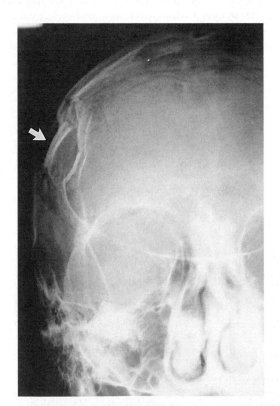

Figure 9.20.   DEPRESSED SKULL FRACTURE. Multiple fracture fragments are seen displaced inward (arrow).

Depressed Fracture

Depressed fractures, which are nearly always located within the cranial vault, result from high-velocity impact by a small object. (4) (Figs. 9.20, 9.21) They represent 15% of all skull fractures. (4) The depression usually effects several fragments of bone, which are usually angulated inward.

This type of fracture may appear *stellate*, due to the radiating pattern of the multiple fragments, and will appear very radiopaque when viewed *en face* due to the overlap of the fractured fragments.

Depressed fractures must be seen in profile to determine the depth of displacement of the fracture fragments. Approximately one third of depressed fragments are associated with dural tears that require surgical repair. (4) Displacement of 5 mm or more of depression beyond the inner table suggests a high probability of dural tear.

Ping Pong Fracture.   This fracture represents a variation of the depressed fracture and is seen most often in the young child, whose skull is very soft and pliable. (4) The skull sustains a deep and broad depression without an associated overt fracture, much like the indentation produced by one's fingers being pushed into a ping pong ball. (5) They are best seen on frontal radiographs, since most lesions occur on the lateral surface of the skull.

Basal Skull Fracture

The skull base is one of the most difficult areas in which to demonstrate a fracture. (6) The most reliable index of the presence of a basal skull fracture is an air/fluid (hemorrhage) level or complete opacification of the sphenoid sinus. (7) This sign is seen in up to 75% of patients with basal skull fractures. (7) Horizontal-beam lateral radiographs of the skull are required in order to demonstrate an air-fluid level in the sphenoid sinus. (7)

Fractures of the occipital condyle are rare and characteristically arise from compression type forces. (8) They can occur as isolated findings, though there is frequently a coexisting fracture of the atlas. These fractures are very rarely visible on conventional radiographic studies and require axial CT with coronal reconstruction for recognition. (8)

Diastatic Fracture

Diastatic fracture represents a traumatic sutural separation, which is usually unilateral and seen most commonly in children. (Fig. 9.22A and B) They account for 5% of all cranial fractures. (9) The lambdoidal and sagittal sutures are the most common areas of diastasis. (9) Unilateral separation of a suture greater than 2 mm is considered a sufficient roentgen sign to make the diagnosis of a *diastatic* fracture.

Complications of Skull Fractures

Leptomeningeal Cyst.   Dural tears may occur beneath an area of fracture adhering to the bone adjacent to the margins of the fracture. (10) Cerebrospinal fluid accumulates, forming a cyst within this relative space. The pulsation within the cyst erodes bone, increasing the size of the bony and dural defect, which, in turn, increases the size of the fracture (''growing'' fracture). (4) Therefore, any widening of a fracture line within the skull suggests the possibility of development of a *leptomeningeal cyst*. The significance of this lesion is not bone erosion, but the pressure on the subadjacent cerebral cortex, leading to focal neurologic deficit.

Pneumocephalus.   When a fracture extends through the bony wall of a paranasal sinus or mastoid air cell, air may dissect its way through to the subarachnoid space, reaching the ventricular system. Less than 3% of all skull fractures are associated with pneumocephalus, with 8% of fractures of the paranasal sinuses resulting in pneumocephalus. (11)

Subdural and Extradural Hematoma.   Only 15% of subdural hematomas and 40% of extradural hematomas have an associated skull fracture. (4) (Fig. 9.18) Computed tomography (CT) is the examination of choice where the collection of blood will be depicted as a crescenteric region of high attenuation in contact with the adjacent internal bony surface. The medial surface of the hematoma is characteristically concave. The side of fracture is not necessarily the side of the hematoma (contre coup injury).

FACIAL BONE FRACTURES
General Considerations

More than 70% of victims of auto accidents sustain facial injury, the majority of which are soft tissue in nature. (4) The standard radiographic evaluation of facial trauma includes four projections—a PA Water's, PA Caldwell, lateral, and submentovertex. These views should include the entire mandible. CT is especially useful in complex injuries and in the evaluation of extension into other structures such as sinuses.

Nasal Bones

Nasal fractures are sustained by high-velocity forces directly impacting in the region of the nasion. They may occur as isolated entities or may be associated with more complex fractures. (12) Most nasal fractures are transverse and tend to depress the distal portion of the nasal bones; however, longitudinal fractures do occur. (4) Nasal bone fractures are best seen on lateral projec-

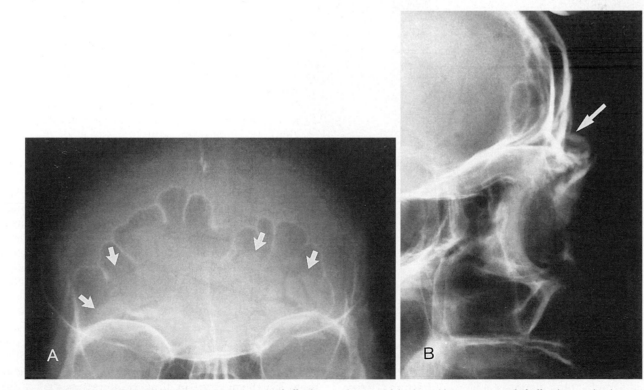

Figure 9.21.   DEPRESSED FRACTURE: FRONTAL BONE. A. PA Skull. The loss of aeration throughout the inferior portions of both frontal sinuses represents accumulated hemorrhage (arrows) associated with a comminuted fracture of the frontal bone. **B. Lateral Skull**. Observe the depressed contour of the frontal bone adjacent to the frontal sinus (arrow). (Courtesy of Richard T. Coade, MIR, DC, Kempsey, New South Wales, Australia)

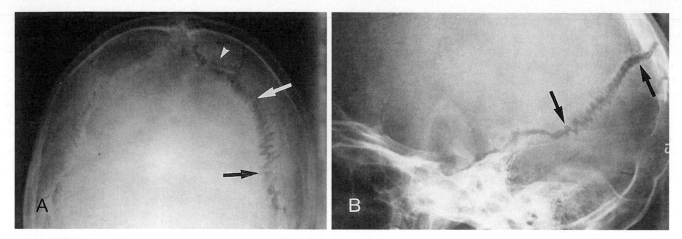

Figure 9.22. DIASTATIC FRACTURES. A. AP Towne's View. A widening of the lambdoidal suture is evident (arrows). A communicating linear fracture extends into the adjacent parietal bone (arrowhead). **B. Lateral Skull.** The lambdoidal suture is widened (arrows).

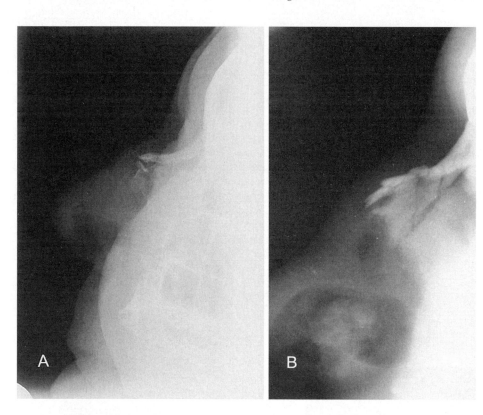

Figure 9.23. NASAL FRACTURES. A. Lateral View. A simple fracture is evident through the nasal bone, with adjacent soft tissue swelling. **B. Lateral Nose.** A comminuted fracture of the nasal bone is observed.

tions, which need to be underexposed to enhance depiction of the fractures. (Fig. 9.23A and B)

Orbital Blowout Fracture

The mechanism of injury in the *blowout* fracture was first described by Smith and Regan in 1957. (13) It is defined as a fracture that disrupts the infraorbital plate of the maxillary bone. The orbital rim may remain intact. Orbital blowout fractures usually occur as a result of a blow by a fist or a ball directly over the globe of the eye or just caudal to it. Additional ocular damage occurs in 30% of cases. (14) The patient often complains of diplopia.

The radiographic presentation of a blowout fracture is dense opacification of the maxillary sinus, with an inverted domelike or polypoid mass (usually representing the inferior rectus mus-

cle) hanging from the roof of the maxillary sinus. (4) Intraorbital emphysema (air) may also be found if the fracture involves an aerated sinus. These findings are best seen on the Water's projection. (4) The opacification of the maxillary sinus is due to hemorrhage or herniated orbital contents, periorbital fat, and the inferior rectus muscle. (14) The inferior orbital rim is usually intact but may be displaced. A thin spicule of bone is often seen caudal to the orbit, representing the depressed portion of the orbital floor.

Tripod Fracture

The tripod fracture is the most common fracture of the facial bones. (4) The mechanism of injury represents a blow over the malar eminence and primarily involves the zygoma. (4) The patient complains of restricted jaw movement due to trapping of the coronoid process of the mandible by the zygoma. The focal points of the fracture affect the three distinct limbs of the zygomatic bone—the zygomatic arch, the orbital process, and the maxillary process surrounding the superior and lateral margins of the maxillary sinus. (Fig. 9.24) Because of the three components of this fracture, it was named *tripod* fracture.

LeFort Fractures

This fracture classification was named for the French investigator Rene LeFort, whose original studies were upon cadavers. (15) By a series of experiments in which he varied the direction and strength of forces upon the face, three consistent patterns of fracture lines emerged—LeFort 1, 2, and 3.

LeFort 1. This type represents a fracture through the midportion of the maxilla and the pterygoid plates. (15)

LeFort 2. This type occurs as a result of a blow to the nasofrontal area. The fracture line extends across the ethmoidal bone obliquely, across the medial maxillary surface of the orbit, and shears obliquely through the lateral maxilla between the inferior orbital fissure and the lateral maxillary wall. (15)

LeFort 3. The fracture line completely separates the facial skeleton from the skull. The actual fracture line extends from the nasofrontal area across the ethmoid posteriorly to the inferior orbital fissures and pterygoid process, then laterally through the lateral wall of the orbit and the zygomatic arches. (15) This is best seen on the Caldwell and Water's projections and is poorly seen on the lateral.

Tomography and CT may be needed to demonstrate and clarify the three types of LeFort fractures. Combinations of the three types are in fact more common than the specific types originally described. (4)

Fractures of the Mandible

Most mandibular fractures occur in automobile and bicycle accidents or fist fights, accounting for approximately 80% of all mandibular fractures. (4,16) The most common site for fracture of the mandible is the body, occurring in 30 to 40% of cases. (17) (Fig. 9.25A and B) Other sites include the mandibular angle (25 to 30%), condyle (15 to 35%), symphysis (7 to 15%), ramus (3 to 9%), coronoid process (1 to 2%), and those limited to the alveolar process (2 to 4%). (16,17) Since the mandible forms a ring, multiple fractures occur in more than 60% of cases. (4) Fractures of

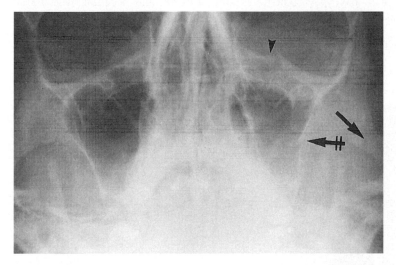

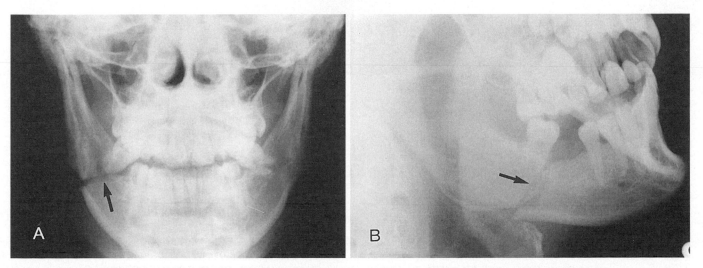

Figure 9.24.   TRIPOD FRACTURE: WATER'S VIEW. Three fracture sites are visible, involving the zygomatic arch (arrow), orbital process (arrowhead), and maxillary process (crossed arrow). Adjacent clouding of the maxillary antrum due to hemorrhage is also apparent.

Figure 9.25.   MANDIBLE FRACTURE. A. AP View. A fracture line is seen to extend through the body of the mandible (arrow). **B. Oblique View.** The fracture line is clearly seen (arrow).

the mandibular condyle are best seen on overpenetrated Towne's views. Notably, the mandible is the slowest healing bone in the body with radiographic union lagging well behind clinical union. (16,17)

FRACTURES AND DISLOCATIONS OF THE SPINE
INTRODUCTION

Fractures of the spinal column are found most commonly at C1-C2, C5-C7, and T12-L2. There has been a significant rise in spinal fractures and spinal cord injuries that appears attributable to an increase in automobile accidents and sports activities. (1) Approximately 20% of spinal fractures are associated with fractures elsewhere. (2) Spinal cord injuries occur in 10 to 14% of spinal fractures and dislocations. (3) Fractures of the cervical spine produce neurologic damage in approximately 40% of cases, whereas the incidence in fractures of the thoracolumbar junction is 4%, and in the thoracic spine it is approximately 10%. (4) The incidence of neurologic deficit is much higher when the fractures affect the neural arch as well as the vertebral body. (4) In 10% of the spinal cord injuries there are no associated fractures. (3,4)

Flexion is the most common line of force in spinal injuries, with extension, rotation, shearing, compression, and distraction occurring less frequently. In order to demonstrate the presence of any fracture or dislocation, the radiographic examination must be comprehensive and of good diagnostic quality. Therefore, a complete series in each region of the spine should be performed,

and, occasionally, pillar views, tomograms, bone scans, or CT may be necessary to demonstrate the presence or absence of a fracture. (5)

FRACTURES AND DISLOCATIONS OF THE CERVICAL SPINE
Fractures of the Atlas

Jefferson's Fracture ("Bursting" Fracture of the Atlas). A bursting fracture of the ring of the atlas, with fractures through the anterior and posterior arches, was first described in 1920 by Sir Geoffrey Jefferson, a British neurosurgeon. (6) (Fig. 9.26A–D) Up to one third of all atlas fractures are of the Jefferson's variety. (7,8)

Jefferson's fracture is a compression injury created by a forceful blow upon the skull vertex, which is transmitted through the occipital condyles to the lateral masses of the atlas. Many of these fractures occur from automobile accidents or diving injuries, usually into too-shallow water. The force displaces the lateral masses laterally, classically producing the fractures on each side of the anterior and posterior arches of the atlas. CT has since demonstrated variations in this fracture pattern. Death or significant neurologic deficit is uncommon, though approximately 50% will have persistent neck pain, stiffness, and occipital dysesthesia. (9,10)

The radiographic signs can be subtle and require an adequate AP open-mouth radiograph, which may be supplemented with

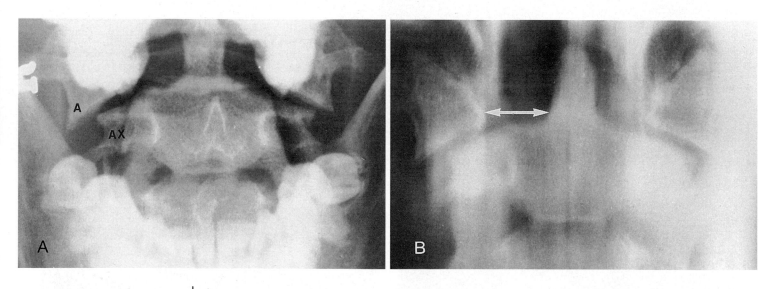

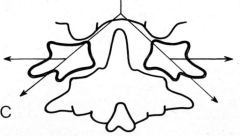

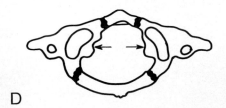

Figure 9.26.   JEFFERSON'S FRACTURE. A. AP Open Mouth. Significant overlap of the lateral masses of the atlas (*A*) upon the axis (*AX*) is present bilaterally. A significant increase has also occurred in both lateral periodontoid spaces. **B. AP Tomogram.** This clearly demonstrates the increased per-

iodontoid spaces (arrows). **C. Mechanism of Jefferson's Fracture.** A compression force applied through the skull results in lateral displacement of the lateral masses of the atlas. **D. Schematic Diagram.** Observe the bilateral fractures through the anterior and posterior arches of the atlas.

CT. (5,8,9) The key signs are linked to the spreading apart of the lateral masses, creating an increased lateral paraodontoid space bilaterally and offset of the lateral edge of the atlas lateral masses and the axis superior articular processes. (9) A total offset of more than 8 mm signifies the transverse ligament is also ruptured. (11) There often is evidence of prevertebral swelling.

Most lesions are bilateral, except when the causative force is eccentrically applied to the skull and is transmitted in greater magnitude to one lateral mass. Unilateral Jefferson's fracture is not as common as the bilateral type. (Fig. 9.27A and B)

Simulation of a Jefferson's fracture (pseudospread) may occur in four circumstances. In children under 10 years of age, most commonly around 4 years, the atlas may grow at a greater rate than the axis. (9,12,13) (Fig. 9.28) Developmental anomalies of the atlas, such as localized lateral mass malformation or combined anterior-posterior spina bifida of the atlas, can produce a similar

appearance. (9,14,15) Rotary atlantoaxial subluxation and torticollis may also mimic a Jefferson's fracture. Such variations usually do not produce lateral offset of more than 2 mm, whereas a Jefferson's fracture typically exceeds 3 mm.

Posterior Arch Fracture of the Atlas. This is the most common fracture of the atlas, accounting for at least 50% of all atlas fractures. (8,10) The fracture is usually a bilateral vertical fracture through the neural arch, through or close to the junction of the arch to the posterior surfaces of the lateral masses. (7) This fracture occurs as a result of the posterior arch of the atlas being compressed between the occiput and the large posterior arch of the axis during severe hyperextension. (7,16) Almost 80% will have another cervical spine fracture. (10) It is best seen on the lateral projection and can easily be overlooked. (17) (Fig. 9.29) Serious complications are unusual, though associated cervical fractures may precipitate spinal cord injury. (10) Close anatomic

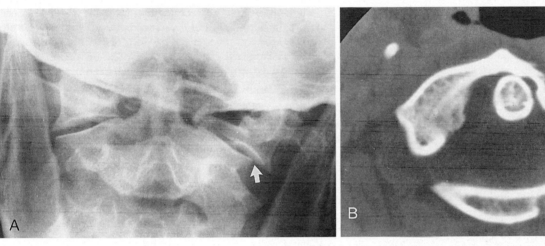

Figure 9.27.   UNILATERAL JEFFERSON'S FRACTURE. A. AP Open Mouth. Significant overlap of the lateral mass of the atlas has occurred unilaterally (arrow). **B. CT Scan.** Fracture sites are evident unilaterally through the anterior and posterior arches (arrows). (Courtesy of Lisa Shelton, BAppSc (Chiropractic), Erina, Australia)

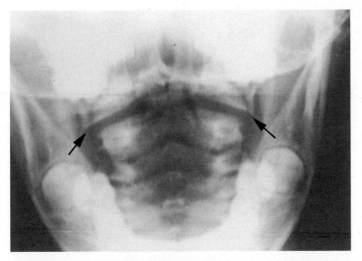

Figure 9.28.   PSEUDOSPREAD OF THE ATLAS. Observe the bilateral overhang of the atlas lateral masses in relation to the axis (arrows). This is a normal variation in some children, which is identical to the appearance of a Jefferson's fracture. It is most frequently found at around age 4. (Courtesy of Appa L. Anderson, DC, DACBR, Fellow, ACCR, Portland, Oregon)

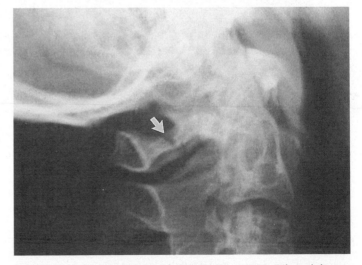

Figure 9.29.   POSTERIOR ARCH FRACTURE: ATLAS. Bilateral fracture lines are seen at the junction of the posterior arch with the lateral masses (arrow). Observe the close proximity of the fracture lines to the course of the vertebral artery, which may be injured in this fracture.

proximity of the vertebral artery to the fracture site may occasionally lead to serious vascular injury.

Anterior Arch Fracture of the Atlas. These fractures are usually horizontal segmental avulsions from hyperextension at the attachment of the anterior longitudinal ligament and longus colli muscle. (18) They constitute less than 2% of neck fractures and often coexist with odontoid fractures. (18) The avulsed fragment is best seen on the lateral film displaced inferiorly from the anterior arch, though a special frontal view with the tube angled cephalad beneath the mandible has been advocated. (19) CT is definitive for diagnosis. (20)

Lateral Mass Fracture of the Atlas. Disruption of the lateral mass is uncommon and often only appreciated on CT examination. Avulsion fracture at the insertion of the transverse ligament at the medial aspect of the lateral mass occasionally is observed. (21) Isolated fracture of the transverse process has been described. (22)

Rupture of the Transverse Ligament. Isolated traumatic disruption of the transverse ligament is infrequent. The ligament is strong, with the odontoid usually breaking before the ligament is completely compromised. Rupture of the ligament is common in association with Jefferson's fracture, inflammatory arthritis (e.g., rheumatoid arthritis, psoriasis, ankylosing spondylitis, and Reiter's syndrome). (23) Additionally, 20% of Down's syndrome patients exhibit laxity or agenesis of this ligament.

A key radiologic feature of a ruptured transverse ligament is an abnormally wide atlantodental interspace (ADI) (more than 3 mm in adults and 5 mm in children), most pronounced in flexion. (Fig. 9.30A and B) The posterior cervical line will also be disrupted. Cord compression may not be clinically apparent until considerable anterior displacement of the atlas (up to 10 mm) has occurred, due to the protective effect of the surrounding tissues of the cord, which make up approximately one third of the diameter of the atlas ring. Steele's Rule of Thirds divides the atlas ring into thirds—one third cord, one third space, and one third odontoid. Consideration of this division is a crucial factor in calculating the amount of atlas displacement possible before cord compression occurs. (Fig. 9.30C and D)

Fractures of the Axis

Hangman's Fracture (Traumatic Spondylolisthesis). Fractures of the neural arch of the axis are among the most common injuries of the cervical spine. Up to 40% of axis fractures are hangman's fractures. (24) They are usually the results of automobile accidents in which there is abrupt deceleration from a high speed,

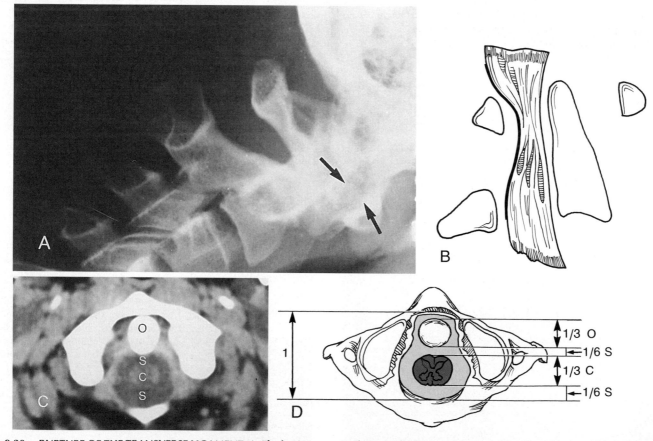

Figure 9.30. RUPTURE OF THE TRANSVERSE LIGAMENT. A. Flexion Lateral Cervical. In flexion the atlantodental interspace increases to approximately 7 mm (arrows), a radiologic sign of transverse ligament instability (arrows). **B. Diagrammatic Representation.** Anterior displacement of the atlas upon the axis due to rupture of the transverse ligament may result in significant cord compression with entrapment between the posterior tubercle and odontoid process (guillotine mechanism). **C. Computerized Tomogram Through the C1-C2 Articulation.** The relationship of the odontoid (*O*), spinal cord (*C*), and soft tissues surrounding the cord (*S*) is clearly depicted. **D. Diagrammatic Representation of the C1-C2 Articulation.** Approximately one third of the atlas ring is occupied by the odontoid (*O*), one third by the spinal cord (*C*), and the remaining one third by the space surrounding the cord (*S*). This anatomic division explains why patients with anterior atlas displacement may be relatively asymptomatic until a large degree of translation has occurred (Steele's Rule of Thirds).

though the fracture occurs during hyperextension. The distribution of the fracture is similar to that resulting from judicial hanging. This has prompted the term *hangman's fracture*. (25) This is actually a misnomer, since the hangman does not receive the fracture. It should more accurately be called the *hangee's fracture*.

The fracture occurs as a bilateral disruption through the pedicles of the axis. (24) The fracture lines are best seen on CT or the lateral view just anterior to the inferior facet, usually in association with anterior displacement of C2 upon C3. (Fig. 9.31A–C) This displacement is usually persistent following osseous union, a sign of previous injury, which should be recognized. Occasionally the axis body will be flexed and distracted superiorly. (26) Prevertebral hemorrhage is common, increasing the retropharyngeal interspace that may compromise the adjacent airway. Up to 25% have an accompanying fracture, usually of the atlas. (27) An avulsion of the anterior-inferior corner of the vertebral body (teardrop fracture) often occurs simultaneously. (25)

There is a surprising lack of neurologic findings in fractures of the neural arch of the axis due to the large spinal canal at this level. (28) Extension of the fracture into the transverse foramen may precipitate vertebral artery injury. (27,29)

Teardrop Fracture. This fracture is an avulsion of a triangular-shaped fragment from the anteroinferior corner of the axis body. (Fig. 9.32A and B) Although teardrop fractures can occur at any cervical body, the lesion is most common at the axis. (30) At this level an acute hyperextension is the usual mechanism of injury, which explains its common occurrence in combination with a hangman's fracture. (25,30)

Odontoid Process Fracture. Fractures of the odontoid process are common traumatic injuries of the cervical spine comprising 40 to 50% of axis fractures. (24,31) Pathologic fracture may complicate metastatic carcinoma, multiple myeloma and other tumors, rheumatoid arthritis, and ankylosing spondylitis as well as other causes for osteopenia. (32,33) Dens fractures are described by Anderson and D'Alonzo on the basis of their location. (34) (Fig. 9.33A–C) (Table 9.6)

Type 1. This type is an avulsion of the tip of the odontoid process as a result of apical or alar ligament stress. It is an uncommon injury that is rarely complicated by nonunion.

Type 2. This is a fracture at the junction of the odontoid process and the body of the axis. This is the most common odontoid process fracture, and the one that most frequently results in nonunion due to reduced vascularity of the separated fragment. (35,36) During union hypertrophic callus may induce myelopathy. (37) Post fracture osteolysis of the dens has been recorded. (38)

Type 3. The fracture is found deep within the vertebral body, below the base of attachment of the odontoid process to the body. This type is almost as common as type 2, though it heals more readily.

Recognition of odontoid fractures is notoriously difficult and demands high-quality radiographic examinations. (39) The most reliable imaging findings consist of the fracture line, odontoid displacement, disrupted axis "ring," enlargement of C2 body and

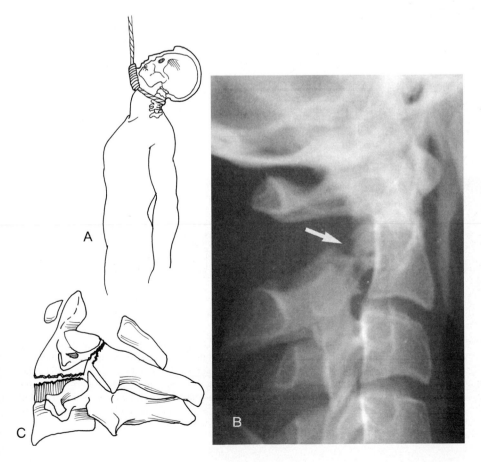

Figure 9.31. HANGMAN'S FRACTURE. A. Mechanism of Injury. During judicial hangings, a hyperextension and rotatory force to the neck directs the impact to the pedicle regions of the C2 segment, resulting in fracture. **B. Radiologic Manifestations.** An irregular fracture line (arrow) is seen to extend through the pedicle of the axis. Minimal anterior displacement of the C2 segment upon C3 is also apparent. **C. Diagrammatic Representation.** In addition to the fracture through the pedicle region, disruption at the discovertebral junction may result in vertebral displacement.

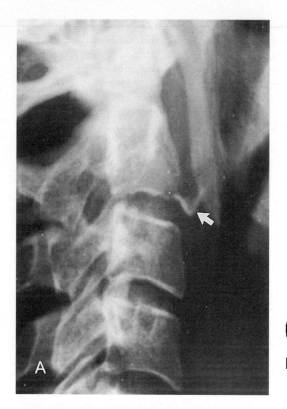

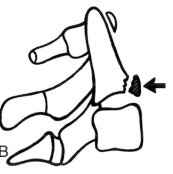

Figure 9.32.　TEARDROP FRACTURE. A. C2. Observe the anteroinferior corner of C2, which has been avulsed, creating a free triangular fragment (teardrop) (arrow). **B. Diagrammatic Representation (arrow).**

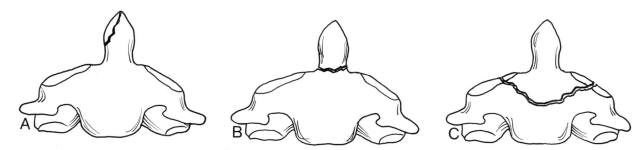

Figure 9.33.　ANDERSON AND D'ALONZO CLASSIFICATION OF ODONTOID FRACTURES. A. Type I. B. Type II. C. Type III.

Table 9.6.	Classification of Odontoid Fractures	
Type	**Location**	**Stability**
I	Odontoid tip	Stable (union)
II	Odontoid base	Unstable (nonunion)
III	Extension into body	Stable (union)

Table 9.7.   Imaging Findings in Odontoid Fractures

Plain Film Radiography
  Lateral Projection
    Fracture line
    Fragmentation
    Anteroposterior displacement
    Disrupted posterior cervical line
    Disrupted axis "ring"
    Enlarged axis body ("fat C2")
    Absent callus
    Retropharyngeal swelling
    Normal anterior arch
  Frontal Projection
    Fracture line
    Tilted odontoid process (> 5°)
    Osteolysis of the odontoid
Computed Tomography
  Axial and Reconstructed Images
    Displacement of odontoid
    Comminution of the axis
    Prevertebral swelling
    Central canal compromise
    Intraspinal hematoma
Magnetic Resonance Imaging
  T1- and T2-Weighted Sagittal and Coronal Images
    Vertebral marrow signal changes
    Spinal canal and cord integrity
    Intraspinal hematoma

retropharyngeal swelling. (Table 9.7) Additional CT and MR imaging investigation is undertaken in equivocal cases or for investigation of the spinal cord. (40) The fracture line is not always visible but is best seen on AP open-mouth radiographs as an irregular radiolucent line. Even CT may not identify the fracture line. (40)

Displacement of the odontoid in either the anterior or posterior position is usually less than 3 mm. (36) This displacement creates an offset of the posterior cervical line (PCL) of the atlas as it relates to the normally positioned axis. Impingement on the spinal cord occurs in isolated rupture of the transverse ligament with an intact odontoid process, creating a "guillotine" or "pincers" effect upon the cord. (Fig. 9.34A–C) A lateral tilt of the odontoid process more than 5° indicates an underlying fracture. (41) (Fig. 9.36C)

Disruption of the anterior axis cortex may be visible in type 3 fractures on the lateral projection. The vertically elongated ring structure formed by a confluence of neural arch and vertebral body structures superimposed over the odontoid may show disruption. (42) When significant comminution extends into the axis body, its sagittal size may increase ("fat C2" sign). (43)

Signs of nonunion consist of smooth sclerotic margins, widening of the fracture line, progressive osteolysis of the dens, mobility across the fracture site in flexion-extension, and the appearance of a "vacuum" within the fracture. (44) Surgical intervention is required in cases of nonunion and is either performed with posterior fusion (Gallie fusion) or screw fixation. (39,45) (Fig. 9.35)

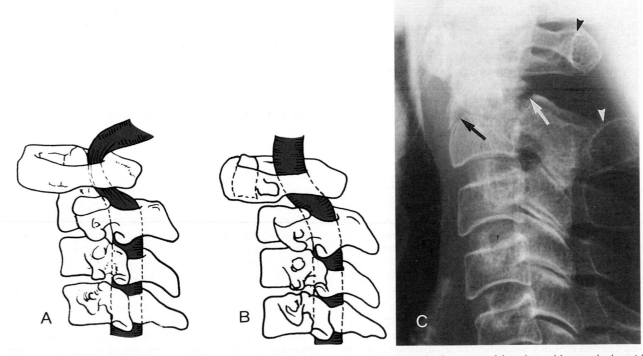

Figure 9.34.   GUILLOTINE EFFECT OF ANTERIOR ATLAS DISPLACEMENT. A. Schematic Diagram. Transverse ligament rupture creates a potential for cord compression between the approximated posterior arch and odontoid process. **B. Schematic Diagram**. Odontoid process fractures result in less compression of the spinal cord, since the odontoid process and atlas move as a unit. **C. Lateral Cervical**. A type III odontoid process fracture (arrows) is present which has disrupted the axis "ring" and the anterior cortex, with anterior displacement of the atlas and fractured odontoid complex (arrowheads). COMMENT: The incidence of isolated transverse ligament rupture following trauma is much less than odontoid process fractures, since the transverse ligament is stronger than the odontoid attachment. However, a transverse ligament rupture represents a more life-threatening situation as a result of the guillotine effect.

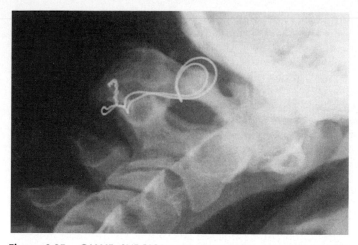

Figure 9.35. GALLIE SURGICAL STABILIZATION FOR ODONTOID FRACTURE. A combination of osseous and wire arthrodesis has been performed, fixing the posterior arch of the atlas to the spinous process of the axis. Note the residual anterior displacement of the atlas.

A number of artifacts and variants can mimic a fracture through the dens, including Mach bands, dentocentral synchondrosis, congenital odontoid tilt, and os odontoideum. Mach bands due to overlap of various structures such as the anterior and posterior atlas arches, tongue, and the teeth can simulate a fracture line at the junction of the base of the odontoid process and the body of the axis. (46) (Fig. 9.36A) Occasionally, an apparent vertical cleft within the odontoid process occurs from the space between the frontal incisors. (Fig. 9.36B) Vertical cleft fractures of the odontoid are virtually impossible to create, and none have been reported. (36) Developmental lateral tilt of the dens is rarely greater than 3° implying that any such observed tilt should be considered due to fracture. (41) (Fig. 9.36C) Posterior tilt of the odontoid is more commonly encountered as a normal variation. (41) (Fig. 9.36D) The radiolucent dentocentral synchondrosis at the junction of the dens and vertebral body in children begins to close by age 5, is fused by age 7, but remnants persist into adolescence. (36) A paraodontoid notch should similarly not be confused with fracture. (Fig. 9.36A)

Os odontoideum represents a developmental failure of the dens to unite with the body of the odontoid but exhibits distinctive radiographic features that allow differentiation from acute fracture. (Fig. 9.37A and B) (Table 9.8) The cleft at the site of nonunion is wide, smooth, and often sclerotic in contradistinction to the closely apposed fragments, and serrated or jagged, nonsclerotic margins of acute fracture. Either odontoid fracture or os odontoideum may coexist with atlantoaxial subluxation. In equivocal cases or for medicolegal purposes a bone scan may show activity of a healing fracture. Additional helpful signs for os odontoideum can be identified in the anterior arch of the atlas. It often is enlarged and densely sclerotic, exhibits a thick cortex, and displays either a rounded or angular posterior surface that may invaginate into the odontoid cleft. (48) These changes appear to be a result of hypertrophy secondary to an abnormal amount of biomechanical stress being placed upon the anterior tubercle of the atlas from the underlying instability of the os odontoideum. This roentgen sign may also be found in association with other upper cervical anomalies such as agenesis or hypoplasia of the posterior arch of the atlas, agenesis or hypoplasia of the odontoid process, and spina bifida of the atlas or axis. Close scrutiny of the

posterior surface of the anterior tubercle will show it to be straight in odontoid fractures and occasionally angular in os odontoideum, the angle having its apex adjacent to the separating odontoid cleft.

Vertebral Body Compression Fractures

Wedge Fracture. This occurs as a result of mechanical compression of the involved vertebra between the adjacent vertebral bodies from forced hyperflexion. This is a stable fracture, because the intervertebral disc, anterior longitudinal ligament, and posterior ligamentous structures are intact. Two thirds of wedge fractures occur at the fifth, sixth, and seventh cervical segments. (49)

The lateral radiograph is diagnostic, demonstrating a sharp, triangular, anterior wedging of the superior vertebral endplate. (Fig. 9.38) If the anterior height of a vertebral body measures 3 mm or more less than the posterior height, a fracture of the vertebral body can be assumed. (36) An increase in the retropharyngeal interspace (RPI) above the normal limit of 20 mm can occur as the result of prevertebral hemorrhage. Displacement of the prevertebral fat strip may also occur secondary to hemorrhage and edema. Occasionally, a fragment of bone may occur near the anterior surface of the vertebral endplate as a remnant of the traumatic incident. The frontal radiograph is usually of little help in evaluation of the fracture. The absence of a vertical fracture line in the vertebral body in a wedge fracture helps distinguish the wedge fracture from the burst fracture on the frontal film.

Burst Fracture. A burst fracture is precipitated by vertical compression to the head propelling the nucleus pulposus through the endplate into the vertebral body. The force fractures the vertebra vertically, causing a comminution of the vertebral body with the fragments migrating centrifugally. (Fig. 9.39A and B) Posteriorly displaced fragments of bone may create extrinsic pressure on the ventral surface of the cord leading to neurologic deficit or paralysis. (50) This is best seen by CT.

The lateral radiograph reveals a comminuted vertebral body, which is usually flattened centrally. The frontal radiograph often demonstrates a vertical fracture line of the vertebral body in the burst fracture, a sign not seen with the simple wedge fracture. Associated fracture in the neural arch is common.

Teardrop Fracture. *Teardrop fracture* is the term used to describe the triangular-shaped bone that has been separated from the anteroinferior corner of a vertebral body. These may occur from a hyperextension injury as an avulsive process (extension teardrop fracture) or from a hyperflexion force that compresses the anterior body corners and shears off a significant anteroinferior fragment (flexion teardrop fracture). (Figs. 9.40A and B, 9.41)

These fractures produce severe and unstable injuries of the cervical spine. Misalignment abnormalities are common and a reflection of the severe underlying ligamentous disruption. Forward dislocation of the involved vertebra occurs frequently, because of complete tearing of the anterior longitudinal ligament and partial tearing of the disc and its attachment to the vertebral endplates. Occasionally, rupture of the posterior ligaments allows unilateral or bilateral facet dislocation to occur, with localized kyphosis and widening of the interlaminar and interspinous interspaces. (51) Disc spaces at the fracture level can be narrowed or even widened.

Teardrop fractures are unstable injuries often associated with the *acute anterior cervical cord syndrome*. (51) This is composed of immediate, complete motor paralysis and loss of the anterior column sensations of pain and temperature. The posterior column sensations of position, vibration, and motion are maintained. In-

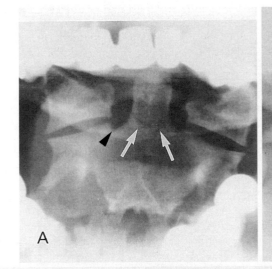

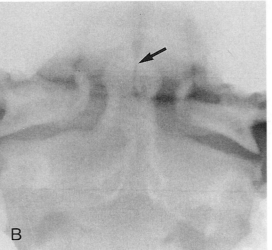

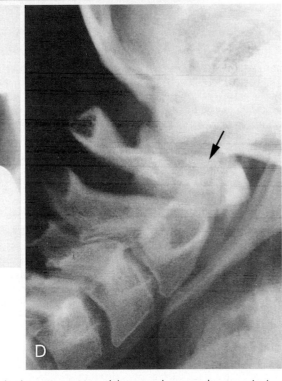

**Figure 9.36.   UPPER CERVICAL ABNORMALITIES SIMULATING ODON-
TOID FRACTURE. A. Mach Band Effect: APOM.** Observe the simulation of
a radiolucent fracture line present at the base of the odontoid process (arrows) as a result of the mach band effect. This pseudoradiolucent line is due
to the superimposition of the arch of the atlas near the base of the odontoid
process. A prominent para-odontoid notch should also not be confused with
a fracture site (arrowhead). **B. Pseudocleft of the Odontoid: APOM.** There
is a radiolucent pseudocleft (arrow) in the odontoid processes noted as a
result of superimposition of the space between the upper incisors. **C. True
Odontoid Fracture: APOM.** Observe the jagged radiolucent line at the base
of the odontoid, representing a true fracture (arrow). Tilting of the odontoid
process more than 5° is an additional reliable roentgen sign of odontoid
fracture. **D. Variant Posterior Odontoid Tilt.** Observe the marked posterior
tilt of the odontoid process (arrow). This is an occasional variant appearance
of the dens and is not to be confused with acute or previous fracture deformity. (Courtesy of Lance M. Thomas, DC, Denver, Colorado)

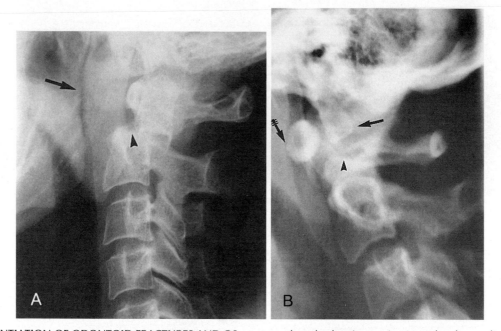

Figure 9.37.   DIFFERENTIATION OF ODONTOID FRACTURES AND OS ODONTOIDEUM. A. Lateral Cervical: Odontoid Fracture. A type II fracture of the odontoid process with posterior displacement of the atlas has occurred. An increase in the prevertebral soft tissue space (arrow) secondary to hemorrhage in association with an irregular fracture line (arrowhead) at the base of the odontoid process is seen. Observe the normal size and shape of the anterior tubercle of C1. **B. Lateral Cervical: Os Odontoideum.** A small bony ossicle represents the separated odontoid ossicle (arrow). The radiolucent space between the odontoid ossicle and base of the axis, and the smooth and sclerotic margins (arrowhead), are distinctive. Significant enlargement and increased density of the anterior tubercle (crossed arrow) is also a frequent finding in os odontoideum. The enlargement of the anterior tubercle with an increase in density is a stress response secondary to chronic upper cervical instability. This radiographic sign is found in chronic instability and is not seen in acute fractures. Close observation of the posterior surface of the anterior tubercle reveals an angular surface with its apex directed posteriorly.

Table 9.8.   Differential Features Between Os Odontoideum and Odontoid Fracture

	Os Odontoideum	Fracture
Zone of separation	Wide	Narrow
Marginal details	Round, smooth, sclerotic	Irregular
Odontoid orientation	Vertical	Often tilted
Posterior cervical line	Interrupted	Interrupted
Anterior tubercle size/ density	Increased	Normal
Anterior tubercle posterior shape	Angular	Straight

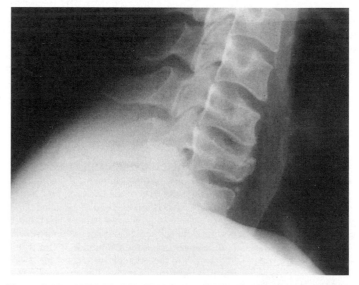

Figure 9.38.   WEDGE COMPRESSION FRACTURE OF THE C7 VERTEBRAL BODY. A characteristic wedge-type deformity with loss of intervertebral height and preservation of the posterior vertebral margins secondary to a hyperflexion injury. COMMENT: The lower cervical spine in the C5 through C7 area is the most common location for these fractures.

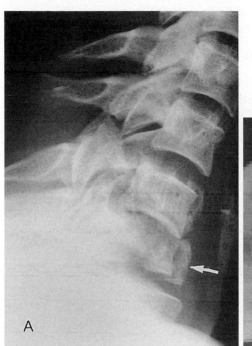

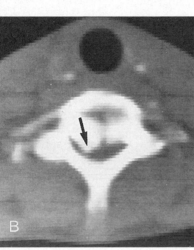

Figure 9.39.   BURST FRACTURE OF THE VERTEBRAL BODY. A. Lateral Cervical. There are multiple fracture fragments of the C7 vertebral body (arrow) that have been displaced in various directions. **B. Computed Tomogram: C7.** The displaced fracture fragments are seen to extend posteriorly, which has resulted in significant spinal stenosis (arrow). This demonstrates the clinical value of computed tomography in vertebral body fractures.

Figure 9.40.   MECHANISMS FOR THE DEVELOPMENT OF TEARDROP FRACTURE. A. Extension Teardrop Fracture. This is an avulsion fracture following a hyperextension injury, which pulls off a small triangular fragment from the anteroinferior corner of the vertebral body. **B. Flexion Teardrop Fracture.** Compression of the anterior vertebral body corners creates a shearing effect which disrupts the triangular fragment from the anteroinferior aspect of the vertebral body following a hyperflexion cervical injury.

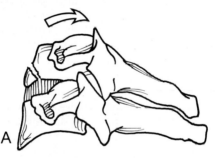

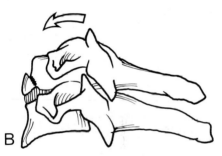

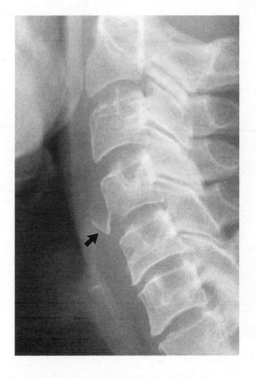

Figure 9.41.   TEARDROP FRACTURE: CERVICAL SPINE. There is a teardrop avulsion fracture noted at the anteroinferior aspect of the C4 vertebral body (arrow). COMMENT: Teardrop fractures are often unstable and may be associated with facet dislocation and an acute anterior cervical cord syndrome. (Courtesy of Margaret A. Seron, DC, DACBR, FACO, Denver, Colorado)

volvement of the upper extremities is greater than that of the lower extremities.

Articular Pillar Fractures

Fractures of the articular pillar are among the most frequently missed fractures of the cervical spine, partly because the pillars are not well seen on standard views. (52,53) The articular pillar is formed by the superior and inferior articular processes, which fuse to form a rhomboidal-shaped structure. Articular pillars are best demonstrated by specific pillar views or on bone window CT images. (54)

Pillar fractures most commonly occur at C4 through C7, with C6 representing the site of approximately 40% of cases. (15) The most common form of pillar fracture is the compression type. Most articular pillar fractures are caused by automobile accidents due to combined compressive hyperextension and lateral flexion of the cervical spine.

Articular pillar fractures exhibit an altered shape with loss of vertical height the most common change. There can be associated anterolisthesis of the segment. (53,55) (Fig. 9.42A and B) It is important to note that congenital developmental asymmetry and flattening of the articular pillars is common. (56) On routine frontal radiographs a fractured pillar can manifest as a recognizable joint space due to rotation of the pillar ("horizontal facet" sign). (36) Bone scan can be helpful in the detection of occult lateral mass fracture.

Clay Shoveler's Fracture

Clay shoveler's fracture (coal-miner's or root-puller's fracture) is an avulsive injury of the spinous process. The injury derives its name from its common occurrence in clay miners in Australia during the 1930s. (57) It results from abrupt flexion of the head, such as is found in automobile accidents, diving, or wrestling injuries, or from repeated stress caused by the pull of the trapezius and rhomboid muscles on the spinous process. The spinous avulsion most commonly occurs at C7, with C6 and T1 also frequently involved. (58) It may also be caused by a direct blow to the base of the neck. This is a stable fracture without neurologic deficit.

On the lateral projection an oblique radiolucent fracture line through the base of the spinous process or distal tip may be visible. (Fig. 9.43A–C) Its margins are rough and serrated, a helpful roentgen sign to differentiate nonunion of the secondary growth center for the spinous process or a nuchal bone. (59) The distal portion of the spinous process that is fractured is often displaced caudally, a sign not seen with nonunion.

The frontal radiograph demonstrates the apparent presence of two spinous processes for a single vertebra which is called the *double spinous process* sign. (60) (Fig. 9.44) This is especially useful when the cervicothoracic junction is poorly visualized on lateral radiographs and may be the only sign present.

Lamina and Transverse Process Fractures

Laminar fractures occur in the mid to lower cervical spine, with C5 and C6 being the most common sites. (61) While difficult to see on standard views, they are readily depicted on CT images. (Fig. 9.45A and B) Transverse process fractures are decidedly rare, with C7 the most exposed protuberance. Severe trauma with lateral flexion is necessary and, as such, these often coexist with other cervical fractures and brachial plexus lesions. (Fig. 9.46A and B) The fracture line tends to localize near its junction with the pedicle and if in continuity with the transverse foramen may produce vertebral artery injury.

Whiplash Syndrome

The so-called *whiplash syndrome* is a common clinical condition that has received a high volume of published material over the last four decades, much of which—when scrutinised scientifically

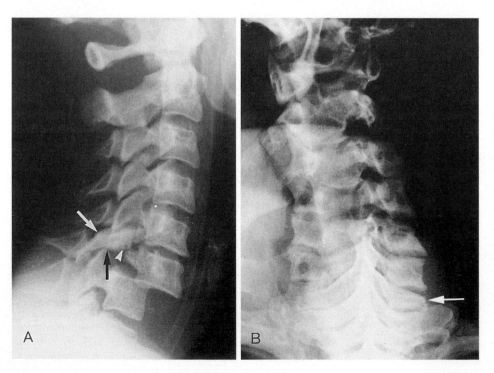

Figure 9.42.   PILLAR FRACTURE. A. Associated with Dislocation. Significant decrease in the vertical height of the articular pillar of C6, along with an increase in density of the compressed articular pillar, is characteristic of a pillar fracture (arrows). A fracture through the pedicle can be seen (arrowhead) and dislocation of the C6 vertebral body has occurred. **B. Pillar Compression Fracture, Pillar View.** On this view in a different patient there is a notable loss of height in the C7 articular pillar (arrow). (Courtesy of Thomas M. Goodrich, DC, DACBR, Indianapolis, Indiana)

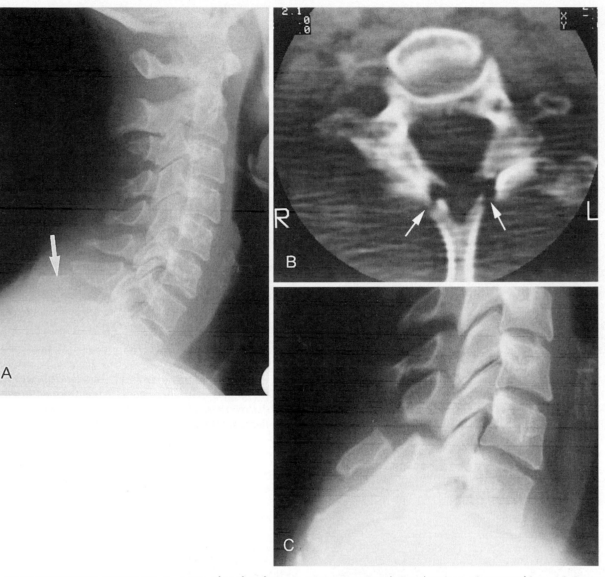

Figure 9.43. CLAY SHOVELER'S FRACTURE. A. Acute Clay Shoveler's Fracture: Lateral Cervical. An avulsion fracture of the spinous process of C7 with inferior displacement of the distal fragment is noted (arrow). Observe the fracture line, which is irregular and exhibits no sclerosis. **B. CT Scan, Acute Clay Shoveler's Fracture.** The sites of fracture at the base of the spi- nous process are depicted (arrows). (Courtesy of Steven P. Brownstein, MD, Springfield, New Jersey) **C. Old Clay Shoveler's Fracture.** The presence of smooth and sclerotic opposing margins indicates an old clay shoveler's frac- ture. (Courtesy of Peter Christensson, DC, Rome, Italy)

for validity—is found flawed. (62) Neck sprains are common in all Western countries and are reported in 20 to 60% of all motor vehicle accidents. (63,64) Classically, the injury follows a forced hyperextension–hyperflexion of the cervical spine most com- monly associated with a rear end motor vehicle collision. The lay press and legal profession have popularized the term *whiplash* as an all-embracing term for a wide variety of soft tissue neck in- juries from a broad spectrum of causes. Synonyms are numerous including *acceleration-deceleration, flexion-extension, hyperflexion-hy- perextension, sprain-strain, myofascial injury,* and *soft tissue injury.* There is no consensus on terminology though the most contem- porary and appropriate term appears to be *cervical sprain-strain injury.*

A broad spectrum of presentations is found, ranging from rel- atively minor complaints to severe incapacitation. Pain in the pos- terior neck is a cardinal manifestation, and that may be either dull and aching with exacerbation on movement, or sharp related to movement, or a combination of the two. (62) Pain may also ra- diate to the head, shoulder, arm, or interscapular region. Asso- ciated stiffness of the neck is common. As many as 85% of these patients may have as their pain source the cervical facet joints. (65,66) Palpation and assessment of joint characteristics can ac- curately isolate the involved painful joints. (67,68) Other common complaints include headache, visual disturbances, memory im- pairment, and dizziness. (62)

Imaging of whiplash injuries is limited to or is dominated by soft tisssue rather than osseous abnormalities. Exclusion of frac- tures and dislocations is a first priority, though frequently unre- warding. Identification of soft tissue injury is often difficult and inherently limited by the technical restraints of the imaging mo-

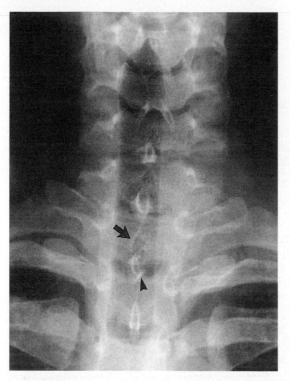

Figure 9.44.   DOUBLE SPINOUS PROCESS SIGN: CLAY SHOVELER'S FRACTURE. Two spinous process shadows are seen at the T1 segment, the first of which shows the intact base of the spinous process (arrow). The second shadow is the caudally displaced distal fragment (arrowhead). (Courtesy of Lawrence C. Pyzik, DC, DACBR, Chicago, Illinois)

dality employed. A number of soft tissue imaging findings have been described. (Table 9.9)

Conventional Imaging.   The standard posttraumatic plain film radiographic series consists of a minimum of frontal, lateral, and oblique projections. (46,69,70) The most important view is the lateral, which is positive in 70 to 90% of cases. (70) Since certain fractures and intersegmental instabilities may not be demonstrated on this survey, clinical consideration should be given to employing the use of flexion-extension studies, once the initial frontal and lateral studies have been scrutinized for contraindications ("Davis series"). (71) A key rule in posttraumatic radiography of the neck is "to see all seven." Especially on the lateral projection, the first to seventh cervical segments should be adequately imaged since serious lesions at each caudad and cephalad extreme may be overlooked.

Three key areas for review for evidence of extraosseous injury are the soft tissues, vertebral alignment, and joints. (72)

Abnormal soft tissues. Perusal of the paravertebral soft tissues should include the prevertebral spaces (retropharyngeal, retrotracheal) and trachea. As many as 20% of motor vehicle accident patients presenting to an emergency department may have prevertebral swelling. (73)

1. *Widened retropharyngeal space.* The tissue immediately anterior to the anteroinferior aspect of the C2 body should not exceed 7 mm in children or adults. (72,74) Hematoma or edema within the longus colli, torn anterior longitudinal ligament, or torn discovertebral junction will manifest as a widening of this soft tissue landmark. (72,75) (Fig. 9.47)

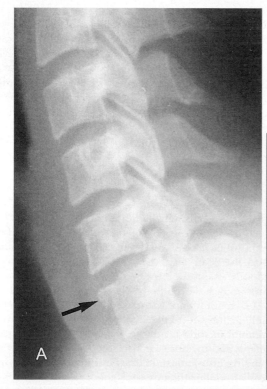

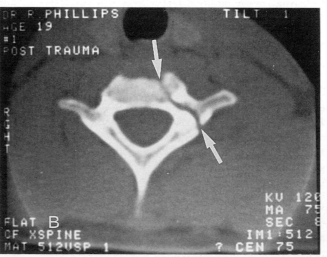

Figure 9.45.   VERTEBRAL BODY AND ASSOCIATED NEURAL ARCH FRACTURE. A. C7 Body Fracture. An anterior compression fracture with a "step defect" is present at the anterosuperior corner of the body of C7 (arrow). **B. Computed Tomogram: C7.** The fracture line is seen to extend through the vertebral body, pedicle, and base of the transverse process (arrows). The extension into the posterior arch could not be appreciated on the plain film radiographs. (Courtesy of Reed B. Phillips, DC, DACBR, PhD, Los Angeles, California)

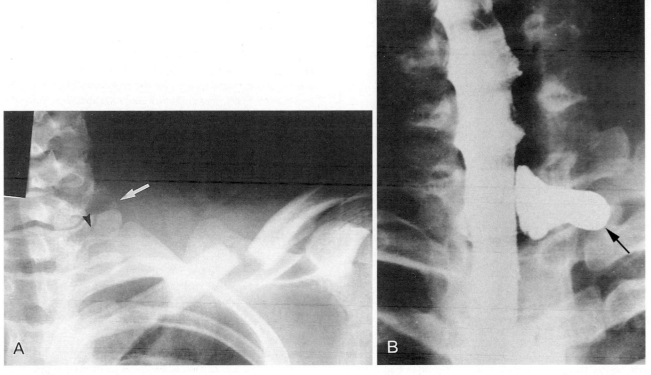

Figure 9.46.   TRANSVERSE PROCESS FRACTURES OF C7 AND T1. A. AP Plain Film. There is a small avulsion fracture noted at the tip of the C7 transverse process (arrow), along with an oblique transverse process fracture of T1 (arrowhead). Additionally noted is a fracture with malalignment of the mid one-third of the clavicle. **B. Nerve Root Avulsion.** Myelogram demonstrates an outpouching of the dural sleeve due to avulsion of the T1 nerve root (arrow). COMMENT: Transverse process fractures in the cervical spine are infrequent and often are markers of brachial plexus injury.

2. *Widened retrotracheal space.* The tissue immediately anterior to the anteroinferior aspect of the C6 body should not exceed 14 mm in children or 22 mm in adults. (72,75) Hematoma or edema within the esophagus, longus colli, anterior longitudinal ligament or discovertebral junction will manifest as a widening of this soft tissue landmark. (72,75)
3. *Displacement of the prevertebral fat stripe.* A thin radiolucent vertical linear shadow corresponding to fatty areolar tissue is frequently observed adjacent to the anterior aspects of the C6-C7 bodies. (76) Hematoma or edema from tears within the longus colli, scalenes, anterior longitudinal ligament, or discovertebral junction will manifest as a widening of this soft tissue landmark. (72) Compression and subtle endplate fractures will also displace the prevertebral fat stripe.
4. *Tracheal deviation and laryngeal dislocation.* Lateral or anterior tracheal displacement following injury may be due to hematoma or torticollis. Elevation of the hyoid bone above the plane of the superior endplate of C3 is found in tracheal transection. (77)
5. *Soft tissue emphysema.* Gas within the neck's soft tissues is indicative of either tracheal laceration or transection, pneumomediastinum, or pneumothorax. (77) Epidural pneumatosis (pneumorrachis, air in the spinal canal) may accompany these air escaping injuries. (78)

Abnormal vertebral alignment. Spatial relationships should be carefully assessed using various lines and angles.

1. *Loss of the lordosis.* This is the most commonly observed finding on postwhiplash radiographs. (72) The significance of alordosis or hypolordosis however remains controversial and on its own cannot be construed to be a strong indicator of underlying soft tissue injury. (73) Traditionally the clinical implication of a reduced lordosis has been that it is secondary to muscle spasm. (72) Reduction of the lordosis is readily reproduced with degenerative disc disease, a small degree of head nodding, or if the exposure is made while recumbent. (72,79–82) (Fig. 9.48)
2. *Acute kyphotic angulation.* At a single level an abrupt angular change in the configuration of the cervical curve ("acute kyphosis sign") with two adjacent spinous processes widely separated ("divergent spinous process sign") is suggestive of disruption of the posterior ligamentous complex. (72,83,84) The C5 and C6 segments are the most common levels of involvement. This deformity can be exaggerated in the flexion view and is always associated with significant facet subluxation almost to the point of dislocation. (Fig. 9.49) The widened interspinous space can be appreciated on frontal radiographs. The incidence of disc degeneration at this level 5 years later may be higher. (84) If found in combination with an absence of cord injury, it requires no special treatment. (73)
3. *Widened interspinous space.* A generalized multisegmental uniform widening of the interspinous space ("fanning") usually coexists with a comparable reversal of the cervical curve ("arcual kyphosis"). (Fig. 9.49, Fig. 9.50) At a single level ("divergent spinous process sign") this may denote significant posterior ligamentous injury and is readily recognised by an abrupt transition to kyphosis ("acute kyphosis sign"). (72,85) This is identifiable by the interspinous space being wider by

Table 9.9.   Soft Tissue Imaging Findings in Whiplash Injuries

Conventional Imaging
  Abnormal soft tissues
    Widened retropharyngeal space
    Widened retrotracheal space
    Displacement of prevertebral fat stripe
    Tracheal deviation and laryngeal dislocation
    Soft tissue emphysema
  Abnormal vertebral alignment
    Loss of the lordosis
    Acute kyphotic angulation
    Widened interspinous space
    Altered flexion patterns
    Vertebral body rotation
    Sagittal translation
    Torticollis
  Abnormal joints
    Widened median atlantoaxial joint (ADI)
    Widened or narrowed intervertebral disc
    Displaced ring epiphysis
    Widening of the zygapophyseal joint
Computed Tomography
  Herniated intervertebral disc
Magnetic Resonance Imaging
  Discovertebral endplate separations
  Anterior longitudinal ligament injuries
  Occult endplate fractures
  Disc herniation
  Cord injury
  Prevertebral edema or hematoma
Nuclear Bone Scan
  Occult fractures
  Negative for post injury inflammatory facet joint
Diagnostic Nerve Blocks
  Facet syndrome
Discography
  Internal disc disruption
  Pain provocation

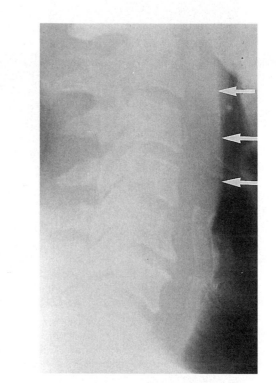

Figure 9.47. POSTTRAUMATIC RETROPHARYNGEAL HEMORRHAGE: CERVICAL SPINE. An abnormally increased retropharyngeal interspace (RPI) from C2 to C4 has occurred in the absence of fracture following a whiplash injury (arrows). (Courtesy of Norman W. Kettner, DC, DACBR, St. Louis, Missouri)

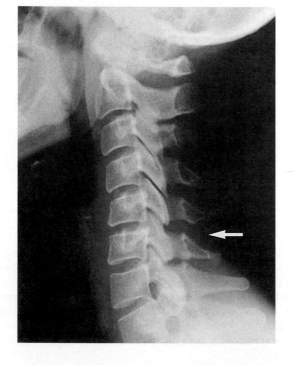

Figure 9.48. LOSS OF THE CERVICAL LORDOSIS. There is a loss of the cervical lordosis. Observe the degenerative disc disease at C5 at the apex of the kyphosis (arrow). COMMENT: Altered cervical patterns of lordosis may occur as a result of patient positioning, muscle spasm, or posterior ligamentous injury. An arcual kyphosis is often associated with muscle spasm, while the acute cervical kyphosis sign indicates localized intersegmental posterior ligamentous damage.

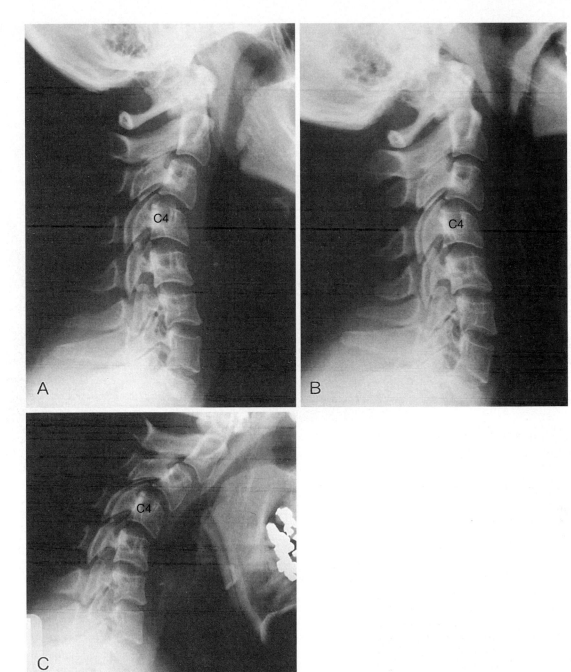

**Figure 9.49.   ARCUAL KYPHOSIS WITH C3-C4 AND C4-C5 INSTABIL-
ITY. A. Neutral Lateral Cervical.** There is marked reversal of the cervical
lordosis. Localized widening of the C3-C4 interspinous space is apparent
("divergent spinous process sign"). **B. Extension Cervical.** The curvature remains fixed with only slight extension of the atlas on the axis. **C. Flexion
Cervical.** At C3-C4 there is anterior translation and increased angular divergence between the segments. At C4-C5 less pronounced but similar changes
are apparent. Observe the distinct lack of intersegmental mobility from C5
to C7. COMMENT: This configuration of cervical curve reversal and isolated
intersegmental increased motion patterns may provide some circumstantial
evidence for ligamentous injury. Care must be taken however to correlate
the findings with the clinical history and presentation as such radiographic
findings can be found in the absence of significant trauma. (Courtesy of W.
Michael Spurlock, DC, Moorehead, Kentucky)

greater than 2 mm compared to other levels. Developmental
variation of the spinous processes can simulate ligamentous
disruption. (Fig. 9.50)
4. *Altered flexion patterns.* Four patterns of cervical flexion have
   been described in studies obtained shortly after trauma. (86)
   No intersegmental motion is seen in up to 25%, only at one
   level in 25%, at two levels in 30%, and at three or more in 20%

of cases. No movement or movement at only one level most
closely correlates with the presence of soft tissue injury. Three
or more levels of motion is a normal pattern.
5. *Vertebral body rotation.* Rotatory deformities can be subtle but
   important as they can accompany serious facet subluxation or
   even dislocation. These may be considered to occur in three
   planes but typically occur as combinations.

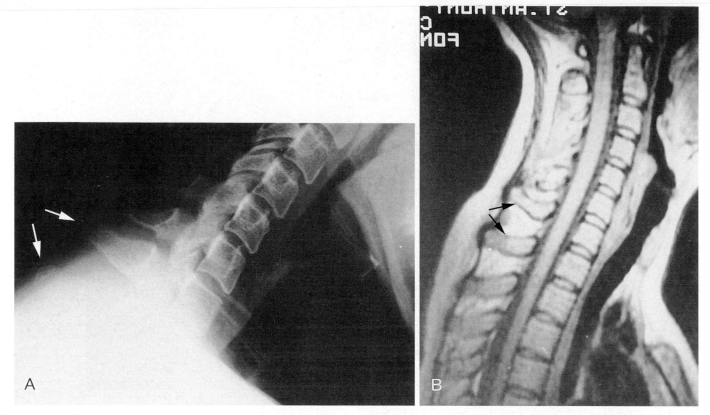

Figure 9.50.   PSEUDODIVERGENT SPINOUS PROCESS SIGN, C7-T1. A. Neutral Lateral Cervical. The interspinous process distance appears significantly increased between C7 and T1 (arrows). **B. MRI**. The increased interspinous distance is again observed though no underlying dislocation, disc or soft tissue injury is identified (arrows). COMMENT: A localized widening of the interspinous space suggests possible underlying instability, such as facet instability even dislocation ("divergent spinous process sign"). In this case developmental variation in spinous process orientation has simulated this finding ("pseudodivergent spinous process sign"). (Courtesy of Norman W. Kettner, DC, DACBR, St. Louis, Missouri)

Sagittal rotations (flexion-extension). Greater than 11.5° of intersegmental angular incongruence constitutes evidence for significant ligamentous injury. (85,87,88)

Coronal rotations (lateral flexion). Divergence of adjacent endplates may indicate facet instability with disruption of the joint capsule or even unilateral facet dislocation.

Axial rotations (rotatory). At mid and lower levels evidence for intersegmental rotation can be established by displacement of the spinous processes from the midline. (72) On the lateral film the articular pillars on the side of anterior rotation will lie superimposed over the vertebral bodies. Additionally the posterior borders of these pillars will be duplicated. Axial rotation may be due to torticollis, artifactual rotation of the head, or the first indication of a unilateral subluxation or even dislocation of a cervical facet joint. Rotatory subluxation of the atlantoaxial joint is often traumatically induced.

6. *Sagittal translation*. On the lateral study four lines ("cervical arc lines") are used. (70) These lines connect the anterior body margins, posterior body margins, spinolaminar junctions, and tips of the spinous processes and serve as useful visual inspection landmarks for identifying anteroposterior displacements. Such displacements are best demonstrated on flexion-extension studies. Greater than a total of 3.5 mm intersegmental excursion identifies clinically significant intersegmental instabilty. (87) (Fig. 9.51)

7. *Torticollis*. On the frontal study there is disparity in the levels of the inferior aspects of the mandible, scoliosis with coupled intersegmental motions of lateral flexion and rotation. (72)

Abnormal joints. Three joint complexes should be scrutinized for abnormal widening—the median atlantoaxial joint, the intervertebral disc spaces, and facet joints.

1. *Widened median atlantoaxial joint*. This is reflected in an increase of the atlantodental interspace (ADI) of more than 3 mm in adults and 5 mm in children. (72) It is due to posttraumatic disruption of the transverse ligament. (89) (Fig. 9.28)

2. *Widened or narrowed intervertebral disc*. Alterations in height and symmetry may signify significant discal injury. (72) Widening of a single space in the neutral position is a potentially serious marker of severe ligamentous disruption. Axial distraction may demonstrate alarming instability not otherwise apparent. On extension anterior "gaping" of a disc may correlate with disruption of the anterior longitudinal ligament. (72,75,90,91) Narrowing of a disc can correlate with disc rupture. (92) In the presence of a vertebral body compression fracture the disc adjacent is often narrowed due to disc disruption.

3. *Vacuum phenomenon*. The presence of a small, smooth lucent cleft ("vacuum phenomenon") adjacent to the anterior vertebral endplate often seen only on the extension lateral has been implicated as evidence of annular avulsion from the discovertebral junction. (93) (Fig.9.52) Contemporary opinion is that

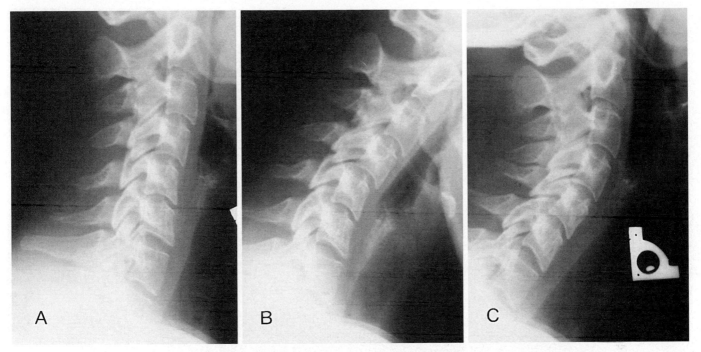

Figure 9.51.   STRESS EVALUATION IN LIGAMENTOUS INSTABILITY. A. Neutral Lateral Cervical. Anterolisthesis of C4 is accompanied by a widened interspinous space. **B. Lateral Cervical Flexion.** There is an increase in the anterolisthesis of C4 in the flexion attitude. **C. Lateral Cervical Extension.** A reduction of the anterolisthesis is noted in the extension position.

COMMENT: Radiologic signs of ligamentous instability may be minimal or absent on neutral cervical films. Flexion and extension radiographs are necessary to demonstrate the presence of intersegmental ligamentous instability which otherwise may be overlooked. (Courtesy of Kenneth E. Yochum, DC, St. Louis, Missouri)

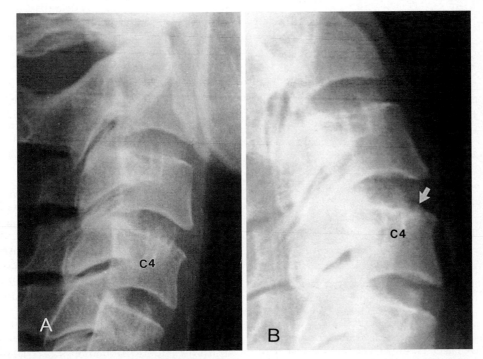

Figure 9.52.   VACUUM CLEFT SIGN. A. Neutral Lateral Cervical. Observe closely the discal area adjacent to the anterosuperior corner of the C4 vertebral endplate. No abnormality is seen. **B. Lateral Cervical Extension.** In the same area a radiolucent linear shadow has appeared due to a focal accumulation of nitrogen within an annular tear of the disc ("vacuum cleft"

sign) (arrow) COMMENT: The formation of this vacuum cleft sign is usually only identified on the extension radiograph. This is a subtle and often overlooked sign of a traumatic intervertebral disc injury, which is primarily seen in instances of whiplash. This may also be seen as a degenerative phenomenon. (Courtesy of Donald M. Kuppe, DC, Denver, Colorado)

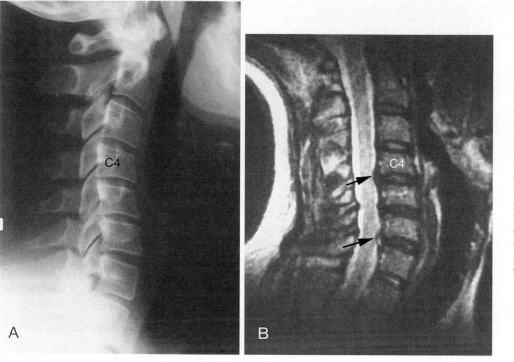

Figure 9.53.   INTERVERTEBRAL DISC HER-NIATION, WHIPLASH INJURY. A. Lateral Cervical Neutral. An arcual kyphosis is evident with generalized loss of intervertebral disc height at all levels. On flexion-extension there was generalized loss of intersegmental movement. **B. MRI.** Two intervertebral disc herniations can be seen indenting the ventral aspect of the thecal sac (arrows). COMMENT: MRI is particularly useful in whiplash patients who exhibit neurologic changes for which a cause cannot be determined. The finding of a disc herniation may not, however, determine if it is the result of the injury as it may have predated the event.

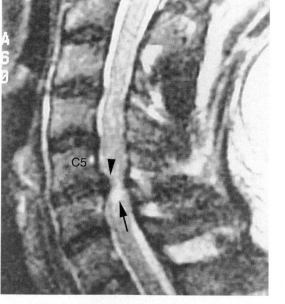

Figure 9.54.   SPINAL CORD EDEMA, MRI DEMONSTRATION. Observe the focal area of increased signal intensity within the cord representing edema (arrow). There is evidence of a disc herniation at C5 (arrowhead). COMMENT: This 35-year-old female had been involved in a motor vehicle accident and developed widespread upper and lower extremity migratory paresthesias. It is most likely that the cord edema has precipitated these symptoms, a finding that only MR imaging can identify.

such a finding is most commonly degenerative in nature and cannot be reliably linked to a traumatic lesion. (94)

4. *Displaced ring epiphysis.* A dislodged anterior ring epiphysis in a young patient is a bony marker of significant discovertebral injury and usually coexists with a prevertebral hematoma. (75,95,96) The superior epiphysis is displaced in flexion injuries while the inferior epiphysis avulses in extension trauma. (96)

5. *Widening of the zygapophyseal joint.* A joint space of more than 2mm may denote tearing of the facet joint capsule. (46,70,72) The tetrad of a wide facet joint, wide interspinous space, compression fracture, and loss of the cervical lordosis may denote significant tearing of the posterior ligamentous complex and instability. (97)

Computed Tomography (CT).   The primary role of CT is in the detection and assessment of fractures, disc herniations, prevertebral lesions and hematomas, relationship of bone fragments to the cord and actual cord lesions. (70)

Magnetic Resonance Imaging (MR).   Utilization of MR in the detection of soft tissue injuries in both the acute and chronic settings is often rewarding. MR clearly shows lesions of the ligaments, discs, cord, prevertebral tissues, and muscles that would otherwise be overlooked. (69,70,90)

Ligamentous lesions include rupture or incomplete tears, especially of the anterior longitudinal ligament. Healing of these structures can also be demonstrated. Discal abnormalities may include separations at the discovertebral junctions, annular avulsions, herniations, and progressive degenerative changes. (Fig. 9.53) Epidural hematomas, myelopathy, and cord edema are well depicted. (Fig. 9.54) Muscle tears, edema, and hematomas similarly can also be identified in other soft tissues.

Nuclear Bone Scan.   In the presence of fracture that may not be depicted by plain films, tomography, or even CT the sensitivity of scintigraphy may allow identification. However, it is not a useful procedure in identifying symptomatic joints that are not fractured, even when augmented by Single Photon Emission Computed Tomography (SPECT). (98) The isolation of anatomical sites of soft tissue injury in acutely injured patients has been demonstrated with technetium-99m scans. (99)

MEDICOLEGAL IMPLICATIONS
Whiplash Syndrome

- The first priority is to exclude the presence of fracture, significant instability, and dislocation. High quality radiographs with sufficient projections are essential. There should be clear differentiation between congenital variations, pseudofractures, artifacts, and positional errors which may be simulating traumatic lesions. (Fig. 9.55)

- Prognosis is multifactorial, embracing clinical, psychosocial, and medicolegal issues. (62,100,101) There is a paucity of meaningful and reliable data upon which to predict an outcome. (62,102,103) Increasing age, cognitive impairment, and severity of initial neck pain have been shown to be predictive for persistent neck pain after 6 months. (104) Other associations, but not predictive of a poor outcome include, objective neurologic signs, degenerative changes, and thoracolumbar pain. (73,105–107) The role of secondary gain ("litigation neurosis") in recovery remains controversial. (62)

- A constellation of imaging findings have been at varying times purported to be of prognostic significance including preexisting degenerative changes, (108) segmentation defects (congenital and acquired block vertebrae, Klippel–Feil syndrome, occipitalisation), (108–110) narrowed central canal, (108) intersegmental instability, (108) altered cervical lordosis, and intervertebral disc vacuum phenomena. Reversal of the lordosis does not appear to be associated with long term disability. (84,107) Prevertebral swelling does not diminish long term prognosis. (73)

- Degenerative changes found on a patient some time after the injury are difficult to evaluate as to whether they were caused by the injury or predated it. Previous films are helpful. It is known that if degenerative changes are present at the time of injury the prognosis is poor. (105,106) In the presence of degenerative spondylosis, hyperextension can precipitate cord edema and hematomyelia due to a pinching mechanism between the anterior protruding disc-osteophyte complex and thickened posterior ligamentum flavum. Current literature supports that whiplash injuries do predispose to premature disc disease. (90,104,109)

- Restricted posttraumatic cervical motion has been shown to develop a high incidence of degenerative changes in the following five years. (84) The earliest plain film findings of degenerative disc disease, including loss of disc height and early osteophyte formation, may be demonstrated as early as 3 months following injury. Patients undergoing discectomy for unresolved discogenic pain following whiplash do so at an average of 8 years post injury. (109)

- Following acute injury, plain films are often normal despite significant disc or cord trauma. MR may show diminished disc hydration within weeks of the injury. (93) Additionally, posttraumatic cord edema may be demonstrated only with MR. (111)

Dislocations of the Cervical Spine

Atlanto-Occipital Dislocation. This is a rare and usually fatal injury following hyperextension and distraction applied to the head. (112) The injury is more prevalent in pediatric patients, who survive three times more often than adults. (113) Most dislocations of the cranium occur in an anterior direction and can be detected by specific measurement methods (See Chapter 2). (114,115) (Fig. 9.56A–C) The injury usually results from motor vehicle accidents—more frequently in pedestrians, though falls from heights and neonatal forceps delivery have been described. (113)

Atlantoaxial Dislocation. Anterior atlantoaxial dislocation has been discussed under "Rupture of the Transverse Ligament."

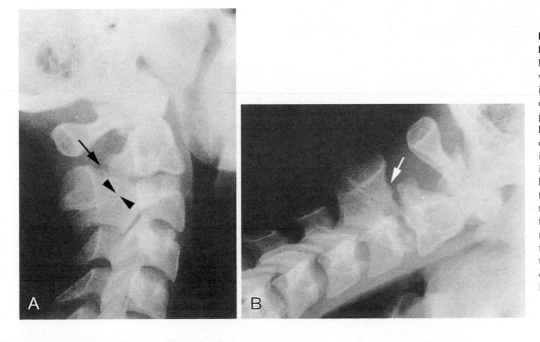

Figure 9.55. CONGENITAL SPONDYLOLYSIS SIMULATING FRACTURE. A. Neutral Lateral Cervical. A wide cleft is visible extending through the pedicle-lamina region of the axis (arrow). Note the congenital fusion of the C2-C3 spinous process, lamina, and facets (arrowheads). **B. Flexion Cervical.** The separating pedicle-lamina cleft widens (arrow), but there is no direct evidence for significant C2-C3 instability. COMMENT: The patient had been in a motor vehicle accident, and on the basis of this film, was initially thought to have developed a hangman's fracture of the axis. The recognition of associated markers for an underlying congenital basis for the appearance, however, confirms that this abnormality was a preexisting condition. (Courtesy of Ted F. Durling, DC, FACO, New Port Richey, Florida)

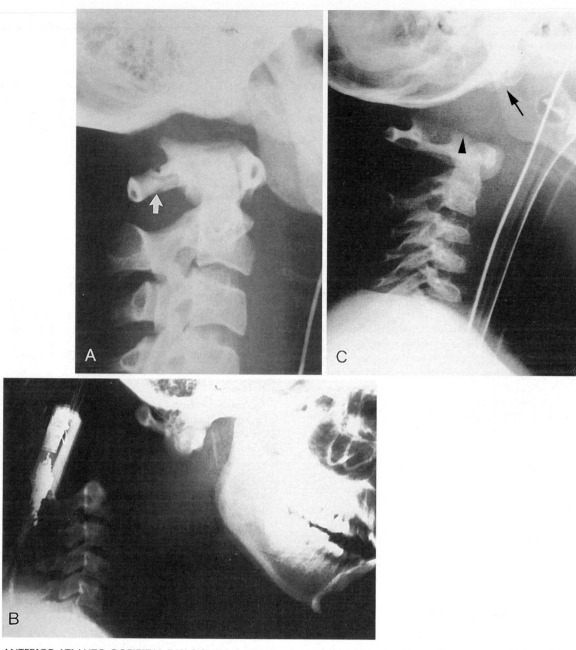

Figure 9.56.   ANTERIOR ATLANTO-OCCIPITAL DISLOCATION: CERVI-CAL SPINE. A. Vertical Translation. Complete vertical dislocation of the occipital condyles upon the atlas has occurred. Note the associated posterior arch fracture of the atlas (arrow). (Courtesy of Steven B. Wasserman, DC, Long Beach, California) **B. Severe Anterior Dislocation.** This extreme degree of translation and distraction has a poor prognosis. (Courtesy of Rebecca Kane, DC, New York, New York) **C. Pediatric Anterior Dislocation.** This 4- year-old was involved in a rollover motor vehicle accident where the neck became entrapped in a shoulder strap exerting a distraction type force. The occipital condyles (arrow) are well displaced from the atlas lateral masses (arrowhead). (Courtesy of Alan Plunkett MD, Denver, Colorado) COMMENT: These injuries are frequently fatal, follow severe trauma—usually motor vehicle accidents—and most frequently are found in pedestrians.

Rotary atlantoaxial fixation (subluxation) is a unique condition of the upper cervical complex that is frequently undiagnosed and poorly understood. (116) First described by Corner in 1907, (117) the exact pathophysiology remains enigmatic though spontaneous occurrence, trauma (even minor), upper respiratory tract infection, oral surgery, and inflammatory arthritis are known precipitants. (118) Proposed theories focus on joint effusion, tearing of the atlantoaxial joint capsule, and the entrapment of intraarticular inclusions (fibroadipose meniscoids, fat pads, synovium, capsular rims). (116,118–120) It is more common in children. Clin- ically the acute patient exhibits torticollis, the head is held in the ''cock robin'' position (lateral flexion, rotated to the opposite side and slight flexion), neck pain is prominent, and there often is subjective upper limb weakness without objective neurologic deficit. Some resolve with no sequelae; others follow a chronic course with persistent head tilt, neck pain and reduced range of motion. Treatment consists of hospitalization with cervical traction for up to 7 weeks followed by a cervical collar for several months. (116) Unresolved cases, especially types II–IV may require posterior Gallie fusion. The efficacy and role of active manipulation has not been investigated though some authors consider it a contraindication. (116)

Four types have been described (118):

Type I: Rotatory fixation without anterior displacement and within the normal range of motion. This is the most common type.

Type II: Rotatory fixation with 3–5 mm anterior dispacement of the atlas.

Type III: Rotatory fixation with more than 5 mm anterior displacement of the atlas.

Type IV: Rotatory fixation with posterior displacement of the atlas. The odontoid needs to be defficient to allow this type.

Diagnosis depends on radiographic findings with adequate views which are technically difficult to obtain due to the head and neck distortion. (Fig. 9.57A–D) On the frontal view the key findings are: (a) on the side of anterior rotation the atlas lateral mass is wider and closer to the dens; (b) on the side of posterior rotation the lateral mass is narrower and away from the dens, while the atlantoaxial joint space is obscured; and (c) the axis spinous process may be rotated. (118) The presence of fixation is demonstrated when these findings remain unchanged with four additional frontal views: views obtained in 15° lateral right & left bending and another pair in 15° of right & left rotation. (119,121)

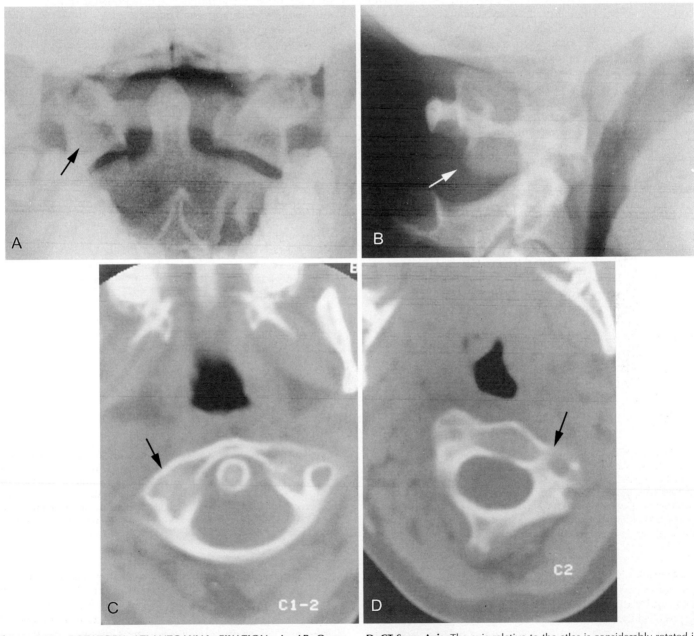

Figure 9.57. ROTATORY ATLANTOAXIAL FIXATION. A. AP Open Mouth. There is a distinct discrepancy in the width of the lateral masses of the atlas with the narrow side posteriorly rotated (arrow). **B. Lateral Cervical Neutral**. Note the altered appearance of the atlas. The posteriorly rotated lateral mass can be seen (arrow). **C. CT Scan, Atlas.** The cranium and atlas maintain their normal alignment with posterior rotation on the left (arrow).

D. CT Scan, Axis. The axis relative to the atlas is considerably rotated in a contralateral direction (arrow). COMMENT: These are characteristic findings of rotatory atlantoaxial fixation. If functional views were obtained in bilateral 15°, lateral bending, and rotation these features would not change. (Courtesy of Thomas Ulmer, DC, Sioux Falls, South Dakota)

On the lateral film the only features may be an increased atlantodental interspace more than 3 mm, visualisation of the entire atlas posterior arch as a ringlike structure, and a lateral flexion-rotation of the cervical spine due to torticollis. CT scan is the definitive method of diagnosis which can employ the same principals of unchanged relationships on right and left rotation in relation to the static position. (121)

Bilateral Interfacetal Dislocation (BID).   Bilateral interfacetal dislocation is the result of a severe hyperflexion injury and is most often found affecting C4 through C7. This injury primarily involves the soft tissues rather than fracture of the skeletal structures. (Fig. 9.58A and B) Those soft tissue structures that are torn are the posterior longitudinal ligament, the posterior ligamentous complex, the annulus fibrosus, and, occasionally, the anterior longitudinal ligament. Disc herniations are common. (122) Bilateral interfacetal dislocation is an unstable lesion that has a high incidence of cord injuries. Dislocation is more prone to occur one segment above a congenitally or surgically fused segment. (123) Anatomically, the superior facets are seen to lie fully anterior to the inferior facets and in such a position are referred to as being "locked" since they will not reposition spontaneously.

In a complete bilateral interfacetal dislocation the facets come to lie within the intervertebral foramina. The body of the dislocated segment is usually displaced anteriorly a distance greater than one half of the anteroposterior diameter of the body below. (124) If the dislocation is incomplete, oblique radiographs will establish the bilaterality of the lesion. On axial CT images the absence of one articular surface at a single facet joint due to dislocation may be seen ("naked facet sign"). Dislocations at the cervicothoracic junction are notoriously difficult and may be suspected on plain films (divergent spinous processes, prevertebral fat stripe displacement, posterior cervical line, widened interspinous distance) and confirmed with CT or MR imaging. (125)

Chip fractures from the tip of the articulating processes are often found in association with bilateral interfacetal dislocation. Surgical arthrodesis is the usual mode of treatment. (Fig. 9.58B)

Unilateral Interfacetal Dislocation (UID).   Unilateral interfacetal dislocation is one of the few injuries caused by a flexion/rotation force. The rotational injury occurs around one of the interfacetal joints, causing it to dislocate into the intervertebral foramen and is sometimes referred to as a "jumped facet." (Fig. 9.59A–C) In this position the dislocated articular mass is mechanically locked in a dislocated position.

On the lateral radiograph, unilateral interfacetal dislocation is characterized by forward displacement of the vertebral body. Alteration in the superimposition of the articular pillars on the lateral view represents a subtle sign of unilateral interfacetal dislocation. (126) The combination of the anteriorly displaced articular pillar with its former opposing pillar produces the "bow tie sign." Frontal radiographs reveal upward rotation of the spinous process of the dislocated segment, the level marked by a sudden intersegmental rotational deformity. (126) Oblique projections are necessary to identify the dislocated facet joint. On axial CT unilateral absence of one facet surface can be present ("naked facet sign") though the appearance of a false joint can be simulated. (127)

MEDICOLEGAL IMPLICATIONS
Cervical Spine Injuries

- The minimum study is an AP open mouth, AP lower cervical, right and left obliques, and a lateral view. Supplemental projections include flexion, extension, and pillar views, as indicated by mechanism of injury, clinical findings, and abnormalities visible on initial studies.

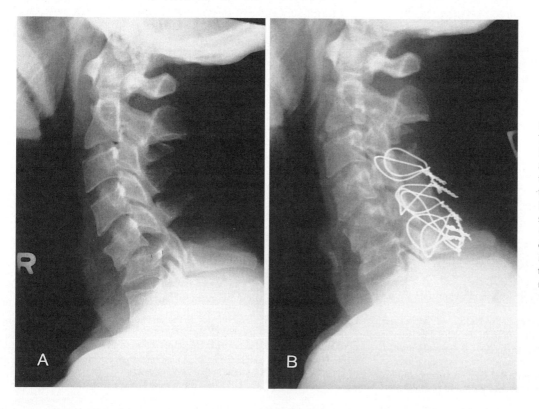

Figure 9.58. BILATERAL INTERFACETAL DISLOCATION. A. Lateral Cervical. Notice the displacement of the superior anterior articular pillar of C5 in conjunction with an acute deflection deformity of the vertebral body. **B. Lateral Cervical.** Postsurgical reduction and wire arthrodesis of the previous interfacetal dislocation. COMMENT: A bilateral interfacetal dislocation frequently remains locked, requiring surgical reduction and fusion. Observe the acute widening of the C5-C6 interspinous space.

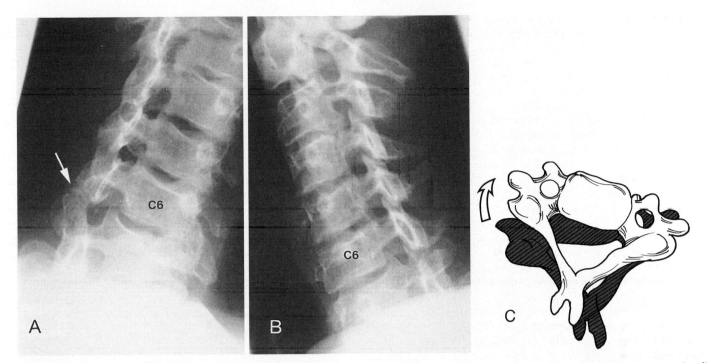

Figure 9.59.   UNILATERAL INTERFACETAL DISLOCATION: C6. A. Cervical Oblique. Observe the altered contour to the C6 IVF, with anterior displacement of the articular pillar and vertebral body (arrow). **B. Opposite Cervical Oblique**. No abnormality is visible, with a normally shaped intervertebral foramen, articular pillar, and vertebral body alignment. **C. Sche-**matic Diagram. Unilateral interfacetal dislocation occurs in an anterior direction, following a severe rotational trauma. COMMENT: Unilateral interfacetal dislocations are frequently overlooked and are best visualized on oblique radiographs.

- Close inspection for odontoid and atlas fractures with adequate AP open mouth or specific odontoid views must be obtained in cervical spine trauma. Consideration should be given to supplemental tomography or reconstructed CT images in questionable cases or to exclude pseudofractures due to overlying structures and mach bands (teeth, tongue, etc.)

- Inclusion of "all seven" vertebrae on lateral views should be attempted as is practicable to identify obscured fractures and dislocations of the cervicothoracic and craniocervical junctions. Supplemental views may be required (e.g., "swimmer's lateral").

- Evidence for intersegmental instabilities clinically and on the lateral view should be searched for prior to performing flexion-extension studies.

- Recognition of preexisting congenital variations (block vertebra, odontoid anomalies), degenerative diseases (disc degeneration, DISH), or other disease states should be made and correlated with the mechanism of trauma and the resultant clinical features.

- In the presence of posttraumatic neurologic deficits, even with normal radiographs consideration of MR imaging (when available) should be contemplated to determine cord or nerve root injury. CT with myelography may be useful if MR is not available.

FRACTURES AND DISLOCATIONS OF THE THORACIC SPINE
Compression Fracture

The most common site for thoracic spine compression fractures is between T11-T12 due to a combination of axial and flexion injury. (128) Compression fractures between the T4 and T8 segments occasionally occur in association with injuries related to convulsions or electric shock therapy as a result of violent contractions of the thoracic and abdominal muscles. Most compression fractures in the thoracic spine are wedge shaped, with few having any associated neurologic deficit unless there is significant retropulsion of fragments into the spinal canal. (Figs. 9.60A–C, 9.61) The presence of a paraspinal mass (edema) may be an indirect clue to the presence of a fracture. Pathologic fractures may be identified by loss of the posterior body height, pedicle and other structures, and a paraspinal mass. On MR imaging, abnormal marrow can be demonstrated. (Fig 9.62) Additional views (swimmer's lateral), tomography, CT, and MR imaging may be necessary in order to demonstrate fractures of the thoracic spine and assess involvement of the spinal cord. (128)

Radiographic signs of compression fracture are covered under "Fractures and Dislocations of the Lumbar Spine."

Fracture Dislocation

Fracture dislocation of the thoracic spine occurs most often in the T4-T7 area. Fractures of the lamina, facets, or vertebral bodies are often associated (Fig. 9.63) and paralysis is a frequent complication since the spinal canal is small and the blood supply is relatively sparse. (129) A great majority of these patients have been in severe automobile accidents; and these injuries are particularly common in motorcyclists who have been catapaulted into stationary objects. (130) Radiographic depiction can be initially difficult and requires an overpenetrated frontal view. Features consist of loss of vertebral body height, displacement, widened interpediculate distance and paraspinal widening. (128,130)

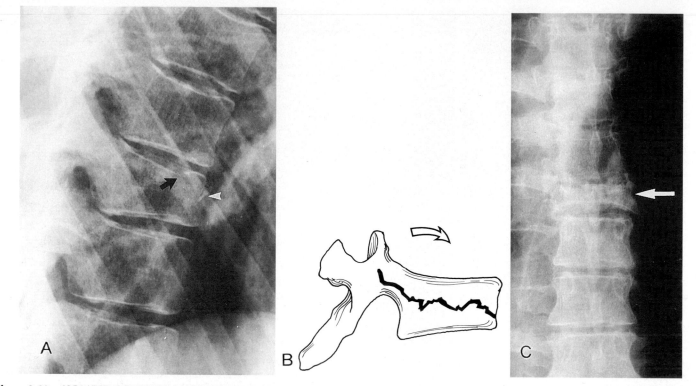

Figure 9.60.   ISOLATED COMPRESSION FRACTURE: THORACIC SPINE. A. Lateral Projection. Focal depression of the superior endplate (arrow) of the T10 vertebral body, with a displaced anterior fracture fragment (arrowhead), is identified. A characteristic trapezoidal vertebral shape has been formed due to anterior compression of the superior vertebral endplate. (Courtesy of Richard M. Nuzzi, DC, Denver, Colorado) **B. Schematic Diagram.** The usual precipitating force is an anterior compression injury focusing the compressive forces to the anterior aspect of the vertebral body. **C. AP Projection.** The most notable features are a decrease in vertebral height, with approximation of the vertebral endplates, and associated lateral displacement of the vertebral body margins (arrow). (Courtesy of Lawrence P. Rosenbaum, MA, DC, MD, Linkoping, Sweden)

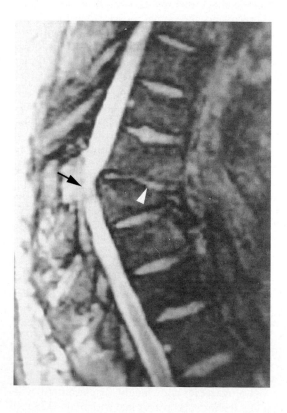

Figure 9.61.   COMPRESSION FRACTURE WITH CORD COMPROMISE, MRI. An anterior wedged compression fracture can be delineated at T7 (arrowhead). There has been retropulsion of the posterior aspect of the vertebral body compromising the spinal canal and distorting the spinal cord (arrow). The patient was rendered paraplegic from the injury, incurred from a motorcycle accident.

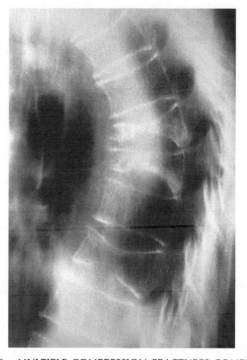

Figure 9.62. MULTIPLE COMPRESSION FRACTURES COMPLICATING OSTEOPOROSIS. Multiple compression fractures are present within the midthoracic spine, as evidenced by decreased anterior body height and biconcave deformities of the vertebral endplates. COMMENT: Thoracic wedge compression fractures are a frequent complications of osteoporosis and may accentuate the kyphotic curvature. The loss of posterior vertebral body height is consistent with a pathologic fracture, the differential diagnosis include causes of osteopenia such as postmenopausal osteoporosis, multiple myeloma, and metastatic carcinoma.

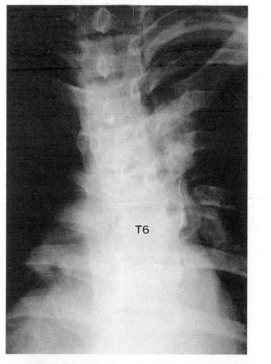

Figure 9.63. FRACTURE DISLOCATION: THORACIC SPINE. There has been a compression deformity of the T5 vertebral body, in combination with a lateral dislocation of the fractured segment. COMMENT: Fracture dislocations of this variety are frequently associated with severe trauma and complicating paralysis.

Associated injuries include fractures elsewhere, aortic arch tears, sternal fractures, thoracic disc herniation, instability and rarely Kummel's disease (delayed posttraumatic vertebral collapse due to complicating avascular necrosis). (128,129)

MEDICOLEGAL IMPLICATIONS
Thoracic Spine Injuries

- Minimum study consists of AP and lateral views. Supplemental projections of the cervicothoracic and thoracolumbar regions are often required to overcome exposure difficulties.

- Instances of persistent pain or neurologic deficits even in the absence of plain film findings may require further imaging such as CT and MRI. Bone scan findings may reveal evidence of subtle compression or other fracture.

- Subtle compression fractures are readily overlooked. Careful attention to the anterior body margin for evidence of a "step" sign and displacement of the paraspinal line may reveal the only clues to the presence of fracture.

- Key variants should not be confused with evidence of fracture—physiologic wedging up to 5°, Schmorl's nodes, Scheuermann's disease, degenerative osteophytes, and Hahn's venous channel.

- Compression fractures in the absence of significant trauma should raise the suspicion of an underlying pathology. Loss of posterior vertebral body height is indicative of pathologic fracture and should instigate a search for its cause including the many etiologies of osteoporosis, multiple myeloma, and metastatic carcinoma.

FRACTURES AND DISLOCATIONS OF THE LUMBAR SPINE
Compression Fractures

Compression fractures are the most common fractures of the lumbar spine. They result from combined flexion and axial compression. (131,132) The most common segmental levels to develop compression fractures are T12-L1. (133) The extent of the vertebral compression and degree of comminution are dependent upon the severity of the force applied and the relative strength of the vertebra. (14) In children they are torus-type fractures. In the elderly, osteoporosis can precipitate spontaneous compression fractures during everyday activities, which technically render them classifiable as insufficiency fractures ("grandma fracture"). Up to 35% of compression fractures in female patients over the age of 45 years may be due to early menopause and 30% to secondary osteopenia, most often from corticosteroids (15%), hyperthyroidism (8%), and malignancy (less than 2%). (134) The disruption of the cortical vertebral endplate causes acute symptoms of only 10–14 days duration, as long as no dislocations accompany the fracture. (135)

Post-fracture stability is determined based on the classification by Denis. (136) Three columns are recognized: anterior column (from the anterior longitudinal ligament to the midvertebral body), middle column (from the midvertebral body to the posterior longitudinal ligament), and the posterior column (from the posterior longitudinal ligament to the supraspinous ligament). If

Table 9.10.   Radiologic/Pathologic Correlation in Compression Fractures

Radiologic	Pathologic
Step defect	Cortical offset
Wedge deformity	Anterior impaction
Linear zone of condensation	Impaction, callus
Endplate displacement	Impaction, disruption
Paraspinal swelling, psoas obliterations	Bleeding, edema
Abnormal small bowel gas	Reflex adynamic ileus

two or more compartments are disrupted the fracture complex is unstable. The likelihood of neurologic injury is high and interventional surgery is likely to be necessary.

Radiographic Signs of Vertebral Compression Fracture. Radiographs of optimum quality are necessary in order to adequately demonstrate these fractures. Lateral radiographs best demonstrate fracture features. Radiographic signs of vertebral compression fracture include a step defect, wedge deformity, linear zone of condensation, displaced endplate, paraspinal edema, and abdominal ileus. (Table 9.10)

The Step Defect. (Fig. 9.64A–C) Since the anterior aspect of the vertebral body is under the greatest stress, the first bony injury to occur is a buckling of the anterior cortex, usually near the superior vertebral endplate. This sign is best seen on the lateral view as a sharp step off of the anterosuperior vertebral margin along the smooth concave edge of the vertebral body. In subtle com-

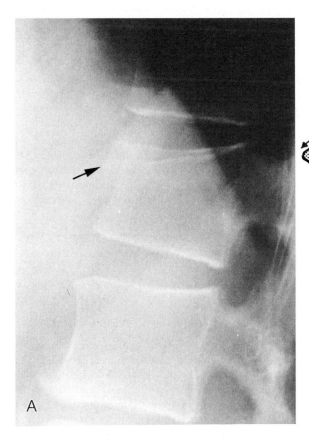

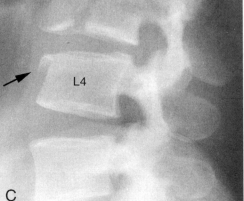

Figure 9.64.   COMPRESSION FRACTURE: STEP DEFECT. A. Single Level. The L1 vertebral body is wedge-shaped with a characteristic "step defect" evident at the anterosuperior border (arrow). **B. Schematic Diagram: Step Defect. C. Lateral Lumbar Spine**. Step defects (arrows) are present at the anterosuperior corners of the L2 and L4 vertebral bodies, along with a minimal decrease in the anterior vertebral body height. There is an unusual vertical fracture line through the vertebral body of L3 ("acquired coronal cleft vertebra"). COMMENT: This step defect may be the only sign of an acute vertebral body fracture. With time, this fracture fragment will be remodeled and will no longer be visible. (Reprinted with permission: Yochum TR, et al: *Compression fractures of L2 and L4: An L3 vertical vertebral body fracture.* ACA J Chiro, Radiology Corner, August 1982)

pression fractures the "step" defect may be the only radiographic sign of fracture. Anatomically, the actual step off deformity represents the anteriorly displaced corner of the superior vertebral cortex. As the superior endplate is compressed in flexion, a sliding forward of the vertebral endplate occurs, creating this roentgen sign. (Fig. 9.64B)

Wedge Deformity. (Fig. 9.65A–D) In most compression fractures an anterior depression of the vertebral body occurs, creating a triangular wedge shape. The posterior vertebral height remains uncompromised, differentiating a traumatic fracture from a pathologic fracture. This wedging may create angular kyphosis in the adjacent area. The superior endplate is far more often involved than the inferior endplate. Up to 30% or greater loss in anterior height may be required before the deformity is readily apparent on conventional lateral radiographs of the spine. (137) Normal variant anterior wedging of 10 to 15% or 1–3 mm is common throughout the thoracic spine, and most marked at T11-L2. (138,139)

In all compression fractures there should be clear differentiation from an underlying pathology that has produced the fracture. Key features of pathologic fractures include loss of the posterior body height, pedicle, and other structures. There may be a paraspinal mass. On MR imaging abnormal marrow can be demonstrated. (140)

Linear White Band of Condensation (Zone of Impaction). Occasionally, a band of radiopacity may be seen just below the vertebral endplate which has been fractured. The radiopaque band represents the early site of bone impaction following a forceful flexion injury where the bones are driven together. (Fig. 9.66A and B) Callus formation adds to the density of the radiopaque band later, in the healing stage of the fracture injury. This radiographic sign

is striking when present; however, it is an unreliable sign, since it is not present as often as might be expected. Its presence, however, denotes a fracture of recent origin (less than 2 months' duration).

Disruption in the Vertebral Endplate. A sharp disruption in the fractured vertebral endplate may be seen with spinal compression fracture. (Fig. 9.67A and B) This may be difficult to perceive on plain films and tomography; CT provides the definitive means of identification. The edges of the disruption are often jagged and irregular. The superior endplate is more commonly fractured than the inferior endplate.

Paraspinal Edema. In cases of extensive trauma unilateral or bilateral paraspinal masses may occur which represent hemorrhage. These are best seen in the thoracic spine on the anteroposterior projection but may occur adjacent to the lumbar spine, creating asymmetrical densities or bulges in the psoas margins.

Abdominal Ileus. This may occur with severe spinal trauma and is a warning sign to the observer that the trauma has been severe and the likelihood of fracture is great. Abdominal ileus is seen radiographically as excessive amounts of small or large bowel gas in a slightly distended lumen. (Fig. 9.68A and B) It occurs as a result of disturbance to the visceral autonomic nerves or ganglia from pain, paraspinal soft tissue injury, edema, or hematoma.

Determining an Old Versus a New Compression Fracture

Differentiation between old and recent compression fracture is often difficult. (Table 9.11) In general the presence of a soft tissue hemorrhage, "step" defect, and the white band of condensation are signs of an active or current fracture (less than 2 months

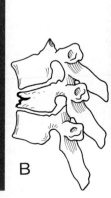
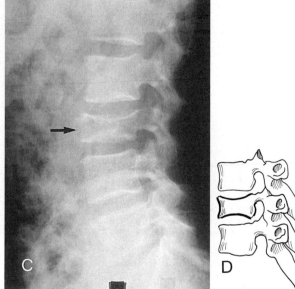

Figure 9.65. TRAUMATIC VERSUS PATHOLOGIC VERTEBRAL BODY COMPRESSION FRACTURES. A. Lateral Thoracolumbar: Traumatic Compression Fracture. A characteristic trapezoidal configuration of the vertebral body is identified. **B. Schematic Diagram: Traumatic Compression Fracture. C. Pathologic Compression Fracture.** Observe the uniform collapse of the L3 vertebral body (arrow). A subtle loss of bone density due to multiple myeloma accompanies this deformity. **D. Schematic Diagram: Pathologic**

Compression Fracture. COMMENT: In all compression fractures of the spine the posterior aspect of the vertebral body must be assessed. A decrease in this posterior dimension, a radiographic sign which is not found in traumatic benign compression fractures signifies underlying bone pathology. The most common causes for pathologic fractures of this nature are metastatic carcinoma and multiple myeloma.

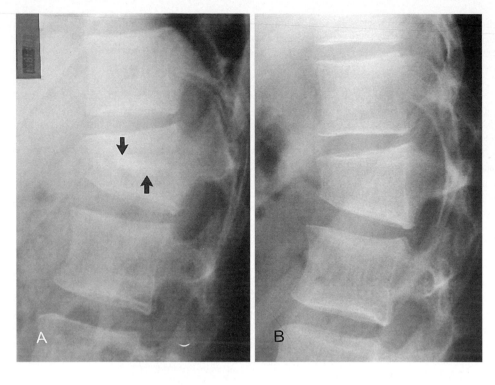

Figure 9.66.   COMPRESSION FRACTURE WITH A ZONE OF IMPACTION. A. Lateral Thoracolumbar Spine. A linear radiopaque band extends through the midportion of the L1 vertebral body (arrows). This represents the area of trabecular impaction, resulting in a trapezoid deformity of the vertebral body. B. Lateral Thoracolumbar Projection: 3 Years Later. Absence of the zone of impaction signifies a resolved compression fracture; however, the trapezoid deformity of the vertebral body remains permanent.

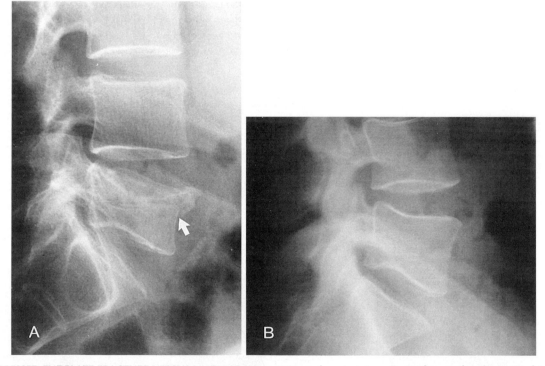

Figure 9.67.   DEPRESSED ENDPLATE FRACTURE VERSUS NUCLEAR IMPRESSION DEFORMITY. A. Compression Fracture: Lateral Lumbar. Significant depression of the superior endplate of the L5 vertebral body, along with a "step defect" (arrow) at the anterosuperior corner, are characteristic signs of acute injury. B. Nuclear Deformity: Lateral Lumbar Spine. The broad-based, smooth indentation of the inferior surface of the L5 vertebral endplate is characteristic of a nuclear impression (notochordal persistence), and no acute disruption of the vertebral endplate is demonstrated.

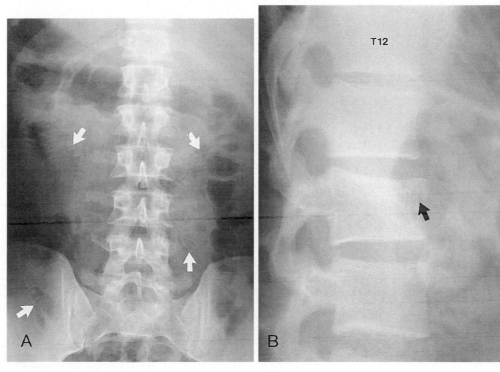

Figure 9.68. ABDOMINAL ILEUS ASSOCIATED WITH VERTEBRAL COMPRESSION FRACTURE. A. AP Lumbar Spine. An excessive amount of small bowel gas is seen (arrows), along with distention of its lumen. **B. Lateral Lumbar Spine**. A wedge type compression fracture, along with a "step"

defect (arrow), is present at the superior vertebral endplate of L2. COMMENT: The paralytic form of abdominal ileus is often seen following severe trauma and, when present, indicates a likelihood of associated fracture.

Table 9.11.   Radiologic Criteria for Determining Old and New Compression Fractures of the Spine

	Old	New
Shape	Wedge	Wedge
Step defect	Absent	Present
Band of condensation	Absent	Present
Degenerative disc	Present	Absent
Bone scan	Negative/Positive	Positive

old). These signs vanish with the healing that may take up to 3 months in the adult spine. The presence of contiguous disc degeneration is common in old compression fractures due to altered discovertebral mechanics.

Radionuclide bone scan may be helpful showing increased uptake ("hot spot") with recent fractures undergoing active repair. (135) These fractures however may remain active for up to 18–24 months following injury, which diminishes its usefulness. (135)

Burst Fractures

A burst fracture is a specific form of compression fracture of the vertebral body wherein a posterosuperior fragment is displaced into the spinal canal. (141) Considerable forces of axial compression and flexion create a burst fracture. Posteriorly displaced bone fragments may cause neurologic injury in up to 50% of cases to the spinal cord, conus medullaris or cauda equina which is best demonstrated by CT and MRI. (133)

On the frontal radiograph a vertical fracture line is often seen,

a characteristic that helps differentiate the simple wedge compression fracture from the burst fracture. (Fig. 9.69A and B) Widening of the interpediculate distance on conventional frontal films signifies a fracture within the neural arch. In patients with relatively normal discs a coronally oriented fracture may separate the vertebral body into anterior and posterior halves ("acquired coronal cleft vertebra"). (142) (Fig. 9.64C) Central depression of the superior and inferior endplates occurs with comminution of the vertebral body and is best seen on the lateral film. Careful examination of the posterior vertebral body surface (posterior vertebral body line, George's line) may identify the posteriorly displaced fragment, though CT is most definitive. (143) On CT images the degree of fragmentation is determined as well as defining any retropulsed fragments and associated neural arch fractures. MR imaging is used in the assessment of neurologic involvement. (Fig. 9.70A and B)

Posterior Apophyseal Ring Fractures

Separation of the posterior vertebral body ring apophysis (posterior limbus bone) is a relatively uncommon abnormality. Though more common in adolescents and young adults, it can be encountered into the fourth decade due to delayed apophyseal fusion. (144) Clinical features include stiffness and spasm, numbness, weakness, neurogenic claudication and, occasionally, cauda eqina syndrome. (144,145) Some will be found with no associated clinical findings. The most common levels are L4-L5 and L5-S1 respectively, though all lumbar levels can be affected, even T12. (144–146) Trauma, including motor vehicle accidents, weight lifting, and gymnastics constitute up to 50% of known precipitants. (144) Surgical removal may be indicated after failure of conser-

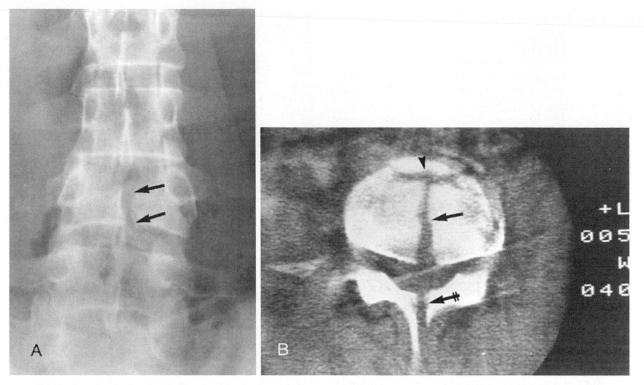

Figure 9.69.   BURST FRACTURE: LUMBAR SPINE. A. AP Lumbar Spine. There is a vertical fracture line through the vertebral body of L4 (arrows). **B. Computed Tomogram: L4.** The vertical fracture line in the body of L4 is observed (arrow). A transverse vertebral body fracture (arrowhead), and a fracture through the lamina (crossed arrow) are well demonstrated on this computed tomogram. (Courtesy of Gary L. Whitehead, DC, Las Vegas, Nevada)

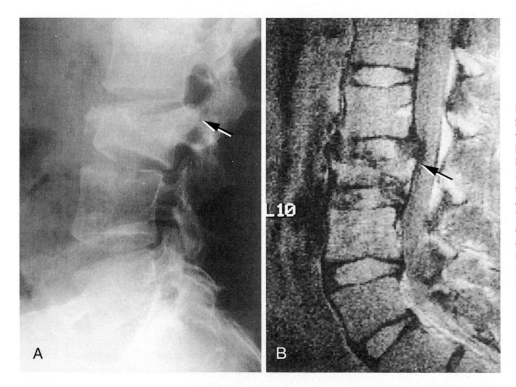

Figure 9.70.   BURST FRACTURE: LUMBAR SPINE. A. Lateral Lumbar Spine. There is a wedged-shaped deformity of the L3 vertebral body with a disruption of the posterior vertebral body line (George's line) due to a retropulsed fragment (arrow). **B. MRI Sagittal Image.** The effect of the retropulsed fragment (arrow) on the adjacent cauda equina can be appreciated. COMMENT: The recognition of the retropulsed fragment is decisive in assessing the neurologic relevance of a compression fracture. This fragment carries a substantial risk for inducing significant neurologic deficits. (Courtesy of Robert M. Kelty, DC, Central Point, Oregon)

vative care and in the presence of significant neurologic compromise. (144,147)

Various morphologic types are described, including simple central separation of the entire posterior rim, the central rim with some underlying vertebral body, posterolateral separations and those that extend well beyond the body margins. (144,146) Co-existing disc herniation is common.

Approximately 15 to 20% will be visible on plain film examination, usually the lateral view. (144) (Fig. 9.71A–C) A thin linear arc of calcification may be seen extending from near the posterior body corner across the intervertebral disc. A posterior focal Schmorl's node may be seen and the disc height can be marginally diminished. CT is the definitive method for identifying the separated fragment, the indentation from its site of origin, the associated disc herniation, and the effective compromise of the spinal canal and neural contents. MR imaging is generally ineffective in identifying the separated rim. (144)

Kummel's Disease

Kummel was the first to describe delayed posttraumatic vertebral collapse, originally describing a rarefying process in the vertebral bodies of an injured patient occurring months after an episode of spinal trauma. (148) The existence of this condition is controversial with few cases reported. (149–151) It appears to be due to complicating avascular necrosis resulting in progessive compression deformity. An intravertebral vacuum phenomenon may be evident on radiographic examination. (151)

Fractures of the Neural Arch

Transverse Process Fractures. Transverse process fractures are the second most common fractures of the lumbar spine, with compression fracture being the most common. They occur from avulsion of the paraspinal muscles usually secondary to a severe hyperextension and lateral flexion blow to the lumbar spine. The

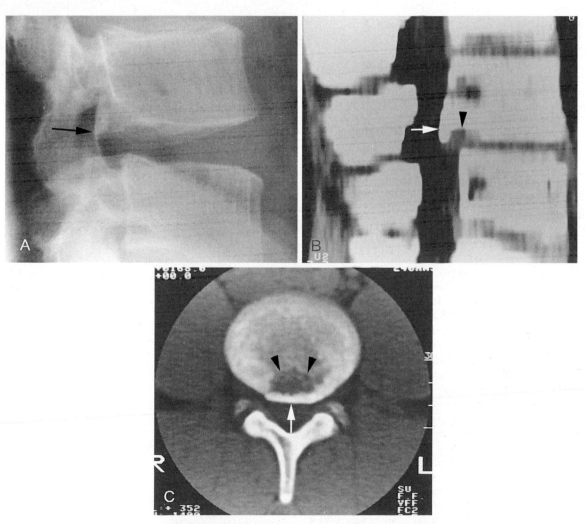

Figure 9.71. POSTERIOR VERTEBRAL APOPHYSEAL RING FRACTURE, L4. A. Lateral Lumbar. An arc of calcification is apparent extending from the posterior-inferior corner of the L4 vertebral body (arrow). Note the discontinuity of the posterior vertebral body cortex. **B. CT, Sagittal Reconstruction.** Observe the uniform posterior arc of calcification of the displaced ring apoph-ysis (arrow). A Schmorl's node is also evident beneath the displaced posterior rim (arrowhead). **C. CT Scan, Axial Image.** The displaced posterior apophyseal rim is clearly delineated (arrow). The Schmorl's node is also evident anterior to the displaced posterior rim (arrowhead). COMMENT: Only 15–20% of these lesions are apparent on conventional radiographs. They are frequently found in adolescents and young adults, often symptomatic, and most likely traumatic in origin. (Courtesy of Kevin A. Szekely, BAppSc (Chiropractic), Henley Beach, Australia)

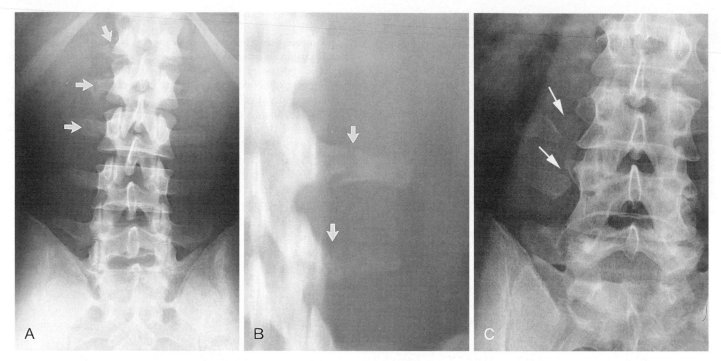

A   B   C

Figure 9.72.   TRANSVERSE PROCESS FRACTURES, LUMBAR SPINE. A. Transverse Process Fractures, AP Tomogram. Irregular fracture lines are seen at the base of the L3 and L4 transverse processes (arrows). These were difficult to identify on the conventional frontal radiograph as part of the investigation for posttraumatic hematuria, a sign of renal damage. (Courtesy of Deborah E. Springer, DC and George E. Springer, DC, Clearwater, Florida)

B. Healing Transverse Process Fractures. The left transverse processes of L1, L2, and L3 display evidence of callus formation adjacent to the fracture lines (arrows). **C. Ununited Transverse Process Fractures.** The left L3 and L4 transverse processes have been previously fractured as evidenced by their characteristic inferior displacement and smooth, sclerotic borders (arrows).

most common segments to suffer transverse process fractures are L2 and L3. (Fig. 9.72A–C)

Radiographically the fracture line appears as a jagged radiolucent separation, usually occurring close to its point of origin from the vertebra. Frequently, the separated fragment is displaced inferiorly. If the fracture line is horizontal, close inspection for a transverse or Chance fracture should be performed. Fractures often occur at multiple levels. Fractures of the fifth lumbar transverse process are frequently found in association with pelvic fractures, particularly fractures of the sacral ala, or disruption of the sacroiliac joint. Occasionally, loss of the psoas shadow may occur secondary to hemorrhage. Ossification within this hemorrhage (myositis ossificans) can result in bony bridging between transverse processes (lumbar ossified bridging syndrome, LOBS). (152) Renal damage may occur which may be associated with hematuria.

A fracture of the transverse process can be simulated by overlying fat lines or intestinal gas or by developmental nonunion, especially at L1, where the psoas margin crosses the tip of the transverse process. (Fig. 9.73) Oblique or tilt views may be necessary to rule out fracture.

Pars Interarticularis Fractures.   Fractures of the pars interarticularis are uncommon. (153) The mechanism of injury is violent hyperextension of the lumbar spine, usually producing the pars fracture at the L4 or L5 level. (Fig. 9.74) The fracture line is seen as a jagged radiolucency that is usually vertically oriented and is best seen on oblique radiographs (''collar'' sign).

Acute fractures of the pars interarticularis should not be confused with spondylolysis of the pars, which is usually the result of a stress fracture. (154) Acute fractures are invariably unilateral,

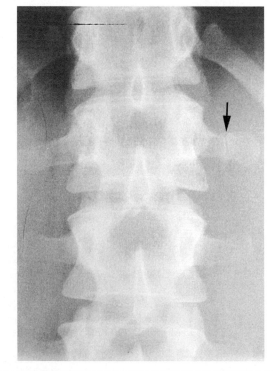

Figure 9.73.   DEVELOPMENTAL NONUNION, TRANSVERSE PROCESS, L1. A characteristic and common developmental variation of the first lumbar transverse process is evident (arrow). The smooth opposing borders, lack of inferior displacement, and incidence of the variant make differentiation from fracture possible.

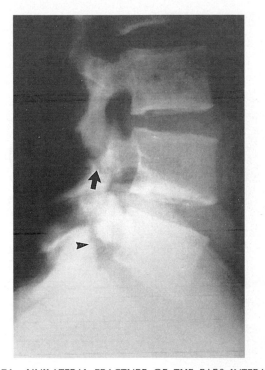

Figure 9.74. UNILATERAL FRACTURE OF THE PARS INTERARTICU-LARIS, L4. The jagged radiolucent fracture line of the L4 pars is demonstrated (arrow). A bilateral spondylolysis of the pars interarticularis is present at the L5 vertebra (arrowhead). COMMENT: Fractures of the pars interarticularis are uncommon and usually follow violent hyperextension of the lumbar spine, as was the case in this 16-year-old male patient, who was "clipped" while playing football. It is of particular interest to note that the force required to fracture the pars at L4 had no effect on the position of the L5 vertebra, which had bilateral spondylolysis present prior to the trauma. For further discussion concerning displacement in spondylolisthesis, see Chapter 5. (Courtesy of Barton W. DuKett, DC, Bigelow, Arkansas)

while spondylolysis is usually bilateral. Acute fractures frequently heal without residual defects or anterior displacement.

Chance or Lap Seat Belt Fracture

In 1948 Chance described a peculiar fracture of the vertebra consisting of "horizontal splitting of the spine and neural arch, ending in an upward curve that usually reaches the upper surface of the body just in front of the neural foramen." (155) Use of lap–type seat belts in the 1950s and 1960s coincided with an increasing occurence of Chance fractures. (156) Severe abrasions can be seen on the lower anterior abdominal wall, outlining the position of the seat belt at the time of impact. Internal visceral damage may also occur, such as rupture of the spleen or pancreas and tears of the small bowel and mesentery. Neurologic deficit occurs in 15% of cases. (157) The most common location for the transverse Chance fracture is in the upper lumbar spine (L1-L3). (157)

This fracture has also been referred to as a *fulcrum* fracture of the lumbar spine. The mechanism of injury is produced by the seat belt acting as a fulcrum over the abdomen, creating flexion and distraction forces in the lumbar spine. The posterior and middle columns fail with different patterns described (133,159): (a) Chance fracture–horizontal splitting of the spinous process and pedicle continuing though into the posterior vertebral body to involve the superior endplate; (b) horizontal splitting fracture–horizontal division of the spinous process, pedicle, and posterior

vertebral body without involvement of the endplate; and (c) Smith injuries–rupture through the interspinous ligaments partially rupturing the intervertebral disc (type A), avulsing the posterior inferior corner of the vertebral body (type B), or fracturing the superior articular process (type C). (133,158)

Radiographic detection of the Chance fracture can be represented by two appearances on the frontal radiograph: (a) a clear transverse fracture through the posterior elements, and (b) rupture of the soft tissue structures and angulation of the superior portion of the fractured vertebra. (Fig. 9.75A and B) This leaves a wide radiolucent gap between the two fractured segments, which has been referred to as the *empty* vertebra. (135) Often, a break in the oval cortex of the pedicles or a split in the spinous process can be seen. (Fig. 9.75C) The lateral radiograph usually demonstrates the radiolucent split through the spinous process, lamina, pedicle, and the upper corner of the posterior aspect of the vertebral body. (Fig. 9.75B) This appearance is characteristic of the Chance or lap seat belt fracture.

Fracture Dislocation

The vast majority of the fracture dislocations of the lumbar spine occur in the thoracolumbar area following a violent flexion injury. (159) Avulsion fractures (teardrop) are commonly found associated with dislocations of the lumbar spine. (Fig. 9.76) Complete luxation with lateral shift of the spine may create cord or cauda equina paralysis. Most dislocations are anterior in position, without lateral displacement. Shearing injuries with disc and ligament rupture and fractures of the posterior arch are common. (Fig. 9.77) On axial CT scans the absence of apposed articular facets is diagnostic of facet dislocation ("naked facet sign"). (159,160)

MEDICOLEGAL IMPLICATIONS
Lumbar Spine Fractures

- Minimum studies of AP and lateral views must be obtained. Supplemental views including obliques, spot, and lumbosacral tilt are often also required.

- Instances of persistent pain or neurologic deficits even in the absence of plain film findings may require further imaging such as CT and MRI. Bone scan may reveal evidence of subtle compression or other fracture.

- Compression fracture in the absence of significant trauma should raise the suspicion of an underlying pathology. Loss of posterior vertebral body height is indicative of pathologic fracture and should instigate a search for its cause including the many etiologies of osteoporosis, multiple myeloma, and metastatic carcinoma.

- Compression fractures must be assessed for the presence of retrolisthesis, anterolisthesis, retropulsed fragment, and widening of the interpediculate distance as markers for possible neurologic complications.

- The differentiation between old and recent fracture is a common contentious issue. Signs of acute fracture include a linear sclerotic zone of impaction or callus (0–8 weeks), angular cortical disruption, normal adjacent disc space, and displacement of the paraspinal line. Bone scan is unhelpful, as it may show activity for at

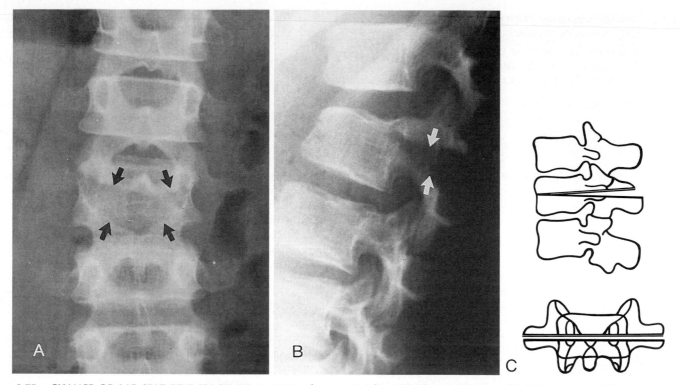

Figure 9.75. CHANCE OR LAP SEAT BELT FRACTURE. A. AP Lumbar Spine. There is a clear transverse fracture through the pedicles, pars inter-articularis, lamina, and spinous process of the L3 vertebra (arrows). **B. Lateral Lumbar Spine.** There is superior angulation of the superior portion of the fractured vertebra, creating a wide radiolucent gap between the two fracture segments (arrows). This has been referred to as the "empty" vertebra.

C. Schematic Diagram. Horizontal Splitting Fracture. This is a variant of a true Chance fracture since it does not involve the superior endplate. COMMENT: The chance or lap seat belt fracture represents an injury caused by the seat belt acting as a fulcrum over which the vertebral body and neural arch are split transversely into two parts in severe motor vehicle accidents. This has also been referred to as a "fulcrum" fracture.

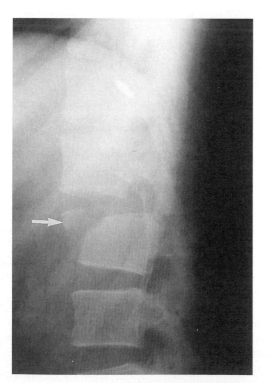

Figure 9.76. FRACTURE DISLOCATION AT THE THORACOLUMBAR JUNCTION. A complete dislocation of T12 upon L1 with an associated tear-drop avulsion fracture at the anterosuperior corner of L1 (arrow) is noted. This injury resulted in severance of the spinal cord and paralysis. (Courtesy of David P. Thomas, MD, Melbourne, Australia)

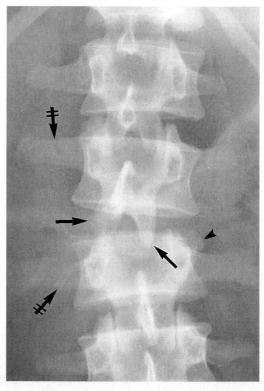

Figure 9.77. FACET DISLOCATION: LUMBAR SPINE. Note the inferior facet dislocations affecting the L2 vertebra (arrows). Associated fractures of the superior vertebral endplate of L3 (arrowhead) and unilateral transverse processes of L2 and L3 (crossed arrows) are present.

least a year after occurence. MR shows high signal intensity on T2-weighted images due to edema.

- Transverse process fractures require assessment by ultrasound, CT, or IVP for renal damage. Persistent hypertension after injury should also invoke investigation for renal involvment.

FRACTURES OF THE PELVIS
SACRAL FRACTURES

Sacral fractures usually occur as a result of a fall upon the buttocks, direct trauma, or in association with pelvic fractures. Isolated fractures of the sacrum are uncommon, and a diligent search for an associated fracture of the pelvic ring or symphysis pubis is often beneficial. Two types are horizontal and vertical.

Horizontal (Transverse) Fractures. These are the most common types of sacral fractures. The most common location is at the level of the third and fourth sacral tubercle, which are near the lower end of the sacroiliac joint. (Fig. 9.78) The fracture line is frequently difficult to identify due to overlying intestinal contents, which may require reexaminatiom or enema. Careful identification of the cortex outlining each sacral foramen ("foraminal lines") should be scrutinized for disruption or distortion. (1,2) (Fig. 9.79A and B) The lateral radiograph occasionally demonstrates the fracture with disruption of the anterior cortex. (Fig. 9.80) Often, the lower segment of the sacrum may be displaced or angled forward. (3) (Fig. 9.81)

A horizontal fracture of the upper sacrum, affecting the first or second sacral segments, may occur from high falls such as attempts at suicide ("suicidal jumper's" fracture). (4)

Vertical Fractures. These usually occur as a result of indirect trauma to the pelvis with more than 50% suffering pelvic organ damage. (5) They are visible in the frontal radiograph but not the lateral view. The cephalic tilt view, tomography, or CT may be necessary in order to demonstrate the vertical fracture line, which usually runs nearly the entire length of the sacrum. (1,5) (Figs. 9.79, 9.82) The normally symmetrical transverse sacral foraminal lines should be carefully scrutinized for detection of the fracture line. (1,2)

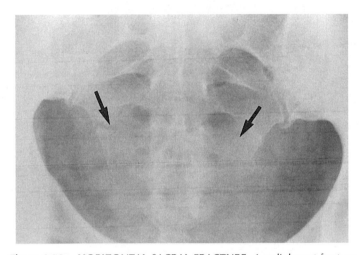

Figure 9.78. HORIZONTAL SACRAL FRACTURE. A radiolucent fracture line is seen just inferior to the fourth sacral foramina (arrows). COMMENT: A horizontal fracture is the most common type of sacral fracture. The most common location is near the lower end of the sacroiliac joints, around the level of the third and fourth sacral tubercle.

COCCYGEAL FRACTURES

Most fractures of the coccyx are transversely oriented, similar to those of the sacrum. Seldom are they seen on the frontal radiograph; the lateral film best demonstrates this type of fracture. The fracture line is usually oblique in presentation, and slight anterior displacement of the distal occyx is quite common. (Fig. 9.83) Developmental variation in the position of the distal coccygeal segment may provide some concern to the inexperienced observer.

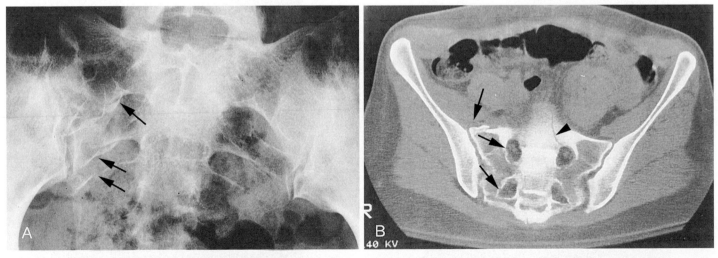

Figure 9.79. SACRAL FRACTURE, DISRUPTION OF FORAMINAL LINES. A. AP Sacrum. On the frontal view no definite fracture line is evident. Scrutiny of the left foraminal cortical outlines ("foraminal" or "arcuate lines") shows disruption at three levels due to a vertical fracture through the sacral ala (arrows). **B. CT Scan.** Disruption of the anterior sacral cortex and foram- inal walls is depicted (arrows). An additional vertical fracture is seen on the contralateral side (arrowhead). COMMENT: Frequently the only evidence for sacral fracture is disruption of the foraminal lines. Many sacral pathologies, including tumors and Paget's disease can also result in alteration to the appearance of these lines. (Courtesy John C. Slizeski, DC, Denver, Colorado)

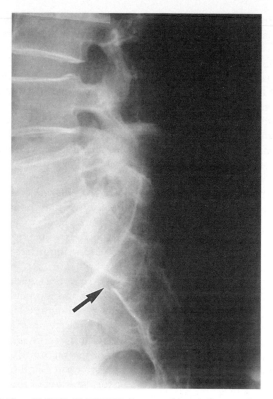

Figure 9.80.   SACRAL FRACTURE. Fracture through the anterior surface of the second sacral segment crates an acute offset of its anterior cortical surface (arrow).

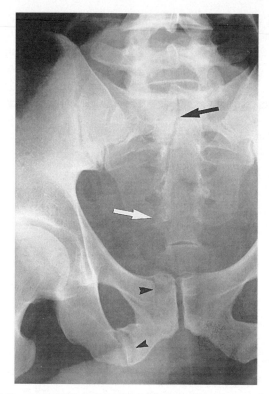

Figure 9.82.   VERTICAL FRACTURE OF THE SACRUM. A radiolucent verticalfracture extends through the entire height of the sacrum (arrows). Fractures of the superior and inferior pubic rami are also noted (arrowheads).

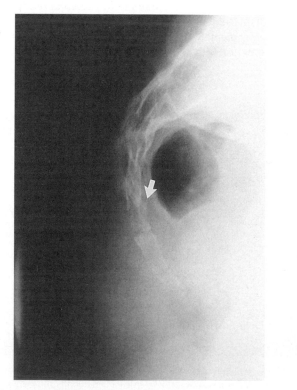

Figure 9.81.   FRACTURE, DISTAL SACRUM. There is a fracture of the distal sacrum, with slight anterior displacement of the fracture fragment (arrow). (Courtesy of Phillip C. Lening, DC, Houston, Texas)

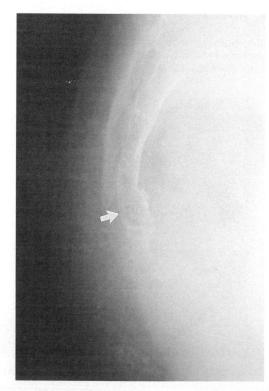

Figure 9.83.   COCCYX FRACTURE. There is an oblique fracture through the distal surface of the coccyx, with minimal anterior displacement (arrow).

FRACTURES OF THE ILIUM
Iliac Wing Fractures

Duverney first described iliac wing fracture which now bears his name. (6) Direct force from a lateral direction causes a splitting of the iliac wing. The fracture line is best seen on oblique views as a single radiolucency (Fig. 9.84A and B) or may appear as a stellate radiating pattern of fracture lines. The surrounding large muscle attachments prevent separation of the fracture fragments. This is a stable fracture.

Malgaigne Fracture

The Malgaigne fracture is a double injury to one hemipelvis. It is defined as an ipsilateral double vertical fracture of the superior pubic ramus and the ischiopubic ramus, with fracture or dislocation of the sacroiliac joint. (Fig. 9.85A and B) There may be superior or posterior displacement of the entire hemipelvis with fracture of the fifth lumbar transverse process. The fracture results from vertical shearing forces to the pelvis (7) and is by far the most common fracture and represents approximately one

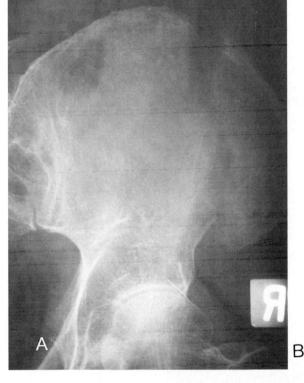
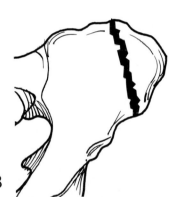

Figure 9.84.   DUVERNY'S FRACTURE OF THE IL-IAC WING. A. AP Pelvis. There is a large radiolucent fracture line visualized through the lateral surface of the iliac wing (Duverney's fracture). **B. Schematic Diagram: Duverny's Fracture.**

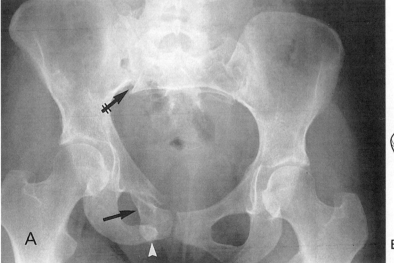
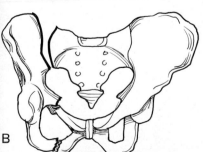

Figure 9.85.   MALGAIGNE FRACTURE OF THE PELVIS. A. AP Pelvis. Observe the unilateral superior pubic ramus fracture (arrow), inferior pubic ramus fracture (arrowhead), and fracture dislocation through the ipsilateral sacroiliac joint (crossed arrows). This patient has an old, healed Malgaigne fracture. (Courtesy of Joseph W. Howe, DC, DACBR, Fellow, ACCR, Los Angeles, California) **B. Schematic Diagram: Malgaigne Fracture.**

third of all pelvic fractures. (8) All features are usually readily appreciated on plain films. (9) It may be complicated by rupture of the diaphragm and bowel, is unstable, and has a high morbidity and mortality rate.

Bucket-Handle Fracture

A bucket-handle fracture represents a fracture through the superior pubic ramus and ischiopubic junction on the side opposite the oblique force of impact to the pelvis. A fracture or dislocation of the sacroiliac joint on the side of impact is part of the injury. (10) (Fig. 9.86A–C) The pubic component of the fracture is usually displaced inward and superiorly. This lesion often results from an automobile or auto/pedestrian accident, and may be associated with injuries to the head, thorax, and abdominal viscera.

Acetabular Fractures

Approximately 20% of all pelvic fractures in adults involve the acetabulum. (11) Most occur in automobile or auto/pedestrian accidents. Almost all acetabular fractures are due to indirect injury, i.e., injury to the foot, knee, or greater trochanter of the fe-

mur. These fractures are affected by the position of the femur at the instant of impact.

Signs of capsular distension may be present in fractures around the acetabulum including displacement of the obturator internus muscle, widening of the teardrop space, and distorted fascial planes of the psoas and gluteus medius muscles. (12) The fat plane overlying the obturator internus muscle should be observed for medial displacement or asymmetry ("obturator internus sign"). This indicates a hematoma beneath or within the obturator internus. (Fig. 9.87A and B) Widening of the teardrop may be seen in children but is unusual in adults.

There are four basic types of acetabular fractures:

Posterior Rim Fracture (Dashboard Fracture).   This type of fracture usually occurs after a blow to the knee while the leg is in flexion and adduction. Often, there is a posterior dislocation of the hip. This fracture represents one-third of all acetabular fractures. (8)

Simple Posterior Column Fracture.   This is an uncommon fracture. The fracture is best seen on an external oblique projection, though the frontal view may also reveal the ilioischial line displaced medially and separated from the teardrop.

Central Acetabular Fracture (Explosion Fracture).   This type of fracture is the most common acetabular fracture. It divides the

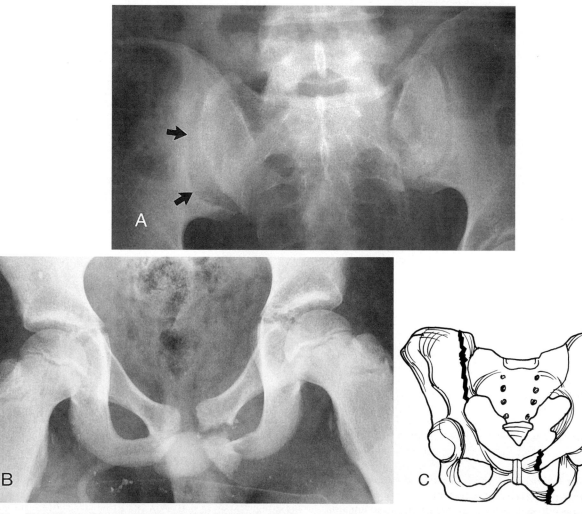

Figure 9.86.   BUCKET-HANDLE FRACTURE OF THE PELVIS. A. AP Sacrum. Diastasis of the sacroiliac joint is present (arrows). **B. AP Pelvis.** A contralateral fracture of the pubic ring. **C. Schematic Diagram.** Bucket-handle fracture of the pelvis.

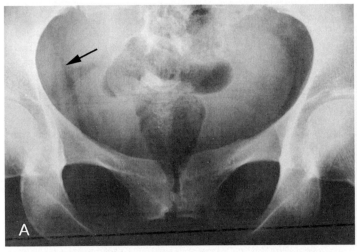

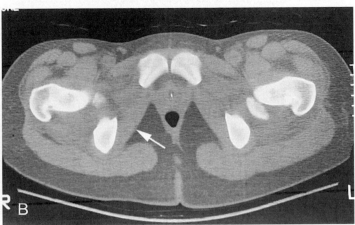

Figure 9.87. OCCULT ACETABULAR FRACTURE, OBTURATOR INTER-NUS SIGN. A. AP Pelvis. Observe the medially displaced fascial fat plane of the obturator internus muscle (arrow). **B. CT Pelvis.** The obturator internus muscle is clearly defined which bulges medially (arrow). No definite fracture line is depicted. COMMENT: Frequently the only evidence for an acetabular fracture is displacement of the obturator internus muscle. Many acetabular pathologies including tumors, infections, as well as fractures can also result in this sign. (Courtesy of Appa L. Anderson, DC, DACBR, Fellow, ACCR, Portland, Oregon)

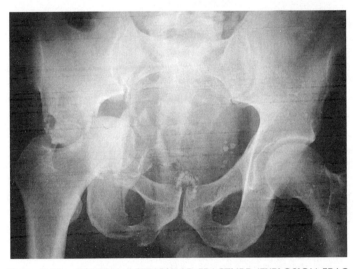

Figure 9.88. CENTRAL ACETABULAR FRACTURE (EXPLOSION FRAC-TURE). Complete dissolution and bony fragmentation of the acetabulum is noted, as the femoral head has been driven through its roof. The bony fragments are also seen, and an associated fracture through the ipsilateral ischium is present. COMMENT: Central acetabular fractures ("explosion" fractures) are the most common acetabular fractures and divide the innominate bone into superior and inferior halves.

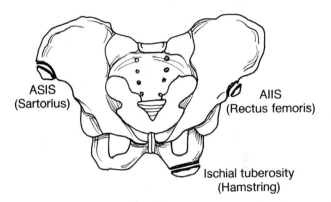

Figure 9.89. AVULSION FRACTURES OF THE PELVIS. This schematic diagram demonstrates the three most common areas of avulsion fractures of the pelvis.

innominate bone into superior and inferior halves. In the transverse type, the fracture line bisects the ischial spine. (Fig. 9.88)

In the oblique variety the fracture extends posterosuperiorly to the sacrosciatic notch. This fracture is difficult to diagnose, and a positive obturator internus sign may be the only roentgen finding. If the fracture is severe, there may be central dislocation of the femoral head.

Simple Anterior Column Fracture. The fracture may terminate anywhere along the pubis or ischiopubic junction. On the frontal view there is a loss of continuity of the iliopubic line and medial displacement of the teardrop. This fracture is best visualized on an internal oblique view.

Avulsion Fractures

An avulsion fracture of the ilium is a separation of a bony fragment usually a tuberosity or bony process (apophysis or epiphysis). They are also referred to as *tug* lesions. These fractures may be due to a single acute episode or the result of chronic, repetitive injury. Adolescents and young adult athletes are especially predisposed, usually prior to fusion of the involved growth center, and lesions are mediated by severe, uncontrolled muscular contractions. (13) They are particularly common in sprinters, long jumpers, gymnasts, hurdlers, and cheerleaders. (8,13) These fractures might be considered the adolescent equivalent of muscle pulls in mature athletes. (8)

Avulsion fractures of the ilium include (Fig. 9.89):

Anterosuperior Iliac Spine (ASIS). This avulsion by the sartorius muscle appears radiographically as the displacement of a curvilinear bony fragment from the anterosuperior iliac spine. (14) (Fig. 9.90A and B) A healed displaced ASIS avulsion may simulate an osteochondroma. Pain is classically relieved by hip flexion following acute injury. Chronic disability is uncommon.

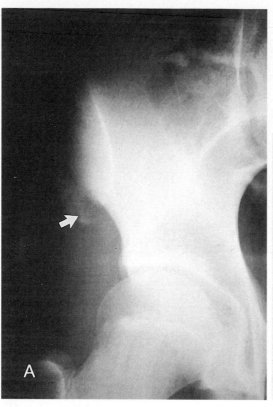

Figure 9.90. AVULSION FRACTURE OF THE ANTEROSUPERIOR ILIAC SPINE. A. AP Pelvis and Hip. Avulsion of the anterosuperior iliac spine (ASIS) has occurred, leaving a bony fragment in the adjacent soft tissues (arrow).

B. Bone Scan. There is a large area of increased radionuclide uptake present in the area of the focal avulsion of the ASIS (arrow). The large semicircular black area near the pubic rami represents the distended urinary bladder.

(13,14) Treatment by open reduction and internal fixation reduces convalescence to three to four weeks. (14)

Anteroinferior Iliac Spine (AIIS). Avulsion by the rectus femoris muscle results in the inferior displacement of a fragment from the anteroinferior iliac spine. (Fig. 9.91A and B) Active flexion of the hip in acute injuries is painfully limited though long-term disability is uncommon. (13) This is a common fracture in rugby, soccer, or football players. (15)

Fractures of the Pubis and Ischium

Straddle Fractures

The straddle fracture, or comminuted fracture, of the pubic arches is the most common type of unstable fracture of the pelvis. (8,11) This double vertical fracture involves both superior pubic rami and ischiopubic junctions bilaterally. (Fig. 9.92A and B) The central fracture fragment is usually displaced posterosuperiorly, placing pressure upon the ventral surface of the bladder. Bladder rupture and urethral tear, which may require diagnosis via urethrography and cystography, occurs in 20% of these patients. (16)

Avulsion Fractures

Symphysis Pubis. Severe acute and recurrent chronic injuries of the major adductor muscles cause a tearing of bone from the superior or inferior pubic rami near the pubic articulation. This injury is common in soccer players. Radiographically there can be unilateral or bilateral irregularity of the symphysis joint surface, roughening of the pubic bone cortex, and localized admixture of sclerosis and lucency. The injury is usually active on isotopic bone scan (17) and it can appear identical to osteitis pubis.

Ischial Tuberosity (Rider's Bone). This type of fracture represents an avulsion of the secondary growth center (apophysis) for the ischial tuberosity as a result of a forceful contraction of the hamstring group of muscles. (13) (Fig. 9.93A–E) These can be acute or chronic injuries and are frequently bilateral. (13) With healing, an unexplained overgrowth of the avulsed apophysis occurs, often leaving a wide radiolucent gap between the avulsed fragment and the parent ischium. This overgrowth may be the effect of hyperemia upon the ischial apophysis. Occasionally, the avulsed ischial apophysis may assume a size larger than the parent ischium. (Fig. 9.93E) This large overgrowth can be confused with an osteochondroma. Usually, the patient's history of a previous severe hamstring injury and the fact that the lesion is asymptomatic secures the proper diagnosis. Reduction in hip mobility is common and surgical intervention has not been encouraging. (13) These fractures are seen most commonly in cheerleaders and hurdlers. Since chronic stress often produces this lesion in horseback riders the residual bony fragment has been called *rider's bone.*

DISLOCATIONS OF THE PELVIS

Sprung Pelvis

The sprung pelvis is a severe injury, representing complete separation of the symphysis pubis and one or both of the sacroiliac joints. (Fig. 9.94A and B) It is often stated that the pelvis is opened like a book, with one or both innominates displaced

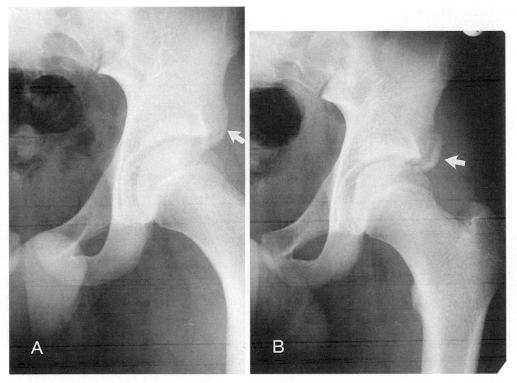

Figure 9.91.   AVULSION FRACTURE OF THE ANTEROINFERIOR ILIAC SPINE. A. AP Hip. Normal anteroinferior iliac spine (AIIS) (arrow). **B. AP Hip.** An avulsion fracture of the anteroinferior iliac spine (AIIS) is noted (arrow).

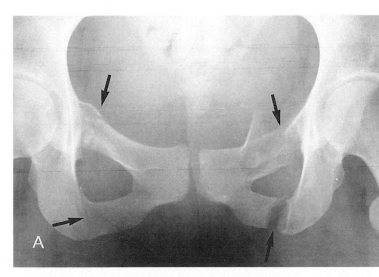 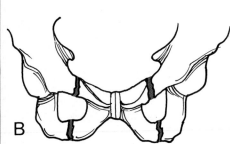

Figure 9.92.   STRADDLE FRACTURE OF THE PELVIS. A. AP Pelvis. Double vertical fractures are present involving both the superior pubic rami and the ischiopubic junctions bilaterally (arrows). **B. Schematic Diagram: Straddle Fracture.**

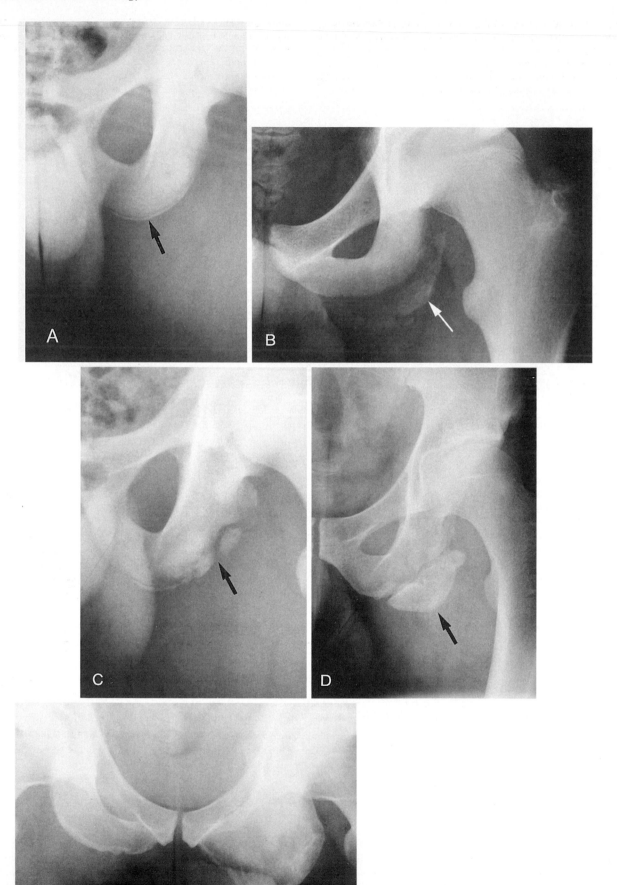

Figure 9.93.

Figure 9.93. AVULSION FRACTURE OF THE ISCHIAL TUBEROSITY. A. Normal Ischial Growth Center. The normal secondary growth center for the ischial apophysis is noted as a thin curvilinear zone of ossification (arrow). **B. Acute Avulsion.** There is displacement of the growth center away from the ischium (arrow). (Courtesy of Laurence A. Cooperstein, MD, Pittsburgh, Pennsylvania) **C. Partial Chronic Avulsion.** Fragmentation of the ischial apophysis is observed (arrow). **D. Old Avulsion.** There is a large bony ossicle noted inferior to the ischial tuberosity, representing the residual avulsed and overgrown ischial apophysis (Rider's bone) (arrow). **E. Old Avulsion Fused to the Ischium.** The entire ischial tuberosity is grossly enlarged due to a previous avulsion and subsequent overgrowth ischial apophysis (arrow). (Courtesy of John R. Kosbau, DC, Roseville, California)

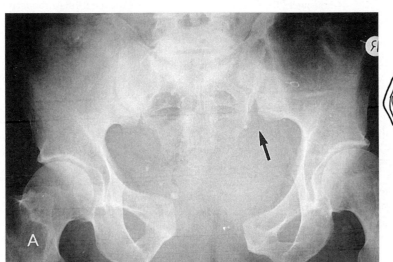

Figure 9.94. SPRUNG PELVIS. A. AP Pelvis. Severe separation of the pubic articulation and right sacroiliac joint (arrow) characterize the radio-graphic presentation of a "sprung" pelvis. **B. Schematic Diagram: "Sprung" Pelvis.**

laterally. (5) Because of this analogy, this particular injury is sometimes known as an *open book* or *sprung* pelvis. (18) Severe pelvic basin visceral damage may occur, such as rupture of the urethra.

Pubic Diastasis

This injury represents a shearing separation of the pubic articulation. (Fig. 9.95) The normal distance betwen the pubic bones should not exceed 8 mm in nonpregnant adults or 10 mm in children. (19) Often associated unilateral dislocation of the sacroiliac joint is overlooked.

ASSOCIATED SOFT TISSUE INJURIES

All fractures of the pelvis may be serious injuries, because of the often associated soft tissue injury.

Common soft tissue complications of pelvic injury include:

Vascular Injuries. Intrapelvic hemorrhage is the most common complication, due to laceration of large blood vessels. Ecchymosis of the scrotum (or labia), inguinal area, and buttocks should make you suspect hemorrhage.

Bladder and Urethral Injuries. These complications are usually due to pubic bone fractures. The incidence is between 10 and 40%, depending upon whether the pubic bone fracture is unilateral or bilateral and if one or both pubic rami have been broken. One of the more common injuries is a laceration or complete rupture of the urethra, bladder, and ureters at the trigone, which leads to serosanguineous fluid accumulation within the lower peritoneal cavity. Bruising in the perineum, retention of urine and, especially, fresh blood at the tip of the urethra are important

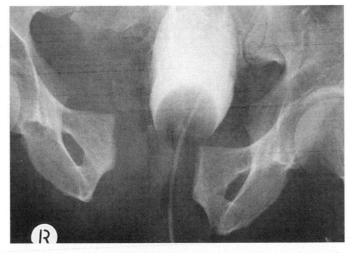

Figure 9.95. PUBIC DIASTASIS. Marked separation of the symphysis pubis is apparent. The bladder is filled with contrast medium in an attempt to evaluate urethral and bladder injury which has not occurred in this case.

signs of urinary tract injury in patients who have had pelvic trauma.

Bowel Injuries. Laceration or obstruction at the rectum is the most frequent bowel complication with pelvic fracture.

Diaphragm Injuries. The diaphragm is quite often traumatically ruptured in patients with pelvic injury. A radiograph of the chest is a must in all patients who have had pelvic trauma. The left diaphragm is most commonly ruptured, due to the protective effect of the liver on the right side.

FRACTURES AND DISLOCATIONS OF THE HIP
FRACTURE OF THE PROXIMAL FEMUR
General Considerations

Fractures around the proximal femur are relatively uncommon in young to middle-aged patients, with a sharp increase in the geriatric patient. (1) Severe forces are necessary to fracture the proximal femur in the young and middle years, while only moderate to minimal trauma may induce a fracture in the osteoporotic bone of the elderly. Certain predisposing factors may allow fractures to occur, such as the presence of Paget's disease, fibrous dysplasia, benign or malignant bone tumors, osteoporosis, osteomalacia, and radiation-induced osteonecrosis.

The overall incidence of all types of fractures of the proximal femur shows a 2 to 1 female-to-male ratio. (2) A 5 to 1 female predominance exists with intracapsular fractures. (2) The average age is approximately 70 years. (3) It has been estimated that 10% of white females and 5% of white males will sustain a fracture of the proximal femur by the age of 80 years. (4) The incidence by the age of 90 years increases to 20% for women and 10% for men. (4) Many elderly patients with fractures of the proximal femur die within six months of the original injury. This occurs secondary to pulmonary or cardiac complications. Therefore, fractures of the proximal femur and their attendant sinister complications are of such proportions that they represent a major health hazard to the elderly and constitute a significant public health issue because of their frequency, morbidity, and cost. (3)

The standard radiographic examination of the hip joint includes an anteroposterior (AP) full pelvis, AP hip spot (involved side), and an oblique or frog-leg projection. A specialized projection such as a groin lateral taken with a horizontal beam and grid cassette may be helpful, particularly with subtle dislocations. CT is especially useful in the detection of obscured fractures, intraarticular fragments, and adjacent soft tissue injury. (5) MR imaging is also proving to be useful in hip trauma especially in the recognition of occult and stress fractures. (6) Isotopic bone scans have their major application in the detection of occult and stress injuries, though as high as 20% of acute fractures are not detected 24 hours after injury and 5 to 10% may not be visible after 72 hours. (7)

Types of Hip Fractures

The types of hip fractures are divided into intracapsular and extracapsular, as determined by the relationship of the fracture line to the joint capsule. (Fig. 9.96) (Table 9.12) In general intracapsular fractures have a high incidence of nonunion and avascular necrosis due to probable disruption of the tenuous blood supply.

Intracapsular Fracture.   Any fracture involving the femoral head or neck proximal to the trochanters is classified as being intracapsular. These are then named according to the fracture location: (a) subcapital (involving the junction of the femoral head and neck; (b) midcervical (through the midportion of the femoral neck); (c) basicervical (traversing the base of the femoral neck and its junction with the trochanters). Most femoral neck fractures are subcapital; midcervical and basicervical fractures are uncommon. (8,9)

Subcapital fractures are either impacted or displaced. (Fig. 9.97A and B) They are often classified by the Garden classification: Stage 1–impaction of the lateral cortex at the head-neck junction without angulation, Stage 2–impaction with no displacement across the width of the entire neck, Stage 3–complete fracture with partial displacement with the surfaces still in apposition, and Stage 4–complete fracture with full displacement without contact between the fracture surfaces. (3,10) The incidence of complications increases progressively with each stage.

Subcapital fractures are readily overlooked due to the common absence of displacement. The fracture line may be difficult to visualize but is most common at the junction of the head and neck, superiorly, spiraling anteriorly and inferiorly to the anteromedial aspect of the femoral neck. The much less common midcervical and basicervical fractures are seen as complete transverse fractures involving both the medial and lateral cortices, with a variable degree of displacement. (3)

Pathologic fractures of the femoral neck are common and tend to occur in a basicervical location. (3) (Fig. 9.98A and B) Nonunion

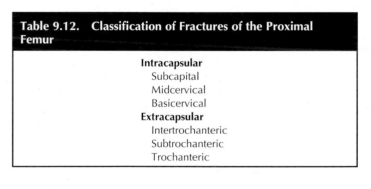

Table 9.12.   Classification of Fractures of the Proximal Femur
Intracapsular
Subcapital
Midcervical
Basicervical
Extracapsular
Intertrochanteric
Subtrochanteric
Trochanteric

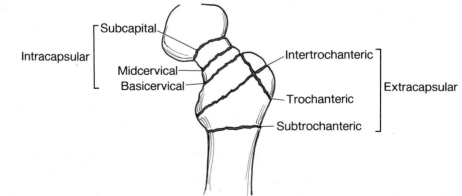

Figure 9.96.   PROXIMAL FEMUR FRACTURE CLASSIFICATION. This schematic diagram demonstrates the various types of intracapsular and extracapsular fractures of the proximal femur.

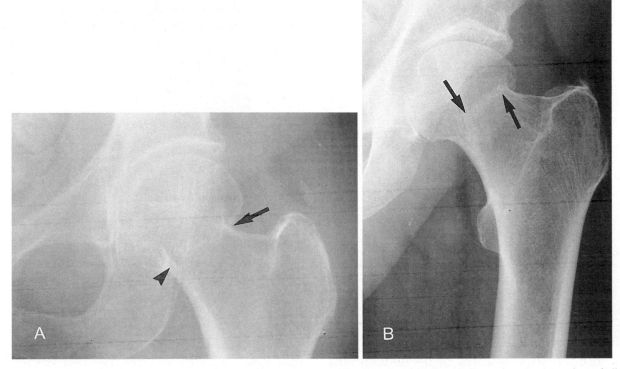

Figure 9.97. SUBCAPITAL FRACTURES. A. Angular Manifestation. An acute angle at the lateral margin of the femoral neck (arrow) has occurred secondary to a subcapital fracture. Sharp attenuation of the medial cortex (arrowhead) signifies offset of the femoral head and neck.

B. Impaction Presentation. A thin radiopacity extends medially from the lateral surface of the femoral neck (arrows), representing the zone of impaction in a subcapital fracture of the femur.

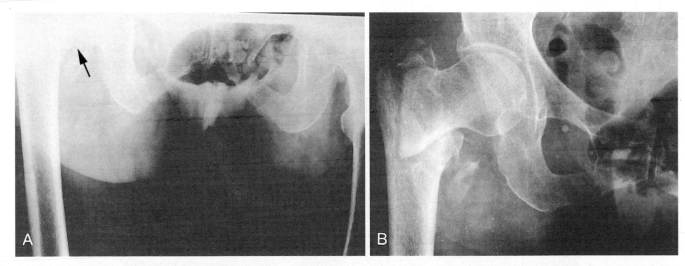

Figure 9.98. BASICERVICAL FRACTURE. A. AP Femurs. This 73-year-old female presented with thigh pain following a fall. This was the only film obtained which, despite the angular deformity at the proximal femur (arrow), was interpreted as normal. **B. AP Hip.** The basicervical fracture of the femur is now readily apparent. COMMENT: This case demonstrates the need to adequately view the entire proximal femur in any case of hip trauma. The primary complaint of thigh pain misdirected the radiographic examination. (Courtesy Dan L. Satterburg, DC, Minneapolis, Minnesota)

occurs in as high as 25% of displaced intracapsular fractures. (3) (Fig. 9.99)

The incidence of avascular necrosis as a complication to femoral neck fractures varies from 8% to as high as 30%, depending upon early detection and degree of displacement. (11) MR imaging has not been able to predict the likelihood for posttraumatic avascular necrosis. (12) The major blood supply of the femoral head arises from branches of the medial and lateral femoral circumflex arteries, which form a vascular ring around the femoral neck. The branches pass under the capsule and are at risk in intracapsular fractures. These are predisposing factors to the development of avascular necrosis. The radiographic changes may appear as early as 3 to 5 months and as late as 2 to 3 years after the fracture. (2,11) The average time of appearance of initial radiographic change is 1 year following the injury. (1)

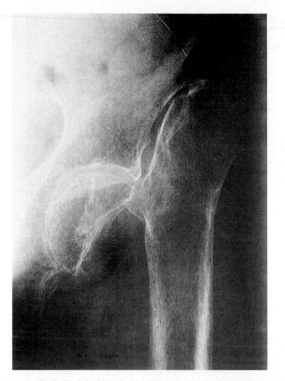

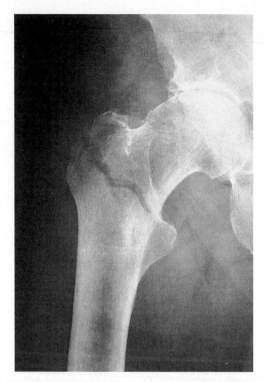

Figure 9.99.   OLD SUBCAPITAL FRACTURE OF THE HIP WITH NON-UNION. Nonunion of the fracture site is recognized by the sclerotic margins, the superior displacement of the femoral shaft, and the formation of a pseudoarthrosis on the lateral surface of the ilium. (Courtesy of David J. Byrnes, DC, Coffs Harbor, New South Wales, Australia)

Figure 9.100.   INTERTROCHANTERIC FRACTURE OF THE PROXIMAL FEMUR. An oblique fracture line extends from the greater trochanter to the lesser trochanter. This fracture line is extracapsular in location. (Courtesy of Phillip S. Bolton, DC, PhD, Newcastle, Australia)

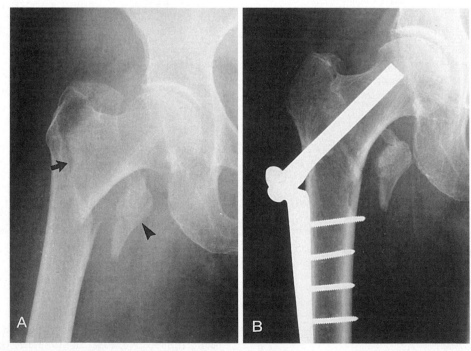

Figure 9.101.   COMMINUTED INTERTROCHANTERIC FRACTURE OF THE PROXIMAL FEMUR. AP Hip. A fracture line from the greater trochanter extends inferiorly (arrow), with displacement of the femoral neck upon the shaft. There is an associated avulsion fracture of the lesser trochanter (arrow-head). **B. AP Hip: Surgical Pinning**. There has been restitution of the normal angle by means of an orthopedic metallic fixation device. The lesser trochanter has not reunited to the femoral shaft.

Extracapsular Fracture.   This type of fracture occurs outside of the joint capsule and includes intertrochanteric, subtrochanteric and avulsion fractures of the greater or lesser trochanters. Avascular necrosis and nonunion are uncommon complications in extracapsular fractures.

The intertrochanteric fractures are usually comminuted, with the greater or lesser trochanter, or both, forming separate fragments. (Figs. 9.100, 9.101A and B) The oblique fracture line usually splits the trochanters, separating the femur into two components. The proximal component consists of the head and neck, and the distal component includes the shaft and the remainder of the trochanter.

The subtrochanteric fracture is found in the area 2 inches below the lesser trochanter. This is an uncommon type of fracture of the proximal femur. Middiaphyseal fractures follow severe trauma and are prone to malalignment unless treated appropriately. (Fig. 9.102) Pathologic fractures of the proximal femur often occur in the subtrochanteric region. Paget's disease and metastatic lesions in the proximal femur may be predisposing factors to the development of a subtrochanteric fracture; thus the presence of a subtrochanteric fracture should be a signal to the observer to look closely for roentgen signs of adjacent bone disease.

Isolated avulsion fractures of the greater trochanters occur most often in the elderly as a result of a fall. Lesser trochanter avulsions usually occur in children or the adolescent athlete. Most adult lesser trochanter avulsions occur as pathologic fractures secondary to a metastatic lesion. (3,13)

DISLOCATIONS OF THE HIP

Most dislocations of the hip are the result of severe trauma, usually in motor vehicle accidents. Hip dislocations represent 5% of all dislocations. (14) They are classified as anterior or posterior, with posterior being the most common type (85%).

Posterior Hip Dislocation

Posterior dislocations occur with the hip in flexion and usually follow a blow to the knee such as that occurring in a dashboard injury. Abduction of the thigh at the time of impact not only induces a posterior dislocation but may result in a fracture of the posterior lip of the acetabulum. This fracture should not be confused with the os acetabuli, a normal variant. Posterior hip dislocation is usually complete, with the entire femoral head out of the acetabulum. (Fig. 9.103A and B) A small fracture from the anterior femoral head is found in up to 13% of cases and if found an associated fracture of the posterior acetabulum will be found in almost 90% of cases. (15) (Fig. 9.103B) These fragments are rarely visible on plain films and require CT for identification.

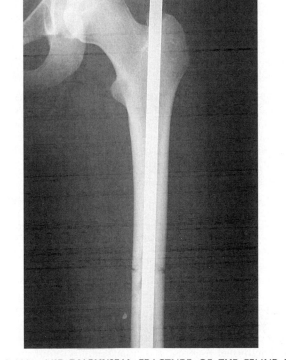

Figure 9.102.   MID-DIAPHYSEAL FRACTURE OF THE FEMUR WITH PLACEMENT OF AN INTRAMEDULLARY ROD. Good alignment of a previous mid-diaphyseal fracture of the femur has been obtained by the placement of an intramedullary rod.

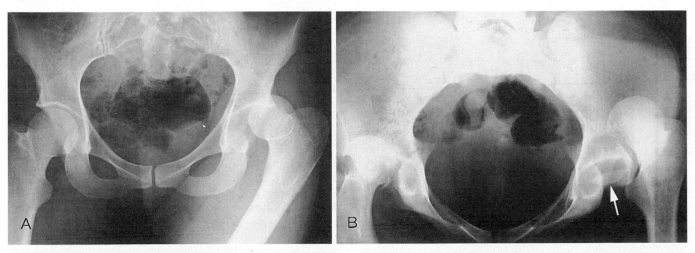

Figure 9.103.   POSTEROSUPERIOR DISLOCATION OF THE HIP. A. Unilateral Presentation. Posterosuperior dislocation of the hip is present and represents the most common form of hip dislocation. **B. Bilateral Presentation with Intraarticular Fragment.** Posterior dislocations are evident at both hip joints. Note the cresenteric bone fragment which has originated from the femoral head (arrow). (Courtesy of Brian Howard, DC, MD, Charlotte, North Carolina)

Anterior Hip Dislocation

Anterior dislocations are caused by forced abduction and extension of the femur. The femoral head usually lies caudal and medial to the acetabulum and near the obturator foramen. (Fig. 9.104)

Complications of Dislocations of the Hip

The most common complication is sciatic nerve paralysis, which occurs in 10 to 15% percent of cases of posterior dislocation of the hip. (16) This paralysis usually occurs secondary to pressure by the femoral head or displaced acetabular fragments. Myositis ossificans and avascular necrosis of the femoral head occur in 10% of cases. (14,16) Posttraumatic degenerative arthritis may occur as a sequela to the previous dislocation.

SLIPPED FEMORAL CAPITAL EPIPHYSIS

General Considerations

Slipped femoral capital epiphysis (SFCE, adolescent coxa vara, epiphyseal coxa vara, epiphyseolisthesis) occurs during the adolescent rapid growth period (10 to 15 years) and is the result of a slipping of the neck on the femoral head as the head remains in the acetabulum. There is upward displacement, external rotation, and adduction of the neck on the head. The result is a varus deformity, adduction, and external rotation of the femur. Males are more commonly affected than females, with the peak incidence in males occurring at age 13 and in females at age 12. Blacks are more commonly affected than whites. The left hip is more often involved than the right, and both hips are involved in 20 to 30% of cases. (17,18) Bilateral involvement is more common in females. Simultaneous bilateral slips are rare, but in cases progressing to bilateral involvement, the second slip usually follows the first within one year. (17) (Fig. 9.105)

The diagnosis of SFCE requires clinical suspicion. It is the most common disorder of the adolescent hip. (19) The onset of a limp accompanied by hip pain referred to the knee in an obese adolescent describes the classic presentation. Pain in the thigh and knee is a more common initial presentation than pain in the hip and SFCE is therefore often overlooked if the hip is not carefully examined. Irritation of the genu branch of the obturator nerve may explain the knee pain before hip pain in slipped femoral

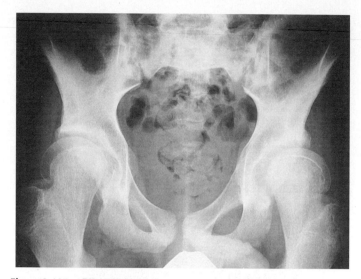

Figure 9.105.   BILATERAL SLIPPED FEMORAL CAPITAL EPIPHYSIS. There is lateral displacement of both femoral capital epiphyses. COMMENT: Slipped femoral capital epiphysis (SFCE) is bilateral in 20–30% of cases and affects males more commonly than females, the peak incidence in males occurring at age 13 and at age 12 for females. When unilateral, the left hip is more often involved than the right.

capital epiphysis. Tenderness around the hip exists, with limitation of motion, particularly abduction and internal rotation.

The lower extremity gradually develops an adduction and external rotation deformity, with a shortening of leg length. When the slippage is extreme, the gluteus medius is rendered inadequate, and the Trendelenburg test is positive. Bilateral severe slippage results in a highly characteristic bilateral gluteus medius gait termed a "waddling gait" and is marked by listing of the trunk toward the affected side with each step. (10)

SFCE can be considered a special form of the type I Salter-Harris epiphyseal fracture, a displacement without visible fracture of either the epiphysis or the metaphysis. (20) Because of the anatomy of the proximal femur, the upper femoral epiphysis is subject to shearing stress, and this may be a predisposing factor to the development of SFCE. About 50% of patients have a history of significant injury prior to its discovery, representing fracture through the growth plate. (17) In some cases the exact etiology of the slipped epiphysis is unknown. An obese body habitus (Fröhlich's body type) is common. Fröhlich's syndrome (adiposogenital dystrophy) is characterized by marked obesity and hypodevelopment of the gonads and is considered a form of hypopituitarism. SFCE is also associated with renal osteodystrophy, rickets, and radiotherapy.

Radiologic Features

Radiographic evaluation must include both anteroposterior and frog-leg (oblique) views bilaterally. Early or minimally slipped epiphysis on an anteroposterior view presents subtle findings, with many cases the slippage is only demonstrable on the frog-leg view. It is important to obtain films of the hips in any adolescent with unexplained knee pain.

Posterior medial slippage of the epiphysis is usually present. The slip may be predominantly posterior, which would be visible on the oblique (frog-leg) view, or may be predominantly medial, which would then best be visualized on the anteroposterior view. Usually, a combination of posteromedial slippage is present.

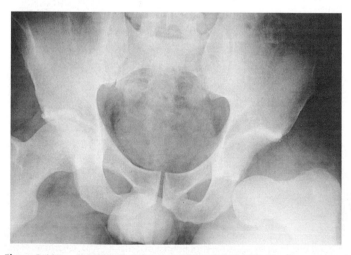

Figure 9.104.   ANTERIOR DISLOCATION OF THE HIP. The femoral head lies caudal and medial to the acetabulum, the characteristic position in anterior dislocation of the hip.

Table 9.13. Radiologic Features of Slipped Femoral Capital Epiphysis

Decreased vertical epiphyseal height
Wide, irregular growth plate
Frayed metaphyseal margin
Beaked inferior-medial epiphysis
Increased teardrop distance
Medial buttressing on the femoral neck
Lateral buttressing on the femoral neck ("Herndon's hump")
Klein's line abnormal
Metaphysis lateral to acetabulum ("Capener's sign")
Curved contour of deformed proximal femur ("Pistol-grip deformity")

The radiographic alterations are usually clearly depicted when the correct signs are searched for in the proper locations. (Table 9.13) This includes apparent widening of the growth plate (metaphyseal radiolucency), reduced epiphyseal height, medial epiphyseal "beaking," abnormal Klein's line, widened teardrop space and medial femoral neck periosteal buttressing. (Figs. 9.106A and B, 9.107A and B)

Early radiographic changes on the anteroposterior view include a widened, ill-defined growth plate with slight metaphyseal deossification. The height of the epiphysis on the slipped side will be less than on the normal side.

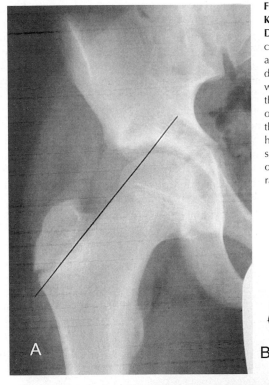

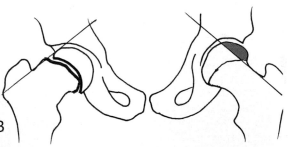

Figure 9.106. SLIPPED FEMORAL CAPITAL EPIPHYSIS: KLEIN'S LINE. A. AP Hip. Normal Klein's line. **B. Schematic Diagram.** Abnormal Klein's line associated with slipped femoral capital epiphysis (SFCE). COMMENT: Klein's line is used on the anteroposterior projection of the hip joint and represents the line drawn along the superior lateral cortex of the femoral neck, which extends through a small portion of the lateral margin of the femoral epiphysis, normally. In slipped epiphysis, the femoral epiphysis on the affected side will align more medially to this line so that no intersection with the epiphysis occurs. It is helpful to compare this with the opposite, uninvolved side. In subtle cases this alteration in Klein's line may be the only sign of slipped femoral capital epiphysis on the anteroposterior radiograph.

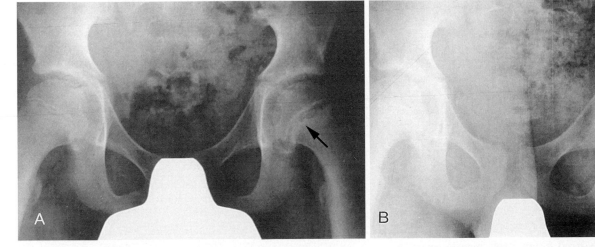

Figure 9.107. SLIPPED FEMORAL CAPITAL EPIPHYSIS: MISSED DIAGNOSIS. A. AP Hips, Metaphyseal Radiolucency. Compare the proximal femurs bilaterally, noting carefully the asymmetrical appearance of the growth plate (arrow). No frog-leg projection was obtained. **B. AP Hips 2 Months Later.** There has been progressive slip with a loss in vertical epiphyseal height, medial "beaking" of the epiphysis (arrowhead). The metaphysis lies lateral to the posterior acetabular margin (Capener's sign) and there is now periosteal buttressing along the medial femoral neck (arrow). COMMENT: This case demonstrates how an SFCE is easily overlooked unless a careful search for signs is systematically applied. Also failure to obtain a frog-leg view greatly diminishes the probability of detection. (Courtesy of Norman W. Kettner, DC, DACBR, St. Louis, Missouri)

Displacement of the epiphysis will be marked by extrusion laterally of the medial one third of the metaphysis from the acetabulum. As the femoral head is displaced medially and downward, the lower margin of the epiphysis becomes beak-shaped ("parrot's beak" appearance). The frog-leg view will show the abnormal relationship of the femoral head to the femoral neck due to the medial and downward displacement of the femoral head in relationship to the femoral neck. The metaphysis lies lateral to the margin of the posterior acetabulum (Capener's sign). (21) Chronic forms exhibit reactive bone along the superolateral aspect of the femoral neck, creating a broad-based protuberance (Herndon's hump) and a sweeping curvature of the femoral neck ("pistol-grip" appearance).

A very helpful way of detecting slipped capital femoral epiphysis is the use of Klein's line. (22) (See Chapter 2) This line is used on the anteroposterior projection and is drawn along the superior lateral cortex of the femoral neck. Normally the line extends through a small portion of the lateral margin of the femoral epiphysis. In SFCE the femoral epiphysis on the affected side will lie medial to this line with no intersection (Trethowan's sign). (21) Asymmetry in the appearance of Klein's line is highly suggestive for SFCE. In subtle cases, the alteration in Klein's line may be the only detectable sign of slipped femoral capital epiphysis on anteroposterior radiographs. (22) (Fig. 9.108A and B)

There is an occasional widening of the medial joint space due to intraarticular effusion. In addition, cases that have had a chronic history with no therapy frequently exhibit a layer of periosteal new bone along the medial surface of the femoral neck (buttressing).

Complications

The usual treatment for slipped femoral capital epiphysis is to prevent further slip by fixation of the femoral epiphysis in relationship to the femoral neck by mechanical means, usually some form of threaded pins. Multiple pins are used in order to obtain several points of fixation. The pins are usually removed after growth plate fusion has occurred. (Fig. 9.109A–C) Union is marked radiographically by the disappearance of the metaphyseal zone of lucency. (23)

Following surgical treatment, radiographic follow-up examinations are required until the epiphyseal plate has closed. The opposite and presumed normal hip should also be examined and radiographed, since bilateral involvement occurs in 20 to 30% of patients in weeks to months after the initial slip.

Complications of slipped femoral capital epiphysis include coxa vara deformity, femoral neck broadening and shortening, avascular necrosis of the femoral head, acute cartilage necrosis (chondrolysis), and degenerative joint disease (osteoarthritis) of the hip. (24) Degenerative joint disease is the most frequent complication. Avascular necrosis or osteonecrosis is an uncommon complication but is more likely to follow if there is operative reduction (forceable manipulation) or if wedge osteotomies of the femoral neck are performed (35% of cases). (24) For these reasons, the displaced slipped femoral capital epiphysis is usually pinned in situ. Corrective operative procedures are carried out at a later date. With in situ fixation utilizing pins, the incidence of avascular necrosis is as low as 1.5% in some studies. (11,12) In view of these complications a more conservative approach of traction followed by treatment in a spica cast has been advocated. (23)

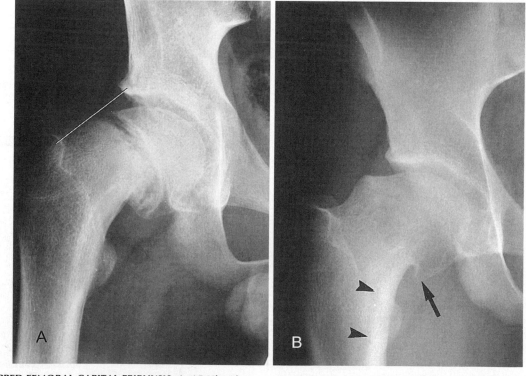

Figure 9.108.   SLIPPED FEMORAL CAPITAL EPIPHYSIS. A. AP Hip. There is a significant posteromedial slip of the femoral capital epiphysis, with an alteration in Klein's line. **B. AP Hip.** A 2-year follow-up radiograph after an intramedullary metallic fixation device was placed within the slipped femoral epiphysis demonstrates premature fusion of the growth plate. Early osteophylic formation is present at the anteromedial aspect of the femoral head (arrow). Cortical buttressing (arrowheads) is noted in the area of the femoral neck and the medial aspect of the proximal shaft of the femur. This is a stress response.

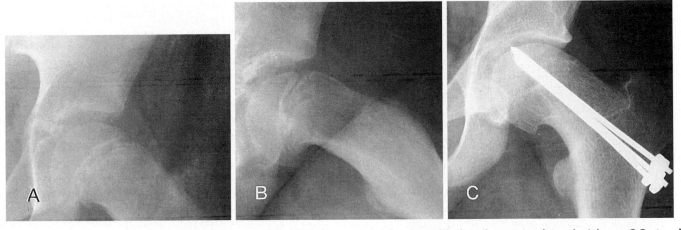

Figure 9.109. TREATMENT FOR SLIPPED FEMORAL CAPITAL EPIPHYSIS. A. AP Hip. B. Frog-Leg Hip. Medial displacement of the femoral capital epiphysis alters the normal relationship of the lateral edge of the femoral epiphysis to Klein's line. The oblique frog-leg projection augments the visualization of the posteromedial epiphyseal slip, and depicts the "pistol-grip" deformity and the lateral convexity of Herndon's hump. **C. Postsurgical Radiograph: AP Hip**. Three threaded metallic pins have been passed through the femoral neck into the area of the epiphysis to prevent further slippage. The metallic fixation has precipitated premature fusion of the growth plate.

FRACTURES AND DISLOCATIONS OF THE KNEE
FRACTURES OF THE KNEE

All bones contributing to the formation of the knee joint may be fractured. (Table 9.14)

Distal Femur

Supracondylar Fractures. These fractures occur distal to the femoral shaft and proximal to the condyles. They present as transverse or oblique fractures, are often comminuted and intraarticular. (1) The supracondylar fracture is occasionally associated with fractures or fracture/dislocations of the hip. (2) Supracondylar fractures occur following severe impaction forces on the femur and may also occur with fractures of the tibial shaft. When this occurs, the knee is left isolated from the remainder of the extremity and has been called the *floating knee*. (3)

Fractures of the Femoral Condyles. These fractures are intraarticular and are either confined to one or include both condyles. (2) These fractures may be "T" or "Y" shaped and, with separation, the joint frequently becomes deformed. Fractures confined to one condyle are usually obliquely oriented. (Fig. 9.110) A fracture of the condylar articular surface may displace a small osteochondral fragment, resulting in an intraarticular loose body.

Fractures of the Proximal Tibia

Fracture of the Tibial Plateau (Bumper or Fender Fracture). This type of fracture results from the impact of the femoral condyles being forced into the weaker tibial plateau. (Fig. 9.111) It is called a *bumper* or *fender* fracture as the tibial plateau is at the approximate height of a car bumper, though only 25% of lateral tibial plateau fractures are due to traffic/pedestrian accidents. (4,5)

Over half of the patients who sustain a fracture of the tibial plateau are 50 years of age or older. (4) Approximately 5 to 10% of tibial plateau fractures are confined to the medial tibial plateau, another 10 to 15% involve both plateaus, and the remaining 80% will be limited to the lateral tibial plateau. (4)

Table 9.14. Sites of Fracture at the Knee

Femur	Patella	Tibia	Fibula
Supracondylar	Waist	Plateau	Styloid
Intercondylar		Condyle	Head
Condylar		Tuberosity	
		Eminences	

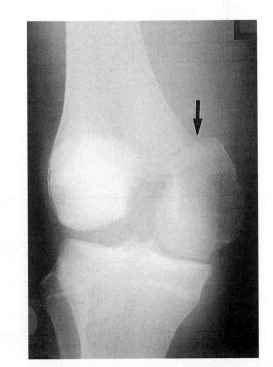

Figure 9.110. FRACTURE OF THE FEMORAL CONDYLE: DISTAL FEMUR. There is a complete fracture affecting the upper margin of the medial condyle of the distal femur (arrow). A large separation between the medial condyle and the remainder of the femur is also present.

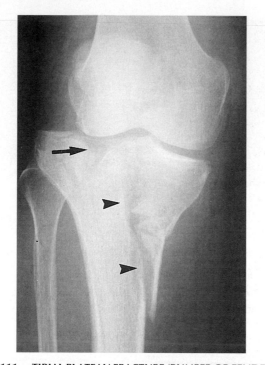

Figure 9.111.   TIBIAL PLATEAU FRACTURE (BUMPER OR FENDER FRACTURE): KNEE. The lateral tibial plateau has been depressed, and a radiolucent fracture line is present (arrow). An oblique fracture through the metaphysis below the medial tibial plateau (arrowheads) has allowed caudal displacement of a portion of the medial surface of the tibial plateau.

The lateral tibial plateau fracture is quite common and is frequently found in elderly patients with osteoporosis. The radiographic appearance is that of depression of the lateral tibial joint surface, with or without a vertical radiolucent split of the joint margin. The fracture line in undisplaced fractures may be obliquely oriented, and it is often difficult to visualize on the routine anteroposterior and lateral views of the knee. Oblique views are frequently necessary to demonstrate the fracture. (6) CT is useful to establish the size, number, and degree of depression of the fracture fragments. (6,7) (Fig. 9.112A and B)

Ligamentous injuries occur in 10 to 12% of tibial plateau fractures and occur as a result of severe valgus stress. (4) The medial or lateral collateral ligaments, or the anterior or posterior cruciate ligaments, may be torn. Stress radiographs may be necessary to establish the diagnosis radiographically. After these fractures heal, follow-up radiographic evaluation will demonstrate degenerative osteoarthritis in 20% of cases. (4)

Avulsion Fracture of the Anterior Tibial Spine.   This fracture occurs at the site of origin of the anterior cruciate ligament. (8) The mechanism of injury is hyperextension of the knee, with internal rotation of the tibia. It is most often found in children, and over half of these injuries occur in a fall from a bicycle. (8) The radiographic appearance varies with the degree of displacement. An undisplaced fracture exhibits a horizontal fracture line at the base of the anterior portion of the tibial spine. Those associated with displacement may allow inversion of the fracture fragment and are usually easier to demonstrate radiographically. (4)

Trampoline Fracture.   Fractures of the proximal tibia occur in young children (2 to 10 years) who jump on a trampoline with another person. As the heavier person jumps, the trampoline mat recoils upward from its stretched downward position with the

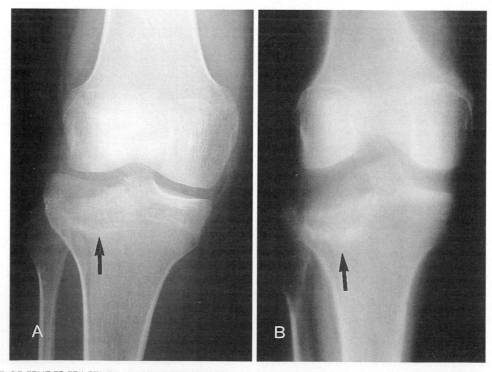

Figure 9.112.   BUMPER OR FENDER FRACTURE: CHARACTERISTIC FEATURES. A. AP Knee. A characteristic depression of the lateral tibial plateau is noted. Impaction of the lateral tibial plateau is demonstrated by an area of radiopacity (arrow). **B. AP Tomogram: Knee.** Tomographic evaluation of the tibia demonstrates significant caudal displacement of the lateral tibial plateau characteristic of the "bumper" or "fender" tibial plateau fracture. The impaction zone of increased radiopacity is once again demonstrated (arrow).

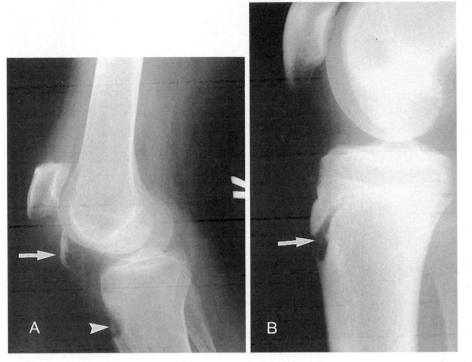

Figure 9.113. AVULSION FRACTURE OF THE TIBIAL TUBEROSITY. A. Lateral Knee. Avulsion of the tibial tuberosity with cephalic displacement is noted (arrow). A radiolucent defect is present in the normal location of the tibial tuberosity (arrowhead). **B. Lateral Knee**. The tibial apophysis during its normal growth may appear to the inexperienced observer to represent an avulsion fracture. The radiolucent area below the tibial growth center represents the cartilaginous plate (arrow). This should not be confused with a fracture or Osgood-Schlatter's disease.

smaller child landing on the upward-moving mat, impacting the descending child's leg. The force applied at just the right time and angle may be sufficient to cause fractures through the proximal tibial metaphysis. (9)

Avulsion Fracture of the Tibial Tuberosity. This type of fracture usually occurs in association with a comminuted or subcondylar fracture of the proximal end of the tibia. (10) It is most common in adolescent boys and may be predisposed by the presence of Osgood–Schlatter disease. (11) An isolated avulsion fracture of the tibial tuberosity allows for proximal displacement of the fractured fragment and, often, an associated rupture of the infrapatellar tendon. (10) (Fig. 9.113A and B) This injury often takes place during athletic activities where the knee is flexed and the quadriceps tendon contracted and firmly resisting further flexion. (10)

Segond's Fracture. This fracture represents an avulsion fracture of the bony insertion of the tensor fascia lata (iliotibial band) at the margin of the lateral tibial condyle. (12) A small bony flake is seen adjacent to the lateral tibia. On MR imaging evidence for avulsion is confirmed with a high signal intense zone at the site of lateral tibial insertion. (13) Up to 75 to 100% are associated with tears of the anterior cruciate ligament and almost 70% with meniscal tears. (13,14) Most disrupt the lateral capsule. (14)

Fractures of the Proximal Fibula

Isolated fractures of the proximal fibula are very rare and are usually found associated with ligamentous injuries of the knee or fractures of the lateral tibial plateau or ankle. (4) Injuries in these locations should be sought when a fracture of the proximal fibula is noted.

Proximal fibular fractures can present as an impacted, comminuted fracture of the head of the fibula, or avulsion of the proximal pole or styloid process of the fibula. The avulsion injury occurs at the site of attachment of the biceps femoris muscle or lateral collateral ligament. (4) This type of injury may be associated with damage to the common peroneal nerve. (15) The association of ruptures of the lateral capsular and ligamentous structures and peroneal nerve injuries resulting from adduction stresses at the knee has been called the *lateral compartment* syndrome of the knee and *ligamentous peroneal nerve* syndrome. (16)

Lipohemarthrosis

Fractures that enter the joint often create a soft tissue radiologic sign of a fat/fluid level secondary to lipohemarthrosis. With an intraarticular fracture, marrow fat may extrude into the joint fluid, along with blood (hemarthrosis). (17) The fat floats upon the superior surface of the blood and synovial joint fluid, creating a fat/fluid level in the suprapatella bursa (FBI sign—F fat, B = blood, I = interface). (18)

A horizontal-beam lateral radiograph of the knee is necessary to demonstrate the subtle fat/fluid level. (4) (Fig. 9.114A–C) The presence of lipohemarthrosis is a helpful radiologic sign signifying the presence of fracture in virtually 100% of patients, even if one is not seen. (19) However not all intraarticular fractures have a lipohemarthrosis so that the absence of an "FBI" sign does not exclude the presence of such a lesion. (19)

The knee is the most common joint to be involved; the shoulder is the second most common site. The most likely site for an easily overlooked fracture in association with the presence of lipohemarthrosis is the lateral tibial plateau. (4,19)

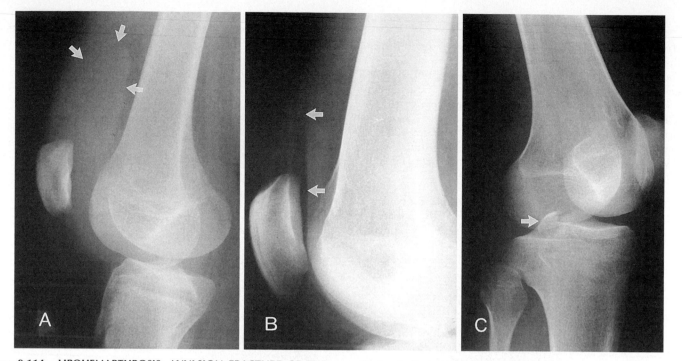

Figure 9.114. LIPOHEMARTHROSIS: AVULSION FRACTURE OF THE TIBIAL EMINENCE. A. Routine Lateral Knee. Observe the anterior displacement of the patella and significant suprapatellar effusion (arrows) in this patient following trauma. No evidence of a fat/blood interface ("FBI" sign) is noted. **B. Cross-Table Lateral: Knee.** A fat/blood interface ("FBI" sign) is noted, with the radiolucent area (arrows) representing the fat and the radiopacity below it representing the sanguinous fluid. **C. Oblique Knee.** Same patient as in **B,** demonstrating a tibial eminence avulsion fracture (arrow). COMMENT: In order to demonstrate the "FBI" sign (F=fat, B=blood, I=interface), a cross-table lateral projection is necessary. The patient in **A** may well have an "FBI" sign; however, this is a routine lateral film and not a cross-table lateral. The presence of the "FBI" sign suggests that an intraarticular fracture has occurred, allowing marrow fat to extrude into the joint fluid, along with blood, creating a lipohemarthrosis.

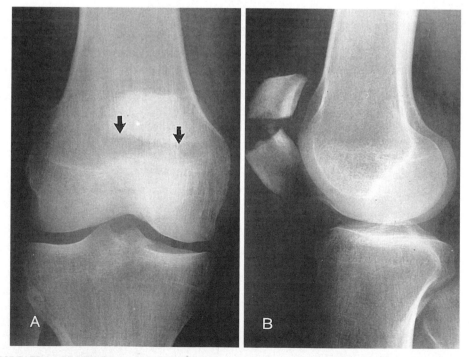

Figure 9.115. TRANSVERSE PATELLA FRACTURE. A. AP Knee. There is a large transverse radiolucent fracture through the patella. This has created a significant radiolucent gap between the superior and inferior pole of the patella (arrows). **B. Lateral Knee.** A transverse fracture of the patella has occurred.

Fractures of the Patella

The patella, because of its superficial position and location within the substance of the quadriceps tendon (which subjects it to the forces of the quadriceps muscle) is susceptible to fracture from both direct and indirect trauma. Fractures of the patella are described by the fracture line orientation. The most common fracture is transverse, or slightly oblique, and involves the midportion of the patella. (20) Transverse patellar fractures represent 60% of all types, with comminuted (stellate) accounting for 25% and vertical fracture for approximately 15%. (20)

Radiographically, the anteroposterior and lateral films will show most patellar fractures. The skyline or tangential view of the patella is the projection that best shows the vertical fracture. A transverse fracture is seen as a radiolucent line, usually through the midportion of the patella on the frontal projection. (Fig. 9.115A and B) The stellate or comminuted fracture of the patella presents as a multidirectional radiolucency leaving the patella in fragments. (Fig. 9.116A and B)

The differential diagnosis of patellar fractures is primarily a developmental bipartite or tripartite patella. (See Chapter 2) These separated ossicles always occur on the superolateral pole,

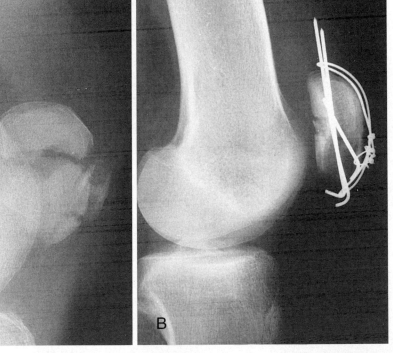

Figure 9.116. COMMINUTED FRACTURE OF THE PATELLA. A. Oblique Knee. There is a comminuted fracture of the patella, creating a stellate appearance with multiple fragments. **B. Lateral Knee.** Surgical fixation with a compression procedure is the treatment of choice in comminuted patellar fractures. (Courtesy of Kevin G. Schwager, BAppSc (Chiropractic), Newcastle, Australia)

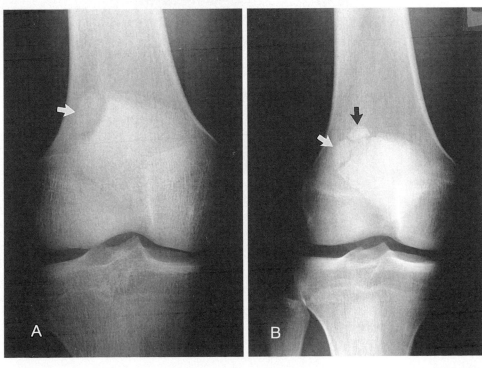

Figure 9.117. NORMAL VARIANT OF THE PATELLA SIMULATING FRACTURE. A. AP Knee: Bipartite Patella. Occasionally, the patella will exhibit a bony ossicle, representing nonunion of an ossification center (arrow). **B. AP Knee: Tripartite Patella.** Two bony ossicles (arrows) represent congenital nonunion of the ossification centers. COMMENT: Bipartite and tripartite patellae always occur on the superolateral margins, a rare site for fracture. Most patellar fractures occur in a transverse fashion through the waist. (Courtesy of Kenneth E. Yochum, DC, St. Louis, Missouri)

a rare site for an isolated avulsion fracture. A bilateral presentation is common in bipartite patellae (80% of cases) and helps confirm the congenital origin. The radiographic appearance of the ossicles are well defined, an appearance uncommon with patellar fractures. (Fig. 9.117A and B)

DISLOCATIONS OF THE KNEE
Patellar Dislocation

The patella may dislocate either laterally, horizontally, or on its vertical axis. (4) Lateral dislocation is by far the most common type. Lateral patellar dislocation occurs when direction is suddenly changed while running or even dancing. (21) Patellar dislocation is often transient and may be reduced immediately by an attendant or the patient.

There is a high incidence of osteochondral fractures associated with patellar dislocation ("flake" fractures). (22) (Fig. 9.118A–C) These occur as the medial facet of the patella impacts the lateral femoral condyle during the dislocation. The small bony fragments are best seen on the tangential view of the patella or CT and, if not removed, could be a predisposing factor to the development of degenerative joint disease.

Femorotibial Joint Dislocation

This type of joint dislocation is either anterior or posterior in presentation. (Fig. 9.119) It usually follows severe injury to the knee such as that found in a fall from a significant height or an automobile accident. In either the anterior or posterior dislocation the cruciate ligaments are often torn, along with injuries to the popliteal artery and peroneal nerve. (23) Tears of the collateral ligaments can be demonstrated by stress radiography. (Fig. 9.120A–C)

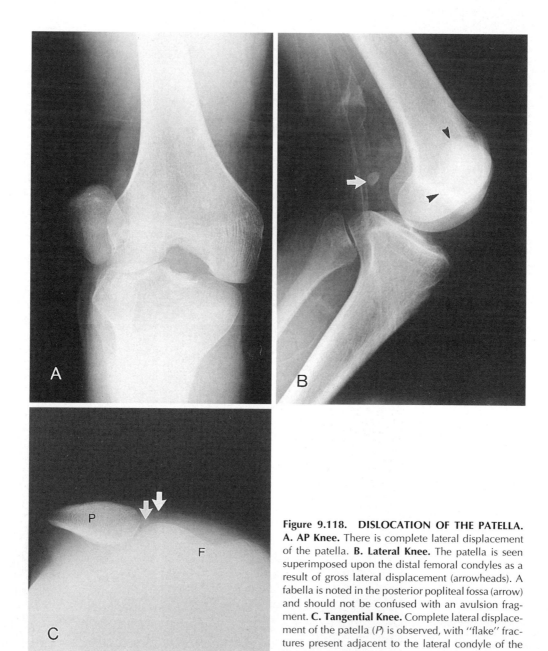

Figure 9.118.   DISLOCATION OF THE PATELLA. A. AP Knee. There is complete lateral displacement of the patella. **B. Lateral Knee.** The patella is seen superimposed upon the distal femoral condyles as a result of gross lateral displacement (arrowheads). A fabella is noted in the posterior popliteal fossa (arrow) and should not be confused with an avulsion fragment. **C. Tangential Knee.** Complete lateral displacement of the patella (*P*) is observed, with "flake" fractures present adjacent to the lateral condyle of the distal femur (*F*) (arrows).

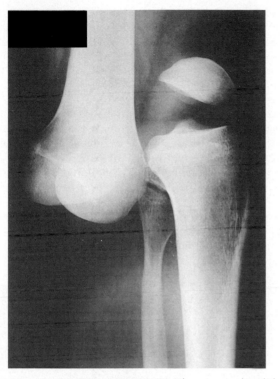

Figure 9.119.   FEMOROTIBIAL LUXATION. There is complete dislocation of the femorotibial articulation without fracture. This patient suffered permanent peroneal nerve damage from this injury. (Courtesy of Geoffrey G. Rymer, DC, Sydney, Australia)

Proximal Tibiofibular Joint Dislocation

Dislocation of the proximal tibiofibular joint is classified as anterior, posterior, or superior and is based on the displacement of the head of the fibula. (24) This is an unusual injury, but the anterolateral dislocation is by far the most common. (24) The typical mechanisms of injury are either a fall (landing in the sitting position with the leg flexed beneath the body) or a twisting injury. (4) It is commonly found as a result of participation in various sports and is particularly frequent in parachutists.

The key radiographic appearance is anterior displacement of the head of the fibula. This is best seen on the lateral radiograph. On the frontal view the head of the fibula is seen almost in its entirety, with very little overlap of the lateral tibial condyle. (2) Normally, there is overlap of the tibial condyle at the head of the fibula in the anteroposterior projection.

EPIPHYSEAL INJURIES

Fractures in the area of the knee in children prior to epiphyseal closure may involve the distal femoral or the proximal tibial epiphyses. These lesions may present as any one of the five types of Salter-Harris epiphyseal injuries. (Fig. 9.121)

SOFT TISSUE INJURIES

Lesions involving the ligaments, menisci, and osteochondral surfaces of the knee are far more common than fractures. Imaging of these abnormalities goes beyond conventional plain film radiography, employing CT and primarily MR imaging. (25)

Ligamentous injuries. Collateral ligaments can be assessed with varus–valgus stress views and noting the width of the

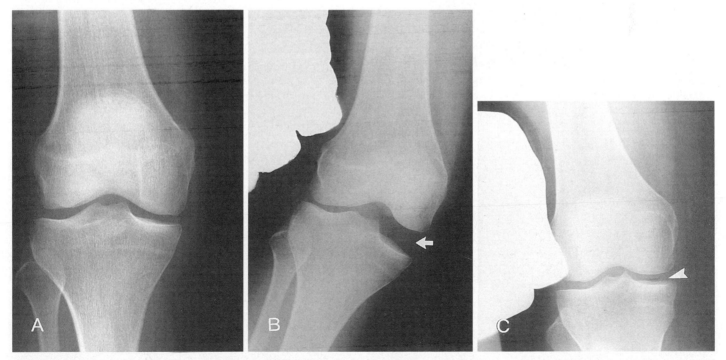

Figure 9.120.   STRESS STUDIES OF THE KNEE: LIGAMENTOUS INSTABILITY. A. AP Knee. A routine AP projection of the knee demonstrates no malalignment or instability. **B. AP Knee: Valgus Stress Position**. In the valgus position there is significant widening of the medial joint compartments (arrow), suggesting medial ligamentous instability. This was not appreciated on the original unstressed AP radiograph. **C. AP Knee: Stress Radiograph**. There is no evidence of malalignment of the medial joint compartment under valgus stress. Observe the normal vacuum phenomenon (arrowhead) present in the medial joint compartment. This is a commonly observed, normal finding with joints under traction.

stressed joint space. (Fig. 9.120) Previous avulsions from the medial collateral attachment at the distal femur may calcify and be visible on plain films (Pelligrini–Stieda disease). Coronal plane MR imaging is most useful for assessing collateral ligaments—grade 1 injuries show ligament thickening, grades 2 and 3 show variable degees of focal discontinuity, and, in the presence of avulsion from a bony attachment, features of osseous contusion may be seen. (25)

Cruciate ligament injuries are reliably imaged by MR imaging with sensitivities and specificities greater than 90%. (25) Signs of abnormality include discontinuity and abnormal caliber, and edema is seen as increased signal on T2-weighted images. (25) Sagittal images are the optimum, though coronal images can also demonstrate the cruciates clearly. (Fig. 9.122) Tears of the anterior cruciate ligament (ACL) often coexist with bone contusion on the anterior lateral femoral condyle and posterolateral tibia. (25)

Meniscal Injuries. Internal derangements involving the menisci can be depicted by MRI in up to 97% of cases. (25) A tear is identified on MR imaging as a linear band of increased signal on T2-weighted images extending from one surface to the other. These tend to be vertical, whereas degenerative tears orient horizontally. (Fig. 9.123A and B) MR imaging dramatically demonstrates meniscal cysts, which most commonly involve the lateral aspect of the joint, coexisting with a tear in the lateral meniscus. (26)

Osteochondral Injuries. Fractures through cancellous bone appear on MR imaging as linear or serpiginous bands of low signal intensity surrounded by high signal intensity edema.

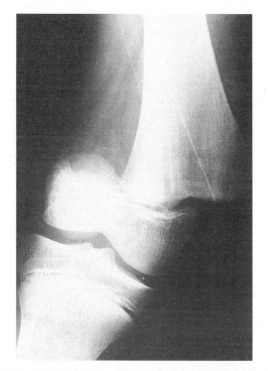

Figure 9.121. SALTER-HARRIS FRACTURE OF THE KNEE: TYPE I. There is complete medial displacement of the distal femur on its distal epiphysis.

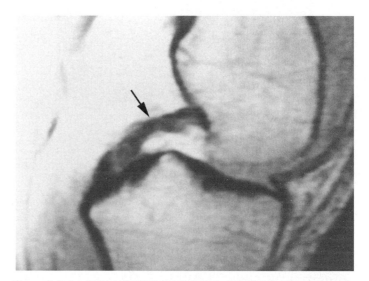

Figure 9.122. MRI, NORMAL POSTERIOR CRUCIATE LIGAMENT. The posterior cruciate ligament is readily depicted on this sagittal T1-weighted image as a uniform low signal curvilinear density (arrow).

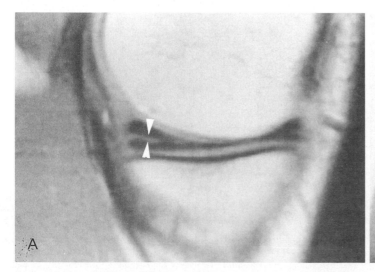

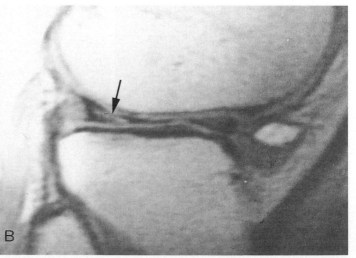

Figure 9.123. MENISCAL TEARS: GRADE III. A. MRI, T1-Weighted Sagittal Knee. Note the linear hyperintense signal intensity traversing through the posterior horn of the medial meniscus (arrowheads). This is consistent with a horizontal cleavage tear. **B. MRI, T1-Weighted Sagittal Knee.** There is an obliquely oriented, linear hyperintensity which extends to the inferior articular surface of the posterior horn of the lateral meniscus (arrow).

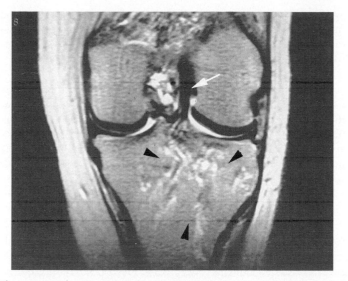

Figure 9.124. MRI, OCCULT FRACTURE. MRI, T-2 Weighted Coronal Knee. Note the numerous, linear, high signal intensity areas (arrowheads) extending from the proximal tibial cortex into the metaphysis. These findings are consistent with an occult tibial plateau fracture and surrounding marrow edema. (Courtesy of The Children's Hospital, Department of Radiology, Denver, Colorado)

(Fig. 9.124) Bone contusions (bone bruises) within the marrow show as decreased signal intensity on T1- and increased signal on T2-weighted images. There is a high association with ligamentous injuries, especially of the ACL. (25, 27) Chondral lesions can be observed as defects in the cartilage surface.

FRACTURES AND DISLOCATIONS OF THE ANKLE

The routine radiographic evaluation of the ankle consists of three views—anteroposterior, lateral, and medial oblique. The medial oblique projection is taken with 35 to 45° of internal rotation of the foot. Special projections (i.e., tomography and stress views) may be helpful in demonstrating subtle fractures, ligamentous instability, and even dislocations.

CT provides excellent bone detail and assessment of the complex articulations of the foot and ankle. It is the technique of choice for examination of the subtalar joint. (1,2) CT is also useful for imaging neoplasms of the foot and ankle. Acute skeletal trauma and posttraumatic arthropathy especially of the hindfoot including the calcaneus are well demonstrated with CT. It is not helpful for soft tissue injury such as ligamentous tears. (3)

MR imaging provides superior soft tissue contrast, multiple image planes, excellent spatial resolution and is noninvasive. It is particularly useful in the demonstration of ligament, tendon, cartilage, soft tissue, and even bony abnormalities. (4)

FRACTURES OF THE ANKLE

A number of classifications of ankle fractures have been developed. The two most commonly used are the Lauge–Hansen and Danis–Weber systems. (5) The Laug–Hansen classification is derived from the forces involved to produce the fracture but is cumbersome. The Danis–Weber classification is the simplest and most frequently used by orthopedic personnel. (6,7)

The Danis–Weber system is based on the position of the fibular fracture in relation to the tibiotalar joint space, with three types

defined: A, B and C. Type A consists of fractures of the fibula below the tibiotalar joint and do not involve the syndesmosis. Type B fractures occur at the joint level producing an oblique fibular fracture. Two categories of type C fractures are described. Type C1 is an oblique fibular fracture above the level of the distal tibiofibular ligaments. Type C2 lesions present with higher fibular fractures and therefore coexist with more extensive rupture of the syndesmosis. Type A injuries can be treated by closed methods while types B and C usually require internal fixation. (7)

Medial Malleolus Fracture

The medial malleolus is the most distal portion of the tibia. (Fig. 9.125) Fractures are usually transverse or oblique in orientation caused by angular forces generated by movement of the talus against the medial malleolus. Fractures of the medial malleolus distal to the ceiling of the tibiotalar joint line ("plafond") are more stable than those that arise proximal. (5) A fracture of the medial malleolus is best seen on the anteroposterior radiograph as a radiolucent line with adjacent soft tissue swelling.

Lateral Malleolus Fracture

The most distal portion of the fibula is the lateral malleolus. The most common fracture of the lateral malleolus is an oblique or spiral fracture extending from the inferior and anterior margin upward and backward to the posterior margin of the shaft of the distal fibula. (5) (Fig. 9.126) This fracture occurs as a result of outward or external rotation of the foot and is best observed on the medial oblique projection as a radiolucent oblique line with adjacent soft tissue swelling (McKenzie's sign). A variety of small

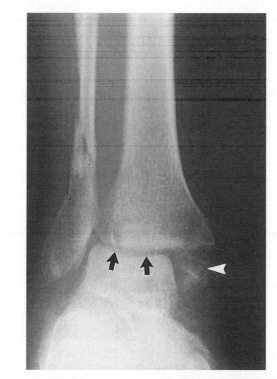

Figure 9.125. MEDIAL MALLEOLUS FRACTURE AND ASSOCIATED DISTAL FIBULA FRACTURE. There is a medial malleolus fracture observed (arrowhead) and an oblique fracture of the distal fibula, along with lateral displacement of the talus. The linear subchondral radiolucency in the talar dome (arrows) is a radiographic sign for an intact blood supply to the talus (Hawkin's sign), which represents the unlikelihood of complicating avascular necrosis.

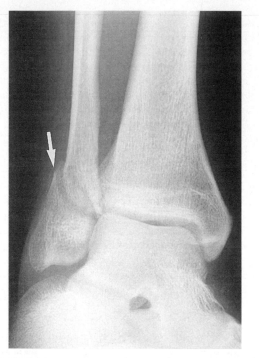

Figure 9.126.   DISTAL FIBULA FRACTURE. The most common fracture of the lateral malleolus is an oblique fracture extending upward (arrow). This fracture is best seen on the medial oblique projection.

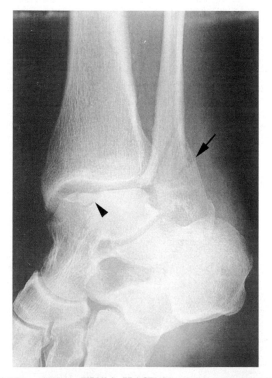

Figure 9.127.   DISTAL FIBULA FRACTURE WITH OSTEOCHONDRAL TALAR FRACTURE. Fracture of the lateral malleolus is evident (arrow). At the medial talar dome an isolated piece of bone contiguous with the articular surface can be seen (arrowhead).

avulsion fractures occur around the tip of the lateral malleolus mediated by the lateral collateral ligaments. Small talar dome osteochondral fractures on occasion accompany lateral malleolar fractures. (Fig. 9.127)

Bimalleolar Fracture

Bimalleolar fracture represents a fracture through both the medial and lateral malleoli. The fracture on one side is transverse, because of tensile forces, and the opposite fracture is oblique or spiral. (8) (Figs. 9.128, 9.129) Diffuse soft tissue swelling over the malleoli is often present, alerting the observer to look closely for fracture.

Trimalleolar Fracture

Trimalleolar fractures affect the posterior lip of the tibia (sometimes called the *third malleolus*) in addition to the medial and lateral malleoli. (9) A trimalleolar fracture has been referred to by some as a *Cotton's* fracture, despite Henderson's first description. (10,11)

Trimalleolar fractures are often found with tibiotalar dislocation. These fractures are due to external rotation of the foot and are therefore laterally and posteriorly displaced. (9) Fracture of the third malleolus is best seen on the lateral radiograph, with the fracture fragment being displaced posteriorly and/or superiorly.

Pott's Fracture

Pott's fracture, as classically described, is a partial dislocation of the ankle, with fracture of the fibula within 6 to 7 cm above the lateral malleolus and rupture of the distal tibiofibular ligaments of the ankle. (12) (Fig. 9.130) Sir Percival Pott described this fracture in 1768 and ascribed the injury to "leaping or jumping."

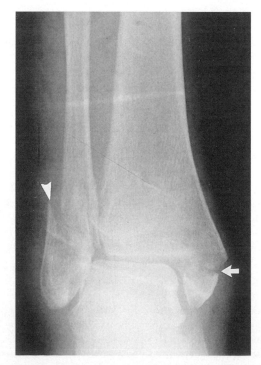

Figure 9.128.   BIMALLEOLAR FRACTURE: ANKLE. A characteristic transverse fracture through the medial malleolus (arrow), along with a spiral fracture of the lateral malleolus (arrowhead).

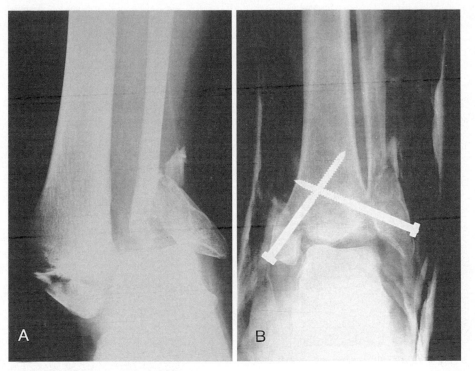

Figure 9.129.   BIMALLEOLAR FRACTURE DISLOCATION: ANKLE. A. AP Radiograph. Observe the gross lateral displacement of the talus, with bimalleolar fractures. **B. AP Ankle: Postsurgical Reduction.** Two surgical metallic screws have been placed through the bimalleolar fractures, with good alignment resulting. COMMENT: Fracture dislocation of this magnitude is invariably associated with permanent ligamentous instability of the ankle mortise joint.

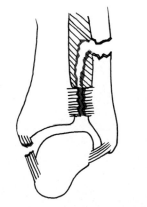

Figure 9.130.   POTT'S FRACTURE: SCHEMATIC DIAGRAM, ANKLE. This fracture is defined as a fracture through the distal fibula, 6 to 7 cm above the lateral malleolus, accompanied by rupture of the distal tibiofibular ligaments of the ankle. Disruption of the medial collateral ligament, while common, is not considered an integral part of this osteoligamentous injury.

The term *Pott's fracture* has been used erroneously to describe a number of fractures, such as the bimalleolar or trimalleolar fractures. The term *Pott's fracture* should be avoided in describing any injury that includes a malleolar fracture.

Dupuytren's Fracture

Dupuytren's fracture was described by Dupuytren based on a single clinical case in 1816 in which a patient who had sustained a fracture of the distal fibula also presented with a widened ankle mortise and medial displacement of the tibia. (13) Dupuytren's fracture, as classically described, is a fracture of the distal fibula (lateral malleolus) with rupture of the distal tibiofibular ligaments, diastasis of the syndemosis, lateral dislocation of the talus, and displacement of the foot upward and outward. (13) Unfortunately, Dupuytren's fracture is used to describe several varieties of bimalleolar fractures and, because of its similarity to Pott's fracture, has created some confusion within the literature. It should only be used as classically described by Dupuytren (13).

Maisonneuve's Fracture

In 1840 Maisonneuve described a fracture of the proximal fibular shaft. (14) This fracture is caused by forceful inversion and external rotation of the ankle. This motion forces the talus laterally against the fibula, initially producing rupture of the inferior tibiofibular syndemosis. As the force is maintained, the fibula, freed from the tibia, continues to be displaced laterally and posteriorly. The superior tibiofibular joint, remaining intact, secures the proximal fibula so that the long lever of the fibula produces a fracture of the fibula in its proximal third.

Maisonneuve's fracture may be easily overlooked because patients rarely complain of pain in the region of the proximal fibula when more painful injuries at the ankle exist. A full view of the entire tibia and fibula should be considered in patients where the mechanism of injury to the ankle is as Maisonneuve described. (14) (Fig. 9.131)

Tillaux's Fracture

This fracture is through the medial malleolus with diastasis of the distal tibiofibular syndemosis. This creates an avulsion of the anterior tubercle of the tibia, and a fracture of the lateral malleolus 6 to 7 cm proximal to the distal end of the fibula. (15) There are

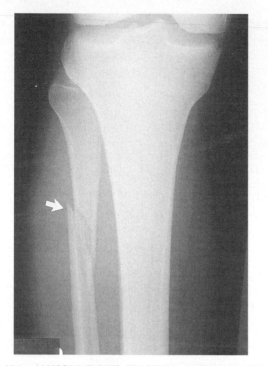

Figure 9.131. MAISONNEUVE'S FRACTURE: PROXIMAL FIBULA. An oblique fracture of the proximal fibula (arrow) has occurred secondary to a forceful inversion and external rotation of the ankle. COMMENT: These fractures are often overlooked, due to the severity of the ankle injury, and close inspection of the proximal fibula should be performed in all instances of ankle trauma.

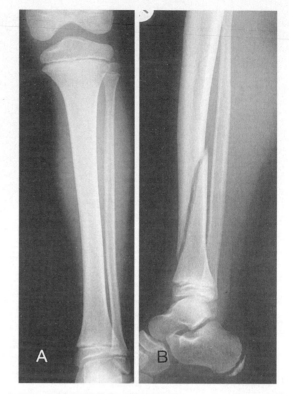

Figure 9.132. TODDLER'S FRACTURE: TIBIA. A. AP Tibia and Fibula. No fracture line is evident. **B. Lateral Tibia and Fibula**. A spiral fracture line is visualized in the distal one-third of the diaphysis of the tibia. COMMENT: This case demonstrates the need for a minimum of AP and lateral radiographs in traumatized patients. The toddler's fracture is often seen in only one of the projections.

three residual fractures: medial malleolus, anterior tibia, and distal fibular shaft. This fracture is best seen on anteroposterior radiographs of the ankle.

Toddler's Fracture

Toddler's fracture, an undisplaced spiral fracture of the tibia, occurs in children from 9 months to 3 years of age. It is caused by a fall, or by the child getting a foot caught between the slats of the crib and then rolling over. The baby, often too young to verbalize its complaints, may evidence only a mysterious refusal to bear weight on the extremity.

Radiographic examination reveals an undisplaced spiral fracture of the tibia, which is usually seen only on one projection—either the anteroposterior or lateral view. (5) (Fig. 9.132A and B) Most toddler's fractures are seen on the anteroposterior view and are not demonstrated on the lateral projection. Rarely, the fibula may be fractured as well. (5) The adult form, where the tibial fracture occurs adjacent to the top of high-top boots, is called a *boot-top* fracture. (Fig. 9.133) If both the tibia and fibula are fractured, these can also be referred to as *BB* or *both bones* fractures.

DISLOCATIONS OF THE ANKLE

Since subluxations and dislocations of the ankle joint associated with malleolar fractures have already been discussed, it remains only to consider the displacements that follow extensive ligamentous and capsular damage without fracture.

The talus may be dislocated at one, two, or all three of its articulations; however, we will consider only those that involve the ankle joint. Dislocation of the talus occurs as an isolated event,

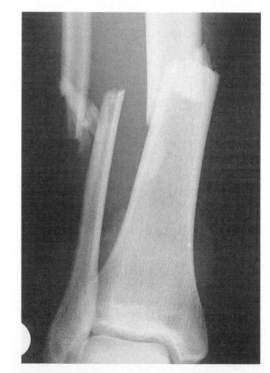

Figure 9.133. BOOT-TOP FRACTURE. Comminuted fractures of the distal tibia and fibula are seen at the level of a skier's boot-top. COMMENT: Fractures of this type may be referred to as "BB," representing both bones. The "BB" fracture can be found in the radius and ulna or in the tibia and fibula.

in association with fracture of the neck of the talus, or as an element in total extrusion of the talus. (16)

Anterior Dislocation

Isolated dislocation of the ankle may occur in either an anterior or posterior direction. Medial or lateral dislocation is commonly associated with a fracture of the tibia or fibula. Anterior dislocation follows a force that results in posterior displacement of the tibia on the fixed foot. All ligamentous and capsular attachments from the tibia and fibula to the talus are torn, with the exception, occasionally, of the posterior talofibular ligament. Clinically, the foot is usually slightly dorsiflexed and appears elongated anteriorly. The depressions on either side of the Achilles tendon are obliterated. The talus is prominent anteriorly, and the dorsalis pedis pulse may be absent. (16)

Posterior Dislocation

Posterior dislocation occurs more often than anterior displacement. Both are rare, and both involve fracture of the corresponding tibial margin. Posterior dislocation of the talus most often follows a blow to the posterior aspect of the tibia and results in plantar flexion of the ankle with apparent shortening of the foot. Reduction is carried out by exerting traction in the long axis of the limb and lifting the heel forward. Subsequent operative repair of the ligaments is an individual decision. (16)

COMPLICATIONS OF ANKLE FRACTURE

Nonunion

Nonunion is most frequent in fracture of the medial malleolus; it occurs in 10 to 15% of patients treated by closed methods. (16) Nonunion of the lateral or posterior malleolus is rare. (16) Nonunion at the level of the plafond is more commonly symptomatic than that below the plafond. (17)

Traumatic Degenerative Arthritis

Traumatic degenerative arthritis occurs in 20 to 40% of ankle fractures, regardless of the method of treatment. (17,18) Predisposing factors are inaccurate reduction of the mortise, comminution of the plafond, and advanced age. (16)

Ligamentous Instability

Often, fractures and dislocations of the ankle are found with complete or incomplete tears of the supporting ligaments. Ligamentous damage unassociated with fracture often goes ignored and is especially dangerous because it may go unrecognized and untreated, leading to permanent disability of the ankle. The important ligaments of the ankle joint are the lateral collateral ligament, the medial (deltoid) collateral, and the tibiofibular ligament (tibiofibular syndemosis). (19) A variety of tears to these ligaments occurs with the numerous types of injuries, which can affect the ankle joint. The most frequent injury is disruption of the lateral ligaments of the ankle.

Routine imaging is not effective in determining ligamentous injury. (20) Signs of soft tissue swelling consist of displacement of the skin line, blurring of the fascial plane lines, infiltration of the pre-Achilles fat, and the presence of a "teardrop" shaped soft tissue density anterior to the ankle mortise on the lateral view. (21) Myositis ossificans is unusual in the foot and ankle but can be observed in the Achilles tendon, interosseous membrane, and intermetatarsals. In the absence of fracture or obvious dislocation, considerable soft tissue swelling is an indication for stress studies to evaluate for ligamentous damage. (22)

Stress views in both the AP and lateral positions are useful examinations. (22–25) Up to 25% of ankles with verified ligament disruption will have normal stress radiographs. (26) On valgus and varus positions normal talar tilt ranges from 5 to 23°. (27,28) Comparison with the normal side is essential with more than 10° greater tilt significant of ligamentous disruption. (28,29) If there is greater than 6° tilt in the neutral position and or 3 mm difference in joint space this is also indicative of probable ligament damage. (26,30–32)

Anteroposterior (drawer) stress views are done in the lateral projection to indicate anterior talofibular ligament injury (positive drawer sign). A difference of 2 mm or more in comparison with the normal side suggests significant injury. (27)

Arthrography can produce diagnostic accuracy close to 95% of all ligament tears. (22,27) CT and MR imaging are useful in evaluating tendons around the ankle but are less effective in visualising the capsule and ligaments. (4)

FRACTURES AND DISLOCATIONS OF THE FOOT

FRACTURES OF THE FOOT

Trauma to the foot with fractures is frequent, with fractures of the feet accounting for approximately 10% of all fractures. (1,2) Direct trauma can be from objects falling on the foot or from movement of the foot against a variety of objects. (1) Indirect trauma occurs from torsion of the joints or avulsion at tendon or capsule attachments. (1) The stress of overuse or unaccustomed activity may result in fatigue fractures. (1) Diabetic neutrophic arthropathy often leads to tarsal fractures and fracture/dislocation of the tarsometatarsal joints. (3)

The routine views of the foot are the dorsoplantar, 35° medial oblique, and lateral. (3) An axial projection is necessary when calcaneal fracture is a major concern. Occasionally, varying oblique projections, tomography and CT may be needed in order to demonstrate the fracture or dislocation. (4,5) MR imaging is more suited to the depiction of effusions and bone bruises, as well as tendon and ligament injuries. (6)

Calcaneal Fractures

The calcaneus is the largest tarsal bone and the one most often fractured. (3,7) It has two major functions—to bear weight and to serve as a springboard for locomotion. (1) Approximately 25% of calcaneal fractures involve the various processes of the bone and spare the subtalar joint; 75% involve the subtalar joint and body of the calcaneus. (8)

There are two basic types of calcaneal fractures—the compressive and the noncompressive (avulsive).

Compression Fracture. This is the result of compression forces generated in crushing injuries as encountered by falling from a height and landing on the feet. (9) Approximately 10% of these fractures are bilateral, and 10% are associated with vertebral body compression or neural arch fracture of the thoracolumbar spine. (10) (Fig. 9.134A–C) The weight of the body is transmitted through the tibia and talus onto the calcaneus. (1) The resultant fracture is comminuted, and the degree of displacement and comminution is directly related to the magnitude of the forces involved. (1) The fracture usually involves the subtalar joint, with

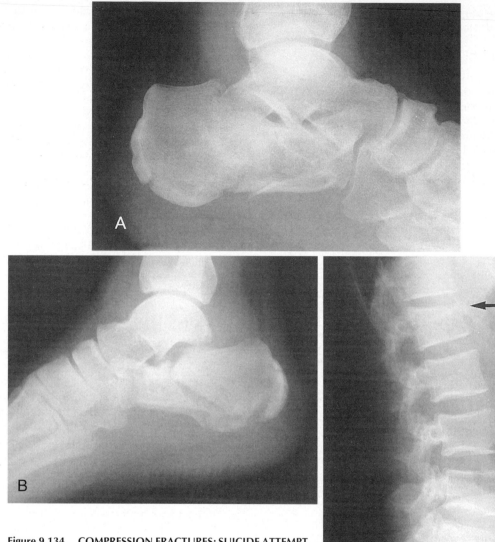

Figure 9.134.   COMPRESSION FRACTURES: SUICIDE ATTEMPT. A and B. Right and Left Calcaneus. Both the right and left calcaneus demonstrate comminution fractures secondary to severe forces occurring upon impact with the ground following a suicide jump from a second-story window. **C. Lateral Lumbar Spine.** Observe the associated compression fractures of the superior endplate of the L1 vertebra with a characteristic "step" defect (arrow).

some degree of depression of the posterior facet. Occasionally, a radiolucent fracture line will be seen; however, most cases do not demonstrate such a line.

Boehler's angle is crucial in the detection of these fractures in the absence of fracture lines, as it may be the only sign of compression fracture. (11) Boehler's angle is formed by a line drawn from the superior posterior margin of the tuberosity through the tip of the posterior facet. (11) A second line is drawn from the tip of the posterior facet through the superior margin of the anterior process of the calcaneus. The normal angle is 28 to 40°. (1,11) A Boehler's angle of less than 28° indicates depression and probable fracture. (Fig. 9.135)

Avulsion Fracture.   Those fractures that spare the subtalar joint are usually of the avulsion type. They involve the anterior process, the sustentaculum tali, the superior portion of the tuberosity, and the medial or lateral surface of the tuberosity. (1) Fractures of the anterior process are the most common form of avulsion fracture of the calcaneus. (12)

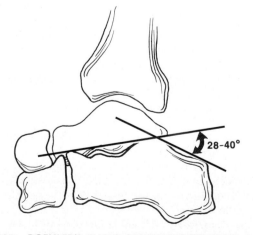

Figure 9.135.   BOEHLER'S ANGLE: SCHEMATIC DIAGRAM. A reduction in Boehler's angle to less than 28° is frequently indicative of a calcaneal compression fracture.

A fracture of the superior portion of the tuberosity of the calcaneus is known as a *beak* fracture. (13) The posterior margin of the tuberosity represents the site of insertion of the Achilles tendon, and the *beak* fracture may be the result of avulsion by the Achilles tendon.

Fractures of the Talus

The talus is the second most common tarsal bone to be fractured, following the calcaneus. The most frequent type of fracture is an avulsion, usually on the anterior surface of the talar neck at the capsular insertion. Fractures are classified according to anatomic site—body, neck, or head. (14)

Talar Body Fractures.   These may be oriented in a transverse or oblique plane. Osteochondral chip fractures of the talar dome occur either at the medial or lateral margins following forceful inversion or eversion injuries, when there is direct contact between the talus and opposing malleolus. (Fig. 9.136)

Talar Neck Fractures.   Avulsions of the anterior surface are the most frequent, followed by vertical fractures. The mechanism of injury in vertical neck fractures is the impact of the anterior lip of the tibia as it is forced downward into the talar neck, which is being forced upward. Vertical neck fractures are most frequently the result of an automobile accident where the driver has the foot firmly applied to the brake pedal at the time of impact. They were first described in World War I when pilots involved in crash landings had the rudder pedal forced into the sole of the foot (aviator's fracture). (15) (Fig. 9.137) These are the fractures most commonly complicated by avascular necrosis of the talus.

Talar Head Fractures.   These fractures are infrequent and are characterized by the fracture line being well forward of the talar neck.

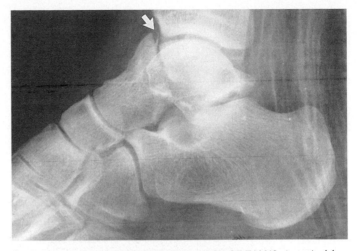

Figure 9.137.   AVIATOR'S FRACTURE: NECK OF TALUS. A vertical fracture line extends through the talar neck (arrow). COMMENT: This type of talar fracture can predispose to avascular necrosis of the body of the talus.

Complications of Talus Fractures

The main concern with talus fractures is the development of avascular necrosis, which usually involves the body and may occur following a talar neck fracture. (16) This may also complicate talar dislocation. The pattern of vascular perfusion to the talar body is such that a neck fracture can significantly compromise its blood supply. Little to no collateral supply exists because over 60% of its external surface is covered by articular cartilage. The main source of blood enters by way of the foramina in the sinus tarsi and tarsal canal. Generally, the more anterior the neck fracture, the greater the likelihood for developing avascular necrosis.

Following a talar fracture, the early formation of a zone of linear lucency beneath the cortex of the dome is a reliable indicator of an intact blood supply with a diminished probability for developing avascular necrosis (Hawkin's sign). (17)

Other Tarsal Fractures

Occasionally, other tarsal bones may fracture.

Navicular Fractures.   Avulsion of its dorsal surface is the most frequent type of tarsal navicular fracture. (18) Acute eversion may also avulse the medial tuberosity because of traction exerted by the tibialis posterior tendon. This infrequent injury must not be confused with the commonly seen accessory ossicle, os tibiale externum. Other navicular fractures are uncommon. (Fig. 9.138)

Cuneiform Fractures.   Isolated fractures are rare. More frequently, fractures of the distal aspects of the cuneiforms are associated with tarsometatarsal dislocation (Lisfranc's injury).

Cuboid Fractures.   Isolated fractures are unusual. (19) The most common site is at the most lateral margin. In children a bone scan may be required to accurately identify the fracture. (19) Care must be taken to not confuse the accessory ossicles seen adjacent to the cuboid (os peroneum, os versalium) as fractures.

Fractures of the Metatarsals

A dropped heavy object is a frequent cause of metatarsal fracture. The majority involve the shaft or neck. The fracture line may be oblique, spiral, or transverse and requires multiple views for visualization. The second and third metatarsals are the most common skeletal sites for stress fractures to occur.

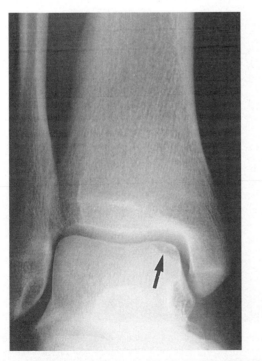

Figure 9.136.   OSTEOCHONDRAL FRACTURE OF THE MEDIAL TALAR DOME. A radiolucent defect with a central bone flake is observed in the medial talar dome (arrow). This represents an osteochondral fracture of the articular surface.

Jones' Fracture (Dancer's Fracture).   Fractures of the base of the fifth metatarsal are among the most common of all bony injuries of the foot. (20) These synonyms are derived from Jones' description, in 1902, of an injury he suffered while dancing. (21) This is a transverse fracture at the proximal end of the fifth metatarsal approximately 15–20 mm from its base. The implicated mechanism is traction exerted from the peroneus brevis tendon or lateral cord of the plantar aponeurosis when the foot is forcefully inverted and plantar flexed. (20) (Fig. 9.139A and B)

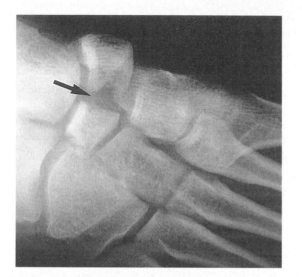

Figure 9.138.   TARSAL NAVICULAR FRACTURE. A fracture through the midportion of the navicular is apparent (arrow). COMMENT: Fractures of the tarsal navicular are relatively uncommon.

In children there is a longitudinally oriented apophysis adjacent to the fracture region which should not be confused with a fracture. (Fig. 9.140A and B)

Clinically and radiographically, these fractures are frequently overlooked, since pain and swelling from the traumatized lateral tendon sheaths and ankle ligaments misdirect the attention to the ankle mortise. The further away the fracture is from the base, the slower it is to heal, and the more it is prone to nonunion due to the intrinsically deficient blood supply. (22)

Fractures of the Phalanges

In the absence of a clinical history and multiple views of the phalanges, these are easily passed over.

Crush Injuries.   Dropping a heavy object on the toe frequently results in a comminuted phalanx, especially the distal phalanx. (Fig. 9.141)

Bedroom Fracture.   A direct blow to the toe such as when striking an object with a bare foot, may produce a fracture of any phalanx, especially those of the first and fifth digits. (Fig. 9.142)

Chip Fracture.   Small fractures of the phalangeal articular margins may follow digital hyperextension or, less frequently, hyperflexion forces.

Hallux Rigidus.   A fracture of the hallux phalanx may produce a stiffened, painful first metatarsophalangeal joint. (Fig. 9.143) Initially the joint may show no alteration but later signs of degenerative arthritis can occur.

Sesamoid Fracture.   Acute fracture may complicate jumping, dancing, and running, especially if done with bare feet. Stress fractures and secondary avascular necrosis can also be found. The medial hallux sesamoid is more frequently involved than the lateral side. Localized pain and swelling over the plantar surface of

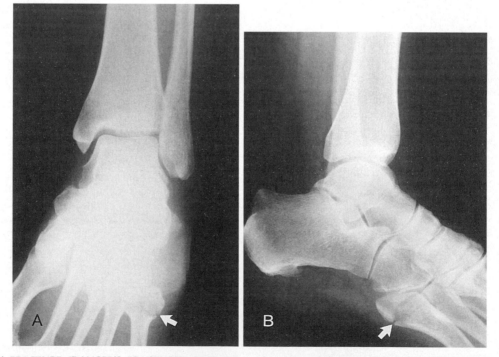

Figure 9.139.   JONES' FRACTURE (DANCER'S FRACTURE): BASE OF FIFTH METATARSAL. A. AP Ankle. B. Lateral Ankle. A transverse fracture line is seen at the base of the fifth metatarsal (arrows). COMMENT: The Jones' or "dancer's" fracture is precipitated by an avulsive force exerted from the peroneus brevis tendon and lateral cord of the plantar aponeurosis when the foot is forcefully inverted and plantar flexed. These fractures are frequently overlooked, since this type of injury causes more noticeable symptoms in the area of the ankle mortise. This is one of the most frequent injuries of the foot.

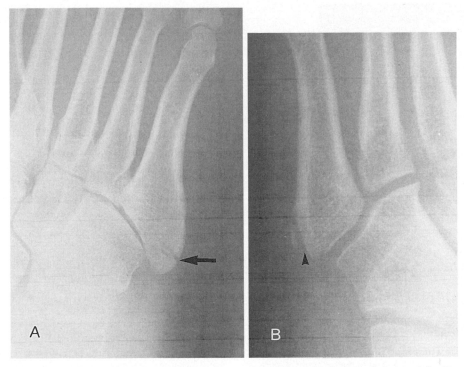

Figure 9.140. JONES' FRACTURE VERSUS NORMAL VARIANT. A. Oblique Foot: Jones' Fracture. Notice the characteristic transverse orientation of the fracture line of the base of the fifth metatarsal (arrow). **B. Oblique Foot: Normal Growth Variation**. The apophysis for the base of the fifth metatarsal is separated by a longitudinally oriented lucent cleft (arrowhead). With skeletal maturation, this radiolucent cleft will eventually ossify and become united to the base of the fifth metatarsal. COMMENT: In the foot of a traumatized young patient recognition of the orientation of the radiolucent cleft will distinguish between transverse fractures of the base of the fifth metatarsal and a normal vertically oriented apophyseal growth.

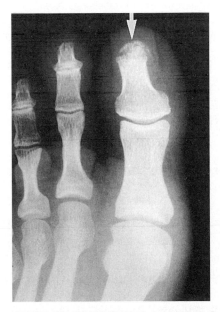

Figure 9.141. CRUSH FRACTURE: DISTAL PHALANX. Comminution of the distal phalanx (arrow) has occurred following a blow from a heavy object. (Courtesy of Robert S. Rowe, Swansea, Australia)

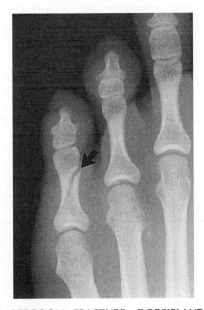

Figure 9.142. BEDROOM FRACTURE: DORSIPLANTAR TOES. An oblique fracture of the shaft of the proximal phalanx of the fifth toe (arrow) has occurred following striking a hard object. (Courtesy of Gaylord H. Hanssen, DC, Doniphan, Nebraska)

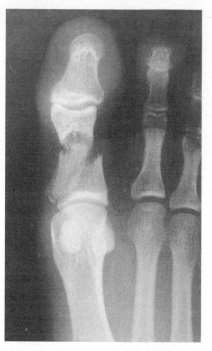

Figure 9.143.   FRACTURE OF THE PROXIMAL PHALANX: GREAT TOE.
There is a comminuted fracture through the shaft of the proximal phalanx of
the great toe, extending immediately distal to the proximal articular surface
of the phalanx. COMMENT: This type of fracture may develop into a stiff,
painful first metatarsal phalangeal joint (hallux rigidus).

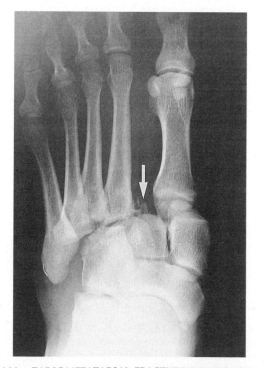

**Figure 9.144.   TARSOMETATARSAL FRACTURE DISLOCATION (LISFR-
ANC'S DISLOCATION).** Displacement of the second through the fifth metatarsal bases has occurred, with associated fractures in the area of diastasis
(arrow) between the bases of the first and second metatarsals. The injury
usually results from a fall with longitudinal compression or a twisting force
through the forefoot. (Courtesy of Gary M. Fieber, DC, Minneapolis,
Minnesota)

the forefoot are the usual findings. The sesamoid may exhibit a
single fracture line or consist of multiple fragments. A specialized
axial submetatarsal view is the best method of depiction. Bone
scan will show increased activity. There should be clear differentiation from the variant bipartite sesamoid which is present in
one third of the population and is bilateral in 85% of these. (23)

DISLOCATIONS OF THE FOOT
Talus Dislocation

The talus is the most common bone in the foot to dislocate. It
may dislocate at three joints—the talotibial, talocalcaneal (subtalar), and talonavicular joints. These may occur singularly or together and also can precipitate avascular necrosis of the talus as
a complication.

Other Tarsal Dislocations

Midtarsal Dislocation (Chopart's Dislocation).   This is a rare
dislocation that separates the foot at the talonavicular and calcaneocuboid joints. (1)

*Tarsometatarsal Fracture Dislocation (Lisfranc's Disloca-
tion).*   The injury has been named after a surgeon in Napoleon's
army—not for his description of the injury but because of his
method of foot amputation through the same region. (24) The site
of separation is at the tarsometatarsal junction. The components
consist of dorsal dislocation of the metatarsal bases in relation to
the opposing tarsals, in combination with fractures at various locations along the site of joint separation. (Fig. 9.144) Additionally,
there may be associated lateral displacement of the metatarsals.
CT is especially useful in the accurate depiction of the injury. (25)
The most common accompanying fractures are at the base of the
second metatarsal and lateral cuboid surface.

Lisfranc injuries, once most common with equestrian accidents, now occur most often in motor vehicle and industrial accidents. The injury usually results from a fall with longitudinal
compression or a twisting force through the forefoot.

Phalangeal Dislocations

These are not as frequent as in the hand and are readily
recognizable.

 MEDICOLEGAL IMPLICATIONS
*Injuries to the Pelvis and Lower
Limbs*

- Injuries to the pelvis may be associated with bladder and urethral
  injuries. Subtle fractures of the pubis and ischium are readily overlooked and frequently require oblique views for demonstration.

- Fractures of the sacrum and coccyx are difficult to identify due to
  angulation and overlying soft tissue. Special views should be employed if fracture is suspected.

- Fractures of the femoral neck and slipped femoral capital epiphysis are common injuries in the elderly and adolescent patients
  respectively, and carry significant morbidity if not detected. These
  injuries require high quality radiographs with AP and frog-leg projections for detection.

- Injuries to the knee most commonly produce ligamentous and meniscal lesions which have few plain film changes. MR imaging is often required in such circumstances. However, AP "tunnel," lateral and "skyline" views should always be obtained initially.

- Ankle injuries requre routine use of AP, AP medial oblique, and lateral views to detect bony lesions. Accessory ossicles at the malleolar tips and the os trigonum can be readily confused variants.

- Growth plate injuries in the developing skeleton should be monitored beyond the healing time to assess for growth deformity. Periodic x-ray examination at 3-, 6-, and 12-month intervals should be considered as clinically indicated.

- Foot injuries can lead to considerable disability if unrecognized. Minimum views of dorsiplantar, medial oblique dorsiplantar, and lateral projections must be performed.

FRACTURES OF THE THORAX
GENERAL CONSIDERATIONS

Significant force is usually required to produce a fractured rib. They are uncommon injuries of childhood, but with advancing age the incidence gradually increases, especially after the third decade, as the bones become more rigid and brittle. (1)

Of all fractures, those involving the ribs are the most difficult to observe due to the curvilinear shape of the rib. They usually require multiple oblique views to orient the fracture line to a plane where the x-ray beam can pass directly through the separation. It is to be expected that rib fractures initially can go undetected, only becoming visible later when enough callus is present.

In general, a single AP radiograph is insufficient for the ac-

curate diagnosis of rib fracture and must be supplemented by multiple oblique projections. Bone scan will demonstrate singular or multiple rib fractures. (Fig. 9.145) Occasionally, the bone scan may assist in the evaluation of the traumatized patient, for medicolegal purposes.

Radiologic Features of Rib Fractures

A number of features should be searched for to aid in locating a rib fracture. (Fig. 9.146) (Table 9.15)

Fracture Line.   When present, the fracture line will usually cross the rib transversely or obliquely and will be radiolucent. Care must be taken to not misinterpret overlying bronchial air shadows as fracture lines, as evidenced by the lung markings continuing beyond the bony rib margin.

Cortical Offset.   This is a most important feature that is frequently seen without visualizing the fracture line. The superior and inferior cortices will be acutely offset at the fracture site, as evidenced by a sharp "step effect."

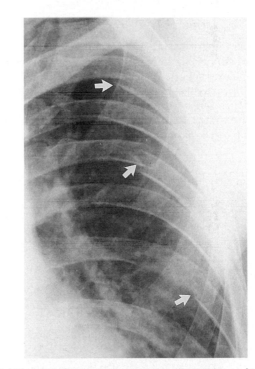

Figure 9.146.   RIB FRACTURES: GENERAL FEATURES. Multiple fracture sites are observed (arrows). Rib fractures can be identified by searching for a fracture line, cortical offset, or altered rib angulation and, when multiple, following along the line of injury looking for additional lesions.

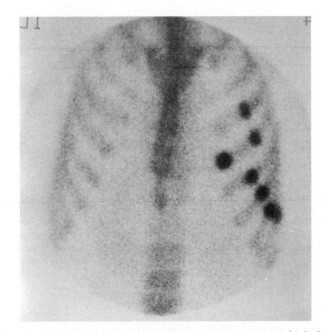

Figure 9.145.   RIB FRACTURES: BONE SCAN FEATURES. Multiple focal areas of increased radioisotopic uptake are present in the anterior ribs. These areas correspond to the sites of rib fractures which were not clearly identifiable on the plain film examination. COMMENT: In view of the difficulty in locating rib fractures, this procedure is particularly useful in medicolegal and equivocal clinical circumstances. (Courtesy of Lawrence A. Cooperstein, MD, Pittsburgh, Pennsylvania)

Table 9.15.   Radiologic Features of Rib Fractures
Radiolucent fracture line
Cortical offset
Altered rib orientation
Pleural deflection
Callus formation
Pleural fluid
Pneumothorax
Subcutaneous emphysema
Diaphragmatic elevation

Rib Orientation.   A sharp deviation in the contour of a single rib may occur at the fracture site. If the distal end of the fractured rib appears hook–like ("costal hook sign"), this may indicate a flail segment.

Callus Formation.   If callus has begun to form, there will be a localized increase in density and a bulbous expansion at the fracture site. (Fig. 9.147)

Pleural Deflection.   A localized hematoma adjacent to the fracture site may displace the pleura inward, indenting into the lung. When the x-ray beam is tangential to the accumulated blood, this will be seen as a radiopaque density that is sharply demarcated, convex toward the lung, gradually blending beyond the fracture site into its normal position (extrapleural sign).

Other Fractures

Multiple rib fractures are usually aligned in a linear fashion along the vector of trauma. The ipsilateral costophrenic recess may be blunted due to sanguineous pleural fluid. Other associations include pneumothorax, subcutaneous emphysema, diaphragmatic elevation, and splenic laceration.

Upper Rib (1–3) Fractures

The upper three ribs rarely fracture due to their inherent strength and supporting musculature. (2) The presence of such upper rib fractures suggests the likelihood of severe trauma with possible injuries to the trachea, aorta, great vessels, brachial plexus, or spine. (Fig. 9.148) Weightlifters may incur fracture of the second rib during heavy bench pressing. (2) Stress fractures of the first rib can occur in throwing athletes. (3)

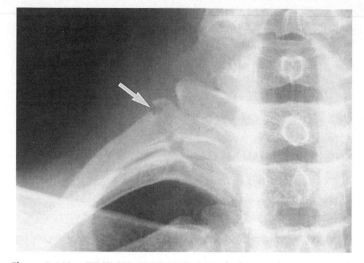

Figure 9.148.   FIRST RIB FRACTURE. A single fracture line traverses the first rib, just distal to the costotransverse joint (arrow). COMMENT: Fractures of the upper ribs are frequently associated with severe trauma and additional injuries to the trachea, aorta, great vessels, brachial plexus, or spine.

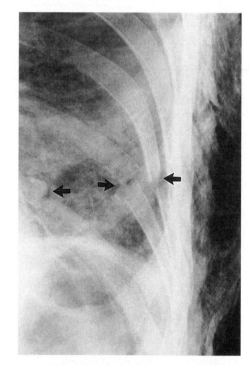

Figure 9.149.   MULTIPLE RIB FRACTURES WITH SUBCUTANEOUS EMPHYSEMA. Multiple rib fractures affecting the posterolateral surface (arrows) are associated with subcutaneous emphysema in the overlying soft tissues. Subcutaneous emphysema is a sign of severe pulmonary injury, allowing direct communication between the bronchial tree and the extrathoracic soft tissues.

Middle Rib (4–9) Fractures

These ribs are the most commonly fractured. The fracture site depends on the mechanism of injury but frequently is found at the lateral aspect of the rib, where it is easily overlooked. (Fig. 9.149) Fractures of these ribs therefore require multiple views for adequate depiction. An extrapleural collection of hematoma may be represented by an inward deflection of the pleara at the site of

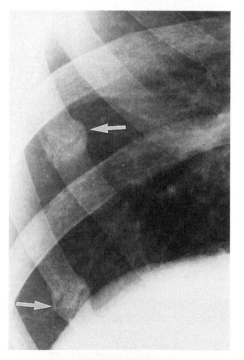

Figure 9.147.   HEALING RIB FRACTURES. Two sites of healing rib fractures are identified (arrows). Radiographic features consist of a localized region of increased density, bony expansion of the rib at the fracture site, and visualization of the fracture line. COMMENT: These rib fractures were not apparent on the initial radiograph examination following a chronic episode of coughing. Follow-up radiographs revealed callus formation, which now localizes the previously unrecognized fracture sites.

fracture. (4) Fractures of the mid to lower anterior ribs should stimulate close scrutiny of the spleen and liver for associated injury.

Flail Chest.   This is the term used to describe the occurrence of two fractures involving the same rib, isolating a section of the rib. Usually, multiple adjacent ribs are affected, which allows these isolated rib fragments ("flail segment") to move during respiration in an opposite direction (paradoxical motion). This reduces ventilation of the underlying lung to interfere with pulmonary gaseous exchange, potentially creating a life-threatening situation. A radiologic clue to a flail chest is the isolated rib section rotates and exhibits a hook–like distal end on the frontal radiograph ("costal hook sign").

Golfer's Fracture.   On occasion a golfer may inadvertently strike the ground rather than the ball. This abrupt termination of the swing is sometimes forceful enough to precipitate a fracture of a rib at its lateral margin.

Passion (Bear Hug) Fracture.   Fracture of a rib can occasionally be precipitated when one is the recipient of an overenthusiastic hug. The presence of osteopenia may predispose the elderly to these fractures.

Lower Rib (10–12) Fractures

These are uncommonly fractured, since they are relatively mobile and yielding; however, if a fracture is observed, associated kidney damage should be evaluated. (Fig. 9.150)

Cough (Post-Tussive) Fracture.   In any condition where persistent and/or violent coughing is experienced, stress fractures of the lower anterior ribs may occur. (5) (Fig. 9.147) The 6 to 7th anterior ribs are the most common sites. (6)

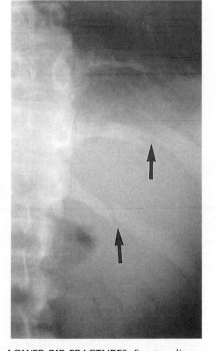

Figure 9.150.   LOWER RIB FRACTURES. Fracture lines are seen through both the 11th and 12th ribs (arrows), with minimal displacement. COMMENT: The presence of fractures of the lower ribs warrants careful examination of the urinary system, especially renal function and structure. This should include an intravenous pyelogram and other more sophisticated imaging modalities.

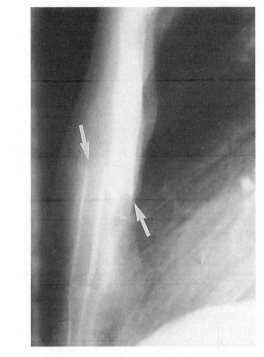

Figure 9.151.   STERNAL FRACTURE WITH DISPLACEMENT. A complete fracture through the body of the sternum, with displacement and overlap (arrows) across the fracture site. COMMENT: Sternal injuries are uncommon and usually follow severe blunt trauma to the anterior thorax.

Costal Cartilage Injuries

Costal cartilage injuries on plain films generally cannot be discerned. If calcified, fractures can be identified as a disruption. Nuclear bone scanning and CT will assist in their evaluation.

Fractures of the Sternum.   Blunt compressive impacts to the chest, such as from the steering wheel in motor vehicle accidents, are the major causes of sternal injury. The most common sites of fracture involve the body or manubriosternal junction and are usually transverse in nature. The best projection is the lateral view, where a fracture line, displacement, and associated hematoma may be observed. (7) (Fig. 9.151) Tomography or computed tomography may be required for optimal visualization of the sternum. All sternal injuries should point to careful evaluation of the thoracolumbar spine for associated abnormalities. (8)

COMPLICATIONS OF THORACIC TRAUMA

Various tissues and organs may suffer damage in association with injuries of the thorax. (8)

Pleural Complications

Traumatic Pneumothorax.   Intrapleural negative pressure functions to maintain lung inflation. When the pleura is torn, this pressure is lost, allowing the lung to collapse.

Hemothorax Complications.   Blood may accumulate in the pleural space from ruptured blood vessels. This can be identified by observing blunt costophrenic sulci, widening of the paraspinal space, and apical "capping." (8)

Chylothorax Complications.   Lymphatic fluid may accumulate in the same manner as does blood.

Lung Complications

Contusion.   Intrapulmonary hemorrhage can produce an irregular, localized lung opacity. This appears shortly after the injury and then gradually resorbs within 3–10 days.

Pneumonia.   This may complicate the immobility of the chest following a rib fracture, due to the inactivation of the normal lung fluid clearing mechanisms.

Other Tissue Complications

Various associated injuries have been reported, including rupture of the spleen, diaphragm, tracheobronchial tree, esophagus, kidney, and heart, as well as formation of aortic aneurysms and lung cysts. (8) Thoracic spine lesions are also common.

FRACTURES AND DISLOCATIONS OF THE SHOULDER GIRDLE

GENERAL CONSIDERATIONS

The shoulder girdle is vulnerable to damage, but the specific site of injury varies with age. Fracture of the clavicle is the most common skeletal injury during birth and childhood. (Fig. 9.152) Between 20 and 40 years of age, dislocation of the shoulder, acromioclavicular joint separation, and clavicle fractures predominate. In the elderly, shoulder dislocations and surgical neck fractures of the humerus become increasingly more common.

Technologically, the shoulder girdle requires specific projections for proper evaluation. A minimum general survey of the shoulder should include anteroposterior views with internal rotation, external rotation, and abduction ("baby arm"). At least one view should include the upper thoracic cage and lung to the spine. Additional specific projections for the acromioclavicular joint, clavicle, and scapula must be performed, as clinically indicated, for optimum evaluation. A "hotlight" should be routinely used to view the shoulder structures, due to inherent overexposure of thinner body areas such as the distal clavicle and acromioclavicular joint.

FRACTURES OF THE CLAVICLE

Technologic Features

The "S" shape and normal overlap with the upper rib cage renders the clavicle a difficult structure to evaluate on straight anteroposterior projections. (Fig. 9.153A and B) The optimal view is an anteroposterior projection with 15° cephalad tube angulation. Weights (10 to 15 pounds) may be held to aid in detecting undisplaced fractures. The exposure factors should be approximately half of that utilized in standard shoulder projections to prevent overexposure.

Radiologic Features

Generally, the clavicle is the bone most commonly fractured during birth and during childhood. Direct trauma to the shoulder is usually involved.

Medial Clavicle Fractures.   This is the least common site, representing only approximately 5% of all clavicle fractures. (1) These are difficult to observe and usually require tomography.

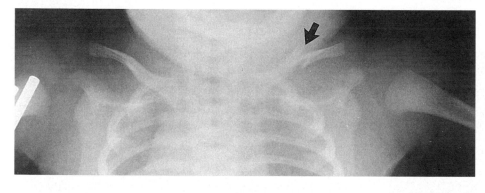

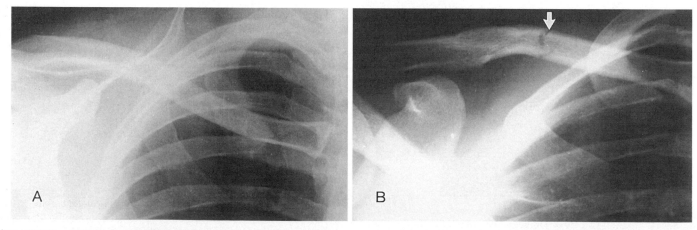

Figure 9.152.   BIRTH FRACTURE OF THE CLAVICLE. A midclavicular fracture (arrow) has occurred during the birth process. COMMENT: Fracture of the clavicle is the most common birth fracture.

Figure 9.153.   CLAVICLE FRACTURE EVALUATION: ANGULATED VERSUS NONANGULATED PROJECTIONS. A. AP Nonangulated Projection. No fracture line is visible. **B. Angulated Projection.** With 15° cephalad tube angulation, the fracture line is clearly evident (arrow). COMMENT: In evaluation of clavicular trauma specific clavicle projections must be obtained to demonstrate fractures, particularly through the midportion of the clavicle. (Courtesy of Kenneth E. Yochum, DC, St. Louis, Missouri)

Middle Clavicle Fractures.   This is the most common site, representing approximately 80% of all clavicle fractures. (1) A force applied to the distal end of the "S" shaped clavicle creates a shearing effect at the middle third, producing the fracture. The fracture is usually complete, with the medial fragment elevated by the action of the sternocleidomastoid muscle and the lateral fragment depressed by the weight of the shoulder and upper extremity. (Fig. 9.154) In addition to malalignment, an overlap at the fracture site is common, with the distal fragment usually lying below the medial fragment. Healing is often associated with extensive callus formation. (Fig. 9.155)

Lateral Clavicle Fractures.   These account for approximately 15% of all clavicle fractures. (1) There are three varieties: (a) undisplaced; (b) displaced, where the distal fragment moves anterior and inferior; and (c) articular surface extension. (Fig. 9.156)

Whenever a fracture of the lateral third is identified, weight-bearing stress views should be obtained to clarify the status of the coracoclavicular ligaments. (2) Notably, fractures that extend

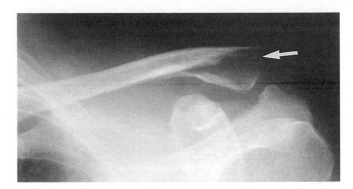

Figure 9.156.   FRACTURE OF THE DISTAL CLAVICLE. A fracture line through the distal surface of the clavicle is identified (arrow). COMMENT: Fractures in this location are frequently overlooked due to technical overexposure. Bright light illumination is required for clear identification. These fractures frequently predispose to degenerative arthritis of the acromioclavicular articulation.

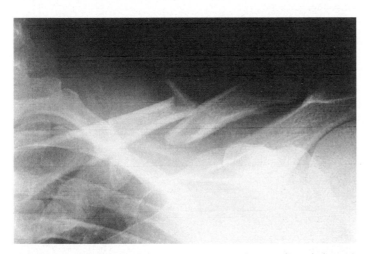

Figure 9.154.   MIDCLAVICULAR FRACTURE. A fracture through the midportion of the clavicle has resulted in superior displacement of the medial portion and inferior displacement of the lateral portion.

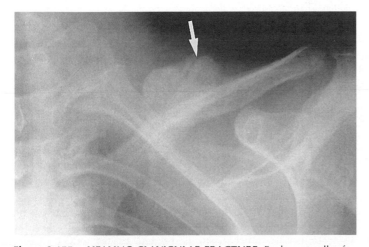

Figure 9.155.   HEALING CLAVICULAR FRACTURE. Exuberant callus formation (arrow) is identified adjacent to a midclavicular fracture. This degree of callus formation is a frequent finding in the healing phase of these injuries. COMMENT: Callus formation of this extent may lead to significant cosmetic disfiguration and compromise of the thoracic outlet.

into the joint frequently precipitate the onset of degenerative arthritis.

Complications of Clavicle Injuries

Childhood clavicular fractures usually heal without sequelae; however, in adults the incidence of complications increases.

Neurovascular Damage.   Associated injury to the underlying neurovascular structures most frequently involves the subclavian artery, less commonly, the vein, and, occasionally, the brachial plexus and sympathetic chain. (3) Compressive effects from the hypertrophic callus can also precipitate pressure-related neurovascular disturbances. (1,4)

Nonunion.   A failure to unite the fracture requires surgical fixation. The key signs of nonunion are located at the fracture margins, where sclerosis, rounding, and a smooth contour will be visible.

Malunion.   In the presence of fragment overlap and massive callus formation, a cosmetic deformity may result. Correction requires osteotomy, realignment, and fixation.

Degenerative Arthritis.   Painful degenerative arthritis frequently follows intraarticular fractures of the clavicle. This is evidenced by loss of joint space, sclerosis, and osteophyte formation.

Posttraumatic Osteolysis.   An injury response peculiar to the clavicle is bone resorption of the distal segment, usually 1–3 mm, but never more than 2–3 cm. (5) This is a commonly overlooked shoulder condition requiring properly exposed radiographs depicting the acromioclavicular joint adequately. (5)

The initiating injury may be relatively minor, often lacking the severity of that required to cause a fracture or dislocation. It first becomes radiologically visible 2–3 months after injury. The precise mechanism is uncertain, although synovial hypertrophy suggests inflammatory osteoclastic activity. (6) Pain is mild to moderate, while the disorder takes a self-limiting course over a number of months.

The earliest radiographic sign in the development of osteolysis is a cystic rarefaction of the clavicular subarticular cortex, followed by cortical dissolution. (6,7) The joint appears wide and the clavicular surface is frayed and irregular or cup-shaped. (5) (Fig. 9.157A and B) With healing, there are varying degrees of bony reconstitution from complete restoration of structure to a permanently tapered distal clavicle and increased joint space.

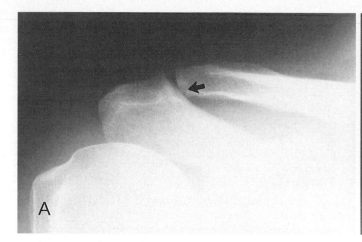

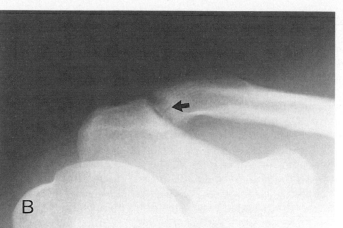

Figure 9.157. POSTTRAUMATIC OSTEOLYSIS OF THE CLAVICLE. A. AP Acromioclavicular Joint. Two months following trauma to the shoulder, a cystic rarefaction (arrow) is present at the inferior aspect of the distal articular surface of the clavicle. **B. AP Acromioclavicular Joint.** There has been extension of the area of rarefaction in the distal clavicle involving the entire distal surface (arrow). Observe the smooth and regular articular margins of the acromial surface, differentiating it from inflammatory joint diseases (rheumatoid arthritis and septic arthritis). COMMENT: This disorder follows a self-limiting course and resolves with varying degrees of reconstitution of the resorbed bone. (Courtesy of Leo J. Bronston, DC, FACO, Sparta, Wisconsin)

FRACTURES OF THE SCAPULA

Severe trauma is usually needed to fracture the scapula. Isolated scapular fractures are infrequent, with approximately 80% demonstrating other injuries. (8,9) Occasionally exercises such as push-ups may cause a fracture. (10) Routine shoulder views usually adequately demonstrate the scapula; however, special projections may be required for a more thorough examination.

Coracoid View (Axillary or Scapular "Y" View). This view is performed anteroposterior, with 25 to 40° of cephalad tube tilt.

Lateral View. This view is performed posteroanterior, with the patient rotated 35°. It produces a tangential depiction of the scapula body and acromion.

Axillary View. This view is performed superior-inferior, with the cassette in the axilla and the arm abducted. It demonstrates the glenoid, acromion, and coracoid process.

Radiologic Features of Scapula Fractures

The majority of fractures involve the scapular body and neck (80%). (8) (Fig. 9.158) When the coracoid or acromion fractures, it is usually in the midportion at the narrowest dimension. An avulsion corresponding to the triceps insertion is often seen at the inferior glenoid rim in association with anterior humeral dislocations (Bankart lesion). (11)

FRACTURES OF THE HUMERUS

Most humeral fractures can be identified on standard anteroposterior views in internal and external rotation.

Radiologic Features

Fractures of the proximal humerus are often described by the Neer classification. (12) There are four categories based on the fracture location: the anatomic neck, greater tuberosity, lesser tuberosity, and surgical neck. Fractures of the proximal shaft are not included. The number of these fractures are then added to each other—one part, two part, three part, or four part. Up to 80% are one-part, 10% two-part, 3% three-part and 4% four-part

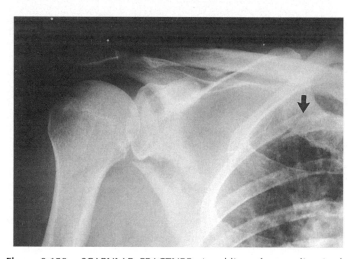

Figure 9.158. SCAPULAR FRACTURE. An oblique fracture line in the subglenoid axillary border of the scapula is visible. An associated rib fracture (arrow) is also seen. COMMENT: The body and neck are the most common sites of scapular fractures. (Courtesy of Gail J. Keilman, DC, Minneapolis, Minnesota)

fractures. (12,13) CT is useful in identifying fragments and articular involvement.

Fractures Proximal to the Anatomic Neck. Isolated fractures through the anatomic neck are uncommon and usually occur in combination with other humeral fractures. There is a high incidence of developing avascular necrosis of the humeral head. (2) Comminuted fractures of the humeral head are referred to as *head-splitting fractures.* (12)

An impaction fracture on the posterolateral surface of the humeral head is commonly associated with anterior shoulder dislocation. The mechanism is related to the effect of the inferior glenoid rim being forcefully pushed into the articular surface of the humeral head (Hill-Sachs defect, "hatchet" defect). (14) The optimal projection to demonstrate the defect is internal rotation.

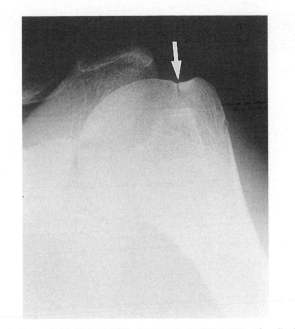

Figure 9.159. FLAP FRACTURE: GREATER TUBEROSITY. The displaced fracture of the greater tuberosity is recognized by the presence of a radiolucent line (arrow). COMMENT: This fracture is best identified in the external rotation view, since the greater tuberosity is brought into profile in this projection.

Fractures of the Greater Tuberosity (Flap Fracture). This structure may be avulsed by the connecting tendons or fractured by direct trauma. (Fig. 9.159) It is frequently fractured during anterior humeral dislocation. (Fig. 9.160) Generally, older patients show a smaller separated fragment than younger individuals.

This fracture is best depicted on the external rotation view. Displacement of more than 1 cm indicates significant rotator cuff disruption. This necessitates open reduction and repair. (4)

Fractures of the Lesser Tuberosity. The lesser tuberosity is not vulnerable to isolated trauma. (15) More commonly it occurs in conjunction with other proximal humeral fractures.

Fractures of the Surgical Neck. This is the most common site of proximal humerus fractures. (Figs. 9.161, 9.162A and B) The site of the fracture is immediately distal to the tuberosities, at the narrowest point of humeral width. These tend to be comminuted, involving the adjacent tuberosities. Anteromedial displacement of the shaft distal to the fracture frequently occurs because of the pull of the pectoralis major muscle. On occasion, injury to the adjacent axillary nerve and artery may complicate the fracture.

Fractures of the Proximal Shaft. Direct trauma is the most common cause for shaft fractures. The relative location of the fracture in relation to muscle insertions determines the type of deformity produced. (4) If the fracture occurs proximal to the pectoralis major attachment, the humeral head will abduct and rotate. Between the pectoralis major and deltoid, the proximal fragment will adduct. Distal to the deltoid, the proximal fragment will abduct.

Complications of Humeral Fractures

Complications of humeral fractures include residual joint stiffness, nonunion, malunion, degenerative joint disease, head avascular necrosis, posttraumatic myositis ossificans, and neurovascular damage.

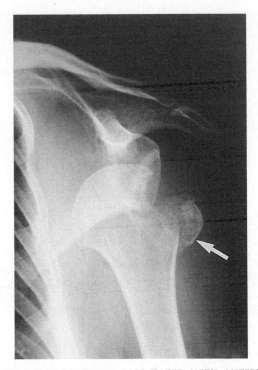

Figure 9.160. FLAP FRACTURE ASSOCIATED WITH ANTERIOR GLENOHUMERAL DISLOCATION. The humeral head is dislocated anteriorly and inferiorly to a subcoracoid position. This is associated with an avulsion fracture of the greater tuberosity of the humerus (flap fracture) (arrow).

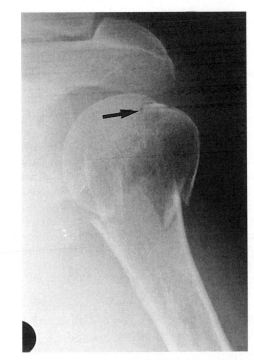

Figure 9.161. SURGICAL NECK FRACTURE: SHOULDER. A transverse comminuted fracture has occurred through the surgical neck of the humerus. There has been extension of the fracture line to involve the greater tuberosity (flap fracture) (arrow).

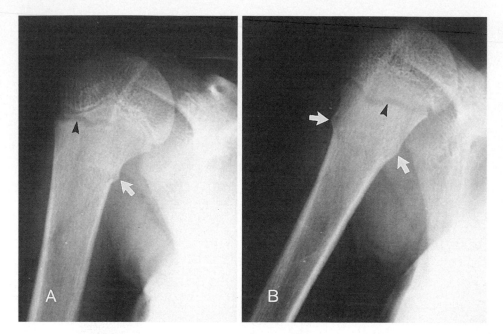

Figure 9.162.   TORUS FRACTURE OF THE PROX-IMAL HUMERUS. A. AP Shoulder: External Rotation. A localized bulging of the cortical surface of the medial metaphysis of the proximal humerus is visible (arrow). **B. AP Shoulder: Internal Rotation.** The cortical bulging is seen to involve both the medial and lateral aspects of the proximal humerus (arrows). This is a characteristic finding of a torus fracture. COMMENT: In young patients the normal cartilaginous growth center (arrowheads) should not be misinterpreted as a fracture line. (Courtesy of Gerald A. Fitzgerald, MD, Sydney, Australia)

DISLOCATIONS OF THE SHOULDER GIRDLE

The shoulder joint is by far the most common joint in the body to dislocate, accounting for over 50% of all joint dislocations. (4) Of the four joint complexes that comprise the shoulder girdle, dislocations at the glenohumeral joint are the most frequent, being involved in 85% of cases. The acromioclavicular joint makes up 12%, the sternoclavicular joint 2%, and the scapulothoracic joint only 1%. (16)

Glenohumeral Joint Dislocations

These are classified further into the direction in which the humeral head has been displaced—anterior, posterior, inferior, and superior.

Anterior Dislocation.   This is the most frequent dislocation of the shoulder, making up approximately 95% of glenohumeral displacements. (Fig. 9.163) Commonly, associated fractures include impaction of the humeral head in 60% of cases (Hill-Sachs defect), fracture of the greater tuberosity in 15% of cases, and, less frequently, avulsion of the inferior glenoid rim (Bankart lesion). (17) (Figs. 9.164A and B, 9.165)

According to where the humeral head comes to rest, positional terms are applied—subglenoid, subcoracoid (most common), subclavicular, and, if trapped between two ribs, intrathoracic. Radiologic signs include inferior and medial humeral displacement, altered humeral head shape, and the Hill-Sachs and Bankart lesions. MR imaging is extremely sensitive and specific in localizing a Hill-Sachs defect. (18)

Posterior Dislocation.   These are uncommon displacements, making up 2 to 4% of glenohumeral dislocations. They follow an epileptic convulsion, electric shock (accidental or therapeutic) or direct trauma. These are difficult lesions to identify radiographically.

The key radiographic signs are widening of the joint space more than 6 mm ("rim" sign), (19) double articlular surface line ("trough line" sign), (20) lack of humeral head/glenoid fossa overlap, (21) lack of close contact at the anterior joint margin (va-

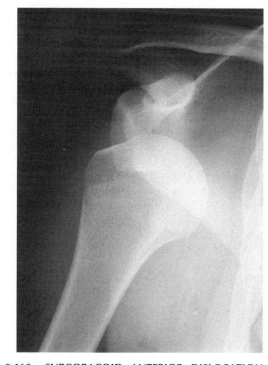

Figure 9.163.   SUBCORACOID ANTERIOR DISLOCATION OF THE SHOULDER. The humeral head has been dislocated anteriorly to lay in a subcoracoid position. COMMENT: This is the most common form of shoulder dislocation.

cant glenoid sign), cystic appearance of the head ("tennis racquet" appearance), and superior displacement. (4) (Fig. 9.166 A and B) Inherent in the displacement is the fact that it is fixed into internal rotation such that no difference in the appearance of the head in the external rotation view is seen.

Inferior Dislocation (Luxatio Erecta).   The lesion follows severe hyperabduction trauma in such a way that the humeral neck

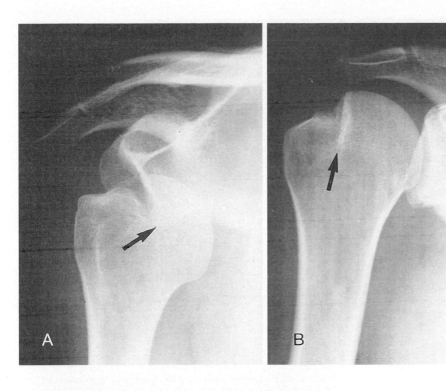

**Figure 9.164.   HILL-SACHS DEFORMITY AS-
SOCIATED WITH ANTERIOR HUMERAL DIS-
LOCATION. A. AP Shoulder.** An anteroinferior
dislocation of the humerus has resulted in an
impaction between the inferior glenoid rim and
opposing humeral head (arrow). The impaction
by the angular surface of the inferior glenoid
rim produces the articular defect that has been
referred to as the ''hatchet'' deformity (Hill-
Sachs defect). **B. AP Shoulder: Postreduction
Radiograph.** Upon repositioning of the humeral head within the glenoid fossa, the residual effect of compression of the articular surface is clearly identified (arrow). COMMENT:
The identification of this Hill-Sachs lesion is a
telltale sign of recurrent anterior shoulder
dislocation.

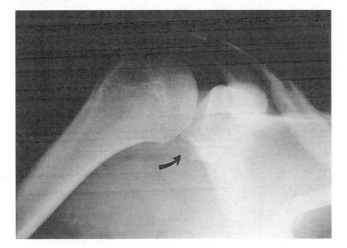

Figure 9.165.   BANKART LESION: SCAPULA. An avulsion fracture of the
inferior glenoid rim (arrow) at the insertion of the triceps muscle frequently
accompanies anterior shoulder dislocations.

contacts the acromion, which acts as a fulcrum to lever the humeral head out and displace it inferiorly. The humerus then locks
into this hyperabduction position, with the humeral head displaced into a subglenoid position.

Occasionally, the humerus may be only partially subluxed inferiorly (drooping shoulder, hanging shoulder). This is seen in
hemarthrosis, joint effusion, stroke, and brachial plexus lesions.
(22)

Superior Dislocation.   This is a rare type of dislocation requiring considerable force, usually with the elbow flexed and the
arm adducted. More commonly experienced is the superior displacement of the humeral head following a tear of the rotator cuff
tendon. This reduces the downward holding power of the infraspinatus tendon, allowing the relatively unopposed action of the

deltoid to elevate the humerus, which, in longstanding cases, may
form a pseudojoint with the undersurface of the clavicle and acromion. If the acromiohumeral distance measures less than 7 mm,
this is an indicator of rotator cuff tear. (23,24)

Rotator Cuff Tears.   Traumatic and degenerative lesions of
the rotator cuff are common injuries, the incidence increasing with age. Diagnosis and treatment are often delayed. Clinical assessment with palpation for the defect may be as high
as 95% accurate. (25) Plain film signs are few and consist
of an elevated humeral head in relation to the glenoid fossa
(unopposed action of the deltoid), narrowing of the acromiohumeral joint space, erosion with sclerosis on the undersurface
of the acromion, and nonspecific roughening with cysts at
the greater tuberosity. Arthrography shows extravasation of
contrast beyond the capsule, with up to 85% sensitivity. (25,26)
Ultrasound, despite being very much operator- and equipment-
dependent and impaired by tendon calcification mimicking
tears, is 60 to 85% sensitive in locating tears. (25,27) MR imaging
is up to 100% sensitive for depicting tears greater than 2 cm.
(25,28)

Glenoid Labral Tears (SLAP Lesions).   These injuries involve
the superior portion of the glenoid labrum and are associated
with shoulder instability. *SLAP* is the abbreviation used to sum-
marise the location of the tear (Superior Labrum Anterior to Posterior). MRI is the imaging modality of choice, demonstrating labral avulsion, absence or a cleft. (29)

Acromioclavicular Joint Separations

The optimal radiographic views are anteroposterior projections with 15° of cephalad tilt and with and without 10 to 15
pounds of weight. These should be done bilaterally, for comparison purposes. An AP view with internal rotation performed
without weights may show grade III tears due to scapular motion.
(30)

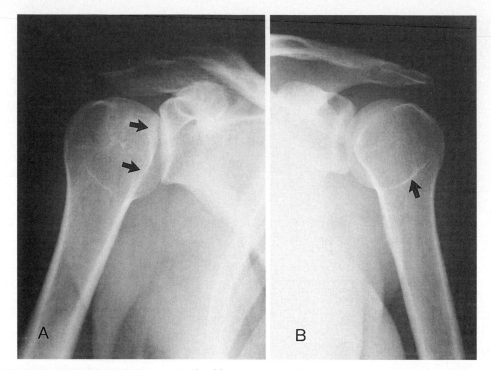

Figure 9.166.   POSTERIOR SHOULDER DISLOCATION. A. AP Shoulder. A double cortical surface is located on the medial aspect of the humeral head (arrows). This is called the "trough line" sign and represents impaction of the humeral head on the posterior glenoid surface. **B. AP Shoulder**. A curvilinear radiopacity spans across the metaphysis of the proximal humerus (arrow) due to severe internal rotation of the humerus ("tennis racquet" appearance). COMMENT: Posterior shoulder dislocations are uncommon, accounting for a 2–4% of glenohumeral dislocations. They most commonly follow either an epileptic convulsion, an electric shock (accidental or therapeutic), or direct trauma.

Radiologic Features.   Three landmarks are assessed on weight-bearing and non-weight-bearing views to evaluate displacement at the acromioclavicular joint.

1. *Acromioclavicular joint space.* Normally, the space is bilaterally symmetrical, within 2–3 mm of each other, and averages between 2–4 mm in absolute width. (31)
2. *Acromioclavicular joint alignment.* The inferior and superior margins of the clavicle and opposing acromion should be in smooth horizontal alignment.
3. *Coracoclavicular distance.* The distance between the inferior margin of the clavicle and the closest surface of the coracoid is normally 11–13 mm. There should be no more than 5 mm difference in the measurement from right to left. (4,32)

Classification of Acromioclavicular Injuries. (4,12)   This is usually based on the degree of injury to the acromioclavicular and coracoclavicular ligaments. (Fig. 9.167) (Table 9.16)

Type I (Mild Sprain).   The acromioclavicular ligament is stretched but not disrupted, and the coracoclavicular ligament is intact. (Fig. 9.168A and B) Even on weight-bearing views, no discernable increase in the joint space or altered alignment is visible. These are treated conservatively.

Type II (Moderate Sprain).   The acromioclavicular ligament is torn, and the coracoclavicular ligaments are stretched but intact. (Fig. 9.168C and D) Radiographically, the joint space is widened and slight elevation of the clavicle has occurred. These are initially treated conservatively, with a brace, but may require surgery. Old injuries to the coracoclavicular ligament may manifest as ligamentous ossifications.

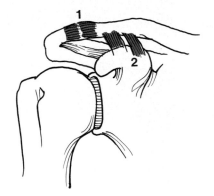

Figure 9.167.   LIGAMENTS OF THE ACROMIOCLAVICULAR JOINT. This schematic diagram demonstrates the locations of (*1*) the acromioclavicular ligaments and (*2*) the coracoclavicular ligaments.

Table 9.16.   Classification of Acromioclavicular Joint Lesions

		Ligament Integrity		
Type	Severity	Acromio-clavicular	Cloraco-clavicular	X-ray Findings
I	Mild	Stretched	Normal	None
II	Moderate	Disrupted	Stretched	Wide joint space Slight clavicle elevation
III	Severe	Disrupted	Disrupted	Wide joint space Severe clavicle elevation

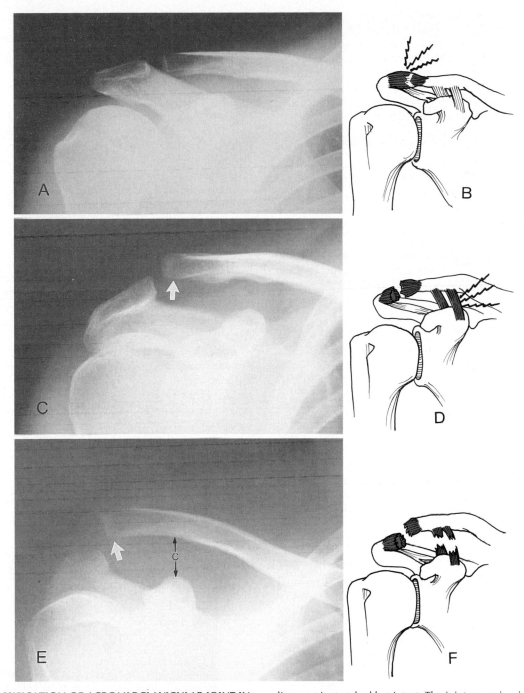

Figure 9.168.   CLASSIFICATION OF ACROMIOCLAVICULAR JOINT IN-JURIES. A. Type I (Mild Sprain): AP Radiograph. B. Type I (Mild Sprain): Schematic Diagram. The acromioclavicular ligament is stretched but not disrupted, and the coracoclavicular ligament is intact. No discernible increase in the joint space or altered alignment is visible. **C. Type II (Moderate Sprain): AP Radiograph** (arrow). **D. Type II (Moderate Sprain): Schematic Diagram**. The acromioclavicular ligament is torn and the coracoclavicular ligament is stretched but intact. The joint space is widened, and slight elevation of the clavicular head has occurred. **E. Type III (Severe Sprain): AP Radiograph** (arrow). **F. Type III (Severe Sprain): Schematic Diagram.** Complete disruption of the acromioclavicular and coracoclavicular ligaments has occurred. There is widening of the joint space, distinct elevation of the clavicle, and widening of the coracoclavicular space (*C*).

Type III (Severe Sprain).   Both the acromioclavicular and cor-acoclavicular ligaments are completely disrupted. (Fig. 9.168E and F) Radiographic signs include widened joint space, distinctive elevation of the distal clavicle above the acromion, and a coracoclavicular space that is widened more than 5 mm more than its contralateral counterpart. The separation can be shown on an AP non-weight-bearing view with internal rotation. (30) These may require joint repair and open fixation.

Sternoclavicular Joint Dislocation

Dislocations of this joint are exceedingly rare and usually follow severe trauma. Anterior displacements of the clavicle are more frequent. Tomography or CT is the technique of choice to demonstrate a sternoclavicular lesion.

Scapulothoracic Joint Dislocation

Severe trauma or thoracoplasty to the upper posterior ribs is required to produce this rare dislocation. Synonyms include locked scapula and scapulothoracic dissociation. (33)

FRACTURES AND DISLOCATIONS OF THE ELBOW AND FOREARM
GENERAL CONSIDERATIONS

Approximately 6% of all fractures and dislocations involve the elbow. (1) The frequency of injury at various sites around the elbow differ between adults and children. (2) (Table 9.17) In adults, approximately 50% of elbow fractures involve the radial head or neck, 20% the olecranon, 10% the supracondylar region of the humerus, and 15% combinations of fracture/dislocations. Unusual sites of fracture involve the humeral condyles, proximal ulna, capitellum, and coronoid process. In children, the most common fracture site is the supracondylar region of the humerus, accounting for approximately 60% of all childhood elbow injuries. The lateral condyle accounts for 15%, and separation of the medial epicondyle ossification center accounts for 10%. The remaining childhood elbow lesions include the olecranon, proximal ulna, radial epiphysis, and dislocations.

Unrecognized elbow fractures frequently produce residual loss of joint mobility and, at times, superimposed degenerative arthritis. The joint and osseous anatomy is complex and requires specific projections for adequate demonstration. (3) A minimum elbow study should include the following views: (a) anteroposterior in full extension; (b) medial oblique; (c) lateral; and (d) axial olecranon projections. In children, confusing growth variations may occasionally be clarified by obtaining similar views of the uninvolved articulation.

Fractures and dislocations of the forearm usually follow significant trauma and are normally readily observable. Standard anteroposterior and lateral projections usually suffice to provide the necessary information required.

Table 9.17. Incidence and Location of Elbow Injuries			
Adults		**Children**	
Location	Incidence	Location	Incidence
Radial head/neck	50%	Supracondylar	60%
Olecranon	20%	Lateral condyle	15%
Supracondylar	10%	Medial epicondyle	10%
Fracture/dislocations	15%		

FRACTURES OF THE ELBOW
Distal Humerus Fractures

These are normally easily recognized. Notably, up to 95% of these fractures extend to disrupt the articular surface. Fractures are classified according to their relationship with the condyles and the shape of the fracture line.

Supracondylar Fractures.   The fracture line extends transversely or obliquely through the distal humerus above the condyles. (Fig. 9.169) This is the most common fracture to occur around the elbow in children (60%). Usually, the distal fracture fragment displaces posteriorly.

Intercondylar Fracture.   The fracture line extends between the medial and lateral condyles and communicates with the supracondylar region. The resultant fracture line may take on a "T" or "Y" configuration. This type of fracture in adults accounts for at least 50% of distal humerus fractures. (4)

The transverse fracture line that passes through both humeral condyles is called a *transcondylar fracture*. A comminuted fracture of the distal humerus, usually with associated ulnar and radial fractures, may occur if an object is struck with the elbow protruding from a car window ("sideswipe" or "baby car" fracture). (1)

Condylar Fracture.   A single condyle may be sheared off due to an angular force through the elbow. Fractures may occur along the articular surfaces of the capitellum and trochlea. The convex surface of the capitellum is particularly susceptible to compression and breakage from forces transmitted from the radial head; the radial head and capitellum are occasionally fractured simultaneously. A small osteochondral fragment may also be sheared off the convex surface of the capitellum, producing an intraarticular loose body (Kocher's fracture, osteochondral fracture, osteochondritis dissecans). (1)

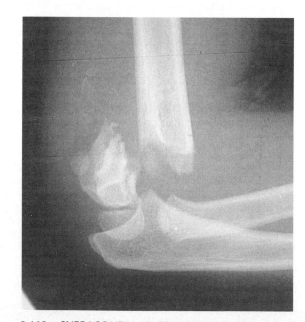

Figure 9.169.   SUPRACONDYLAR FRACTURE OF THE HUMERUS. A complete comminuted fracture is present through the supracondylar region of the humerus. Significant posterior displacement of the distal fragment has also occurred. COMMENT: This is the most common fracture of the elbow in children.

Epicondylar Fracture. These are usually avulsive injuries from traction of the respective common flexor or extensor tendons and collateral ligaments on the medial or lateral epicondyles. Separation of the medial epicondyle is a common injury in sports where strong throwing actions are performed, such as in baseball, especially in adolescents before the apophysis unites to the humerus at between 18 and 19 years of age (Little Leaguer's Elbow). (5) (Fig. 9.170)

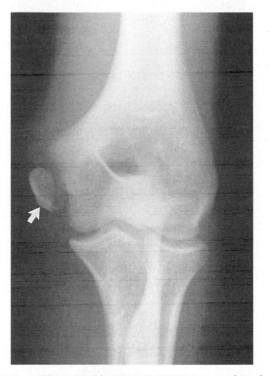

Figure 9.170.   MEDIAL EPICONDYLE FRACTURE. An avulsion fracture of the medial epicondyle has occurred (arrow). A similar injury in a developing child or adolescent has been called "Little Leaguer's" elbow, and is usually associated with sports requiring strong throwing motions.

Fractures of the Proximal Ulna

The two most common sites for fracture are the olecranon and coronoid process.

Olecranon Fracture. Fractures of the olecranon account for approximately 20% of adult elbow fractures, ranking second in frequency to radial neck or head fractures. (2) They may follow direct trauma or an acute flexion avulsion from the triceps insertion. The fracture line is usually best seen on the lateral projection adjacent to the inferior convex surface of the trochlea, but may be proximal or distal to this site. Distraction of the separated fragment may be considerable and requires surgical fixation. (Fig. 9.171A and B) Swelling in the adjacent olecranon bursa is a common associated finding.

Coronoid Process Fracture. The coronoid process may be avulsed by the brachialis muscle or by impaction into the trochlea fossa. (Fig. 9.172) As an isolated fracture, this type of fracture is uncommon. It is fractured frequently in combination with posterior elbow dislocation and usually entails a small fracture fragment that is difficult to identify. The optimal projection for visualizing this fracture is the oblique view.

Fractures of the Proximal Radius

Fractures of the radial neck and head are the most common fractures of the adult elbow, accounting for approximately 50% of all injuries to this region. (2) In children and adolescents, the incidence is significantly lower, with a frequency of approximately 15%. (6) The majority of proximal radius fractures are due to a fall on an outstretched hand, transmitting a longitudinal axis of force to create impaction of the radial head into the capitellum. An incomplete fracture of the radial head which extends from the center of the articular surface for approximately 10 mm, is called a "chisel" fracture. (7) (Fig. 9.173) In the presence of a positive fat-pad sign, if a fracture is not identified specific radial head views may demonstrate a fracture of the radial head. (8)

Radial Head Fracture. The fracture line may be subtle and easily overlooked, so the observer must search for the various signs that indicate an occult fracture. (Fig. 9.174)

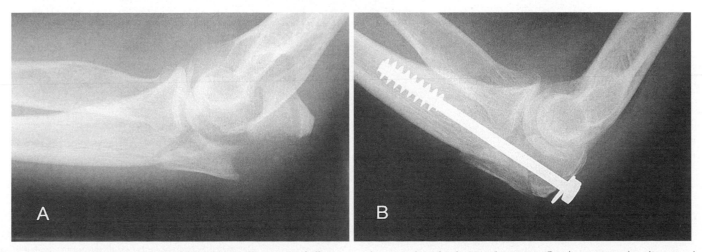

Figure 9.171.   OLECRANON FRACTURE WITH REPAIR. A. Lateral Elbow. Two fracture lines have occurred through the olecranon process. The proximal fragment has retracted due to the pull of the triceps muscle. **B. Lateral Elbow.** A surgical pin has been placed longitudinally through the proximal ulna to realign the fracture fragments. Good appositional realignment has been obtained. COMMENT: The olecranon represents the second most common site for elbow fractures in the adult. The radial head is the most common site.

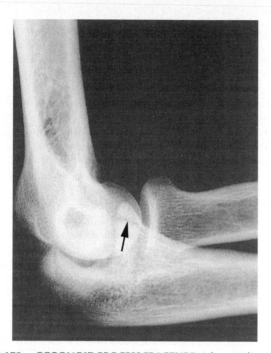

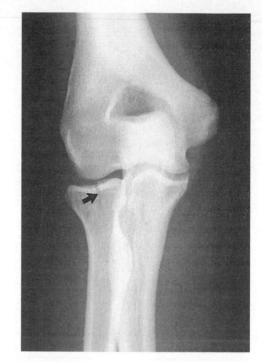

Figure 9.172.   CORONOID PROCESS FRACTURE. A fracture line is clearly visible through the tip of the coronoid process (arrow). COMMENT: This fracture was incurred following acute hyperextension of the elbow as part of an exercise conducted for training for manual spinal adjusting ("toggle recoil"). It healed with no residual functional impairment. (Courtesy of Sandra M. O'Connor, DC, DACBR, Toronto, Canada)

Figure 9.173.   CHISEL FRACTURE: RADIAL HEAD. A vertical fracture line extends through the articular surface of the radial head, with minimal offset of the articular contour (arrow).

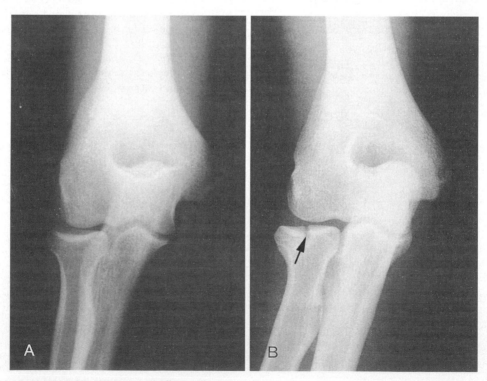

Figure 9.174.   OCCULT RADIAL HEAD FRACTURE. A. AP Elbow. This 17-year-old baseball pitcher developed elbow pain following throwing a "fast ball" pitch. No evidence of fracture is apparent in the radial head. **B. AP Elbow, 2 Months Later.** A vertical fracture line is now apparent ("chisel fracture") (arrow). COMMENT: Radial head fractures can be difficult to identify initially since the fracture line may be but a mere crack. This is one of the most common fractures of the elbow and may require specific radial head views for depiction.

Fracture Line. A radiolucent line is seen usually oriented vertically and penetrating the articular cortex toward the lateral side of the head. (Fig. 9.175)

Cortical Disruption. At the fracture site, the cortex will be broken.

Cortical Deformity. At the fracture site, a sharp step-off or angulation is common, due to fragment displacement. Depression of the fracture's fragment may produce a "double cortical" sign, which is seen as a linear opacity paralleling the normal articular cortex of the radial head. (9) (Fig. 9.176)

Altered Supinator Fat Line. On a normal lateral film, a linear radiolucent line representing the outer fascial plane of the supinator muscle, 1 cm above the anterior radial surface, will be observed. In fractures of the radial head or neck the fat line may be obliterated, blurred, or ventrally displaced by more than 1–2 cm. (10)

Fat Pad Sign. A useful sign of an intraarticular fracture of the elbow is the clear depiction of displaced humeral capsular fat-pads. (11) In the normal elbow a layer of fat ("fat-pad") lies between the synovial and fibrous layers of both the anterior and posterior joint capsule. In the lateral projection of the normal elbow the anterior fat-pad is seen as an obliquely oriented radiolucency. When acute intracapsular swelling is present from any origin (hemorrhagic, inflammatory, or traumatic), the anterior fat-pad is elevated to be oriented horizontally, while the posterior fat-pad will now be visible ("fat-pad" sign). (12) In joint distensions the elevated fat pads, especially anteriorly, may be obliterated due to hemorrhage or edema; therefore, the posterior fat-pad, when visible, is the most reliable sign of intraarticular effusion. In children and adolescents, 90% of posterior fat-pad signs will have an associated fracture. (11) In adults the sign is less frequently seen, and its absence does not exclude the presence of a fracture. (12) (Fig. 9.177)

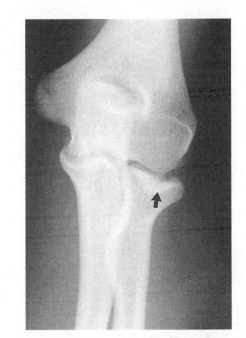

Figure 9.176. RADIAL HEAD FRACTURE: DOUBLE CORTICAL SIGN. Observe the increased density of the articular cortex of the radial head, with projection of the opacity below the articular surface (arrow). Posteriorly, a fracture line is identified as a linear radiolucency. COMMENT: This "double cortical" sign is the result of an impaction fracture from the capitellum into the radial head, which displaces the cortex distally. Frequently, this is the only sign of a radial head fracture.

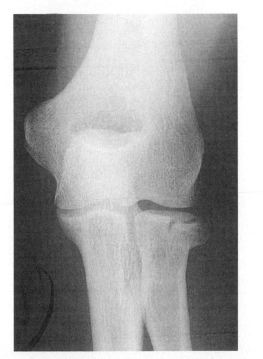

Figure 9.175. DISPLACED RADIAL HEAL FRACTURE. A fracture through the lateral portion of the radial head has occurred, with minimal depression of the articular cortex and lateral displacement of the isolated fragments.

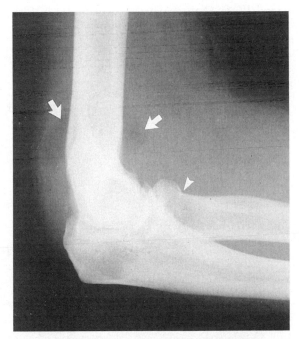

Figure 9.177. FAT-PAD SIGN: SUBTLE RADIAL NECK FRACTURE. Two triangular areas of radiolucency are seen to project away from the distal humeral shaft at the anterior and posterior aspects (arrows). A subtle fracture of the radial neck is also identified (arrowhead). COMMENT: Whenever both the anterior and posterior fat-pads are visible in this projection, a careful search must be performed to rule out a subtle intraarticular fracture. The most common fracture associated with a fat-pad sign is a radial head or neck fracture. The posterior fat-pad is a more reliable indicator of fracture, since the anterior fat-pad may be poorly visualized or present in normal patients.

Radial Neck Fracture.   The most common fracture is an impaction at the junction of the head and neck. The only sign may be a sharpened angle on the anterior surface, best depicted on the lateral projection. (Figs. 9.177, 9.178) Complete fractures will be readily seen as a transverse lucent line with varying degrees of displacement. A comminuted fracture of the radial head in combination with dislocation of the distal radioulnar joint is called an Essex-Lopresti fracture. (13)

FRACTURES OF THE FOREARM

Forearm fractures may involve the radius or ulna singularly, but, more commonly, they are both affected.

Fractures of Both the Radius and Ulna

As in any bony ring structure such as the pelvis, a fracture in one location is frequently associated with a disruption or another fracture or dislocation somewhere else in the ring. Approximately 60% of all forearm fractures will involve both bones (''B-B'' fractures), most commonly in the mid-third of the shaft. (14) (Figs. 9.179, 9.180) Almost all fractures of these bones have asociated displacement with angulation and rotation. These almost always require open surgery and fixation.

Isolated Fractures of the Ulna

Two types of fractures of the ulnar shaft have been described—distal and proximal.

Distal Ulnar Shaft Fracture (Nightstick or Parry Fracture). These fractures occur from direct trauma to the forearm, which is raised to protect the head during an assault with a club or hard object. (15) (Fig. 9.181)

Proximal Ulnar Shaft (Monteggia) Fracture.   In 1814 Monteggia first described fractures of the proximal ulna with associated anterior dislocation of the proximal radius. (Fig. 9.182) This definition has been widened to include all fractures of the ulnar shaft associated with displacement of the radius in any direction. (16) In children, the ulnar component of this lesion is often a green-stick fracture.

Isolated Fractures of the Radius

The most frequent fracture site is toward the distal shaft of the radius. Other sites are rare.

Distal Radial Shaft (Galeazzi, Piedmont, or Reversed Monteggia Fracture).   This is a rare but serious traumatic injury of the forearm. It is defined as a fracture of the radius at the junction

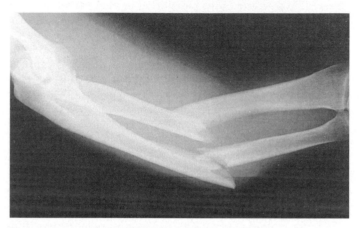

Figure 9.179.   RADIUS AND ULNA SHAFT FRACTURES. Oblique comminuted fractures have occurred through the mid-diaphyseal portions of the radius and ulna, with significant angulation and rotational deformity. COMMENT: These are unique fractures that usually follow significant direct trauma to the forearm.

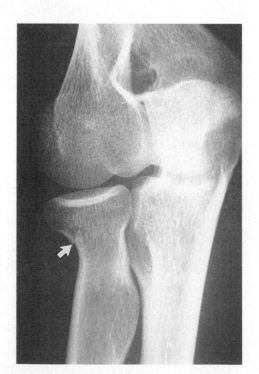

Figure 9.178.   RADIAL NECK FRACTURE. A thin fracture line disrupts the lateral aspect of the cortex (arrow).

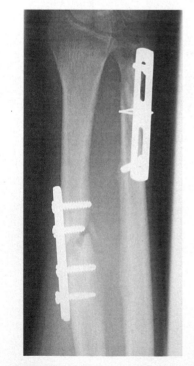

Figure 9.180.   SURGICAL FIXATION: RADIUS AND ULNA FRACTURES. Metallic plates have been placed across the fracture sites of the radius and ulna to realign the fracture fragments and reduce the amount of residual deformity.

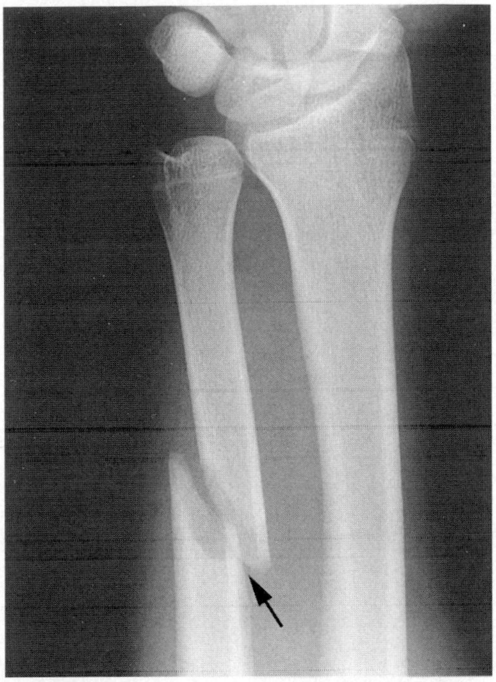

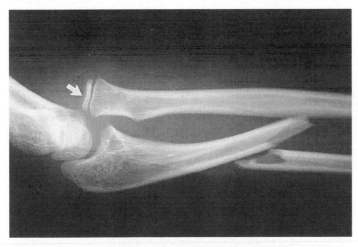

Figure 9.181.   NIGHTSTICK FRACTURE: ULNAR FRACTURE. A fracture is evident in the distal ulna. COMMENT: This type of ulnar fracture can be associated with an attempt at self-protection of the head during an assault with a hand-held object. Since assaults often occur at night and a stick may be used as the attack weapon, this fracture has been called a "nightstick" fracture.

Figure 9.182.   MONTEGGIA FRACTURE OF THE FOREARM. A fracture through the proximal one-third of the ulna is present, with associated anterior angulation of the proximal fracture fragment. The radial head has also been displaced anteriorly, with dislocation at the elbow (arrow).

of the middle and distal thirds, with dislocation of the distal radioulnar joint. (17,18) (Fig. 9.183) Despite treatment, this fracture is frequently complicated by nonunion and has a tendency to redislocate.

Dislocations of the Elbow

The elbow is the third most common site of dislocation in adults, the shoulder and interphalangeal joints of the fingers be-

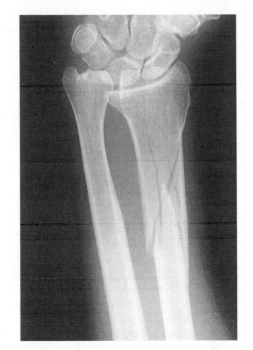

Figure 9.183.   GALEAZZI'S FRACTURE. A comminuted fracture of the radius is present at the junction of the middle and distal thirds, with an associated dislocation of the distal radioulnar joint. There has been an overall shortening of the distal radius, which is a common finding in this fracture/dislocation.

ing first and second, respectively. In children, it is the most common dislocation. (19,20) It is classified according to the displacement of the radius and ulna relative to the humerus—posterior, posterolateral, anterior, medial, and anteromedial.

Posterior and Posterolateral Dislocations. These are the most common dislocations of the elbow, comprising up to 85 to 90% of all such lesions. (19) In practically all elbow dislocations both the radius and ulna will be displaced. More than 50% of elbow dislocations will have associated fractures, most commonly of the medial epicondyle and radial head or neck. (21) In children, an avulsed medial epicondyle may become entrapped in the joint. A small percentage of posterior dislocations will develop posttraumatic myositis ossificans at the anterior aspect of the joint, usually in the brachialis muscle.

Pulled Elbow. Children between 2 to 5 years of age are vulnerable to this unique, transient injury. It occurs when the hand of the child is tractioned, such as in lifting the child from the floor. The child begins to cry immediately, holds the forearm held in midpronation, and does not allow it to be moved. The lesion is due to the radial head slipping out from under the annular ligament, trapping the ligament in the radiohumeral articulation. (22) No radiographic signs of the displacement will be evident. The ligament is easily replaced, often inadvertently or during the radiographic examination, by supinating the hand, producing immediate relief of symptoms. Recurrence is common in the ensuing weeks.

FRACTURES AND DISLOCATIONS OF THE WRIST

GENERAL CONSIDERATIONS

The wrist is one of the most frequent sites for fractures. Dislocations are less common. Many eponyms have been applied to various fractures and their related deformities to honor those who either first described, or most accurately defined, the entity.

The bone and joint anatomy of the wrist is complex and requires specific projections for adequate demonstration. A minimum study of the wrist should include posteroanterior neutral, posteroanterior with ulnar flexion, oblique, and lateral projections. More precise definition of the individual carpal bones and their related soft tissue components requires specialized projections. CT of the wrist is especially useful in identifying occult and complex fractures. (1,2)

FRACTURES OF THE WRIST

Distal Radius Fractures

The distal radius is one of the most common sites of fracture in the wrist. Care must be taken to search all projections for these fractures, many of which are often subtle and obscure. In the absence of an obvious fracture, close observation of the lateral projection for displacement of the pronator quadratus fat line is a useful indicator for the presence or absence of fracture. (Fig. 9.184) Normally, this fat line appears as a well-defined linear lucency oriented parallel with the plane of the radius, 2 to 5 mm from its anterior surface. In almost all cases of distal radius fractures the pronator quadratus fat line will be altered. (3) These alterations include anterior displacement, blurring, irregularity, and obliteration of the line.

Colles' Fracture.   In 1814 Abraham Colles wrote the definitive desription of this fracture, which consequently bears his name. (4) The injury is defined as a fracture of the distal radius approximately 20 to 35 mm proximal to the articular surface, with posterior angulation of the distal fragment. (Fig. 9.185A and B) More than 60% will have an accompanying fracture of the ulnar styloid process. (4) The usual mechanism is a fall on an outstretched, extended hand. The physical appearance of the fractured distal

forearm and wrist has led to its being called the *dinner fork* deformity. The incidence of the fracture increases with age, and this increase is so rapid in women that by age 65 the lesion is six times more common in women than in men. (5) Osteoporosis appears to be the underlying influencing factor. Complications are common and may be severe. (6)

The radiologic features are distinctive and relatively consistent.

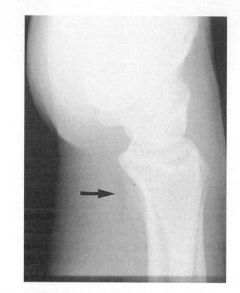

Figure 9.184.   NORMAL QUADRATUS FAT LINE. Observe the clearly defined linear radiolucency (arrow) on the anterior aspect of the forearm in relatively close apposition to the distal radius. This fat line represents the outer surface of the pronator quadratus muscle. COMMENT: In the presence of distal radius fractures this fat line may become obliterated, blurred, or displaced away from the radial surface.

Figure 9.185.   COLLES' FRACTURE: DISTAL RADIUS, WITH POSTERIOR ANGULATION. A. PA Wrist. The fracture line is obscured by a zone of impaction, seen as a transverse linear opacity. However, cortical offset is apparent at the lateral radial margin. **B. Lateral Projection**. This view demonstrates the comminuted fracture of the distal radius with impaction on the posterior surface (arrow). The distal articular surface of the radius is angulated dorsally. The external skin contour displays the typical ''dinner fork'' deformity.

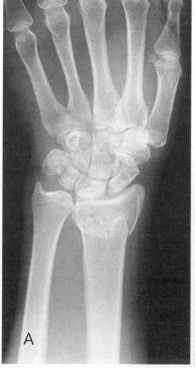

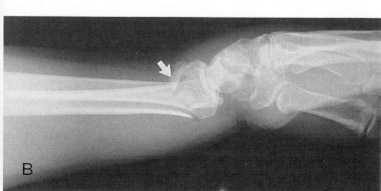

Fracture Line. Usually transverse and comminuted, it is normally readily visible. A variable degree of impaction is apparent on the dorsal surface at the fracture site.

Radial Contour. A sharp cortical overlap is seen at the fracture site, especially visible on the frontal projection due to the proximal migration of the distal fragment.

Radial Length. The overall length of the radius is decreased due to the proximal migration of the distal fragment.

Angulation. The distal fragment is tilted dorsally, as evidenced by the altered angle of the articular surface, which is seen on the lateral projection. Normally, there is 5 to 15° palmar angulation of the articular surface.

Soft Tissue. The distorted skin contour is apparent. The pronator quadratus fat plane will usually be altered.

Smith's Fracture (Reversed Colles Fracture).   In 1854 Smith described a fracture of the distal radius with anterior angulation of the distal fragment. (7) The usual mechanism of injury is a direct blow or fall with the wrist being forced into hyperflexion. This mechanism and resultant angular deformity is the direct opposite of a Colles' fracture, and, hence, the synonym *reverse Colles' fracture.* Smith's fracture is far less common than Colles' fracture.

Radiologically, the same signs as the Colles' fracture will be visible to varying degrees, except there will be anterior angulation of the distal fragment. (Fig. 9.186A–C)

Barton's (Rim) Fracture.   In 1838 Barton described a posterior rim fracture of the distal radial articulating surface with associated proximal dislocation of the carpus (8). The usual mechanism is forceful hyperextension of the wrist to produce the posterior rim fracture. A fracture of the anterior rim has been called a *reverse Barton's fracture.*

Radiologically, on the frontal projection the proximal carpal row overlaps the articulating surface of the radius. On the lateral view the posterior rim fracture will be visible, along with the posterior and proximal displacement of the carpals. (Fig. 9.187A and B)

Chauffeur's (Backfire, Hutchinson's) Fracture.   These fractures were formerly encountered as a result of a backfire that occurred when attempting to start a car engine with a hand crank,

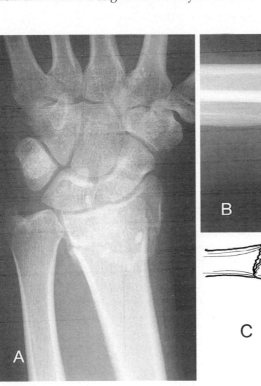

Figure 9.186.   SMITH'S FRACTURE. A. PA Wrist. A transverse fracture line extends through the distal radius, with an associated linear density at the fracture site. **B. Lateral Wrist.** The fracture line is clearly identified through the distal radius, with impaction at the fracture site on the anterior surface (arrow). Associated anterior angulation of the distal fragment has altered the articular plane in this same direction. **C. Schematic Diagram.** The combination of a distal radius fracture with anterior angulation of the articular surface characterizes this fracture deformity.

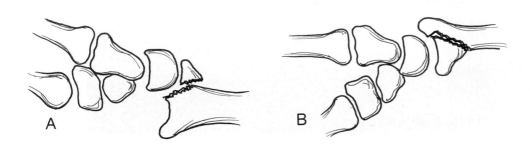

Figure 9.187. RIM FRACTURES OF THE DISTAL RADIUS. A. Barton Fracture. A fracture of the posterior rim of the distal radial articular surface with associated posterior and proximal migration of the entire carpus is referred to as a "Barton fracture." **B. Reversed Barton Fracture.** The fracture line extends through the anterior rim of the articular cortex with anterior displacement of the carpus.

with the crank striking the dorsal surface of the wrist. (9) The fracture involves the radial styloid process as an avulsion or radial impaction by the adjacent scaphoid. The fracture line is either transverse or oblique, and, usually, there is no displacement. (Fig. 9.188)

Moore's Fracture. In 1880 Moore described, in association with Colles' fracture, a fracture of the ulnar styloid process and dislocation of the distal ulna. (10)

Torus Fracture (Fig. 9.189A and B). This is the most common fracture of the wrist between 6 and 10 years of age. Typically, the

fracture is located 2 to 4 cm from the distal growth plate. A torus fracture can occur in any long bone and is the term applied to a buckled cortex following trauma. As such, the key radiologic sign is a localized cortical bulge or bump.

Slipped Radial Epiphysis (Fig. 9.190A and B). This injury is the childhood equivalent of the Colles' fracture. The mechanism involved is a shearing force across the growth plate following a forceful hyperextension injury. The radial epiphysis is usually displaced posteriorly and will almost always have a small, displaced metaphyseal fragment ("corner" sign), classifying it as a Salter-Harris Type II epiphyseal injury. Practically all of these epiphyseal separations are treated successfully by closed reduction, with no effects on growth.

Distal Ulnar Fractures

Ulnar Styloid Process Fracture (Fig. 9.191). As an isolated fracture, this is an uncommon injury and is usually an avulsion through the ulnar collateral ligament. More frequently, it is found in combination with other fractures and dislocations of the wrist.

Distal Ulnar Shaft (Nightstick) Fracture. (See "Fractures of the Forearm.") (Page 754)

Scaphoid Fractures

The scaphoid is the most common carpal bone to fracture. The usual age of occurrence is between 15 and 40 years. Scaphoid fractures are distinctly rare in children. The mechanism of injury is complex, but it essentially consists of various degrees of hyperextension and radial flexion, such as falling on an outstretched hand. These fractures are frequently overlooked and exhibit a significant incidence of complications. The scaphoid is the most common site for occult fracture. (11)

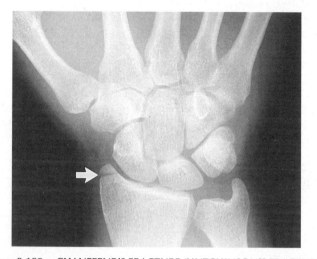

Figure 9.188.   CHAUFFEUR'S FRACTURE (HUTCHINSON'S FRACTURE): FRACTURE OF THE RADIAL STYLOID. A small fracture is seen to extend through the distal radial styloid process (arrow). It may be due to an avulsion or impaction by the adjacent scaphoid.

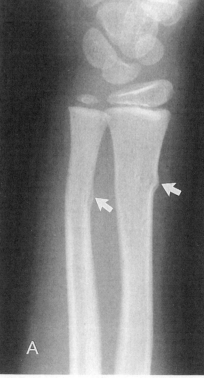

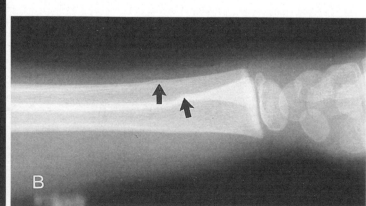

Figure 9.189.   TORUS FRACTURE: DISTAL RADIUS AND ULNA. A. PA Wrist. A discrete area of cortical bulging is apparent at the lateral margins of the radius and ulna (arrows). **B. Lateral Wrist.** The cortical bulges are visualized as acute angulations in the posterior cortical contours (arrows). COMMENT: This is the most common fracture of the wrist between the ages of 6 and 10. The bulging of the cortex is due to a buckling of the bone, and is the key radiologic sign of this injury.

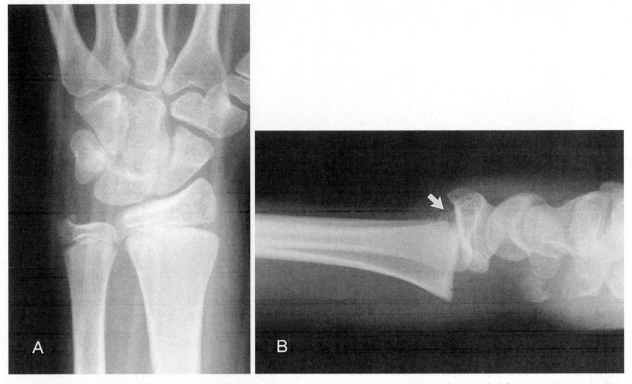

Figure 9.190.   SLIPPED RADIAL EPIPHYSIS. A. PA Wrist. There is a subtle separation of the radial growth plate, with ulnar displacement of the distal epiphysis. **B. Lateral Wrist**. The posterior epiphyseal displacement is clearly demonstrated. A small displaced metaphyseal fragment from the radius ("corner" sign) (arrow) is also noted. COMMENT: Diagnosis of slipped radial epiphysis requires a minimum of two projections. This injury is the childhood equivalent of the adult Colles' fracture.

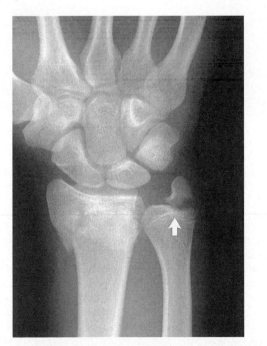

Figure 9.191.   ULNAR STYLOID FRACTURE. An avulsion fracture of the ulnar styloid process is clearly visible. The radiolucent line through the distal ulna (arrow) should not be confused with a fracture line, as this represents an unfused epiphyseal growth plate. There is an associated fracture through the distal radius. COMMENT: Isolated ulnar styloid fractures are infrequent. These lesions are usually associated with other fractures of the wrist, especially the distal radius, as is the case here.

Fracture Classification and Incidence.   The scaphoid is divided into three regions—the distal pole, waist, and proximal pole. Some add a fourth segment, the tuberosity, which is part of the distal pole. Approximately 70% of fractures involve the waist, 20% the proximal pole, and 10% the distal pole. (11)

Radiologic Features.   The optimum routine view is the ulnar flexion projection, since it eliminates foreshortening of the scaphoid and may distract the fracture fragments and widen the fracture line. The major radiologic sign is identifying the fracture line, which is often difficult. (Fig. 9.192A and B) If no fracture is seen initially, yet the clinical picture is suspicious, then precautionary immobilization should be applied and the wrist x-rayed in 7 to 10 days. A fracture, if present, will be visible by 20 days post injury. (12) Bone scans in equivocal circumstances within 24 to 72 hours following injury can show a false positive rate of 6 to 16% but no false negative. (12) After this time period, the fracture line widens, due to resorption along the fracture margins (occult fracture). The fracture line is usually transverse or, less commonly, oblique in relation to the long axis of the scaphoid. (Fig. 9.193)

A useful soft tissue sign of a subtle scaphoid fracture can be found in alterations to the adjacent scaphoid fat stripe. The normal fat stripe is a linear collection of fat betwen the radial collateral ligament and tendon sheaths of the extensor pollicus brevis and abductor pollicus longus. In almost 90% of fractures involving the radial compartment of the wrist the fat strip will be displaced laterally or totally obliterated ("navicular fat stripe" sign). (13)

Healing occurs without periosteal callus, the fracture line just gradually disappearing. Healing time varies according to the frac-

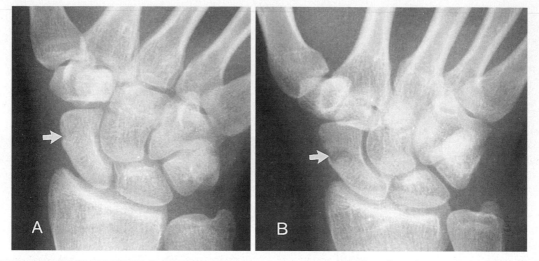

Figure 9.192.   OCCULT SCAPHOID FRACTURE. A. PA Wrist: Initial Radiograph. A subtle fracture line is visible through the distal waist region of the scaphoid (arrow). Observe the absence of the navicular fat stripe adjacent to the fracture site. **B. PA Wrist: 3 Weeks Postinjury.** The fracture line is now clearly evident, due to bony resorption of the fracture margins (arrow). COMMENT: The scaphoid is the most common site for occult fracture. Follow-up radiographs, normally within 7 to 10 days of the injury, will usually demonstrate the fracture line as resorption occurs.

ture site. The more distal the fracture, the faster the healing and the less likely the development of complications. The converse applies to those fractures occurring proximally. (Fig. 9.193) The actual time required for healing ranges between 6 and 20 weeks and will vary with the individual. (6)

Complications.   The major complications consist of avascular necrosis, nonunion, carpal instability, and radiocarpal degenerative arthritis.

Avascular Necrosis.   This complication is encountered in approximately 1 to 15% of scaphoid fractures. (14) The scaphoid is anatomically predisposed to avascular necrosis following fracture due to the patterns of nutrient blood supply.

The scaphoid receives a dual blood supply. A small artery enters and perfuses the distal pole and tuberosity. A larger vessel, with an entry site that may be proximal or distal to the scaphoid waist, is resposible for perfusing the remaining areas of the bone. (Fig. 9.194A–D)

In the development of complicating avascular necrosis, the position of the fracture relative to the principal artery is the most crucial factor. If the fracture is distal to the major vessel, then avascular necrosis is unlikely; if proximal, then the probability for avascular necrosis increases significantly. In general, the more proximal the fracture line, the greater the probability for avascular necrosis.

Radiologic signs of the avascular segment include increased density and fragmentation. The fracture line will appear wider and is often cystic in appearance. (Fig. 9.195) All of the signs will take a variable time after the fracture incident to appear, ranging from months to years.

Nonunion.   Nonunion occurs in approximately 30% of fractures involving the waist of the scaphoid. (15) As with avascular necrosis, the major variable that determines the development of nonunion, or even delayed union, is the relationship of the fracture line to the principal artery. If there is delayed diagnosis or inappropriate immobilization, that may also predispose to this complication. Nonunion is associated with the progressive development of radiocarpal degenerative joint disease. (12)

Radiologic features of nonunion include widening of the frac-

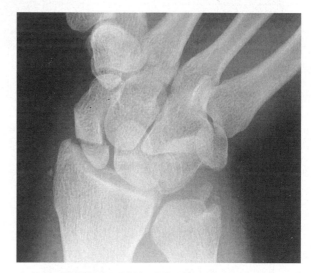

Figure 9.193.   PROXIMAL SCAPHOID FRACTURE. An oblique fracture line extends through the proximal portion of the scaphoid. There are associated fractures of the ulnar and radial styloid processes. COMMENT: Fractures of the proximal pole are more likely to result in major complications, such as avascular necrosis, nonunion, and radiocarpal degenerative arthritis.

ture line, cyst formation, and development of opposing sclerotic surfaces along the fracture line. (Fig. 9.196)

Carpal Instability.   Carpal instability is manifested by changes in alignment of the capitate, lunate, radius, and scaphoid. These may occur in concert with fractures, dislocations, isolated ligament rupture, repetitive stress injury, and degenerative and rheumatoid arthritis. (15,16) A number of instabilities have been described—dorsal intercalated segment instability (DISI), ventral (volar) intercalated segmental instability (VISI), scapholunate dissociation, ulnar translocation, dorsal or palmar carpal subluxation, capitolunate instability, and midcarpal instability. (15) The three most common instabilities are DISI, VISI, and scapholunate dissociation.

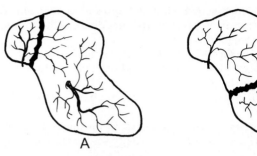 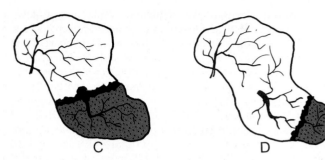

Figure 9.194. SCAPHOID FRACTURE AND BLOOD SUPPLY DISTRIBUTION: SCHEMATIC DIAGRAM. A. Distal Pole Fracture. B. Distal Waist Fracture. C. Proximal Waist Fracture. D. Proximal Pole Fracture. COMMENT: Fractures distal to the entrance of the main supplying artery have a significantly reduced incidence of avascular necrosis and nonunion. Those fractures proximal to this artery are frequently complicated by these abnormalities. The shaded regions indicate the location for complicating avascular necrosis.

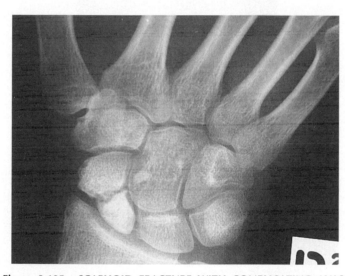

Figure 9.195. SCAPHOID FRACTURE WITH COMPLICATING AVASCULAR NECROSIS. A wide fracture line can be seen passing through the waist of the scaphoid. The proximal pole is homogeneously sclerotic, with no evidence of fragmentation. These findings are consistent with an ununited scaphoid fracture with associated avascular necrosis of the proximal pole.

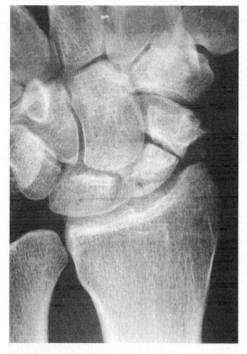

Figure 9.196. SCAPHOID FRACTURE WITH NONUNION. A smooth fracture line traverses the waist of the scaphoid. The opposing margins of the fracture line are sclerotic and well defined. These findings are distinctive for fracture nonunion.

Scapholunate dissociation (rotary subluxation of the scaphoid). This is the most common instability of the wrist, usually following an acute dorsiflexion injury of the wrist. (15) Pain, crepitus, and weakened grip strength are typical. The fundamental defect is disruption of the scapholunate ligament, though other ligaments are commonly incompetent, including other interosseous ligaments (capitate, lunate, scaphoid) and the dorsal radiocarpal ligament. The radiographic features consist of a wide scapholunate joint space ("Terry Thomas sign"), foreshortening of the scaphoid due to rotation ("ring sign") and loss of parallel joint surfaces. (15,17) A scapholunate space of 2 mm is suspicious, with greater than 4 mm definitely abnormal (15) (see "Scaphoid Dislocation"). A wide scapholunate space occurs as a normal variant in almost 50% of lunotriquetral coalitions. (18) These changes are often best depicted on PA ulnar deviation and "clenched fist" views, as routine views may not show evidence of instability. Surgery may only be indicated in symptomatic cases though there is a link with the development of radiocarpal arthritis. (19)

Dorsal intercalated segment instability (DISI). The lunate tilts dorsally and the capitate displaces slightly dorsally to lie posterior to the longitudinal axis of the radius. This is best appreciated on the lateral view of the wrist such that the lunate tilts at an angle greater than 80° to the radius. (15) DISI is more common than VISI. (20)

Ventral (volar) intercalated segment instability (VISI). The lunate tilts ventrally with the capitate extended or tilted dorsally. This is best appreciated on the lateral view of the wrist.

Radiocarpal Degenerative Arthritis. This may follow a healed scaphoid fracture, nonunion or avascular necrosis of the scaphoid, and radius fracture. A decreased radiocarpal joint space, subchondral sclerosis, osteophytes, and subchondral cysts characterize this complication. (Fig. 9.197) Overgrowth of Lister's tubercle on the dorsum of the distal radius as seen on CT may cause atrophy and/or rupture of the extensor pollicus longus tendon. (21) In the absence of trauma, the presence of these radiocarpal changes should suggest the diagnosis of calcium pyrophosphate dihydrate crystal deposition disease (CPPD). Scapholunate advanced collapse (SLAC) may follow where there is severe loss of the radiocarpal joint and scapholunate dissociation with proximal migration of the capitate. (Fig. 9.198)

Fractures of the Triquetrum

This is the second most common carpal bone to fracture. (6) The most common type of fracture is an avulsion from the dorsal surface at the site of attachment of the radiocarpal ligament. (Fig. 9.199) This has been called a *Fischer's fracture.* (22,23) These fractures usually follow hyperflexion injuries and present with swelling and localized pain on the dorsum of the wrist. Radiologically, they are best identified on the lateral projection as a small, displaced flake of bone.

Fractures of Other Carpal Bones

Fractures of the remaining carpals are unusual and are typically related to a specific type of injury.

Pisiform Fracture (Fig. 9.200). A direct, impacting blow, such as a fall on an outstretched hand, is the usual mechanism. The most common fracture is a vertical fracture dividing the bone into approximate halves.

Trapezium Fracture (Fig. 9.201). These most commonly follow hyperabduction thumb trauma and typically fracture the radial portion of the bone.

Trapezoid Fracture. This is the least commonly fractured carpal bone.

Capitate Fracture. The capitate is an uncommon carpal to fracture, and, when it occurs, it is usually associated with scaph-

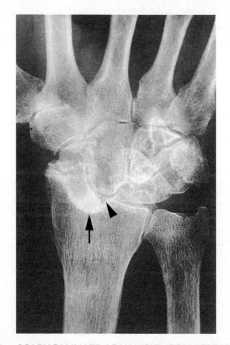

Figure 9.198. SCAPHOLUNATE ADVANCED COLLAPSE (SLAC). Severe loss of radiocarpal joint space with erosion of the radius by the scaphoid is apparent (arrow). There is scapholunate dissociation as evidenced by the widened interosseous space (arrowhead). Note the proximity of the capitate (c) to the distal radius. COMMENT: This is a marked complication of previous wrist trauma. (Courtesy of Ian Chen, MD, Denver, Colorado)

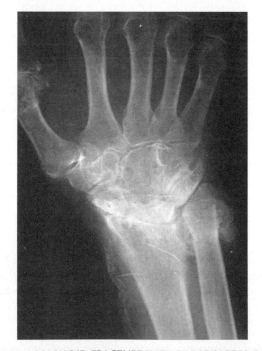

Figure 9.197. SCAPHOID FRACTURE WITH RADIOCARPAL DEGENERATIVE ARTHRITIS. Severe loss of radiocarpal joint space, osteophytes, subchondral sclerosis, and associated cyst formation are visible throughout the carpal and distal radius articulations. Careful scrutiny of the proximal pole of the scaphoid demonstrates its resorption, most likely secondary to mechanical deformation and avascular necrosis. COMMENT: This is a severe form of posttraumatic radiocarpal degenerative arthritis in a retired professional boxer. His opposite hand appeared similar. (Courtesy of Stephen W. Hayman, DC, DeLand, Florida)

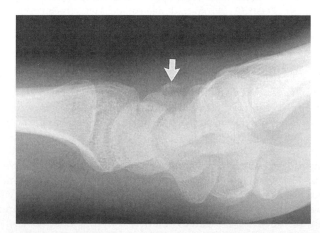

Figure 9.199. AVULSION FRACTURE OF THE TRIQUETRUM (FISCHER'S FRACTURE). A small avulsed fragment can be seen displaced posteriorly from the surface of the triquetrum (arrow). Some minimal overlying soft tissue swelling is also appreciated. COMMENT: This fracture is the second most common fracture of the wrist, with the scaphoid being the most common.

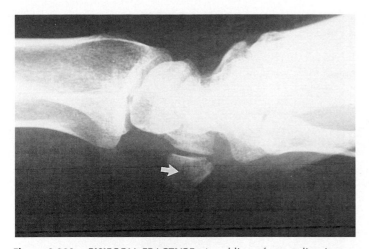

Figure 9.200. PISIFORM FRACTURE. An oblique fracture line is seen through the midportion of the pisiform (arrow). These fractures usually are the result of a direct blow to the pisiform from falling on a hyperextended hand, which typically divides the pisiform in half. (Courtesy of Klaus W. Weber, MD, Fort Wayne, Indiana)

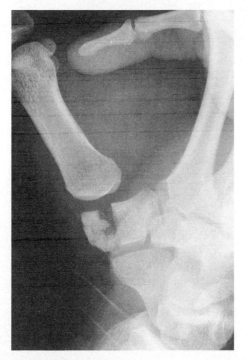

Figure 9.201. TRAPEZIUM FRACTURE. A comminuted fracture of the lateral portion of the trapezium has occurred. Significant widening of the first metacarpal trapezium articulation is also identified, due to severe ligamentous injury.

oid or perilunate dislocations. (6) The most frequent fracture is transverse, through the waist.

Hamate Fracture. This bone may fracture in various areas. The hook is a common site of fracture, which occurs as a result of a direct blow such as may occur in club or racquet sports where the butt end strikes directly over the protuberance. (24,25) On the frontal view the circular contour of the hamate may not be seen. (26) Fracture of its dorsal surface often accompanies posterior dislocation or subluxation of the fourth or fifth metacarpal and is seen as an oblong shaped bone fragment near the articulation.

(27) A special tangential view with the wrist in hyperextension is usually needed for diagnosis.

Lunate Fracture. This fracture is uncommon, since it tends to dislocate before it fractures. If a fracture is seen in the lunate, the diagnosis of Keinböch's disease (avascular necrosis) is likely.

DISLOCATIONS OF THE WRIST

Dislocations of the wrist are relatively uncommon but involve predictable locations. The classification of these injuries identifies two patterns: (a) a single bone that dislocates relative to the remaining carpals, and (b) a single bone that remains in normal position, but with the surrounding bones dislocating.

A useful guideline in evaluating the carpal relationship on the posteroanterior projection is to visually inspect the three carpal arcs. (28) (Fig. 9.202) Arc 1 is formed by connecting the proximal articular surfaces of the proximal carpal row; arc 2 connects the distal articular surfaces of the proximal row; and arc 3 connects the proximal surfaces of the distal carpals (capitate, hamate). These arcs should be smooth and demonstrate proper intercarpal alignment. Disruptions of these arcs indicate a carpal displacement.

Single Carpal Dislocations

Lunate Dislocation (Fig. 9.203). This is the most common carpal to dislocate, usually following a hyperextension injury. When the lunate dislocates, it tilts forward and anterior, disrupting its articulation with the capitate but maintaining close approximation with the anterior rim of the distal radius. This is best seen on the lateral view. On the posteroanterior view the lunate is altered in shape to appear triangular, with the apex pointing distally ("pie" sign). Inspection of the three carpal arcs will demonstrate disruption of arcs 2 and 3 at the midcarpal joint.

Scaphoid. This is the second most common carpal to be dis-

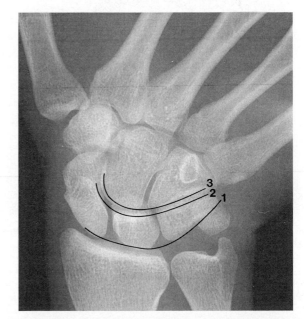

Figure 9.202. THE THREE ARCS OF CARPAL ALIGNMENT. Three curvilinear lines are constructed along the articular margins at the midcarpal and radiocarpal joints. In a normal PA view of the wrist these lines should be smooth and continuous across the connecting joint spaces. COMMENT: Visual inspection of these three arcs is a useful method for detecting carpal displacements.

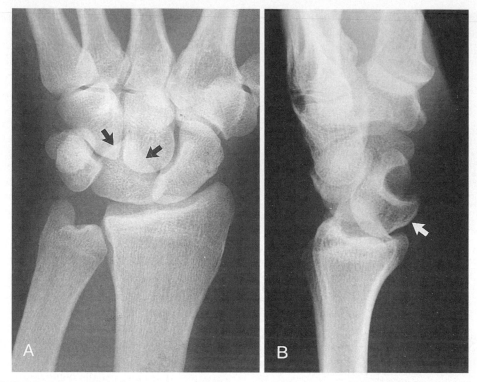

Figure 9.203.   LUNATE DISLOCATION. A. PA Wrist. Note the overlap of the distal lunate with the capitate. The triangular shape ("pie" sign) (arrows) is characteristic of anterior dislocation. **B. Lateral Wrist.** The lunate can be seen displaced anteriorly and tilted forward at its superior aspect (arrow).

COMMENT: Anterior lunate dislocation is the most common carpal displacement. The characteristic findings are well demonstrated with the triangular appearance on the PA film and the anterior forward displacement on the lateral projection.

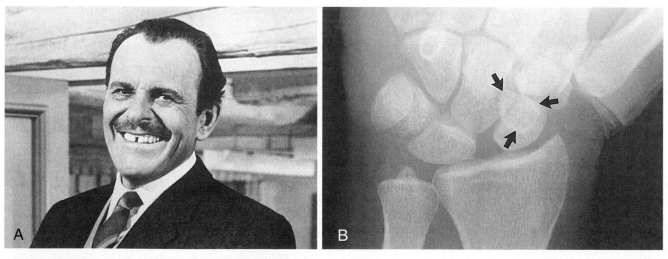

Figure 9.204.   SCAPHOLUNATE DISSOCIATION (ROTARY SCAPHOID SUBLUXATION). A. Terry Thomas. His dental diastema (front incisor gap) provides the basis for the analogy of the widened scapholunate space as a manifestation of instability. (Courtesy of The Bettmann Archive) **B. PA Wrist, "Clenched Fist" View.** The scaphoid is considerably shortened in its longitudinal dimension, with the formation of a rounded cortical contour at its distal margin ("ring" sign) (arrows). A widening of the scapholunate space ("Terry Thomas" sign) has occurred due to disruption of the interconnecting ligament. COMMENT: The scaphoid is the second most common bone to be displaced in the wrist. The combination of the "ring" and "Terry Thomas" signs renders the diagnosis.

placed. Complete dislocation is infrequent, with lesser degrees of subluxation being more common. As the scaphoid displaces, it moves laterally and rotates anteriorly (rotary subluxation). On the posteroanterior view this will be seen as a small, foreshortened scaphoid that appears circular in shape ("ring" or "signet ring" sign). (17) Additionally, there will be an increase in the space between the scaphoid and lunate of more than 4 mm ("Terry Thomas" sign). (17,29) (Fig. 9.204A and B)

Other Carpal Dislocations. These are distinctively unusual and require the occurrence of severe trauma. (Fig. 9.205)

Multiple Carpal Dislocations

Perilunate Dislocations. These usually are comprised of dorsal displacements of all the carpal bones except the lunate, which maintains its normal position with the radius. This is best seen on the lateral projection. On the posteroanterior projection the capitate will be seen to overlie the lunate.

Trans-scaphoid Perilunate Dislocations (Figs. 9.206, 9.207). This is virtually the same injury as the perilunate dislocation, except there is an associated fracture through the waist of the scaphoid. The proximal fragment stays in its normal position with the lunate, while the distal portion displaces with other carpal bones dorsally.

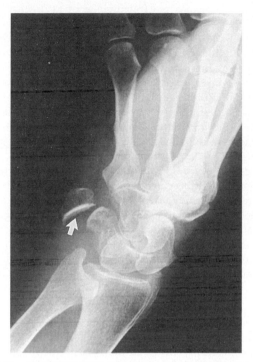

Figure 9.205. PISIFORM DISLOCATION. Displacement of the pisiform away from the triquetrum is clearly seen (arrow). This is an uncommon site for carpal dislocation.

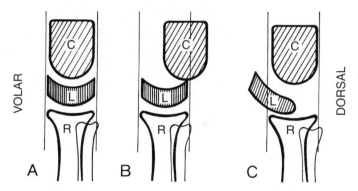

Figure 9.207. LUNATE AND PERILUNATE DISLOCATIONS: SCHEMATIC DIAGRAM REPRESENTING ALIGNMENT OF THE CAPITATE, LUNATE, AND DISTAL RADIUS FROM A LATERAL (SAGITTAL) PERSPECTIVE. A. Normal Alignment. B. Perilunate Dislocation. Note the dorsal displacement of the capitate relative to the normally aligned lunate and distal radius. **C. Lunate Dislocation.** Note the volar dislocation of the lunate bone relative to the normally aligned capitate and distal radius (C=capitate, L=lunate, R=distal radius).

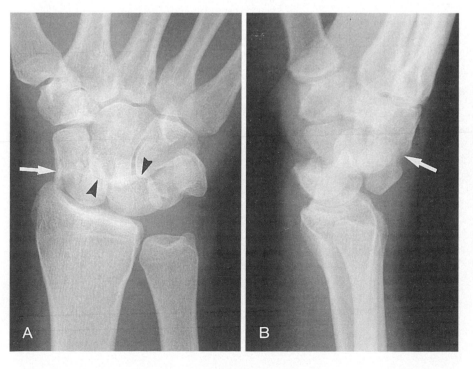

Figure 9.206. TRANS-SCAPHOID FRACTURE AND PERILUNATE DISLOCATION. A. PA Wrist. A transverse fracture through the waist of the scaphoid (arrow) has occurred in association with posterior dislocation of the distal fragment and distal carpal bones. The superimposed densities of the hamate and capitate (arrowheads) signify this posterior dislocation and proximal migration. **B. Lateral Wrist.** The posterior displacement of the distal carpal row can be identified, especially the capitate (arrow). COMMENT: Trans-scaphoid fracture and perilunate dislocations follow severe traumatic injury to the wrist. Characteristically, the fracture is through the midwaist of the scaphoid, with associated posterior displacement of the distal fragment and distal carpal row.

deQuervain's Fracture Dislocation.   Described in 1907 by de-Quervain, this consists of anterior dislocation of the lunate, along with the proximal fragment of a fractured scaphoid. (30)

FRACTURES AND DISLOCATIONS OF THE HAND

GENERAL CONSIDERATIONS

The phalanges and metacarpals are the most common sites of skeletal injury in the entire skeleton. (1) Phalangeal fractures are more common than metacarpal fractures. In the majority of cases only a single bone or joint will be affected. Most can be treated conservatively, with only a few requiring open reduction and soft tissue repair or pin fixation.

Radiologic examination routinely should have no less than three projections, including posteroanterior, oblique, and lateral views. If a single digit is involved, collimated views in these positions should be done to enhance detail. Examination of the thumb requires specialized projections. Knowledge of the locations and appearances of the many sesamoid bones and nutrient canals will reduce the probability of misdiagnosis.

FRACTURES OF THE HAND

Second to Fifth Metacarpal Fractures

Of all the metacarpals, the fifth is the most commonly fractured, the majority of which occur in the distal half.

Boxer's Fracture.   This is a transverse fracture of the neck of the second or third metacarpal, the result of a straight, jabbing type of blow with the fist. (2)

Bar Room Fracture.   This type of fracture is also transverse in nature, involving the neck of the fourth or fifth metacarpals and is the result of a "roundhouse" type of blow characteristic of the inexperienced fighter. (2,3) (Fig. 9.208A and B) This exposes the fourth and fifth metacarpal heads to absorption of the force of the delivered blow.

In most metacarpal neck fractures, there will be anterior an-gulation of the metacarpal head, with variable degrees of shortening and rotation of the fracture fragment.

Shaft Fracture.   These usually involve the third and fourth metacarpals, often simultaneously. Dorsal angulation and displacement across the fracture site quite commonly occurs. (Fig. 9.209A and B)

Base Fracture.   These fractures are rarely seen.

First Metacarpal Fractures

Most thumb metacarpal fractures occur at or near the base. Four distinct patterns are found—Bennett's, Rolando's, transverse, and a Salter-Harris type II that occurs in adolescents.

Bennett's Fracture.   This injury actually is a fracture/dislocation that was first described by Bennett in 1882. (4,5) It commonly follows an injury where there is a grip applied to an object such as a ski pole or handle bar. (5) This type of fracture is defined as an intraarticular fracture through the base of the first metacarpal, with dorsal and radial displacement of the shaft. A small medial fragment remains closely aligned to the trapezium. (Fig. 9.210A and B)

Rolando's Fracture (Comminuted Bennett's Fracture).   In 1910 Rolando described a comminuted intraarticular fracture at the base of the first metacarpal. (6) (Fig. 9.211) This is a difficult fracture to treat and is the least common of all first metacarpal fractures. (1,7)

Transverse Fracture.   This is the most common fracture of the first metacarpal. (8) (Fig. 9.209A) On occasion, the fracture line may be oblique, but it remains articular.

Phalangeal Fractures

Fractures of the phalanges are collectively more common than metacarpal fractures. Distal phalangeal fractures are the most common, comprising 50% of all phalangeal fractures, while 15% affect the proximal phalanges, and 10% the middle phalanges. (9)

Fractures of the Distal Phalanges.   The middle finger is the most common site of fracture. (9) Four types of fracture occur—transverse, longitudinal, comminuted, and chip.

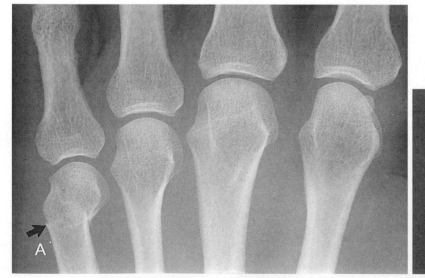

Figure 9.208. BAR ROOM FRACTURE (FIFTH METACARPAL NECK FRACTURE). A. PA Hand. A transverse fracture is seen at the junction of the fifth metacarpal head and shaft (arrow). Some slight radial displacement of the head is also present. **B. PA Oblique Hand.** The oblique view reveals the significant anterior displacement of the metacarpal head, common in these injuries. COMMENT: These metacarpal head fractures are common following a direct blow to the metacarpal phalangeal joints, particularly on the ulnar side of the hand.

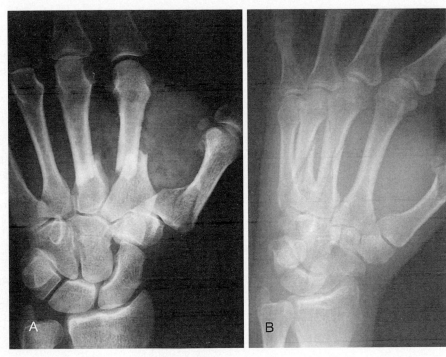

Figure 9.209.   METACARPAL SHAFT FRACTURES. A. PA Hand. Transverse fractures are visualized through the first, second, and third metacarpal shafts. There has been a considerable degree of displacement and overlap, particularly at the second and third metacarpals. **B. Oblique Hand.** Multiple oblique fractures are seen extending through the shafts of the third and fourth metacarpals, as well as the proximal phalanx of the fifth digit. (Courtesy of James R. Brandt, DC, FACO, Coon Rapids, Minnesota)

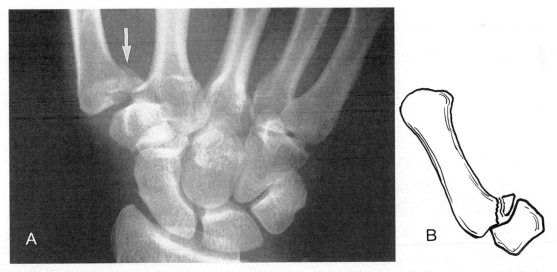

Figure 9.210.   BENNETT'S FRACTURE. A. Oblique Wrist. An oblique intra-articular fracture is present (arrow), extending through the base of the first metacarpal, with associated posterior and radial displacement of the adjacent shaft. **B. Schematic Diagram.**

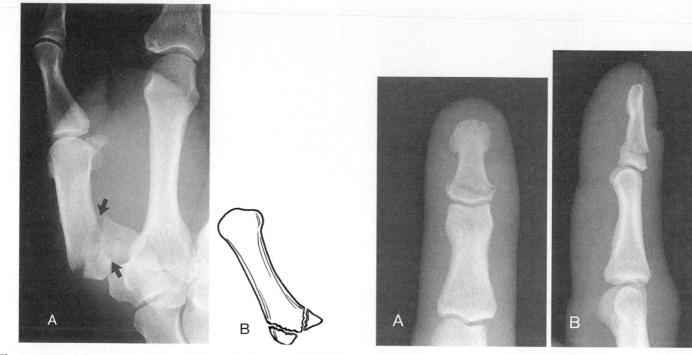

Figure 9.211. ROLANDO'S FRACTURE (COMMINUTED BENNETT'S FRACTURE). A. PA Thumb. A comminuted intraarticular fracture (arrows) is evident at the base of the first metacarpal, which is associated with posterior and radial displacement of the distal metacarpal shaft. **B. Schematic Diagram.**

Figure 9.212. DISTAL PHALANX FRACTURE. A. PA Distal Phalanx. A transverse fracture is present through the base of the distal phalanx. **B. Lateral Distal Phalanx.** There is little displacement across the fracture line.

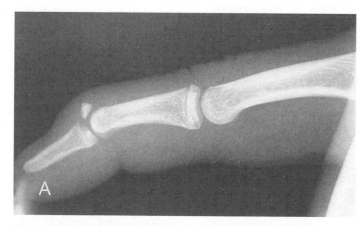

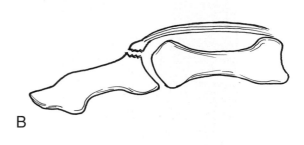

Figure 9.213. POSTERIOR CHIP FRACTURE OF THE DISTAL PHALANX ("MALLET" FINGER OR "BASEBALL" FINGER). A. Lateral Finger. A posterior chip fracture at the base of the distal phalanx is clearly seen. Also, observe the inability to extend the distal interphalangeal joint.

B. Schematic Diagram. COMMENT: These posterior chip fractures are usually secondary to sudden forced flexion of the articulation, with resultant avulsion of the attachment of the extensor tendon.

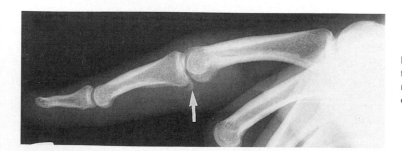

Figure 9.214. VOLAR PLATE FRACTURE. A small chip fracture is seen at the anterior aspect of the distal phalanx (arrow). Because of the small fragment, these fractures are frequently overlooked and may require specific oblique films for identification.

Transverse fractures occur toward the base (Fig. 9.212A and B). Longitudinal fractures may split the phalanx in half and extend all the way to the joint. Comminuted fractures are the most common and are usually limited to the distal tuft. Chip fractures involve the posterior or anterior corners at the phalangeal base. A posterior chip fracture inactivates extension of the distal interphalangeal joint and produces a flexion deformity ("mallet" or "baseball" finger). (Fig. 9.213A and B)

Fractures of the Middle Phalanges.   Most fractures occur in the distal shaft. Another common fracture is one that occurs on the anterior surface, at the base of the phalanx, and is called a "volar plate" fracture. (Fig. 9.214)

Fractures of the Proximal Phalanges.   Most fractures involve the middle and proximal shafts. (Fig. 9.215) These infrequently continue into the adjacent joint.

Turret Exostosis.   This represents a bony protuberance, usually on the ulnar and dorsal aspects of the base of the proximal or middle phalanx. (10) The exostosis represents organization of a traumatic subperiosteal hemorrhage. The hematoma first appears as a soft tissue mass and then ossifies. It produces a painful lump on the dorsal aspect of the fingers and may interfere with flexion. Often, a healed scar of a previous laceration may be identified in the overlying skin. Recurrence rate following surgical removal is high. It may radiographically simulate a sessile osteochondroma, with the clinical history being the key to the differential diagnosis.

Dislocations of the Hand
Metacarpophalangeal Joint Dislocation

Dislocations are usually readily apparent. (Fig. 9.216) The index and little fingers are most commonly dislocated. This type of dislocation is classified by two subgroups—simple and complex. Simple dislocations are easily reducible; complex dislocations have an entrapped, avulsed volar plate within the joint and require open reduction. A diagnostic sign of a complex dislocation is the presence of a sesamoid bone within a widened joint space. (11)

At the first metacarpophalangeal joint a tear or complete rupture of the ulnar collateral ligament results in an instability that has been called *gamekeeper's* thumb. (Fig. 9.217A and C) In 1955 Campbell noted the common occurrence of the injury in English gamekeepers who killed rabbits by breaking their necks between their thumb and forefinger. (12) The term has subsequently lingered in the literature to describe any injury associated with ulnar collateral ligament instability. A more modern mechanism of injury occurs from incorrect placement of a ski pole, producing abduction and extension of the thumb as the skier's momentum carries him downhill.

Radiographic examinations are usually negtive, unless an abduction stress view is taken where a widening of the ulnar joint compartment and radial shaft of the proximal phalanx will be apparent. (1) Occasionally, a small fragment from the radial margin of the base of the proximal phalanx will be avulsed. MR imaging may demonstrate tears of the ulnar collateral ligament. (13) Partial tears and sprains are treated with immobilization, complete tears with open repair, and avulsion fractures by pinning.

Interphalangeal Dislocations

The majority of interphalangeal dislocations follow acute hyperextension and result in posterior displacement of the phalanx. (Fig. 9.218) Anterior dislocations are rare. Usually, only one joint of the same digit will be dislocated and, infrequently, two joints.

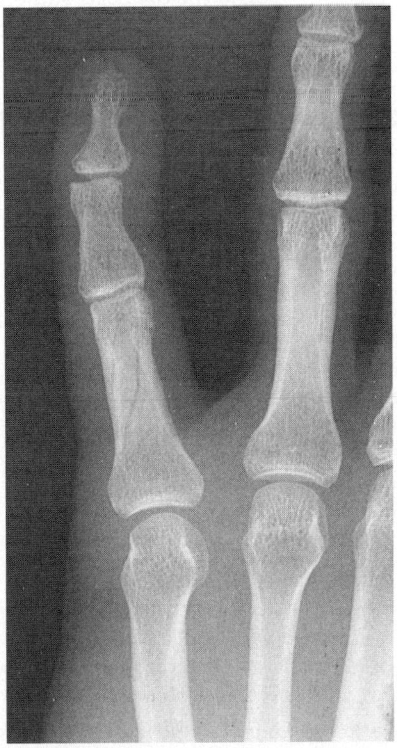

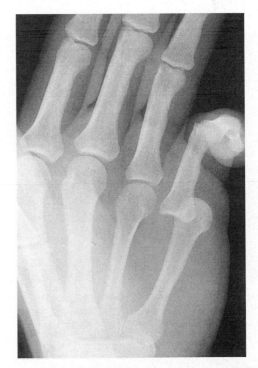

Figure 9.215.   PROXIMAL PHALANGEAL FRACTURE. A spiral fracture is visible in the proximal phalanx of the fifth digit. No significant displacement or intraarticular extension is seen.

Figure 9.216.   METACARPOPHALANGEAL JOINT DISLOCATION. Complete dislocation of the fifth metacarpal phalangeal joint has occurred, with posterior displacement of the proximal phalanx.

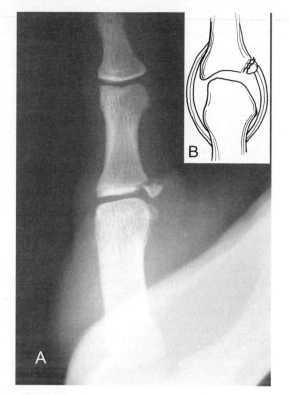

Figure 9.217.   GAMEKEEPER'S THUMB. A. PA Thumb. A small avulsed triangular fragment is evident at the ulnar side at the base of the proximal phalanx. **B. Schematic Diagram.** The avulsion of the phalangeal base is secondary to severe abduction at the first metacarpal phalangeal joint. COMMENT:Gamekeeper's thumb does not always have an associated fractured phalangeal base. Frequently, on plain films no abnormality will be seen. Specific abduction stress views will, however, demonstrate ligamentous instability.

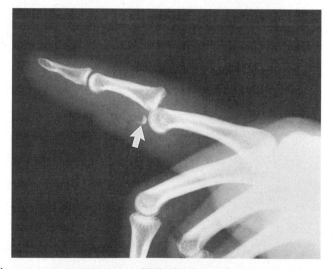

Figure 9.218.   INTERPHALANGEAL JOINT DISLOCATION. A characteristic posterior displacement of the middle phalanx has occurred, with an associated volar plate fracture (arrow). COMMENT:These interphalangeal joint dislocations are the most common encountered.

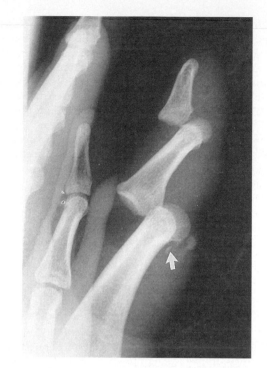

Figure 9.219.   DOUBLE INTERPHALANGEAL JOINT DISLOCATION. Posterior dislocation has occurred at both the distal and proximal interphalangeal joints. There is an associated small volar plate fracture, with the fragment adjacent to the anterior aspect of the metacarpal head (arrow). COMMENT:Double interphalangeal joint dislocations are exceedingly rare. (Courtesy of Gerald A. Fitzgerald, MD, Sydney, Australia)

(Fig. 9.219) In association with the dislocation there frequently is a small volar plate fracture that may become entrapped in the joint and prevent closed reduction.

MEDICOLEGAL IMPLICATIONS
Shoulder Girdle and Upper Limb Injuries

• Any radiographed region should have a minimum of frontal and lateral views. It is preferable that additional projections be obtained to extend this basic examination to detect more subtle lesions. In the shoulder, external rotation places the greater tuberosity into profile revealing an otherwise obscured fracture line ("flap" fracture); in the elbow, the oblique film renders another surface of the radial head visible to identify fracture; in the wrist, an ulnar deviation position may show an otherwise invisible fracture through the scaphoid.

• Follow-up radiographs at appropriate intervals are important if the injury is prone to instability, was compound in nature, or if symptoms persist or worsen. If a fever occurs, the presence of osteomyelitis must be assumed and treated promptly with an antibiotic.

• In cases where the radiologic appearances are normal or equivocal, but the clinical suspicion is high, the site should be treated as if it has a fracture and appropriately immobilized.

• Periodic radiographic examination in patients with recurrence of symptoms may be indicated, especially in sites where there is known to be a high inccidence for complications such as the shoulder (post traumatic osteolysis of the clavicle, degenerative joint disease), radial head (degenerative joint disease) and scaphoid (avascular necrosis, non union).

STRESS FRACTURES

GENERAL CONSIDERATIONS

The term *stress fracture* is applied to a bone injury incurred as the result of repetitive stress of lower magnitude than that required for an acute traumatic fracture. These can occur in normal or abnormal bone. Radiographs can be relatively insensitive in the early course of the disorder, with the bone scan the modality of choice. MR imaging is particularly useful in the differential diagnosis between neoplasm and stress fracture. (1)

Definitions

Fatigue Fracture. Fatigue fractures occur secondary to an abnormal amount of stress or torque applied to a bone with normal integrity. Classically these are found in military recruits, runners, and dancers.

Insufficiency Fracture. Insufficiency fractures occur with normal stress placed upon a bone which has an underlying weakness or pathologic process present. The cause of insuficiency fractures are diverse and include Paget's disease, osteoporosis, osteomalacia or rickets, osteopetrosis, fibrous dysplasia, and osteogenesis imperfecta. (2)

Etiology of Stress Fractures

The major cause of stress fracture is an abnormal degree of repetitive trauma. This often is related to increased physical exertion as is found in sports activities. Stress fractures may also occur due to an altered muscular imbalance placed upon the skeletal structures. Stress may follow certain surgical procedures such as bunionectomy (metatarsals), (3) in the pubic rami following hip replacement, (4) or in knee surgery. (5) Deformity from arthritis, especially at the knee, can precipitate a stress fracture. (6)

Common Sites for Stress Fractures

The metatarsals are the most common lower extremity site, with the middle and distal portions of the shaft of the second and third metatarsals being most frequently affected. (5) (Figs. 9.220A–C, 9.221A–C) These are frequent in military recruits ("march fracture," Deutchlanders disease). Stress fractures of the second and third metatarsals may complicate Morton's syndrome, a congenitally shortened first metatarsal. (7)

The proximal tibia is also a common location, with a high incidence in joggers, marchers, and ballet dancers. (8) (Figs. 9.222A and B, 9.223A and B, 9.224A–C, 9.225) Stress fractures of the calcaneus are found in military recruits and long-distance runners. (9) (Fig. 9.226) The proximal or distal metaphyses of the fibula

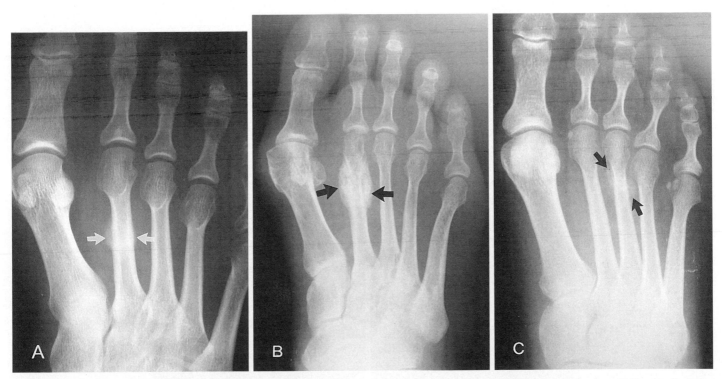

Figure 9.220.   STRESS FRACTURE METATARSALS. A. Dorisplantar Foot. A thin layer of periosteal bone formation is present adjacent to the midshaft of the second metatarsal (arrows). This is frequently the first radiographic manifestation of stress fracture In this location. **B. Dorsiplantar Foot.** A thick layer of solid periosteal new bone is present adjacent to the distal metatarsal shaft (arrows). This represents a longstanding stress fracture with significant callus formation. **C. Dorsiplantar Foot.** A cloudy, veil-like density is seen adjacent to the distal third metatarsal (arrows). This represents periosteal callus formation due to the presence of a stress fracture. COMMENT: The earliest manifestations of stress fractures are often subtle and consist primarily of periosteal callus formation at the fracture site. It is very unusual to see the fracture line in these injuries in the earliest phases.

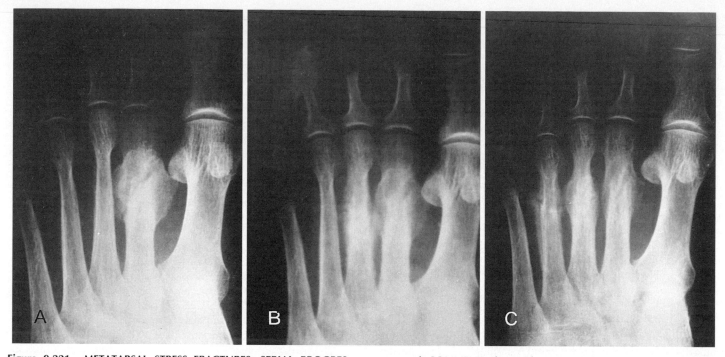

Figure 9.221.   METATARSAL STRESS FRACTURES: SERIAL PROGRESSION. A. Dorsiplantar View: Initial Film. An oblique radiolucent fracture is seen through the second metatarsal shaft. This is surrounded by extensive proliferative callus formation. **B. Dorsiplantar View: 2 Months After Initial Film.** A second stress fracture is visualized in the shaft of the third metatarsal adjacent to the original fracture site. Residual callus formation is noted surrounding the initial stress fracture. **C. Dorsiplantar View: 6 Months After Initial Film**. A third stress fracture is observed in the shaft of the fourth metatarsal. COMMENT: The serial progression of the stress fractures in this case is somewhat unique, since the patient was a 60-year-old energetic gardener who refused to quit the extensive stooping involved in her gardening. The stress related to that position created the serial stress fractures over a period of 6 months. (Courtesy of Donald B. Tomkins, DC, DACBR, Canistota, South Dakota. Special thanks to James F. Winterstein, DC, DACBR, Chicago, Illinois, for his help in obtaining this case)

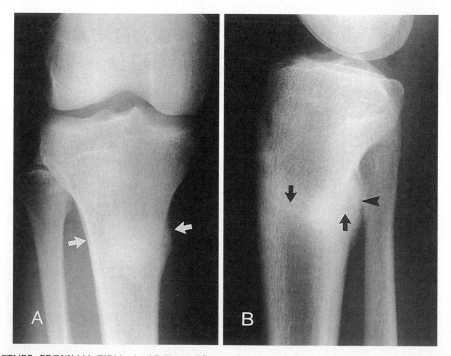

Figure 9.222.   STRESS FRACTURE: PROXIMAL TIBIA. A. AP Knee. Observe the exuberant callus formation surrounding the proximal diaphysis of the tibia (arrows). **B. Lateral Knee**. A horizontal radiolucent fracture line is demonstrated through the area of stress fracture (arrows). Extensive callus formation is noted on the posterior surface of the tibia adjacent to the fracture line (arrowhead). COMMENT: The proximal tibia is a common location for stress fractures, which are found in joggers, marchers, and ballet dancers.

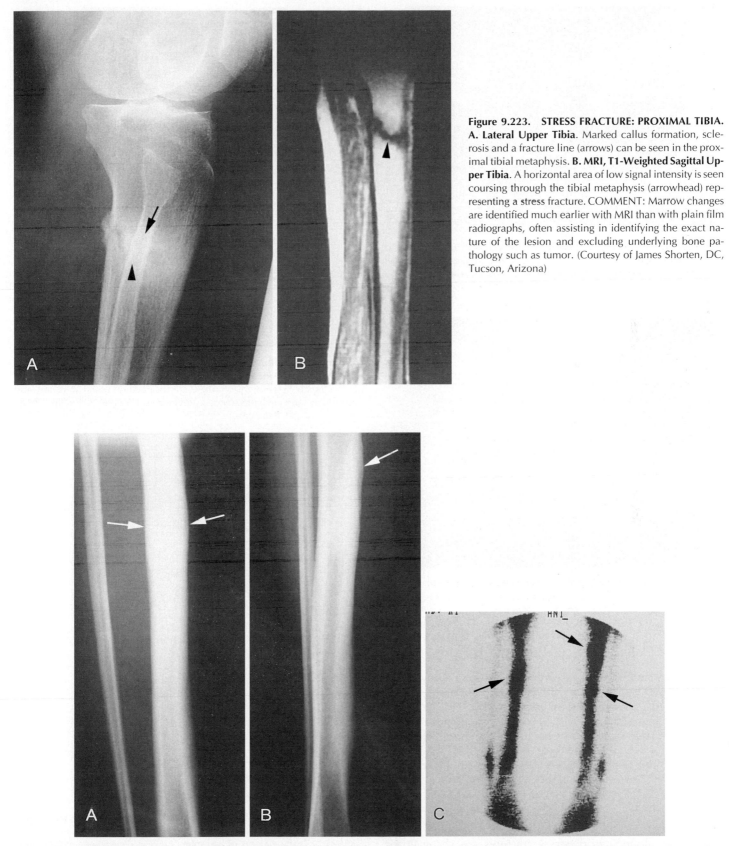

Figure 9.223.   STRESS FRACTURE: PROXIMAL TIBIA. A. Lateral Upper Tibia. Marked callus formation, sclerosis and a fracture line (arrows) can be seen in the proximal tibial metaphysis. **B. MRI, T1-Weighted Sagittal Upper Tibia**. A horizontal area of low signal intensity is seen coursing through the tibial metaphysis (arrowhead) representing a stress fracture. COMMENT: Marrow changes are identified much earlier with MRI than with plain film radiographs, often assisting in identifying the exact nature of the lesion and excluding underlying bone pathology such as tumor. (Courtesy of James Shorten, DC, Tucson, Arizona)

Figure 9.224.   BILATERAL TIBIAL STRESS FRACTURES. A. AP Tibia. There is diffuse periosteal new bone in the upper tibia (arrows). No fracture line is visible. **B. Lateral Tibia**. A similar periosteal response is present (arrow). **C. Delayed Bone Scan, AP View**. Focal regions of increased uptake are present bilaterally, corresponding to the sites of fracture (arrows). COMMENT: This aerobics instructor demonstrates the characteristic findings of stress fractures—minimal plain film changes with an impressive bone scan. Bone scan is the modality of choice in the diagnosis of stress fractures. (Courtesy of Richard L. Green, DC, Winthrop, Massachusetts)

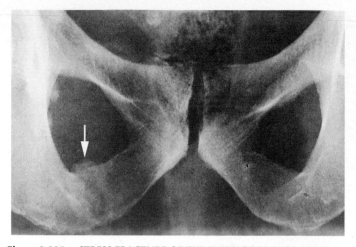

Figure 9.225.   STRESS FRACTURE OF THE INFERIOR PUBIC RAMUS. Localized callus is present (arrow) and a lucent fracture zone can be seen (arrowhead). (Courtesy of Richard M. Nuzzi, DC, Boulder, Colorado)

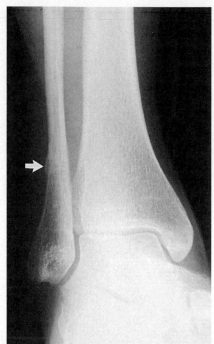

Figure 9.227.   STRESS FRACTURE: DISTAL FIBULA. Periosteal new bone formation, along with a radiolucent fracture line, is seen in the distal diaphysis of the fibula (arrow). COMMENT: Stress fractures of the fibula are most commonly found in ballet dancers and joggers. (Courtesy of Phillip C. Huyler, DC, Nassau, Bahamas)

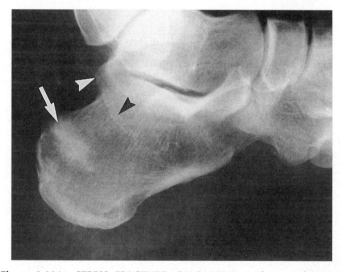

Figure 9.226.   STRESS FRACTURE: CALCANEUS. A dense radiopaque band is present in the posterosuperior portion of the calcaneus (arrow). This is a typical location for stress fracture affecting the calcaneus. Of incidental note is a vascular calcification in the posterior tibial artery (arrowheads).

are not uncommon sites for stress fractures, usually being found in runners and ballet dancers. (10) The distal portion is affected more often than the proximal aspect. (Fig. 9.227)

The pars interarticularis of the lower lumbar spine (L4, L5) is the most common site for stress fracture of the entire skeleton. It may be found with or without spondylolisthesis. (11) (Fig. 9.228) Other sites and their associated activities are outlined. (Figs. 9.229A and B, 9.230A and B) (Table 9.18)

CLINICAL FEATURES

The clinical findings of stress fractures are characteristic. Pain, which is related to activity and is relieved by rest, is typical. Soft tissue swelling with localized tenderness over the area of stress fracture is observed. Almost any bone can be affected, with the bones of the lower extemity being most

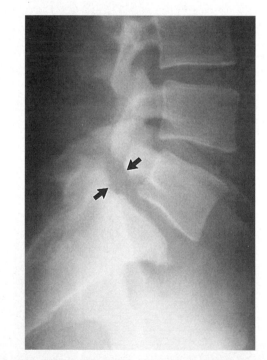

Figure 9.228.   STRESS FRACTURE: LUMBAR PARS INTERARTICULARIS. Spondylolysis of the pars interarticularis of L5 upon the sacrum is noted. COMMENT: The majority of pars interarticularis defects seen in the lumbar spine are the result of stress fractures.

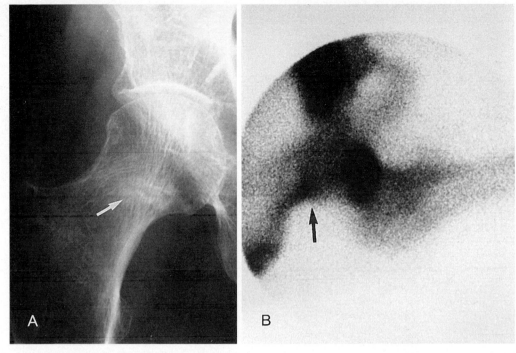

Figure 9.229.   STRESS FRACTURE: PROXIMAL FEMUR. A. AP Hip. The stress fracture can be appreciated by the radiopaque transverse band which is present in the area of the femoral neck (arrow). **B. Bone Scan**. There is a focal area of increased radionuclide uptake in the area of the stress fractures of the femoral neck (arrow).COMMENT: Stress fractures of the femoral neck are a frequent complication of osteoporosis and are also found in marathon runners.

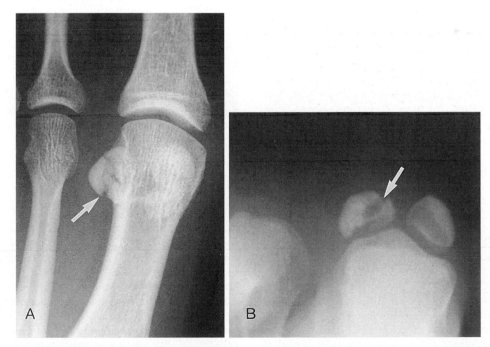

Figure 9.230.   STRESS FRACTURE: SESAMOID BONE OF THE GREAT TOE. A. Dorsiplantar View: Great Toe. There is fragmentation and radiopacity noted within the lateal sesamoid bone on the plantar surface of the great toe (arrow). **B. Axial Metatarsal Head View**. A stress fracture with radiopacity and fragmentation of the sesamoid bone is observed (arrow). COMMENT: This stress fracture occurred in a female marathon runner who experienced severe plantar foot pain while training. (Courtesy of Gary M. Guebert, DC, DACBR, St. Louis, Missouri)

Table 9.18.   Activity-Related Sites for Stress Fractures

Calcaneus	Posterior, plantar portion	Jumping, parachuting, marching, prolonged standing
Clavicle	Outer one third	Persistent tic, radical neck surgery
Femur		
(a) Shaft	Distal one third	Ballet, long distance running
(b) Neck	Midcervical, subcapital	Ballet, marching, long distance running, gymnastics
Fibula	Distal shaft	Long distance running
	Proximal shaft	Jumping, parachuting
Hamate	Hook	Equipment holding (tennis, golf, baseball)
Humerus	Distal shaft	Throwing sports
Metatarsals		
(a) First	Base	Marching, ground stomping
(b) Second	Distal and midshaft	Marching, ground stomping, ballet
(c) Third	Distal metaphysis	Morton's syndrome
(d) Fifth	Shaft, base	Running on banked track fields
Navicular (Tarsal)	Distal one half	Ground stomping, marching, long distance running
Patella	Proximal pole	Hurdling
Pelvis	Obturator ring	Stooping, bowling, gymnastics
Phalanx	Tuft	Guitar players
Ribs		
(a) First	Posterior	Pack carrier, chronic dyspnea
(b) 7-9	Posterolateral	Coughing, golf
Scapula	Coracoid process	Trap shooting
	Inferior glenoid tip	Baseball players
Sesamoids	First metatarsal	Standing, jumping, running
Spine		
(a) Lower cervical	Spinous process	Clay shoveling
(b) Upper thoracic	Spinous process	Clay shoveling
(c) Lower lumbar	Pars interarticularis	Ballet, gymnasts, polevaulters, football players, cricket bowlers, weight lifters, divers
Tibial Shaft	Mid and distal	Long distance running, ballet
	Proximal	Jumping, parachuting, basketball
Ulna	Coronoid process	Throwing sports
	Olecranon	Throwing sports
	Shaft	Pitchfork work, wheelchair

frequently involved. More than one site can be present, with serial radiographs showing fractures at various stages. (Fig. 9.221A–C)

RADIOLOGIC FEATURES

The initial radiographic examination may fail to reveal the fracture line. This is influenced by the location of the fracture and the interval between the time of injury and that of the radiographic examination. The minimum radiographic latent period is 10 to 21 days. Tomography may be helpful in demonstrating the fracture line.

Bone scan is the modality of choice for demonstration. (2,12,13) Focal uptake at the site of fracture on delayed images is characteristic but not specific. The scan may remain active for up to 12 months after healing. (14,15) Combination bone scan with tomography (SPECT) is especially useful in the demonstration of an active stress fracture of the pars interarticularis. By demonstrating a fracture line, CT is a useful tool when the diagnosis is in doubt. MR imaging similarly can detect subtle fractures and aid in the differential diagnosis. (13,16) Occult fracture lines may show as a low signal on T1 and high signal on T2 sequences if local hemorrhage is present or in its absence remain low in signal on T1 and T2. (12,16)

Table 9.19.   Radiologic Features of Stress Fractures

Localized solid periosteal/endosteal new bone
Subtle or absent fracture line
Narrow, poorly defined, opaque band
Positive bone scan

Roentgen Signs of Stress Fractures

Periosteal Response.   The most frequently seen and reliable roentgen sign of stress fracture is periosteal and endosteal cortical thickening. (Table 9.19) The degree of new bone formation can be extreme and usually assumes a solid pattern of periosteal response. This cortical thickening is localized to the area of stress fracture, creating an eccentric protuberance of the cortex.

Fracture Line.   Frequently, the exuberant periosteal new bone will obscure the radiolucent fracture line within the cortex. At other times, the fracture is too thin to be depicted on the radiograph. Oblique fractures are most common though transverse and rare longitudinal varieties do occur. Tomography often will demonstrate the fracture line through the dense sclerosis, when plain films do not.

Transverse Opaque Bands.   When the stress fracture is viewed *en face*, the periosteal callus forms a linear, transverse, radiopaque band. The margins of this density are hazy and poorly defined, which differentiates it from a growth arrest line.

The calcaneus is a characteristic site to visualize such a dense radiopaque line traversing vertically through the bone. (Fig. 9.226)

DIFFERENTIAL DIAGNOSIS

Osteomyelitis

Since osteomyelitis may create a significant periosteal response, an early infectious focus can resemble a stress fracture. The lack of bone destruction adjacent to the periosteal callus is the key roentgen sign, since infectious lesions will produce lytic bone destruction.

Osteosarcoma

Early lesions of osteosarcoma may be confused with stress fractures. Both produce periosteal response, with stress fracture assuming a solid pattern and osteosarcoma creating a spiculated pattern. Bone destruction will be seen with osteosarcoma, a roentgen sign not present with stress fractures. Often, tomography will demonstrate a linear radiolucent fracture line, securing the diagnosis of stress fracture.

Osteoid Osteoma

The radiographic appearance of osteoid osteoma and stress fracture are very similar. The key roentgen sign that allows differntial diagnosis is usually seen on tomographic views and overpenetrated plain films. This sign is the oval radiolucent nidus of osteoid osteoma versus the linear radiolucent fracture line in stress fractures.

Growth Arrest Lines

These present as discrete radiopaque lines through the metaphysis of the bone. The radiopaque line of stress fracture is broader, with a hazy, ill-defined margin to its edge. Additionally, growth arrest lines are usually found in other bones as bilateral, symmetrical, well-defined radiopaque bands.

NON-ACCIDENTAL TRAUMA IN CHILDREN

A number of terms have been applied to encompass the controversial topic of childhood injuries from abuse. Caffey, in 1946, was the first to describe multiple fractures in the long bones of patients who were suffering from subdural hematomas and he coined the phrase *parent-infant traumatic stress syndrome*. (1) The term *battered child syndrome* was offered by Kempe and others in 1962, and stimulated public debate. (2) Other descriptions include *infant abuse syndrome, shaken infant syndrome* and, more recently, *non-accidental trauma of children (NAT)*. Usually, those who inflict the injuries are parents or guardians.

The hallmark of this syndrome is clinical and radiologic evidence of repeated injury. (3) Clinically, multiple bruises or burns of varying degrees of severity are the usual findings. The history is often incompatible with the observed injuries. Unsuspected fractures are uncommon over the age of two, while children older than five rarely sustain a fracture from abuse. (4) Up to 80% of fractures in abused children occur under the age of 18 months. (5) This contrasts with non-abused children, where 85% of their fractures occur over the age of five.

A number of imaging findings have been described. The *shaken infant syndrome* (whiplash shaking syndrome) includes injuries incurred as sequelae to vigorous shaking while clutching the chest. (6) The average age is six months. Injuries include retinal hemorrhages, subdural hemorrhages, cerebral edema, and skull fractures.

A spectrum of skeletal injuries may be observed. In long bones the key findings are fractures in varying stages of healing, multiple closely approximated fractures, metaphyseal corner fractures, epiphyseal displacements, and exuberant periosteal new bone. (Table 9.20) The key to the radiographic diagnosis is the demonstration of multiple fractures at varying stages of healing. (1,3) Quite often, a fresh fracture may be seen next to a callused, deformed bone.

Other common sites involving occurrence of this syndrome are the ribs, skull, clavicle, and scapula. Spinal fractures are uncommon. Since many of these children are severely shaken while held by their arms, bilateral humeral fractures are also common. (Fig. 9.231)

Table 9.20.   Radiologic Features of Non-Accidental Trauma in Children

Fractures in different stages of healing
Multiple closely approximated fractures
Metaphyseal corner fractures
Epiphyseal displacements
Exuberant periosteal new bone

Figure 9.231. NON-ACCIDENTAL TRAUMA OF CHILDHOOD: MULTIPLE FRACTURES OF THE SHOULDER. A recent fracture of the middiaphysis of the humerus is observed. A fracture of older origin is present in the distal aspect of the clavicle, with exuberant callus formation (arrow). COMMENT: The key to the radiographic diagnosis of battered child syndrome is the demonstration of multiple fractures at varying stages of healing, as is seen in this case. The classic radiographic signs are fractures in the corners of the metaphyses, with or without associated epiphyseal displacement, and exuberant periosteal new bone formation along the diaphyses and metadiaphyses of the long bones.

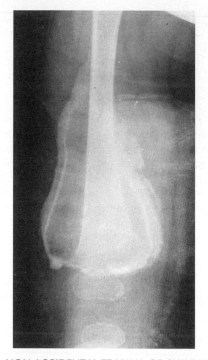

Figure 9.232. NON-ACCIDENTAL TRAUMA OF CHILDHOOD: THIGH. Extensive hemorrhage has lifted the periosteum, creating large, wavy periosteal new bone formation. No fractures are identified on this femoral radiograph.

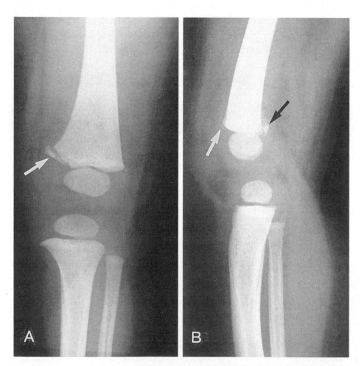

Figure 9.233. NON-ACCIDENTAL TRAUMA OF CHILDHOOD: CORNER FRACTURE. A. AP Knee. A characteristic corner fracture is observed affecting the medial aspect of the metaphysis of the distal femur (arrow). **B. Lateral Knee.** Multiple fracture fragments of the distal metaphysis of the femur are identified (arrows).

The classic radiographic sign is fractures of the corners of the metaphyses with or without associated epiphyseal displacement (*corner fractures*). (3,7) (Fig. 9.232) Corner fractures usually are observed around the knee, especially at the medial aspect of the metaphysis of the distal femur. (Fig. 9.233A and B) These lesions represent avulsion microfractures from the immature metaphysis from traction of the periosteum. (6,7) Separation of the metaphysis in a circumferential manner are called *bucket–handle fractures.* Such metaphyseal lesions often provide the initial clue to suspicion of abuse. The cluster of radiologic findings, which has a high degree of specificity in child abuse, include these metaphyseal lesions (corner fractures), posterior rib, scapular, spine, and sternal fractures. (6,8) Spinal fractures include vertebral body compression, spinous process avulsions, hangman's, and odontoid synchondrosis fractures. (6,9)

Other conditions such as infantile cortical hyperostosis, congenital syphilis, scurvy, and osteogenesis imperfecta may be considered in the differential diagnosis. (10) In general, they are readily excluded by clinical and radiographic signs.

Imaging of suspected child abuse requires meticulous technique and detail. A skeletal survey should include AP and lateral chest, AP humerii and forearms, PA hands, AP pelvis, lateral lumbar spine, AP femora, tibiae, feet, and AP and lateral skull. (6,9) All positive sites should be viewed by at least two projections. Repeat imaging in 7 to 10 days may provide evidence for fracture healing not apparent on the initial study. Bone scan may be useful in difficult cases. CT of the head in children with neurologic abnormality should be performed.

POSTTRAUMATIC MYOSITIS OSSIFICANS
GENERAL CONSIDERATIONS

Traumatic myositis ossificans (myositis ossificans posttraumatica, ossifying hematoma, traumatic ossifying myositis, or heterotopic posttraumatic bone formation) is a condition characterized by heterotopic bone formation in the soft tissues following trauma. The process occurs most often in muscle but may also occur in fascia, tendons, joint capsules, and ligaments. Most occur following any local injury sufficient to cause bruising of the muscle or a frank hemorrhage within it. The most common sites are the brachialis anterior (elbow) (Fig. 9.234A and B), quadriceps femoris (thigh), (Fig. 9.235) adductor muscles of the thigh, medial collateral ligament of the knee (Pellegrini-Stieda disease), (Fig. 9.236) and in cases of rupture of the coracoclavicular ligament of the shoulder. (1,2) Other lesser-known sites are the deltoid in foot soldiers, due to the trauma caused by carrying a rifle. The constant pressure of the saddle against the adductors in riders may cause ossification in the adductor magnus and is known as *Prussian's disease* or, erroneously, as a *saddle tumor.* (Fig. 9.237) Bedridden and wheelchair-confined patients frequently produce heterotopic bone at areas of gravitational stress, most commonly found at the ischial tuberosities. (Fig. 9.238) Up to 50% of paraplegic and quadraplegics exhibit paravertebral ossification (3).

Lumbar Ossified Bridge Syndrome (LOBS). Hematoma within the psoas muscle may ossify and produce complete or incomplete bony union between two or more lumbar transverse processes. (4) (Fig. 9.239) The bony bar consists of mature osseous tissue with cortex, medullary bone and contains marrow. (5) Removal of the bony bridge in symptomatic cases may relieve a pain syndrome. (5)

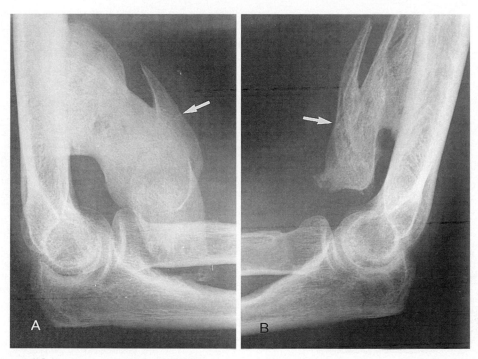

Figure 9.234. POSTTRAUMATIC MYOSITIS OSSIFICANS: ELBOWS. A and B. Bilateral Lateral Elbows. The large ossified masses present anterior to the distal humerus represent posttraumatic ossificans (arrows). The bra-chialis anterior is the most common muscle involved in the area of the elbow.

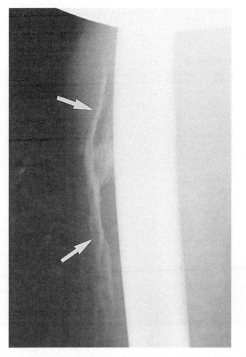

Figure 9.235. POSTTRAUMATIC MYOSITIS OSSIFICANS: ANTERIOR THIGH. There is a wavy, ossific density present in the anterior thigh involving the quadriceps femoris (arrows). (Courtesy of Mark J. Lieffring, DC, Cloquet, Minnesota)

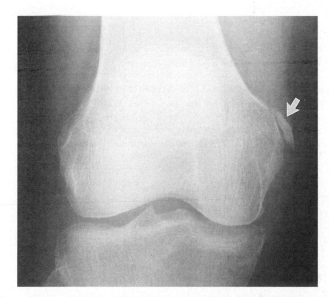

Figure 9.236. MEDIAL COLLATERAL LIGAMENT OSSIFICATION. There is ossification in the area of the medial collateral ligament following avulsion (arrow). This has been referred to as Pellegrini-Stieda disease. (Courtesy of James R. Brandt, DC, MSc, FACO, Coon Rapids, Minnesota)

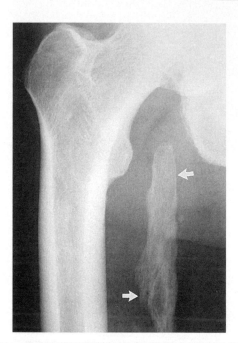

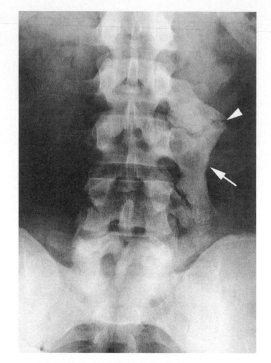

Figure 9.237.   MYOSITIS OSSIFICANS: PRUSSIAN'S DISEASE. There is a large, well-organized ossifying hematoma present in the adductor magnus muscle (arrows). Observe the dense cortical margin, with a relatively radiolucent center. COMMENT: This has been referred to as Prussian's disease and is the result of the constant pressure of the saddle against the adductor muscles, which were found frequently in Prussian soldiers who were horseback riders.

Figure 9.239.   MYOSITIS OSSIFICANS: LUMBAR SPINE (LOBS). Observe the exuberant bridging ossification between the lumbar transverse processes (arrow). There is evidence of pseudojoint formation (arrowhead). COMMENT: This pattern of ossification may follow trauma or sudden paraplegia and has been referred to as *lumbar ossified bridge syndrome* (LOBS). (Courtesy of Joseph W. Howe, DC, DACBR, Fellow, ACCR, Los Angeles, California)

Figure 9.238.   POSTTRAUMATIC MYOSITIS OSSIFICANS: PARAPLEGIA. There are ossifying hematomas below both ischial tuberosities (arrows). These represent sites of myositis ossificans posttraumatica in a nonambulatory patient restricted to a wheelchair. It occurred as a result of constant mechanical pressure on the soft tissues. Because of the lack of activity and urinary stasis, multiple bladder calculi have developed (arrowheads). These may be differentiated from phleboliths by the lack of a radiolucent center (crossed arrow).

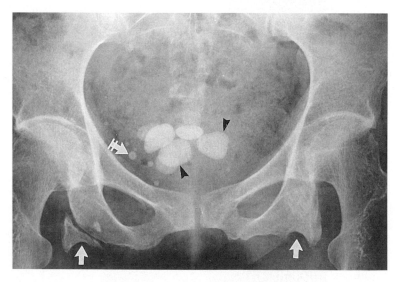

Ossification of the Achilles Tendon. The most common cause is surgery followed by trauma as the second most common cause. Additional causes include DISH, fluorosis, ochronosis, Wilson's disease, renal failure, Reiter's syndrome, gout, and ankylosing spondylitis. (6) The ossific mass lies within the tendon and consists of mature bone containing marrow and may fracture. (Fig. 9.240)

Cortical Irregularity Syndrome. Young adults may show roughening of the posterior femoral surface which has been previously described as a *periosteal desmoid.* (Fig. 9.241A–D) It represents chronic or previous tearing of the musculotendinous insertion along the distal linea aspera. It is commonly confused with osteosarcoma, which can be excluded on the basis of location, appearance, and a failure to show underlying marrow disease on bone scan or MR imaging.

PATHOLOGIC FEATURES

The process can be divided into three stages—pseudosarcoma, differentiation, and maturation.

Stage One: Pseudosarcoma

The sequence of events begins with a traumatic incident in which tissue is crushed or torn. Blunt trauma is common. The precise stimulus that causes metaplastic formation of bone instead of normal repair and scar formation is unknown. Following crushing of the muscle, there is extensive damage and cell death. Holes appear in the sarcolemmal sheath and fluid acumulates. The sarcolemmal nuclei proliferate, the sarcolemma disappears, and the fluid diffuses into the tissues. Phagocytes invade and remove the fibers, enlarging the holes. The capillary bed dilates, as in fracture, producing the clinical symptoms of heat, swelling, and tenderness ("charley horse"). Since the damage is greatest in the center of the traumatized area, these tissues may totally liquefy or be replaced by sheets of nonspecific cells. The breakdown of cellular material in the traumatized area induces a transient inflammatory infiltrate ("myositis").

Unless further trauma is added by injudicious massage, excessive stretching, surgery, or other activity, the stage of degeneration lasts approximately 15 days. It is followed by a phase of activity with extensive proliferation of all mesenchymal cell types. Identifiable osteoid formation is minimal at this stage. A biopsy during this 2- to 4-week period can lead to an erroneous diagnosis of neoplasia. It is a period of indecision for the clinician, radiologist, and pathologist. The clinical history of blunt trauma at the appropriate time is essential in reaching a proper diagnosis.

During the initial 6- to 7-week period the lesion has identifiable zones only if excised in its entirety. The center of the lesion is necrotic, surrounded by zones with less tissue damage.

Stage Two: Differentiation

During the second and third months following injury, the mesenchymal cells differentiate into fibroblasts, osteoblasts, chondroblasts, and so forth. Giant cells are numerous and remove the necrotic debris. Fibrous tissue formation and some primitive osteoid deposition occur. Blood supply to the center of the lesion is precarious. Most of the necrotic cells undergo liquefactive necrosis and resorption—which may leave a cyst filled with fluid—or the area may fill with sheets of nonspecific cells.

Near the periphery of the lesion, where the damage is least, repair is more prompt and complete, leading to mineralization. The matrix will proceed to ossification, with the best developed, mature trabecular bone at the periphery and progressively less differentiated zones in the central portion. This characteristic zoning of the myositis ossificans, with the more mature tissue at the periphery, distinguishes it from neoplasms of bone in which the best-differentiated portions are in the center of the lesion and the least differentiated are at the periphery.

Stage Three: Maturation

As the lesion matures, it shrinks in size, and the periphery becomes heavier and more developed, as is the case with fracture callus. It develops a "periosteum" that separates it from the surrounding tissue, although muscle fibers are frequently attached to the peripheral portion. The inner central area may become entirely cystic, showing removal of liquefied debris, or it may become demarcated as in an infarct and never become replaced. Eventually, the activity subsides and the lesion becomes stable.

Once the periosteum develops, it is easier to remove the lesion surgically. Surgical removal of immature lesions is contraindicated because of the high incidence of recurrence, often with involvement of a larger area than that included in the original lesion. Some ossifications completely disappear, and the smaller ones regress because of osteoclastic resorption within the muscle belly. There is complete restoration of muscle contour, but muscle function is never totally normal. (7)

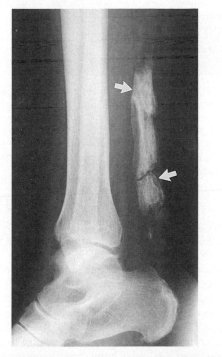

Figure 9.240.   MYOSITIS OSSIFICANS: ACHILLES TENDON. There is ossification of a large hematoma present within the Achilles tendon (arrows). This is sometimes associated with rupture of the tendon.

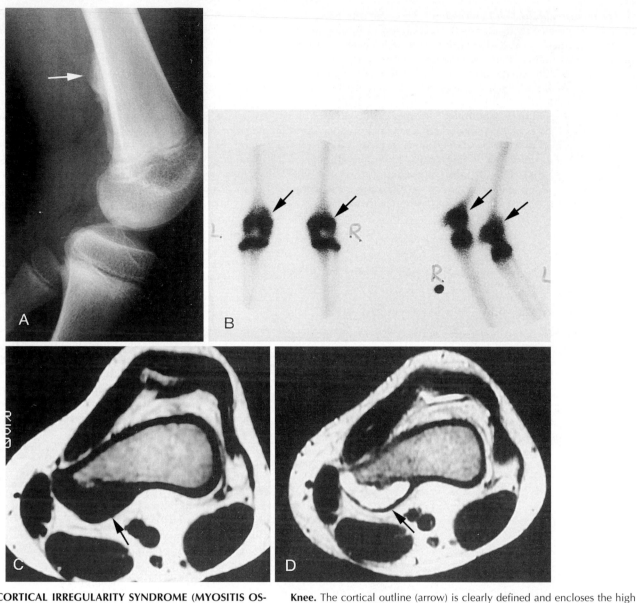

Figure 9.241.   CORTICAL IRREGULARITY SYNDROME (MYOSITIS OS-SIFICANS). A. Lateral Knee. Observe the solid, wavy periosteal new bone formation along the posterior surface of the distal femoral metaphysis (arrow). **B. Bone Scan, Bilateral Knee.** There is a small area of abnormal radiopharmaceutical uptake within the left distal femur (arrows). **C. MRI, T1-Weighted Axial Knee.** Note the eccentric, homogeneous, low signal intensity mass on the posterior surface of the femur (arrow). This region is well encapsulated and is suggestive of a benign process. **D. MRI, T2-Weighted Axial**

Knee. The cortical outline (arrow) is clearly defined and encloses the high signal intensity hemorrhagic edema. These findings are consistent with cortical irregularity syndrome, a condition resulting from traumatic periostitis. COMMENT: A presumptive diagnosis of osteosarcoma was initially made and the patient was scheduled for a biopsy. MRI confirms a fluid signal intensity with no underlying marrow abnormality. (Courtesy of Frank Sivo, DC, North Miami, Florida)

RADIOLOGIC FEATURES

The ossifying hematoma may be visible radiographically within 3 to 4 weeks after the initial injury. (1,8) MR imaging may show the intramuscular hematoma from an early stage. (9) (Fig 9.242) Initially, the roentgen appearance is a fine, lacy radiopacity, which is followed later by a cloudy ossification within a well-defined mass. Its size depends upon the degree of initial trauma and the overall size of the hematoma. Eventually, sequential studies demonstrate a bony mass that is very radiopaque in its peripheral margins, with the center of the lesion appearing relatively radiolucent. (Fig. 9.240) The bony mass usually measures

4 to 5 cm but may be as large as 25 cm on occasion. The soft tissue osseous mass distinctively has no direct connection with the closest bone. (Table 9.21)

Radiologic diagnosis is essential, since biopsy of this mass in its early stages may show what would appear to be a sarcomatous change centrally. A radiologic sign important in making the distinction between this and a bone neoplasm is the characteristic lucent zone (cleavage plane) between the calcified mass and the subadjacent cortex. (10,11) The mass is usually located adjacent to the diaphysis of a tubular bone, but the cortex of the bone is intact. Other important confirmatory properties are a dense periphery with a more lucent center and decrease in volume with

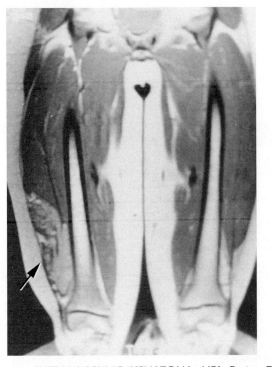

Figure 9.242. INTRAMUSCULAR HEMATOMA. MRI, Proton Density-Weighted Coronal Femora. Observe the prominent inhomogeneous increased signal intensity region within the vastus lateralis muscle (arrow). This finding is consistent with post-traumatic hematoma. (Courtesy of Kenneth B. Heithoff, MD, Minneapolis, Minnesota)

time. (Fig. 9.243A and B) Increased uptake of bone-seeking radionuclide may be noted which diminishes with maturity and inactivity of the lesion. (12)

DIFFERENTIAL DIAGNOSIS

Extraskeletal sarcoma may be difficult to differentiate from myositis ossificans. This condition is rare and tends to occur in older adults. Synovioma, in one third of cases, may calcify and can be located remote from the joint due to its association with tendon sheaths; therefore, this tumor must be given consideration when evaluating a calcified soft tissue mass. A parosteal sarcoma may have a similar appearance, but no lucent zone between it and the diaphysis should be visible. Other soft tissue calcifications such as tumoral calcinosis may present as a densely calcified mass but have an amorphous calcific rather than maturely ossific nature. (13)

Table 9.21.	Radiologic Features of Posttraumatic Myositis Ossificans
EARLY FEATURES	
Hazy soft tissue mass	
Cloudy ossification	
LATER FEATURES	
Round or linear	
Smooth, dense, outer border	
Relatively lucent center	
No connection with adjacent bone	

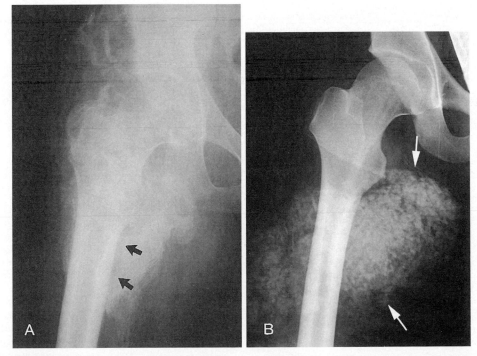

Figure 9.243. PSEUDOSARCOMA APPEARANCE OF MYOSITIS OSSIFICANS POSTTRAUMATIC. A. Proximal Thigh. A large soft tissue mass is present adjacent to the proximal femur. Observe the dense peripheral cortical rim, with a more radiolucent center, which suggests myositis ossificans rather than sarcoma. A clearly defined margin between the soft tissue mass and the cortex of the femur aids in the differential diagnosis (arrows). **B. Proximal Thigh**. A similar lesion is seen though it appears less confluent (arrow). Heat was placed on the injury which probably has not assisted in preventing myositis ossificans developing. (Courtesy of John J. Danchik, DC, CCSP, Belmont, Massachusetts)

SUMMARY TABLES

To follow is a tabulated compilation of named fractures and their eponyms, (Tables 9.22–9.34) named radiologic signs associated with trauma, (Table 9.35) and the most common fracture sites. (Table 9.36)

Table 9.22.   Named and Eponymic Fractures General Terms

AVULSION	Separated bone fragment from a muscle, tendon, or ligament.
BUTTERFLY FRAGMENT	Isolated triangular-shaped cortical fragment in a comminuted fracture.
BANANA-LIKE FRACTURE	Transverse pathologic fracture through a bone affected with Paget's disease.
CHIP (CORNER) FRACTURE	A small bone fragment originating from a joint margin.
CLOSED FRACTURE	Fracture does not penetrate the skin.
COMMINUTED FRACTURE	Two or more bony fragments.
DIASTATIC FRACTURE	Separation of a partly movable joint.
IMPACTION FRACTURE	Trabecular telescoping.
(a) Depressed	Inward bulging of the outer cortex.
(b) Compression	Decreased bone size due to trabecular telescoping.
INCOMPLETE FRACTURE	Fracture only extends partially across the bone.
(a) Greenstick	Buckled trabeculae.
(b) Torus	Buckled trabeculae with a cortical bulge.
INFRACTION FRACTURE	A small impaction fracture.
INSUFFICIENCY FRACTURE	Stress fracture through diseased bone.
OBLIQUE FRACTURE	Fracture line at 45° to the long axis.
OCCULT FRACTURE	A subtle, unidentifiable fracture, usually seen on follow up x-rays 7–10 days after trauma.
OPEN FRACTURE	Fracture penetrates the skin.
PATHOLOGIC FRACTURE	Fracture through diseased bone.
POSTTRAUMATIC ARTHRITIS	Secondary degenerative joint disease due to altered joint mechanics following trauma.
PSEUDOARTHROSIS	Residual motion between fracture fragments, creating a false joint.
PSEUDOFRACTURE	An incomplete pathologic fracturelike defect.
SALTER-HARRIS CLASSIFICATION	Growth plate injuries.
SPIRAL FRACTURE	Fracture line bends circumferentially and longitudinally along the bone.
STRESS (FATIGUE) FRACTURE	Microfracture due to repetitive stress.
THURSTON-HOLLAND FRAGMENT	Metaphyseal fragment in a Salter-Harris Type II epiphyseal injury.
TRANSVERSE FRACTURE	Fracture line at 90° to the long axis.

Table 9.23.   Named and Eponymic Fractures of the Skull and Facial Bones

BLOWOUT FRACTURE	Fracture through the infraorbital plate.
DIASTATIC FRACTURE	Fracture with separation of a suture.
GROWING FRACTURE	Widening of the sutural space due to leptomeningeal cyst.
LEFORT I-III FRACTURE	Facial bone fracture/separations.
PING PONG FRACTURE	A depressed skull fracture in a child.
STELLATE FRACTURE	A depressed skull fracture lines radiate from its center.
TRIPOD FRACTURE	Three fractures through the zygomatic arch, orbital and maxillary processes.

Table 9.24.   Named and Eponymic Fractures of the Cervical Spine

BURSTING FRACTURE OF THE ATLAS	Synonym for Jefferson's fracture.
BURST FRACTURE OF THE BODY	Comminuted vertebral body fracture.
CARROT STICK FRACTURE	Fracture through the ankylosed discovertebral junction in ankylosing spondylitis.
CLAY SHOVELER'S FRACTURE	Avulsion of a lower cervical segment spinous process.
COALMINER'S FRACTURE	Synonym for clay shoveler's fracture.
HANGMAN'S FRACTURE (HANGEE'S FRACTURE)	Bipedicular fracture of the axis.
JEFFERSON'S FRACTURE	Fractured anterior and posterior arch of the atlas.
PILLAR FRACTURE	Fractured articular pillar.
TEARDROP FRACTURE	A displaced, triangular fragment from the anteroinferior body corner.
TRAUMATIC SPONDYLOLISTHESIS	Synonym for hangman's fracture.
WEDGE FRACTURE	Compressed anterior vertebral body fracture.

Table 9.25. Named and Eponymic Fractures of the Lumbar Spine

CHANCE FRACTURE (SEATBELT FRACTURE)	Horizontal fracture through a single body and posterior arch.
FULCRUM FRACTURE	Synonym for a Chance fracture.

Table 9.26. Named and Eponymic Fractures of the Pelvis

BUCKET HANDLE FRACTURE	Superior and inferior pubic ramus fracture with a fracture or separation of the contralateral sacroiliac joint.
DASHBOARD FRACTURE	Posterior acetabular rim fracture.
DUVERNEY'S FRACTURE	Iliac wing fracture.
EXPLOSION FRACTURE	Central acetabular fracture.
MALGAIGNE'S FRACTURE	Superior and inferior pubic ramus fracture with a fracture near or separation of the ipsilateral sacroiliac joint.
OPEN BOOK FRACTURE	Synonym for a sprung pelvis.
PRUSSIAN'S DISEASE	Myositis ossificans of the adductor muscles from horseback riding.
RIDER'S BONE	Avulsion of the secondary growth center of the ischium which subsequently does not unite and dramatically enlarges.
SPRUNG PELVIS	Separation of the pubic symphysis and both sacroiliac joints.
STRADDLE FRACTURE	Bilateral superior pubic rami and ischiopubic fractures.
SUICIDAL JUMPER'S FRACTURE	Horizontal fracture through the first or second sacral segments associated with falls from a height.

Table 9.27. Named and Eponymic Fractures of the Knee

BUMPER (FENDER) FRACTURE	Medial or lateral tibial plateau fracture from a severe varus/valgus stress.
FLAKE FRACTURE	Osteochondral fragment separated from the medial facet of the femoral surface of the patella following dislocation.
FLOATING KNEE	Supracondylar femur fracture in combination with proximal tibia fracture.
LIPOHEMOARTHROSIS	Fat and blood in a joint due to an intraarticular fracture.
SEGOND'S FRACTURE	Avulsion of the lateral tibia at the insertion of the tensor fascia lata.
TRAMPOLINE FRACTURE	Proximal tibial metaphysis in children (2–10).

Table 9.28. Named and Eponymic Fractures of the Ankle

B-B FRACTURE	Both bones of the leg or forearm are fractured simultaneously (tibia and fibula; radius and ulna).
BIMALLEOLAR	Medial and lateral malleolar fractures.
BOOT-TOP FRACTURE (SKIER'S FRACTURE)	Distal diaphyseal/metaphyseal spiral fracture of the tibia and fibula in an adult.
COTTON'S FRACTURE	Erroneous synonym for trimalleolar fractures.
DUPUYTREN'S FRACTURE	Distal fibula fracture 6–7 cm above the malleolus, disrupted distal tibiofibular ligament, diastasis, lateral talus dislocation, up and out foot displacement.
MAISSONEUVE FRACTURE	Proximal fibula fracture due to an inversion and external rotation injury of the ankle.
POTT'S FRACTURE	Distal fibula fracture 6–7 cm above the malleolus with disruption of the distal tibiofibular ligament.
TILLAUX'S FRACTURE	Fractures of the medial malleolus, anterior tibial tubercle, and lateral malleolus 6–7 cm from its tip with diastasis of the distal tibiofibular joint.
TODDLER'S FRACTURE	Distal diaphyseal/metaphyseal spiral fracture of the tibia in an infant.

Table 9.29. Named and Eponymic Fractures of the Foot

AVIATOR'S ASTRAGALUS	Synonym for aviator's fracture.
AVIATOR'S FRACTURE	Fracture through the neck of the talus.
BEAK FRACTURE	Avulsion of the posterior calcaneal tubercle.
BEDROOM FRACTURE	Phalangeal fracture from striking an object.
CHOPART'S DISLOCATION	Dislocation between the talonavicular and calcaneonavicular joint.
DANCER'S FRACTURE	Synonym for Jones' fracture.
JONES' FRACTURE	Avulsion fracture of the styloid of the fifth metatarsal base.
LISFRANC FRACTURE/DISLOCATION	Dorsal dislocation of the metatarsal bases with associated fractures.
MARCH FRACTURE	Stress fracture of the second and third metatarsals.

Table 9.30. Named and Eponymic Fractures of the Thorax

COUGH FRACTURE	Stress fracture of a rib due to repetitive coughing episodes.
FAIL CHEST	Two fractures of the same rib which isolates a fragment, allowing paradoxical motion during respiration.
GOLFER'S FRACTURE	Lateral rib fracture incurred from striking the ground rather than the ball.
HUG FRACTURE	Synonym for passion fracture.
PASSION FRACTURE	Rib fracture following an overenthusiastic hug.

Table 9.31. Names and Eponymic Fractures of the Shoulder

BANKART LESION	Avulsion of the triceps insertion of a small fragment from the inferior glenoid rim.
DROOPING SHOULDER	Inferior subluxation of the humeral head due to hemarthrosis, infection, effusion, stroke, and brachial plexus lesions.
FLAP FRACTURE	Avulsion fracture of the greater tuberosity of the humerus.
HATCHET DEFECT	Synonym for Hill-Sachs defect.
HILL-SACHS DEFECT	An impaction fracture at the posterosuperior surface of the humeral head from the inferior glenoid rim following recurrent anterior shoulder dislocation.
SEPARATED SHOULDER	Acromioclavicular joint dislocation.
SUBLUXIO ERECTA	Inferior dislocation of the humerus with the humerus fixed in abduction.

Table 9.32. Named and Eponymic Fractures of the Elbow and Forearm

BABY CAR FRACTURE	Synonym for sideswipe fracture.
CHISEL FRACTURE	Vertical fracture of the radial head extending 10 mm from the articular surface.
ESSEX-LOPRESTI FRACTURE	Radial head comminuted fracture with distal radioulnar dislocation.
GALEAZZI FRACTURE	Fracture of the junction of the distal and middle third of the radial shaft and dislocation of the inferior radioulnar joint.
KOCHER'S FRACTURE	Osteochondral fracture of the capitellum.
LITTLE LEAGUER'S ELBOW	Avulsion of the medial epicondyle.
MONTEGGIA FRACTURE	Fracture of the proximal ulnar shaft with dislocation of the radial head.
NIGHTSTICK FRACTURE	Fracture of the ulnar shaft when the arm is raised to protect the head from a blow.
PARRY FRACTURE	Synonym for nightstick fracture.
PIEDMONT FRACTURE	Synonym for Galeazzi fracture.
PULLED ELBOW	Radial head pulled out from under the annular ligament.
REVERSE MONTEGGIA FRACTURE	Synonym for Galeazzi fracture.
SIDESWIPE FRACTURE	Fracture of the distal humerus, proximal radius, and ulna when an elbow protruding from a car window is struck by an object.
TRAFFIC FRACTURE	Synonym for sideswipe fracture.

Table 9.33. Named and Eponymic Fractures of the Wrist

BARTON'S FRACTURE	Posterior rim fracture of the distal radius.
CHAUFFEUR'S FRACTURE	Fracture of the radial styloid.
COLLES' FRACTURE	Fracture of the radius within 20–35 mm of the joint and posterior angulation of the distal fragment.
DE QUERVAIN'S FRACTURE/ DISLOCATION	Anterior dislocation of the lunate, along with the proximal fragment of a fractured scaphoid.
FISHER'S FRACTURE	Dorsal avulsion of the triquetrum.
MOORE'S FRACTURE	Colles' fracture in conjunction with fractured ulnar styloid process and ulnar dislocation.
REVERSE BARTON'S FRACTURE	Anterior rim fracture of the distal radius.
REVERSE COLLES' FRACTURE	Synonym for Smith's fracture.
RIM FRACTURE	Synonym for Barton's fracture.
SMITH'S FRACTURE	Fracture of the radius within 20–35 mm of joint and anterior angulation of the distal fragment.

Table 9.34. Named and Eponymic Fractures of the Hand

BAR ROOM FRACTURE	Fourth or fifth metacarpal neck fracture with anterior displacement of the head.
BENNETT'S FRACTURE	Intraarticular fracture through the base of the first metacarpal, with dorsal and radial displacement of the shaft.
BOXER'S FRACTURE	Second or third metacarpal neck fracture with anterior displacement of the head.
GAMEKEEPER'S FRACTURE	Disruption of the ulnar collateral ligament at the first metacarpophalangeal joint.
ROLANDO'S FRACTURE	Comminuted intraarticular fracture at the base of the first metacarpal.
VOLAR PLATE FRACTURE	Fractured anterior articular margin at the base of the middle phalanx.

Table 9.35. Named Radiologic Signs in Association with Trauma

Acute Kyphosis Sign	Lateral	Cervical	Kyphotic angulation localized to one level indicates damage to the posterior spinal ligaments and potential vertebral instability following a hyperflexion injury.
Collar Sign	Oblique	Lumbar	Lucent defect through the pars interarticularis simulating a collar on the scotty dog.
Corner Sign	Any	Any	Small metaphyseal fractures, especially found in multiple locations, suggesting "battered child" syndrome.
Corner Sign	Lateral	Wrist	Metaphyseal fragment of the radius associated with slipped epiphysis.
Divergent Spinous	Lateral	Cervical	Due to cervical kyphosis, in spinous processes are divergently orientated to each other as a result of posterior ligamentous damage.
Double Cortical Sign	AP	Elbow	Double cortex to the articulating surface of the radial head due to a depressed fracture.
Double Spinous Sign	AP	Cervical	Double contour to a lower cervical spinous due to a clay shoveler's fracture.
Empty Vertebra Sign	AP	Lumbar	A split in the pedicle creates an open space due to the presence of a Chance fracture.
Extrapleural Sign	Tangential	Thorax	Opaque, convex, well-defined soft tissue density arising adjacent to a rib. A sign of rib disease or traumatic injury such as a hematoma following fracture or metastases.
FBI Sign	Cross-Table	Knee	F = fat; B = blood; I = interface. Usually seen in the knee as a sign of intraarticular fracture.
Fat-Pad Sign	Lateral	Elbow	Visualization of posterior fat-pad seen in intraarticular fractures, most commonly the radial head.
Half Moon Sign	AP	Shoulder	Lack of the normal semilunar overlap density of the humerus and scapula due to posterior shoulder dislocation.
Hawkin's Sign	AP	Ankle	The presence of a linear subcortical zone of radiolucency in the talar dome following fracture of the talus. This is a good sign of an intact blood supply and a decreased likelihood for avascular necrosis.
Lucent Cleft Sign	Extension	Cervical	Small linear radiolucency adjacent to the anteroinferior endplate, representing a region of avulsion of some annular fibers.
Navicular Fat Stripe Sign	PA	Wrist	Obliteration or displacement of the navicular fat stripe due to fracture of the radial styloid, scaphoid, or trapezium.
Pie Sign	PA	Wrist	Triangular shape of the lunate due to anterior lunate dislocation.
Pronator Quadratus Fat Line Sign	Lateral	Wrist	Obliteration or displacement of the pronator quadratus fat line due to fracture of the distal radius.
Rim Sign	AP	Shoulder	Widened glenohumeral joint space greater than 6 mm in posterior humeral dislocation.
Ring Sign	PA	Wrist	Circular configuration of the scaphoid due to dislocation.
Signet Ring Sign	PA	Wrist	Synonym for ring sign.
Supinator Fat Line	Lateral	Elbow	Obliteration or displacement of the supinator fat line due to fracture of the proximal radius.
Terry Thomas Sign	PA	Wrist	Widened scapholunate space more than 4 mm due to scapholunate disassociation with ligament rupture.
Trough Line Sign	AP	Shoulder	Double cortical contour to the superomedial humeral head is visible due to compression fracture associated with posterior shoulder dislocation.
Vacant Glenoid Sign	AP	Shoulder	Absent humeral head in anterior compartment of the joint due to posterior humeral dislocation.
Vertebral Body Step Defect	Lateral	Cervical Thoracic Lumbar	Sharp offset of the cortex due to compression fracture.

Table 9.36. Most Common Fracture Sites

GENERAL		ANKLE	
Nonunion	Spondylolysis, clavicle, ulna, tibia	Tibia	Medial malleolus
Compression	Vertebral bodies	Fibula	Lateral malleolus
Posttraumatic arthritis	Hip, knee, ankle	Talus	Dome margins
SKULL AND FACIAL BONES		Dislocation	Posterior
Skull: Linear Fracture	Cranial vault	FOOT	
Depressions	Parietal, temporal	Tarsal	Calcaneus
Facial	Tripod	Calcaneus	Compression
Mandible	Body	Talus	Neck
CERVICAL SPINE		Metatarsals	Base of the fifth metatarsal
Atlas	Posterior arch	SHOULDER GIRDLE	
Axis	Base of the odontoid (type II)	Clavicle	Mid third
Body	C5–C7	Scapula	Body, neck
Pillar	C6	Humerus	Surgical neck
Spinous	C7	Dislocation	Anterior
Transverse Process	C7	ELBOW	
Lamina	C5, C6	Child	Supracondylar
Facet Dislocation	C4–C7	Adult	Radial head/neck
THORACIC SPINE		Humerus	Supracondylar
Body	T9–T12	Ulna	Olecranon
LUMBAR SPINE		Radius	Head/neck
Chance Fracture	L1–L3	Dislocation	Posterior
Body Fracture	L1, L2	WRIST	
TVP Fracture	L2–L3	Carpal	Scaphoid
Pars Fracture	L4, L5	Scaphoid	Waist
PELVIS		Radius	Colles' fracture
Hemipelvis	Malgaigne's fracture	Ulna	Styloid process
Acetabulum	Central fracture	Dislocation	Lunate
Avulsions	ASIS, AIIS	HAND	
HIP		Metacarpal	4th, 5th metacarpal necks
Proximal Femur	Subcapital	Phalanges	Distal phalanx
Hip Dislocation	Posterior	Thumb	Transverse
KNEE		Dislocation	Posterior
Femur	Supracondylar		
Tibia	Lateral plateau		
Fibula	Styloid process		
Patella	Transverse		

REFERENCES

INTRODUCTION

1. **Peltier LF:** *The impact of Roentgen's discovery upon the treatment of fractures.* Surgery 33:579, 1953.

TYPES OF FRACTURES

1. **Felson B:** *Roentgenology of Fractures and Dislocations,* New York, Grune & Stratton, 1978.
2. **Rogers LF:** *Radiology of Skeletal Trauma.* Vols. 1 and 2, ed 2. New York, Churchill Livingstone, 1992.
3. **Steinbach HL, Kolb FO, Giljilan R:** *A mechanism for the production of pseudofractures in osteomalacia (Milkman's syndrome).* Radiology 62:388, 1954.
4. **Salter RB, Harris WR:** *Injuries involving the epiphyseal plate.* J Bone Joint Surg (Am) 45:587, 1963.
5. **Holland CT:** *Radiographical note on injuries to distal epiphyses of radius and ulna.* Proc R Soc Med 22:23, 1929.
6. **Juhl JH:** *Paul and Juhl's Essentials of Roentgen Interpretation,* ed 4. Philadelphia, Harper & Row, 1981.
7. **Cruess RL, Dumont J:** *Current concepts, fracture healing.* Can J Surg 18:403, 1975.
8. **Schenk R, Willenegger H:** *On the morphological findings in primary fracture healing.* Symp Biol Hung 7:75, 1967.
9. **Gossling HR, Pelligrini VD:** *Fat embolism syndrome: A review of the pathophysiology and physiological basis of treatment.* Clin Orthop 165:68, 1982.
10. **Gurd AR, Wilson RI:** *The fat embolism syndrome.* J Bone Joint Surg (Br) 56:408, 1974.
11. **Stevens DB:** *Postoperative orthopedic infections.* J Bone Joint Surg (Am) 46:96, 1964.
12. **Dellinger EP, Miller SD, Wertz MJ, et al:** *Risk of infection after open fracture of the arm or leg.* Arch Surg 123:1320, 1988.

13. **Lyons FA, Rockwood CA:** *Migration of pins used in operations of the shoulder.* J Bone Joint Surg (Am) 72:1262, 1990.
14. **Rowe LJ, Cardin A:** *Post traumatic osteolysis of the clavicle.* Chiro Sports Med 1:2, 1987.
15. **Cahill BR:** *Osteolysis of the distal part of the clavicle in male athletes.* J Bone Joint Surg (Am) 64:1053, 1982.
16. **Linden MA, Manton WI, Stewart RM, et al:** *Lead poisoning from retained bullets: pathogenesis, diagnosis, and review of the literature.* Ann Surg 195:305, 1982.
17. **Bonakdarpour A, Levy WM, Aegerter E:** *Primary and secondary aneurysmal bone cyst: A radiological study of 75 cases.* Radiology 126:75, 1978.
18. **Kushner DC, Vance Z, Kirkpatrick JA Jr:** *Post-traumatic aneurysmal bone cyst affecting third and fourth ribs.* Skeletal Radiol 4:240, 1979.

FRACTURES OF THE SKULL AND FACIAL BONES

1. **Bell RS, Loop JW:** *The utility and futility of radiographic skull examination for trauma.* N Engl J Med 284:236, 1971.
2. **Alker GJ, Oh YS, Leslie EV, et al:** *Postmortem radiology of head and neck injuries in fatal traffic accidents.* Radiology 114:611, 1975.
3. **Taveras JM, Wood EH:** *Diagnostic Neuroradiology,* ed 2. Baltimore, Williams & Wilkins, 1976.
4. **Rogers LF:** *Radiology of Skeletal Trauma,* Vols. 1 and 2, ed. 2. New York, Churchill Livingstone, 1992.
5. **Genieser NB, Becker MH:** *Head trauma in children.* Radiol Clin North Am 12:333, 1945.
6. **Carlson CO, Haverling M, Molin C:** *Isolated fracture of the base of the skull within the sella region.* Acta Radiol 14:662, 1973.
7. **Reynolds DF:** *Traumatic effusion of the sphenoid sinus.* Clin Radiol 12:171, 1961.
8. **Stroobants J, Seynaeve P, Fidlers L, et al:** *Occipital condyle fracture must be considered in the pediatric population: A case report.* J Trauma 36:440, 1994.
9. **Grossart KWM, Samuel E:** *Traumatic diastasis of cranial sutures.* Clin Radiol 12:164, 1961.

10. **Felson B:** *Roentgenology of Fractures and Dislocations.* New York, Grune & Stratton, 1978.
11. **North JW:** *On the importance of intracranial air.* Br J Surg 58:826, 1971.
12. **Mallew R:** *Fractures of the nasofrontal complex.* Otolaryngol Clin North Am 29:335, 1969.
13. **Smith B, Regan WF Jr:** *Blow-out fracture of the orbit.* Am J Ophthalmol 44:733, 1957.
14. **Milauskas AT, Fueger GF:** *Serious ocular complications associated with blowout fracture of the orbit.* Am J Ophthalmol 62:670, 1966.
15. **LeFort R:** *Etude experimentale sur les fractures de la machoire superieure.* Rev Chir 23:208, 1901.
16. **Henry FA:** *Fractures of the jaw.* Semin Roentgenol 6:397, 1971.
17. **Melmed EP, Loonin AJ:** *Fractures of the mandible: A review of 909 cases.* Plast Reconstr Surg 56:323, 1975.

FRACTURES AND DISLOCATIONS OF THE SPINE

1. **Gehrig R, Michaelis LS:** *Statistics of acute paraplegia and tetraplegia on a national scale.* Paraplegia 6:93, 1968.
2. **Stauffer ES, Kaufer H:** *Fractures and Dislocations of the Spine.* In: Rockwood CA Jr, Green DP, ed.: *Fractures,* vol 2. Philadelphia, JB Lippincott, 1975.
3. **Riggins RS, Kraus JF:** *The risk of neurological damage with fractures of the vertebrae.* J Trauma 17:126, 1977.
4. **Castellano V, Bococoni FL:** *Injuries of the cervical spine with spinal cord involvement (myelic fractures): Statistical considerations.* Bull Hosp Joint Dis 31:188, 1970.
5. **Kettner NW, Guebert GM:** *The radiology of cervical spine injury.* J Manipulative Physiol Ther 14:518, 1991.
6. **Jefferson G:** *Fracture of the atlas vertebra. Report of four cases, and a review of those previously recorded.* Br J Surg 7:407, 1920.
7. **Sherk K, Nicholson JT:** *Fractures of the atlas.* J Bone Joint Surg (Am) 52:1017, 1970.
8. **Levine AM, Edwards CC:** *Fractures of the atlas.* J Bone Joint Surg (Am) 73:680, 1991.
9. **Rowe LJ:** *A clinico-radiologic correlation in cervical trauma- Jefferson's fracture.* J Aust Chiro Assoc 19:5, 1989.
10. **Landells CD, van Peteghem PK:** *Fractures of the atlas: Classification, treatment and morbidity.* Spine 13:450, 1988.
11. **Heller JG, Viroslav S, Hudson T:** *Jefferson fractures: the role of magnification artifact in assessing transverse ligament integrity.* J Spinal Disord 6:392, 1993.
12. **Wirth RL, Zatz LM, Parker BR:** *CT detection of a Jefferson fracture in a child.* AJR 149:1001, 1987.
13. **Suss RA, Zimmerman RD, Leeds NE:** *Pseudospread of the atlas: false sign of Jefferson fracture in young children.* AJR 4:183, 1983.
14. **Gehweiler JA Jr, Daffner RH, Roberts L Jr:** *Malformations of the atlas simulating the Jefferson fracture.* AJR 140:1083, 1983.
15. **Lipson SJ, Mazur J:** *Anteroposterior spondyloschisis of the atlas revealed by computerized tomography scanning.* J Bone Joint Surg (Am) 60:1104, 1978.
16. **Sinbert SE, Berman MS:** *Fracture of the posterior arch of the atlas.* JAMA 114:1996, 1940.
17. **Munro DS:** *Missed C1 posterior arch fracture: A case report.* J Can Chiro Assoc 34:27, 1990.
18. **Stewart GC, Gehweiler JA, Laib RH, et al:** *Horizontal fracture of the anterior arch of the atlas.* Radiology 122:349, 1977.
19. **England AC, Shippel AH, Ray M:** *A simple view for demonstration of fractures of the anterior arch of C1.* AJR 144:763, 1985.
20. **Probousta IR, Sancho RN, Alonso JR, et al:** *Horizontal fracture of the anterior arch of the atlas.* Spine 12:615, 1987.
21. **Barker EG, Krumpelman J, Long JM:** *Isolated fracture of the medial portion of the lateral mass of the atlas: A previously undescribed entity.* AJR 126:1053, 1976.
22. **Clyburn TA, Lionberger DR, Tullos HS:** *Bilateral fracture of the transverse process of the atlas.* J Bone Joint Surg (Am) 64:948, 1982.
23. **Yochum TR, Rowe LJ:** *Arthritides of the upper cervical complex.* ACA J Chiro January, 1981.
24. **Burke JT, Harris JH:** *Acute injuries of the axis vertebra.* Skeletal Radiol 18:335, 1989.
25. **Elliott JM, Rogers LF, Wissinger JP, et al:** *The hangman's fracture.* Radiology 104:303, 1972.
26. **Barros TE, Fielding W:** *Traumatic spondylolisthesis of the axis with unusual distraction.* J Bone Joint Surg (Am) 72:124, 1990.
27. **Mirvis SE, Young JWR, Lim C, Greenberg J:** *Hangman's fracture: Radiologic assessment in 27 cases.* Radiology 163:713, 1987.
28. **Cornish BL:** *Traumatic spondylolisthesis of the axis.* J Bone Joint Surg (Br) 50:31, 1968.
29. **Jeannert B, Magerl F, Stanisic M:** *Thrombosis of the vertebral artery. A rare complication following traumatic spondylolisthesis of the second cervical vertebra.* Spine 11:179, 1986.
30. **Garger WN, Fischer RG, Halfmann HW:** *Vertebrectomy and fusion for "tear-drop fracture" of the cervical spine: Case report.* J Trauma 9:887, 1969.
31. **Hadley MN, Sonntag VKH, Graham TW, et al:** *Axis fractures resulting from motor vehicle accidents. The need for occupant restraints.* Spine 11:861, 1986.
32. **Lally JF, Cossrow JI, Dalinka MK:** *Odontoid fractures in metastatic breast carcinoma.* AJR 128:817, 1977.
33. **Montileone ML:** *Solitary plasmacytoma. A case report.* Roentgenological Briefs. Am Chiro Assoc Council Roentgenol, August, 1981.
34. **Anderson LD, D'Alonzo RT:** *Fractures of the odontoid process of the axis.* J Bone Joint Surg (Am) 56:1663, 1974.

35. **Schatzker J:** *Fractures of the dens (odontoid process): an analysis of thirty-seven cases.* J Bone Joint Surg (Br) 53:392, 1971.
36. **Rogers LF:** Radiology of Skeletal Trauma, Vol. 1, ed 2. New York, Churchill Livingstone, 1992.
37. **Moskovich R, Crockard HA:** *Myelopathy due to hypertrophic nonunion of the dens: Case report.* J Trauma 30:222, 1990.
38. **Freiberger RH, Wilson PD Jr, Nicholas JA:** *Acquired absence of the odontoid process.* J Bone Joint Surg (Am) 47:1231, 1965.
39. **Kitchen RG:** *Nonunion (Type II) odontoid fracture: a case report of a motor vehicle accident.* J Can Chiro Assoc 30:189, 1986.
40. **Nepper-Rasmussen J:** *CT of dens fractures.* Neuroradiology 31:104, 1989.
41. **Thomeier WC, Brown DC, Mirvis SE:** *The laterally tilted dens: a sign of subtle odontoid fracture on plain radiography.* AJNR 11:605, 1990.
42. **Harris JH, Burke JT, Ray RD, et al:** *Low (Type III) odontoid fracture: A new radiographic sign.* Radiology 153:353, 1984.
43. **Smoker WRK, Dolan KD:** *The "fat" C2: A sign of fracture.* AJR 148:609, 1987.
44. **Williams AL, Carrera GF, Grogan JP, et al:** *Vacuum phenomenon as a sign of an ununited, unstable dens fracture.* AJNR 8:1144, 1987.
45. **Esses SI, Bednar DA:** *Screw fixation of odontoid fractures and nonunions.* Spine 16:S483, 1991.
46. **Daffner RH:** *Pseudofracture of the dens: mach bands.* AJR 128:607, 1977.
47. **Swischuk LE, Hayden CK, Sarwar M:** *The posteriorly tilted dens. A normal variation mimicking a fractured dens.* Pediatr Radiol 8:27, 1979.
48. **Holt RG, Helms CA, Munk PL, et al:** *Hypertrophy of C-1 anterior arch: useful sign to distinguish os odontoideum from acute dens fracture.* Radiology 173:207, 1989.
49. **Miller MD, Gehweiler JA, Marintez, et al:** *Significant new observations on cervical spine trauma.* AJR 130:659, 1978.
50. **Bhatia S, Sharma BS, Mathuriya SN, et al:** *Complete dislocation with burst fracture of the lower cervical spine. Case report.* Paraplegia 31:542, 1993.
51. **Kim KS, Chen HH, Russell EJ, et al:** *Flexion teardrop fracture of the cervical spine: radiographic characteristics.* AJR 152:319, 1989.
52. **Smith GR, Beckly DE, Abel MS:** *Articular mass fracture: a neglected cause of posttraumatic neck pain?* Clin Radiol 27:335, 1976.
53. **Nykoliation JW, Cassidy JD, Dupuis P, et al:** *Missed cervical spine fracture-dislocations prior to manipulation: A review of three cases.* J Can Chiro Assoc 30:69, 1986.
54. **Daffner RH:** *Evaluation of cervical vertebral injuries.* Semin Roentgenol 27:239, 1992.
55. **Lee C, Woodring JH:** *Sagittally orientated fractures of the lateral masses of the cervical vertebrae.* J Trauma 31:1638, 1991.
56. **Vines FS:** *The significance of "occult" fractures of the cervical spine.* AJR 107:493, 1969.
57. **Harris JH Jr:** *Acute injuries of the spine.* Semin Roentgenol 13:53, 1978.
58. **Cancelmo JJ Jr:** *Clay shoveler's fracture: A helpful diagnostic sign.* AJR 115:540, 1972.
59. **Rowe LJ:** *Clay shoveler's fracture.* Am Chiro Assoc J 21:83, 1987.
60. **Scher AT:** *The value of the anteroposterior radiograph in "hidden" fractures and dislocations of the lower cervical spine—a case report.* S Afr Med J 55:221, 1979.
61. **Abel MS:** *Occult traumatic lesions of the cervical spine.* Crit Rev Clin Radiol and Nucl 7:469, 1975.
62. **Barnsley L, Lord S, Bogduk N:** *The pathophysiology of whiplash.* State Art Rev (3):329, 1993.
63. **Taylor JR, Twomey LT:** *Acute injuries to cervical joints. An autopsy study of neck Sprain.* Spine 18:1115, 1993.
64. **Porter KM:** *Neck sprains after car accidents: a common cause of long term disability.* Br Med J 298:973, 1989 (Editorial).
65. **Aprill C, Bogduk N:** *The prevalence of cervical zygapophyseal joint pain: A first approximation.* Spine 17:744, 1992.
66. **Lord S, Barnsley L, Bogduk N:** *Cervical zygapophyseal joint pain in whiplash.* State Art Rev 7(3):355, 1993.
67. **Jull G, Bogduk N, Marsland A:** *The accuracy of manual diagnosis for cervical zygapophyseal joint syndromes.* Med J Aust 148:233, 1988.
68. **Lenhart LJ:** *Post traumatic cervical syndrome.* J Manipulative Physiol Ther 11:409, 1988.
69. **Harris JH, Yeakley JW:** *Hyperextension dislocation of the cervical spine. Ligament injuries demonstrated by magnetic resonance imaging.* J Bone Joint Surg 74A:567, 1992.
70. **Murphey MD, Batitzky S, Bramble JM:** *Diagnostic imaging of spinal trauma.* Radiol Clin N Am 27:855, 1989.
71. **Davis AG:** *Injuries of the cervical spine.* JAMA 127:149, 1945.
72. **Clark WM, Gehweiler JA, Laib R:** *Twelve significant signs of cervical spine trauma.* Skeletal Radiol 3:201, 1979.
73. **Miles KA, Maimaris C, Finlay D, et al:** *The incidence and prognostic significance of radiological abnormalities in soft tissue injuries of the cervical spine.* Skeletal Radiol 17:493, 1988.
74. **Wholey MH, Bruwer AJ, Baker HL:** *The lateral roentgenogram of the neck.* Radiology 71:350, 1958.
75. **Edeiken-Monroe B, Wagner LK, Harris JH:** *Hyperextension dislocation of the cervical spine.* AJR 146:803, 1986.
76. **Whalen JP, Woodruff CL:** *The cervical prevertebral fat stripe.* AJR 109:455, 1970.
77. **Polansky A, Resnick D, Sofferman RA, et al:** *Hyoid bone elevation: a sign of tracheal transection.* Radiology 150:117, 1984.
78. **Place JN, Pezzuti RT:** *Clinical significance of traumatic pneumorrachis.* AJR 153:655, 1989.

79. **Weir DC:** *Roentgenographic signs of cervical injury.* Clin Orthop 109:9, 1975.

80. **Fineman S, Borrelli FJ, Rubinstein BM, et al:** *The cervical spine: transformation of the normal lordotic pattern into a linear pattern in the neutral posture.* J Bone Joint Surg 45A: 1179, 1963.

81. **Juhl JH, Miller SM, Roberts GW:** *Roentgenographic variations in the normal cervical spine.* Radiology 78:591, 1962.

82. **Macnab I:** *Cervical spondylosis.* Clin Orthop Rel Res 109:69, 1975.

83. **Scher AT:** *Ligamentous injury of the cervical spine—two radiological signs.* S Afr Med J 55:221, 1978.

84. **Hohl M:** *Soft tissue injuries of the neck in automobile accidents.* J Bone Joint Surg 56A:1675, 1974.

85. **Scher AT:** *Radiographic indicators of traumatic cervical spine instability.* S Afr Med J 62:562, 1982.

86. **Bohrer SP, Chen YM, Sayers DG:** *Cervical spine flexion patterns.* Skeletal Radiol 19:521, 1990.

87. **White AA, Johnson RM, Panjabi MM, et al:** *Biomechanical analysis of clinical instability of the cervical spine.* Clin Orthop 109:85, 1975.

88. **McGregor M, Mior S:** *Anatomical and functional perspectives of the cervical spine: Part III: The "unstable" cervical spine.* J Can Chiro Assoc 34:145, 1990.

89. **Feilding JW, Cochran GVB, Lawsing JF, et al:** *Tears of the transverse ligament of the atlas.* J Bone Joint Surg 56A:1683, 1974.

90. **Davis SJ, Teresi LM, Bradley WJ, et al:** *Cervical spine hyperextension injuries: MR findings.* Radiology 180:245, 1991.

91. **Cintron E, Gilula LA, Murphy WA, et al:** *The widened disc space—a sign of cervical spine hyperextension injury.* Radiology 141:639, 1981.

92. **Harris W, Hamblen D, Ojemann R:** *Traumatic disruption of the cervical disc from hyperextension injury.* Clin Orthop 60:163, 1968.

93. **Reymond RD, Wheeler PS, Prerovic M, et al:** *The lucent cleft, a new radiographic sign of cervical disc injury or disease.* Clin Radiol 23:188, 1972.

94. **Bohrer SP, Chen YM:** *Cervical spine annulus vacuum.* Skeletal Radiol 17:324, 1988.

95. **Jonsson K, Niklasson J, Josefsson PO:** *Avulsion of the cervical spinal ring apophyses: acute and chronic appearance.* Skeletal Radiol 20:207, 1991.

96. **Keller RN:** *Traumatic displacement of the cartilaginous rim: a sign of intervertebral disc prolapse.* Radiology 110:21, 1974.

97. **Webb JK, Broughton RBK, McSweeney T, et al:** *Hidden flexion injury of the cervical spine.* J Bone Joint Surg 58B:322, 1976.

98. **Barnsley L, Lord S, Thomas P, et al:** *SPECT bone scans for the diagnosis of symptomatic cervical zygapophyseal joints.* Br J Rheumatol 32(Suppl 2: Abstracts):52, 1993.

99. **Barton D, Allen M, Finlay D, et al:** *Evaluation of whiplash injuries by technetium 99 m scanning.* Arch Emerg Med 10:197, 1993.

100. **Chapman-Smith D:** *Whiplash—current management and systems of prognosis.* Chiropractic Report 2(6):1, 1988.

101. **Chapman-Smith D:** *The biomechanical basis of whiplash injuries.* Chiropractic Report 8(2):1, 1994.

102. **Ameis A:** *Cervical whiplash: considerations in the rehabilitation of cervical myofascial injury.* Can Fam Physician 32:1871, 1986.

103. **Livingstone M:** *Whiplash injury: misconceptions and remedies.* Aust Fam Physician 21(11):1646, 1992.

104. **Radanov BP, Dvorak J, Valach L:** *Cognitive deficits in patients after soft tissue injuries of the cervical spine.* Spine 17:127, 1992.

105. **Norris SH, Watt I:** *The prognosis of neck injuries from rear-end vehicle collisions.* J Bone Joint Surg 65B:608, 1983.

106. **Watkinson A, Gargan MF, Bannister GC:** *Prognostic factors in soft tissue injuries of the cervical spine.* Injury 22:307, 1991.

107. **Maimaris C, Barnes MR, Allen MJ:** *"Whiplash injuries" of the neck: A retrospective study.* Injury 19:393, 1988.

108. **Torg JS, Pavlov H, Genuario SE, et al:** *Neuropraxia of the cervical spinal cord with transient quadriplegia.* J Bone Joint Surg 68A:1354, 1986.

109. **Nagib MG, Maxwell RE, Chou SN:** *Identification and management of high risk patients with Klippel-Feil syndrome.* J Neurosurgery 61:523, 1984.

110. **Scher AT:** *Cervical spine fusion and the effects of injury.* S Afr Med J 56:525, 1979.

111. **Flanders AE, Schaefer DM, Doan HT, et al:** *Acute cervical spine trauma: Correlation of MR imaging findings with degree of neurologic deficit.* Radiology 177:25, 1990.

112. **Woodring JH, Selke AC, Duff DE:** *Traumatic atlantooccipital dislocation with survival.* AJR 137:21, 1981.

113. **Maves CK, Souza A, Prenger EC, et al:** *Traumatic atlanto—occipital disruption in children.* Pediatr Radiol 21:504, 1991.

114. **Harris JH, Carson GC, Wagner LK:** *Radiologic diagnosis of traumatic occipitovertebral dissociation: 1. normal occipitovertebral relationships on lateral radiographs of supine subjects.* AJR 162:881, 1994.

115. **Harris JH, Carson GC, Wagner LK, et al:** *Radiologic diagnosis of traumatic occipitovertebral dissociation: 2. comparison of three methods of detecting occipitovertebral relationships on lateral radiographs of supine subjects.* AJR 162:887, 1994.

116. **Ono K, Yonenobu K, Fuji T, et al:** *Atlantoaxial rotatory fixation. Radiographic study of its mechanism.* Spine 10:602, 1985.

117. **Corner EM:** *Rotatory dislocations of the atlas.* Ann Surg 45:9, 1907.

118. **Fielding JW, Hawkins RJ:** *Atlanto-axial rotatory fixation. Fixed rotatory subluxation of the atlantoaxial joint.* J Bone Joint Surg (Am) 59:37, 1977.

119. **Wortzman G, Dewar FP:** *Rotary fixation of the atlanto-axial joint: rotational atlantoaxial subluxation.* Radiology 90:479, 1968.

120. **Mercer S, Bogduk N:** *Intraarticular inclusions of the cervical synovial joints.* Br J Rheumatol 32:705, 1993.

121. **Murray JB, Ziervogel M:** *The value of computed tomography in the diagnosis of atlanto--axial rotatory fixation.* Br J Radiol 63:894, 1990.

122. **Eismont FJ, Arena MJ, Green BA:** *Extrusion of an intervertebral disc associated with traumatic subluxation or dislocation of cervical facets.* J Bone Joint Surg (Am) 73:1555, 1991.

123. **Whitehill R, Stowers SF, Ruch WW, et al:** *Cervical dislocation adjacent to a fused motion segment.* Spine 12:396, 1987.

124. **Beatson TR:** *Fractures and dislocations of the cervical spine.* J Bone Joint Surg (Br) 45:21, 1963.

125. **Goldberg AL, Rothfus WE, Deeb ZL, et al:** *The impact of magnetic resonance on the diagnostic evaluation of acute cervicothoracic spinal trauma.* Skeletal Radiol 17:89, 1988.

126. **Scher AT:** *Unilateral locked facet in cervical spine injuries.* AJR 129:45, 1977.

127. **Kornberg M:** *The computed tomographic appearance of a unilateral jumped facet cervical facet (the "false" facet joint sign).* Spine 11:1038, 1986.

128. **Meyer S:** *Thoracic spine trauma.* Semin Roentgenol 27:254, 1992.

129. **El-Khoury GY, Whitten CG:** *Trauma to the upper thoracic spine: Anatomy, biomechanics, and unique imaging features.* AJR 160:95, 1993.

130. **Daffner RH, Deeb ZL, Rothfus WE:** *Thoracic fractures and dislocations in motorcyclists.* Skeletal Radiol 16:280, 1987.

131. **Gertzbein SD:** *Spine update: Classification of thoracic and lumbar fractures.* Spine 19:626, 1994.

132. **Roaf R:** *A study of the mechanics of spinal injuries.* J Bone Joint Surg (Br) 42:810, 1960.

133. **Kricun ME, Kricun R:** *Fractures of the lumbar spine.* Semin Roentgenol 27:262, 1992.

134. **Caplan GA, Scane AC, Francis RM:** *Pathogenesis of vertebral crush fractures.* J Royal Soc Med 87:200, 1994.

135. **Gehweiler JA, Osborne RL Jr, Becker RF:** *The Radiology of Vertebral Trauma.* Philadelphia, WB Saunders, 1980.

136. **Denis F:** *Spinal stability as defined by the three column concept in acute spinal trauma.* Clin Orthop 189:65, 1984.

137. **Dibos PE, Wagner HN Jr:** *Atlas of Nuclear Medicine—Bone.* Philadelphia, WB Saunders, 1978.

138. **Fletcher GH:** *Anterior vertebral wedging.* AJR 57:232, 1947.

139. **Luridsen KN, De Carvalho A, Holst, et al:** *Degree of vertebral wedging of the dorsolumbar spine.* Acta Radiol 25:29, 1984.

140. **Baker LL, Goodman SB, Perkash I, et al:** *Benign versus pathologic compression fractures of the vertebral bodies: Assessment with conventional spin–echo, chemical shift, and STIR MR imaging.* Radiology 174:495, 1990.

141. **Atlas SW, Regenbogen V, Rogers LF, et al:** *The radiographic characterization of burst fractures of the spine.* AJR 147:575, 1986.

142. **Wilson ARM, Preston BJ, Cassar-Pullicino V, et al:** *Acquired coronal cleft vertebra.* Clinical Radiol 40:167, 1989.

143. **Daffner RH, Deeb ZL, Rothfus WE:** *The posterior vertebral body line: Importance in the detection of burst fractures.* AJR 148:93, 1987.

144. **Epstein NE, Epstein JA:** *Limbus lumbar vertebral fractures in 27 adolescents and adults.* Spine 16:962, 1991.

145. **Dietemann JL, Runge M, Badoz, et al:** *Radiology of posterior lumbar apophyseal ring fractures: report of 13 cases.* Neuroradiol 30:337, 1988.

146. **Takata K, Inoue S, Takahashi K, et al:** *Fracture of the posterior margin of a lumbar vertebral body.* J Bone Joint Surg (Am) 70:589, 1988.

147. **Thiel HW, Clements DS, Cassidy JD:** *Lumbar apophyseal ring fractures in adolescents.* J Manipulative Physiol Ther 15:250, 1992.

148. **Kummel H:** *Uber die traumatischen erkrankunger der wirbels aule.* Deutsch Med Wchnschr 21:180, 1895.

149. **Schinz HR, et al:** *Roentgen Diagnostics,* Vol 2, ed 2. New York, Grune & Stratton, 1967.

150. **Brower AC, Downey EF:** *Kummell disease: Report of a case with serial radiographs.* Radiology 141:363, 1981.

151. **Kumpan W, Salomonowitz E, Seidl G:** *The intravertebral vacuum phenomenon.* Skeletal Radiol 15:444, 1986.

152. **Osti OL, Fraser RD:** *Osseous bridging of lumbar intertransverse processes after trauma.* Spine 17:362, 1992.

153. **Melamed A:** *Fracture of pars interarticularis of lumbar vertebra.* AJR 94:584, 1965.

154. **Wiltse LL, Widell EH, Jackson DW:** *Fatigue fracture: The basic lesion in isthmus spondylolisthesis.* J Bone Joint Sur (Am) 57:17, 1975.

155. **Chance GQ:** *Note on type of flexion fracture of spine.* Br J Radiol 21:452, 1948.

156. **Dehner JR:** *Seatbelt injuries of the spine and abdomen.* AJR 111:833, 1971.

157. **Rogers LF:** *The roentgenographic appearance of transverse or Chance fractures of the spine. The seat belt fracture.* AJR 111:844, 1971.

158. **Smith WS, Kaufer H:** *Patterns and mechanisms of lumbar injuries associated with lap seat belts.* J Bone Joint Surg (Am) 51:239, 1969.

159. **Gellad FE, Levine AM, Joslyn JN, et al:** *Pure thoracolumbar facet dislocation: clinical features and CT appearance.* Radiology 161:505, 1986.

160. **O'Callaghan JP, Ullrich CG, Yuan HA, et al:** *CT of facet distraction in flexion injuries of the thoracolumbar spine: The "naked" facet.* AJNR 1:97, 1980.

FRACTURES AND DISLOCATIONS OF THE PELVIS

1. **Jackson H, Kam J, Harris JH, et al:** *The sacral arcuate lines in upper sacral fractures.* Radiology 145:35, 1982.

2. **Jackson H, Burke JT:** *The sacral foramina.* Skeletal Radiol 11:282, 1984.

3. **Furey WW:** *Fractures of the pelvis with special reference to associated fractures of the sacrum.* AJR 47:89, 1942.

4. **Roy-Camile R, Saillant G, Gagna G, et al:** *Transverse fracture of the upper sacrum—Suicidal jumpers fracture.* Spine 10:838, 1985.

5. Ebraheim NA, Savolaine ER, Skie MC, et al: *Longitudinal fracture of the sacrum: Case report.* J Trauma 36:447, 1994.
6. Duverney JG: *Traite des maladies de os.* Vol. 1. Paris: DeBure l'Aine, 1751.
7. Malgaigne JF: *Treatise on Fractures,* Philadelphia, JB Lippincott, 1959.
8. Rogers LF: Radiology of Skeletal Trauma, Vols. 1 and 2, ed 2. New York, Churchill Livingstone, 1992.
9. Pitt MJ, Ruth JT, Benjamin JB: *Trauma to the pelvic ring and acetabulum.* Seminars Roentgenol 27:299, 1992.
10. Dunn AW, Morris HD: *Fractures and dislocations of the pelvis.* J Bone Joint Surg (Am) 50:1639, 1968.
11. Lansinger O: *Fractures of the acetabulum.* Acta Orthop Scan 165:1, 1977.
12. Olive RJ, Marsh HO: *Occult central acetabular fracture resulting in fracture—dislocation.* Clin Orthop 248:240, 1988.
13. Sundar M, Carty H: *Avulsion of the pelvis in children: a report of 32 fractures and their outcomes.* Skeletal Radiol 23:85, 1994.
14. Veselko M, Smrkolj V: *Avulsion of the anterior—superior iliac spine in athletes: Case reports.* J Trauma 36:444, 1994.
15. Albers VL: *Avulsion fracture of the anterior inferior iliac spine.* ACA J Chiro 18:67, 1984.
16. Conolly WB, Hedberg EA: *Observations on fractures of the pelvis.* J Trauma 9:104, 1969.
17. Schneider R, Kaye JJ, Ghelman B: *Adductor avulsive injuries near the symphysis pubis.* Radiology 120:567, 1976.
18. Trunkey DD, Chapman MW, Lim RC, et al: *Management of pelvic fractures in blunt trauma injury.* J Trauma 14:912, 1974.
19. Muecke EC, Currarino G: *Congenital widening of the pubic symphysis.* AJR 103:179, 1968.

FRACTURES AND DISLOCATIONS OF THE HIP

1. Stevens L, Freeman PA, Nordin BEC, et al: *The incidence of osteoporosis in patients with femoral neck fracture.* J Bone Joint Surg (Br) 44:520, 1962.
2. Barnes R, Brown JT, Garden RS, et al: *Subcapital fractures of the femur. A prospective review.* J Bone Joint Surg (Br) 58:2, 1976.
3. Rogers LF: *Radiology of Skeletal Trauma,* Vol. 1, ed 2. New York, Churchill Livingston, 1992.
4. Alffram PA: *An epidemiologic study of cervical and trochanteric fractures of the femur in an urban population. Analysis of 1,664 cases with special reference to etiologic factors.* Acta Orthop Scand 65:11, 1964.
5. Norris MA, De Smet AA: *Fractures and dislocations of the hip and femur.* Semin Roentgenol 24:100, 1994.
6. Rubin DA, Dalinka MK, Kneeland JB: *Magnetic resonance imaging of lower extremity injuries.* Semin Roentgenol 24:194, 1994.
7. Holder LE, Schwartz C, Wernicke PG, et al: *Radionuclide bone imaging in the early detection of fractures in the proximal femur: Multifactorial analysis.* Radiology 174:509, 1990.
8. Klenerman L, Marcuson RW: *Intracapsular fractures of the neck and femur.* J Bone Joint Surg (Br) 52:514, 1970.
9. Brown JT, Abrami G: *Transcervical femoral fracture.* J Bone Joint Surg (Br) 46:648, 1964.
10. Garden RS: *Low-angle fixation in fractures of the femoral neck.* J Bone Joint Surg (Br) 43:647, 1961.
11. Baylis AP, Davidson JK: *Traumatic osteonecrosis of the femoral head following intracapsular fracture. Incidence and earliest radiological features.* Clin Radiol 28:407, 1977.
12. Speer KP, Spritzer CE, Harrelson JM, et al: *Magnetic resonance imaging of the femoral head after acute intracapsular fracture of the femoral neck.* J Bone Joint Surg (Am) 72:98, 1990.
13. Phillips CD, Pope TL, Jones JE, et al: *Non-traumatic avulsion of the lesser trochanter: a pathognomonic sign of metastatic disease?* Skeletal Radiol 17:106, 1988.
14. Epstein HC: *Traumatic dislocations of the hip.* Clin Orthop 92:116, 1973.
15. Richardson P, Young JWR, Porter D: *CT detection of cortical fracture associated with posterior hip dislocation.* AJR 155:93, 1990.
16. Hunter GA: *Posterior dislocation and fracture—dislocation of the hip. A review of fifty-seven patients.* J Bone Joint Surg (Br) 51:38, 1969.
17. Ratliff HHC: *Traumatic separation of the upper femoral epiphysis in young children.* J Bone Joint Surg (Br) 50:757, 1969.
18. Bloom ML, Crawford AH: *Slipped capital femoral epiphysis. An assessment of treatment modalities.* Orthopedics 8:36, 1985.
19. Crawford AH: *Current concepts review. Slipped capital femoral epiphysis.* J Bone Joint Surg (Am) 70:1422, 1988.
20. Rogers LF, Poznanski AK: *Imaging of epiphyseal injuries.* Radiology 191:297, 1994.
21. Albers VL, Yochum TR: *Slipped femoral capital epiphysis. Case report.* ACA J Chiro April:45, 1981.
22. Klein A, et al: *Roentgenographic features of slipped capital femoral epiphysis.* AJR 66:361, 1951.
23. Betz RR, Steel HH, Emper WD, et al: *Treatment of slipped capital femoral epiphysis.* J Bone Joint Surg (Am) 72:587, 1990.
24. Rowe LJ, Nook BC: *Avascular necrosis as a complication to previous slipped femoral capital epiphysis.* ACA J Chiro, Radiology Case Report May, 1985.

FRACTURES AND DISLOCATIONS OF THE KNEE

1. Neer CS, Shelton ML: *Supracondylar fracture of the adult femur. A study of one hundred and ten cases.* J Bone Joint Surg (Am) 49:591, 1967.
2. Seinsheimer F: *Fractures of the distal femur.* Clin Orthop 153:169, 1980.

3. Blake R, McBryde A: *The floating knee: Ipsilateral fractures of the tibia and femur.* South Med J 68:13, 1975.
4. Rogers LF: *Radiology of Skeletal Trauma,* Vols. 1 and 2, ed 2, Churchill Livingston, 1982.
5. Reibel DB, Wade PA: *Fractures of the condyles of the tibia.* J Trauma 2:337, 1962.
6. Newberg AH, Greenstein R: *Radiographic evaluation of tibial plateau fracture.* Radiology 126:319, 1978.
7. Rafii M, Firooznia H, Golimbu C, et al: *Computed tomography of tibial plateau fractures.* AJR 142:1181, 1984.
8. Roberts JM, Lovel WW: *Fractures of the intercondylar eminence of the tibia.* J Bone Joint Surg (Am) 52:827, 1970.
9. Boyer RS, Jaffe RB, Nixon GW, et al: *Trampoline fracture of the proximal tibia in children.* AJR 146:83, 1986.
10. Hand WL, et al: *Avulsion fractures of the tibial tubercle.* J Bone Joint Surg (Am) 53:1579, 1971.
11. Frankl U, Wasilewski SA, Healy WL: *Avulsion fracture of the tibial tubercle with avulsion of the patellar ligament.* J Bone Joint Surg (Am) 72:1411, 1990.
12. Schultz RJ: *The Language of Fractures.* Baltimore, Williams & Wilkins, 1976.
13. Weber WN, Neumann CH, Barakos JA, et al: *Lateral tibial rim (Segond) fractures: MR imaging characteristics.* Radiology 180:731, 1991.
14. Goldman AB, Pavlov H, Rubenstein D: *The Segond fracture of the proximal tibia: a small avulsion that reflects major ligamentous damage.* AJR 151:1163, 1988.
15. Platt H: *On the peripheral nerve complications of certain fractures.* J Bone Joint Surg (Am) 10:403, 1928.
16. Towne LC, et al: *Lateral compartment syndrome of the knee.* Clin Orthop 76:160, 1971.
17. Saxon HM: *Lipohemarthrosis.* Br J Radiol 35:122, 1962.
18. Wenzel WW: *The FBI sign.* Rocky Mount Med J 69:71, 1972.
19. Lee JH, Weissman BN, Nikpoor et al: *Lipohemarthrosis of the knee: a review of recent experiences.* Radiology 173:189, 1989.
20. Bostrom A: *Longitudinal fractures of the patella.* Reconstr Surg Traumatol 14:136, 1974.
21. Scheller F, Martenson L: *Traumatic dislocation of the patella.* Acta Radiol Suppl 336:5, 1974.
22. Rogers LF, Hendrix RW: *Sports-related knee injuries.* Contemp Diag Radiol 11:1, 1979.
23. Levitsky KA, Berger A, Nicholas GG, et al: *Bilateral open dislocation of the knee joint.* J Bone Joint Surg (Am) 70:1407, 1988.
24. Ogden JA: *Subluxation and dislocation of the proximal tibiofibular joint.* J Bone Joint Surg (Am) 56:145, 1974.
25. Rubin DA, Dalinka MK, Kneeland JB: *Magnetic resonance imaging of lower extremity injuries.* Semin Roentgenol 24:194, 1994.
26. Burke DL Jr, Dalinka ML, Kanal E, et al: *Meniscal and ganglion cysts of the knee: MR evaluation.* AJR 150:331, 1988.
27. Vellet AD, Marks PH, Fowler PJ, et al: *Occult posttraumatic osteochondral lesions of the knee: Prevalence, classification, and short-term sequelae evaluated with MR imaging.* Radiology 178:271, 1991.

FRACTURES AND DISLOCATIONS OF THE ANKLE

1. Solomon MA, Gilula LA, Oloff LM, et al: *CT scanning of the foot and ankle: 1. normal anatomy.* AJR 146:1192, 1986.
2. Solomon MA, Gilula LA, Oloff LM, et al: *CT scanning of the foot and ankle: 2. clinical applications and a review of the literature.* AJR 146:1204, 1986.
3. Rosenburg ZS, Feldman F, Singson RD: *Peroneal tendon injuries: CT analysis.* Radiology 161:743, 1986.
4. Roberts DK, Pomeranz SJ: *Current status of magnetic resonance in radiologic diagnosis of foot and ankle injuries.* Orthop Clin N Am 25:61, 1994.
5. Rogers LF: *Radiology of Skeletal Trauma,* Vols. 1 and 2, ed. 2. New York, Churchill Livingstone, 1992.
6. Arimoto HR, Forrester DM: *Classification of ankle fractures: An algorithm.* AJR 135:1057, 1980.
7. Rowe LJ: *Imaging of the Foot and Ankle.* In: Logan R, ed.: *The Foot and Ankle.* Chapter 4. *Clinical Applications.* Rockville, Aspen Publishers, 1995.
8. Kleiger B: *Mechanisms of ankle injury.* Orthop Clin North Am 5:127, 1974.
9. McDaniel WJ, Wilson FC: *Trimalleolar fractures of the ankle.* Clin Orthop 122:37, 1977.
10. Cotton FJ: *A new type of ankle fracture.* JAMA 64:318, 1915.
11. Henderson MS: *Trimalleolar fracture of the ankle.* Surg Clin North Am 12:867, 1932.
12. Pott P: *Some Few General Remarks on Fractures and Dislocations.* London, Hawes Clarke & Collins, 1768.
13. Dupuytren G: *Of fractures of the lower extremity of the fibula, and luxations of the foot.* [Reprinted in] Medical Classics 4:151, 1939.
14. Maisonneuve JG: *Recherches sur la fracture du petone.* Arch Gen de Med 7:165, 1840.
15. Protas JM, Kornblatt BA: *Fractures of the lateral margin of the distal tibia, the Tillaux fracture.* Radiology 138:55, 1981.
16. Rockwood CA, Green DP: *Fractures.* Philadelphia, JB Lippincott, 1975.
17. Burwell HN, Charnley AD: *The treatment of displaced fractures at the ankle by rigid internal fixation and early joint movement.* J Bone Joint Surg (Br) 47:634, 1965.
18. Klossner O: *Late results of operative and nonoperative treatment of severe ankle fractures.* Acta Chir Scan [Suppl] 293:1, 1962.
19. Edeiken J, Cotler JM: *Ankle.* In: Felson B. *Roentgenology of Fractures and Dislocations.* New York, Grune & Stratton, 1978.

20. **Simon RR, Hoffman JR, Smith M:** *Radiographic comparison of plain films on second- and third-degree ankle sprains.* Am J Emergency Med 4:387, 1986.
21. **Towbin R, Dunbar JS, Towbin J:** *Teardrop sign: Plain film recognition of ankle effusion.* AJR 134:985, 1980.
22. **Ala-Ketola L, Puronen J, Koivisto E, et al:** *Arthrography in the diagnosis of ligament injuries and classification of ankle injuries.* Radiology 125:63, 1977.
23. **Edeiken J, Cotler JM:** *Ankle injury. The need for stress films.* JAMA 240:1182, 1978.
24. **Horsefield D, Murphy G:** *Stress views of the ankle joint in lateral ligament injury.* Radiography 51:224, 1986.
25. **Harper MC:** *Stress radiographs in the diagnosis of lateral instability of the ankle and hindfoot.* Foot Ankle 13:435, 1992.
26. **Johannsen A:** *Radiologic diagnosis of lateral ligament lesions of the ankle. A comparison between talar tilt and anterior drawer sign.* Acta Orthop Scand 49:259, 1978.
27. **Berquist TH:** *Radiology of the Foot and Ankle.* New York, Raven Press, 1989.
28. **Rubin G, Witten M:** *The talar tilt angle and the fibular collateral ligaments. A method for the determination of talar tilt.* J Bone Joint Surg 42A:311, 1960.
29. **Shereff MJ:** *Radiographic Analysis of the Foot and Ankle.* In: MH Jahss.: *Disorders of the Foot and Ankle.* Philadelphia, WB Saunders, 1991.
30. **Olson RW:** *Ankle arthrography.* Radiol Clin North Am 19:255, 1981.
31. **Frolich H, Gotzen L, Adam D:** *Evaluation of stress roentgenograms of the upper ankle joint.* Unfallheilunde 83:457, 1980.
32. **Larson E:** *Experimental instability of the ankle: A radiographic investigation.* Clin Orthop 204:193, 1986.

FRACTURES AND DISLOCATIONS OF THE FOOT

1. **Rogers LF:** *Radiology of Skeletal Trauma*, Vols. 1 and 2, ed 2. New York, Churchill Livingstone, 1992.
2. **Zatkin HR:** *Trauma in the Foot.* Semin Roentgenol 5:419, 1970.
3. **Kraft E, Spyropoulos E, Finby N:** *Neurogenic disorders of the foot in diabetes mellitus.* AJR 124:17, 1975.
4. **Karasick D:** *Fractures and dislocations of the foot.* Semin Roentgenol 24:152, 1994.
5. **Rowe LJ:** *Imaging of the Foot and Ankle.* In: Roy Logan, ed.: *The Foot and Ankle. Clinical Applications*, Chapter 4, Rockville, Aspen Publishers, 1995.
6. **Rubin DA, Dalinka MK, Kneeland JB:** *Magnetic resonance imaging of lower extremity injuries.* Semin Roentgenol 24: 194, 1994.
7. **Rockwood CA, Green DP:** *Fractures.* JB Lippincott, Philadelphia, 1975.
8. **Essex-Lopresti P:** *The mechanism, reduction technique, and results in fractures of the os calcis.* Br J Surg 39:395, 1952.
9. **Caue EF:** *Fractures of the os calcis—the problem in general.* Clin Orthop 30:64, 1963.
10. **Rowe CR, Sakellarides T, Freeman PA, et al:** *Fractures of the os calcis.* JAMA 184:98, 1963.
11. **Boehler L:** *Diagnosis, pathology, and treatment of fractures of the os calcis.* J Bone Joint Surg (Am) 13:75, 1931.
12. **Dachtler HW:** *Fractures of the anterior superior portion of the os calcis due to indirect violence.* AJR 25:629, 1931.
13. **Thomas HM:** *Calcaneal fracture in childhood.* Br J Surg 56:664, 1969.
14. **Pennal GF:** *Fractures of the talus.* Clin Orthop 30:53, 1963.
15. **Coltart WD:** *Aviator's astralgus.* J Bone Joint Surg (Br) 34:545, 1952.
16. **Canale ST, Kelly FB Jr:** *Fractures of the neck of the talus.* J Bone Joint Surg (Am) 60:143, 1978.
17. **Hawkins LG:** *Fractures of the neck of the talus.* J Bone Joint Surg (Am) 52:991, 1970.
18. **Sangeorzan BJ, Benirschke SK, Mosca V, et al:** *Displaced intra—articular fractures of the tarsal navicular.* J Bone Joint Surg (Am) 71:1504, 1989.
19. **Blumberg K, Patterson RJ:** *The toddler's cuboid fracture.* Radiology 179:93, 1991.
20. **Richli WR, Rosenthal DI:** *Avulsion fracture of the fifth metatarsal: Experimental study of the pathomechanics.* AJR 143:889, 1984.
21. **Jones R:** *Fracture of the base of fifth metatarsal bone by indirect violence.* Ann Surg 35:697, 1902.
22. **Smith JW, Arnoczky DVM, Hersh A:** *The intraosseous blood supply of the fifth metatarsal: implications for proximal fracture healing.* Foot Ankle 13:143, 1992.
23. **Taylor JAM, Resnick D:** *Acute foot pain during an aerobics class.* J Musculoskel Med April:81, 1993.
24. **Foster SC, Foster RR:** *Lisfranc's tarsometatarsal fracture dislocation.* Radiology 120:79, 1976.
25. **Goiney RC, Connell DG, Nichols DM:** *CT evaluation of tarsometatarsal fracture–dislocation injuries.* AJR 144:985, 1985.

FRACTURES OF THE THORAX

1. **Reynolds J, Davis JT:** *Injuries of the chest wall, pleura, lungs, bronchi, and esophagus.* Radiol Clin North Am 4:383, 1966.
2. **Goeser CD, Aikenhead JA:** *Rib fracture due to bench pressing.* J Manipulative Physiol Ther 13:26, 1990.
3. **Lankenner PA, Micheli LJ:** *Stress fracture of the first rib.* J Bone Joint Surg (Am) 67:159, 1985.
4. **Sellers T:** *The extrapleural sign.* ACA J Chiro 22:65, 1988.
5. **Rogers LF:** *Radiology of Skeletal Trauma*, Vols. 1 and 2, ed 2. New York, Churchill Livingstone, 1992.
6. **Garrett KD, Doughty R:** *Cough fracture of a rib: A case report.* ACA J Chiro 29:55, 1992.
7. **Kattan KR:** *Trauma of the bony thorax.* Semin Roentgenol 13:69, 1978.
8. **Groskin SA:** *Selected topics in chest trauma.* Radiology 183:605, 1992.

FRACTURES AND DISLOCATIONS OF THE SHOULDER GIRDLE

1. **Pavlov H, Freiberger RH:** *Roentgenology of Fractures and Dislocations. Shoulder.* Felson B. ed. New York, Grune & Stratton, 1978.

2. **Heppenstall RB:** *Fractures and dislocations of the clavicle.* Orthop Clin North Am 6:477, 1975.
3. **Yates OW:** *Complications of fractures of the clavicle.* Injury 7:189, 1975.
4. **Rockwood CA, Green DP:** *Fractures*, Philadelphia, Lippincott, 1975.
5. **Rowe LJ, Cardin A:** *Posttraumatic osteolysis of the clavicle.* Chiro Sports Med 1:2, 1987.
6. **Levine HL, Pais MJ, Schwartz EE:** *Posttraumatic osteolysis of the distal clavicle, with emphasis on early radiologic changes.* AJR 127:781, 1976.
7. **Madsen B:** *Osteolysis of the acromial end of the clavicle following trauma.* Br J Radiol 36:822, 1963.
8. **Imatani RJ:** *Fractures of the scapula: a review of 53 fractures.* J Trauma 15:473, 1975.
9. **Harris RD, Harris JH:** *The prevalence and significance of missed scapular fractures in blunt chest trauma.* AJR 151:747, 1988.
10. **Deltoff MN, Bressler HB:** *Atypical scapular fracture. A case report.* Am J Sports Med 17:292, 1989.
11. **Bankart ASB:** *Recurrent or habitual dislocation of the shoulder joint.* Br Med J 1:1132, 1923.
12. **Neer CS II:** *Displaced proximal humeral fractures. Part I. Classification and evaluation.* J Bone Joint Surg (Am) 52:1077, 1970.
13. **Rogers LF:** *Radiology of Skeletal Trauma*, Vols. 1 and 2, ed 2. New York, Churchill Livingstone, 1992.
14. **Hill HA, Sachs MD:** *The grooved defect of the humeral head—A frequent unrecognized complication of dislocations of the shoulder joint.* Radiology 35:690, 1940.
15. **Ross GJ, Love MB:** *Isolated avulsion fracture of the lesser tuberosity of the humerus: report of two cases.* Radiology 172:833, 1989.
16. **Rowe CR:** *An atlas of anatomy and treatment of mid-clavicular fractures.* Clin Orthop 58:29, 1968.
17. **Rockwood CA, Green DP:** *Fractures.* Philadelphia, JB Lippincott, 1975.
18. **Workman TL, Burkhard TK, Resnick D, et al:** *Hill–Sachs lesion: comparison of detection with MR imaging, radiography, and arthroscopy.* Radiology 185:847, 1992.
19. **Amdt JH, Sears AD:** *Posterior dislocation of the shoulder.* AJR 94:639, 1965.
20. **Cistermino S, Rogers LF, Stufflebaum BC, et al:** *The trough line: A radiographic sign of posterior shoulder dislocation.* AJR 130:951, 1978.
21. **Nobel W:** *Posterior traumatic dislocation of the shoulder.* J Bone Joint Surg (Am) 44:523, 1962.
22. **Lev-Toaf AS, Karasick D, Rao VM:** *Drooping shoulder—nontraumatic causes of glenohumeral subluxation.* Skeletal Radiol 12:34, 1984.
23. **Alexander C:** *The acromiohumeral distance in health and disease.* Proc Coll Radiol Aust 3:102, 1959.
24. **Peterson CJ, Redlund-Johnell I:** *Joint space in normal glenohumeral radiographs.* Acta Orthop Scand 54:274, 1983.
25. **Lyons AR, Tomlinson JE:** *Clinical diagnosis of tears of the rotator cuff.* J Bone Joint Surg (Br) 74:414, 1992.
26. **Drakeford MK, Quinn MJ, Simpson SL, et al:** *A comparative study of ultrasonography and arthrography in evaluation of the rotator cuff.* Clin Orthop 253:118, 1990.
27. **Vick CW, Bell SA:** *Rotator cuff tears: diagnosis with sonography.* AJR 154:121, 1990.
28. **Ianotti JP, Zlatkin MB, Esterhai JL, et al:** *Magnetic resonance imaging of the shoulder: Sensitivity, specificity, and predictive value.* J Bone Joint Surg (Am) 73:17, 1991.
29. **Smith AM, McCauley TR, Jokl P:** *SLAP lesions of the glenoid labrum diagnosed with MR imaging.* Skeletal Radiol 22:507, 1993.
30. **Vanarthos WJ, Ekman EF, Bohrer SP:** *Radiographic diagnosis of acromioclavicular joint separation without weight bearing: importance of internal rotation of the arm.* AJR 162:120, 1994.
31. **Allman FL Jr:** *Fractures and ligamentous injuries of the clavicle and its articulations.* J Bone Joint Surg (Am) 49:774, 1963.
32. **Prolass JJ, Stampfli FW, Osmer JC:** *Coracoid process fracture diagnosis in acromioclavicular separation.* Radiology 116:61, 1975.
33. **Ward WG, Weaver JP, Garrett WE:** *Locked scapula.* J Bone Joint Surg (Am) 71:1558, 1989.

FRACTURES AND DISLOCATIONS OF THE ELBOW AND FOREARM

1. **Rockwood CA, Green DP:** *Fractures*, Philadelphia, JB Lippincott, 1975.
2. **Conn J Jr, Wade PA:** *Injuries of the elbow. A ten year review.* J Trauma 1:248, 1961.
3. **Karasick D, Burk DL Jr, Gross GW:** *Trauma to the elbow and forearm.* Semin Roentgenol 26:318, 1991.
4. **Knight RA:** *Fractures of the humeral condyles in adults.* South Med J 48:1165, 1955.
5. **Brogdon BG, Crow NE:** *Little leaguer's elbow.* AJR 83:671, 1960.
6. **Rogers LF:** *Radiology of Skeletal Trauma*, Vols. 1 and 2, ed 2. New York, Churchill Livingstone, 1992.
7. **Schultz RJ:** *The Language of Fractures*, Baltimore, Williams & Wilkins, 1976.
8. **Hall-Craggs MA, Shorvon PJ, Chapman M:** *Assessment of the radial head–capitellum view and the dorsal fat-pad sign in acute elbow trauma.* AJR 145:607, 1985.
9. **Nelson S:** *Some important diagnostic and technical fundamentals in the radiology of trauma, with particular emphasis on skeletal trauma.* Radiol Clin North Am 4:241, 1966.
10. **Rogers SL, MacEwan DW:** *Changes due to trauma in the fat plane overlying the supinator muscle: a radiologic sign.* Radiology 128:643, 1969.
11. **Norell HG:** *Roentgenologic visualization of the extracapsular fat. Its importance in the diagnosis of traumatic injuries to the elbow.* Acta Radiol 42:205, 1954.
12. **Hunter RD:** *Swollen elbow following trauma.* JAMA 230:1573, 1974.
13. **Essex-Lopresti P:** *Fractures of the radial head with distal radioulnar dislocation.* J Bone Joint Surg (Br) 33:244, 1951.

14. **Smith H, Sage FP:** *Medullary fixation of forearm fractures.* J Bone Joint Surg (Am) 39:91, 1957.
15. **DuToit FP, Grabe RP:** *Isolated fractures of the shaft of the ulna.* S Afr Med J 56:21, 1957.
16. **Bado JL:** *The Monteggia lesion.* Clin Orthop 50:71, 1967.
17. **Reckling FW, Pellier LF:** *Ricardo Galeazzi and Galeazzi's fracture.* Surgery 58:453, 1965.
18. **Hughston JC:** *Fracture of the distal radial shaft.* J Bone Joint Surg (Am) 39:249, 1957.
19. **Linscheid RL, Wheeler DK:** *Elbow dislocations.* JAMA 194:1171, 1965.
20. **Asher MA:** *Dislocations of the upper extremity in children.* Orthop Clin North Am 7:583, 1976.
21. **Neviager JS, Wickstrom JK:** *Dislocation of the elbow. A retrospective study of 115 patients.* South Med J 70:172, 1977.
22. **Salter RB, Zaltz C:** *Anatomic investigations of the mechanisms of injury and pathologic anatomy of the "pulled elbow" in young children.* Clin Orthop 77:134, 1971.

FRACTURES AND DISLOCATIONS OF THE WRIST

1. **Stewart NR, Gilula LA:** *CT of the wrist: a tailored approach.* Radiology 183:13, 1992.
2. **Hindman BW, Kulik WJ, Lee G, et al:** *Occult fractures of the carpals and metacarpals: demonstration by CT.* AJR 153:529, 1989.
3. **MacEwen DW:** *Changes due to trauma in the fat plane overlying the pronator quadratus muscle. A radiologic sign.* Radiology 82:879, 1964.
4. **Colles A:** *On the fracture of the carpal extremity of the radius.* Edinb Med Surg J 10:182, 1814.
5. **Alfram P, Bauer GCH:** *Epidemiology of fractures of the forearm.* J Bone Joint Surg (Am) 44:105, 1962.
6. **Rockwood CA, Green DP:** *Fractures,* Philadelphia, JB Lippincott, 1975.
7. **Smith RW:** *A treatise on fractures in the vicinity of joints, and on certain forms of accidental and congenital dislocations.* Dublin, Hodges & Smith, 1854.
8. **Barton JR:** *Views and treatment of an important injury to the wrist.* Med Examiner 1:365, 1838.
9. **Edwards HC:** *Mechanism and treatment of backfire fracture.* J Bone Joint Surg (Am) 8:701, 1926.
10. **Moore EM:** *Three cases illustrating luxation of the ulna in connection with Colles' fracture.* Med Record 17:305, 1880.
11. **Mazet R Jr, Hohl M:** *Fractures of the carpal navicular.* J Bone Joint Surg (Am) 45:82, 1963.
12. **Gelberman RH, Wolock BS, Siegel DB:** *Current concepts review. Fractures and non-unions of the carpal scaphoid.* J Bone Joint Surg (Am) 71:1560, 1989.
13. **Terry DW Jr, Ramin JE:** *The navicular fat stripe. A useful roentgen fracture for evaluating wrist trauma.* AJR 124:25, 1975.
14. **Graham J, Wood SK:** *Aseptic necrosis of bone following trauma.* In: Davidson JK ed.: *Aseptic necrosis of bone.* Amsterdam, Excerpta Medica, 1976.
15. **Rogers LF:** *Radiology of Skeletal Trauma.* Vols. 1 and 2, ed. 2. New York, Churchill Livingstone, 1992.
16. **Watson HK, Black DM:** *Instabilities of the wrist.* Hand Clin 3:103, 1987.
17. **Hudson TM, Caragol WJ, Kaye JJ:** *Isolated rotatory subluxation of the carpal navicular.* AJR 126:601, 1976.
18. **Metz VM, Schimmerl SM, Gilula LA, et al:** *Wide scapholunate joint space in lunotriquetral coalition: A normal variant?* Radiology 188:557, 1993.
19. **Mior SA, Dombrowsky N:** *Scapholunate failure: a long term follow–up.* J Manipulative Physiol Ther 15:255, 1992.
20. **Linscheid RL:** *Kinematic considerations of the wrist.* Clin Orthop 202:27, 1986.
21. **Quinn SF, Murray W, Watkins T, et al:** *CT for determining the results of treatment of fractures of the wrist.* AJR 149:109, 1987.
22. **Kohler A, Zimmer EA:** *Borderlands of the Normal and Early Pathologic in Skeletal Roentgenology,* ed 3. New York, Grune & Stratton, 1968.
23. **Bartone NF, Grieco RV:** *Fractures of the triquetrum.* J Bone Joint Surg (Am) 38:353, 1956.
24. **Bowen TL:** *Injuries of the hamate bone.* Hand 4:235, 1973.
25. **Carter PR, Eaton RG, Littler JW:** *Ununited fracture of the hook of the hamate.* J Bone Joint Surg (Am) 59:583, 1977.
26. **Norman A, Nelson J, Green S:** *Fractures of the hook of the hamate: Radiographic signs.* Radiology 154:49, 1985.
27. **Gillespy T, Stork JJ, Dell PC:** *Dorsal fracture of the hamate: Distinctive radiographic appearance.* AJR 151:351, 1988.
28. **Gilula LA:** *Carpal injuries: analytic approach and case exercises.* AJR 133:503, 1979.
29. **Frankel VH:** *The Terry Thomas sign.* Clin Orthop Rel Res (Letter) 129:321, 1977.
30. **deQuervain F:** Spezielle chirugische diagnostik fur studierende und aertze. Leipzig, FCW Vogel, 1907.

FRACTURES AND DISLOCATIONS OF THE HAND

1. **Rockwood CA, Green DP:** *Fractures,* Philadelphia, JB Lippincott, 1975.
2. **Brown PS:** *Management of phalangeal and metacarpal fractures.* Surg Clin North Am 53:1393, 1973.
3. **Terrett AGJ, Molyneaux TP:** *Hit or miss? The impact of three cases.* J Aust Chiro Assoc 14(4):153, 1984.
4. **Bennett EH:** *Fractures of the metacarpal bones.* Dublin J Med Sci 73:72, 1882.
5. **Rowe LJ:** *Bennett's fracture. A case study.* ACA Council Roent. Roentgen Brief. November, 1983.
6. **Rolando S:** *Fracture de la base du premier metacarpein et princpalement sur une variete non encore decrite.* Presse Med 33:303, 1910.
7. **Proubasta IR:** *Rolando's fracture of the first metacarpal. Treatment by external f fixation.* J Bone Joint Surg (Am) 74:416, 1992.

8. **Gedda KO:** *Studies on Bennett's fracture. Anatomy, roentgenology, and therapy.* Acta Chir Scand 193:1, 1954.
9. **Butt WB:** *Fractures of the hand.* Can Med Assoc J 86:371, 1962.
10. **Wissinger HA, McClain EJ, Boyes JH:** *Turrett exostosis: ossifying hematoma of the phalanges.* J Bone Joint Surg (Am) 48:105, 1966.
11. **Green DP, Terry GC:** *Complex dislocation of the metacarpophalangeal joint.* J Bone Joint Surg (Am) 55:1480, 1972.
12. **Campbell CS:** *Gamekeeper's thumb.* J Bone Joint Surg (Br) 37:148, 1955.
13. **Spaeth HJ, Abrams RA, Bock GW, et al:** *Gamekeeper thumb: Differentiation of nondisplaced tears of the ulnar collateral ligament with MR imaging.* Radiology 188:553, 1993.

STRESS FRACTURES

1. **Stafford SA, Rosenthal DI, Gebhardt MC, et al:** *MRI in stress fracture.* AJR 147:553, 1986.
2. **Daffner RH:** *Stress fractures: current concepts.* Skeletal Radiol 2:221, 1978.
3. **Michetti M:** *March fracture following a McBride bunionectomy.* J Am Podiatry Assoc 60L:286, 1970.
4. **Resnick D, Guerra J Jr:** *Stress fractures of the inferior pubic ramus following hip surgery.* Radiology 137:335, 1980.
5. **Drez D Jr, Young JC, Johnston RD, et al:** *Metatarsal stress fractures.* Am J Sports Med 8:123, 1980.
6. **Martin LM, Bourne RB, Rorabeck CH:** *Stress fracture associated with osteoarthritis of the knee.* J Bone Joint Surg (Am) 70:771, 1988.
7. **Morton D:** *The Human Feet,* New York, Columbia University Press, 1948.
8. **Burrows HJ:** *Fatigue infraction of the middle of the tibia in ballet dancers.* J Bone Joint Surg (Br) 38:83, 1956.
9. **Winfield AC, Dennis JM:** *Stress fractures of the calcaneus.* Radiology 72:415, 1959.
10. **Symeonides PP:** *High stress fracture of the fibula.* J Bone Joint Surg (Br) 62:192, 1980.
11. **Wiltse LL, Widell EH Jr, Jackson DW:** *Fatigue fracture: the basic lesion in isthmic spondylolisthesis.* J Bone Joint Surg (Am) 57:17, 1975.
12. **Daffner RH, Pavlov H:** *Stress fractures: Current concepts.* AJR 159:245, 1992.
13. **Ulmans H, Pavlov H:** *Stress fractures of the lower extremities.* Semin Roentgenol 29:176, 1994.
14. **Roug IK, Kettner NW:** *Radiology of stress fracture.* Topics Diagn Radiol Adv Imag (Spring):4, 1993.
15. **Martire JR:** *The role of nuclear medicine scans in the evaluation of pain in athletic injuries.* Clin Sports Med 6:713, 1987.
16. **Lee JK, Yao L:** *Stress fractures: MR imaging.* Radiology 169:217, 1988.

NON-ACCIDENTAL TRAUMA OF CHILDREN

1. **Caffey J:** *Multiple fractures in the long bones of infants suffering from chronic subdural hematoma.* AJR 56:163, 1946.
2. **Kempe CH, Silverman FN, Steele BF, et al:** *The battered-child syndrome.* JAMA 181:17, 1962.
3. **Kogutt MS, Swischuk LE, Fagan CJ:** *Patterns of injury and significance of uncommon fractures in the battered-child syndrome.* AJR 121:143, 1974.
4. **Rogers LF:** *Radiology of Skeletal Trauma,* Vols 1 and 2, ed 2. New York, Churchill Livingstone, 1992.
5. **Worlock P, Staner M, Barbor P:** *Patterns of fracture in accidental and non accidental injury in children: a comparative study.* Br Med J 293:100, 1986.
6. **Kleinman PK:** *Diagnostic imaging in infant abuse.* AJR 155:703, 1990.
7. **Kleinman PK, Marks SC, Blackbourne B:** *The metaphyseal lesion in abused infants: a radiologic histopathologic study.* AJR 146:895, 1986.
8. **Kleinman PK, Marks SC, Adams VI, et al:** *Factors affecting visualization of posterior rib fractures in abused infants.* AJR 150:635, 1988.
9. **Kleinman PK, Zito JL:** *Avulsion of the spinous processes caused by infant abuse.* Radiology 151:389, 1984.
10. **Ablin DS, Greenspan A, Reinhart M, et al:** *Differentiation of child abuse from osteogenesis imperfecta.* AJR 154:1035, 1990.

POSTTRAUMATIC MYOSITIS OSSIFICANS

1. **Thompson HC, Garcia A:** *Myositis ossificans.* Clin Orthop 50:129, 1967.
2. **Danchik JJ, Yochum TR, Aspergren DD:** *Myositis ossificans traumatica.* J Manipulative Physiol Ther 16:605, 1993.
3. **Park YH, Huang GS, Taylor JT, et al:** *Patterns of vertebral ossification and pelvic abnormalities in paralysis: a study of 200 patients.* Radiology 188:561, 1993.
4. **Yoslow W, Becker MH:** *Osseous bridges between the transverse processes of the lumbar spine.* J Bone Joint Surg (Am) 50:513, 1968.
5. **Osti OL, Fraser RD:** *Osseous bridging of lumbar intertransverse processes after trauma.* Spine 17:362, 1992.
6. **Yu JS, Witte D, Resnik D, et al:** *Ossification of the Achilles tendon: imaging abnormalities in 12 patients.* Skeletal Radiol 23:127, 1994.
7. **Thorndike A:** *Myositis ossificans traumatica.* J Bone Joint Surg (Am) 22:315, 1940.
8. **Ackerman LV:** *Extra-osseous localized nonneoplastic bone and cartilage formation (so-called myositis ossificans)* J Bone Joint Surg (Am) 40:279, 1958.
9. **Kransdorf MJ, Meis JM, Jelinek JS:** *Myositis ossificans: MR appearance with radiologic-pathologic correlation.* AJR 157:1243, 1991.
10. **Yochum TR, et al:** *Posttraumatic myositis ossificans.* ACA J Chiro Radiology Corner, July 1982.
11. **Goldman AB:** *Myositis ossificans circumscripta, a benign lesion with a malignant differential diagnosis.* AJR 126:32, 1976.
12. **Drane WE:** *Myositis ossificans and the three-phase bone scan.* AJR 142:179, 1984.
13. **Norman A, Dorfman HD:** *Juxtacortical circumscribed myositis ossificans: evolution and radiographic features.* Radiology 96:301, 1970.

Appendix MNEMONICS
A Learning Aid for Students of Skeletal Radiology

INTRODUCTION

All students of radiology have struggled to remember extensive lists for the differential diagnosis of various roentgen signs. The following encyclopedic list of roentgen signs with mnemonics is offered as an aid to assist the student in quick recall of some of these entities.

A **MNEMONIC** is defined by Webster's Dictionary as "something which assists or intends to assist one's memory, of or relating to memory, a technique of improving the memory, a device or code to assist memory recall."

The following list of mnemonics is divided into eight skeletal categories:

1. *Congenital—Chapter 3*
2. *Skeletal Dysplasias—Chapter 8*
3. *Trauma—Chapter 9*
4. *Arthritis—Chapter 10*
5. *Tumor and Tumorlike Processes—Chapter 11*
6. *Infection—Chapter 12*
7. *Vascular—Chapter 13*
8. *Nutritional, Metabolic, and Endocrine—Chapter 14*

These mnemonics are presented in alphabetical order based on the roentgen signs within the appropriate category of bone disease.

A CATEGORICAL APPROACH TO BONE DISEASE
mnemonic: **"CAT BITES"**
Congenital
Arthritis
Trauma

Blood
Infection
Tumor
Endocrine/metabolic
Soft tissues

Chapter 3—Congenital

BASILAR INVAGINATION
mnemonic: **"COOP"**
Congenital
Osteogenesis imperfecta
Osteomalacia
Paget's disease

BILATERAL MADELUNG DEFORMITY
mnemonic: **"RED HOT"**
Radial ray dysplasias
Epiphyseal dysplasias
Dyschondrosteosis

Hereditary multiple exostosis (HME) (bayonet deformity)
Ollier's disease
Thalidomide

Chapter 8—Skeletal Dysplasias

METACARPAL SIGN (short 4th metacarpal)
mnemonic: **"Ping Pong Is Tough To Teach"**
Pseudohypoparathyroidism
Pseudopseudohypoparathyroidism
Idiopathic
Trauma
Turner's syndrome
Trisomy 13-18

RADIAL RAY DYSPLASIA (hypoplastic or agenetic radius)
mnemonic: **"I FETCH"**
Idiopathic
Fanconi syndrome
Ellis-van Creveld syndrome
Thrombocytopenia
Cornelia De Lange syndrome
Holt-Oram syndrome

SOLITARY LYTIC DEFECT IN SKULL
mnemonic: **"M T HOLE"**
Metastasis, Myeloma

Tuberculosis, Trauma

Histiocytosis X
Osteomyelitis
Leptomeningeal cyst
Epidermoid/dermoid, Enigma (fibrous dysplasia)

WORMIAN BONES
mnemonic: **"PORK CHOPS"**
Pyknodysostosis
Osteogenesis imperfecta
Rickets in healing phase
Kinky hair syndrome

Cleidocranial dysplasia
Hypothyroidism/Hypophosphatasia
Otopalatodigital syndrome
Primary acro-osteolysis (Hajdu-Cheney)/
    Pachydermoperiostosis
Syndrome of Down

Chapter 9—Trauma

ROTATOR CUFF MUSCLES
mnemonic: **"SITS"**
Supraspinatus
Infraspinatus
Teres minor
Subscapularis

Chapter 10—Arthritis

ARTHRITIS WITH DEMINERALIZATION
mnemonic: **"HORSE"**
Hemophilia
Osteomyelitis
Rheumatoid arthritis, **R**eiter's syndrome
Scleroderma
Erythematosus, systemic lupus

CHONDROCALCINOSIS
mnemonic: Three **"Cs"**
Cation: copper—Wilson's disease
    iron—hemochromatosis
    calcium—hyperparathyroidism
Crystal: CPPD—pseudogout
    urate—gout
Cartilage: HADD

CHONDROCALCINOSIS
mnemonic: **"WHIP A DOG"**
Wilson's disease
Hemochromatosis, **H**emophilia, **H**ypothyroidism,
    Hyperparathyroidism (Primary, 15%),
    Hypophosphatasia, Familial **H**ypomagnesemia
Idiopathic (aging)
Pseudogout (CPPD)

Amyloidosis

Diabetes mellitus
Ochronosis
Gout

CAUSES OF SECONDARY OSTEOARTHRITIS
mnemonic: **"NOT A PHOWIE"**
Neurogenic arthropathy
Ochronosis
Trauma

Acromegaly, **A**vascular necrosis

Pseudogout (CPPD)
Hemochromatosis, **H**emophilia
Occupational
Wilson's disease
Idiopathic
Erosive osteoarthritis

EARLY OSTEOARTHRITIS
mnemonic: **"Early OsteoArthritis"**
Epiphyseal dysplasia, multiple
Ochronosis
Acromegaly

NEUROTROPHIC ARTHROPATHY
mnemonic: **"6 Ds"**
Distension (earliest finding due to effusion)
Density (increase in subchondral bone sclerosis)
Debris (bony intraarticular fragments)
Dislocation (joint surfaces often malaligned)
Disorganization (joint components usually disrupted
    "bag of bones")
Destruction (articular bone shows loss of bone
    substance)

PREMATURE OSTEOARTHRITIS
mnemonic: **"COME CHAT"**
Calcium pyrophosphate dihydrate arthropathy
Ochronosis
Marfan's syndrome
Epiphyseal dysplasia

Charcot joint = neurotrophic arthropathy
Hemophilic arthropathy
Acromegaly
Trauma

PROTRUSIO ACETABULI
mnemonic: **"PORT"**
Paget's disease
Osteomalacia
Rheumatoid arthritis
Trauma

SPOTTY CARPAL BONES
mnemonic: **"GS RAT"**
Gout
Sudeck's atrophy

Rheumatoid
Arthritis
Tuberculosis

Chapter 11—Tumor and Tumorlike Processes

ABSENT GREATER WING OF SPHENOID
mnemonic: **"M FOR MARINE"**
Meningioma

Fibrous dysplasia
Optic glioma
Relapsing hematoma

Metastasis
Aneurysm
Retinoblastoma
Idiopathic
Neurofibromatosis
Eosinophilic granuloma

BLOW OUT LESION OF POSTERIOR ELEMENTS (SPINE)
mnemonic: **"GO APE"**
Giant cell tumor
Osteoblastoma

Aneurysmal bone cyst
Plasmacytoma
Eosinophilic granuloma

BONE TUMORS FAVORING VERTEBRAL BODIES
mnemonic: **"CALL HOME"**
Chordoma
Aneurysmal bone cyst
Leukemia
Lymphoma

Hemangioma
Osteoid osteoma, Osteoblastoma
Myeloma, Metastasis
Eosinophilic granuloma

CALCIFYING METASTASES
mnemonic: **"BOTTOM"**
Breast
Osteosarcoma
Testicular
Thyroid
Ovary
Mucinous adenocarcinoma of GI tract

DESTRUCTION OF MEDIAL END OF CLAVICLE
mnemonic: **"MILERS"**
Metastases
Infection
Lymphoma
Eosinophilic granuloma
Rheumatoid arthritis
Sarcoma

DIAPHYSEAL LESIONS
mnemonic: **"FEMALE"**
Fibrous dysplasia
Ewing's sarcoma
Metastasis
Adamantinoma
Lymphoma, Leukemia
Eosinophilic granuloma

DIFFUSE OSTEOSCLEROSIS
mnemonic: **"FROM"**
Fluorosis
Renal osteodystrophy
Osteopetrosis
Myelosclerosis, Metastases (blastic),
   Mastocytosis

EPIPHYSEAL LESIONS
mnemonic: **"DELCO"**
Degenerative subchondral cyst (geode)
Enchondroma
Lipoma
Cyst, Chondroblastoma
Osteomyelitis

EXPANSILE RIB LESION
mnemonic: **"THELMA"**
Tuberculosis
Hematopoiesis
Eosinophilic granuloma, Ewing's sarcoma,
   Enchondroma
Leukemia, Lymphoma
Myeloma, Metastases
Aneurysmal bone cyst (ABC)

INCREASE IN SKULL THICKNESS
mnemonic: **"HIPFAM"**
Hyperostosis frontalis interna
Idiopathic
Paget's disease
Fibrous dysplasia
Anemia (sickle cell, iron deficiency, thalassemia,
   spherocytosis)
Metastases

IVORY VERTEBRA
mnemonic: **"My Only Sister Left Home On Friday Past"**
Myelosclerosis
Osteoblastic metastasis
Sickle-cell disease
Lymphoma
Hemangioma
Osteoporosis
Fluorosis
Paget's disease

METASTATIC LESIONS INVOLVING BONE
mnemonic: **"BLT with a Kosher Pickle 'N Hot Sauce**
Breast
Lung
Thyroid
Kidney
Prostate
Neuroblastoma
Hodgkin's disease
Sarcoma, Squamous cell

MOTH-EATEN BONE DESTRUCTION
mnemonic: **"H LEMMON"**
Histiocytosis X
Lymphoma
Ewing's sarcoma
Metastasis
Multiple myeloma
Osteomyelitis
Neuroblastoma

OSTEOBLASTIC METASTASES
mnemonic: "5 Bees Lick Pollen"
Brain (medulloblastoma)
Bronchus
Breast
Bowel (especially carcinoid)
Bladder

Lymphoma
Prostate

POSTERIOR VERTEBRAL BODY SCALLOPING
mnemonic: "HAMENTS"
Hurler's syndrome, Hydrocephalus
Achondroplasia, Acromegaly
Marfan syndrome
Ehlers-Danlos syndrome
Neurofibromatosis
Tumor (meningioma, ependymoma)
Syringohydromyelia

ROUND CELL TUMORS
mnemonic: "LEMON"
Leukemia, Lymphoma
Ewing's sarcoma, Eosinophilic granuloma
Multiple myeloma
Osteomyelitis
Neuroblastoma

SKELETAL METASTASES IN ADULT
mnemonic: "Common Bone Lesions Can Kill The Patient"

Colon
Breast
Lung
Carcinoid
Kidney
Thyroid
Prostate

SOAP BUBBLE LESIONS
mnemonic: "FEGNOMASHIC"
Fibrous dysplasia
Enchondroma
Giant cell tumor
Nonossifying fibroma
Osteoblastoma
Multiple myeloma, Metastasis
Aneurysmal bone cyst
Simple bone cyst
Hyperparathyroidism, Hemophilic pseudotumor
Infection
Chondroblastoma

TRANSVERSE LUCENT METAPHYSEAL LINES
mnemonic: "LINING"
Leukemia
Illness, systemic (rickets, scurvy)
Normal variant
Infection, transplacental (congenital syphilis)
Neuroblastoma metastases
Growth lines

Chapter 12—Infection

BUTTON SEQUESTRUM
mnemonic: "TORE ME"
Tuberculosis
Osteomyelitis
Radiation
Eosinophilic granuloma

Metastasis
Epidermoid

Chapter 13—Vascular

ACQUIRED ACRO-OSTEOLYSIS
mnemonic: "RADISH"
Raynaud's disease
Arteriosclerosis
Diabetes
Injury (burns, frostbite)
Scleroderma, Sarcoidosis
Hyperparathyroidism

ANTERIOR VERTEBRAL BODY SCALLOPING
mnemonic: "LAT"
Lymphadenopathy
Aortic aneurysm
Tuberculosis

ASEPTIC NECROSIS
mnemonic: "ASEPTIC"
Alcoholism, Atherosclerosis
Sickle cell, Storage diseases
Endogenous and Exogenous corticosteroids
Pancreatitis
Trauma
Idiopathic (Legg-Calvé-Perthes)
Caisson disease

AVASCULAR NECROSIS
mnemonic: **"PLASTIC RAGS"**
Pancreatitis, Pregnancy
Lupus
Alcoholism
Steroids
Trauma
Idiopathic
Caisson disease, Collagen disease (SLE)

Rheumatoid arthritis, Radiation
Amyloid
Gaucher disease
Sickle cell disease

OSTEOCHONDRITIS DISSECANS OF KNEE
mnemonic: **"LAME"**
Lateral
Anterior
Medial
Epicondyle

SCHMORL NODE
mnemonic: **"SHOOT"**
Scheuermann disease
Hyperparathyroidism
Osteoporosis
Osteomalacia
Trauma

Chapter 14—Nutritional, Metabolic, and Endocrine (NME)

DENSE METAPHYSEAL BANDS
mnemonic: **"Heavy Cretins Sift Scurrilously through Rickety Systems"**

Heavy metal poisoning (lead, bismuth, phosphorus)
Cretinism
Syphilis, congenital
Scurvy
Rickets (healed)
Systemic illness
    also: normal variant; methotrexate therapy

DIFFUSE PERIOSTEAL REACTION IN CHILDREN
mnemonic: **"PERIOSTEAL"**
Physiologic, Pachydermoperiostosis
E Prostaglandin E
Rickets (esp. healing phase)
Idiopathic (Caffey's disease)
Osteoarthropathy (hypertrophic)
Syphilis, Scurvy
Thyroid acropachy
Excess fluorine (fluorosis)
A hypervitaminosis A, Abuse (child)
Leukemia

FRAYED METAPHYSES
mnemonic: **"CHARMS"**
Congenital infections (rubella, syphilis)
Hypophosphatasia
Achondroplasia
Rickets
Metaphyseal dysostosis
Scurvy

GENERALIZED SCLEROSIS OF BONE
mnemonic: **"MARBLE"**
Myelosclerosis, Mastocytosis, Metabolic
    (hypervitaminosis D, fluorosis, hypothyroidism,
    phosphorus poisoning)
Anemia (sickle cell)
Renal osteodystrophy
Blastic metastasis
Lymphoma
Enigmas (Paget's disease, osteopetrosis,
    melorheostosis, pyknodysostosis, tuberous
    sclerosis)

HEEL PAD THICKENING
= heel pad thickening > 25 mm (normal < 21 mm)
mnemonic: **"MAD COP"**
Myxedema
Acromegaly
Dilantin therapy

Callous
Obesity
Peripheral edema

PENCILED DISTAL END OF CLAVICLE
mnemonic: **"SHIRT Pocket"**
Scleroderma
Hyperparathyroidism
Infection
Rheumatoid arthritis
Trauma

Progeria

VERTEBRA PLANA
mnemonic: **"FETISH"**
Fracture
Eosinophilic granuloma
Tumor (metastasis, myeloma)
Infection
Steroids
Hemangioma

Index

Page numbers in **color** indicate main discussions; those followed by *t* and *f* indicate tables and figures, respectively.

in epiphyseal dysplasia multiplex, 597, 598f
epiphyseal injury, 660f
fractures, 729–732
  BB fracture, 732, 732f, 785t
  bimalleolar, 730, 730f–731f, 785t
  boot-top fracture, 732, 732f, 785t
  both bones fracture, 732, 732f
  complications, 733
  Cotton's fracture, 730, 785t
  Danis-Weber classification, 729
  Dupuytren's fracture, 731, 785t
  lateral malleolus, 729–730, 730f
  Laug-Hansen classification, 729
  ligamentous instability with, 733
  Maisonneuve's fracture, 731, 732f, 785t
  medial malleolus, 729, 729f
  named and eponymic, 785t
  nonunion, 733
  Pott's fracture, 730–731, 731f, 785t
  sites, 788t
  Tillaux's fracture, 731–732, 785t
  toddler's fracture, 732, 732f, 785t
  traumatic degenerative arthritis with, 733
  trimalleolar, 730
in hemophilia, 1253, 1254f–1255f
in hydroxyapatite deposition disease, 954
infection, 578f
in juvenile rheumatoid arthritis, 875f
lateral collateral ligament injury, magnetic
      resonance imaging, 454–455
ligamentous injury, magnetic resonance
      imaging, 454
magnetic resonance imaging, 455–461, 729
neurotrophic arthropathy in, 845f, 849f
nonossifying fibroma, 1113, 1114f
pain, 531f
radiographic anatomy
  anteroposterior projection, 72–73, 73f
  lateral projection, 76–77, 77f
  medial oblique projection, 74–75, 75f
radiographic evaluation, 729
radiographic projections
  anteroposterior, 72f, 72–73, 73f
  lateral, 76f, 76–77, 77f
  medial oblique, 74f, 74–75, 75f
in Reiter's syndrome, 906, 907f–908f
in rheumatoid arthritis, 870
in rickets, 1345f
synoviochondrometaplasia, 854f
tendon injury, magnetic resonance imaging,
      454
in thalassemia, 1249f
tubercular arthritis, 1222, 1224f
Ankylosing spondylitis, 877–892, 1514f, 1522f,
      1524f
  Andersson lesion in, 885, 890f, 890–891,
      891t
  aneurysms in, 1308
  ankylosis of joint prosthesis in, 892
  arachnoid diverticula in, 891f, 891–892
  atlantoaxial instability in, 885, 888f
  atlantoaxial rotary subluxation in, 892
  atlantodental interspace in, 148, 885, 888f
  bamboo spine in, 885, 887f, 891t
  barrel-shaped vertebrae in, 882, 884f, 891t
  calcaneus in, 889
  capsule summary, 892
  cardiac involvement in, 878
  carrot stick fracture in, 890, 890f, 891t
  cartilage articulations in, 879
  cervical spine in, 885, 888f–889f
  clinical features, 877–878
  complications, 890–892
  computed tomography, 489, 490f

dagger sign in, 885, 888f, 891f, 891t
endplate erosion in, 885, 887f
entheses in, 879, 879f
enthesopathy in, 889, 890f, 891t
erythrocyte sedimentation rate in, 878
hips in, 889, 889f
HLA-B27 in, 148
ischium in, whiskering, 879f, 890f, 891t
laboratory findings in, 878
ocular involvement in, 878
pathology, 878–879
peripheral joints in, 885–889
pulmonary manifestations, 878
radiologic/diagnostic/technologic correlation
      in, 883t
radiologic features, 879f–885f, 879–880
Romanus lesion in, 879f, 882, 884f, 891t
sacroiliac joint in, 880, 880f–883f, 881t
shiny corner sign in, 882, 884f–885f, 891t
shoulder in, 889
skeletal distribution, 878, 878f
spinal involvement in, 880–885, 883f–889f,
      883t
  apophyseal joints, 885, 887f–888f
  costovertebral joints, 885, 887f–888f
  discovertebral junction (syndesmophyte
      formation), 882f–887f, 882–885, 891t
  squared vertebrae in, 882, 884f, 891t
symphysis pubis width and, 174
synonyms for, 877, 877t
synovial articulations in, 879, 879f
temporomandibular joint involvement in,
      885
trolley track sign in, 885, 888f, 891t
whiskering in, 879f, 889, 890f, 891t
Ankylosis
in end-stage tubercular arthritis, 1230f, 1231
of joint prosthesis, in ankylosing spondylitis,
      892
in juvenile rheumatoid arthritis, 874, 875f
in psoriatic arthritis, 896, 899f
with septic arthritis, 1214, 1217f
Annihilation radiation, 508
Annular fissure, definition, 501
Annulus fibrosus
  bulging. See Disc(s), intervertebral, bulging
  normal, 413
Anterior cervical cord syndrome, acute, 676–
      680, 679f
Anterior C1 spondyloschisis, 262f
Anterior drawer sign, 442
Anterior rachischisis, 204f
Anterolisthesis. See also Spondylolisthesis
  George's line and, 149
  lumbar spine, 162, 162f
  posterior cervical line and, 150
Anteroposterior position, definition, 3, 5f
Antibiotic balls, in femoral shaft, 1438f
Anticonvulsants, prenatal exposure to, and
      Conradi-Hunermann syndrome, 593
Aorta, atherosclerosis, 1306, 1306f
Aortic aneurysm(s), 1308–1310
Aortic arch
  aneurysm, 1310, 1313f
  thumbnail sign, 274f
Aortic knob, prominent, 274f
Aortic valve prosthesis, radiographic
      appearance, 1437f
AP. See Anteroposterior
Apical vertebra, 309
Apophyseal joints
  in ankylosing spondylitis, 885, 887f–888f
  degeneration, 807, 808f, 812–813, 814f–815f
  in rheumatoid arthritis, 868

Apophysis, 559f
  definition, 7
  lesions predisposed to, 564, 564t, 565f
Apophysis sign, 310
Appa's view, 62, 63f
Apple core defect, 452
Apple core deformity, 855, 962, 964f
Arachnodactyly. See also Marfan's syndrome
  in Marfan's syndrome, 608, 608f
Arachnoid diverticula, in ankylosing
      spondylitis, 891f, 891–892
Arachnoiditis
  clinical features, 426
  definition, 495
  etiology, 426
  magnetic resonance imaging in, 426f, 426–427
  signs and symptoms, 426
Arch-body line, measurement, 150, 150f
Arcual kyphosis, 683, 685f
Arcuate lines (of the sacrum), 705, 705f
Arnold-Chiari malformation, 202
  left thoracic scoliosis and, 311, 313f
  magnetic resonance imaging, 386, 388f
  medicolegal implications, 202
  scoliosis and, 386–388
  syrinx and, 201f, 202, 386–388, 388f–389f
  type I, 202
    clinical features, 386
    magnetic resonance imaging, 386, 388f
  type II, 202
    clinical features, 386
    magnetic resonance imaging, 386
  type III, 202
    clinical features, 386
    magnetic resonance imaging, 386
  type IV
    clinical features, 386
    magnetic resonance imaging, 386
Arterial disorder(s), 1306–1318
  capsule summary, 1320
Arterial injury, 663
Arteriogram, 552
Arteriolosclerosis, 1307
  capsule summary, 1320
Arteriosclerosis, 1306–1307
  capsule summary, 1320
Arteritis, aneurysms in, 1308
Arthritis
  computed tomography in, 485–489
  degenerative
    with ankle fractures, 733
    with clavicular fractures, 743
    with hip dislocation, 718
    hip joint space width and, 173
    radiocarpal, with scaphoid fracture, 762, 762f
    spinal, scoliosis and, 313, 317f
  degenerative disorders, 802–855. See also
      specific disorder(s)
  enteropathic, 893–894
  gouty. See Gout
  inflammatory disorders, 855–929
    enthesopathy in, 889, 890f, 890t–891t
  metabolic disorders, 929–965. See also specific
      disorder(s)
  monostotic versus polyostotic, 563t
  posttraumatic, 784t
  psoriatic, 895–904
  Reiter's syndrome. see Reiter's syndrome
  septic, 561–562, 1211–1218
    ankylosis as sequela to, 1214, 1217f
    bone scan in, 1211, 1213f
    capsule summary, 1218
    clinical course, 1211, 1212f
    clinical features, 172, 1211

Osteoarthropathy
  barotraumatic. *See* Caisson disease
  hypertrophic, developing from osteosarcoma,
    1021, 1022*f*
  pressure-induced. *See* Caisson disease
Osteoblastoma, 1093–1097
  age distribution, 1093
  capsule summary, 1097
  clinical features, 1093–1094
  in extremity, 1097
  historical perspective on, 1093
  incidence, 1093
  pathology, 1094–1095
  prognosis for, 1097
  radiologic features, 1095*t,* 1095–1097
  sex distribution, 1093
  signs and symptoms, 1094
  skeletal distribution, 564*t,* 1094, 1094*f*–1095*f,*
    1128*t*
  spinal, radiologic features, 1094*f*–1095*f,*
    1095–1097, 1096*f*
  time of occurrence, 1127*t*
  treatment, 1097
Osteochondral fractures, 659, 750
Osteochondral talar fracture, 730, 730*f*
Osteochondritis dissecans, 750, 1279*t,* 1295–
    1301
  capsule summary, 1301
  classic, 1297*f*
  clinical features, 1295, 1295*t,* 1296*f*
  degenerative joint disease secondary to, 1298
  displaced, 1296–1301, 1297*t*
  elbow in, 1300*f,* 1300–1301
  extended classic, 1297*f*–1298*f*
  femoral locations, 1297*f,* 1297–1298, 1298*f*–
    1299*f*
  foot in, 1300
  hips in, 1300
  lateral talar, 1299–1300, 1300*f*
  Legg-Calvé-Perthes disease and, 1284
  loose bodies in, 1296, 1296*f*
  magnetic resonance imaging, 450–451, 451*f,*
    460–461, 461*f,* 468, 468*f,* 1298*f*
  medial talar, 1298–1299, 1299*f*
  patellar, 1300, 1300*f*
  pathologic-radiologic correlation in, 1296,
    1297*t*
  pathology, 1296, 1296*f*
  radiologic features, 1296–1301, 1297*t*
  shoulder in, 1300
  sites of involvement, 1295, 1295*t,* 1296*f,* 1297–
    1301
  in situ, 1296–1301, 1297*t*
  skeletal distribution, 1295, 1295*t,* 1296*f*
  spontaneous osteonecrosis of knee versus,
    1270, 1270*t*
  talar involvement in, 1298–1300, 1299*f*–1300*f*
  temporomandibular joint in, 1301
  wrist in, 1301
Osteochondritis juvenilis dorsi. *See*
    Scheuermann's disease
Osteochondrodystrophy. *See* Hurler's
    syndrome
Osteochondroma
  age distribution, 1060
  bayonet hand deformity with, 1066, 1068*f*
  cauliflower, 1062*f,* 1063, 1063*f*
  clinical features, 1060–1061
  fracture, 1063, 1063*f*
  incidence, 1060
  malignant degeneration, 1029, 1032
  multiple, 1060*f,* 1060–1061, 1066, 1068*f*
  with osteocartilaginous cap, 1061, 1062*f*
  position in bone, 564*t*

  pressure erosion from, 1066, 1068*f*
  prognosis for, 1063
  radiation-induced, 1276
  radiologic features, 1061*f*–1064*f,* 1061–1063,
    1064*t*
  sessile, 1063, 1064*f,* 1069*f*
  sex distribution, 1060
  signs and symptoms, 1060
  skeletal distribution, 564*t,* 1060*f,* 1060–1061,
    1061*f,* 1128*t*
  solitary, 1060–1065
    capsule summary, 1065
    historical perspective on, 1060
    malignant degeneration, 1061, 1061*t,* 1182*t*
    skeletal distribution, 1060–1061, 1061*f*
  spinal, radiation-induced, 1276
  subungual exostosis, 1063, 1065*f*
  treatment, 1063
Osteochondrosis
  Blount's disease, 1279*t,* 1280*f,* 1301, 1302*f*
  Calvé's disease, 1279*t,* 1301
  capsule summary, 1305
  Diaz's disease, 1279*t,* 1280*f,* 1301, 1302*f*
  Hass's disease, 1279*t,* 1280*f,* 1301–1303,
    1302*f*–1303*f*
  Kohler's disease, 1279*t,* 1280*f,* 1303, 1303*f*
  Kummel's disease, 701, 1279*t,* 1280*f,* 1303–
    1304
  Mauclaire's disease, 1279*t,* 1280*f,* 1304
  miscellaneous, 1301–1305
  Panner's disease, 1279*t,* 1280*f,* 1304, 1304*f*
  Preiser's disease, 1279*t,* 1280*f,* 1304, 1304*f*
  Sever's disease, 1279*t,* 1280, 1280*f,* 1304,
    1305*f*
  Sinding-Larsen-Johansson disease, 1279,
    1279*t,* 1280*f,* 1304
  Thiemann's disease, 1279*t,* 1280*f,* 1305
  van Neck's disease, 1279*t,* 1280, 1280*f,* 1305,
    1305*f*
Osteochondrosis dissecans, 1295
Osteoclast-activating factor, 535
Osteoclastoma. *See* Brown tumors
Osteogenesis imperfecta, 618–622, 1514*f*
  classification, 618, 620
  clinical features, 618–619, 643*t*
  complications, 643*t*
  congenita, 618
  diagnostic criteria, 618
  generalized osteoporosis and, 1337
  genetics, 618
  medicolegal implications, 622
  pathologic features, 619
  radiologic features, 619–621, 620*f*–621*f,*
    645*t*
  tarda, 618
    clinical features, 618, 619*f*
  type I, 618
  type II, 618
  type III, 618
  type IV, 618
Osteogenic sarcoma. *See* Osteosarcoma
Osteoid osteoma, 487*f,* 1086–1093
  age distribution, 1087
  cancellous, 1088
  capsule summary, 1093
  clinical features, 1087
  cortical, 1088
  differential diagnosis, 777, 1085, 1092–1093
  en bloc excision, 1092*f,* 1093
  historical perspective on, 1086
  incidence, 1087
  pathology, 1088, 1088*f*
  pedicle, 358*f*
  periosteal response with, 575*t*

  position in bone, 564*t*
  prognosis for, 1093
  radiologic features, 1088*f*–1092*f,* 1088–1092,
    1092*t*
  scoliosis produced by, 316*f*
  sex distribution, 1087
  signs and symptoms, 1087
  skeletal distribution, 564*t,* 1087, 1087*f*–1088*f,*
    1128*t*
  subperiosteal, 1088
  time of occurrence, 1127*t*
  treatment, 1092*f,* 1093
Osteoid seams, 1341, 1343
Osteology, 6
Osteolysis
  acromioclavicular joint space and, 185
  posttraumatic, 663
    with clavicular fractures, 743, 744*f*
Osteolytic bone lesions, 568–570, 570*t,* 571*f*
  geographic, 568, 570*t,* 571*f*–572*f*
  motheaten, 568–570, 570*t,* 571*f*
  permeative, 570, 570*t*
Osteoma, 574*f,* 1078. *See also* Gardner's
    syndrome; Osteoid osteoma
  differential diagnosis, 1085–1086
  frontal sinus, 1078, 1079*f*–1080*f*
  giant, 1078, 1078*f*
  radiologic features, 1078, 1078*f*–1081*f,*
    1079*t*
  skeletal distribution, 564*t,* 1078, 1078*f*–1079*f*
  sphenoid sinus, 1078, 1079*f*
Osteomalacia, 1337, 1340–1343
  capsule summary, 1343
  clinical features, 1340–1341
  deformities in, 1342, 1343*f*
  etiology, 1340, 1341*t*
  pathology, 1341, 1341*t*
  pseudofractures in, 1341–1342, 1342*f*–1343*f*
  radiologic features, 1341*f*–1343*f,* 1341*t,* 1341–
    1342
  skull in, 143–145
Osteomyelitis, 532*f,* 561–562
  bone scan in, 521*f*
  chronic, 1205, 1210*f*–1211*f*
  in Cushing's disease, 1359
  in diabetic, 513*f*
  differential diagnosis, 777
  fracture-related, 663, 664*f*
  Garré's sclerosing osteomyelitis, 1201*f,* 1205
    differential diagnosis, 1092
  of ischiopubic synchrosis, 520*f*
  mycotic, 1238–1240
  nonsuppurative, 1219–1235
    capsule summary, 1235
    and suppurative, comparison, 1231, 1231*t*
  periosteal response with, 576*f*
  postsurgical, 1198*f*
  radionuclide scintigraphy in, 529–533, 531*f*–
    532*f*
  Salmonella, sickle cell anemia and, 1243, 1246,
    1246*t*
  in sickle cell anemia, 1243, 1246, 1246*t*
  suppurative, 1193–1204
    bone destruction in, radiologic features,
      1196, 1198*f*
    capsule summary, 1204
    clinical features, 1193–1194
    end-stage ankylosis, 1200, 1203*f*
    etiology, 1193
    extremity involvement, radiologic features,
      1195–1196, 1196*f*–1197*f,* 1197*t*
    historical perspective on, 1193
    incidence, 1193
    medicolegal implications, 1204

Signs, radiographic—*continued*
  signet ring, 764*f*, 765, 787*t*
  snowcap, in spontaneous osteonecrosis of
    femoral head, in adults, 1268
  tennis racquet appearance, 746, 748*f*
  Terry Thomas, 761, 764*f*, 765, 787*t*, 857*t*, 864
  thumbnail, 274*f*
  trolley track, 885, 888*f*, 891*t*
  vacuum cleft. *See* Intravertebral vacuum cleft
  Waldenstrom's, 172–173, 821, 1214, 1214*f*
Silicone breast implant(s), artifacts caused by,
    1420*f*, 1427*f*
Silver dollar vertebra, 1516, 1516*f*
Simple bone cyst, 1117–1121
  age distribution, 1117
  capsule summary, 1121
  clinical features, 1117
  fallen fragment sign, 1118, 1119*f*
  hinged fragment sign with, 1118, 1120*f*
  incidence, 1117
  pathology, 1117–1118
  position in bone, 564*t*
  prognosis for, 1120
  radiologic features, 1118*f*–1120*f*, 1118–1120,
    1120*t*
  sex distribution, 1117
  signs and symptoms, 1117
  skeletal distribution, 564*t*, 1117, 1118*f*
  treatment, 1120, 1120*t*
Sinding-Larsen-Johansson disease, 1279, 1279*t*,
    1280*f*, 1304
  Osgood-Schlatter's disease with, 1304
Single-photon absorptiometry, in osteoporosis,
    1328
Single photon emission computed tomography,
    347, 350*f*, 509, 514–515, 515*f*–516*f*, 555
  bone scan, 350*f*, 3347
  of pars interarticularis, 351*f*, 347
  in spondylolysis and/or spondylolisthesis,
    347–353
    patient management and, 351, 352*f*
    technique, 347–351
  of stress fractures, 776
  for surgical spine, 351
Sinography
  applications, 555
  technical considerations, 555
Six Ds, of neurotrophic arthropathy, 844, 845*f*
Skeletal age, 310
Skeletal anatomy, 6–8, 559–561
Skeletal development, 559
Skeletal dysplasia(s), 585–651. *See also specific
    disorder(s)*
Skeletal maturity, radiographic determination,
    321*f*, 321–322
Skeletal physiology, 559–561
Skeletal tumor(s). *See also* Bone tumor(s);
    specific tumor(s)
  medicolegal implications, 1183–1184
Skeletal variant(s). *See also* Congenital
    anomalies
  normal, 252–302
Skier's fracture, 732, 732*f*, 785*t*
Skin
  in acromegaly, 1352, 1353*f*
  in Ehlers-Danlos syndrome, 611–612, 612*f*
  fibrous dysplasia and, 1159–1160
  in neurofibromatosis, 1173
Skin cancer, skeletal metastases, radiologic
    presentation, 981*t*
Skinner's line
  clinical significance, 179, 192*t*
  measurement, 179, 179*f*, 192*t*
Skin rash, in systemic lupus erythematosus,
    910

Skull
  in acquired syphilis, 1238, 1238*f*
  in acromegaly, 1352, 1353*f*–1354*f*
  in cleidocranial dysplasia, 589, 590*f*
  computed tomography, 665*f*
  with eosinophilic granuloma, 1362
  in fibrous dysplasia, 1170, 1170*f*
  fracture, 665*f*–668*f*, 665–667
    basal, 666–667
    complications, 667
      extradural hematoma, 667
      leptomeningeal cyst, 667
      pneumocephalus, 667
      subdural hematoma, 667
    depressed, 666, 666*f*–667*f*
    diastatic, 667, 668*f*, 784*t*
    growing, 667, 784*t*
    linear, 665, 666*f*
    named and eponymic, 784*t*
    ping pong, 666, 784*t*
    sites, 788*f*
    stellate, 666, 784*t*
  geographic, 1362, 1362*f*
  hemangioma, 1074*f*, 1075, 1075*f*
  in hyperparathyroidism, 1350, 1350*f*
  imaging, 665
  lines and angles of, 188*t*
  in Marfan's syndrome, 608
  measurements, 141–147
  metastatic disease, 996, 996*f*, 1002*f*, 1002–1003
  in multiple myeloma, 1006, 1006*f*–1009*f*
  in neurofibromatosis, 1173, 1179–1180
  with osteogenesis imperfecta, 621, 621*f*
  osteoma, 1078, 1080*f*–1081*f*
  in osteopetrosis, 626, 632*f*
  in osteoporosis, 1334–1335
  in Paget's disease, 1146*f*, 1147, 1148*f*–1149*f*
    malignant degeneration, 1137*f*
  pepper pot, 1347, 1350*f*
  radiographic anatomy
    anteroposterior Towne's projection, 14–15,
      15*f*
    lateral projection, 11, 11*f*
    posteroanterior Caldwell projection, 12–13,
      13*f*
  radiographic projections
    anteroposterior Towne's, 14*f*, 14–15, 15*f*
    lateral, 10, 10*f*
    posteroanterior Caldwell, 12, 12*f*
  raindrop, 1006, 1008*f*
  salt and pepper, 1347, 1350*f*
  in thalassemia, 1248, 1249*f*
  in tuberous sclerosis, 639, 639*f*
SLAP lesions, 466–467, 747
SLE. *See* Systemic lupus erythematosus
Slipped femoral capital epiphysis, 718–720
  bilateral, 718
  clinical features, 718
  complications, 720
  diagnosis, 718
  epidemiology, 718
  iliofemoral line and, 178
  Klein's line and, 179, 719, 719*f*, 720, 720*f*
  predisposing factors, 718
  radiologic features, 718–720, 719*f*, 719*t*
  Shenton's line and, 177
  treatment, 720, 721*f*
Slipped radial epiphysis, 758, 759*f*
  corner sign with, 758, 759*f*, 787*t*
Smith's fracture, 757, 757*f*, 786*t*
Smoky appearance of bone, 1165, 1165*f*
Snowball appearance, 570, 572*f*
  with metastatic bone tumor, 981
Snow-cap epiphysis, in Legg-Calvé-Perthes
    disease, 1282, 1282*f*

Snowcap sign, in spontaneous osteonecrosis of
    femoral head, in adults, 1268
SNR. *See* Signal-to-noise ratio
Soap bubble appearance, 436
Soap bubble lesion, 568, 572*f*, 1014, 1018*f*
Soap bubble pattern, with giant cell tumor,
    1057, 1058*f*
Soap bubble vertebra, 1524
Soft disc, 413
Soft tissue
  abnormalities, with venous insufficiency, 1320
  in bone disease, 575, 578*f*
  calcification. *See also* Myositis ossificans
    differential diagnosis, 783
  cavernous hemangiomas, in Maffucci's
    syndrome, 1105
  with Ewing's sarcoma, 578*f*
  fibromas, in Gardner's syndrome, 1079
  hemangioma, 1076*f*, 1077
  in hemophilia, 1251, 1252*f*
  in hyperparathyroidism, 1349
  in hypertrophic osteoarthropathy, 929
  injury
    cervical spine. *See* Whiplash syndrome
    in Cushing's disease, 1359
    knee, 728–729
    with pelvic fractures, 713
  in Legg-Calvé-Perthes disease, 1281
  lipoma, 573*f*, 1125, 1126*f*
  with malignant synovioma, 578*f*
  mass, with fibrosarcoma, 1041*f*
  metastatic disease, 1001, 1001*f*
  prevertebral
    cervical
      clinical significance, 155, 189*t*
      masses, 155
      measurement, 155, 155*f*, 155*t*, 189*t*
    cervical spine trauma and, 155
  in scleroderma, 917–918, 918*f*
  in septic arthritis, 1214, 1214*f*–1215*f*
  in suppurative osteomyelitis, 1196, 1197*f*
    radiologic features, 1196, 1197*f*
  swelling, in psoriatic arthritis, 896, 896*f*
  in systemic lupus erythematosus, 911, 912*f*
  in tuberculous spondylitis (Pott's disease),
    1220–1222
Soft tissue window, 475
Solitary bone cyst, time of occurrence, 1127*t*
Solitary enchondroma, 1098–1102
Solitary osteochondroma, 1060–1065
Solitary plasmacytoma. *See* Plasmacytoma,
    solitary
SONK. *See* Osteonecrosis, spontaneous, of
    knee
Spatulated ribs, in Hurler's syndrome, 614,
    615*f*–616*f*
SPECT. *See* Single photon emission computed
    tomography
Sphenobasilar angle, measurement, 142, 142*f*,
    142*t*
Sphenoid sinus
  air-fluid level in, 666
  osteoma, 1078, 1079*f*
Spheno-occipital chordoma
  capsule summary, 1047
  radiologic features, 1044–1045, 1045*f*
  signs and symptoms, 1043
Spherocytosis, hereditary. *See* Hereditary
    spherocytosis
Spider-like fingers, in Marfan's syndrome, 608,
    608*f*
Spider spine, 1226*f*
Spina bifida
  occulta, 231
  of atlas and axis, 210*f*–211*f*

in progressive diaphyseal dysplasia, 636, 636*f*
in thalassemia, 1249*f*
Upright position, definition, 3
Uptake, radiopharmaceutical, 509
Ureteric colic, in Paget's disease, 1132
Urethral injury, with pelvic fracture/
    dislocation, 713
Uric acid
  in blood, in multiple myeloma, 1005
  normal laboratory values, 580*t*
Urinary tract, in hyperparathyroidism, 1349
Urine, Bence Jones proteoses, in multiple
    myeloma, 1005
Uterine cancer, skeletal metastases, 994*f*
  radiologic presentation, 981*t*
Uterine fibroid, 1454*f*

—V—

Vacant glenoid sign, 746, 787*t*
Vacuum cleft sign. *See* Intravertebral vacuum
    cleft sign
Vacuum phenomenon, 821*f*. *See also* Vacuum
    sign (of Knuttson)
  anatomic/radiologic correlation, 818*t*
  in cervical spondylosis, 808, 810*f*, 812*f*
  in whiplash syndrome, 686–688, 687*f*
Vacuum sign (of Knuttson)
  in lumbar spine spondylosis, 816*f*, 816–817,
    817*f*
  in peripheral joints, 817, 817*f*–818*f*
  physiologic, 817*f*
Vagina, foreign bodies in, radiographic
    appearance, 1507*f*. *See also* Tampon(s)
Vagotomy clips, artifacts caused by, 1433*f*
Van Akkerveeken's measurement of lumbar
    instability, 164, 164*f*, 190*t*
  clinical significance, 164, 190*t*
Vanishing bone disease. *See* Massive osteolysis
    of Gorham
van Neck's disease, 1279*t*, 1280, 1280*f*, 1305,
    1305*f*
Vascular anatomy, of bone, 1194, 1194*f*
Vascular disorder(s), 1306–1320. *See also specific*
    disorder(s)
  capsule summary, 1320
  computed tomography in, 484*f*, 485
  generalized osteoporosis and, 1337
Vascular injury, with pelvic fracture/
    dislocation, 713
Vasectomy, radiographic appearance, 1451*f*,
    1455*f*
Vastine–Kinney method, of pineal gland
    localization, 141, 141*f*, 188*t*
VATER syndrome, 227–231
Velvety skin, in Ehlers–Danlos syndrome, 612
Venogram, 552
Venous disorder(s), 1318–1320. *See also specific*
    disorder
  capsule summary, 1320
Venous insufficiency, 1319–1320
  capsule summary, 1320
  radiologic features, 1319*f*, 1319*t*, 1319–1320
  soft tissue abnormalities with, 1320
Ventral (volar) intercalated segment instability,
    with scaphoid fracture, 761
Ventriculoperitoneal shunt, radiographic
    appearance, 1422*f*
Vertebra, pig snout, 283*f*
Vertebra/vertebrae
  acquired coronal cleft, 696*f*, 699
  anomalies, congenital scoliosis and, 311
  apical, 309
  barrel–shaped, 1514, 1514*f*

in ankylosing spondylitis, 882, 884*f*, 891*t*
beaked, 1514
biconcave (lens), 621, 621*f*, 1514, 1514*f*
  in osteoporosis, 1331*f*, 1331–1332, 1332*f*
blind, 985, 988*f*–989*f*, 1514, 1514*f*
block, 1525*f*
  cervical, 210–214, 211*f*–216*f*
  congenital, 949, 951*f*
  lumbar, 223*f*–225*f*
  Paget's disease in, 1151, 1155*f*
bottle–like, 1515, 1515*f*
bullet–nosed, 1515, 1515*f*
  in achondroplasia, 587, 588*f*
butterfly, 222–223, 225*f*–226*f*, 1515, 1515*f*
chordoma
  capsule summary, 1047
  radiologic features, 1045, 1046*f*
  signs and symptoms, 1043
clover leaf, 1516
codfish, 1518, 1518*f*
  in osteoporosis, 1331*f*, 1331–1332, 1332*f*
coin on edge, with eosinophilic granuloma,
    1363, 1363*f*
coin–on–end, 1516, 1516*f*
collapse, in steroid–induced osteonecrosis in
    Cushing's disease, 1357, 1357*f*–1358*f*
compression fracture
  acute, magnetic resonance imaging, 394*f*–
    395*f*
  benign versus malignant, magnetic
    resonance imaging, 396
  magnetic resonance imaging, 382, 384*f*
  old versus new, magnetic resonance
    imaging, 388, 394*f*–395*f*
corduroy cloth, 403, 1070, 1073*f*, 1516, 1516*f*
corner, 1516
cupped, 1516, 1517*f*
empty, 703, 704*f*, 787*t*, 1516, 1517*f*
end, 309
fibrous dysplasia, 1170, 1171*f*
fish, 1244, 1246, 1518, 1518*f*
  in Cushing's disease, 1358
  in Gaucher's disease, 1367
  in osteoporosis, 1331*f*, 1331–1332, 1332*f*
  in sickle cell anemia, 1244, 1246
fishbone, 1518, 1518*f*
fishmouth, in osteoporosis, 1331*f*, 1331–1332,
    1332*f*
flame–shaped, 1518, 1518*f*
fractures
  age determination, magnetic resonance
    imaging for, 388, 395*f*
  computed tomography, 388, 393*f*
  magnetic resonance imaging, 388, 393*f*–394*f*
  in osteoporosis, 1331*f*, 1332
framelike, 1518
frog head, 1518
fused
  degenerative, 215*f*
  posttraumatic, 216*f*
ghost, 1275*f*, 1518, 1518*f*
"H," 1516, 1517*f*
  in Gaucher's disease, 1367
  in sickle cell anemia, 1244, 1245*f*
heaping–up, 599, 600*f*, 1518, 1519*f*
hemangioma, magnetic resonance imaging,
    403, 405*f*–406*f*
hemivertebra. *See* Hemivertebra
hooked, 1514
hourglass, in osteoporosis, 1331*f*, 1331–1332,
    1332*f*
hump–shaped, 599, 600*f*
interpediculate distance, measurement, 168,
    168*f*, 168*t*, 190*t*
inverted "U" or "H," 1519

isolated endplate deformities, in osteoporosis,
    1331*f*, 1332
ivory, 983*f*–984*f*, 986*f*, 989–992, 990*f*–992*f*,
    991*t*, 1200, 1519, 1519*f*
  causes, 1149
  differential diagnosis, 1150*t*, 1151*f*
  with Hodgkin's lymphoma of bone, 1050,
    1051*f*
  malignant, 1151*f*
  in Paget's disease, 1134*f*, 1149, 1151*f*
  solitary, 1150*t*
jigsaw, 844, 847*f*, 848*t*, 1520, 1520*f*
keel–shaped, 1520
limbus, 1520, 1521*f*
long, 1520, 1521*f*
  in tuberculous spondylitis, 1227, 1227*f*
lozenge–shaped, 1520
lumbar, static vertebral malpositions, 162, 162*f*
named, 1513–1526
neoplasm, marrow replacement with,
    magnetic resonance imaging, 401, 405*f*
notched, 1514, 1520
occipital, 198–199, 1520
one–eyed, 1520, 1521*f*
osseous tumors of. *See also specific tumor(s)*
  magnetic resonance imaging, 401–403
  metastatic, magnetic resonance imaging,
    401, 403*f*–405*f*
pancake, in osteoporosis, 1331, 1331*f*
pear–shaped, 1518, 1519*f*
picture–frame, 1520, 1521*f*
  in Paget's disease, 1147, 1150*f*
pig snout, 1522, 1522*f*
sail, 1522, 1523*f*
sandwich, 626, 630*f*, 1522, 1523*f*
sawtooth, in actinomycosis, 1239
scalloped, 1522–1523, 1523*f*
  in neurofibromatosis, 1175, 1176*f*–1178*f*
shape changes, in osteoporosis, 1329–1332,
    1331*f*–1332*f*
shiny corner, 1524, 1524*f*
silver dollar, 1516, 1516*f*
soap bubble, 1524
solitary plasmacytoma, 1014, 1015*f*
spool–shaped, in pyknodysostosis, 638
square, 1524, 1524*f*
squared, in ankylosing spondylitis, 882, 884*f*,
    891*t*
squared–off, 1524, 1524*f*
step–off. *See* Corner vertebra
striated, 403, 1516, 1516*f*
surgically fused, 214*f*–215*f*
tall, 1525
tongue–shaped, 1525
transitional, 234–235, 236*f*–237*f*
wafer–like, 1525
wafer thin, 1516, 1516*f*
wasp waist, 1525, 1525*f*
wedge, 1525
wedged, in osteoporosis, 1331, 1331*f*–1332*f*
window–like, 1520, 1521*f*
winking owl, 1520, 1521*f*
wrinkled, 1008, 1525, 1525*f*
Vertebral artery
  aneurysm, 1314*f*, 1314–1315, 1315*f*–1317*f*
  displacement, by osteophytes, 808, 809*f*
  tortuosity, with erosion of axis, 1315, 1316*f*–
    1317*f*
Vertebral body
  definition, 7
  lumbar, trapezoid, 283*f*
  metastatic disease, 985, 985*f*–986*f*, 986*t*
  osteoid osteoma, 1092, 1092*f*
  in Paget's disease, 1129*f*
  step defect, 696*f*, 696–697, 787*t*